Robert A. Adler
Editor

OSTEOPOROSIS

Pathophysiology and Clinical Management

Second Edition

Humana Press

Editor
Robert A. Adler, MD
McGuire Veterans Affairs
Medical Center
Section of Endocrinology
1201 Broad Rock Blvd.
Richmond VA 23249
USA
robert.adler@va.gov

Series Editor
P. Michael Conn, PhD
Oregon Health & Science University
Beaverton, OR

ISBN 978-1-934115-19-0 (hardcover) ISBN 978-1-59745-459-9 (eBook)
ISBN 978-1-61779-518-3 (softcover)
DOI 10.1007/978-1-59745-459-9
Springer New York Heidelberg Dordrecht London

Library of Congress Control Number: 2009937295

Printed on acid-free paper

Humana Press is a brand of Springer
Springer is part of Springer Science+Business Media (www.springer.com)

Preface

The first edition of *Osteoporosis: Pathophysiology and Clinical Management* was edited by Eric Orwoll and Michael Bliziotes. It was a successful compilation in which one could learn the science behind clinical care by reading a chapter on the basic aspects followed by a chapter on clinical aspects. In this second edition, I have tried to keep to this same strategy for most topics in the ever-growing literature of osteoporosis. Some new chapters have been added. With her colleagues, Dr. Sharmila Majumdar has provided information on new bone imaging methods that hold great promise. Dr. Margaret Gourlay has tackled the important topic of screening for osteoporosis. We will be hearing more about screening as performance measures for osteoporosis are instituted. My colleagues, Drs. Valentina Petkov and Melissa Williams provided a new chapter on adherence to therapy, a major problem in the care of patients with osteoporosis. Finally, I took the editor's prerogative in adding my own chapter on osteoporosis in men, despite the presence of chapters on basic and clinical aspects of androgens in bone. While clearly less at risk for fracture than women, men are living long enough to fracture; and we finally have some data upon which management can be based.

Every book suffers from the potential for being out of date by the time of publication. Getting all authors to write chapters expeditiously is challenging, and when the field moves as quickly as that of osteoporosis, the final product can be stale upon arrival. In editing the book, I have strived to make the chapters as current as possible. I want to thank three authors in particular for their timeliness. Dr. Robert Lindsay wrote his chapter on relatively short notice. Both Dr. Michael Maricic and Dr. Ann Cranney, two authors who sent in their chapters quickly, provided updated versions when there were major advancements in their fields. These authors clearly went the extra mile.

However, I need to thank all the contributors for producing quality work. In an era when time is precious and all of us are stretched, writing a chapter is not usually high on the priority list. Therefore, the tremendous work of the contributors to this volume, all recognized experts in their fields, is greatly appreciated.

Robert A. Adler

Contents

Contributors

ROBERT A. ADLER, MD • *McGuire Veterans Affairs Medical Center, Departments of Internal Medicine and Epidemiology and Community Health, Virginia Commonwealth University School of Medicine, Richmond, VA, USA*

MARIA SCHULLER ALMEIDA, PhD • *Division of Endocrinology and Metabolism, UAMS Center for Osteoporosis and Metabolic Bone Disease, University of Arkansas for Medical Sciences, Little Rock, AR, USA*

MOISE AZIRA, PhD • *Novartis Pharma AG, Basel, Switzerland*

SUCHANDRIMA BANERJEE, PhD • *Musculo-skeletal and Quantitative Imaging Research Group, Department of Radiology, University of California, San Francisco, CA, USA*

BELINDA R. BECK, PhD • *School of Physiotherapy and Exercise Science, Gold Coast Campus, Griffith University, Southport, Australia*

JOHN P. BILEZIKIAN, MD • *Metabolic Diseases, Department of Medicine, Columbia University, College of Physicians and Surgeons, New York, NY, USA*

GLEN M. BLAKE, PhD • *Division of Imaging Sciences, King's College London Osteoporosis Unit, Guy's Hospital, London, UK*

JEAN-PHILIPPE BONJOUR, MD • *Department of Bone Disease, University Hospital of Geneva, Geneva, Switzerland*

CHARLES H. CHESNUT III, MD • *Osteoporosis Research Group, University of Washington, Seattle, WA, USA*

JACQUELINE H. COLE, PhD • *Department of Chemistry, University of Michigan, Ann Arbor, MI, USA*

ANN CRANNEY, MSC • *Department of Medicine, Ottawa Hospital, Ottawa, Ontario, Canada*

STEFAN GOEMAERE, MD • *Unit for Osteoporosis and Metabolic Bone Diseases, Department of Rheumatology and Endocrinology, Ghent University Hospital, Ghent, Belgium*

MARGARET GOURLAY, MD, MPH • *Department of Family Medicine, University of North Carolina, Chapel Hill, NC, USA*

ROBERT P. HEANEY, MD • *Department of Medicine, Creighton University, Omaha, Nebraska*

JANET M. HOCK, BDS, PhD • *Maine Institute for Human Genetics and Health, Brewer, ME, USA*

STEFAN JUDEX, PhD • *Department of Biomedical Engineering, State University of New York at Stony Brook, Stony Brook, NY, USA*

JEAN-MARC KAUFMAN, MD, PhD • *Department of Endocrinology and Laboratory of Hormonology and Andrology, University Hospital of Ghent, Ghent, Belgium*

MARIUS E. KRAENZLIN, MD • *Division of Endocrinology, Diabetes and Clinical Nutrition, University Hospital Basel, Basel, Switzerland*

ROLAND KRUG, PhD • *Musculo-skeletal and Quantitative Imaging Research Group, Department of Radiology, University of California at San Francisco, San Francisco, CA, USA*

THOMAS F. LANG, PhD • *Department of Radiology, Center for Molecular and Functional Imaging, University of California at San Francisco, San Francisco, CA, USA*

ROBERT LINDSAY, MBCHB, PhD, FRCP • *Regional Bone Center, Helen Hayes Hospital, West Haverstraw, NY, USA*

SHARMILA MAJUMDAR, PhD • *Musculo-skeletal and Quantitative Imaging Research Group, Department of Radiology, University of California, San Francisco, San Francisco, CA, USA*

MICHAEL MARICIC, MD • *University of Arizona, Catalina Pointe Rheumatology, Tucson, AZ, USA*

CHRISTIAN MEIER, MD • *Division of Endocrinology, Diabetes and Clinical Nutrition, University Hospital Basel, Basel, Switzerland*

VALENTINA I. PETKOV, MD, MPH • *Research Service, McGuire Veterans Affairs Medical Center, Virginia Commonwealth University, Richmond, VA, USA*

SVEN PREVRHAL, PhD • *Musculo-skeletal and Quantitative Imaging Research Group, Department of Radiology and Biomedical Imaging, University of California at San Francisco, San Francisco, CA, USA*

RICHARD L. PRINCE, MD, FRACP • *Department of Endocrinology, Sir Charles Gardner Hospital, University of Western Australia, Perth, Australia*

IAN REID, MD, MBChB • *Professor of Medicine and Endocrinology, Faculty of Medical and Health Sciences, University of Auckland, Auckland, New Zealand*

ALFRED A. RESZKA, PhD • *Corporate Licensing, Merck & Co., Inc, Whitehouse Station, NJ*

RENE RIZZOLI, MD • *Division of Bone Diseases, Department of Rehabilitation and Geriatrics, World Health Organisation Collaborating Center for Osteoporosis Prevention, Geneva University Hospitals and Faculty of Medicine, Geneva, Switzerland*

CLINTON T. RUBIN, PhD • *Department of Biomedical Engineering, Center for Biotechnology, State University of New York at Stony Brook, Stony Brook, NY*

MARKUS J. SEIBEL, MD, PhD, FRACP • *Endocrinology, Bone Research Program, ANZAC Research Institute, University of Sydney, Sydney, Australia*

ELIZABETH SHANE, MD • *Department of Medicine, Columbia University, College of Physicians and Surgeons, New York, NY*

GLORIA SIDHOM, MD, PhD • *Departments of Nutritional Sciences, and Laboratory Medicine and Pathobiology, University of Toronto, and Pathology and Laboratory Medicine, Mount Sinai Hospital, Toronto, Canada*

EMILY M. STEIN, MD, MS • *Department of Medicine, Columbia University, College of Physicians and Surgeons, New York, NY*

GUY T'SJOEN, MD, PhD • *Department of Endocrinology, University Hospital of Ghent, Ghent, Belgium*

MARJOLEIN C.H. VAN DER MEULEN, PhD • *Sibley School of Mechanical and Aerospace Engineering, Cornell University, Ithaca, NY*

REINHOLD VEITH, PhD, FCACB • *Department of Pathology and Laboratory Medicine, Mount Sinai Hospital Toronto, Ontario, Canada*

MELISSA I. WILLIAMS, PharmD • *Pharmacy Service, McGuire Veterans Affairs Medical Center, Virginia Commonwealth University School of Pharmacy, Richmond, VA*
KERRI M. WINTERS-STONE, PhD • *Department of Nutrition and Exercise Science, Oregon State University, Corvallis, OR*
KRISTINE M. WIREN, PhD • *Bone and Mineral Unit, Oregon Health & Science University, Portland Veterans Affairs Medical Center, Portland, OR*

1 Determinants of Peak Bone Mass Acquisition

René Rizzoli and Jean-Philippe Bonjour

CONTENTS

Key Words: Osteoporosis, fracture, adolescence, bone strength

DEFINITION AND IMPORTANCE OF PEAK BONE MASS

Peak bone mass (PBM) corresponds to the amount of bony tissue present at the end of skeletal maturation. It is a major determinant of the risk of fractures later in life, because there is an inverse relationship between fracture risk and areal bone mineral density, in women as well as in men. From epidemiological studies it can be assumed that an increase of 10% of PBM in the female population, corresponding to approximately 1 standard deviation, would be associated with a 50% decrease in the risk of fracture. Hence, exploring ways of increasing PBM could be considered as a valuable measure in the primary prevention of osteoporosis. Bone mineral accumulation from infancy to postpuberty is a complex process. It can be appreciated with the availability of noninvasive techniques able to accurately measure areal (a) or volumetric (v) bone mineral density (BMD) at several sites of the skeleton by either dual X-ray absorptiometry (DXA) or quantitative computed tomography (QCT). Noninvasive specific evaluations of the cancellous and cortical bone compartments, even of trabecular microstructure, are also becoming available (see Chapter 3). These techniques allow one to capture part of the change in the macroarchitecture or geometry of the bones which along with the mineral mass strongly influence the resistance to the mechanical strain. This chapter attempts to summarize some of the knowledge that has accumulated

From: *Contemporary Endocrinology: Osteoporosis: Pathophysiology and Clinical Management*
Edited by: R. A. Adler, DOI 10.1007/978-1-59745-459-9_1,

over the past few years on the characteristics of normal bone mass development from infancy to the end of the skeleton maturation and the genetic and environmental factors influencing bone mass accrual, hence PBM.

CHARACTERISTICS OF PEAK BONE MASS ACQUISITION

Measurement of Bone Mass Development

Most of the information on the characteristics of skeletal growth during childhood and adolescence has been obtained thanks to the availability of noninvasive techniques allowing one to quantify with great precision and accuracy bone mass at various sites of the skeleton *(1,2)*. The bone mass of a part of the skeleton is directly dependent on both its volume or size and the density of the mineralized tissue contained within its periosteal envelope. The mean volumetric mineral density of bony tissue (BMD in g of hydroxyapatite per cm^3) can be determined noninvasively by quantitative computed tomography (QCT). The technique of either single or dual X-ray (SXA, DXA) absorptiometry provides measurement of the areal or surface bone mineral density (BMD in g of hydroxyapatite per cm^2). The values generated by this technique are directly dependent on both the size and the integrated mineral density of the scanned skeletal tissue. This second variable is made of several components including the cortical thickness, the number and thickness of the trabeculae, and the "true" mineral density corresponding to the amount of hydroxyapatite per unit volume of the bone organic matrix. The term bone mineral *density* without the additional "areal" qualification has been widely used with the general understanding that neither SXA nor DXA techniques provide a measurement of volumetric density. This notion, which should be obvious to bone biologists using DXA technology in either experimental or clinical settings, has not always been fully appreciated leading to mis- or overinterpretation of the data generated by this noninvasive technology *(3)*. Therefore, it has to be reemphasized that aBMD is the summation of several structural components which may evolve differently in response to genetic and environmental factors. Nevertheless, areal BMD remains of clinical relevance in the context of osteoporosis. Indeed, the values of areal BMD have been shown to be directly related to bone strength, i.e., to the resistance of the skeleton to mechanical stress both in vivo and in vitro *(4–7)*. There is an inverse relationship between areal BMD values and the prevalence of osteoporotic fractures *(8)*.

At the spinal level, the total mineral content (BMC in g of hydroxyapatite) of the vertebrae, including the posterior arch, can be measured using the classical antero-posterior (frontal) projection. BMC and areal BMD of the vertebral body "isolated" from the vertebral arch can also be obtained by using DXA in the lateral projection *(9)*. Low accuracy and precision preclude this measurement to be performed in routine clinical practice. The so-called bone mineral "apparent" density (BMAD in g/cm^3) is an indirect and rather imprecise estimate of the volumetric skeletal density *(10)*. This extrapolated variable can be expected to be less related to bone strength than areal BMD, because it does not take into account the important size component that influences the mechanical resistance.

Therefore, in terms of overall bone strength prediction, areal BMD/BMC values are more informative than the isolated measurement of volumetric trabecular density, since the former variable includes both bone geometry, thickness and its integrated volumetric density. This statement does not mean that other variables which are more difficult to accurately assess, such as the microarchitecture of the trabecular network and/or the intrinsic "quality" of the mineralized tissue, do not contribute to the resistance to mechanical force. Furthermore, it is obvious that a full understanding of the fundamental mechanisms that underlie the marked interindividual variability observed in bone mass gain will require separate analysis of how bone size, cortical thickness, volumetric trabecular density, and microstructure evolve during growth. This will also allow one to identify which are the main respective genetic and environmental factors that determine the development of each of these three important contributors to bone strength in adulthood.

Bone Mass Development

Before puberty, no substantial gender difference in bone mass of either axial or appendicular skeleton has been reported. There is no evidence for a gender difference in bone mass at birth. Likewise, the volumetric bone mineral density appears to be also similar between female and male newborns *(11)*. This absence of substantial sex difference in bone mass is maintained until the onset of pubertal maturation *(12,13)*. During puberty the gender difference in bone mass becomes expressed. This difference appears to be mainly due to a bone maturation period more prolonged in males than in females, with a larger increase in bone size and cortical thickness *(14)*. Puberty affects much more the bone size than the volumetric mineral density *(15,16)*. There is no significant sex difference in the volumetric trabecular density at the end of pubertal maturation *(13,16)*. During puberty, areal BMD changes at both the lumbar spine and the femoral neck levels increase four- to six-fold over 3- and 4-year period in females and males, respectively *(14)*. The change in bone mass accumulation rate is less marked in long bone diaphysis *(14)*. There is an asynchrony between the gain in standing height and the growth of bone mineral mass during pubertal maturation *(12,14,17)*. This phenomenon may be responsible for the occurrence of a transient fragility that may contribute to the higher incidence of fracture known to occur when the dissociation between the rate of statural growth and mineral mass accrual is maximal *(18–20)*.

Time of Peak Bone Mass Attainment

In female adolescents the rate of bone mass gain declined rapidly after menarche *(14)* to become not statistically different from 0 to 2 years later *(14)*. In male adolescents, the gain in BMD/BMC which was particularly high from 13 to 17 years markedly declined thereafter, although it remained significant between 17 and 20 years in both L2–L4 BMD/BMC and midfemoral shaft BMD *(14)*. In contrast, no significant increase was observed for femoral neck BMD. In subjects having reached pubertal stage P5 and growing less than 1 cm/year, a significant bone mass gain was still present in male but not in female individuals. This suggests the existence of an important sex difference in the magnitude and/or duration of the consolidation phenomenon that contributes to the PBM value.

Observations made with QCT technology also indicate that the maximal volumetric bone mineral density of the lumbar vertebral body will be achieved soon after menarche since no difference was observed between the mean values of 16-year-old and 30-year-old subjects *(21,22)*. This is in keeping with numerous observations indicating that bone mass does not significantly increase from the third to the fifth decade. The balance of all available data does not sustain the concept that bone mass at any skeletal site, in both genders, in all races and in any geographical area continues to substantially accumulate until the fourth decade. In other words, the fact that peak bone mass would be reached in the mid-30s does not seem to be a constant phenomenon of human physiology. On the contrary, numerous cross-sectional studies suggest that proximal femur areal BMD begins to decline already during the third decade.

Bone outer dimensions can become larger during the adult life. This phenomenon has been documented by measuring the external diameter of several bones by radiogrammetry *(23–25)*. It may be the consequence of an increased endosteal bone resorption with enlargement in the internal diameter. Such a modeling phenomenon would be a response to bone loss, tending to compensate the reduction in the mechanical resistance *(26)*.

Peak Bone Mass Variance

At the beginning of the third decade, there is a large variability in the normal values of areal BMD in axial and appendicular skeleton *(15)*. This large variance, which is observed at sites particularly susceptible to osteoporotic fractures such as lumbar spine and femoral neck, is barely reduced after correction for standing height and does not appear to substantially increase during adult life. The height-independent broad variance in bone mineral mass which is already present before puberty appears to increase further during pubertal maturation at sites such as lumbar spine and femoral neck *(12,14)*. In young healthy adults, the biological variance in lumbar spine BMC is four to five times larger than that of standing height; the latter does not increase during puberty *(17)*.

CALCIUM PHOSPHATE METABOLISM DURING GROWTH

Several physiological functions influence bone accumulation during growth. Animal studies have identified physiological mechanisms that sustain increased bone mineral demand in relation to variations in growth velocity. In this context, two adaptive mechanisms affecting calcium phosphate metabolism appear to be particularly important, namely the increase in the plasma concentration of 1,25-dihydroxyvitamin D_3 (calcitriol), and the stimulation of the renal tubular reabsorption of inorganic phosphate (Pi). The increased production and higher plasma level of calcitriol enhance the capacity of the intestinal epithelium to absorb both calcium and Pi. The increase in the tubular reabsorption of Pi results in a rise in its extracellular concentration. Without these two concerted adaptive responses, growth and mineralization would not be optimal. The increase in tubular Pi reabsorption is not mediated by a rise in the renal production or in the plasma level of calcitriol.

Analysis of cross-sectional studies suggests that these two adaptive mechanisms could be essential to cope with the increased bone mineral demand during the pubertal growth spurt. An increase in plasma calcitriol concentrations has been reported during pubertal maturation *(27)*. Both the pattern of this response and its consequence for intestinal calcium absorptive capacity in relation to pubertal bone mass acquisition remain difficult to document, since it would require a time-integrated estimate of the controlling (calcitriol and intestinal calcium absorption) elements. A tight relationship exists between tubular reabsorption of Pi, plasma Pi level, and growth velocity in children *(28)*. A rise in plasma Pi during puberty has been reported *(29,30)*. Precise quantitation of the relationship between changes in regulatory component of tubular Pi reabsorption and plasma concentration of Pi, and bone mass gain during puberty remains to be done. However, similar to the calcitriol–intestinal calcium absorption regulatory pathway, a correct evaluation would require a time-integrated assessment of the changes in the tubular reabsorption and plasma concentration of Pi during the period of accelerated bone mass gain.

The mechanism underlying the parallel rise in calcitriol and the tubular reabsorption of Pi has been recently clarified. Experimental studies indicate that one single factor, namely insulin-like growth factor-I (IGF-I), could be responsible for the stimulation of both calcitriol production and tubular Pi reabsorption (TmPi/GFR) in relation to the increased calcium and Pi demand associated with bone growth *(31)*. In humans, the plasma IGF-I level rises transiently during pubertal maturation, to reach a peak during mid-puberty. Its maximal level thus occurs at an earlier chronological age in females than in males *(32)*. IGF-I, whose production is influenced by dietary protein intakes, enhances longitudinal and radial bone growth, increases renal tubular reabsorption of phosphate and stimulates calcitriol synthesis (Fig. 1). The rise in IGF-I, calcitriol, and Pi plasma levels

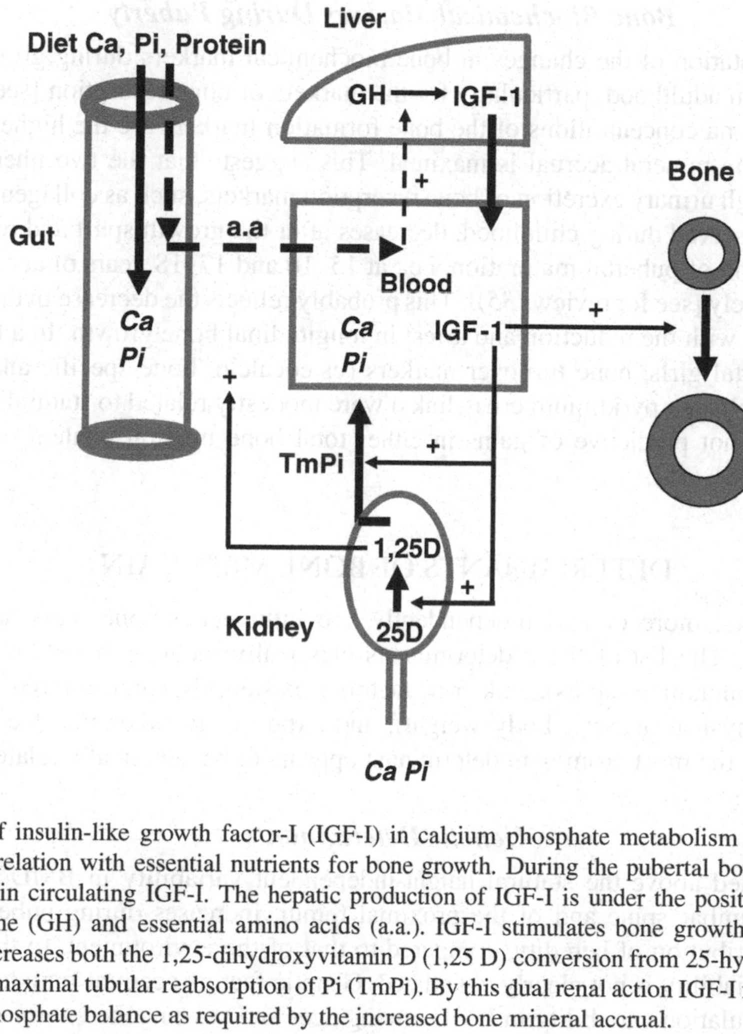

Fig. 1. Role of insulin-like growth factor-I (IGF-I) in calcium phosphate metabolism during pubertal maturation in relation with essential nutrients for bone growth. During the pubertal bone growth spurt there is a rise in circulating IGF-I. The hepatic production of IGF-I is under the positive influence of growth hormone (GH) and essential amino acids (a.a.). IGF-I stimulates bone growth. At the kidney level, IGF-I increases both the 1,25-dihydroxyvitamin D (1,25 D) conversion from 25-hydroxyvitamin D (25D) and the maximal tubular reabsorption of Pi (TmPi). By this dual renal action IGF-I favors a positive calcium and phosphate balance as required by the increased bone mineral accrual.

is correlated with elevation in indices of the bone appositional rate such as alkaline phosphatase *(33)* and osteocalcin *(34,35)*. Plasma concentrations of gonadal sex hormones, as well as those of adrenal androgens (dehydroepiandrosterone and androstendione), which increase before and during pubertal maturation, are not associated with the accelerated bone mass gain *(36)*. Whether differences in the adaptive responses which control calcium and phosphate homeostasis could play a role in the increased variance in lumbar spine or femoral neck BMD/BMC remains to be explored. As recently reviewed, the interaction between the growth hormone-IGF-I axis and sex steroids is quite complex *(35)*. The effect of these interactions on the gains in bone size and mass during pubertal maturation, independent of their influence on the rate and duration of longitudinal growth, remains largely unknown. A bone-derived factor, FGF23, has been suggested to contribute to the bone–kidney link, whose presence has been proposed for many years, as it influences renal tubular transport of inorganic phosphate and calcitriol synthesis *(37)*. In young adults, serum FGF23 concentrations appear to be influenced by dietary phosphorus intakes *(38)*.

Bone Biochemical Markers During Puberty

The interpretation of the changes in bone biochemical markers during growth is more complex than in adulthood, particularly for the markers of bone resorption [see for review *(35)*]. The plasma concentrations of the bone formation markers are the highest when the velocity of bone mineral accrual is maximal. This suggests that the two phenomena are related. The high urinary excretion of bone resorption markers, such as collagen pyridinium cross-links, observed during childhood, decreases after the growth spurt and reaches adult values at the end of pubertal maturation, i.e., at 15–16 and 17–18 years of age in girls and boys, respectively [see for review *(35)*]. This probably reflects the decrease in the resorption rate associated with the reduction and arrest in longitudinal bone growth. In a longitudinal study in pubertal girls, bone turnover markers (osteocalcin, bone-specific alkaline phosphatase, and collagen pyridinium cross-links) were modestly related to statural height gain, but they were not predictive of gains in either total bone mineral content or density as assessed by DXA *(39)*.

DETERMINANTS OF BONE MASS GAIN

Many factors, more or less independently, are influencing bone mass accumulation during growth. The list of these determinants classically includes heredity, sex, dietary components (calcium, proteins), endocrine factors (sex steroids, calcitriol, IGF-I), mechanical forces (physical activity, body weight), and exposure to other risk factors *(40,41)*. Quantitatively, the most prominent determinant appears to be genetically related (Fig. 2).

Genetic Determinants

As mentioned above the statural height-independent variability in BMD/BMC at the level of the lumbar spine and of the proximal femur, increases during pubertal maturation. The contribution of heredity, compared to that of the environment, to this increased bone mass variability is not clearly elucidated. Genetic factors account for a large percentage of the population variability in BMD among age- and sex-matched normal individuals

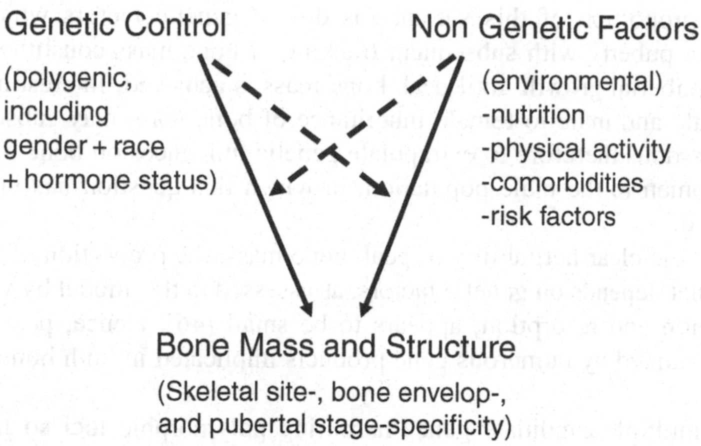

Fig. 2. Interaction between genetic and non-genetic factors on bone mineral mass and structure changes during puberty. Genetic factors are either acting directly on bone or indirectly by modulating the sensitivity to environmental factors. Similarly, environmental factors are acting either directly on bone or indirectly by modulating the genetic potential. The various influences are variable according to the skeletal site, even the bone envelop at a given skeletal site, and according to pubertal stage.

(40,41). Daughters of osteoporotic women have a low BMD *(42)*. To investigate the proportion of the BMD variance across the population explained by genetic factors, known as its heritability, two human models mainly have been used. In the twin model, within-pair correlations for BMD are compared between monozygotic (MZ) twins, who by essence share 100% of their genes, and dizygotic twins, who have 50% of their genes in common. Stronger correlation coefficients among adult MZ as compared to DZ twins are indicative of the genetic influence on peak bone mass. Genetic factors could explain as much as 80% of lumbar spine and proximal femur BMD variance. Lean and fat mass are also genetically determined *(43)*, since it appears that 80 and 65% of variance of lean and fat mass, respectively, are attributable to genetic factors. However, genetic factors affecting lean and fat mass have only little influence on lumbar spine or femoral neck BMD.

Parents–offspring comparisons have also shown significant relationships for BMD, albeit heritability estimates have been somewhat lower (in the range of 60%) than in the twin model. Actually, the magnitude of direct genetic effects on peak bone mass as evaluated in both human models may be overestimated by similarities in environmental covariates *(44)*. Bone mineral content, areal and volumetric bone mineral density, and bone area in the lumbar spine and femur (neck, trochanter, and diaphysis) were compared in premenopausal women and in their prepubertal daughters *(45)*. Regressions were adjusted for height, weight, and calcium intake, to minimize the impact of indirect genetic effects as well as of dietary influences on bone mineral mass resemblance among relatives. Despite great disparities in the various constituents of bone mass before puberty with respect to peak adult values, heredity by maternal descent is detectable at all skeletal sites and affected virtually all bone mass constituents, including bone size and volumetric mineral density. Moreover, when daughters' bone values were reevaluated 2 years later, while puberty had begun and bone mineral mass had considerably increased, measurements were highly correlated with prepubertal values and mother–daughter correlations had remained unchanged.

Thus, a major proportion of this variance is due to genetic factors which are already expressed before puberty with subsequent tracking of bone mass constituent through the phase of rapid pubertal growth until peak bone mass is achieved. Interestingly, it appears that male to male and male to female inheritance of bone mass may substantially differ. It might be hazardous therefore to extrapolate genetic influences on bone mineral mass as identified in women to the male population, in which this question has virtually not yet been investigated.

In contrast to the clear heritability of peak bone mass, the proportion of the variance in bone turnover that depends on genetic factors, as assessed in this model by various markers of bone formation and resorption, appears to be small *(46)*. Hence, peak bone mass is very likely determined by numerous gene products implicated in both bone modeling and remodeling.

Among the multiple candidate genes harboring polymorphic loci so far investigated in relation to BMD and/or BMD changes, vitamin D receptor alleles provide controversial results. A large meta-analysis including 26242 subjects has reviewed the association between VDR polymorphisms, BMD and fractures in postmenopausal women *(47)*. Whereas *Fok*I, *Bsm*I, *Apa*I, and *Taq*I VDR polymorphisms were associated with neither BMD nor fractures, a Cdx2 polymorphism could be associated with vertebral fracture risk. Several independent investigators have shown the importance of age, gene–environment, and gene–gene interactions to explain the inconsistent relationship between bone mineral mass and VDR genotypes. Thus, significant BMD differences between VDR-3′ *Bsm*I genotypes were detected in children *(48,49)* but were absent in premenopausal women from the same genetic background *(48)*. Moreover, the latter study found that BMD gain in prepubertal girls was increased at several skeletal sites in Bb and BB subjects in response to calcium supplements whereas it remained apparently unaffected in bb girls, who had a trend for spontaneously higher BMD accumulation on their usual calcium diet *(48,50)*. Accordingly, a model taking into account the early influence of VDR-3′ polymorphisms, calcium intake and puberty on BMD gain has been proposed to explain the relation between these genotypes and peak bone mass. Interestingly also, several investigators have noted a significantly lower height among women and men with the VDR-3′ BB compared to Bb or bb genotypes *(48,51)*. Altogether, these observations provide a possible physiological mechanism for the relationship between VDR gene polymorphisms and bone mass and emphasize the methodological limitations of earlier studies focusing on the association between VDR genotypes and BMD regardless of age and environmental factors. Thus, VDR-3′ and 5′-alleles are possibly weak determinants of bone mineral density, their effects being easily confounded by the influence of many other genes and environmental factors. Hence, VDR gene polymorphisms alone are not clinically useful genetic markers of peak bone mass, but could be one significant factor to explain some of the variability observed in the population.

Independent genomewide quantitative trait locus studies have suggested a locus for bone mineral density and stature, on chromosome 11q12–13, a region in which the low-density lipoprotein receptor-related protein 5 (LRP5) gene is located. Mutations in the LRP5 gene were recently implicated in osteoporosis-pseudoglioma and "high-bone-mass" syndromes. Polymorphisms in the LRP5 gene appear to contribute to bone mass variance in the general population. Indeed, in a cross-sectional cohort of 889 healthy Caucasian subjects of both sexes, significant associations were found for a missense substitution in exon 9 (c.2047G→A) with lumbar spine BMC, with bone scanned projected area, and with stature

(52). The associations were observed mainly in adult men, in whom LRP5 polymorphisms accounted for close to 15% of the traits' variances. Results of haplotype analysis of five single-nucleotide polymorphisms in the LRP5 region suggest that additional genetic variation within the locus might also contribute to bone mass and size variance. LRP5 haplotypes were also associated with 1-year gain in vertebral bone mass and size in 386 prepubertal children. Again, significant associations were observed for changes in BMD and in bone area in relation to LRP5 gene polymorphisms in males but not females.

Physical Activity

The responsiveness to either an increase or a decrease in mechanical strain is probably greater in growing than adult bones. Hence, the concept of public health programs aimed at increasing physical activity among healthy children and adolescents in order to maximize peak bone mass has been proposed. Several recent reports in children or adolescents involved in competitive sport or ballet dancing indicate that intense exercise is associated with an increase in bone mass accrual in weight-bearing skeletal sites *(53–55)*. The question arises whether this increase in BMD/BMC resulting from intense exercise is translated into greater bone strength. A recent cross-sectional study in male elite-tennis players using peripheral QCT and side-to-side arm comparison indicates that the increase in BMC reflected an increased bone size which was associated with an augmentation in an index of bone strength. By contrast, no change in either cortical or trabecular vBMD was observed *(56)*. Whether the same type of structural changes beneficial for bone strength is observed at other skeletal sites, such as vertebral bodies and proximal femur, in response to different kinds of intense exercise during childhood and adolescence, is not established. In terms of general public health, observations made in elite athletes cannot be the basis of recommendations for the general population, since intense exercise is beyond the reach of most individuals. Much more relevant is information on the effect of *moderate* exercise on bone mass acquisition. Some, but not all cross-sectional studies have found a slightly positive association between physical activity and bone mass values in children and adolescents. However, the positive association found cross-sectionally was not consistently confirmed by observational longitudinal studies relating bone mass gain to physical activity. Measurements of the duration, intensity, and type of physical activity that are based on recall are not very accurate, particularly in children. Therefore, it is possible that negative findings could be ascribed to poor validity in the methods used to estimate physical activity. Controlled prospective studies carried out in prepubertal girls *(57)* or boys *(58)* indicate that exercise programs undertaken in schools, and considered on the average as *moderate*, can increase bone mineral mass acquisition [for review, see *(59)*]. These indicate that the growing skeleton is certainly sensitive to exercise and suggest that prepuberty would be an opportune time for implementing physical education programs consisting in various moderate weight-bearing exercises. Nevertheless, it remains uncertain to what extent the greater aBMD gain in response to moderate and readily accessible weight-bearing exercise is associated with a commensurate increase in bone strength *(58)*. The magnitude of benefit in terms of bone strength will depend on the nature of the structural change, and possibly on the gender. Indeed, increasing levels of physical activity were associated with higher response weight-bearing BMD in boys than in girls before puberty *(60)*. An effect consisting primarily of an increased periosteal apposition and consecutive diameter will confer greater mechanical resistance than a response limited to the endosteal apposition rate leading essentially to a reduction in the endocortical diameter. There is a need for further studies aimed at examining the effects of mechanical loading components, such as magnitude and frequency of various types of exercise on the mass and geometry of bones in children and adolescents *(61)*.

Studies in adult elite athletes strongly indicate that increased bone mass gains resulting from intense physical activity during childhood and adolescence are maintained after training decreases or even completely ceases *(53,62,63)*. Finally, the question whether the increased peak bone mass induced by physical exercise will be maintained in old age and lead to a reduction in fracture rate remains open. A recent cross-sectional study of retired Australian elite soccer players suggests that this may not be the case *(64)*. However, the lack of information on the peak bone mass values of these men does not allow one to draw firm conclusion about this observation.

Nutritional Factors

Puberty is considered to be a period with major behavioral changes and alterations in lifestyle. It is also assumed that important modifications in food habits occur during pubertal maturation, particularly in affluent societies. To what extent variations in the intakes of some nutrients in healthy, apparently well-nourished, children and adolescents can affect bone mass accumulation, particularly at sites susceptible to osteoporotic fractures, has received increasing attention over the last 15 years. Most studies have focused on the intake of calcium. However, other nutrients such as protein should also be considered.

Calcium

It is usually accepted that increasing the calcium intake during childhood and adolescence will be associated with a greater bone mass gain and thereby a higher peak bone mass *(65,66)*. However, a survey of the literature on the relationship between dietary calcium and bone mass indicates that some *(67–69)*, but not all studies *(70,71)*, have found a positive correlation between these two variables. As with physical activity, several sets of cross-sectional and longitudinal data, including our own results on dietary calcium intake and bone mass accrual in female and male subjects aged 9–19, are compatible with a "two-threshold model." On one side of the normal range one can conceive the existence of a "low" threshold, set at a total calcium intake of about 400–500 mg/day, below which a positive relationship can be found. Within this low range the positive effect of calcium would be explained merely by its role as a necessary substrate for bone mass accrual. On the other side of the normal range, there would be a "high" threshold, set at about 1600 mg/day, above which the calcium intake through another mechanism could exert a slightly positive influence on bone mass accrual. In addition, the levels of the two thresholds could vary according to the stage of pubertal maturation. In our own cross-sectional and longitudinal study, a significant positive relationship between total calcium intake as determined by two 5-day diaries was found in females in the pubertal subgroup P1–P4, but not in the P5 subgroup *(12,14)*.

Several intervention studies have been carried out in children and adolescents *(72–75)*. Overall, these trials indicate greater bone mineral mass gain in children and adolescents receiving calcium supplementation over periods varying from 12 to 36 months. The benefit of calcium supplementation has been mostly detected in the appendicular rather than in the axial skeleton *(72–77)*. In prepubertal children, calcium supplementation is more effective on cortical appendicular bone (radial and femoral diaphysis) than on axial trabecular-rich bone (lumbar spine) or on the hip (femoral neck, trochanter) [for review, see *(78)*]. The skeleton appears to be more responsive to calcium supplementation before the onset of pubertal maturation *(75)*. In 8-year-old prepubertal girls with baseline low calcium intake, increasing the daily calcium intake from about 700 to 1400 mg augmented the mean gain in aBMD of six skeletal sites by 58% as compared to the placebo group, after 1 year of supplementation. This difference corresponds to a gain of +0.24 standard deviation (SD) *(72)*. If sustained over a period of 4 years such an increase in the calcium intake could augment mean aBMD by 1 SD. Thus, milk calcium supplementation could modify the bone growth trajectory and thereby increase peak bone mass. In this regard it is interesting to note that an intervention influencing calcium phosphate metabolism and limited to the first year of life may also modify the trajectory of bone mass accrual. A 400 IU/day vitamin D-supplementation given to infants for an average of 1 year was associated with a significant increase in aBMD measured at the age of 7–9 years *(79)*. The aBMD difference between the vitamin D-supplemented and non-supplemented group was particularly significant at the femoral neck, trochanter, and radial metaphysis. These observations are compatible with the "programming" concept, according to which environmental stimuli during critical periods of early development can provoke long-lasting modifications in structure and function *(80,81)*.

Another aspect to consider is that the type of the supplemented calcium salt could modulate the nature of the bone response. Thus, the response to a calcium phosphate salt from milk extract appears to differ from those recorded with other calcium supplements. Indeed, the positive effect on aBMD was associated with an increase in the projected bone area at several sites of the skeleton *(72)*. Interestingly, this type of response was similar to the response to whole milk supplementation *(82)*. But in the latter study, the positive effect on bone size could be ascribed to other nutrients contained in whole milk, such as protein, whereas in the former study the tested calcium-enriched foods had the same energy, lipid, and protein content as those given to the placebo group *(72)*.

It is important to consider whether or not the gain resulting from the intervention will be maintained after discontinuation of the calcium supplementation. One year and 3.5 years after discontinuing the intervention, differences in the gain in aBMD and in the size of some bones were still detectable, but at the limit of statistical significance *(15,72)*. These results need additional confirmation by long-term follow-up of the cohort, ideally until PBM has been attained, as well as by other prospective studies. Bone mineral density was also measured 7.5 years after the end of calcium supplementation. In these young adult girls, it appeared that menarche occurred earlier in the calcium-supplemented group, and that persistent effects of calcium were mostly detectable in those subjects with an earlier puberty *(74)*.

A recent meta-analysis has reviewed 19 calcium intervention studies involving 2859 children *(78)*, with doses of calcium supplementation varying between 300 and 1200 mg per day, from calcium citrate–malate, calcium carbonate, calcium phosphate, calcium lactate–gluconate, calcium phosphate milk extract, or milk minerals. Calcium supplementation had a positive effect on total body bone mineral content and upper limb bone mineral density, with standardized mean differences (effect size) of 0.14 for both. At the upper limb, the effect persisted after cessation of calcium supplementation. Analyzing 17 studies involving 2088 children, the same authors concluded that calcium supplementation has no significant effect on weight, height, or body fat.

Despite a positive effect on mean aBMD gain there is still wide interindividual variability in the response to calcium supplementation. As discussed above, it is possible that part of the variability in the bone gain response to calcium supplementation could be related to VDR gene polymorphisms *(83)*. Indeed, the response to calcium supplementation in terms of bone mineral mass accrual was preferentially observed in subjects with a given VDR genotype.

PROTEIN

Among nutrients other than calcium, various experimental and clinical observations point to the existence of a relationship between the level of protein intake and either calcium phosphate metabolism or bone mass, or even osteoporotic fracture risk *(84,85)*. Nevertheless, any long-term influence of dietary protein on bone mineral metabolism and skeletal mass so far has been difficult to identify. Apparently contradictory information suggests that either a deficient or an excessive protein supply could negatively affect calcium balance and the amount of bony tissue contained in the skeleton *(84,85)*.

Despite these uncertainties, multiple animal and human studies indicate strongly that low protein intake per se could be particularly detrimental for both the acquisition of bone mass and the conservation of bone integrity with aging. During growth, undernutrition, including inadequate supply of energy and protein, can severely impair bone development. Studies in experimental animals indicate that isolated protein deficiency leads to reduced bone mass and strength without histomorphometric evidence of osteomalacia *(86)*. Thus, inadequate supply of protein appears to play a central role in the pathogenesis of the delayed skeletal growth and reduced bone mass observed in undernourished children *(87)*.

Low protein intake could be detrimental for skeletal integrity by lowering the production of IGF-I. Indeed, the hepatic production and plasma concentration of this growth factor, which exerts several positive effects on the skeleton, are under the influence of dietary protein *(88–90)*. Protein restriction has been shown to reduce circulating IGF-I by inducing resistance to the hepatic action of growth hormone. In addition, protein restriction appears to decrease the anabolic actions of IGF-I on some target cells *(91)*. In this regard, it is important to note that growing rats maintained on a low protein diet failed to restore growth when IGF-I was administered at doses sufficient to normalize its plasma concentrations.

Variations in the production of IGF-I could explain some of the changes in bone and calcium phosphate metabolism that have been observed in relation to intake of dietary protein. Indeed, the plasma level of IGF-I is closely related to the growth rate of the organism. In humans, circulating IGF-I, of which the major source is the liver, progressively increases from 1 year of age to reach peak values during puberty. As described above, this factor appears to play a key role in calcium phosphate metabolism during growth by stimulating two kidney processes, Pi transport and the production of calcitriol *(92)*. IGF-I is considered an essential factor for bone longitudinal growth, as it stimulates proliferation and differentiation of chondrocytes in the epiphyseal plate *(93,94)*. It also has an effect on trabecular and cortical bone formation. In experimental animals, administration of IGF-I also positively affects bone mass *(95)*, increasing the external diameter of long bone, probably by enhancing the process of periosteal apposition. Therefore, during adolescence a relative deficiency in IGF-I or a resistance to its action that could be due to an inadequate protein supply may result not only in a reduction in the skeletal longitudinal growth, but also in an impairment in widthwise or cross-sectional bone development.

In well-nourished children and adolescents, the question arises whether variations in the protein intake within the "normal" range can influence skeletal growth and thereby modulate the genetic potential in peak bone mass attainment. There is a positive relationship between protein intake, as assessed by two 5-day dietary diary methods with weighing most food intakes *(86,96)*, and bone mass gain, particularly from pubertal stage P2 to P4. The correlation remained statistically significant even after correcting for the influence of either age or calcium intake. The association between bone mass gain and protein intake was observed in both sexes at the lumbar spine, the proximal femur, and the femoral mid-shaft.

In prepubertal boys, BMD/BMC changes were positively associated with spontaneous protein intake *(97)*. In addition, this study also suggested that protein intake modulates the effect of calcium supplementation on bone mineral mass gain. Hence, in prepubertal boys, the favorable effects of calcium supplements were mostly detectable in those with a lower protein intake. At higher protein intake, the effect of calcium was not significant, suggesting that less stringent calcium requirements are necessary for optimal bone growth with high dietary protein. Thus, it appears that nutritional environmental factors could affect bone accumulation at specific periods during infancy and adolescence.

In a prospective longitudinal study performed in healthy children and adolescents of both genders, between the age of 6 and 18, dietary intakes were recorded over 4 years, using a yearly administered 3-day diary *(98)*. Bone mass and size were measured at the radius diaphysis using peripheral computerized tomography. A significant positive association was found between long-term protein intakes, on one hand, and periosteal circumferences, cortical area, bone mineral content, and with a calculated strength strain index, on the other hand. These children had relatively high mean protein intakes due to a western style diet. Indeed, protein intakes were around 2 g/kg body weight × day in prepubertal children, whereas they were around 1.5 g/kg × day in pubertal individuals. The minimal requirements for protein intakes in the corresponding age groups are 0.99 and 0.95, respectively *(99)*. There was no association between bone variables and intakes of nutrients with high sulfur-containing amino acids or intake of calcium. Overall, protein intakes accounted for 3–4% of the bone parameters variance *(98)*. However, even when they are prospective and longitudinal, observational studies do not allow one to draw conclusion on a causal relationship. Indeed, it is quite possible that protein intake could be to a large extent related to growth requirement during childhood and adolescence. Only intervention studies could reliably address this question. To our knowledge, there is no large randomized controlled trial having tested the effects of dietary protein supplements on bone mass accumulation, except for milk or dairy products.

In addition to calcium, phosphorus, calories, and vitamins, 1 L of milk provides 32–35 g of protein, mostly casein, but also whey protein which contains numerous growth-promoting elements. The correlation between dairy products intake and bone health has been investigated in both cross-sectional and longitudinal observational studies, and in intervention trials. In growing children, long-term milk avoidance is associated with smaller stature and lower bone mineral mass, either at specific sites or at the whole body levels

(100–108). Low milk intake during childhood and/or adolescence increases the risk of fracture before puberty (+2.6-fold), and possibly later in life *(109,110)*. In a 7-year observational study, there was a positive influence of dairy products consumption on bone mineral density at the spine, hip, and forearm in adolescents, leading thereby to a higher peak bone mass *(69)*. In addition, higher dairy products intakes were associated with greater total and cortical proximal radius cross-sectional area. Based on these observations, it was suggested that whereas calcium supplements could influence volumetric BMD, thus the remodeling process, dairy products may have an additional effect on bone growth and periosteal bone expansion, i.e., a modeling influence *(69)*. In agreement with this observation, milk consumption frequency and milk intake at age 5–12 and 13–17 years were significant predictors of the height of 12–18-year-old adolescents, studied in the NHANES 1999–2002 *(111)*.

A variety of intervention trials have confirmed a favorable influence of dairy products on bone health during childhood and adolescence *(82,112–123)*. In an open randomized intervention trial, Cadogan et al. *(82)* studied the effects of 568 ml/day milk supplement for 18 months in 12-year-old girls. With this milk supplement, the differences between the treated and control groups in calcium and protein intakes at the end of the study were around 420 mg/day and 14 g/day, respectively, taking into consideration the spontaneous consumption. In the milk supplemented group, serum IGF-I levels were significantly higher (+17%). Compared to the control group, the intervention group had greater increases of whole body bone mineral density and bone mineral content.

In another study, cheese supplements appeared to be more beneficial for cortical bone accrual than a similar amount of calcium supplied under the form of tablets *(113)*. This could also be compatible with a favorable effect of dairy products provided protein. Again, the positive influence of milk on cortical bone thickness may be related to an effect on the modeling process, since metacarpal periosteal diameter was significantly increased in Chinese children receiving milk supplements *(121)*.

Only prospective interventional studies will establish whether variations in protein intake within the range recorded in our Western "well-nourished" population can affect bone mass accumulation during growth. Such prospective intervention studies should delineate the crucial years during which modifications in nutrition would be particularly effective for bone mass accumulation in children and in adolescents. This kind of information is of importance in order to make credible and well-targeted recommendations for osteoporosis prevention programs aimed at maximizing peak bone mass.

CONDITIONS IMPAIRING PEAK BONE MASS ATTAINMENT

Various genetic and acquired disorders can impair optimal bone mass acquisition during childhood and adolescence *(124,125)*. In some endocrine disorders, such as Turner's syndrome, Klinefelter's syndrome, glucocorticoid excess, hyperthyroidism or growth hormone deficiency, low bone mass has been attributed to abnormalities in a single hormone system. In diseases such as anorexia nervosa and exercise-associated amenorrhea, malnutrition, sex steroid deficiency, and other factors combine to increase the risk of osteopenia or low bone mass. This is probably also the case of various chronic diseases, which in addition may require therapies that can affect bone metabolism. Impaired bone growth has been frequently observed in chronic rheumatoid arthritis, chronic renal failure, cystic fibrosis, inflammatory bowel diseases, hematologic malignancies, and hemoglobinopathies such as thalassemia major.

Delayed Puberty

Epidemiological studies have provided suggestive evidence that late menarche is a risk factor for osteoporosis through a negative effect on PBM. In a cohort of men with a history of delayed puberty, osteopenia has been reported *(126)*. There is an inverse correlation between distal radius or tibia cortical thickness or cortical density, and menarcheal age *(127,128)*. The causes of delayed adolescence have been classified into permanent and temporary disorders *(129)*. The permanent ones can be due to either hypothalamo-pituitary or gonadal failure *(129)*. Among the temporary disorders, some can be explained by the presence of chronic systemic diseases, nutritional disorders, psychological stress, intensive competitive training, or hormonal disturbances such as hyposecretion of thyroid hormones or growth hormone or hypercortisolism *(129)*. However, the most common cause of delayed adolescence is the so-called constitutional delay of growth and puberty (CDGP). It is a transient disorder with, in some cases, a familial history of late menarcheal age of the mother or sisters or a delayed growth spurt in the father. This condition has been considered as an extreme form of the physiological variation of the timing of the onset of puberty for which the "normal" range is about 8–12 and 9–13 years of age in girls and boys, respectively. The onset of puberty is a complex process involving the activation of the hypothalamic–pituitary–gonadal axis and other endocrine systems such as the growth hormone–IGF axis of which the targets include factors influencing the bone mineral balance and the growth rate of the skeleton. Several mechanisms whereby CDGP may lead to a low peak bone mass have been suggested *(130)*.

Anorexia Nervosa

Significant deficits in trabecular and cortical bone, which may result in osteoporotic fractures, have been observed in young adult women with chronic anorexia nervosa. Several factors can contribute to the reduced bone mass acquisition, including low protein intake resulting in a reduction in IGF-I production and thereby decreasing bone formation; low calcium intake enhancing bone resorption; estrogen deficiency; and glucocorticoid excess which interrupts normal acquisition of bone mineral and may contribute to increased bone loss *(131)*.

Exercise-Associated Amenorrhea

Impaired bone mass acquisition can occur when hypogonadism and low body mass accompany intensive physical activity. As in anorexia nervosa, both nutritional and hormonal factors probably contribute to this impairment. Intake of energy, protein and calcium may be inadequate as athletes go on diets to maintain an idealized physique for their sport. Intensive training during childhood may contribute to a later onset and completion of puberty. Hypogonadism, as expressed by the occurrence of oligomenorrhea or amenorrhea, can lead to low bone mass in females who begin training intensively after menarche *(124)*. Oligo-amenorrhea in long-distance runners was found to be associated with a decrease in BMD affecting more the lumbar spine than the proximal and mid-shaft femur *(132)*.

CONCLUSION

Peak bone mass is an important determinant of osteoporotic fracture risk. Hence, the interest of exploring ways of increasing peak bone mass in the primary prevention of osteoporosis. Bone mineral mass accumulation from infancy to postpuberty is a complex process implicating interactions of genetic, endocrine, mechanical, and nutritional factors. From birth to peak bone mass (PBM), which is attained in axial skeleton and in the proximal femur by the end of the second decade, the increase in mass and strength is essentially due to an increment in bone size, vBMD changing very little during growth. Therefore, clinically the best simple estimate of bone strength is aBMD rather than vBMD which does not take into account the size of the bone. It can be estimated that in women an increase of PBM by 10%, i.e., by approximately 1 standard deviation (SD), could decrease the risk of fragility fracture by 50%. Like standing height in any individual bone mineral mass during growth follows a trajectory corresponding to a given percentile or standard deviation from the mean. Nevertheless, this trajectory can be influenced by the environmental factors. On the negative side various chronic diseases and their treatment can shift downward this trajectory. On the positive side and most important in the context of primary prevention of adult osteoporosis, prospective randomized controlled trials strongly suggest that increasing the calcium intake or mechanical loading can shift upward the age–bone mass trajectory. Prepuberty appears to be an opportune time for obtaining a substantial benefit of increasing either the calcium intake or the physical activity. Further studies should demonstrate that changes observed remain substantial by the end of the second decade and thus are translated in a greater peak bone mass. In this long-term evaluation of the consequence of modifying the environment, it will be of critical importance to assess whether any change in densitometric and morphometric bone variables observed at PBM confers a greater resistance to mechanical strain.

ACKNOWLEDGMENTS

Research by the authors of this chapter is supported by the Swiss National Science Foundation (Grant Nos. 32-49757.96, 32-58880.99, and 32-58962.99), Nestec Ltd, Cerin, Novartis, Institut Candia.

REFERENCES

1. Bachrach LK. Assessing bone health in children: who to test and what does it mean? Pediatr Endocrinol Rev 2005;2(Suppl 3):332–336.
2. Binkovitz LA, Sparke P, Henwood MJ. Pediatric DXA: clinical applications. Pediatr Radiol 2007;37(7):625–635.
3. Seeman E, Hopper JL. Genetic and environmental components of the population variance in bone density. Osteoporos Int 1997;7(Suppl 3):S10–16.
4. Ammann P, Rizzoli R. Bone strength and its determinants. Osteoporos Int 2003;14(Suppl 3):S13–18.
5. Engelke K, Gluer CC. Quality and performance measures in bone densitometry: part 1: errors and diagnosis. Osteoporos Int 2006;17:1283–1292.
6. Gluer CC, Lu Y, Engelke K. Quality and performance measures in bone densitometry. Part 2: fracture risk. Osteoporos Int 2006;17:1449–1458.
7. Kanis JA, Gluer CC. An update on the diagnosis and assessment of osteoporosis with densitometry. Committee of Scientific Advisors, International Osteoporosis Foundation. Osteoporos Int 2000;11: 192–202.

8. Kanis JA. Diagnosis of osteoporosis and assessment of fracture risk. Lancet 2002;359:1929–1936.
9. Slosman DO, Rizzoli R, Donath A, Bonjour JP. Vertebral bone mineral density measured laterally by dual-energy X-ray absorptiometry. Osteoporos Int 1990;1:23–29.
10. Katzman DK, Bachrach LK, Carter DR, Marcus R. Clinical and anthropometric correlates of bone mineral acquisition in healthy adolescent girls. J Clin Endocrinol Metab 1991;73:1332–1339.
11. Trotter M, Hixon BB. Sequential changes in weight, density, and percentage ash weight of human skeletons from an early fetal period through old age. Anat Rec 1974;179:1–18.
12. Bonjour JP, Theintz G, Buchs B, Slosman D, Rizzoli R. Critical years and stages of puberty for spinal and femoral bone mass accumulation during adolescence. J Clin Endocrinol Metab 1991;73: 555–563.
13. Gilsanz V, Boechat MI, Roe TF, Loro ML, Sayre JW, Goodman WG. Gender differences in vertebral body sizes in children and adolescents. Radiology 1994;190:673–677.
14. Theintz G, Buchs B, Rizzoli R, Slosman D, Clavien H, Sizonenko PC, Bonjour JP. Longitudinal monitoring of bone mass accumulation in healthy adolescents: evidence for a marked reduction after 16 years of age at the levels of lumbar spine and femoral neck in female subjects. J Clin Endocrinol Metab 1992;75:1060–1065.
15. Bonjour JP, Rizzoli R. Bone acquisition in adolescence. In: Marcus R, Feldman D, Kelsey J, eds. Osteoporosis. Vol. 1, Chapter 25. San Diego: Academic Press, 2001:621–638.
16. Seeman E. Clinical review 137: sexual dimorphism in skeletal size, density, and strength. J Clin Endocrinol Metab 2001;86:4576–4584.
17. Fournier PE, Rizzoli R, Slosman DO, Theintz G, Bonjour JP. Asynchrony between the rates of standing height gain and bone mass accumulation during puberty. Osteoporos Int 1997;7:525–532.
18. Bailey DA, Wedge JH, McCulloch RG, Martin AD, Bernhardson SC. Epidemiology of fractures of the distal end of the radius in children as associated with growth. J Bone Joint Surg Am 1989;71:1225–1231.
19. Ferrari SL, Chevalley T, Bonjour JP, Rizzoli R. Childhood fractures are associated with decreased bone mass gain during puberty: an early marker of persistent bone fragility? J Bone Miner Res 2006;21: 501–507.
20. Landin LA. Fracture patterns in children. Analysis of 8682 fractures with special reference to incidence, etiology and secular changes in a Swedish urban population 1950–1979. Acta Orthop Scand Suppl 1983;202:1–109.
21. Gilsanz V, Gibbens DT, Carlson M, Boechat MI, Cann CE, Schulz EE. Peak trabecular vertebral density: a comparison of adolescent and adult females. Calcif Tissue Int 1988;43:260–262.
22. Wren TA, Kim PS, Janicka A, Sanchez M, Gilsanz V. Timing of peak bone mass: discrepancies between CT and DXA. J Clin Endocrinol Metab 2007;92:938–941.
23. Garn SM, Rohmann CG, Wagner B, Ascoli W. Continuing bone growth throughout life: a general phenomenon. Am J Phys Anthropol 1967;26:313–317.
24. Garn SM, Wagner B, Rohmann CG, Ascoli W. Further evidence for continuing bone expansion. Am J Phys Anthropol 1968;28:219–221.
25. Seeman E. Invited review: pathogenesis of osteoporosis. J Appl Physiol 2003;95:2142–2151.
26. Turner CH. Toward a cure for osteoporosis: reversal of excessive bone fragility. Osteoporos Int 1991;2:12–19.
27. Rosen JF, Chesney RW. Circulating calcitriol concentrations in health and disease. J Pediatr 1983;103: 1–17.
28. Corvilain J, Abramow M. Growth and renal control of plasma phosphate. J Clin Endocrinol Metab 1972;34:452–459.
29. Krabbe S, Transbol I, Christiansen C. Bone mineral homeostasis, bone growth, and mineralisation during years of pubertal growth: a unifying concept. Arch Dis Child 1982;57:359–363.
30. Round JM, Butcher S, Steele R. Changes in plasma inorganic phosphorus and alkaline phosphatase activity during the adolescent growth spurt. Ann Hum Biol 1979;6:129.
31. Caverzasio J, Bonjour JP. IGF-I, a key regulator of renal phosphate transport and 1,25-dihydroxyvitamin D3 production during growth. News Physiol Sci 1991;6:206–210.
32. Underwood LE, D'Ercole AJ, Van Wyk JJ. Somatomedin-C and the assessment of growth. Pediatr Clin North Am 1980;27:771–782.
33. Krabbe S, Christiansen C, Rodbro P, Transbol I. Pubertal growth as reflected by simultaneous changes in bone mineral content and serum alkaline phosphatase. Acta Paediatr Scand 1980;69:49–52.

34. Delmas PD, Chatelain P, Malaval L, Bonne G. Serum bone GLA-protein in growth hormone deficient children. J Bone Miner Res 1986;1:333–338.
35. Szulc P, Seeman E, Delmas PD. Biochemical measurements of bone turnover in children and adolescents. Osteoporos Int 2000;11:281–294.
36. Krabbe S, Christiansen C. Longitudinal study of calcium metabolism in male puberty. I. Bone mineral content, and serum levels of alkaline phosphatase, phosphate and calcium. Acta Paediatr Scand 1984;73:745–749.
37. Fukumoto S, Yamashita T. FGF23 is a hormone-regulating phosphate metabolism-Unique biological characteristics of FGF23. Bone 2007;40:1190–1195.
38. Ferrari SL, Bonjour JP, Rizzoli R. Fibroblast growth factor-23 relationship to dietary phosphate and renal phosphate handling in healthy young men. J Clin Endocrinol Metab 2005;90:1519–1524.
39. Cadogan J, Blumsohn A, Barker ME, Eastell R. A longitudinal study of bone gain in pubertal girls: anthropometric and biochemical correlates. J Bone Miner Res 1998;13:1602–1612.
40. Pocock NA, Eisman JA, Hopper JL, Yeates MG, Sambrook PN, Eberl S. Genetic determinants of bone mass in adults. A twin study. J Clin Invest 1987;80:706–710.
41. Rizzoli R, Bonjour JP, Ferrari SL. Osteoporosis, genetics and hormones. J Mol Endocrinol 2001;26: 79–94.
42. Seeman E, Hopper JL, Bach LA, Cooper ME, Parkinson E, McKay J, Jerums G. Reduced bone mass in daughters of women with osteoporosis. N Engl J Med 1989;320:554–558.
43. Nguyen TV, Howard GM, Kelly PJ, Eisman JA. Bone mass, lean mass, and fat mass: same genes or same environments? Am J Epidemiol 1998;147:3–16.
44. Slemenda CW, Christian JC, Williams CJ, Norton JA, Johnston CC. Genetic determinants of bone mass in adult women: a reevaluation of the twin model and the potential importance of gene interaction on heritability estimates. J Bone Miner Res 1991;6:561–567.
45. Ferrari S, Rizzoli R, Slosman D, Bonjour JP. Familial resemblance for bone mineral mass is expressed before puberty. J Clin Endocrinol Metab 1998;83:358–361.
46. Garnero P, Arden NK, Griffiths G, Delmas PD, Spector TD. Genetic influence on bone turnover in postmenopausal twins. J Clin Endocrinol Metab 1996;81:140–146.
47. Uitterlinden AG, Pols HA, Burger H, Huang Q, Van Daele PL, Van Duijn CM, Hofman A, Birkenhager JC, Van Leeuwen JP. A large-scale population-based study of the association of vitamin D receptor gene polymorphisms with bone mineral density. J Bone Miner Res 1996;11:1241–1248.
48. Ferrari SL, Rizzoli R, Slosman DO, Bonjour JP. Do dietary calcium and age explain the controversy surrounding the relationship between bone mineral density and vitamin D receptor gene polymorphisms? J Bone Miner Res 1998;13:363–370.
49. Sainz J, Van Tornout JM, Loro ML, Sayre J, Roe TF, Gilsanz V. Vitamin D-receptor gene polymorphisms and bone density in prepubertal American girls of Mexican descent. N Engl J Med 1997;337: 77–82.
50. Ferrari S, Bonjour JP, Rizzoli R. The vitamin D receptor gene and calcium metabolism. Trends Endocrinol Metab 1998;9:259–265.
51. Lorentzon M, Lorentzon R, Nordstrom P. Vitamin D receptor gene polymorphism is associated with birth height, growth to adolescence, and adult stature in healthy caucasian men: a cross-sectional and longitudinal study. J Clin Endocrinol Metab 2000;85:1666–1670.
52. Ferrari SL, Deutsch S, Choudhury U, Chevalley T, Bonjour JP, Dermitzakis ET, Rizzoli R, Antonarakis SE. Polymorphisms in the low-density lipoprotein receptor-related protein 5 (LRP5) gene are associated with variation in vertebral bone mass, vertebral bone size, and stature in whites. Am J Hum Genet 2004;74:866–875.
53. Bass S, Pearce G, Bradney M, Hendrich E, Delmas PD, Harding A, Seeman E. Exercise before puberty may confer residual benefits in bone density in adulthood: studies in active prepubertal and retired female gymnasts. J Bone Miner Res 1998;13:500–507.
54. Kannus P, Haapasalo H, Sankelo M, Sievanen H, Pasanen M, Heinonen A, Oja P, Vuori I. Effect of starting age of physical activity on bone mass in the dominant arm of tennis and squash players. Ann Intern Med 1995;123:27–31.
55. Khan KM, Bennell KL, Hopper JL, Flicker L, Nowson CA, Sherwin AJ, Crichton KJ, Harcourt PR, Wark JD. Self-reported ballet classes undertaken at age 10–12 years and hip bone mineral density in later life. Osteoporos Int 1998;8:165–173.

56. Haapasalo H, Kontulainen S, Sievanen H, Kannus P, Jarvinen M, Vuori I. Exercise-induced bone gain is due to enlargement in bone size without a change in volumetric bone density: a peripheral quantitative computed tomography study of the upper arms of male tennis players. Bone 2000;27:351–357.
57. Morris FL, Naughton GA, Gibbs JL, Carlson JS, Wark JD. Prospective ten-month exercise intervention in premenarcheal girls: positive effects on bone and lean mass. J Bone Miner Res 1997;12:1453–1462.
58. Bradney M, Pearce G, Naughton G, Sullivan C, Bass S, Beck T, Carlson J, Seeman E. Moderate exercise during growth in prepubertal boys: changes in bone mass, size, volumetric density, and bone strength: a controlled prospective study. J Bone Miner Res 1998;13:1814–1821.
59. Hind K, Burrows M. Weight-bearing exercise and bone mineral accrual in children and adolescents: a review of controlled trials. Bone 2007;40:14–27.
60. Kriemler S, Zahner L, Puder JJ, Braun-Fahrländer C, Schindler C, Farpour-Lambert NJ, Kränzlin M, Rizzoli R. Weight-bearing bones are more sensitive to physical exercise in boys than in girls during pre- and early puberty: a cross-sectional study. Osteoporos Int 2008;19: 1749–1758.
61. Marcus R. Exercise: moving in the right direction. J Bone Miner Res 1998;13:1793–1796.
62. Karlsson MK, Johnell O, Obrant KJ. Is bone mineral density advantage maintained long-term in previous weight lifters? Calcif Tissue Int 1995;57:325–328.
63. Kontulainen S, Kannus P, Haapasalo H, Heinonen A, Sievanen H, Oja P, Vuori I. Changes in bone mineral content with decreased training in competitive young adult tennis players and controls: a prospective 4-yr follow-up. Med Sci Sports Exerc 1999;31:646–652.
64. Karlsson MK, Linden C, Karlsson C, Johnell O, Obrant K, Seeman E. Exercise during growth and bone mineral density and fractures in old age. Lancet 2000;355:469–470.
65. Bonjour JP, Rizzoli R. Bone acquisition in adolescence. In: Marcus R, Feldman D, Kelsey J, eds. Osteoporosis. San Diego, CA: Academic Press, 1996:465–476.
66. Weaver CM. Calcium requirements of physically active people. Am J Clin Nutr 2000;72:579S–584S.
67. Chan GM. Dietary calcium and bone mineral status of children and adolescents. Am J Dis Child 1991;145:631–634.
68. Lloyd T, Rollings N, Andon MB, Demers LM, Eggli DF, Kieselhorst K, Kulin H, Landis JR, Martel JK, Orr G, et al. Determinants of bone density in young women. I. Relationships among pubertal development, total body bone mass, and total body bone density in premenarchal females. J Clin Endocrinol Metab 1992;75:383–387.
69. Matkovic V, Landoll JD, Badenhop-Stevens NE, Ha EY, Crncevic-Orlic Z, Li B, Goel P. Nutrition influences skeletal development from childhood to adulthood: a study of hip, spine, and forearm in adolescent females. J Nutr 2004;134:701S–705S.
70. Cheng JC, Maffulli N, Leung SS, Lee WT, Lau JT, Chan KM. Axial and peripheral bone mineral acquisition: a 3-year longitudinal study in Chinese adolescents. Eur J Pediatr 1999;158:506–512.
71. Uusi-Rasi K, Haapasalo H, Kannus P, Pasanen M, Sievanen H, Oja P, Vuori I. Determinants of bone mineralization in 8 to 20 year old Finnish females. Eur J Clin Nutr 1997;51:54–59.
72. Bonjour JP, Carrie AL, Ferrari S, Clavien H, Slosman D, Theintz G, Rizzoli R. Calcium-enriched foods and bone mass growth in prepubertal girls: a randomized, double-blind, placebo-controlled trial. J Clin Invest 1997;99:1287–1294.
73. Chevalley T, Bonjour JP, Ferrari S, Hans D, Rizzoli R. Skeletal site selectivity in the effects of calcium supplementation on areal bone mineral density gain: a randomized, double-blind, placebo-controlled trial in prepubertal boys. J Clin Endocrinol Metab 2005;90:3342–3349.
74. Chevalley T, Rizzoli R, Hans D, Ferrari S, Bonjour JP. Interaction between calcium intake and menarcheal age on bone mass gain: an eight-year follow-up study from prepuberty to postmenarche. J Clin Endocrinol Metab 2005;90:44–51.
75. Johnston CC, Miller JZ, Slemenda CW, Reister TK, Hui S, Christian JC, Peacock M. Calcium supplementation and increases in bone mineral density in children. N Engl J Med 1992;327:82–87.
76. Matkovic V, Goel PK, Badenhop-Stevens NE, Landoll JD, Li B, Ilich JZ, Skugor M, Nagode LA, Mobley SL, Ha EJ, Hangartner TN, Clairmont A. Calcium supplementation and bone mineral density in females from childhood to young adulthood: a randomized controlled trial. Am J Clin Nutr 2005;81: 175–188.
77. Nowson CA, Green RM, Hopper JL, Sherwin AJ, Young D, Kaymakci B, Guest CS, Smid M, Larkins RG, Wark JD. A co-twin study of the effect of calcium supplementation on bone density during adolescence. Osteoporos Int 1997;7:219–225.

78. Winzenberg T, Shaw K, Fryer J, Jones G. Effects of calcium supplementation on bone density in healthy children: meta-analysis of randomised controlled trials. BMJ 2006;333:775.
79. Zamora SA, Rizzoli R, Belli DC, Slosman DO, Bonjour JP. Vitamin D supplementation during infancy is associated with higher bone mineral mass in prepubertal girls. J Clin Endocrinol Metab 1999;84: 4541–4544.
80. Barker DJ. Intrauterine programming of adult disease. Mol Med Today 1995;1:418–423.
81. Cooper C, Westlake S, Harvey N, Javaid K, Dennison E, Hanson M. Review: developmental origins of osteoporotic fracture. Osteoporos Int 2006;17:337–347.
82. Cadogan J, Eastell R, Jones N, Barker ME. Milk intake and bone mineral acquisition in adolescent girls: randomised, controlled intervention trial. BMJ 1997;315:1255–1260.
83. Ferrari S, Rizzoli R, Manen D, Slosman D, Bonjour JP. Vitamin D receptor gene start codon polymorphisms (FokI) and bone mineral density: interaction with age, dietary calcium, and 3'-end region polymorphisms. J Bone Miner Res 1998;13:925–930.
84. Orwoll ES. The effects of dietary protein insufficiency and excess on skeletal health. Bone 1992;13: 343–350.
85. Rizzoli R, Bonjour JP. Dietary protein and bone health. J Bone Miner Res 2004;19:527–531.
86. Rizzoli R, Bonjour JP, Chevalley T. Dietary protein intakes and bone growth. In: Nutritional Aspects of Osteoporosis 2006, First Edition, International Congress Series 1297, pp. 50–59. P. Burckhardt B. Dawson-Hughes and R.P. Heaney, eds. Elsevier B.V., Amsterdam, 2007.
87. Bonjour JP, Ammann P, Chevalley T, Rizzoli R. Protein intake and bone growth. Can J Appl Physiol 2001;26(Suppl):S153–S166.
88. Isley WL, Underwood LE, Clemmons DR. Dietary components that regulate serum somatomedin-C concentrations in humans. J Clin Invest 1983;71:175–182.
89. Thissen JP, Ketelslegers JM, Underwood LE. Nutritional regulation of the insulin-like growth factors. Endocr Rev 1994;15:80–101.
90. Ammann P, Bourrin S, Bonjour JP, Meyer JM, Rizzoli R. Protein undernutrition-induced bone loss is associated with decreased IGF-I levels and estrogen deficiency. J Bone Miner Res 2000;15: 683–690.
91. Bourrin S, Ammann P, Bonjour JP, Rizzoli R. Dietary protein restriction lowers plasma insulin-like growth factor I (IGF-I), impairs cortical bone formation, and induces osteoblastic resistance to IGF-I in adult female rats. Endocrinology 2000;141:3149–3155.
92. Caverzasio J, Montessuit C, Bonjour JP. Stimulatory effect of insulin-like growth factor-1 on renal Pi transport and plasma 1,25-dihydroxyvitamin D3. Endocrinology 1990;127:453–459.
93. Rosen CJ. Insulin-like growth factor I and bone mineral density: experience from animal models and human observational studies. Best Pract Res Clin Endocrinol Metab 2004;18:423–435.
94. Yakar S, Rosen CJ. From mouse to man: redefining the role of insulin-like growth factor-I in the acquisition of bone mass. Exp Biol Med (Maywood) 2003;228:245–252.
95. Ammann P, Rizzoli R, Muller K, Slosman D, Bonjour JP. IGF-I and pamidronate increase bone mineral density in ovariectomized adult rats. Am J Physiol 1993;265:E770–E776.
96. Clavien H, Theintz G, Rizzoli R, Bonjour JP. Does puberty alter dietary habits in adolescents living in a Western society? J Adolesc Health 1996;19:68–75.
97. Chevalley T, Bonjour JP, Ferrari S, Rizzoli R. High-protein intake enhances the positive impact of physical activity on BMC in prepubertal boys. J. Bone Miner. Res 23; 131–142, 2008.
98. Alexy U, Remer T, Manz F, Neu CM, Schoenau E. Long-term protein intake and dietary potential renal acid load are associated with bone modeling and remodeling at the proximal radius in healthy children. Am J Clin Nutr 2005;82:1107–1114.
99. Young VR, Borgonha S. Nitrogen and amino acid requirements: the Massachusetts Institute of Technology amino acid requirement pattern. J Nutr 2000;130:1841S–1849S.
100. Black RE, Williams SM, Jones IE, Goulding A. Children who avoid drinking cow milk have low dietary calcium intakes and poor bone health. Am J Clin Nutr 2002;76:675–680.
101. Bounds W, Skinner J, Carruth BR, Ziegler P. The relationship of dietary and lifestyle factors to bone mineral indexes in children. J Am Diet Assoc 2005;105:735–741.
102. Chan GM, Hoffman K, McMurry M. Effects of dairy products on bone and body composition in pubertal girls. J Pediatr 1995;126:551–556.

103. Henderson RC, Hayes PR. Bone mineralization in children and adolescents with a milk allergy. Bone Miner 1994;27:1–12.
104. Hidvegi E, Arato A, Cserhati E, Horvath C, Szabo A. Slight decrease in bone mineralization in cow milk-sensitive children. J Pediatr Gastroenterol Nutr 2003;36:44–49.
105. Infante D, Tormo R. Risk of inadequate bone mineralization in diseases involving long-term suppression of dairy products. J Pediatr Gastroenterol Nutr 2000;30:310–313.
106. Jensen VB, Jorgensen IM, Rasmussen KB, Molgaard C, Prahl P. Bone mineral status in children with cow milk allergy. Pediatr Allergy Immunol 2004;15:562–565.
107. Opotowsky AR, Bilezikian JP. Racial differences in the effect of early milk consumption on peak and postmenopausal bone mineral density. J Bone Miner Res 2003;18:1978–1988.
108. Rockell JE, Williams SM, Taylor RW, Grant AM, Jones IE, Goulding A. Two-year changes in bone and body composition in young children with a history of prolonged milk avoidance. Osteoporos Int 2005;16:1016–1023.
109. Goulding A, Rockell JE, Black RE, Grant AM, Jones IE, Williams SM. Children who avoid drinking cow's milk are at increased risk for prepubertal bone fractures. J Am Diet Assoc 2004;104:250–253.
110. Teegarden D, Lyle RM, Proulx WR, Johnston CC, Weaver CM. Previous milk consumption is associated with greater bone density in young women. Am J Clin Nutr 1999;69:1014–1017.
111. Wiley AS. Does milk make children grow? Relationships between milk consumption and height in NHANES 1999–2002. Am J Hum Biol 2005;17:425–441.
112. Baker IA, Elwood PC, Hughes J, Jones M, Moore F, Sweetnam PM. A randomised controlled trial of the effect of the provision of free school milk on the growth of children. J Epidemiol Community Health 1980;34:31–34.
113. Cheng S, Lyytikainen A, Kroger H, Lamberg-Allardt C, Alen M, Koistinen A, Wang QJ, Suuriniemi M, Suominen H, Mahonen A, Nicholson PH, Ivaska KK, Korpela R, Ohlsson C, Vaananen KH, Tylavsky F. Effects of calcium, dairy product, and vitamin D supplementation on bone mass accrual and body composition in 10–12-y-old girls: a 2-y randomized trial. Am J Clin Nutr 2005;82:1115–1126; quiz 1147–1148.
114. Du X, Zhu K, Trube A, Fraser DR, Greenfield AH, Zhang Q, Ma G, Hu X. Effects of school-milk intervention on growth and bone mineral accretion in Chinese girls aged 10–12 years: accounting for cluster randomisation. Br J Nutr 2005;94:1038–1039.
115. Du X, Zhu K, Trube A, Zhang Q, Ma G, Hu X, Fraser DR, Greenfield H. School-milk intervention trial enhances growth and bone mineral accretion in Chinese girls aged 10–12 years in Beijing. Br J Nutr 2004;92:159–168.
116. Ho SC, Guldan GS, Woo J, Yu R, Tse MM, Sham A, Cheng J. A prospective study of the effects of 1-year calcium-fortified soy milk supplementation on dietary calcium intake and bone health in Chinese adolescent girls aged 14 to 16. Osteoporos Int 2005;16:1907–1916.
117. Lau EM, Lynn H, Chan YH, Lau W, Woo J. Benefits of milk powder supplementation on bone accretion in Chinese children. Osteoporos Int 2004;15:654–658.
118. Merrilees MJ, Smart EJ, Gilchrist NL, Frampton C, Turner JG, Hooke E, March RL, Maguire P. Effects of diary food supplements on bone mineral density in teenage girls. Eur J Nutr 2000;39: 256–262.
119. Volek JS, Gomez AL, Scheett TP, Sharman MJ, French DN, Rubin MR, Ratamess NA, McGuigan MM, Kraemer WJ. Increasing fluid milk favorably affects bone mineral density responses to resistance training in adolescent boys. J Am Diet Assoc 2003;103:1353–1356.
120. Zhu K, Greenfield H, Du X, Zhang Q, Fraser DR. Effects of milk supplementation on cortical bone gain in Chinese girls aged 10–12 years. Asia Pac J Clin Nutr 2003;12(Suppl):S47.
121. Zhu K, Greenfield H, Zhang Q, Ma G, Zhang Z, Hu X, Fraser DR. Bone mineral accretion and growth in Chinese adolescent girls following the withdrawal of school milk intervention: preliminary results after two years. Asia Pac J Clin Nutr 2004;13:S83.
122. Zhu K, Du X, Cowell CT, Greenfield H, Blades B, Dobbins TA, Zhang Q, Fraser DR. Effects of school milk intervention on cortical bone accretion and indicators relevant to bone metabolism in Chinese girls aged 10–12 y in Beijing. Am J Clin Nutr 2005;81:1168–1175.
123. Zhu K, Zhang Q, Foo LH, Trube A, Ma G, Hu X, Du X, Cowell CT, Fraser DR, Greenfield H. Growth, bone mass, and vitamin D status of Chinese adolescent girls 3 y after withdrawal of milk supplementation. Am J Clin Nutr 2006;83:714–721.

124. Bachrach LK. Malnutrition, endocrinopathies, and deficits in bone mass acquisition. In: Bonjour JP, Tsang RC, eds. Nutrition and Bone Development. Vol. 41. Philadelphia, PA: Lippincott-Raven, 1999:261–277.
125. Baroncelli GI, Bertelloni S, Sodini F, Saggese G. Osteoporosis in children and adolescents: etiology and management. Paediatr Drugs 2005;7:295–323.
126. Finkelstein JS, Neer RM, Biller BM, Crawford JD, Klibanski A. Osteopenia in men with a history of delayed puberty. N Engl J Med 1992;326:600–604.
127. Chevalley T, Bonjour JP, Ferrari S, Rizzoli R. Influence of age at menarche on forearm bone microstructure in healthy young women. J Clin Endocrinol Metab 2008; 93: 2594–2601.
128. Chevalley T, Bonjour JP, Ferrari S, Rizzoli R. Deleterious effect of late menarche on distal tibia microstructure in healthy 20-year-old and premenopausal middle-aged women. J Bone Miner Res 2009; 24: 144–152.
129. Bourguignon JP. Delayed puberty and hypogonadism. In: Bertrand J, Rappaport R, Sizonenko PC, eds. Pediatric Endocrinology, Physiology, Pathophysiology, and Clinical Aspects. Baltimore, MD: Williams & Wilkins, 1993:404–429.
130. Bonjour JP. Delayed puberty and peak bone mass. Eur J Endocrinol 1998;139:257–259.
131. Misra M, Klibanski A. Evaluation and treatment of low bone density in anorexia nervosa. Nutr Clin Care 2002;5:298–308.
132. Gremion G, Rizzoli R, Slosman D, Theintz G, Bonjour JP. Oligo-amenorrheic long-distance runners may lose more bone in spine than in femur. Med Sci Sports Exerc 2001;33:15–21.

2 Bone Mineral Assessment of the Axial Skeleton: Technical Aspects

Thomas F. Lang

CONTENTS

SUMMARY

The goal of this chapter is to describe the underlying principles and error sources associated with X-ray based bone densitometry methods used to assess the central skeleton. The first portion of the chapter focuses on projectional densitometry measurements which are most widely used in the clinical setting. The concepts of single and dual photon absorptiometry are used to provide a simple and clear explanation of the physical principles underlying dual X-ray absorptiometry (DXA). The section then describes the error sources associated with DXA, including precision errors, bone size dependence and the effect of adipose tissue distribution. The second portion of the chapter describes quantitative X-ray computed tomography (QCT), an adaptation of clinical computed tomography imaging for assessment of skeletal integrity. This section describes how CT images are acquired and the physical meaning of the image units as they relate to bone mineral content and density. The section then describes the use of QCT of the hip and spine to assess cortical and trabecular bone mineral density, the physical errors associated with those assessments, and the application of QCT to assess measures of bone quality such as bone geometry and whole bone strength.

Key Words: Axial skeleton, bone mineral, X-ray absorptiometry, quantitative computed tomography

INTRODUCTION

The purpose of the bone density measurement is to quantify the density or mass of bone mineral (calcium hydroxyapatite) in a medium consisting not only of the mineral itself but also fat, muscle, and bone marrow constituents as well as other biological materials.

From: *Contemporary Endocrinology: Osteoporosis: Pathophysiology and Clinical Management*
Edited by: R. A. Adler, DOI 10.1007/978-1-59745-459-9_2,

Measurements at central sites, such as the hip and spine, are inherently more complex than peripheral measurements because the bones are embedded in greater tissue thicknesses of more variable composition. Compared to peripheral sites (e.g., the calcaneus and forearm), where single-energy X-ray absorptiometry (SXA) and ultrasound measurements are available, central measurements require multiple-energy projection imaging techniques such as dual X-ray absorptiometry (DXA) or quantitative computed tomography (QCT).

The purpose of this chapter is to describe the underlying physical principles and principal error sources of DXA and QCT measurements as they apply to the central skeleton. In addition to describing the underlying principles and error sources, which have remained relatively constant since the inception of these techniques, this chapter will also provide information on the currently available whole-body DXA and QCT systems and some of the new approaches used by these systems to reduce cost and scan times and to improve precision and ease of use.

All X-ray-based bone densitometry systems operate by comparing the X-ray attenuation of the tissue being measured to the attenuation of a reference system containing a mineral sample of known composition. In most systems, the mineral used in the reference sample is calcium hydroxyapatite ($Ca_{10}(PO_4)_6OH_2$). The comparison to a reference of fixed composition assumes that the composition of the mineral in the tissue does not vary significantly. Although this assumption is violated in a few disease conditions, it is generally not considered a problem for the clinical application of bone densitometry.

The term X-ray attenuation refers to the removal of X-ray photons from the incident beam of X-rays impinging on the tissue. At the X-ray energies common in bone mineral density measurements, the two common mechanisms are the photoelectric effect, in which an atom absorbs the incident photon, and Compton scattering, in which the photon is deflected by a collision with an atomic electron and loses an amount of energy which is a function of both the incident energy and the deflection angle. Photoelectric absorption and Compton scattering depend on the energy of the incident photon, the density of electrons in the tissue, and the mean atomic number of the atoms in the tissue. Photoelectric absorption depends particularly strongly on the atomic number (Z) of the tissue and is more important in bone than in soft tissue because the bone contains a larger proportion of the higher-Z elements such as calcium ($Z=20$) and phosphorus ($Z=15$). The fractional attenuation of incident X-ray photons as a function distance L in centimeters of tissue traversed is

$$\frac{I}{I_0} = \exp(-(\mu \cdot L)) \tag{1}$$

where I is the measured X-ray intensity exiting the tissue, I_0 is the incident X-ray intensity, and μ is called the linear attenuation coefficient and is typically given in units of cm^{-1}. It is also possible to write this equation using the mass attenuation coefficient μ_m, which is typically given in cm^2/g, and which depends *only* on the photon energy and the elemental composition of the tissue:

$$\frac{I}{I_0} = \exp(-(\mu_m \cdot \rho L)) \tag{2}$$

ρ is the density in g/cm^3 of the tissue. As we will see later, if the μ_m of the tissue is known, it is possible to measure the areal density, ρL (g/cm^2), which is the primary measurement provided by DXA. ρL is the mineral mass per unit cross-sectional area measured at a given point in the two-dimensional DXA image. On the other hand, QCT images are cross-sectional maps of the linear attenuation coefficient (μ), which are converted to maps of bone-equivalent density (typically mg calcium hydroxyapatite per cm^3 of tissue) by comparison to a calibration standard scanned in the CT system.

PROJECTIONAL ABSORPTIOMETRY

In a DXA system, the areal density of bone mineral is measured at a specific location in the image based on the differential attenuations of two X-ray beams of different energies. Before discussing the procedure by which the areal density is calculated from the absorptiometric measurements, we will explore two simple examples, single-photon absorptiometry (SPA) *(1–3)* and dual-photon absorptiometry (DPA) *(4–6)*. These two techniques are based on measurement of attenuation of monoenergetic radionuclide sources (DPA employed a ^{153}Gd radionuclide source with 44 and 100 keV photon energies) and were employed prior to the introduction of DXA. However, the simple physics employed in SPA and DPA devices can be readily extended to understand the basic underlying principle of DXA, which utilizes a poly-energetic X-ray source.

Figure 1 shows a cross section through an idealized limb consisting of an outer cylinder containing concentric rings consisting of subcutaneous fat, muscle, and bone. An intensity I_0 of photons of known energy E is emitted from the radionuclide source and impinges on the limb. On the other side, the output intensity I is measured. The fractional attenuation of the photon beam is given by

$$\frac{I}{I_0} = \exp\left(-\left(\mu_{\mathrm{m}}^{\mathrm{fat}} \cdot (\rho L)^{\mathrm{fat}} + \mu_{\mathrm{m}}^{\mathrm{muscle}} \cdot (\rho L)^{\mathrm{muscle}} + \mu_{\mathrm{m}}^{\mathrm{bone}} \cdot (\rho L)^{\mathrm{bone}}\right)\right) \tag{3}$$

It is clear that to measure the areal density $(\rho L)^{\mathrm{bone}}$, we must know the areal densities of the other components, assuming a priori knowledge of the mass attenuation coefficients for muscle, fat, and bone at the photon energy E. In an SPA or in a single-energy X-ray system (SXA), this is accomplished by assuming a constant thickness of soft tissue of known composition around the bone of interest. Such an assumption may be realized experimentally by placing the limb of interest in a water bath to obtain a soft-tissue baseline, a known and constant attenuation of soft tissue. In this setting (Fig. 1), the composition of soft tissue is considered to be water equivalent, and of negligible thickness compared to the thickness of the water bath.

In projectional densitometry of central sites such as the spine or hip, it is not possible to use a single-energy approach in combination with a water bath because of high variability in the thickness and composition of the surrounding soft tissue. In this case, soft tissue attenuation is determined by measuring the differential attenuation of two photon energies *(4–6)*. Figure 2 illustrates the principle of DPA by showing a cross section through a segment of torso containing a lumbar vertebral body. The fractional attenuations of the two photon energies are given by two equations:

$$\begin{aligned}\left(\frac{I}{I_0}\right)_{\mathrm{LE}} &= \exp\left(-\left(\mu_{\mathrm{m,LE}}^{\mathrm{ST}} \cdot (\rho L)^{\mathrm{ST}} + \mu_{\mathrm{m,LE}}^{\mathrm{bone}} \cdot (\rho L)^{\mathrm{bone}}\right)\right)\\ \left(\frac{I}{I_0}\right)_{\mathrm{HE}} &= \exp\left(-\left(\mu_{\mathrm{m,HE}}^{\mathrm{ST}} \cdot (\rho L)^{\mathrm{ST}} + \mu_{\mathrm{m,HE}}^{\mathrm{bone}} \cdot (\rho L)^{\mathrm{bone}}\right)\right)\end{aligned} \tag{4}$$

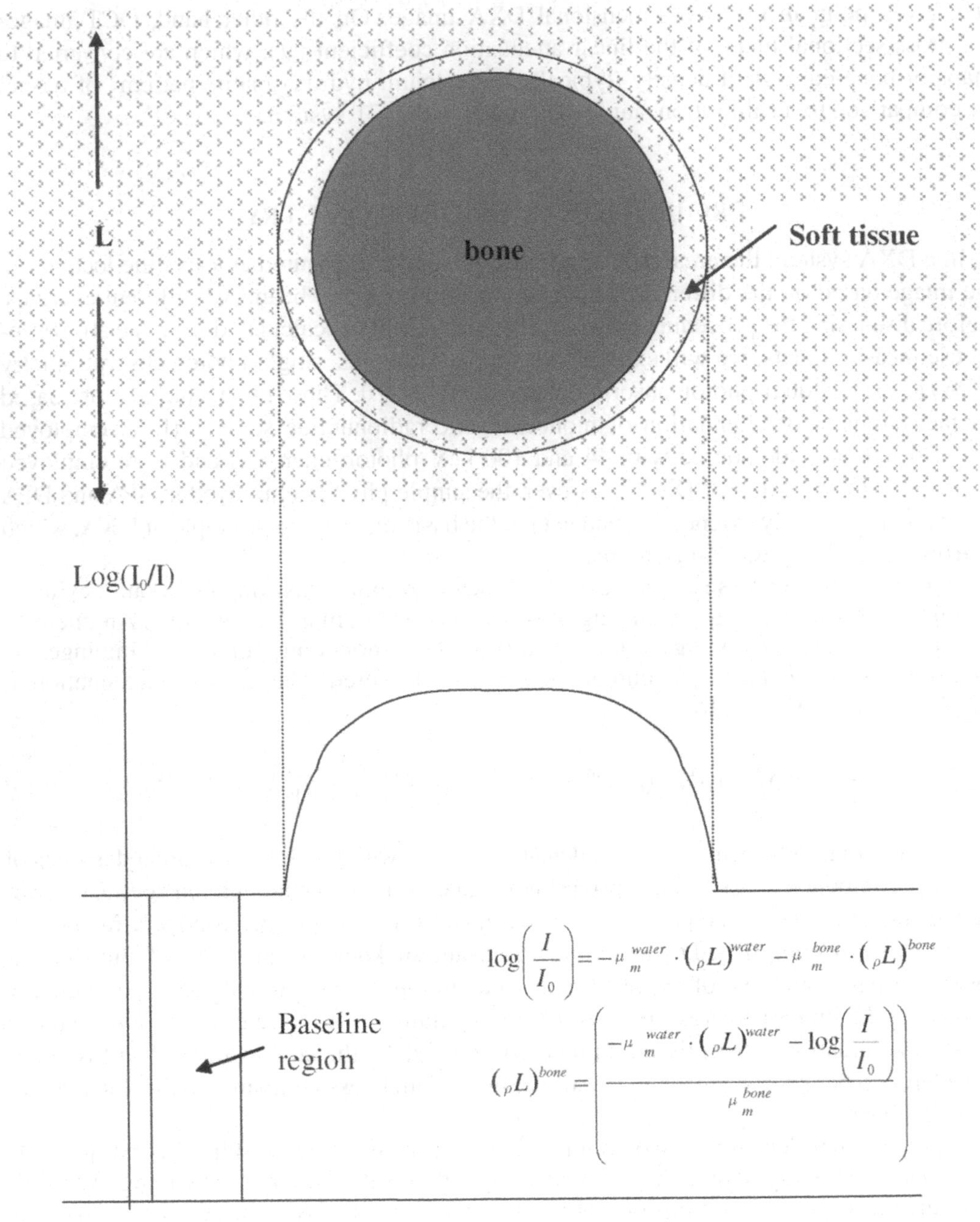

Fig. 1. Profile of photon attenuation across idealized bone.

The fractional attenuation on the left-hand side is measured experimentally, and the mass attenuation coefficients μ_m^{bone} and μ_m^{ST} are known a priori at the two energies. We can simplify this by calculating the log attenuation factors (LA), where $(LA)_{LE} = \log(I/I_0)_{LE}$ and $(LA)_{HE} = \log(I/I_0)_{HE}$

$$\begin{aligned} (LA)_{LE} &= -\mu_{m,LE}^{ST} \cdot (\rho L)^{ST} - \mu_{m,LE}^{bone} \cdot (\rho L)^{bone} \\ (LA)_{HE} &= -\mu_{m,HE}^{ST} \cdot (\rho L)^{ST} - \mu_{m,HE}^{bone} \cdot (\rho L)^{bone} \end{aligned} \quad (5)$$

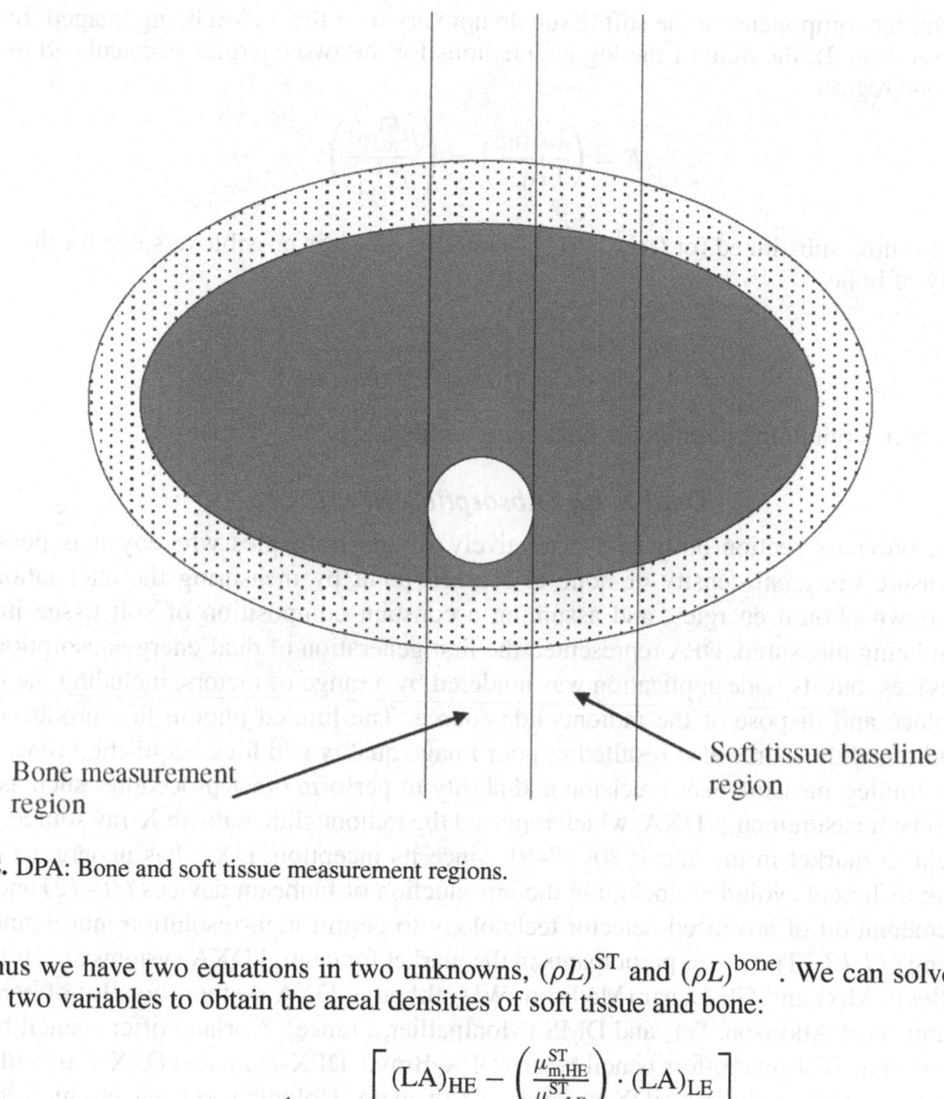

Fig. 2. DPA: Bone and soft tissue measurement regions.

Thus we have two equations in two unknowns, $(\rho L)^{\mathrm{ST}}$ and $(\rho L)^{\mathrm{bone}}$. We can solve for these two variables to obtain the areal densities of soft tissue and bone:

$$
\begin{aligned}
(\rho L)^{\mathrm{bone}} &= \left[\frac{(\mathrm{LA})_{\mathrm{HE}} - \left(\frac{\mu^{\mathrm{ST}}_{\mathrm{m,HE}}}{\mu^{\mathrm{ST}}_{\mathrm{m,LE}}}\right)\cdot(\mathrm{LA})_{\mathrm{LE}}}{\mu^{\mathrm{bone}}_{\mathrm{m,HE}} - \left(\frac{\mu^{\mathrm{ST}}_{\mathrm{m,HE}}}{\mu^{\mathrm{ST}}_{\mathrm{m,LE}}}\right)\cdot\mu^{\mathrm{bone}}_{\mathrm{m,LE}}}\right] \\
(\rho L)^{\mathrm{ST}} &= \left[\frac{-(\mathrm{LA})_{\mathrm{HE}} + \left(\frac{\mu^{\mathrm{bone}}_{\mathrm{m,HE}}}{\mu^{\mathrm{bone}}_{\mathrm{m,LE}}}\right)\cdot(\mathrm{LA})_{\mathrm{LE}}}{-\mu^{\mathrm{ST}}_{\mathrm{m,HE}} + \left(\frac{\mu^{\mathrm{bone}}_{\mathrm{m,HE}}}{\mu^{\mathrm{bone}}_{\mathrm{m,LE}}}\right)\cdot\mu^{\mathrm{ST}}_{\mathrm{m,LE}}}\right]
\end{aligned}
\tag{6}
$$

Thus, from measuring attenuation values at a given point using two photon energies, it is possible to measure the areal densities of the soft tissue and bone tissue components. However, this assumes that the mass attenuation coefficients for the bone and soft tissue components are known at the photon energy. While this may be readily measured or estimated for bone material, the composition of the soft tissue (proportion of lean and fat) is highly variable. This may be estimated by performing a log attenuation measurement in a region where there are no bone elements and assuming that the relative proportions of lean and fat components in the soft tissue do not vary over the region being imaged. In this case (see Fig. 2), the ratio of the log attenuations for the two energies is calculated in this non-bone region

$$R = \left(\frac{\mathrm{LA_{HE}}}{\mathrm{LA_{LE}}}\right) = \left(\frac{\mu^{\mathrm{ST}}_{\mathrm{m,HE}}}{\mu^{\mathrm{ST}}_{\mathrm{m,LE}}}\right) \tag{7}$$

If R is now substituted for $(\mu^{\mathrm{ST}}_{\mathrm{mHE}}/\mu^{\mathrm{ST}}_{\mathrm{mLE}})$ into Eq. (6), it is possible to solve for the areal density of bone,

$$(\rho L)^{\mathrm{bone}} = \left[\frac{(\mathrm{LA})_{\mathrm{HE}} - R \cdot (\mathrm{LA})_{\mathrm{LE}}}{\mu^{\mathrm{bone}}_{\mathrm{m,HE}} - R \cdot \mu^{\mathrm{bone}}_{\mathrm{m,LE}}}\right] \tag{8}$$

at any bone containing point in the dual-energy image.

Dual X-Ray Absorptiometry (DXA)

The previous section outlined the relatively simple principles whereby it is possible to measure the areal density of bone at a given point by measuring the attenuation of two known photon energies, and assuming a constant composition of soft tissue in the region being measured. DPA represented the first generation of dual-energy absorptiometric devices, but its wide application was hindered by a range of factors, including the need to replace and dispose of the radionuclide source. The limited photon flux produced by the radionuclide source also resulted in poor image quality and long acquisition times and which limited measurement precision and ability to perform other procedures such as lateral spine measurements. DXA, which replaced the radionuclide with an X-ray source, was brought to market in the late 1980s *(7–9)*. Since its inception, DXA has undergone continuing technical evolution, including the introduction of fanbeam devices *(10–12)* and the implementation of advanced detector technology to permit high-resolution morphometric imaging *(11,13)*. The major participants in the market for central DXA systems are Hologic (Waltham, MA) and GE-Lunar (Madison, WI), although DXA systems are also offered by Norland (Fort Atkinson, WI) and DMS (Montpellier, France). Norland offers pencil beam systems and GE-Lunar offers pencil beam (DPX-Bravo, DPX-Duo, and DPX-Pro) and rectilinear scanning fanbeams (iDXA, Prodigy Advance). Hologic's current product line is based entirely on a linear fanbeam geometry. The range in system cost is large, with purchase costs of roughly US $40,000 for basic pencil beam systems and ranging up to US $200,000 for fanbeam systems offering a C-Arm capability for lateral measurements for vertebral fracture evaluation.

Figure 3 shows a schematic of a DXA system. An X-ray tube is mounted on a gantry, as is a detector system. The dual-peak energy spectrum provides an approximation of the dual-photon condition and such dual-energy X-ray spectra are generated by a range of approaches, depending on the manufacturer. With GE-Lunar systems, a Cerium K-edge filter is placed at the tube aperture, with the K-edge absorption resulting in a bi-modal X-ray spectrum. All Hologic systems use a rapid switching of the X-ray tube kilovoltage to change the X-ray effective energy. Norland DXA systems use dynamic Samarium filtration of the tube aperture to achieve this purpose. The detector system measures the intensity I of X-rays transmitted through the tissue being imaged. An air calibration, typically performed daily or several times per day, provides a reference value I_0, which is divided into

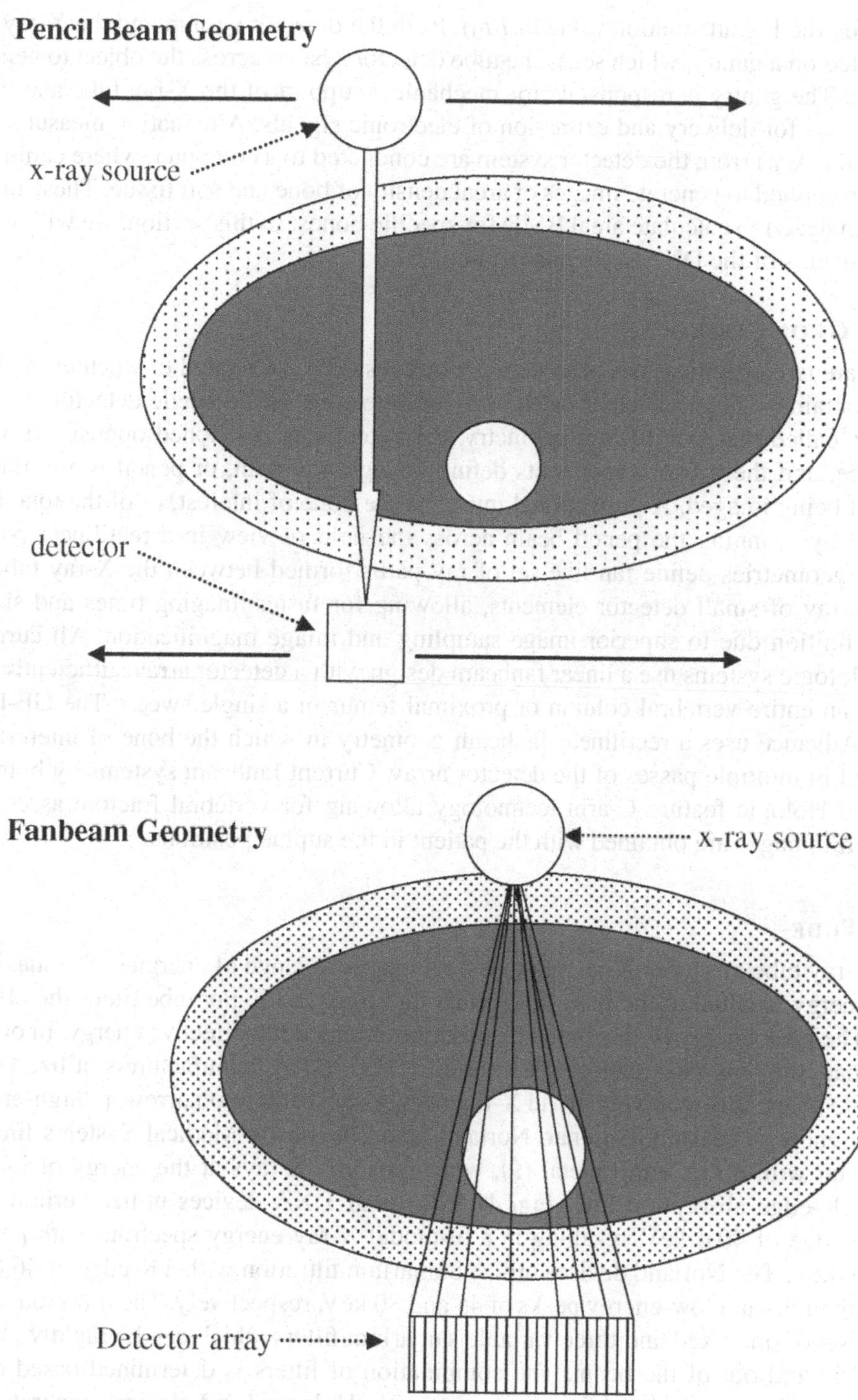

Fig. 3. DXA: Pencil and fanbeam geometry.

I to provide the log attenuation value $\ln(I/I_0)$. Both the detector system and the X-ray tube are mounted on a gantry, which scans the tube detector system across the object to generate the image. The gantry is responsible for mechanical support of the X-ray tube and detector, as well as for delivery and extraction of electronic signals. Attenuation measurements (LA_{HE} and LA_{LE}) from the detector system are conducted to a computer, where calibration factors are applied to generate images of areal density of bone and soft tissue. These images are then analyzed to calculate areal BMD for specific bones. In this section, we will discuss the components of the DXA system in detail.

System Geometries

There are two specific types of system geometries (Fig. 3), related to whether the DXA system contains a single detector or an array of detectors. In the single detector scanning geometry, called the pencil beam geometry, the detector is positioned opposite from the X-ray tube, and these two components define a single ray path, or pencil beam, through the object being imaged. A projectional image of the bone of interest, or of the total body, is formed by scanning the pencil beam across the field of view in a rectilinear pattern. Fanbeam geometries define fan-like set of ray paths formed between the X-ray tube and a linear array of small detector elements, allowing for faster imaging times and sharper image definition due to superior image sampling and image magnification. All currently offered Hologic systems use a linear fanbeam design with a detector array sufficiently wide to image an entire vertebral column or proximal femur in a single sweep. The GE-Lunar Prodigy Advance uses a rectilinear fanbeam geometry in which the bone of interest may be imaged in multiple passes of the detector array. Current fanbeam systems by both GE-Lunar and Hologic feature C-arm technology allowing for vertebral fracture assessment from lateral images are obtained with the patient in the supine positions.

X-Ray Tube

The X-ray tube produces X-ray photons having a wide range of energies. The maximum photon energy is equal to the peak kilovoltage (kVp) of the X-ray tube times the electron charge. The peak energy of this broad distribution is called the effective energy. In order to approximate the dual-peak energy spectrum of ^{153}Gd, DXA manufacturers utilize various methods to shape this relatively broad X-ray energy spectrum into narrower "high-energy" and "low-energy" peaks. GE-Lunar, Norland, and Diagnostic Medical Systems filter the X-ray beam with a rare earth metal *(9)*, which absorbs X-rays at the energy of its characteristic K-edge absorption line (Fig. 4). GE-Lunar DXA devices utilize cerium filters with a K-edge of 40.4 keV, resulting in a bi-modal X-ray energy spectrum with peaks at 38 and 70 keV. The Norland devices utilize Samarium filtration with a K-edge of 46.8 keV, generating high- and low-energy peaks of 45 and 80 keV, respectively. The filtration assembly consists of one fixed and three variable samarium filters which can be rapidly (11 ms) switched in and out of the beam. The combination of filters is determined based on the soft tissue thickness measured for a given ray path. Hologic DXA devices generate dual-energy X-ray spectra by switching the X-ray tube voltage on a rapid timescale *(8)*. The current Hologic devices generate a bi-modal X-ray energy spectrum by rapidly switching the X-ray tube voltage between 100 and 140 kV on an 8-ms timescale (Fig. 4).

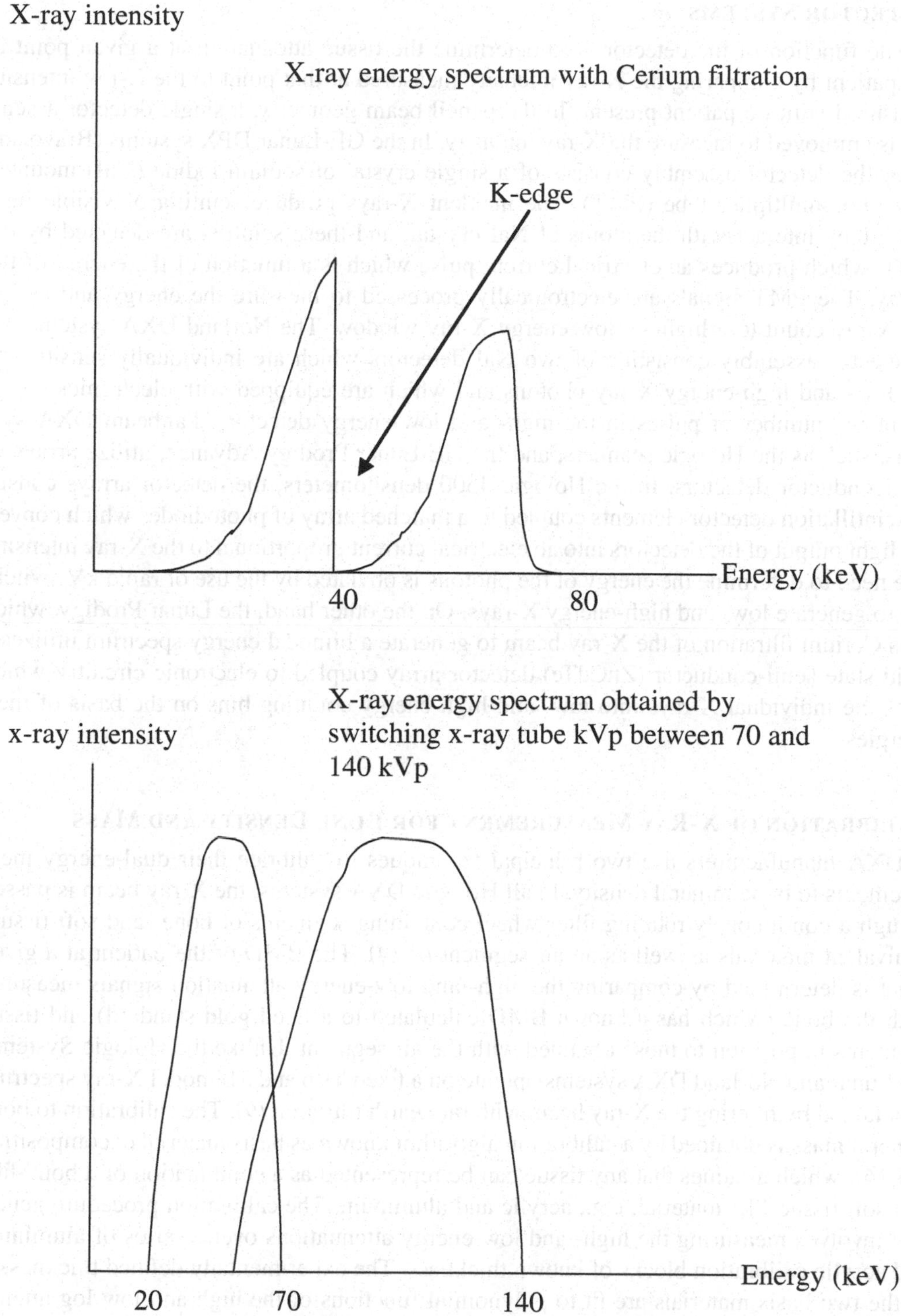

Fig. 4. Illustration of X-ray spectrum obtained with Cerium filtration (*top*) and kVp switching (*bottom*).

Detector Systems

The function of the detector is to determine the tissue attenuation at a given point in the patient by comparing the X-ray intensity measured at that point to the X-ray intensity measured with no patient present. In the pencil beam geometry, a single detector assembly is employed to measure the X-ray intensity. In the GE-Lunar DPX systems (Bravo and Duo) the detector assembly consists of a single crystal of sodium iodide (NaI) mounted to a photomultiplier tube (PMT). The incident X-rays produce scintilla of visible light when they interact with the atoms of NaI crystal, and these scintilla are detected by the PMT, which produces an electrical current pulse which is a function of the energy of the X-ray. The PMT signals are electronically processed to measure the energy and assign the X-ray count to a high- or low-energy X-ray window. The Norland DXA systems use a detector assembly consisting of two NaI detectors which are individually sensitive to the low- and high-energy X-ray photons and which are equipped with electronics which count the number of pulses in the high- and low-energy detectors. Fanbeam DXA systems, such as the Hologic scanners, and the GE-Lunar Prodigy Advance, utilize arrays of semiconductor detectors. In the Hologic 4500 densitometers, the detector arrays consist of scintillation detector elements coupled to a matched array of photodiodes which convert the light output of the detectors into an electrical current proportional to the X-ray intensity. The need to determine the energy of the photons is obviated by the use of rapid kV switching to generate low- and high-energy X-rays. On the other hand, the Lunar Prodigy, which uses Cerium filtration of the X-ray beam to generate a bimodal energy spectrum utilizes a solid state semi-conductor (ZnCdTe) detector array coupled to electronic circuitry which sorts the individual X-rays into low- and high-energy counting bins on the basis of their energies.

Calibration of X-Ray Measurement for Bone Density and Mass

DXA manufacturers use two principal techniques to calibrate their dual-energy measurements to bone mineral density. In all Hologic DXA systems, the X-ray beam is passed though a continuously rotating filter wheel containing segments of bone- and soft tissue-equivalent materials as well as an air segment *(8,14)*. The BMD of the patient at a given point is determined by comparing the high- and low-energy attenuation signals measured with the bone (which has a known BMD calculated to a fixed gold standard) and tissue segments in position to those obtained with the air segment. Unlike the Hologic Systems, the Lunar and Norland DXA systems operate on a fixed kVp and a bimodal X-ray spectrum is obtained by filtering the X-ray beam with rare earth filtration *(9)*. The calibration to bone mineral mass is obtained by a calibration algorithm known as basis material decomposition *(15,16)*, which assumes that any tissue can be represented as a combination of a bone-like and soft tissue-like material, e.g., acrylic and aluminum. The calibration procedure generally involves measuring the high- and low-energy attenuations over a series of aluminum and acrylic calibration blocks of known thickness. The experimentally defined thicknesses of the two basis materials are fit to polynomial functions of the high and low log attenuation measurements and the patient count rate data are mapped to equivalent thicknesses of aluminum and acrylic using these calibration relationships. The equivalent thicknesses of aluminum and acrylic are mapped to bone mineral density using a special calibration block containing a bone mineral reference with precise bone mineral content. Fat content is measured by applying the basis material decomposition method to a soft tissue area near the bone, with the fat content then being subtracted from the soft tissue thickness estimate.

Determination of BMC and BMD Values

DXA images are acquired and transferred to a computer system for analysis. The computer system has the tasks of extracting the bone mineral information from the dual-energy images, storing the values in a database and generating a report of the results. The low- and high-energy images are combined to generate a two-dimensional map of areal BMD. To carry out these computations, the computer software must segment the bone in the image, i.e., discriminate the bone from the soft tissue and then determine the location of key anatomic landmarks to select specific regions for calculation of areal BMD, BMC, and projected area measures. The algorithms used to segment the bone tissue vary with the manufacturer and each represent many years of technical development and refinement. The segmentation software employed by the GE-Lunar devices uses a "gradient search" algorithm which computes the gradient in density values across the images, with the high contrast between the bone and the soft tissue generally ensuring that the edges are consistent with sharp local increases in the gradient. Hologic devices utilize an approach based on computation of density histograms in local neighborhoods of the image. To divide the bone tissue areas into anatomic sub-regions, the software detects anatomic landmarks. In the spine, the software automatically determines default locations for the intervertebral spaces, which may be translated or rotated if appropriate by the operator. Typically, four regions of interest corresponding to the L1–L4 vertebral bodies are delineated. Each individual region of interest is bounded by the edges of the spinal column and the intervertebral boundaries. For the hip, the analysis involves determination of a central axis through the femoral neck. Once this is carried out the manufacturers vary in their approaches to divide the proximal femur into sub-regions. The GE-Lunar software centers its femoral neck region on the lowest density section through the neck. For the Hologic software, the lateral aspect of the neck region is determined by the boundary point between the trochanter and the neck. The BMC is calculated by computing the mean areal BMD within the region of interest and then multiplying by the projected area. The data are reported as the BMD, BMC, and areas of the individual vertebral bodies, as well as the total value corresponding to the summed BMC and Area values for the total number of bodies scanned. A fat correction is applied to the bone pixels based on a soft tissue baseline performed in the area adjacent to the bone. The spinal and proximal femoral regions of interest and their clinical application are presented in Chapter 3

Radiation Dose

The radiation doses for DXA are quite small and are generally equivalent to the radiation exposure level associated with a few days of background radiation *(17–19)*. Effective doses on the order of 1–2 μSv have been reported for pencil beam DXA of the spine and hip *(20)*. The radiation dose from fanbeam measurements is higher by about a factor of 10, potentially ranging up to 62 μSv *(21)*.

Sources of Error

Precision and Accuracy Errors Literature reports on the accuracy error of DXA in studies of excised bone samples vitro have ranged from 2 to 4% *(22–27)*. The precision of DXA depends on both machine, patient- and operator-dependent factors *(9,11,23,24,28–32)*. Machine-dependent factors include changes in the effective energy of the X-ray tube, which may affect the stability of the BMD calibration and instabilities in the detector and associated electronics. However, this source of precision error is generally quite small, and for well-maintained systems the long-term precision in vitro is typically on the order of 0.5%. In pencil beam systems, statistical uncertainties in the mean BMD in a region of interest are a source of random precision error in BMD measurements. This is more of a problem with the photon counting systems than for the current-integrating systems because photon counting requires a low X-ray beam intensity to operate properly. Precision error in vivo is dominated by patient positioning, since the projected area of the spine or hip is affected by the rotation of the bone. Other sources of precision error include inconsistencies in the bone edges as determined by computer algorithms, as well as user interaction in the placement of anatomic markers (e.g., vertebral markers). For PA spine measurements, published values for the short-term in vivo precision vary between 0.7 and 1.5%. Reported precision errors for lateral spine measurements are higher and have been reported to range up to 3%. Precision values for AP hip measurements range from 0.8 to 1.8%, with the lowest precision errors found for the total femur region. Precision errors are typically higher in the elderly than in younger subjects, because reduced bone density results in poorer bone edge definition as well as difficulty in placement of intervertebral markers.

Inherent Error in Measurement of Areal BMD–Bone Size Dependence The first limitation is that both DXA BMC and areal BMD measurements scale with bone volume *(33,34)*. Of two bones with the same volumetric density, the larger bone will have a higher areal density. Thus, the bone densities of two populations having different skeletal sizes and shapes are not directly comparable. Several literature reports have examined the impact of this technical problem on comparisons of DXA BMD between ethnic groups *(35,36)* as well as measurement of BMD in children *(37–40)*. To address this issue, Carter et al. *(34)* devised an approach, called bone mineral apparent density (BMAD) to estimate volumetric BMD based on dividing the BMC by an estimated vertebral volume computed from the vertebral height and width extracted from the AP image. For this size correction approach, the estimated volume was taken as the projected area in the AP plane multiplied by the vertebral width. Another method used vertebral dimensions estimated from paired AP and lateral scans to estimate the volumetric density *(33)*. This involved dividing the vertebral body BMC in the lateral dimension by the vertebral volume estimated by multiplying the projected lateral area by the AP width. A subsequent investigation found that the BMAD estimated from the paired AP and lateral scans was more highly correlated to the true volumetric BMD than the AP-based estimate *(41)*. A similar BMAD approach was proposed for the femoral neck, in which the BMC was divided by an estimated volume computed by multiplying the projected neck area by the width of the femoral neck box *(42)*. This investigation, which was based on the Study of Osteoporotic Fractures, found that use of the femoral neck BMAD did not improve discrimination of hip fractures compared to femoral neck BMD alone.

Dependence on Fat Distribution The bone mineral calculation of DXA assumes that human tissue is a two-component system consisting of bone and a soft tissue component of uniform composition. DXA systems resolve this problem by acquiring a soft tissue baseline in a region adjacent to the bone of interest, and using Eqs. (7) and (8) to correct for the admixture of adipose tissue. This approach assumes uniformity in the proportion of adipose material in the soft tissue. However, this assumption may not be correct for all body shapes, and thus the fat content overlying the bone may be different from that estimated from the soft tissue sample. If the amount of fat in the beam path is underestimated, this may artificially lower the BMD value. If it is less, it may artificially increase the BMD value. This problem has been extensively examined in the literature *(43–45)*. Several studies have utilized CT images to delineate the distribution of adipose tissue and employed this information to check the assumptions of DXA. Tothill found that inhomogenities in the adipose distribution resulted in errors up to approximately 5% in AP spinal BMD and larger errors for lateral imaging *(43)*. Svendsen et al. *(44)* performed a similar study and found accuracy errors of 5% for the AP spine, 10% for the lateral spine, and 6% for the femoral neck and total femur regions.

Variable Magnification Images acquired by a fanbeam system are magnified by a system- and patient-dependent magnification factor *(11–*13,46,*47)*. For a DXA image, the size of this magnification factor is a function of the distance of the bone from the detector and of the source detector distance. Because the magnification has similar effects on both the projected area and the BMC, its effect on the diagnostic value of areal BMD is not considered to be significant. However, the patient-dependent magnification factor should be taken into account for studies in which geometric variables such as femoral neck width or the hip axis length are measured from DXA images.

Beam Hardening Beam hardening is a phenomenon which results in a dependence of the BMD measurement on the total thickness of tissue. Beam hardening results from the fact that the radiation source is not monoenergetic but is fact a distribution of X-ray energies. As the poly-energetic X-ray beam traverses the body, the lower energy photons in the continuous spectrum are preferentially absorbed. Thus, for particularly large body sizes, the energies of the X-ray beam, and thus, the log attenuations, are different than those obtained during the calibration measurement, which may involve a much smaller overall thickness of tissue. While the dual-energy calibration is able to account for most of the range of fat and lean tissue thicknesses, the fact it is that at the extreme end, the effective shape of the X-ray spectrum differs from that used across the calibration measurement. Reports have investigated the magnitude of this effect on BMD measurements in conditions appropriate to hip and spine studies *(11,25,48–50)*. Blake et al. *(48)* performed at phantom study with body thicknesses varied between 15 and 25 cm and found a maximum BMD deviation BMD from the known value of 0.23 g/cm^2, with an RMS deviation on the order of 0.01 g/cm^2, which is approximately equal to the measurement precision.

Patient-Related Sources of Error Several error sources may falsely elevate AP spinal BMD values. These include aortic calcium deposits, osteophytic growth near the endplates, hypertrophy of the posterior elements, hemangiomas and vertebral wedge and crush fractures. Some of these error sources may be circumvented by performing spinal DXA measurements in the lateral projection. While lateral vertebral BMD measurements do show greater ability to discriminate vertebral fractures than AP measurements *(51,52)*, they have limitations as well. These include higher precision errors, as well as potential superposition of the L1 and L4 vertebral bodies by the ribs and ilium, respectively *(33)*.

Fracture Risk Assessment According to the World Health Organization (WHO) criterion established in 1994, osteoporosis is defined in white women as a BMD value at least 2.5 SD below the young normal BMD value for white women *(53)*. However, fracture risk not only is a function of BMD but also comprises diminished bone quality and multiple factors related to the risk of falling, and thus individuals with high BMD may also be at high risk for fracture *(54)*. Thus, application of the WHO criterion without taking into account other risk factors results in reduced diagnostic sensitivity and a high number of false positives *(55)*. Thus, the WHO, acting in concert with other organizations, has recommended the combination of BMD with clinical risk factors into a 10-year absolute fracture risk score *(56)*. Seven clinical risk factors which predict fracture independently of BMD were chosen in addition to age and sex, including prior fragility fractures, a parental history of hip fracture, smoking, system corticosteroid use, excessive alcohol use, body mass index, and rheumatoid arthritis *(56)*. The impact on osteoporosis prevalence of incorporating multiple risk factors in addition to BMD is now being studied, but a recent publication indicates that this approach appears to increase the prevalence of elderly women considered to be at high risk for fracture *(57)*. Eventually, it is expected that such multi-risk factor absolute fracture risk scores will be incorporated into future DXA reports.

QUANTITATIVE COMPUTED TOMOGRAPHY

Computed tomography (CT) is a three-dimensional X-ray absorptiometric measurement which provides the distribution of linear attenuation coefficient in a thin cross section of tissue. Figure 5 depicts the geometry of a CT measurement. The patient cross section is contained within a fan of X-rays defined between the edges of the detector array and an X-ray point source. The X-ray attenuation of the patient is measured along ray paths corresponding the lines defined between individual detector elements and the X-ray source. Along the patient's length, the X-ray beam is shaped to radiate a relatively thin "slice" of tissue typically ranging from 1 to 10 mm. The fan of X-rays circumscribes a circular field of view, which itself is contained within a square image matrix, which typically consists of 512 $\times$ 512 square pixel elements or "pixels." Because the image represents a slice of tissue, the picture elements have a thickness and thus are volume elements or "voxels." The dimensions of the voxels may be adjusted depending on the size of the organ being imaged. The voxel dimensions in the slice plane typically range from 0.9 to 0.2 mm, with slice thicknesses varying from 10 to 1 mm. The CT image is acquired when the X-ray source and detector rotate around the patient, and the absorption is continuously measured for each detector element. Through a 360°C source -detector rotation, each voxel is intersected by several ray paths. The X-ray absorption measurements taken at the different angles are recorded in a computer and combined in a process known as back-projection to calculate the linear attenuation coefficient at each voxel. In the resulting CT image, the voxel values are based on the linear attenuation coefficients. Because these linear attenuation coefficients depend on the effective X-ray energy (which varies between CT scanner models and different kVp settings of the same scanner), a simple scale, known as the Hounsfield scale, is

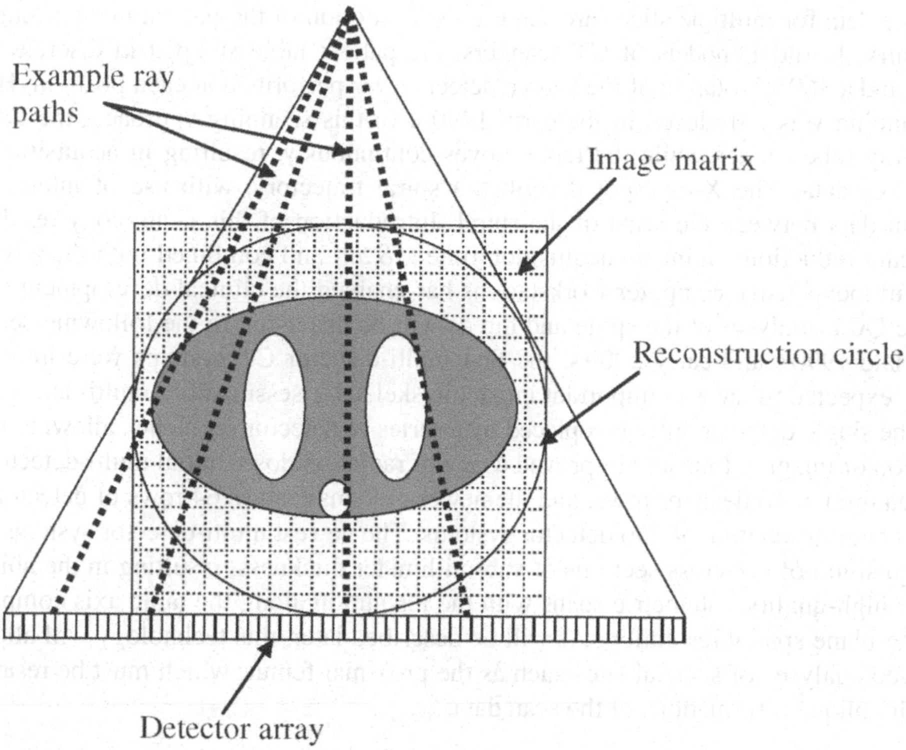

Fig. 5. Diagram illustrating geometry of a CT scan.

used to standardize them. The gray-scale value of each voxel is represented as a Hounsfield Unit, given by

$$HU_T \equiv \left(\frac{\mu_T - \mu_W}{\mu_W}\right) \times 1000$$

where HU_T is the HU of a volume element of tissue and μ_T and μ_W are the linear attenuation coefficients of the tissue and of water, respectively. The HU scale is a linear scale in which air has a value of –1000, water 0, muscle 30, with bone typically ranging from 300 to 3000 units.

The value of the Hounsfield unit for a given tissue type depends on several technical factors. First, if the sizes of the structures in the tissue are smaller than the dimensions of the voxel, the HU value is subject to partial volume averaging, in which the HU value is the average HU of the constituent tissues of the voxel, weighted by their volume fractions. For example, a 0.78 mm × 0.78 mm × 10 mm voxel of trabecular bone is a mixture of bone, collagen, cellular marrow, and fatty marrow, and HU is the volume-weighted average of these four constituents. Beam hardening is a second source of variation in HU. In a CT image, the result of this is that for the same tissue, attenuation coefficients at the outside of the patient are systematically higher than those in the interior. Although manufacturers of CT equipment have implemented beam-hardening corrections, the efficacy of these corrections varies between manufacturers and between technical settings on different machines.

Image data for multiple slices are acquired with motion of the patient table through the CT gantry. In older models of CT scanners, the patient table stepped in discrete increments, and a 360°C rotation of the source/detector was performed at each position. Helical CT scanning was introduced in the early 1990 s. In this scanning approach, the detector and X-ray tube rotates while the table moves continuously, resulting in acquisition of a volume of data. The X-ray spot describes a spiral trajectory, with use of interpolation to fill in data between the arms of the spiral. Introduction of this technology resulted in significant reductions in image acquisition time *(58,59)* and combined with the advent of powerful inexpensive computer workstations has enabled the clinical development of volumetric QCT analyses of the spine and hip as will be discussed in the following sections. In the late 1990 s and early 2000 s, the first multi-detector CT systems were introduced and are expected to have an important impact in skeletal assessment. In multi-detector systems, the single detector array is replaced by a series of detector segments, allowing for the reduction of imaging time and improved usage of radiation dose. Initial multi-detector systems featured 4–16 detector rows, and the newer systems feature 64 rows of detector data, with recent introduction of 256 detector systems. The newest multi-detector systems allow for acquisition of CT cross sections of sub-millimeter thickness, resulting in the ability to acquire high-quality volumetric scans with the resolution along the table axis comparable to the in-plane spatial resolution. As will be described later, this technology will allow for improved analyses of skeletal sites such as the proximal femur, which must be resampled through oblique reformations of the scan data.

Physical Significance of QCT Measurements

CT BMD assessment is based on quantitative analysis of the HU in volumes of bone tissue. Typically, the BMD is quantified using a bone mineral reference phantom which is scanned simultaneously with the patient. In order to minimize the impact of beam hardening, the calibration phantom is placed as close as possible to the vertebrae and is normally located under the lumbar spine of the patient. The calibration standard originally developed by Cann et al. *(60)* at UCSF and which is currently marketed by Mindways (South San Francisco, CA, USA) consists of an acrylic wedge containing cylinders of solutions with varying concentrations (200, 100, 50, and 0 mg/cm^3) of dipotassium hydrogen phosphate in water. An additional cylinder contained alcohol as a reference material for fat. A solid calcium hydroxyapatite-based calibration standard was later developed by Image Analysis (Columbia, KY, USA) and by Siemens Medical Systems (Erlangen, Germany). The Image Analysis standard consists of rods with varying concentrations (200, 100, and 50 mg/cm^3) of calcium hydroxyapatite mixed in a water-equivalent solid resin matrix *(61)*. During the analysis of the QCT image, regions of interest are placed (Fig. 6) in each of the calibration objects, and linear regression analysis is used to determine a relationship between the mean HU measured in each region and the known concentrations of bone-equivalent material. This calibration relationship is then used to convert the mean HU in the patient region of interest (e.g., vertebra or proximal femur) into a concentration (reported in mg/cm^3, i.e., the *mass of bone per unit tissue volume*) of bone-equivalent material in the region of interest. Unlike areal bone mineral density, the QCT density measurement is independent of bone size and thus is more robust measure for comparisons of bone density between populations and potentially for growing children as well.

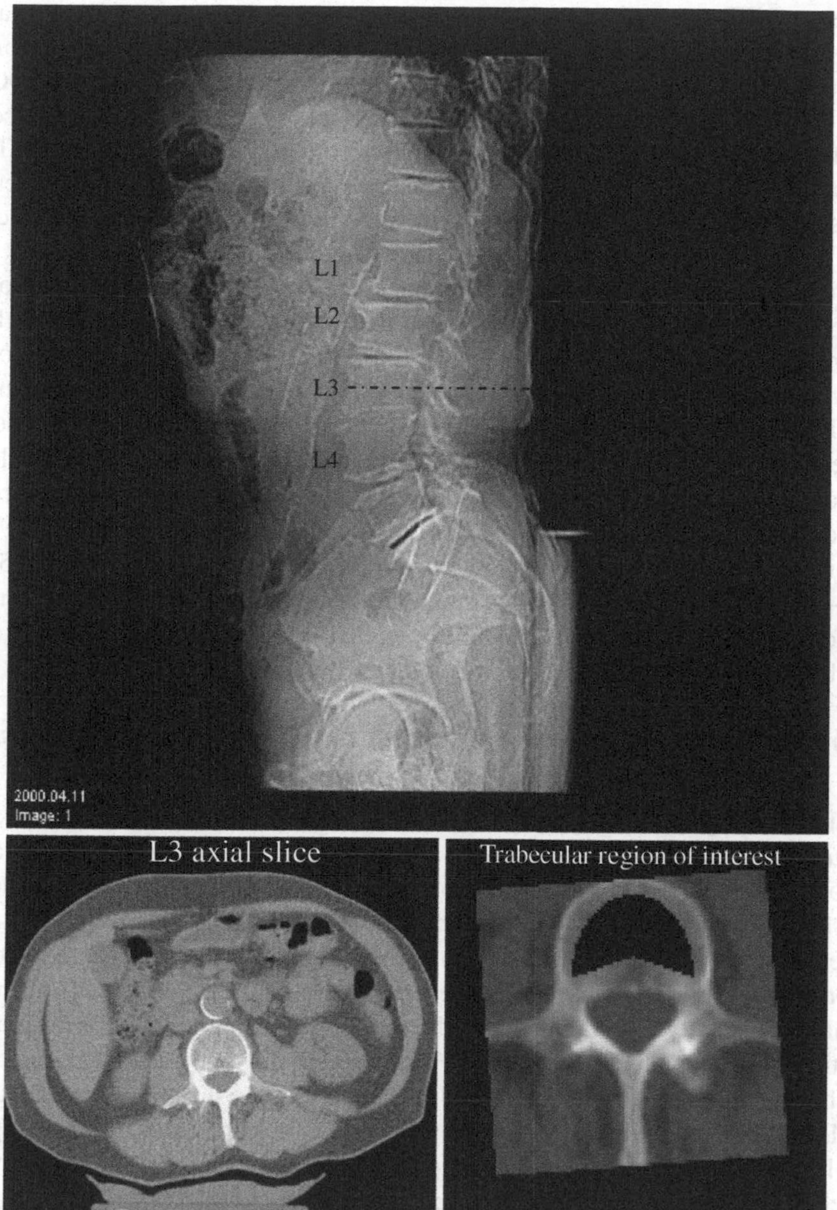

Fig. 6. Lateral scoutview. L1–L4 verebrae are labeled. *Bottom left*: Axial slice through L3 vertebral body. *Bottom right*: Trabecular region of interest in L3 vertebral body.

The major source of error in the QCT bone measurement is the phenomenon of partial volume averaging. Because the voxel dimensions in QCT measurements (0.8–1.0 mm in the imaging plane, 3–10 mm slice thicknesses) are larger than the dimensions and spacing of trabeculae, a QCT voxel includes both bone and marrow constituents. Thus a QCT measurement is the mass of bone in a volume containing bone, red marrow, and marrow fat. A single-energy QCT measurement is capable of determining the mass of bone in a volume consisting of two components (e.g., bone and red marrow), but not in a three-component system. Resolving the mass fractions of bone, red marrow, and marrow fat in the QCT voxel requires a dual-energy QCT measurement. Because fat has an HU value of –200, compared to 30 HU for red marrow and 300–3000 HU for bone, the presence of fat in the QCT volume reduces the HU measurement. Thus, the presence of marrow fat causes single-energy QCT to underestimate the mass of bone per unit tissue volume, an error which can be corrected using dual-energy acquisitions. The effect of marrow fat on QCT measurements is larger at the spine than at the hip or peripheral skeletal sites. Whereas the conversion from red to fatty marrow tends to finish by the mid-20 s in the hip and peripheral skeleton, the vertebrae show a gradual age-related increase in the proportion of fat in the bone marrow which starts in youth and continues through old age *(62)*. The inclusion of fatty marrow in the vertebral BMD measurement results in accuracy errors ranging from 5 to 15% depending on the age group. However, because the increase in marrow fat is age-related, single-energy CT data can be corrected using age-related reference databases, and the residual error is not considered to be clinically relevant. Provided that the QCT scan is acquired at low effective energies (i.e., 80–90 kVp), the population SD in marrow fat accounts for roughly 5 mg/cm^3 of the 25–30 mg/cm3 population SD in spinal trabecular BMD. This residual error is not considered large enough to merit clinical use of dual-energy techniques, which are more accurate, but which have larger radiation doses and precision errors.

Trabecular Bone Mineral Assessment Based on Scanning of Cross Sections Through the Lumbar Mid-vertebrae

Quantitative computed tomography (QCT) was developed in the late 1970 s as a method for measuring BMD in the metabolically active trabecular bone in the vertebral bodies *(60,63–65)*. In this approach, a lateral projection scan is utilized to localize the lumbar vertebral bodies and scans of 8–10 mm thickness are acquired through 2–4 contiguous lumbar vertebral levels (Fig. 6). The patient is imaged simultaneously with a bone mineral calibration standard, which is used to convert the native HU scale of the CT image to units of bone mineral density. The CT image is then processed using a software program which analyzes the calibration phantom to convert HU to BMD and then places a region of interest in the trabecular bone of the vertebral body *(41,65,66)*. The program then calculates the mean BMD of the vertebral region of interest. This is either presented as an average of 2–4 vertebral levels. The radiation dose for this procedure has been reported as 80 μSv, a value which includes the dose of the lateral localizer scan *(19)*.

Precision errors ranging from 1 to 2% have been reported for spinal QCT *(41,66)*. This precision error is attributable to several sources including the reproducibility of slice and region of interest positioning as well as scanner instabilities *(67)*. Simultaneous calibration corrects to some extent for scanner instabilities, as well as for variable beam hardening depending on patient size and shape. Using a simultaneous calibration technique, the long-term CV of a well-maintained CT scanner should be close to 1%. The effect of variable patient positioning can be minimized by careful review of lateral localizer scans to ensure consistent slice placement and gantry angulations. Computer programs that place the region of interest automatically or semi-automatically may also be used to reduce precision errors.

Measurement of BMD Using Volumetric CT Images of the Spine and Hip

Three-dimensional CT scanning and image analysis procedures have become feasible with the advent of fast helical and multi-detector CT scanners and the cost reduction in computer processing power, which allows for inexpensive processing of the large volumes of CT data acquired in helical scans. Procedures have been developed for three-dimensional scanning of the spine and hip. In typical spine and hip protocols, the lumbar vertebrae and proximal femora (from superior aspect of femoral head to inferior aspect of lesser trochanter) are scanned with a helical protocol using reconstructed sections of 1–3 mm thickness *(41,68)*. The earliest scanning protocols used settings of 80 kVp and 140 and 280 mAs for hip and spine respectively, with 3-mm section thicknesses. Using a radiation dose calculation developed by Kalender et al. *(69)*, the radiation doses for these procedures have been estimated at 350 and 1200 μSv for spine and hip protocols, respectively. Many research protocols now employ higher radiation dose scanning protocols for better image quality, with 120 kVp, 150–250 mAs, and 1-mm section thicknesses. These higher dose procedures result in radiation doses ranging up to 3–6 mSv for spine and hip assessments.

One of the most powerful applications of helical CT scanning and three-dimensional image analysis is for assessment of bone mineral density, geometry, and strength of the proximal femur. Analysis approaches range from assessment of density, geometry, and macro-structural processes based on reconstruction of cross sections and volumes of femoral neck tissue to finite element modeling approaches to model the strength of the hip based on bone geometry and material properties mapped from CT image values.

Densitometric and structural assessments based on volume reconstructions of the proximal femur based on CT scans have been developed at the University of California, San Francisco *(68,70)* and the University of Erlangen *(71,72)*. These approaches involve reformatting of the QCT scans along the femoral neck axis and segmentation of the entire proximal femoral envelope, with combinations of mathematical morphology and thresholding, and edge detection approaches to derive the cortical envelope for volume and thickness assessments. The computer algorithm described by Kang et al. *(71,72)* carries out volumetric analyses of the femoral neck and the approach described by Lang et al. *(68,70)* at UC San Francisco processes three-dimensional CT images of the proximal femur to measure bone mineral density in the femoral neck, the total femur, and in a region which combines the trochanteric and intertrochanteric sub-regions similar to those of DXA systems (Fig. 7). Within each anatomic sub-region, the density, mass, and volume are computed for the cortical and trabecular components as well as for the integral bone envelope. For trabecular BMD measurements, the precision of this method in vivo was found to range from 0.6 to 1.1% depending on the volume of interest assessed. Both the Erlangen and UCSF approaches carry out geometric and structural analyses of the minimum femoral neck cross section, computing cross-sectional area, and moments of inertia for strength estimation. In addition to the two approaches described above, a program for proximal femoral analysis has also been developed at the Mayo clinic *(73)*. In this approach, rather than reconstruct the whole proximal femoral volume, a single cross section of the femoral neck is reconstructed, and measures of integral, cortical and medullary density, and cross-sectional area are computed in addition to bending and axial compressive strength indices. The various QCT proximal femoral density and strength indices are predictors of proximal femoral strength in vitro *(68)*, and recent studies have delineated the correlation of these

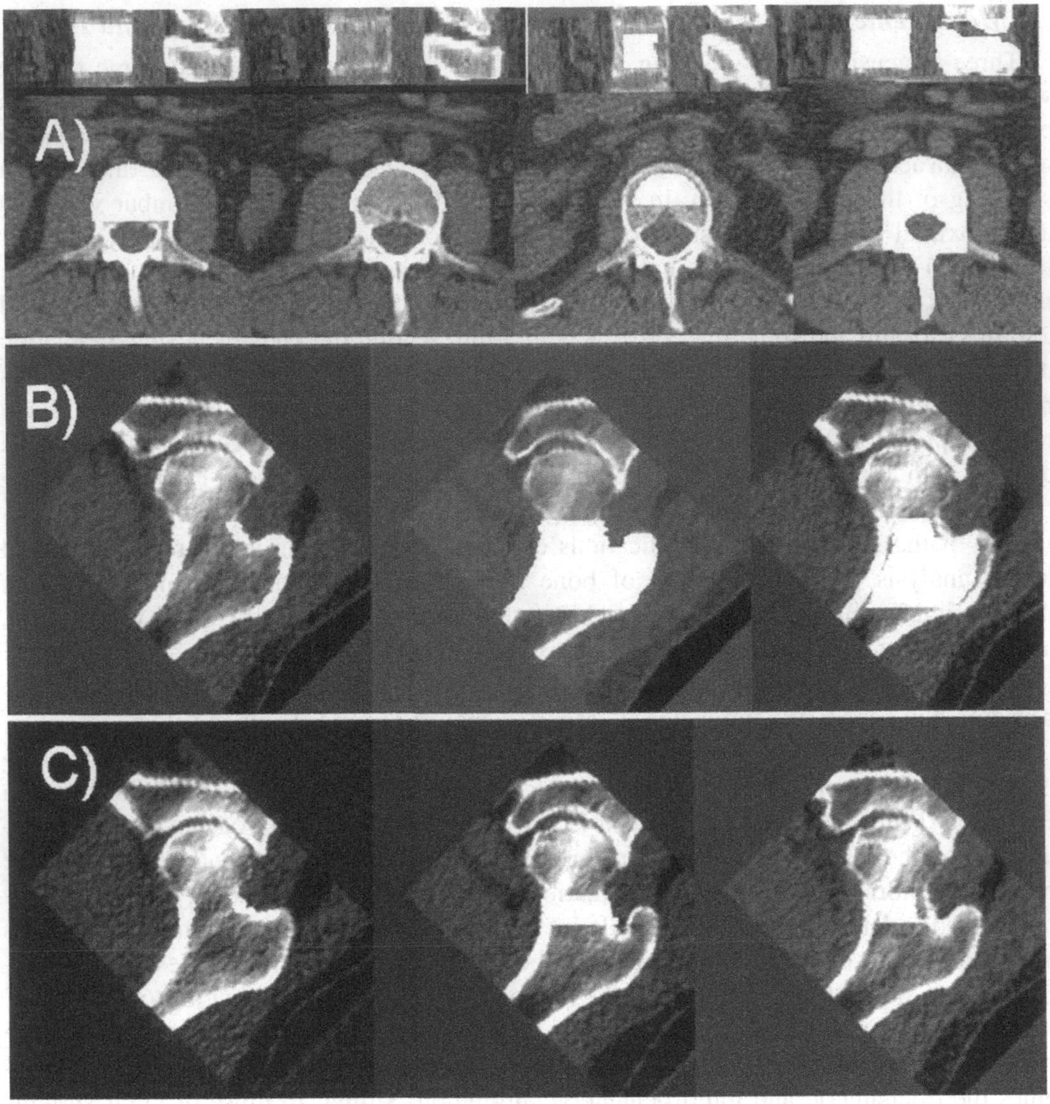

Fig. 7. Integral, trabecular and cortical regions of interest overlaid as white pixels on CT images. (A) Spine (B) Total femur (C) Femoral Neck.

measures to age *(73,74)*, changes in mechanical loading *(75)*, treatment *(76,77)*, and fracture status *(78)*. Several cross-sectional studies of the effect of aging on proximal femoral geometry have shown the positive association of age with femoral neck cross-sectional area, supporting the idea of periosteal apposition as a compensation for age-related bone loss *(73,79,80)*. These findings were supported by a recently published longitudinal study using QCT of the hip, in which a cohort of astronauts was followed for a year after conclusion of spaceflights of 4–6 months length *(75)*. Crew of long-duration spaceflight lose on average 1–2.7% of their proximal femoral bone mass per month of spaceflight, depending on anatomic sub-region and compartment, and this longitudinal study showed that the total tissue volumes and the femoral neck cross-sectional area increased in the year after the mission. These data were consistent with a periosteal apposition as a protective response to resumed mechanical loading after a prolonged period of skeletal atrophy. In addition to studies of aging and spaceflight, there are several reports describing the employment of QCT to quantify the differential response of cortical and trabecular bone in the hip to parathyroid hormone and alendronate. PTH studies show concurrent decreases in cortical BMD and increases in trabecular BMD, with cortical tissue volume measures consistent with increased volume of cortical tissue having low mineralization *(76,77)*. Finally, recent data have confirmed that in addition to association with mechanical strength in vitro, QCT measures are associated with hip fracture in vivo. A recent cross-sectional study comparing women imaged within 48 h of a hip fracture to age and body-size matched controls, showed that hip fracture was significantly associated with reduced vBMD in the cortical, integral, and trabecular compartments, as well as reduced measures of cortical volume and thickness *(78)*. Two interesting findings of the study were that fracture status was associated with increased femoral neck cross-sectional area, consistent with an earlier finding of increased proximal femoral intertrochanteric width from pelvic radiographs in the Study of Osteoporotic Fractures *(81)*. The study also found that measures of cortical geometry and trabecular vBMD were independently associated with hip fracture. QCT was also employed to characterize the association of femoral neck density and geometry parameters with incident hip fracture in men in the prospectively designed Mr. Os study. Orwoll et al. found that the percentage of proximal femoral tissue volume occupied by cortical tissue, a measure of cortical thickness, was associated with incident hip fracture in men aged 69–90 and that the association was undiminished by adjustment of the data either for trabecular volumetric BMD or areal integral BMD of the femoral neck (Orwoll et al., 2006 American Society of Bone and Mineral Research, Philadelphia 2006).

In the spine, the use of volumetric QCT measurements impacts precision more than discriminatory capability. Their ability to improve the precision of spinal measurements relates to the use of three-dimensional anatomic landmarks to guide the placement of volumes of interest and to correct for differences in patient positioning which affect single-slice scans. Currently, single-slice QCT techniques are highly operator dependent, requiring careful slice positioning and angulation as well as careful region of interest placement. Lang et al. *(82)* developed a volumetric spinal QCT approach in which an image of the entire vertebral body is acquired and anatomic landmarks such as the vertebral endplates and the spinous process are used to fix the three-dimensional orientation of the vertebral body, allowing for definition of new trabecular and integral regions which contain most of the bone in the vertebral centrum, as shown in Fig. 7. Although measuring a larger volume of tissue may enhance precision, these new regions are highly correlated with the mid-vertebral sub-regions assessed with standard QCT techniques and may not contain significant new information about vertebral strength. Consequently, volumetric studies of regional BMD, which examine specific sub-regions of the centrum that may vary in their contribution to vertebral strength, and studies of the cortical shell, the condition of which may be important for vertebral strength in osteoporotic individuals, are of interest for future investigation.

Finite Element Modeling

FEM is a mathematical technique used by engineers to evaluate the strength of complex structures such as engine parts, bridges, and, more recently, bones. The structure is divided into "finite elements" (discrete pieces of the structure) to form an "FE mesh" so that it can be analyzed. The advantage of using FE modeling in this study is that this method can account for the material heterogeneity and irregular geometry of the femur, factors that cannot be considered using other approaches. Until recently, it has not been possible to analyze individual bones due to the extraordinary amount of labor involved in generating the FE mesh. Not only does the complex three-dimensional geometry needs to be defined, but the material properties, which vary dramatically within the bone, must be specified. As a result, researchers have often spent months, or even years, to create just one FE model, and even then, the model often lacked adequate refinement. To address this problem, researchers have developed methods to derive finite element models from CT scans of the hip and spine. These methods involve volumetric QCT whole hip *(83–87)* or whole vertebra images *(88–90)* obtained with 1- or 3-mm slice thickness. The finite element modeling application involves three steps. First, the bone geometry information is obtained by determining the outer boundaries of the proximal femora or vertebra on each imaged cross section on the stack of cross sections which encompass the bone. Next, material properties, such as elastic modulus and strength, are computed for each voxel within the bone boundaries. These are computed using parametric relationships between BMD and material properties obtained by scanning and then mechanically testing samples of trabecular and cortical bone. Once the material properties and bone geometry have been defined, load vectors are applied, which simulate the forces applied to bone in normal loading, or in traumatic events such as falls. Keyak et al. *(83–85)* have developed an automated, CT scan-based method of generating patient-specific FE models of the hip. This method takes advantage of the voxel-based nature of quantitative CT scan data to achieve fully automated mesh generation and, more significantly, to allow heterogeneous material properties to be specified. The FE models can be analyzed using a loading condition simulating a load on the femur in a single-legged gait or a fall backward and to the side with an impact on the greater trochanter. For each voxel, elastic modulus and strength are estimated as material properties and the factor of safety (FOS) is determined as the strength at each element divided by the stress, with FOS < 1 representing mechanical failure. A fracture is considered to occur if 15 contiguous elements fail. The outcome variable produced by the modeling technique is failure load, which is defined as the load magnitude required to produce a fracture. This procedure has been extensively tested in vitro, with high correlations to measure failure load for both loading conditions ($r = 0.95$ and 0.96 for fall and stance loading conditions, respectively) *(83)*. In addition to their close correlation with fracture load, the FE models depict areas of high strain which occur at the sites where the bones fracture in vitro and where fractures occur in vivo (Fig. 8). The application of FEM to clinical studies has been limited in the past, but is now growing with the wide employment of CT scanning in clinical osteoporosis research. Keaveny et al. *(88)* recently applied FEM to compare the effects of teriparatide and alendronate on estimated vertebral strength and vertebral bone density and Lian et al. *(91)* employed FEM to compare estimated proximal femoral strength between subjects with glucorticoid-induced osteoporosis and age-matched controls.

Commercially Available Equipment for Spinal QCT Measurements

QCT equipment typically includes a bone mineral reference phantom and software to process the CT images and report the results. All manufacturers of CT equipment offer

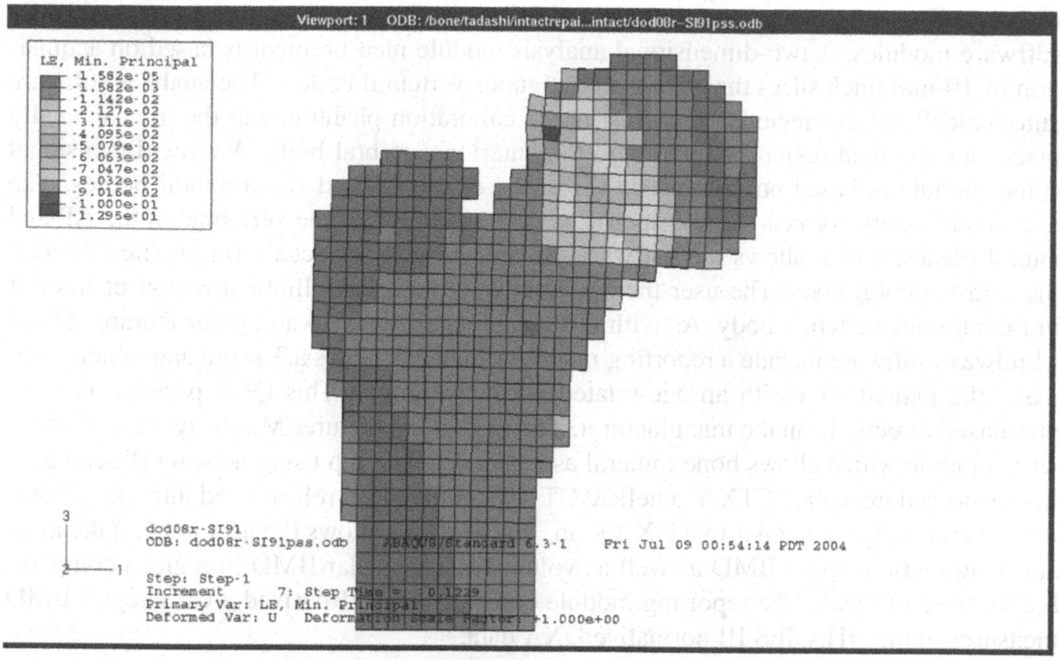

Fig. 8. Stress plot of hip from finite element model loaded under simulated single-legged stance loading condition (J. Keyak, University of California, Irvine).

a QCT option which may be purchased during installation or upgrade of the CT scanner. Alternatively, a QCT package may be purchased from one of the manufacturers of specialized QCT equipment. The price for a QCT package can range between $5000 and $35,000, depending on whether the package only includes a calibration phantom or whether it also includes an analysis computer and software. The following vendors offer QCT systems:

Image Analysis (Columbia, KY, USA) offers a package which includes a bone mineral calibration reference standard incorporating 200, 100, and 50 mg/cm^3 concentrations of calcium hydroxyapatite in a water-equivalent resin matrix, an anthropometric torso phantom for longitudinal scanner QC, and computer software to analyze spinal CT images, report BMD results, and analyze longitudinal QC scans. The BMD measurement is based on acquisition of 10-mm thick slices through the T12-L3 vertebral bodies. The analysis software automatically places regions of interest in the calibration phantom and an elliptical region of interest in the anterior vertebral body. Other features of the Image Analysis software include a reporting module which calculates a T-score and which compares the patient data with an age-related normative curve. This QCT package may be purchased directly from the manufacturer or as an add-on in installation and upgrade of selected CT scanner models.

MINDWAYS (San Francisco, CA, USA) offers a package which include a bone mineral calibration reference standard incorporating four solutions of different concentrations of dipotassium hydrogen phosphate as well as a sample of fat-equivalent material encased in a Lexan framework. Mindways also provides an anthropometric torso phantom for longitudinal scanner QC and computer software modules to analyze spinal CT images, report BMD results and analyze longitudinal QC scans. There are two different spinal BMD software modules. A two-dimensional analysis module measurement is based on acquisition of 10-mm thick slices through 2–4 contiguous vertebral bodies. The analysis software automatically places regions of interest in the calibration phantom and the user manually places an elliptical region of interest in the anterior vertebral body. A three-dimensional spine module is based on volumetric CT scans of the L1 and L2 vertebral bodies. The user interactively corrects the volumetric scans for rotation of the vertebrae in the AP and lateral planes, which allows the software to reconstruct a corrected 10-mm slice through the mid-vertebral body. The user then interactively places an elliptical region of interest in the anterior vertebral body. As with the Image Analysis software, other features of the Mindways software include a reporting module which calculates a T-score and which compares the patient data with an age-related normative curve. This QCT package may be purchased directly from the manufacturer. The QCT manufacturer Mindways offers a software module which allows bone mineral assessment of the hip using helical CT scanning. In this procedure, called CTXA, a helical CT scan of the hip is reformatted into the AP projection and analyzed similar to a DXA scan. The program allows the user to compute areal and volumetric integral BMD as well as volumetric trabecular BMD in regions comparable to those of DXA. The reporting module compares the CT-derived areal integral BMD measures to the NHANES III normative DXA data.

CIRS (Norfolk, VA, USA) offers a non-simultaneous calibration reference which consists of vertebra-shaped calcium hydroxyapatite inserts inside a simulated human torso. The user scans and analyzes images of the phantom to derive a scanner dependent but not patient-specific relationship between concentration of calcium hydroxyapatite and HU. The analysis software applies this relationship to the mean HU inside a vertebral ellipse placed interactively by the user. The package includes reporting software which allows comparison of the patient BMD to a normative curve.

REFERENCES

1. Madsen M. Vertebral and peripheral bone mineral content by photon absorptiometry. Invest Radiol 1977;12(2):185–188.
2. Cameron EC, Boyd RM, Luk D, McIntosh HW, Walker VR. Cortical thickness measurements and photon absorptiometry for determination of bone quantity. Can Med Assoc J 1977;116(2):145–147.
3. Naftchi NE, Viau AT, Marshall CH, Davis WS, Lowman EW. Bone mineralization in the distal forearm of hemiplegic patients. Arch Phys Med Rehabil 1975;56(11):487–492.
4. Mazess RB, Peppler WW, Chesnut CH, Nelp WB, Cohn SH, Zanzi I. Total body bone mineral and lean body mass by dual-photon absorptiometry. II. Comparison with total body calcium by neutron activation analysis. Calcif Tissue Int 1981;33(4):361–363.
5. Mazess RB, Peppler WW, Harrison JE, McNeill KG. Total body bone mineral and lean body mass by dual-photon absorptiometry. III. Comparison with trunk calcium by neutron activation analysis. Calcif Tissue Int 1981;33(4):365–368.
6. Peppler WW, Mazess RB. Total body bone mineral and lean body mass by dual-photon absorptiometry. I. Theory and measurement procedure. Calcif Tissue Int 1981;33(4):353–359.
7. Borders J, Kerr E, Sartoris DJ, et al. Quantitative dual-energy radiographic absorptiometry of the lumbar spine: in vivo comparison with dual-photon absorptiometry. Radiology 1989;170(1 Pt 1):129–131.
8. Stein J, Hochberg AM, Lazetawsky L. Quantitative digital radiography for bone mineral analysis. In: Dequeker JV, Geusens P, Wahner HW, eds. Bone mineral measurements by photon absorptiometry: methodological problems. Louvain, Belgium: Leuven University Press; 1988:411–414.1

9. Mazess RB, Collick B, Trempe J, Barden H, Hanson J. Performance evaluation of a dual energy X-ray bone densitometer. Calcif Tissue Int 1989;44:228–232.
10. Steiger P, von Stetten E, Weiss H, Stein JA. Paired AP and lateral supine dual X-ray absorptiometry of the spine: initial results with a 32 detector system. Osteoporosis Int 1991;1(3):190.
11. Lang T, Takada M, Gee R, et al. A preliminary evaluation of the Lunar Expert-XL for bone densitometry and vertebral morphometry. J Bone Miner Res 1997;12(1):136–143.
12. Mazess RB, Hanson JA, Payne R, Nord R, Wilson M. Axial and total-body bone densitometry using a narrow-angle fan-beam. Osteoporos Int 2000;11(2):158–166.
13. Crabtree N, Wright J, Walgrove A, et al. Vertebral morphometry: repeat scan precision using the Lunar Expert-XL and the Hologic 4500A. A study for the 'WISDOM' RCT of hormone replacement therapy. Osteoporos Int 2000;11(6):537–543.
14. Stein JA, Lazewatsky JL, Hochberg AM. Dual energy X-ray bone densitometer incorporating an internal reference system. Radiology 1987;165(P):313.
15. Lehmann LA, Alvarez RE, Macovski A, Brody WR. Generalized image combinations in dual-kVp-digital radiography. Med Phys 1981;8:659–667.
16. Cardinal HN, Fenster A. An accurate method for direct dual-energy calibration and decomposition. Med Phys 1990;17(3):327–341.
17. Bezakova E, Collins PJ, Beddoe AH. Absorbed dose measurements in dual energy X-ray absorptiometry (DXA). Br J Radiol 1997;70(835):172–179.
18. Njeh CF, Samat SB, Nightingale A, McNeil EA, Boivin CM. Radiation dose and in vitro precision in paediatric bone mineral density measurement using dual X-ray absorptiometry. Br J Radiol 1997;70(835):719–727.
19. Kalender WA. Effective dose values in bone mineral measurements by photon absorptiometry and computed tomography. Osteoporosis Int 1992;2:82–87.
20. Adams JE. Single- and dual-energy: X-ray absorptiometry. In: Genant HK, Guglielmi, G, Jergas, M, eds. Bone densitometry and osteoporosis. Berlin: Springer-Verlag; 1998:305–347.
21. Eiken P, Kolthoff N, Bärenholdt O, Hermansen F, Pors Nielsen S. Switching from DXA pencil-beam to fan-beam. II: studies in vivo. Bone 1994;15(6):671–676.
22. Kuiper JW, van Kuijk C, Grashuis JL, Ederveen AG, Schütte HE. Accuracy and the influence of marrow fat on quantitative CT and dual-energy X-ray absorptiometry measurements of the femoral neck in vitro. Osteoporos Int 1996;6(1):25–30.
23. Kolta S, Ravaud P, Fechtenbaum J, Dougados M, Roux C. Accuracy and precision of 62 bone densitometers using a European Spine Phantom. Osteoporos Int 1999;10(1):14–19.
24. Khan KM, Henzell SL, Broderick C, et al. Instrument performance in bone density testing at five Australian centres [see comments]. Aust N Z J Med 1997;27(5):526–530.
25. Pors Nielsen S, Bärenholdt O, Diessel E, Armbrust S, Felsenberg D. Linearity and accuracy errors in bone densitometry. Br J Radiol 1998;71(850):1062–1068.
26. Pouilles JM, Collard P, Tremollieres F, et al. Accuracy and precision of in vivo bone mineral measurements in sheep using dual-energy X-ray absorptiometry. Calcif Tissue Int 2000;66(1):70–73.
27. Lochmuller EM, Miller P, Burklein D, Wehr U, Rambeck W, Eckstein F. In situ femoral dual-energy X-ray absorptiometry related to ash weight, bone size and density, and its relationship with mechanical failure loads of the proximal femur. Osteoporos Int 2000;11(4):361–367.
28. Engelke K, Glüer CC, Genant HK. Factors influencing short-term precision of dual X-ray bone absorptiometry (DXA) of spine and femur. Calcif Tissue Int 1995;56(1):19–25.
29. Gluer CC, Blake G, Lu Y, Blunt BA, Jergas M, Genant HK. Accurate assessment of precision errors: how to measure the reproducibility of bone densitometry techniques. Osteoporos Int 1995;5(4):262–270.
30. Mazess RB, Nord R, Hanson JA, Barden HS. Bilateral measurement of femoral bone mineral density. J Clin Densitom 2000;3(2):133–140.
31. Patel R, Blake GM, Rymer J, Fogelman I. Long-term precision of DXA scanning assessed over seven years in forty postmenopausal women. Osteoporos Int 2000;11(1):68–75.
32. Ravaud P, Reny JL, Giraudeau B, Porcher R, Dougados M, Roux C. Individual smallest detectable difference in bone mineral density measurements. J Bone Miner Res 1999;14(8):1449–1456.
33. Jergas M, Breitenseher M, Gluer CC, Yu W, Genant H. Estimates of volumetric density from projectional estimates improve the discriminatory capability of dual X-ray absorptiometry. J Bone Miner Res 1995;10:1101–1110.

34. Carter DR, Bouxsein ML, Marcus R. New approaches for interpreting projected bone densitometry data. J Bone Miner Res 1992;7:137–145.
35. Cummings SR, Cauley JA, Palermo L, et al. Racial differences in hip axis lengths might explain racial differences in rates of hip fractures. Osteoporos Int 1994;4:226–229.
36. Yoshikawa T, Turner CH, Peacock M, et al. Geometric structure of the femoral neck measured using dual-energy X-ray absorptiometry. J Bone and Miner Res 1994;9(7):1053–1064.
37. Schönau E. Problems of bone analysis in childhood and adolescence. Pediatr Nephrol 1998;12(5):420–429.
38. Sievänen H, Backström MC, Kuusela AL, Ikonen RS, Mäki M. Dual energy X-ray absorptiometry of the forearm in preterm and term infants: evaluation of the methodology. Pediatr Res 1999;45(1):100–105.
39. Koo WW. Body composition measurements during infancy. Ann N Y Acad Sci 2000;904(4):383–392.
40. Lapillonne A, Braillon PM, Delmas PD, Salle BL. Dual-energy X-ray absorptiometry in early life. Horm Res 1997;48 Suppl 1(3):43–49.
41. Lang TF, Li J, Harris ST, Genant HK. Assessment of vertebral bone mineral density using volumetric quantitative CT. J Comput Assist Tomogr 1999;23(1):130–137.
42. Cummings SR, Marcus R, Palermo L, Ensrud KE, Genant HK. Does estimating volumetric bone density of the femoral neck improve the prediction of hip fracture? A prospective study. Study of Osteoporotic Fractures Research Group. J Bone Miner Res 1994;9(9):1429–1432.
43. Tothill P, Avenell A. Errors in dual-energy X-ray absorptiometry of the lumbar spine owing to fat distribution and soft tissue thickness during weight change. Br J Radiol 1994;67(793):71–75.
44. Svendsen OL, Hassager C, Skødt V, Christiansen C. Impact of soft tissue on in vivo accuracy of bone mineral measurements in the spine, hip, and forearm: a human cadaver study. J Bone Miner Res 1995;10(6):868–873.
45. Formica C, Loro ML, Gilsanz V, Seeman E. Inhomogeneity in body fat distribution may result in inaccuracy in the measurement of vertebral bone mass. J Bone Miner Res 1995;10(10):1504–1511.
46. Ruetsche AG, Lippuner K, Jaeger P, Casez JP. Differences between dual X-ray absorptiometry using pencil beam and fan beam modes and their determinants in vivo and in vitro. J Clin Densitom 2000;3(2):157–166.
47. Griffiths MR, Noakes KA, Pocock NA. Correcting the magnification error of fan beam densitometers. J Bone Miner Res 1997;12(1):119–123.
48. Blake GM, McKeeney DB, Chhaya SC, Ryan PJ, Fogelman J. Dual energy X-ray absorptiometry: the effects of beam hardening on bone density measurements. Med Phys 1992;19(2):459–465.
49. Pietrobelli A, Gallagher D, Baumgartner R, Ross R, Heymsfield SB. Lean R value for DXA two-component soft-tissue model: influence of age and tissue or organ type. Appl Radiat Isot 1998;49(5–6):743–744.
50. Gluer CC, Steiger P, Selvidge R, Elliesen-Kliefoth K, Hayashi C, Genant HK. Comparative assessment of dual-photon-absorptiometry and dual-energy-radiography. Radiology 1990;174:223–228.
51. Grampp S, Genant H, Mathur A, et al. Comparisons of noninvasive bone mineral measurements in assessing age-related loss, fracture discrimination and diagnostic classification. J Bone Miner Res 1997;12(5):697–711.
52. Pacifici R, Rupich R, Griffin M, Chines A, Susman N, Avioli LV. Dual energy radiography versus quantitative computer tomography for the diagnosis of osteoporosis. J Clin Endocrinol Metab 1990;70(3):705–710.
53. Assessment of fracture risk and its application to screening for postmenopausal osteoporosis. Report of a WHO Study Group. World Health Organ Tech Rep Ser 1994;843:1–129.
54. Wainwright SA, Marshall LM, Ensrud KE, et al. Hip fracture in women without osteoporosis. J Clin Endocrinol Metab 2005;90(5):2787–2793.
55. Marshall D, Johnell O, Wedel H. Meta-analysis of how well measures of bone mineral density predict occurrence of osteoporotic fractures. BMJ 1996;312(7041):1254–1259.
56. Kanis JA, Borgstrom F, De Laet C, et al. Assessment of fracture risk. Osteoporos Int 2005;16(6): 581–589.
57. Richards JB, Leslie WD, Joseph L, et al. Changes to osteoporosis prevalence according to method of risk assessment. J Bone Miner Res 2007;22(2):228–234.
58. Kalender WA, Polacin A. Physical performance of spiral CT scanning. Med Phys 1991;18(5):910–915.
59. Kalender WA, Seissler W, Klotz E, Vock P. Spiral volumetric CT with single-breath-hold technique, continuous transport and continuous scanner rotation. Radiology 1990;176:181–183.

60. Cann CE, Genant HK. Precise measurement of vertebral mineral content using computed tomography. J Comp Assist Tomogr 1980;4:493–500.
61. Faulkner KG, Glüer CC, Grampp S, Genant HK. Cross calibration of liquid and solid QCT calibration standards: corrections to the UCSF normative data. Osteo Int 1993;3:36–42.
62. Dunnill M, Anderson J, Whitehead R. Quantitative histological studies on age changes in bone. J Pathol Bacteriol 1967;94:275–291.
63. Cann CE. Low-dose CT scanning for quantitative spinal mineral analysis. Radiology 1981;140:813–815.
64. Genant HK, Cann CE, Boyd DP, et al. Quantitative computed tomography for vertebral mineral determination. In: Frame B, Potts JT, eds. Clinical disorders of bone and mineral metabolism. Amsterdam–Oxford–Princeton: Excerpta Medica; 1983:40–47.
65. Kalender WA, Klotz E, Süss C. Vertebral bone mineral analysis: an integrated approach. Radiology 1987;164:419–423.
66. Steiger P, Block JE, Steiger S, et al. Spinal bone mineral density by quantitative computed tomography: effect of region of interest, vertebral level, and technique. Radiology 1990;175:537–543.
67. Laval-Jeantet AM, Genant HK, Wu C, Glüer CC, Faulkner K, Steiger P. Factors influencing long-term in vivo reproducibility of QCT (vertebral densitometry). JCAT 1993;17(6):915–921.
68. Lang TF, Keyak JH, Heitz MW, et al. Volumetric quantitative computed tomography of the proximal femur: precision and relation to bone strength. Bone 1997;21(1):101–108.
69. Kalender WA, Schmidt B, Zankl M, Schmidt M. A PC program for estimating organ dose and effective dose values in computed tomography. Eur Radiol 1999;9(3):555–562.
70. Lang T, LeBlanc A, Evans H, Lu Y, Genant H, Yu A. Cortical and trabecular bone mineral loss from the spine and hip in long-duration spaceflight. J Bone Miner Res 2004;19(6):1006–1012.
71. Kang Y, Engelke K, Kalender WA. A new accurate and precise 3-D segmentation method for skeletal structures in volumetric CT data. IEEE Trans Med Imaging 2003;22(5):586–598.
72. Kang Y, Engelke K, Fuchs C, Kalender WA. An anatomic coordinate system of the femoral neck for highly reproducible BMD measurements using 3D QCT. Comput Med Imaging Graph 2005;29(7):533–541.
73. Riggs BL, Melton Iii LJ, III, Robb RA, et al. Population-based study of age and sex differences in bone volumetric density, size, geometry, and structure at different skeletal sites. J Bone Miner Res 2004;19(12):1945–1954.
74. Meta M, Lu Y, Keyak JH, Lang T. Young-elderly differences in bone density, geometry and strength indices depend on proximal femur sub-region: a cross sectional study in Caucasian-American women. Bone 2006;39(1):152–158.
75. Lang TF, Leblanc AD, Evans HJ, Lu Y. Adaptation of the proximal femur to skeletal reloading after long-duration spaceflight. J Bone Miner Res 2006;21(8):1224–1230.
76. Black DM, Greenspan SL, Ensrud KE, et al. The effects of parathyroid hormone and alendronate alone or in combination in postmenopausal osteoporosis. N Engl J Med 2003;349(13):1207–1215.
77. McClung MR, San Martin J, Miller PD, et al. Opposite bone remodeling effects of teriparatide and alendronate in increasing bone mass. Arch Intern Med 2005;165(15):1762–1768.
78. Cheng X, Li J, Lu Y, Keyak J, Lang T. Proximal femoral density and geometry measurements by quantitative computed tomography: association with hip fracture. Bone 2007;40(1):169–174.
79. Sigurdsson G, Aspelund T, Chang M, et al. Increasing sex difference in bone strength in old age: the age, gene/environment susceptibility-reykjavik study (AGES-REYKJAVIK). Bone 2006;39(3):644–651.
80. Marshall LM, Lang TF, Lambert LC, Zmuda JM, Ensrud KE, Orwoll ES. Dimensions and volumetric BMD of the proximal femur and their relation to age among older U.S. men. J Bone Miner Res 2006;21(8):1197–1206.
81. Gluer CC, Cummings SR, Pressman A, et al. Prediction of hip fractures from pelvic radiographs: the study of osteoporotic fractures. The Study of Osteoporotic Fractures Research Group. J Bone Miner Res 1994;9(5):671–677.
82. Lang TF, Li J, Harris ST, Genant HK. Assessment of vertebral bone mineral density using volumetric quantitative CT. J Comput Assist Tomogr 1999;23(1):130–137.
83. Keyak JH, Kaneko TS, Tehranzadeh J, Skinner HB. Predicting proximal femoral strength using structural engineering models. Clin Orthop Relat Res 2005(437):219–228.
84. Keyak JH. Improved prediction of proximal femoral fracture load using nonlinear finite element models. Med Eng Phys 2001;23(3):165–173.

85. Keyak JH, Rossi SA, Jones KA, Les CM, Skinner HB. Prediction of fracture location in the proximal femur using finite element models. Med Eng Phys 2001;23(9):657–664.
86. Cody DD, Gross GJ, Hou FJ, Spencer HJ, Goldstein SA, Fyhrie DP. Femoral strength is better predicted by finite element models than QCT and DXA. J Biomech 1999;32(10):1013–1020.
87. Cody DD, Hou FJ, Divine GW, Fyhrie DP. Short term in vivo precision of proximal femoral finite element modeling. Ann Biomed Eng 2000;28(4):408–414.
88. Keaveny TM, Donley DW, Hoffmann PF, Mitlak BH, Glass EV, San Martin JA. Effects of teriparatide and alendronate on vertebral strength as assessed by finite element modeling of QCT scans in women with osteoporosis. J Bone Miner Res 2007;22(1):149–157.
89. Crawford RP, Rosenberg WS, Keaveny TM. Quantitative computed tomography-based finite element models of the human lumbar vertebral body: effect of element size on stiffness, damage, and fracture strength predictions. J Biomech Eng 2003;125(4):434–438.
90. Faulkner KG, Cann CE, Hasegawa BH. Effect of bone distribution on vertebral strength: assessment with patient-specific nonlinear finite element analysis. Radiology 1991;179(3):669–674.
91. Lian KC, Lang TF, Keyak JH, et al. Differences in hip quantitative computed tomography (QCT) measurements of bone mineral density and bone strength between glucocorticoid-treated and glucocorticoid-naive postmenopausal women. Osteoporos Int 2005;16(6):642–650.

3 New Imaging Techniques for Bone

Suchandrima Banerjee, PhD, Roland Krug, PhD, Sven Prevrhal, PhD, and Sharmila Majumdar, PhD

CONTENTS

SUMMARY

This chapter provides a comprehensive review of the existing imaging techniques for assessing trabecular and cortical architecture as well as emerging advances in these areas. A brief description of the physics behind X-ray computed tomography and magnetic resonance imaging is provided to lay the foundation for review of image acquisition techniques. Next, the authors review at length image analysis algorithms that are used to derive measurements of bone structure from these images. Finally, to present the diagnostic capabilities of

From: *Contemporary Endocrinology: Osteoporosis: Pathophysiology and Clinical Management*
Edited by: R. A. Adler, DOI 10.1007/978-1-59745-459-9_3,

the imaging methods, the authors discuss published in vitro and in vivo studies on the relationships of the image-derived bone measures with bone strength, biomechanics, fracture discrimination, and osteoporotic status.

Key Words: Micro-architecture, micro-computed tomography, high-resolution peripheral computed tomography, magnetic resonance imaging

INTRODUCTION

Osteoporosis is characterized by decreased bone strength and an increased propensity to fracture. The routine assessment of skeletal integrity by dual X-ray absorptiometry, although widespread, does not capture all the factors contributing to bone strength. In addition to the bone mass, density, and content, the trabecular and cortical bone architecture, mineralization, micro-fracture, and damage repair also contribute to bone strength.

Considerable effort is being expended in developing techniques to assess trabecular bone micro-architecture non-invasively. Heterogeneity in the micro-architecture of trabecular bone is governed by physiological function and mechanical loading on the skeleton. This results in bone micro-architecture being dependent on the anatomic site, as well as having a directional anisotropy of the mechanical properties and architecture. Thus, site-specific bone structure information would significantly contribute to understanding the results of different therapeutic interventions and potentially assist in optimizing the course of treatment.

Three-dimensional techniques that reveal trabecular bone structure are emerging as important candidates for defining bone quality, at least partially. Techniques such as micro-computed tomography (μCT) have recently been developed and provide high-resolution images of the trabecular architecture. This method is routinely used in specimen evaluation and has recently been extended to in vivo animal and human extremity imaging. A more recent development in the assessment of trabecular bone structure is the use of magnetic resonance (MR) imaging techniques that make it possible to obtain non-invasive bone biopsies at multiple anatomic sites. Using such μCT and MR images, multiple different image processing and image analysis algorithms have been developed. The goal of all of these is to quantify the trabecular bone structure in two or three dimensions. The measures that have been derived so far are many, some of them synonymous with the histomorphometric measures such as trabecular bone volume fraction (BV/TV), trabecular thickness (Tb.Th), trabecular spacing (Tb.Sp), and trabecular number (Tb.N). Others include connectivity or Euler number, fractal dimension, tubularity, and maximal entropy. This chapter provides comprehensive coverage on the image acquisition and analysis methodologies for assessing trabecular and cortical architecture, relationships of the measures with biomechanics, osteoporotic status, as well as emerging advances in these areas.

MICRO-COMPUTED TOMOGRAPHY, HIGH-RESOLUTION PERIPHERAL COMPUTED TOMOGRAPHY

Assessment of trabecular bone structure with X-ray imaging techniques is based on the higher X-ray absorption of bone, in particular its constituent calcium, compared to surrounding tissue such as marrow, fat, and muscle. Because the logarithm of the measured absorption roughly scales linearly with the length of material the beam has penetrated, simultaneous quantitative measurements of bone density are possible. X-ray computed tomography (CT) provides truly three-dimensional image data of bone structure with high contrast and high spatial resolution. Techniques with resolution between 1 and 100 μm are referred to as micro-CT (μCT) and offer the promise of replacing tedious serial staining techniques required by histomorphometric analysis of thin sections and the possibility of longitudinal in vivo investigations in small animals such as mice and rats. Many of the early μCT approaches used Synchrotron radiation *(1)*, which is still the method of choice for ultra high-resolution applications. Obviously, the use of desktop laboratory scanners equipped with X-ray tubes is much more convenient than setting up an experiment at one of the few Synchrotron facilities available. Thus, after the initial and still ongoing university-based research during the last decade, a large variety of X-ray tube-based commercial μCT scanners have been developed. The first in vitro μCT scanner specifically targeted for bone analysis with a spatial resolution of 15–20 μm was developed by Rüegsegger et al. *(2,3)* and has been used extensively in laboratory investigations (Fig. 1). Its high accuracy in relation to standard two-dimensional histomorphometry as well as to serial grindings and their derived three-dimensional parameters triggered a wide distribution of this scanner type. Three-dimensional data sets from μCT systems with this resolution can be used for

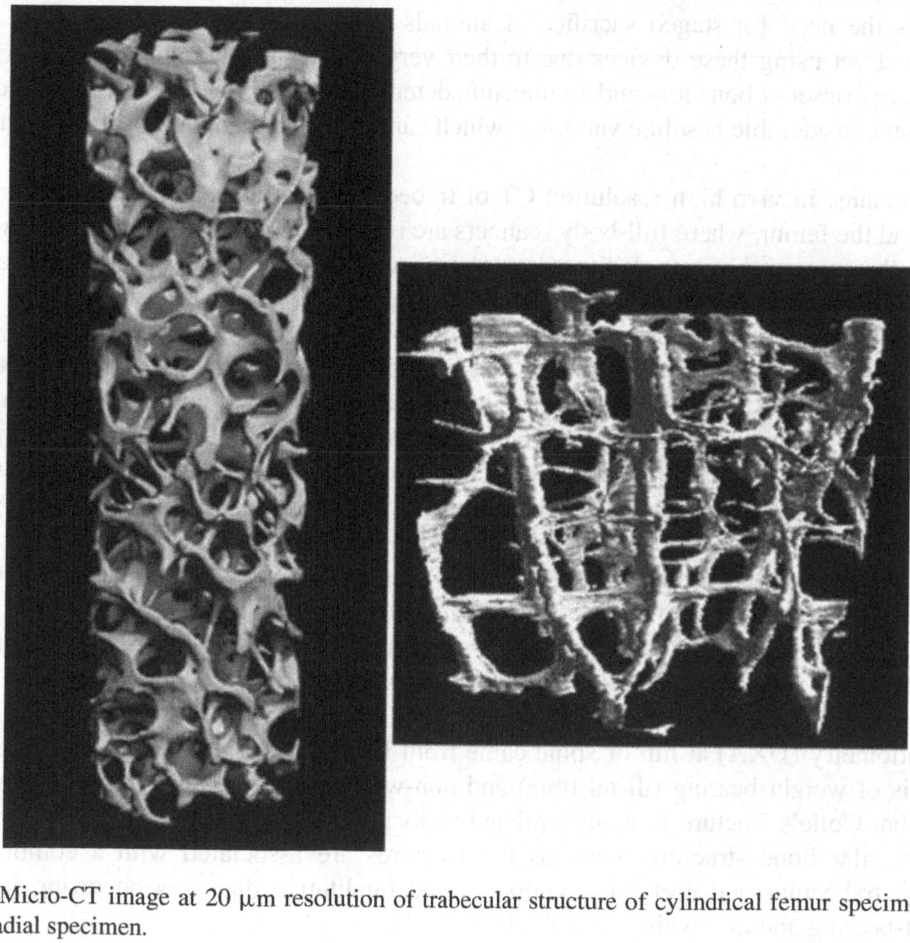

Fig. 1. Micro-CT image at 20 μm resolution of trabecular structure of cylindrical femur specimen and cubic radial specimen.

calculating classical histomorphometric parameters like trabecular thickness and separation as well as for determining topological measurements like the Euler number and connectivity *(4–6)*. Early on, comparison of structural parameters of specimens scanned with these systems and results from mechanical testing showed that not only the amount of bone but also the architecture of trabecular bone contributed to mechanical strength *(7)*. However, other studies failed to show an explanatory power of structural parameters independent of bone mass *(8)*. With the latest generation of in vitro μCT systems approaching spatial resolution of 10 μm or better *(9)*, μCT has found wide application in both preclinical animal studies and clinical research settings *(10)*, for instance in the assessment of skeletal phenotype in gene knock-out or knock-in mice *(11–13)* and in osteoporotic *(14)* or arthritic rodents *(15)*. While μCT-based structure measurements do not rely on accuracy of CT numbers, quantitative density measurements at the microstructural level should be possible, provided artifacts and inaccuracies caused by beam hardening due to preferred attenuation of lower-energy X-rays and partial voluming due to insufficient spatial resolution can be reduced. Prevrhal *(16,17)* showed that the use of an iterative postexposure correction method could reduce beam hardening by an order of magnitude and should allow quantitative bone density measurements.

μCT has more recently been extended to in vivo imaging of small animals, which allows longitudinal study of trabecular bone, for instance in preclinical intervention studies and obviates the need for staged sacrifice of animals *(18,19)*. Not many studies have been published yet using these devices due to their very recent introduction. Boyd et al. *(20)* report early onset of bone loss and architecture deterioration in ovariectomized rats and also point out considerable baseline variation, which cannot be handled well by cross-sectional studies.

In humans, in vivo high-resolution CT of trabecular structure has been applied to the spine and the femur, where full-body scanners are required *(21–26)*, and with greatest success to the forearm because dedicated extremity scanners use narrow bores and are thus able to provide much better spatial resolution. The first to pursue this successfully were Durand and Rüegsegger and coworkers *(3,27)* who built a thin-slice high-resolution laboratory peripheral quantitative CT (pQCT) scanner for in vivo applications with an isotropic voxel size of 170 μm. This work culminated in the XtremeCT, a commercially available in vivo pQCT scanner for the forearm and the tibia (Fig. 2) *(28,29)*. A critical step in the analysis of follow-up scans in order to detect longitudinal changes of bone structure within a given subject is the registration of baseline and follow-up scans with an accuracy that should be in the order of 100 μm. Thus during the scans even slight motions of the forearm must be avoided. While not many studies using this device have been reported yet, Khosla et al. *(28,30)* examined age- and sex-related bone loss cross-sectionally and speculated as to the different patterns of bone loss in men and women. The first extremity CT indication that peripheral trabecular structure assessment is indeed useful to differentiate women with an osteoporotic fracture history from controls better than dual-energy X-ray absorptiometry (DXA) at hip or spine came from Boutroy et al. *(29)*. Three-dimensional analysis of weight-bearing (distal tibia) and non-weight-bearing (distal radius) sites suggests that Colle's fracture is mainly related to local cortical low mineral density instead of trabecular bone structure, whereas hip fractures are associated with a combination of both trabecular and cortical quantitative and qualitative damages occurring in both weight-bearing and non-weight-bearing bones *(31)*.

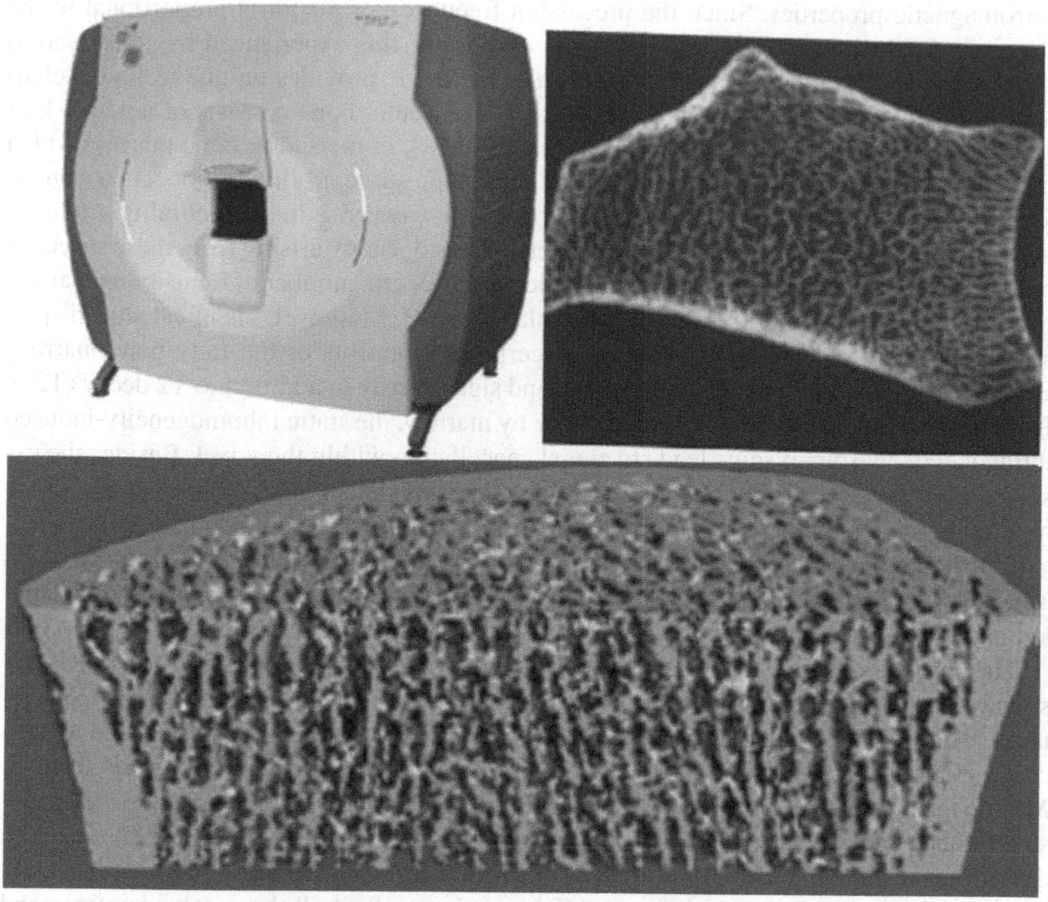

Fig. 2. In vivo micro-CT device and cross-sectional image of distal radius (*top row*). Three-dimensional rendering of tibial bone structure.

MAGNETIC RESONANCE IMAGING

Magnetic resonance imaging (MRI) is a non-ionizing imaging modality that is evolving as a non-invasive tool for monitoring trabecular bone structure in specimens as well as in vivo human studies. Magnetic resonance imaging is based on the interaction between an atom and the external magnetic field. Atoms with odd number of protons/ neutrons, i.e., atoms with unpaired spins, are visible to MRI. In MR experiments, the external static magnetic field (~Tesla) is used to polarize and a radio-frequency (rf) pulse is used to perturb the spin system in the imaging sample. The MR signal is received when the spins release the energy absorbed from the rf pulse and return to their initial state. The spatial position of spins in the imaging sample is generally encoded by two or three perpendicular spatially linearly varying magnetic fields known as gradients. The image intensities in an MR image depend among other things on the density of spins and the spin–spin (T2) and spin–lattice (T1) relaxation rates of the tissues. In MRI, bone marrow yields high signal intensity, whereas trabecular bone has very low signal intensity because it has a very short T2 relaxation. The magnetic field experienced by an atomic spin in the MR magnet also depends on the electronic shielding of the nucleus which causes diamagnetic, paramagnetic, and ferromagnetic properties. Since the precession frequency of a spin is proportional to the magnetic field strength, differences in local magnetic fields experienced by spins lead to off-resonance. The tissue composition of trabecular bone provides unique technical challenges to MR imaging of its micro-architecture. Trabecular bone consists of a network of rod-like elements interconnected by plate-like elements, immersed in bone marrow which is comprised partly of water and partly of fat. Magnetic susceptibility of trabecular bone is substantially different from that of bone marrow. This gives rise to susceptibility gradients at every bone–bone marrow interface. Magnetic inhomogeneity arising from these susceptibility gradients depends on the static magnetic field strength, number of bone–bone marrow interfaces, and the size of individual trabeculae *(32–34)*. Moreover, chemical shift dispersion arises from chemically different triglyceride components of the fatty bone marrow. Both these effects cause dephasing of spins and signal decay in addition to T2 decay (T2*). In a voxel partly occupied by bone and partly by marrow, the static inhomogeneity-induced intravoxel dephasing of spins leads to signal cancellation within the voxel. Besides the tissue composition, the small dimensions of the trabecular elements ($\sim$100 μm) require very high imaging resolutions. The suitability of an MR imaging method (acquisition and analysis) for depicting trabecular micro-structures depends on its ability to yield images with a high enough signal in a reasonable acquisition time and its ability to derive trabecular structural measurements from the images accurately and reproducibly.

The three competing factors to be considered in high-resolution MRI (HR-MRI) are signal-to-noise ratio, spatial resolution, and imaging time. Spatial resolution and signal-to-noise ratio (SNR) are both directly related to imaging time but are inversely related to each other. High spatial resolution is necessary to distinguish the trabecular elements from an MR image. A minimum SNR (>8–10) is required to be able to run computerized analysis of trabecular structure from the images. Acquisition times longer than 15–20 min cause discomfort in patients and motion-induced artifacts and blurring in the images. Recent technique developments in trabecular bone MRI technique reflect all these considerations and have been aiming for increasing SNR and accelerating acquisition.

Signal-to-noise ratio of an MR acquisition can be improved by employing (a) pulse sequences with high magnetization yield, (b) higher static magnetic field strength, and (c) array of small surface coils instead of a single coil with similar coverage for signal reception.

PULSE SEQUENCES

MR pulse sequences can be broadly classified into spin-echo and gradient-echo sequences. In spin-echo sequences the signal decay due to static dephasing over and above T2 decay is recovered at the time of the echo, whereas in gradient-echo sequences it is not. So ideally, three-dimensional spin-echo (SE) sequences are better suited for imaging of trabecular bone micro-architecture than gradient-echo (GE)-based sequences because they are less sensitive to static dephasing and off-resonance effects. However, GE sequences can be employed with short repetition time (TR) because of their higher SNR efficiency and can thus acquire a three-dimensional volume in shorter scan time and avoid patient motion artifacts. As a result, three-dimensional GE sequences such as 3D fast gradient recalled echo (FGRE) are widely employed for HR-MRI of trabecular bone *(35,36)*. However, because of their robustness to off-resonance effects, spin-echo sequences have also been employed for trabecular bone imaging *(37–40)*. In order to reduce long scan times, fast spin-echo (FSE) imaging usually employs multiple rf spin echoes to sample multiple phase-encoding lines in one repetition time *(41)*. However, the long echo train length causes T2 blurring which broadens the point spread function (PSF), and consequently decreases effective image resolution *(42)*. Thus, this type of sequence is not suitable for HR-MRI of small structures. Although a three-dimensional (3D) SE pulse sequence employing only one echo per excitation would be optimal, long imaging time and low SNR efficiency limit its clinical use. To address these problems 3D-SE type pulse sequences with variable flip angle-like rapid SE excitation (RASEE) *(43,44)*, large-angle spin-echo imaging *(45)*, and subsequently fast 3D large-angle spin-echo imaging (FLASE) *(37)* were introduced. The general idea of these approaches was to apply either composite rf pulses (RASEE) or only one large-angle rf pulse (FLASE) so that the longitudinal magnetization is partly tipped to the negative axis. The subsequent 180° phase reversal pulse, while generating an echo, restores the longitudinal magnetization. Even with this scheme, the TR has to be sufficiently long, on the order of 80 ms *(37)*, to avoid saturation. Another approach was recently published introducing a new fully balanced steady-state 3D-spin-echo (bSSSE) pulse sequence in which all applied gradients are fully rewound over one repetition time *(46)*. This scheme represents the most SNR effective SE sequence suited for trabecular bone imaging.

Fully balanced steady-state free-precession (bSSFP) sequences are a class of fully refocused GE sequences that employ very short repetition times (TR << T2). They have found diverse clinical applications because of their high SNR efficiency. Recently, employing bSSFP for HR-MRI of trabecular bone, significant gain in SNR efficiency (~60–140%) compared to FGRE was found in all skeletal sites imaged at 1.5 and 3 T *(47)*. However, the magnetization response to bSSFP is highly sensitive to off-resonance frequencies. The attenuated response from regions of off-resonance may cause dark bands ("banding artifact") to appear in an SSFP image. Due to increased susceptibility effects at higher field (3 T), the range of off-resonance frequencies in a voxel is much larger at 3 T than at 1.5 T, and the selective attenuation of frequencies by the bSSFP magnetization response makes this a more severe problem. Therefore, multiple bSSFP techniques are employed at higher field strengths *(48)*. In this method, data are acquired multiple times with different phases of the rf pulse and combined. Although multiple acquisitions prolong scan time and partly reduce the SNR efficiency of the bSSFP method, this pulse sequence was found to yield highest SNR efficiency compared to FGRE and all spin-echo type sequences used for trabecular imaging *(46)*.

The right choice of pulse sequence for trabecular bone imaging is still a topic of active research. Trade-offs exist for different sequences. For example, although the trabecular thickness can be depicted more accurately using SE pulse sequences, the number of trabeculae is better represented using bSSFP. Availability of the sequences at multiple centers, their robustness, total imaging time versus the anatomical coverage are also considerations.

MAGNETIC FIELD STRENGTH

SNR is linearly proportional to the static magnetic field strength, B_0 in the sample noise dominance regime, making 3 T preferable over 1.5 T magnets. Other factors such as different relaxation times and increased susceptibility effects also affect the SNR gain from a lower to higher field strength. Banerjee et al. *(47)* measured about a 1.6-fold increase in SNR efficiency in high-resolution imaging of trabecular bone with bSSFP when going from 1.5 to 3 T. The 60% gain in SNR can alternatively be utilized to increase the through-plane resolution by 60%. Phan et al. *(49)* imaged the trabecular micro-architecture in 40 cadaveric calcaneus specimens from donors with and without vertebral fractures with MRI at 1.5 and 3 T and compared them with μCT as the gold standard. Correlations between trabecular structural parameters derived from 3 T MR images and μCT were significantly higher ($p < 0.05$) than correlations between structural parameters obtained from 1.5 T MR imaging and μCT. However, the trabecular thickness parameter was significantly overestimated at 3 T compared to 1.5 T due to susceptibility-induced broadening effects. The authors also reported a trend for better differentiation between the population with and without osteoporotic vertebral fractures at 3 T than at 1.5 T. In vivo images may be obtained both at 1.5 and 3 T at the radius, tibia, calcaneus, and proximal femur. In Fig. 3, representative images from different skeletal sites are shown for both 1.5 and 3 T acquisitions.

Preliminary experiments conducted on a 7 T GE Signa Scanner yielded a two-fold increase in SNR for HR-MRI of trabecular bone with a multiple bSSFP sequence. In these experiments, the distal tibia of six volunteers was imaged on 7 and 3 T GE Signa MRI scanners and on a new in vivo three-dimensional peripheral quantitative CT (3D-pQCT) system (XtremeCT, Scanco Medical). As expected the trabecular thickness measured at 7 T was overestimated (~25%) compared to 3 T due to increased susceptibility effects, which also led to an overestimation of the bone fraction. However, imaging at high field strengths has many technical challenges. First, magnetic inhomogeneity induced by susceptibility gradients and chemical shift artifacts increases proportionally with field strength, which leads to more pronounced intravoxel dispersion. As a result, the relaxation time T2* decreases with increasing magnetic field strength. Gradient-echo acquisitions should be employed with shorter echo times to avoid additional signal losses from intravoxel dephasing. Higher readout bandwidth is also warranted in view of larger chemical shifts. Improved shimming routines are required at higher fields to ensure acceptable field homogeneity. Heating issues related to specific absorption rate (SAR) pose serious concerns at high field strengths such as 7 T, especially for spin-echo sequences.

Imaging with an Array of Small Coils

Use of small surface coils that are optimized for the geometry of the body part being imaged can play a very important role in improving the SNR of an MR acquisition. The SNR for a circular loop of surface coil is inversely proportional to the radius of the coil. However, the sensitivity of a surface coil decreases with distance from the surface as $a^2/\sqrt{(a^2+z^2)^3}$, where a is the radius of the coil and z the depth from surface. So the coil geometry should be optimized to the depth of the object of interest being imaged. Employing an array of coils can also ensure sufficient coverage *(50)*. Although receiver setups in musculoskeletal imaging are mostly single coils, phased array coils have recently been designed for imaging at the knee, hip, and extremities *(51,52)*.

Scan Time Reduction with Parallel Imaging

Traditionally, acceleration of MR acquisitions has involved faster coverage of *k*-space such as projection reconstruction techniques or employment of tailored short rf pulses. Parallel imaging offers a different approach to faster acquisition by utilizing the spatial encoding in receiver arrays. In conventional phased-array applications, an array of multiple coil elements is used to receive the MR signal, instead of a single coil with the same

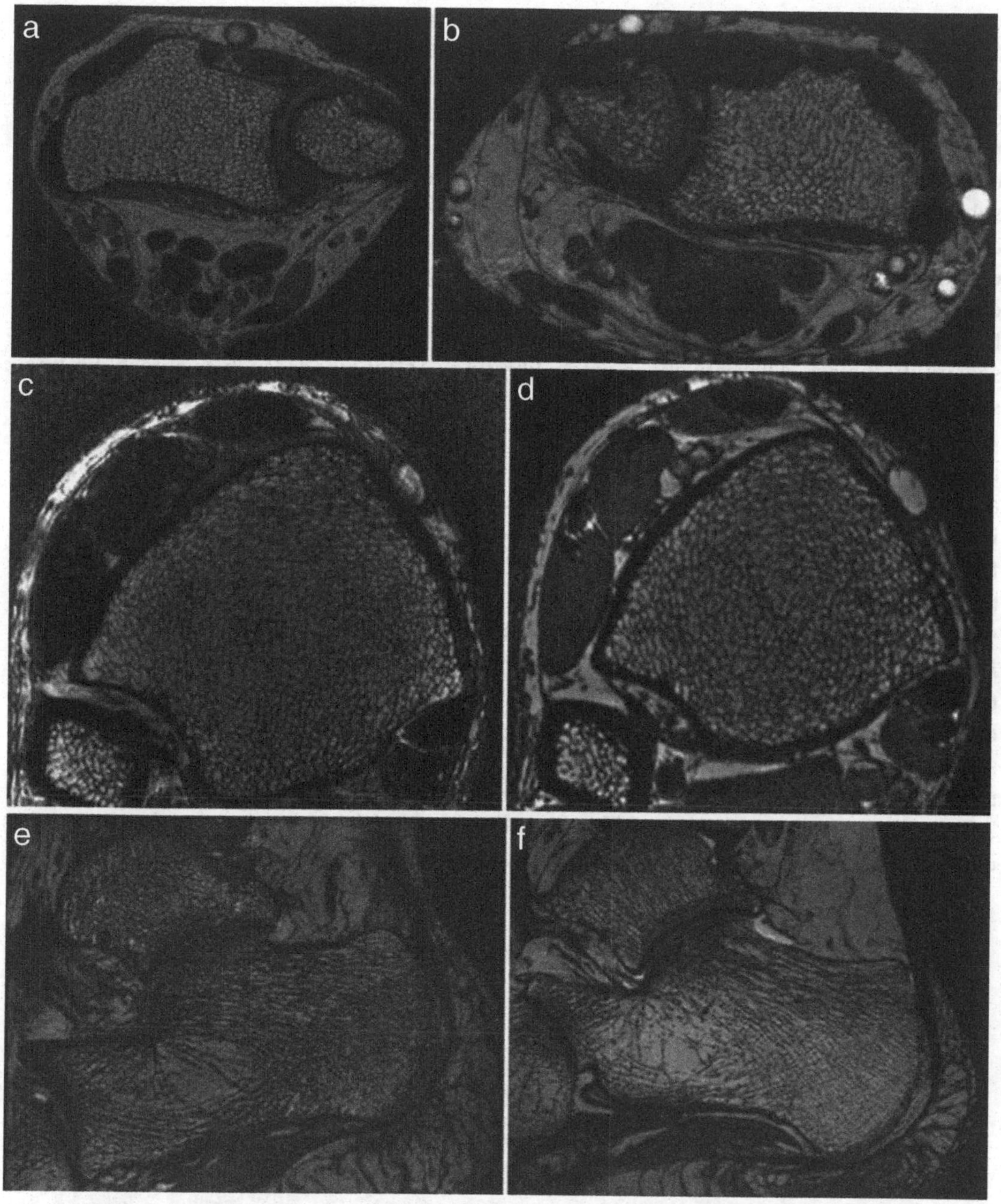

Fig. 3. Axial image of the distal radius acquired at (**a**) 1.5 T using a gradient-echo sequence and TR/TE = 17/4.7 ms, total imaging time 14 min, and spatial resolution of $156 \times 156 \times 500\ \mu m^3$. (**b**) 3 T using a bSSFP sequence TR/TE = 13.8/4.3 ms, total imaging time 9.5 min, and spatial resolution of $156 \times 156 \times 500\ \mu m^3$. Axial images of the distal tibia acquired at (**c**) 1.5 T using a bSSFP sequence TR/TE = 15/4 ms, total imaging time 10.36 min, and spatial resolution of $156 \times 156 \times 500\ \mu m^3$; and (**d**) 3 T using a nSSFP sequence TR/TE = 11/4 ms, total imaging time 9.3 min, and spatial resolution of $156 \times 156 \times 500\ \mu m^3$. Sagittal images of the calcaneus acquired at (**e**) 1.5 T using a bSSFP sequence TR/TE = 15/4 ms, total imaging time 15.2 min, and spatial resolution of $195 \times 195 \times 500\ \mu m^3$ (**f**) 3 T using a bSSFP sequence TR/TE = 12/4 ms, total imaging time 14.5 min, and spatial resolution of $195 \times 195 \times 500\ \mu m^3$.

coverage as the array, because of signal-to-noise ratio (SNR) advantages *(50)*. The final MR image is obtained by calculating the square root of the weighted sum of squares or by optimal pixel-by-pixel combination of the MR images obtained from each array element. Partially parallel imaging (PPI) exploits the over-determinedness of such a system. In PPI, the signal space is undersampled in the phase-encoding/partition-encoding direction to reduce imaging time *(53–55)*. The aliased images due to undersampling are subsequently unfolded using the localized spatial sensitivity information of the receiver array elements. Since the MR signal from the same object is received by the different array elements at spatially distinct locations, it is spatially encoded. The sensitivity encoding matrix can be computed from estimated reception profiles of the coil elements based on a short calibration scan and unfolding can be achieved by direct inversion of the sensitivity matrix. Alternatively, in autocalibrating (AC) methods, such as autocalibrating-simultaneous acquisition of spatial harmonics (AUTO-SMASH) *(56)*, variable density AUTO-SMASH (VD-AUTO-SMASH) *(57)*, and generalized autocalibrating partially parallel acquisitions (GRAPPA) *(58)*, a small set of additional phase-encoding lines is acquired at the Nyquist sampling frequency. These lines serve as training lines for the estimation of interpolation weights, which are then used to synthesize the skipped phase-encoding lines from the acquired lines. GRAPPA has proved to be particularly flexible since it unfolds the full field-of-view (FOV) image of each individual coil element allowing subsequent weighted sum-of-squares array combination and is robust to small FOV imaging situations. Recently, a modified GRAPPA technique was applied to accelerate MR imaging of the three-dimensional trabecular bone micro-architecture *(59)*. The effects of the GRAPPA-based reconstruction on image characteristics and on the measurement of trabecular bone structural parameters were evaluated. Image quality and structural detail were preserved up to four-fold acceleration, which is equivalent to a four-fold reduction in scan time, at 3 T. Preliminary experiments at 7 T indicated that even higher acceleration factors can be employed at 7 T. Figure 4a shows the trabecular architecture at the knee acquired for 48

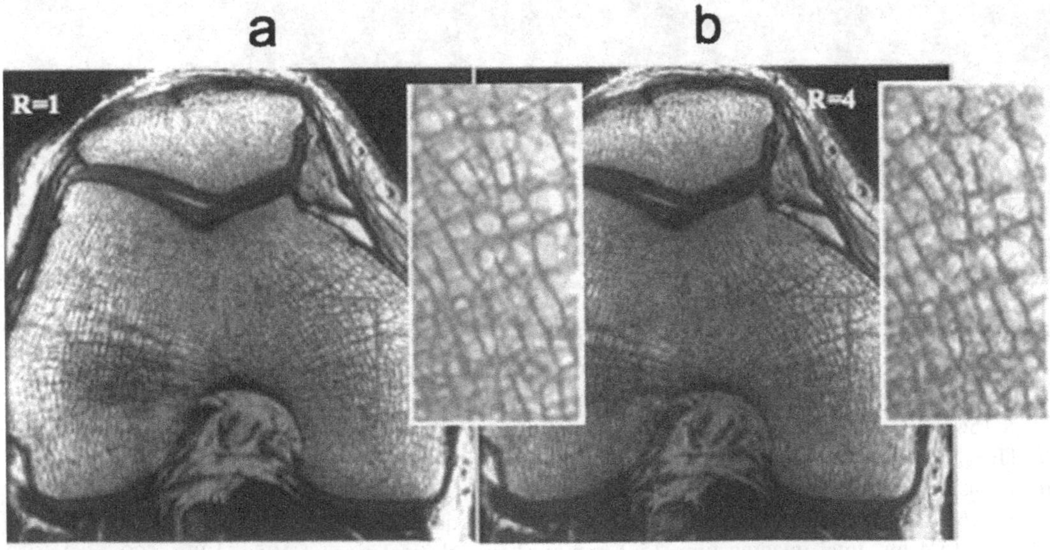

Fig. 4. Axial images of the knee acquired at 7 T without (**a**) and with (**b**) parallel imaging.

slices with in-plane and through-plane resolutions of 190 and 1000 μm, respectively, in a scan time of 10 min 45 s. Figure 4b shows the image of the same knee acquired with four-fold acceleration using PPI in a scan time of only 2 min 52 s. Although the PPI scan has been acquired over a very short time, the structural detail in the trabecular architecture is preserved in the image. However, an overestimation of structural measures such as bone fraction and trabecular number was observed in the accelerated images. After regularization reconstruction was incorporated in the modified GRAPPA reconstruction and standardization techniques were applied to the histograms of the accelerated images, the percent deviation of the measurement values in the accelerated images from conventional images was seen to lie within acceptable limits of the coefficient of variation (unpublished data). PPI technique can also be used to increase the flexibility in protocol design, for example, the scan time saved by PPI can be utilized to increase slice coverage or to improve the resolution.

IMAGE ANALYSIS OF TRABECULAR BONE

Inspired by thin-section microscopy-based bone histomorphometry techniques, MR image analysis techniques probing several properties of the trabecular structural organization such as interelement spacing, anisotropy, connectivity, texture, and lacunarity have been developed over the last two decades to identify all aspects of structural deterioration in trabecular bone associated with osteoporosis. These developments were motivated by reports in the literature that bone mass could only account for around 60% of the bone strength, while an understanding of the spatial distribution of the mass was needed to account for the rest *(60)*. Due to SNR and acquisition time constraints, the best spatial resolution that can be achieved with the most advanced MR sequences is in the order of the average trabecular thickness of 100–200 μm. However, since the intertrabecular spacing is typically much larger than that and is increased in osteoporosis, it is still possible to derive some structural measures from MR images reproducibly. Image intensity variations caused by inhomogeneities in receiver sensitivity usually need to be removed before extraction of the structural measurements.

Most structural parameters are derived from a processed image that has been binarized into bone and non-bone phases, which is typically done by thresholding. However, the choice of threshold is complicated by partial voluming because voxels typically are partly occupied by bone and partly by bone marrow. Majumdar et al. *(61)* proposed a dual-threshold technique in which the bone reference intensity is chosen by sampling regions of the cortical shell from the image, and the marrow intensity is empirically chosen as the upper value at which the histogram has half of the maximum peak height. Alternatively, image processing techniques can be performed to directly generate a bone volume fraction map (BVF), i.e., an image in which the bone fraction of a voxel is assigned as its intensity. Some of the methods belonging to this category are histogram deconvolution analysis (HDA) and local threshold analysis (LTA). Hwang and Wehrli *(62)* proposed HDA in which Riccian noise is convolved with an initial estimate of an ideal histogram that consists of two peaks corresponding to bone and marrow intensities, and the error between the estimate and the experimentally observed histogram was iteratively subtracted from the estimate. Recently, Vasilic and Wehrli *(63)* proposed LTA in which the marrow intensity threshold in the neighborhood of a voxel is determined by nearest neighbor statistics. A Bayesian classification of bone and marrow voxels by computation of maximum likelihood bone fraction for each voxel was also proposed by Hwang et al. *(64)*. Subvoxel processing can be applied to improve the resolution of the bone volume fraction (BVF) map prior to binarization of the image. Subvoxel processing consists of distributing the BVF in a voxel to its subvoxels based on the BVF outside the voxel but adjacent to the subvoxel *(65)*. Unlike conventional interpolation techniques, it also allows a subvoxel to have a higher BVF than its parent voxel. While most image analysis techniques operate on binarized images, fuzzy-based analyses, spatial autocorrelation analyses, and wavelet transformation operate on grayscale images obviating the need for threshold operations.

The most common structural measures analogous to quantitative histomorphometry derived from MR images include app.Tb.N, app.Tb.Sp, and app.Tb.Th *(66,67)*. These measures are generally analyzed by a two-dimensional plate-like model using the mean intercept length (MIL) method *(61)*. In the MIL method, a set of parallel rays is passed through the ROI over different angles. The number of mean intercepts over all the angles gives a measure of the trabecular number, whereas the mean intercept length gives a measure of the intertrabecular spacing. Since the MR images are not acquired at true microscopic resolutions, Majumdar et al. *(68)* described these measures derived from MR images as "apparent" measurements. However, the authors also noted that the apparent structure reflected by the limited-resolution MR images is highly correlated to the "true" structure. Laib et al. *(69)* applied three-dimensional distance transform (DT3D) techniques to derive structural measures without any model assumptions. In DT3D, Tb.Th is computed as the mean diameter of the maximal spheres that can fill the bone phases in a binarized image. After skeletonization of the binary image, Tb.N is computed as the inverse of the mean distance between structuring elements of the skeleton.

Since binarization of a MRI image is not a trivial task, mainly because of partial volume effects, multiple techniques have been developed which operate directly on the grayscale image. Recognizing the fuzzy nature of the images due to partial voluming, Saha and Wehrli *(70)* applied a fuzzy distance transform (FDT) technique for computing trabecular thickness and observed an improved robustness in the computation against loss of resolution. Recently, Krug et al. *(71)* applied wavelet analysis for computing thickness. In wavelet analysis, signal responses according to varying sizes of the wavelet filter are observed. A maximum response is obtained when the filter size matches the mean thickness of the trabecular elements. Probabilistic approaches have also been assumed for extracting the structural measurements *(64,72)*. Relying on the periodicity of the 3D trabecular architecture, spatial autocorrelation analysis was employed to grayscale MR images of trabecular bone *(72)*. The full width at half maximum of the autocorrelation function (ACF) represented the trabecular thickness. Periodicity along a direction which in this case is equivalent to trabecular spacing was represented by the distance to the first maximum of the ACF computed along that particular direction. Contiguity, a measure of the continuity of trabecular structure in the imaging plane, and Tubularity, a measure of trabecular continuity transverse to the imaging plane, were also derived in the autocorrelation analysis.

Trabecular bone structure and the loss of trabecular bone are both anisotropic. So, measures of structural anisotropy and its relation to loading directions of the bone have received attention in the context of mechanical competence of bone. The preferred orientations of trabecular bone can be measured by principal component analysis of the covariance matrix of measurement data. Majumdar et al. *(73)* computed the three preferred orientations by fitting an ellipsoid to the MIL data. Structural anisotropy has also been derived from ACF analysis *(72)*. Anisotropy is generally computed for trabecular spacing and thickness measures and its relation to biomechanical properties have been widely studied. The connectivity of the three-dimensional trabecular architecture is generally described by the Euler number. Feldkamp et al. *(74)* proposed an algorithm for computing the Euler number from a network topology as the number of branches subtracted from the number of nodes. The better connected the network, the more negative is its corresponding Euler number. Digital topological analyses (DTA) such as the Euler number require a skeletonized input image. The Euler characteristic () is computed from the three Betti numbers as $\chi = \beta_0 - \beta_1 + \beta_2$, where β_0, β_1, and β_2 represent the number of objects, handles, and cavities, respectively, of the network that are invariant to homeomorphic transformation. DTA techniques have been applied to quantify the number of surface and curved edges, junctions, and interiors in the trabecular network *(75)*. The composite parameter surface-to-curve ratio (S/C), which is computed as the ratio of the sum of all surface-type voxels and the sum of all curve-type voxels, has received increased attention as an indicator of plate-to-rod conversion in the trabecular network.

Texture is an image feature frequently used for differentiating between healthy and diseased tissue. Most of the texture features used to classify trabecular bone structure have been based on spatial image statistics. These include variance of the gray-level histogram, variance of the gradient matrix, run-length statistics, and cocurrence matrices *(76)*. Cocurrence matrices are based on the joint probability of two pixels assuming two gray levels. Fractal dimension has been computed to characterize variations in the structural network of trabeculae from CT and radiographic images *(77,78)*. Fractal lacunarity analysis with a trivariate hyperbolic lacunarity function has also been employed on MR images of trabecular bone *(79)*. The authors were able to differentiate between healthy, premenopausal, and osteoporotic population on the basis of a lacunarity parameter. Since trabecular bone is believed to become more porous with disease progression, the physical significance of the lacunarity measure can be expected to be relevant. A scaling index method (SIM) was recently applied by Boehm et al. *(80)* to describe the texture of trabecular bone structure assuming that the micro-structure of trabecular bone also has nonlinear properties. SIM uses local scaling properties to characterize these nonlinear correlations in MR images. It provides a measure for local complexity at each point with respect to its structural surrounding and therefore allowing differentiation between cluster, rot, and plate-like structure existent in cancellous bone. It operates directly on the gray values of the image and thus no binarization step is required. Significant correlations between mechanical strength and SIM were reported.

Recently, Carballido-Gamio et al. *(81)* introduced fuzzy parameters to characterize the trabecular structure. In contrast to conventional clustering where image features are assigned to only one cluster category, fuzzy compactness measurements allow partial membership. Thus in MRI where partial volume effects are present, voxels can be assigned partly to bone and partly to bone marrow tissue. The fuzzy output of this segmentation is defined as a fuzzy bone volume fraction (f-BVF) map. Three-dimensional fuzzy geometrical parameters like fuzzy perimeter and fuzzy compactness and measures of fuzziness like linear index of fuzziness, quadratic index of fuzziness, logarithmic fuzzy entropy, and exponential fuzzy entropy can then be computed from f-BVF maps and statistically compared to standard trabecular bone microstructural indexes. Analyzing fuzzy BVF maps obtained from MR and micro-CT images, a good correlation of measures of fuzziness to trabecular number parameters was observed by the authors.

As already mentioned the image resolution is a limiting factor for the determination of structural parameters. This is especially true for in vivo imaging where the scan time is limited because of patient comfort. Kothari et al. *(82)* looked at the dependence of traditional histomorphometric measures on slice thickness for both femur and vertebral body specimens. High accuracy was found up to an image resolution of 100 μm in-plane and 500 μm slice thickness for trabecular spacing and number. Trabecular thickness increased rapidly with slice thickness. Magland et al. *(83)* investigated the resolution dependence of structural parameters in vivo in ten male subjects with severe hypogonadism, matched by age and race to ten normal men. In this study the trabecular thickness was computed as the fuzzy distance transform *(70,83)*. Images were downsampled to in-plane resolutions ranging from 137 to 800 μm with a full resolution of $137 \times 137 \times 410\ \mu m^3$. Trabecular thickness improved for the treatment group, while no significant change in trabecular thickness was detected in the normal men. Although the absolute thickness increased with voxel size, the statistical significance was maintained at all resolutions and for all parameters. They concluded that a reduced resolution is adequate for this type of longitudinal studies.

MAGNETIC RESONANCE IMAGING-DERIVED TRABECULAR STRUCTURE AND RELATION TO MECHANICAL STRENGTH

In Vitro Studies in Specimens

Several studies relating the measures of trabecular structure obtained using MR imaging to the measures of bone strength in vitro have been conducted. In an early study *(84)* involving cubes from the distal radius, MR images were obtained at a resolution comparable to that achievable in vivo ($156 \times 156 \times 300\ \mu m^3$). X-ray tomographic (XTM) images using a synchrotron source were used to assess trabecular bone structure at resolutions of 18 μm isotropic. It was found that trabecular width, area fraction, number, fractal dimension, and number/volume (a measure of trabecular connectivity) measured from the XTM and MR images increase, while trabecular spacing decreases as the bone mineral density and elastic modulus increase. A bivariate analysis showed that in addition to bone mineral density alone, the Betti number, trabecular number, and spacing contributed to the prediction of the elastic modulus.

In another study of excised radial bone, a probability-based method for extracting bone volume fraction from images at a spatial resolution of $156 \times 156 \times 391\ \mu m^3$, it was shown that the same measures account for 91% of the variation in Young's modulus *(85)*. Pothuaud et al. *(86)* conducted a study where 13 trabecular bone mid-sagittal of lumbar vertebrae sections were imaged by MR imaging at the resolution of $117 \times 117 \times 300\ \mu m^3$. Topological parameters were evaluated in applying the 3D-line skeleton graph analysis (LSGA) technique to the binary MR images. The same images were used to estimate the elastic moduli by finite element analysis (FEA). In addition to the mid-sagittal section, two cylindrical samples were cored from each vertebra along vertical and horizontal directions. Monotonic compression tests were applied to these samples to measure both vertical and horizontal ultimate stresses. In this study, BV/TV was found as a strong predictor of the mechanical properties, accounting for 89–94% of the variability of the elastic moduli and for 69–86% of the variability of the ultimate stresses. Topological parameters and BV/TV were combined following two analytical formulations, based on (1) the normalization of the topological parameters and (2) an exponential fit model. The normalized parameters accounted for 96–98% of the variability of the elastic moduli, and the exponential model accounted for 80–95% of the variability of the ultimate stresses. High-resolution MR images and peripheral quantitative computed tomography images were obtained, in addition to measures of bone mineral density, for a set of nine isolated radii. Each bone was subjected to a mechanical load consistent with a fall from a standing height. In the nine bones tested, measures of bone mineral density explained approximately 50% of the variability with load ($0.52 < r^2 < 0.57$, $p < 0.03$), and indices relating to the size of the marrow spaces explained an additional 25–30% of the variance. This held true whether the indices quantifying the marrow space were derived from the MR images ($r^2 = 0.70$, $p = 0.03$) or the pQCT images ($r^2 = 0.82$, $p = 0.006$) *(87)*.

In a study of a total of 94 specimens, 7 from the calcaneus, 15 from distal femur, 47 from the proximal femur, and 25 from the vertebral bodies imaged at 1.5 T at a resolution of 117 μm in-plane and 300 μm in slice thickness, structure measures contributed in addition to bone mineral density to the prediction of bone mechanical properties *(88)*. In addition, there were significant differences in the BMD, trabecular architectural measures, elastic modulus, and strength at the different skeletal sites. The primary orientation axis for most of the specimens was the anatomic superior–inferior (axial) direction.

High-resolution MR images of specimens have been used for micro-finite element analysis by Borah et al. *(108)* and by Van Rietbergen et al. Van Rietbergen *(36)* has shown correlations between MR-derived measures of elastic modulus and those derived from μCT images and also demonstrated the reproducibility of the measures of 4–9%.

In Vitro Studies in Whole Bones

Intact right arms obtained from 73 formalin-fixed cadavers (age 80 ± 11 years, 43 women, 30 men) were imaged using MR (156 μm in-plane resolution) by Hudelmaier et al. *(89)* and trabecular structural indices (app.BV/TV, app.Tb.N, app.Tb.Sp, app.Tb.Th) and fractal dimension (Frac.Dim) were assessed. BMD was measured with DXA and the radius was tested to failure. In addition to differences between the trabecular bone structure between men and women, they found that app.BV/TV, app.Tb.Th, and fractal dimension provided information independent from BMD in the prediction of radial failure loads in multiple regression models. Link et al. *(90)* used HR-MRI combined with structure analysis to investigate the trabecular structure of the human proximal femur. Thirty-one fresh human proximal femur specimens were examined with HR-MRI (voxel size: $0.195 \times 0.195 \times 0.9$ mm^3 and $0.195 \times 0.195 \times 0.3$ mm^3). In these images, structural parameters analogous to standard bone histomorphometry were obtained in a femoral head, neck, and trochanteric regions of interest. In addition, BMD measurements were obtained using DXA and finally, all specimens were tested biomechanically and maximum compressive strength (MCS) was determined. Correlations between BMD and MCS were significant ($p < 0.01$) with R values up to 0.74. Correlating structure parameters and MCS, R values up to 0.69 ($p < 0.01$) were obtained. Using multivariate regression analysis, combining structure parameters and BMD improved correlations versus MCS substantially (up to $R = 0.93$; $p < 0.01$). The highest correlations, however, were obtained combining BMD and structure measures.

In Vitro Studies Showing Relationship to Vertebral Deformities

In a comprehensive study *(91)*, high-resolution magnetic resonance images of the calcaneus, the distal radius, thin-section computed tomographic images of thoracic and lumbar vertebrae, BMD of the spine using quantitative computed tomography, and of the calcaneus using dual X-ray absorptiometry were obtained from 74 cadavers. Spine radiographs of these cadavers were assessed concerning vertebral deformities. Structure analysis was performed using parameters analogous to standard histomorphometry. The diagnostic performance in differentiating fracture and non-fracture subjects was highest for structure parameters in the spine and slightly lower for these parameters in the distal radius.

Using 49 calcaneus specimens from this set of cadaveric bones (mean age, 79.5 ± 11 years, 26 male, 23 female) MR imaging studies were conducted at 3 and 1.5 T *(92)*. After spatial coregistering of images acquired at 3-T and 1.5-T MR imaging, the signal-to-noise ratios and structural parameters obtained at each magnetic field strength were compared in corresponding sections. Micro-CT was performed on calcaneus cores obtained from the corresponding regions in 40 specimens. Vertebral deformities of the thoracic and lumbar spine were radiographically classified by using the spinal fracture index. Diagnostic performance of the structural parameters in differentiating donors with vertebral fractures from those without was assessed by using receiver operator characteristic (ROC) analysis, including area under the ROC curve ($A(z)$). Correlations between structural parameters at 3-T MR imaging and those at μCT were significantly higher ($p<0.05$) than correlations between structural parameters at 1.5-T MR imaging and those at μCT (trabecular thickness, $r=0.76$ at 3 T versus $r=0.57$ at 1.5 T). Trabecular dimensions were amplified at 3 T because of increasing susceptibility artifacts. Also, higher ROC values were found for structural parameters at 3 T than at 1.5 T, but differences were not significant (trabecular thickness, $A(z)=0.75$ at 3 T versus $A(z)=0.66$ at 1.5 T, $p>0.05$).

IN VIVO MAGNETIC RESONANCE IMAGING-DERIVED TRABECULAR STRUCTURE

High-resolution magnetic resonance images of the distal radius were obtained at 1.5 T in premenopausal normal, postmenopausal normal, and postmenopausal osteoporotic women *(93)*. The image resolution was 156 μm in-plane and 700 μm in the slice direction; the total imaging time was approximately 16 min. Trabecular bone mineral density and cortical bone mineral content (BMC) were measured in the distal radius using peripheral quantitative computed tomography , while in a subset of patients, spinal trabecular BMD was measured using quantitative computed tomography (QCT). Cortical BMC and trabecular BMD at the distal radius, spinal BMD, trabecular bone volume fraction, trabecular thickness, trabecular number, and fractal dimension all decreased with age. Trabecular spacing showed the greatest percentage change and increased with age. In addition, significant differences were evident in spinal BMD, radial trabecular BMD, trabecular bone volume fraction, trabecular spacing, and trabecular number between the postmenopausal non-fracture and the postmenopausal osteoporotic subjects. Trabecular spacing and trabecular number showed moderate correlation with radial trabecular BMD but correlated poorly with radial cortical BMC.

High-resolution magnetic resonance imaging has also been used to visualize the bone micro-structure in the finger phalanges in vivo and to assess the topological three-dimensional connectivity of the trabecular network and the shape of the trabeculae in young and elderly healthy volunteers with a spatial resolution of $152 \times 152 \times 280\ \mu m^3$ *(94)*. The results represent a quantitative description of the rarefication of the trabecular network when moving from the epiphysis to the diaphysis.

Three-dimensional MR imaging was performed on 17 healthy volunteers and 6 osteoporotic patients. Two different MR sequences were used to evaluate the impact on MR acquisition on texture analysis results. Images were analyzed with four automated methods of texture analysis (gray-level histogram, co-occurrence, run-length, and gradient matrices) enabling quantitative analysis of gray-level intensity and distribution within three different regions of interest (ROI). Principal component analysis (CFA) and hierarchical ascending classification (HAC) were used to show that age and osteoporotic effects on trabecular bone structure could be determined *(76)*.

Until recently, in vivo MRI of trabecular micro-architecture was limited to peripheral sites such as distal tibia and femur, radius, and calcaneus because of SNR limitations. However, the main sites of osteoporotic fractures are non-peripheral regions such as the vertebral bodies (spine) and the proximal femur (hip). High-resolution magnetic resonance imaging has only recently been applied to the proximal femur *(95)* by using SNR-efficient bSSFP sequences, high magnetic field strength (3 T), and phased array coils. In these initial studies, a relatively large slice thickness had to be applied in order to obtain sufficient SNR. Most recently, the axial resolution could be considerably increased by applying new parallel imaging techniques while reducing scan time. Furthermore, more sophisticated coil and subject positioning (coil holding belt and foot alignment devices) improved image quality. It is now possible to depict the trabecular micro-architecture in the proximal femur in vivo with a slice thickness of 1 mm and an in-plane resolution of 234 μm obtained in a scan time below 10 min (Fig. 5).

Although significant work has been done using MRI to measure trabecular bone structure, there is little work on the macro-architectural geometry of the cortex which may play an equally important role for bone strength. Recently, Newitt and coworkers *(96)* investigated cortical shell geometry of the distal radius in postmenopausal women using the earlier mentioned 3D FGRE pulse sequence. By means of a semi-automatic technique they segmented the cortex from surrounding soft tissue and the internal marrow/bone region. Then cortical volume and mean cortical thickness were calculated. Two methods were applied in order to determine the thickness. The direct DT3D commonly used to determine trabecular thickness *(97)* and the average of the inner and outer contour length both yielded the cortical thickness. A trend of decreasing thickness with increasing age was found.

RELATIONSHIP WITH POSTMENOPAUSAL STATUS AND FRACTURE

Distance transformation techniques were applied to the three-dimensional image of the distal radius of postmenopausal patients, and structural indices such as app.Tb.N, app.Tb.Th, and app.Tb.Sp were determined without model assumptions *(98)*. A new metric index, the apparent intraindividual distribution of separations (app.Tb.Sp.SD), was introduced. The reproducibility or coefficient of variation was found to be 2.7–4.6% for the mean values of structural indices and 7.7% for app.Tb.Sp.SD. It was found that app.Tb.Sp.SD

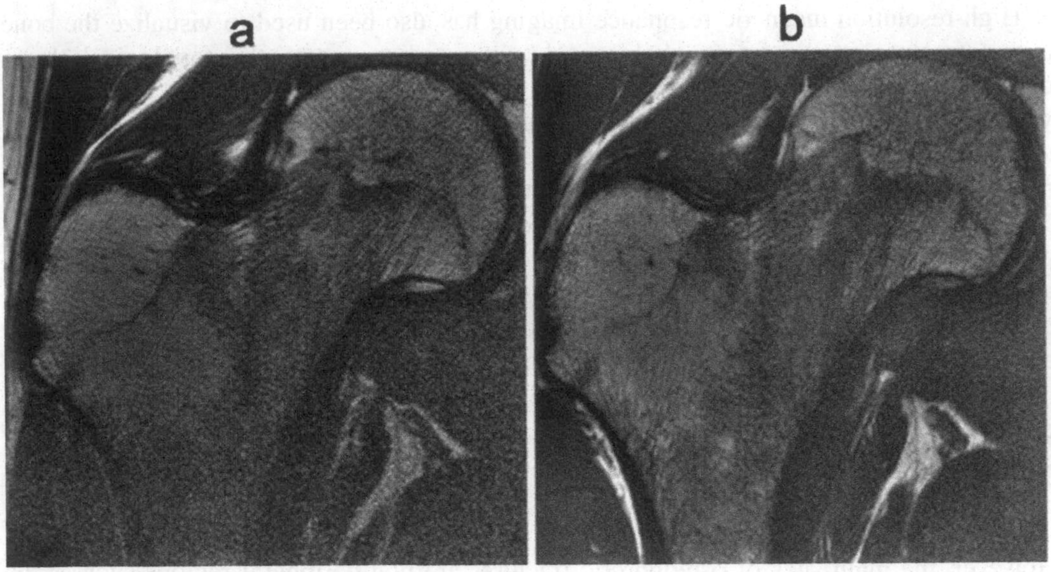

Fig. 5. Coronal images of the proximal femur acquired at (**a**) 1.5 T using a bSSFP sequence TR/TE = 10.3/4.2 ms, total imagine time 6.2 min, and spatial resolution of 234 × 234 × 1000 μm^3 and (**b**) 3 T using a bSSFP sequence TR/TE = 11.3/2.9 ms, total imaging time 9.75 min, and spatial resolution of 234 × 234 × 1000 μm^3.

discriminates fracture subjects from non-fracture patients as well as DXA measurements of the radius and the spine, but not as well as DXA of the hip. Using receiver operating characteristic analysis, the area under the curve (AUC) values were 0.67 for app.Tb.Sp.SD, 0.72 for DXA radius, 0.67 for DXA spine, and 0.81 for DXA of the hip. A combination of MR indices reached an AUC of 0.75. Age-adjusted odds ratio ranged from 1.85 to 2.03 for app.Tb.N, app.Tb.Sp, and app.Tb.Sp.SD ($p<0.003$).

Magnetic resonance (MR)-derived measures of trabecular bone architecture in the distal radius *(99)* and calcaneus *(100)* were obtained in 20 subjects with hip fractures and 19 age-matched postmenopausal controls, in addition to bone mineral density measures at the hip (DXA) and the distal radius (peripheral quantitative computed tomography, pQCT). Measures of app.Tb.Sp and app.Tb.N in the distal radius showed significant ($p<0.05$) differences between the two groups, as did hip BMD measures. However, radial trabecular BMD measures showed only a marginal difference ($p = 0.05$). In the calcaneus, significant differences between both patient groups were obtained using morphological parameters and fractal analysis. Odds ratios for the calcaneus parameters apparent (app.) bone volume/total volume and app.trabecular separation were higher than for hip BMD. Receiver operator characteristic values of calcaneus structure and hip BMD were comparable. The area under the curve (AUC) for total hip BMD was 0.73 and for radial trabecular BMD was 0.69. The AUC for combined BMD (hip) and structure measures was higher (0.87) when radius and calcaneus structure were included.

IN VIVO μFE

In addition, in vivo images have also been combined with micro-finite element analysis in a limited set of subjects. Newitt et al. *(101)* studied subjects in two groups: postmenopausal women with normal bone mineral density (BMD) ($n = 22$, mean age 58 ± 7 years) and postmenopausal women with spine or femur BMD –1 to –2.5 SD below young normal ($n = 37$, mean age 62 ± 11 years). From these images, the directional Young's moduli (E1, E2, and E3), shear moduli (G12, G23, and G13), and anisotropy ratios such as E1/E3 were determined. BMD at the distal radius, lumbar spine, and hip were assessed using DXA. All three directional measures of elastic and shear moduli were lower in the osteopenic group compared with the normal group. Anisotropy of trabecular bone microarchitecture, as measured by the ratios of the MIL values (MIL1/MIL3, etc.), and the anisotropy in elastic modulus (E1/E3, etc.) were greater in the osteopenic group.

THERAPEUTIC RESPONSE USING TRABECULAR BONE STRUCTURE MEASURES IN POSTMENOPAUSAL OSTEOPOROSIS

Topological 3D-LSGA-based measurements *(102)* were evaluated in a set of seven volunteers, and coefficients of variations ranged from 3.5 to 6%. High-resolution MR images of the radius in 30 postmenopausal women from a placebo controlled drug study (Idoxifene), divided into placebo ($n = 9$) and treated ($n = 21$) groups, were obtained at baseline (BL) and after 1 year of treatment (follow-up, FU). In addition, DXA measures of BMD were obtained in the distal radius. Standard morphological measurements based on the MIL technique as well as 3D-LSGA-based measurements were applied to the three-dimensional MR images. Significant changes from BL to FU were detected in the treated group using the topological 3D-LSGA-based measurements, morphological measures of volume of connected trabeculae, and app Tb.N from MIL analysis. In addition, mechanical parameters of a trabecular volume of interest in the calcaneus were calculated using micro-finite element analysis *(103)*. Although there were no significant differences between the mean changes in the treated groups and the placebo group, there were significant changes from baseline within groups after 1 year of treatment. Significant changes, however, were found only for mechanical parameters and only in the treated groups. This was the first demonstration that longitudinal changes in bone mechanical properties due to trabecular micro-architectural changes may be quantified in long-term clinical studies. However, the study duration was short and the number of patients small; thus, these results cannot be interpreted with regard to a true therapeutic response.

Ninety-one postmenopausal osteoporotic women were followed for 2 years ($n = 46$ for nasal spray calcitonin, $n = 45$ for placebo); all women received 500 mg calcium daily *(104)*. MRI measurements of trabecular structure were obtained at distal radius, and calcaneus in addition to DXA-BMD at spine/hip/wrist/os calcis (obtained yearly). MRI assessment of trabecular micro-architecture at individual regions of the distal radius revealed preservation (no significant loss) in the treated group compared with significant deterioration in the placebo control group, as reflected in app.BV/TV ($p < 0.03$), app.Tb.N ($p < 0.01$), and app.Tb.Sp ($p < 0.01$). There was a significant increase in app.Tb.N in the treated group in the calcaneus.

TRABECULAR BONE STRUCTURE IN MEN

Sagittal MR images of the calcaneus were obtained in 50 men (26 patients with osteoporosis and 24 age-matched healthy control subjects) *(105)*. Twenty structural measurements were obtained from these images. Thirteen of 20 structural parameters, especially connectivity parameters, showed significant differences between control subjects and patients (p <.05). Differences between the two groups were more significant (p <.001) for apparent bone marrow skeleton length, apparent node count, apparent node-to-node strut count, and apparent terminus-to-terminus strut count. Odds ratios for 11 of 13 structural parameters but not for calcaneus density were significant ($p < 0.05$). After adjustment for calcaneus density, these parameters were still significant predictors of osteoporotic fracture.

Trabecular bone structure of the tibia was studied in ten men with severe, untreated hypogonadism and age and race matched eugonadal men. Two composite topological indices were determined: the ratio of surface voxels (representing plates) to curve voxels (representing rods), which is higher when architecture is more intact; and the erosion index, a ratio of parameters expected to increase upon architectural deterioration to those expected to decrease, which is higher when deterioration is greater. The surface/curve ratio was 36% lower ($p = 0.004$), and the erosion index was 36% higher ($p = 0.003$) in the hypogonadal men than in the eugonadal men *(106)*. In contrast, bone mineral density of the spine and hip were not significantly different between the two groups. The hypogonadal

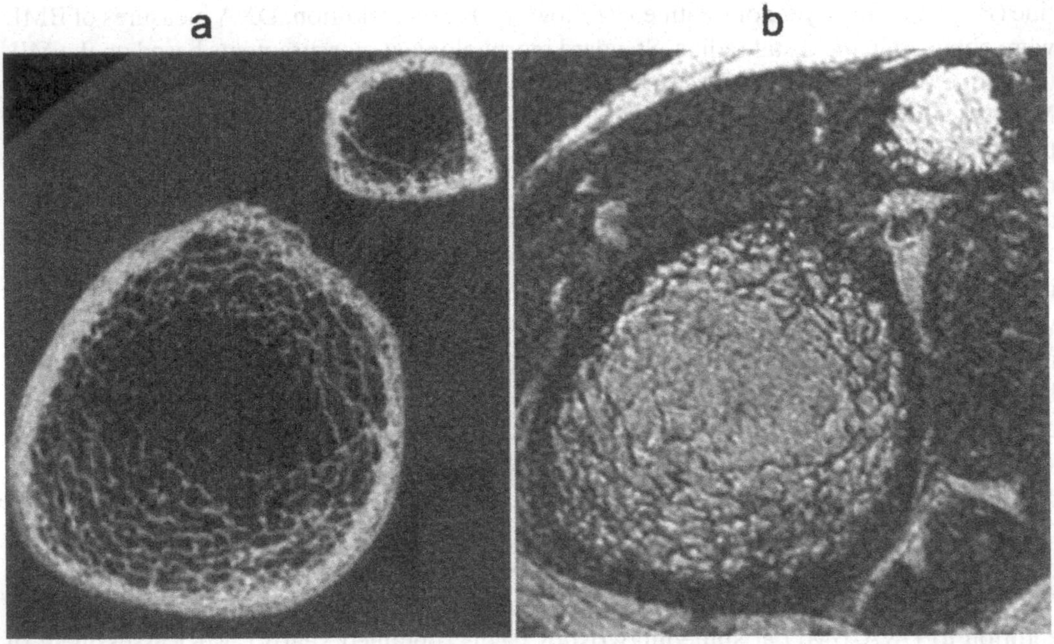

Fig. 6. Images of the distal tibia acquired with (**a**) extremity CT at a pixel resolution of 80 μm isotropic depicts cortical shell and trabeculae in *white* (**b**) and obtained using MR at 3 T at a resolution of a $195 \times 195 \times 500\ \mu m^3$ depicting the cortical shell and trabeculae as signal voids and marrow is bright contrary to (**a**). Visually the differences in trabecular structure, cortical porosity in both images show similar characteristics.

men were followed after 6, 12, and 24 months of testosterone treatment. Serum testosterone concentrations increased to mid-normal after 3 months of treatment and remained normal thereafter. After 24 months of testosterone treatment, BMD of the spine increased 7.4% ($p<0.001$) and of the total hip increased 3.8% ($p=0.008$). Architectural parameters assessed by micro-MRI also changed: the surface-to-curve ratio increased 11% ($p=0.004$) and the topological erosion index decreased 7.5% ($p=0.004$) *(107)*.

SUMMARY

Imaging trabecular and cortical micro-architecture, characterizing the features of trabecular and cortical bone has been an area of fertile and ongoing research. Beyond relating micro-architecture to the biomechanical properties of bone in specimens, advances have been made to extend these measures in vivo in human subjects. In this context, relationship between age, fracture status, and even posttherapeutic response has been studied. New advances in peripheral CT and MR are ongoing and evolving at a rapid pace. Both imaging technologies provide similar data, in fact Fig. 6 shows a peripheral CT and MR image through the tibia and features of similarity may be seen qualitatively. These modalities are being developed, and with the establishment of robust analysis methodologies and normative databases, both have the potential for further clinical utilization in the coming years.

REFERENCES

1. Graeff W, Engelke K. Microradiography and microtomography. In: Ebashi E, Koch M, Rubenstein E, eds. Handbook on synchrotron radiation. Amsterdam: North-Holland, 1991:361–405.
2. Rüegsegger P, Koller B, Müller R. A microtomographic system for the nondestructive evaluation of bone architecture. Calcif Tissue Int 1996;58(1):24–29.
3. Muller R, Hildebrand T, Rüegsegger P. Non-invasive bone biopsy: a new method to analyze and display three-dimensional structure of trabecular bone. Phys Med Biol 1994;39:145–164.
4. Parfitt AM, Mathews CH, Villanueva AR, Kleerekoper M, Frame B, Rao DS. Relationships between surface, volume, and thickness of iliac trabecular bone in aging and in osteoporosis. Implications for the microanatomic and cellular mechanisms of bone loss. J Clin Invest 1983;72(4):1396–1409.
5. Parfitt A. The stereologic basis of bone histomorphometry. Theory of quantitative microscopy and reconstruction of the third dimension. In: Recker R, ed. Bone histomorphometry: techniques and interpretations. Boca Raton: CRC Press, 1983:53–87.
6. Odgaard A, Gundersen HJ. Quantification of connectivity in cancellous bone, with special emphasis on 3-D reconstructions. Bone 1993;14(2):173–182.
7. Goulet RW, Goldstein SA, Ciarelli MJ, Kuhn JL, Brown MB, Feldkamp LA. The relationship between the structural and orthogonal compressive properties of trabecular bone. J Biomech 1994;27(4):375–389.
8. Uchiyama T, Tanizawa T, Muramatsu H, Endo N, Takahashi HE, Hara T. Three-dimensional microstructural analysis of human trabecular bone in relation to its mechanical properties. Bone 1999;25(4): 487–491.
9. Engelke K, Karolczak M, Schaller S, Felsenberg D, Kalender W. A cone beam micro-computed tomography (μCT) system for imaging of 3D trabecular bone structure. In: 13th International bone Densitometry Workshop 1998; Wisconsin, USA; 1998.
10. Jiang Y, Zhao J, Liao EY, Dai RC, Wu XP, Genant HK. Application of micro-CT assessment of 3-D bone microstructure in preclinical and clinical studies. J Bone Miner Metab 2005;23(Suppl):122–131.
11. Sohaskey M, Jiang Y, Zhao J, et al. Insertional mutagenesis of osteopotentia, a novel transmembrane protein essential for skeletal integrity. J Bone Miner Res 2004;19(Suppl 1):S21.
12. Sorocéanu M, Miao D, Jiang Y, et al. Pthrp haploinsufficiency impairs bone formation but potentiates the bone anabolic effects of PTH (1–34). J Bone Miner Res 2004;19(Suppl 1):S97

13. Takeshita S, Namba N, Zhao JJ, et al. SHIP-deficient mice are severely osteoporotic due to increased numbers of hyper-resorptive osteoclasts. Nat Med 2002;8(9):943–949.
14. Bergo MO, Gavino B, Ross J, et al. Zmpste24 deficiency in mice causes spontaneous bone fractures, muscle weakness, and a prelamin A processing defect. Proc Natl Acad Sci USA 2002;99(20): 13049–13054.
15. Jiang Y, Zhao J, Mangadu R, Medicherla S, Protter A, Genant H. Assessment of 3D cortical and trabecular bone microstructure and erosion on micro CT images of a murine model of arthritis. J Bone Miner Res 2004;19(Suppl 1):S474.
16. Prevrhal S. Beam hardening correction and quantitative micro-CT. Proceedings of SPIE 2004;5535: 152–161.
17. Prevrhal S. Simulation of trabecular mineralization measurements in micro-CT. Proc SPIE 2006;6318:631808-1-10.
18. David V, Laroche N, Boudignon B, et al. Noninvasive in vivo monitoring of bone architecture alterations in hindlimb-unloaded female rats using novel three-dimensional microcomputed tomography. J Bone Miner Res 2003;18(9):1622–1631.
19. Gasser JA, Ingold P, Grosios K, Laib A, Hammerle S, Koller B. Noninvasive monitoring of changes in structural cancellous bone parameters with a novel prototype micro-CT. J Bone Miner Metab 2005;23(Suppl):90–96.
20. Boyd SK, Davison P, Muller R, Gasser JA. Monitoring individual morphological changes over time in ovariectomized rats by in vivo micro-computed tomography. Bone 2006;39(4):854–862.
21. Chevalier F, Laval-Jeantet AM, Bergot C. CT image analysis of the vertebral trabecular network in vivo. Calcif Tissue Int 1992;51(1):8–13.
22. Ito M, Ohki M, Hayashi K, Yamada M, Uetani M, Nakamura T. Trabecular texture analysis of CT images in the relationship with spinal fracture. Radiology 1995;194:55–59.
23. Gordon C, Lang T, Augat P, Genant H. Image-based assessment of spinal trabecular bone structure from high-resolution CT images. Osteoporos Int 1998;8:317–325.
24. Timm W, Graeff C, Vilar J, et al. In vivo assessment of trabecular bone structure in human vertebrae using high resolution computed tomography. J Bone Miner Res 2005;20(Suppl 1):S336.
25. Graeff C, Timm W, Farrerons J, et al. Structural analysis of vertebral trabecular bone structure allows to assess the effect of teriparatide treatment independently of BMD. J Bone Miner Res 2005;20(Suppl 1):S411.
26. Ito M, Ikeda K, Nishiguchi M, et al. Multi-detector row CT imaging of vertebral microstructure for evaluation of fracture risk. J Bone Miner Res 2005;20(10):1828–1836.
27. Durand EP, Rüegsegger P. High-contrast resolution of CT images for bone structure analysis. Med Phys 1992;3(19):569–573.
28. Khosla S, Riggs BL, Atkinson EJ, et al. Effects of sex and age on bone microstructure at the ultradistal radius: a population-based noninvasive in vivo assessment. J Bone Miner Res 2006;21(1): 124–131.
29. Boutroy S, Bouxsein ML, Munoz F, Delmas PD. In vivo assessment of trabecular bone microarchitecture by high-resolution peripheral quantitative computed tomography. J Clin Endocrinol Metab 2005;90(12):6508–6515.
30. Khosla S, Melton LJ, III, Achenbach SJ, Oberg AL, Riggs BL. Hormonal and biochemical determinants of trabecular microstructure at the ultradistal radius in women and men. J Clin Endocrinol Metab 2006;91(3):885–891.
31. Zouch M, Gerbay B, Thomas T, Vico L, Alexandre C. Patients with hip fracture exhibit bone microarchitectural deterioration compared to patients with Colle's fracture as assessed with in vivo high resolution 3D micro-pQCT. European Advanced Detection of Bone Quality (ADOQ) Study. J Bone Miner Res 2005;20(Suppl 1):S45.
32. Majumdar S. Quantitative study of the susceptibility difference between trabecular bone and bone marrow: computer simulations. Magn Reson Med 1991;22(1):101–110.
33. Weisskoff RM, Zuo CS, Boxerman JL, Rosen BR. Microscopic susceptibility variation and transverse relaxation: theory and experiment. Magn Reson Med 1994;31(6):601–610.
34. Ford JC, Wehrli FW, Chung HW. Magnetic field distribution in models of trabecular bone. Magn Reson Med 1993;30(3):373–379.

35. Majumdar S, Link TM, Augat P, et al. Trabecular bone architecture in the distal radius using magnetic resonance imaging in subjects with fractures of the proximal femur. Magnetic Resonance Science Center and Osteoporosis and Arthritis Research Group. Osteoporos Int 1999;10(3):231–239.
36. Newitt DC, van Rietbergen B, Majumdar S. Processing and analysis of in vivo high-resolution MR images of trabecular bone for longitudinal studies: reproducibility of structural measures and micro-finite element analysis derived mechanical properties. Osteoporos Int 2002;13(4):278–287.
37. Ma J, Wehrli FW, Song HK. Fast 3D large-angle spin-echo imaging 3D FLASE. Magn Reson Med 1996;35(6):903–910.
38. Gomberg BR, Wehrli FW, Vasilic B, et al. Reproducibility and error sources of micro-MRI-based trabecular bone structural parameters of the distal radius and tibia. Bone 2004;35(1):266–276.
39. Wehrli FW, Hwang SN, Song HK, Gomberg BR. Visualization and analysis of trabecular bone architecture in the limited spatial resolution regime of in vivo micro-MRI. Adv Exp Med Biol 2001;496:153–164.
40. Krug R, Han ET, Banerjee S, Majumdar S. Fully balanced spin-echo SSFP for in-vivo measurements of trabecular bone at 3 Tesla, In: ISMRM 2006; Seattle, 2006.
41. Hennig J, Nauerth A, Friedburg H. RARE imaging: a fast imaging method for clinical MR. Magn Reson Med 1986;3(6):823–833.
42. Constable RT, Gore JC. The loss of small objects in variable TE imaging: implications for FSE, RARE, and EPI. Magn Reson Med 1992;28(1):9–24.
43. Jara H, Wehrli FW, Chung H, Ford JC. High-resolution variable flip angle 3D MR imaging of trabecular microstructure in vivo. Magn Reson Med 1993;29(4):528–539.
44. Bogdan AR, Joseph PM. RASEE: a rapid spin-echo pulse sequence. Magn Reson Imaging 1990;8(1): 13–19.
45. DiIorio G, Brown JJ, Borrello JA, Perman WH, Shu HH. Large angle spin-echo imaging. Magn Reson Imaging 1995;13(1):39–44.
46. Krug R, Han ET, Banerjee S, Majumdar S. Fully balanced steady-state 3D-spin-echo (bSSSE) imaging at 3 Tesla. Magn Reson Med 2006;56(5):1033–1040.
47. Banerjee S, Han ET, Krug R, Newitt DC, Majumdar S. Application of refocused steady-state free-precession methods at 1.5 and 3 T to in vivo high-resolution MRI of trabecular bone: simulations and experiments. J Magn Reson Imaging 2005;21(6):818–825.
48. Bangerter NK, Hargreaves BA, Vasanawala SS, Pauly JM, Gold GE, Nishimura DG. Analysis of multiple-acquisition SSFP. Magn Reson Med 2004;51(5):1038–1047.
49. Phan CM, Matsuura M, Bauer JS, et al. Trabecular bone structure of the calcaneus: comparison of MR imaging at 3.0 and 1.5 T with micro-CT as the standard of reference. Radiology 2006;239(2):488–496.
50. Roemer PB, Edelstein WA, Hayes CE, Souza SP, Mueller OM. The NMR phased array. Magn Reson Med 1990;16(2):192–225.
51. Morze C, Banerjee, S., Tropp, J., Karponidis, K., Carvajal, L., Vigneron, DB., Majumdar, S. A non-overlapping phased array coil for parallel imaging of the hip at 3.0 T. In: ISMRM; 6–12 May 2006; Seattle: Intl Soc Mag Reson Med; 2006.
52. Kwok WE, Zhong J, You Z, Seo G, Totterman SM. A four-element phased array coil for high resolution and parallel MR imaging of the knee. Magn Reson Imaging 2003;21(9):961–967.
53. Pruessmann KP, Weiger M, Scheidegger MB, Boesiger P. SENSE: sensitivity encoding for fast MRI. Magn Reson Med 1999;42(5):952–962.
54. Sodickson DK, Griswold MA, Jakob PM. SMASH imaging. Magn Reson Imaging Clin N Am 1999;7(2):237–254, vii–viii.
55. Sodickson DK, McKenzie CA. A generalized approach to parallel magnetic resonance imaging. Med Phys 2001;28(8):1629–1643.
56. Jakob PM, Griswold MA, Edelman RR, Sodickson DK. AUTO-SMASH: a self-calibrating technique for SMASH imaging. Simultaneous acquisition of spatial harmonics. MAGMA 1998;7(1):42–54.
57. Heidemann RM, Griswold MA, Haase A, Jakob PM. VD-AUTO-SMASH imaging. Magn Reson Med 2001;45(6):1066–1074.
58. Griswold MA, Jakob PM, Heidemann RM, et al. Generalized autocalibrating partially parallel acquisitions (GRAPPA). Magn Reson Med 2002;47(6):1202–1210.
59. Banerjee S, Choudhury S, Han ET, et al. Autocalibrating parallel imaging of in vivo trabecular bone microarchitecture at 3 Tesla. Magn Reson Med 2006;56(5):1075–1084.

60. Siffert RS, Luo GM, Cowin SC, Kaufman JJ. Dynamic relationships of trabecular bone density, architecture, and strength in a computational model of osteopenia. Bone 1996;18(2):197–206.
61. Majumdar S, Newitt D, Jergas M, et al. Evaluation of technical factors affecting the quantification of trabecular bone structure using magnetic resonance imaging. Bone 1995;17(4):417–430.
62. Hwang SN, Wehrli FW. Estimating voxel volume fractions of trabecular bone on the basis of magnetic resonance images acquired in vivo. Int J Imag Syst Technol 1999;10:186–198.
63. Vasilic B, Wehrli FW. A novel local thresholding algorithm for trabecular bone volume fraction mapping in the limited spatial resolution regime of in vivo MRI. IEEE Trans Med Imaging 2005;24(12):15741585.
64. Hwang SN, Wehrli FW, Williams JL. Probability-based structural parameters from three-dimensional nuclear magnetic resonance images as predictors of trabecular bone strength. Med Phys 1997;24(8):1255–1261.
65. Hwang SN, Wehrli FW. Subvoxel processing: a method for reducing partial volume blurring with application to in vivo MR images of trabecular bone. Magn Reson Med 2002;47(5):948–957.
66. Parfitt AM. Assessment of trabecular bone status. Henry Ford Hosp Med J 1983;31(4):196–198.
67. Parfitt AM, Mathews CH, Villanueva AR, Kleerekoper M, Frame B, Rao DS. Relationships between surface, volume, and thickness of iliac trabecular bone in aging and in osteoporosis. Implications for the microanatomic and cellular mechanisms of bone loss. J Clin Invest 1983;72(4):1396–1409.
68. Majumdar S, Newitt D, Mathur A, et al. Magnetic resonance imaging of trabecular bone structure in the distal radius: relationship with X-ray tomographic microscopy and biomechanics. Osteoporos Int 1996;6(5):376–385.
69. Laib A, Newitt DC, Lu Y, Majumdar S. New model-independent measures of trabecular bone structure applied to in vivo high-resolution MR images. Osteoporos Int 2002;13(2):130–136.
70. Saha PK, Wehrli FW. Measurement of trabecular bone thickness in the limited resolution regime of in vivo MRI by fuzzy distance transform. IEEE Trans Med Imaging 2004;23(1):53–62.
71. Krug R, Carballido-Gamio J, Burghardt AJ, et al. Wavelet based characterization of vertebral trabecular bone structure from specimens at 3 Tesla compared to MicroCT In: IEEE Engineering in Medicine and Biology, 2005; Sanghai.
72. Wald M, Vasilic B, Saha PK, Wehrli FW. Study of trabecular bone microstructure using spatial autocorrelation analysis. In: Amini AAMA, ed. SPIE Conference in Medical Imaging; 2005; San Diego. p. 291–302.
73. Majumdar S, Kothari M, Augat P, et al. High-resolution magnetic resonance imaging: three-dimensional trabecular bone architecture and biomechanical properties. Bone 1998;22(5):445–454.
74. Feldkamp LA, Goldstein SA, Parfitt AM, Jesion G, Kleerekoper M. The direct examination of three-dimensional bone architecture in vitro by computed tomography. J Bone Miner Res 1989;4(1):3–11.
75. Gomberg BR, Saha PK, Song HK, Hwang SN, Wehrli FW. Topological analysis of trabecular bone MR images. IEEE Trans Med Imaging 2000;19(3):166–174.
76. Herlidou S, Grebe R, Grados F, Leuyer N, Fardellone P, Meyer ME. Influence of age and osteoporosis on calcaneus trabecular bone structure: a preliminary in vivo MRI study by quantitative texture analysis. Magn Reson Imaging 2004;22(2):237–243.
77. Majumdar S, Lin J, Link T, et al. Fractal analysis of radiographs: assessment of trabecular bone structure and prediction of elastic modulus and strength. Med Phys 1999;26(7):1330–1340.
78. Majumdar S, Weinstein RS, Prasad RR. Application of fractal geometry techniques to the study of trabecular bone. Med Phys 1993;20(6):1611–1619.
79. Zaia A, Eleonori R, Maponi P, Rossi R, Murri R. MR imaging and osteoporosis: fractal lacunarity analysis of trabecular bone. IEEE Trans Inf Technol Biomed 2006;10(3):484–489.
80. Boehm HF, Raeth C, Monetti RA, et al. Local 3D scaling properties for the analysis of trabecular bone extracted from high-resolution magnetic resonance imaging of human trabecular bone: comparison with bone mineral density in the prediction of biomechanical strength in vitro. Invest Radiol 2003;38(5): 269–280.
81. Carballido-Gamio J, Phan C, Link TM, Majumdar S. Characterization of trabecular bone structure from high-resolution magnetic resonance images using fuzzy logic. Magn Reson Imaging 2006;24(8): 1023–1029.
82. Kothari M, Keaveny TM, Lin JC, Newitt DC, Genant HK, Majumdar S. Impact of spatial resolution on the prediction of trabecular architecture parameters. Bone 1998;22(5):437–443.

83. Benito M, Vasilic B, Wehrli FW, Bunker B, Wald M, Gomberg B, Wright AC, Zemel B, Cucchiara A, Snyder PJ. Effect of testosterone replacement on bone architecture in hypogonadal men. J Bone and Miner Res 2005;20:1785.
84. Majumdar S, Newitt D, Mathur A, et al. Magnetic resonance imaging of trabecular bone structure in the distal radius: relationship with X-ray tomographic microscopy and biomechanics. Osteoporos Int 1996;6(5):376–385.
85. Hwang SN, Wehrli FW, Williams JL. Probability-based structural parameters from three-dimensional nuclear magnetic resonance images as predictors of trabecular bone strength. Med Phys 1997;24(8):1255–1261.
86. Pothuaud L, Laib A, Levitz P, Benhamou CL, Majumdar S. Three-dimensional-line skeleton graph analysis of high-resolution magnetic resonance images: a validation study from 34-microm-resolution microcomputed tomography. J Bone Miner Res 2002;17(10):1883–1895.
87. Gordon CL, Webber CE, Nicholson PS. Relation between image-based assessment of distal radius trabecular structure and compressive strength. Can Assoc Radiol J 1998;49(6):390–397.
88. Majumdar S, Kothari M, Augat P, et al. High-resolution magnetic resonance imaging: three-dimensional trabecular bone architecture and biomechanical properties. Bone 1998;22:445–454.
89. Hudelmaier M, Kollstedt A, Lochmuller EM, Kuhn V, Eckstein F, Link TM. Gender differences in trabecular bone architecture of the distal radius assessed with magnetic resonance imaging and implications for mechanical competence. Osteoporos Int 2005;16(9):1124–1133.
90. Link TM, Vieth V, Langenberg R, et al. Structure analysis of high resolution magnetic resonance imaging of the proximal femur: in vitro correlation with biomechanical strength and BMD. Calcif Tissue Int 2003;72(2):156–165.
91. Link TM, Bauer J, Kollstedt A, et al. Trabecular bone structure of the distal radius, the calcaneus, and the spine: which site predicts fracture status of the spine best? Invest Radiol 2004;39(8):487–497.
92. Phan C, Matsuura M, Bauer J, et al. Trabecular bone structure of the calcaneus: comparison of high resolution MR imaging at 1.5 and 3 Tesla using microCT as a standard of reference. Radiology 2005; Accepted.
93. Majumdar S, Genant H, Grampp S, et al. Correlation of trabecular bone structure with age, bone mineral density and osteoporotic status: in vivo studies in the distal radius using high resolution magnetic resonance imaging. J Bone Miner Res 1997;12:111–118.
94. Stampa B, Kuhn B, Liess C, Heller M, Gluer C. Characterization of the integrity of three-dimensional trabecular bone microstructure by connectivity and shape analysis using high-resolution magnetic resonance imaging in vivo. Top Magn Reson Imaging 2002;13(5):357–363.
95. Krug R, Banerjee S, Han ET, Newitt DC, Link TM, Majumdar S. Feasibility of in vivo structural analysis of high-resolution magnetic resonance images of the proximal femur. Osteoporos Int 2005; 16: 1307–1314.
96. Hyun B, Newitt DC, Majumdar S. Assessment of cortical bone structure using high-resolution magnetic resonance imaging, ISMRM Conference Abstract #1985, Miami, USA 2005.
97. Hildebrand T, Reugsegger P. A new method for the model independent assessment of thickness in three dimensional images. J Microsc 1997;185:67–75.
98. Laib A, Newitt DC, Lu Y, Majumdar S. New model-independent measures of trabecular bone structure applied to in vivo high-resolution MR images. Osteoporos Int 2002;13(2):130–136.
99. Majumdar S, Link T, Augat P, et al. Trabecular bone architecture in the distal radius using MR imaging in subjects with fractures of the proximal femur. Osteoporosis Int 1999;10:231–239.
100. Link TM, Majumdar S, Augat P, et al. In vivo high resolution MRI of the calcaneus: differences in trabecular structure in osteoporosis patients. J Bone Miner Res 1998;13(7):1175–1182.
101. Newitt DC, Majumdar S, van Rietbergen B, et al. In vivo assessment of architecture and micro-finite element analysis derived indices of mechanical properties of trabecular bone in the radius. Osteoporos Int 2002;13(1):6–17.
102. Pothuaud L, Newitt DC, Lu Y, MacDonald B, Majumdar S. In vivo application of 3D-line skeleton graph analysis (LSGA) technique with high-resolution magnetic resonance imaging of trabecular bone structure. Osteoporos Int 2004;15(5):411–419.
103. van Rietbergen B, Majumdar S, Newitt D, MacDonald B. High-resolution MRI and micro-FE for the evaluation of changes in bone mechanical properties during longitudinal clinical trials: application to

calcaneal bone in postmenopausal women after one year of idoxifene treatment. Clin Biomech (Bristol, Avon) 2002;17(3):81–88.

104. Chesnut CH, III, Majumdar S, Newitt DC, et al. Effects of salmon calcitonin on trabecular microarchitecture as determined by magnetic resonance imaging: results from the QUEST study. J Bone Miner Res 2005;20(9):1548–1561.
105. Boutry N, Cortet B, Dubois P, Marchandise X, Cotten A. Trabecular bone structure of the calcaneus: preliminary in vivo MR imaging assessment in men with osteoporosis. Radiology 2003;227(3): 708–717.
106. Benito M, Gomberg B, Wehrli FW, et al. Deterioration of trabecular architecture in hypogonadal men. J Clin Endocrinol Metab 2003;88(4):1497–1502.
107. Benito M, Vasilic B, Wehrli FW, et al. Effect of testosterone replacement on trabecular architecture in hypogonadal men. J Bone Miner Res 2005;20(10):1785–1791.
108. Borah B, Gross GJ, Dufresne TE, Smith TS, Cockman MD, Chmielewski PA, Lundy MW, Hartke JR, Sod EW. Three-dimensional microimaging (MRmicroI and microCT), finite element modeling, and rapid prototyping provide unique insights into bone architecture in osteoporosis. Anat Rec. 2001;265(2): 101–110.

4 The Clinical Role of Bone Density Scans in the Diagnosis and Treatment of Osteoporosis

Glen M. Blake

CONTENTS

SUMMARY

Dual energy X-ray absorptiometry (DXA) measurements of hip and spine bone mineral density (BMD) have an important role in the evaluation of individuals at risk of osteoporosis and in helping clinicians advise patients about the appropriate use of antifracture treatment. Compared with alternative bone densitometry techniques, hip and spine DXA examinations have a number of advantages that include a consensus that BMD results can be interpreted using the World Health Organisation (WHO) *T*-score definition of osteoporosis, a proven ability to predict fracture risk, proven effectiveness at targeting antifracture therapies and the ability to monitor response to treatment. This chapter discusses the evidence for these and other clinical aspects of DXA scanning, including its role in the new WHO algorithm for treating patients on the basis of their individual fracture risk.

Key Words: Bone density scans, osteoporosis, activities of daily living, fragility fractures, bone mineral density (BMD), fracture intervention trial, selective oestrogen receptor modulators, human parathyroid hormone, strontium ranelate

From: *Contemporary Endocrinology: Osteoporosis: Pathophysiology and Clinical Management*
Edited by: R. A. Adler, DOI 10.1007/978-1-59745-459-9_4,

Osteoporosis is widely recognised as an important public health problem because of the significant morbidity, mortality, and costs associated with its complications, namely fractures of the hip, spine, forearm, and other skeletal sites *(1)*. It is estimated that every year 1.5 million people in the United States experience an osteoporosis-related fracture, including 300,000 cases of hip fracture *(2)*. One in every two white women will suffer an osteoporosis-related fracture in her lifetime and one in six will have a hip fracture *(3)*. There is particular concern about hip fractures because these have the greatest effect on an individual's quality of life and incur the greatest cost for health services *(4)*. However, other fractures are also associated with significant morbidity and costs *(5)* and both hip and vertebral fractures are associated with an increased risk of death *(6,7)* and increased dependence on nursing homes and private and public care services for the basic activities of daily living. Because of the aging population and the previous lack of attention to bone health, the annual number of hip fractures in the United States is set to double by the year 2020 *(2)*.

Although for many years there was awareness of the morbidity and costs associated with fragility fractures, real progress only came with the ability to diagnose osteoporosis before any fractures occur, and with the development of preventive treatments. Bone density scanning played an important role in both these developments. Until the mid-1980 s measurements of bone mineral density (BMD) were used mainly in research, and it was only with the introduction of dual-energy X-ray absorptiometry (DXA) scanners in 1987 that they entered routine clinical practice *(8)*. Further significant developments included the first study showing that bisphosphonate treatment can prevent bone loss *(9)*, the publication of the World Health Organisation (WHO) report defining osteoporosis in terms of a BMD *T*-score at the spine, hip, or forearm of –2.5 or less *(10)* (Table 1), and the Fracture Intervention Trial confirming that bisphosphonate treatment reduced fracture risk *(11)*. Since then a number of international trials have demonstrated the effectiveness of bisphosphonates (BPs) *(12–16)*, selective oestrogen receptor modulators (SERMs) *(17)*, recombinant human parathyroid hormone (PTH) *(18)*, and strontium ranelate *(19–21)* in the prevention of fragility fractures.

Table 1
The WHO Definitions of Osteoporosis and Osteopenia *(10)*

Terminology	T-*score definition*
Normal	$T \geq -1.0$
Osteopenia	$-2.5 < T < -1.0$
Osteoporosis	$T \leq -2.5$
Established osteoporosis	$T \leq -2.5$ in the presence of one or more fragility fractures

THE CLINICAL ROLE OF BONE DENSITY MEASUREMENTS

Bone density measurements have an important clinical role in the evaluation of patients at risk of osteoporosis and in ensuring the appropriate use of antifracture treatment *(22–25)*. A helpful list of clinical indications for performing a bone density examination was published by the International Society for Clinical Densitometry (ISCD) and is summarised in

Table 2
Indications for Bone Mineral Density (BMD) Testing *(26)*

Women aged 65 and older
Postmenopausal women under age 65 with risk factors
Men aged 70 and older
Adults with a fragility fracture
Adults with a disease or condition associated with low bone mass or bone loss
Adults taking medication associated with low bone mass or bone loss
Anyone being considered for pharmacologic therapy
Anyone being treated to monitor treatment effect
Anyone not receiving therapy in whom evidence of bone loss would lead to treatment

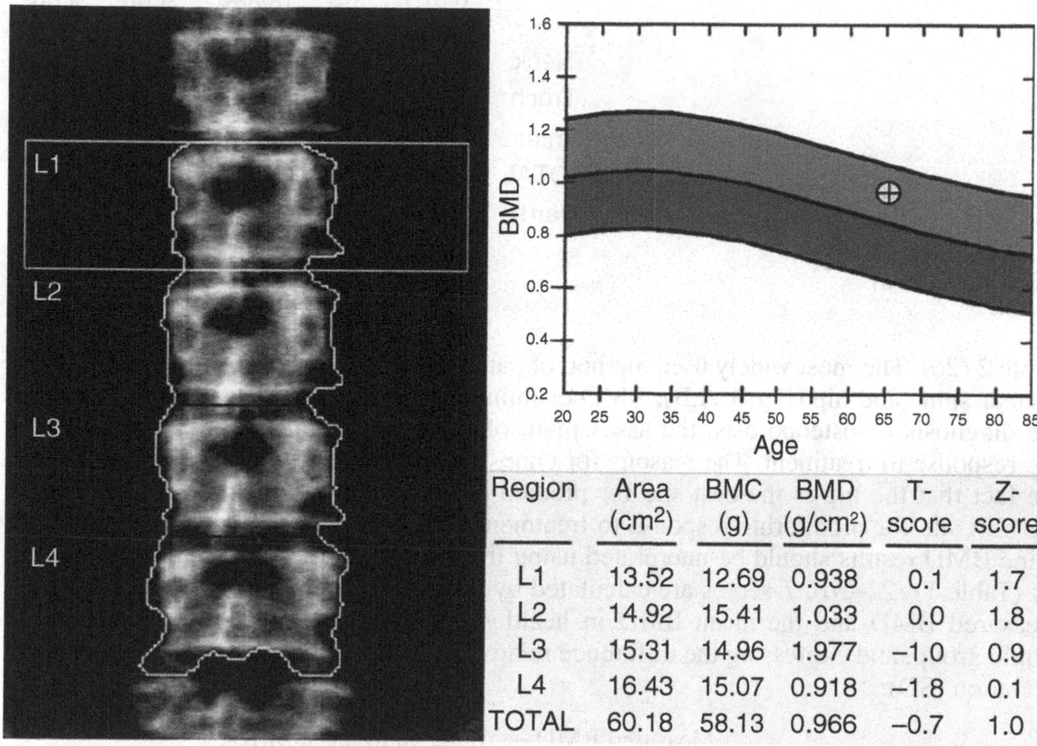

Region	Area (cm²)	BMC (g)	BMD (g/cm²)	T-score	Z-score
L1	13.52	12.69	0.938	0.1	1.7
L2	14.92	15.41	1.033	0.0	1.8
L3	15.31	14.96	1.977	−1.0	0.9
L4	16.43	15.07	0.918	−1.8	0.1
TOTAL	60.18	58.13	0.966	−0.7	1.0

Fig. 1. (**A**) Scan printout of a spine dual-energy X-ray absorptiometry (DXA) examination. The printout shows (*left*) scan image of the lumbar spine; (*top right*) patient's age and bone mineral density (BMD) plotted with respect to the manufacturer's reference range; (*bottom right*) BMD figures for individual vertebrae and total spine (L1–L4), together with the interpretation in terms of *T*-scores and *Z*-scores. (**B**) Scan printout of a hip DXA examination. The printout shows (*left*) scan image of the hip; (*top right*) patient's age and total hip BMD plotted with respect to the National Health and Nutrition Examination Survey (NHANES III) reference range *(40)*; (*bottom right*) BMD figures for five different regions of interest in the hip (femoral neck, greater trochanter, intertrochanteric, total hip, and Ward's triangle), together with the interpretation in terms of *T*-scores and *Z*-scores using the NHANES III reference range.

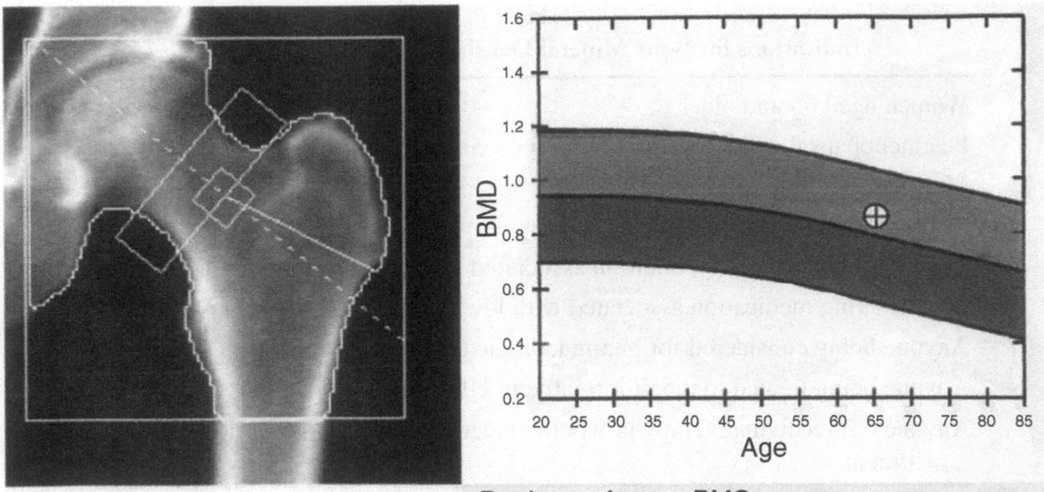

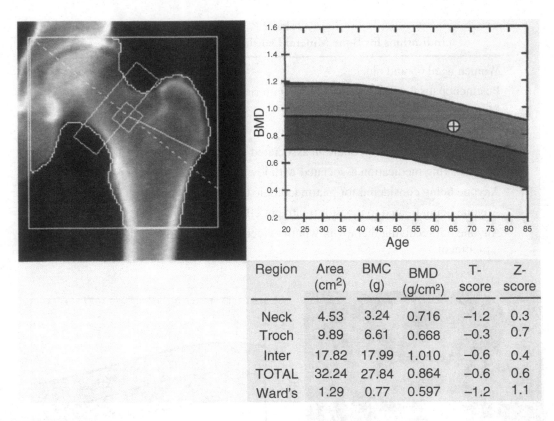

Region	Area (cm^2)	BMC (g)	BMD (g/cm^2)	T-score	Z-score
Neck	4.53	3.24	0.716	−1.2	0.3
Troch	9.89	6.61	0.668	−0.3	0.7
Inter	17.82	17.99	1.010	−0.6	0.4
TOTAL	32.24	27.84	0.864	−0.6	0.6
Ward's	1.29	0.77	0.597	−1.2	1.1

Fig. 1. (continued)

Table 2 *(26)*. The most widely used method of patient investigation is DXA scanning of the lumbar spine and hip (Fig. 1 A,B). BMD examinations have three principal roles, namely the diagnosis of osteoporosis, the assessment of patients' risk of fracture, and monitoring response to treatment. The reasons for choosing to measure the hip and spine include the fact that the hip is the best site for predicting hip fracture risk *(27–29)*, the spine is the best site for monitoring response to treatment *(30,31)* and the consensus that hip and spine BMD results should be interpreted using the WHO *T*-score definition of osteoporosis (Table 1) *(22–26)*. *T*-scores are calculated by taking the difference between a patient's measured BMD and the mean BMD in healthy young adults, matched for gender and ethnic group, and expressing the difference relative to the young adult population standard deviation (SD):

$$T\text{-score} = \frac{\text{Measured BMD} - \text{Young adult mean BMD}}{\text{Young adult population SD}} \quad (1)$$

Other practical advantages of DXA scanning include short scan times, easy patient set-up, low radiation dose, and good measurement precision. These and other advantages of spine and hip DXA are summarised in Table 3. Most of the rest of this chapter is devoted to discussing these advantages in greater detail.

In addition to central DXA systems that measure the spine and hip, a wide variety of other types of bone densitometry equipment are also available *(8,32)*. These include

Table 3
Clinical Advantages of Hip and Spine DXA

Proven ability to predict fracture risk
Consensus that BMD results can be interpreted using WHO *T*-scores
Proven for effective targeting of antifracture treatments
Effective for monitoring response to treatment
Basis of new WHO algorithm for predicting fracture risk
Many systems can perform vertebral fracture assessment
Short scan times
Easy patient set-up
Low radiation dose
Good precision
Availability of reliable reference ranges
Stable calibration
Effective instrument quality control procedures

quantitative computed tomography (QCT) measurements of the spine and hip *(33,34)*, peripheral DXA (pDXA) systems for measuring the forearm, heel or hand *(35)*, and quantitative ultrasound (QUS) devices for measurements of the heel and other peripheral sites *(36)*. In principle pDXA and QUS devices offer a quick, cheap and convenient way of evaluating skeletal status that makes them attractive for widespread use. In practice, however, these alternative types of measurement correlate poorly with hip and spine BMD, with correlation coefficients in the range $r = 0.5–0.7$ *(37)*. This lack of agreement with measurements made using hip and spine DXA has proved a barrier to reaching a consensus on the best way of introducing these other methods into wider clinical practice *(37,38)*.

WHICH MEASUREMENT IS BEST?

Given the choice of so many different types of measurement, how do we decide which technique is the most effective for decisions about patient treatment? Fundamental to the clinical use of any type of bone densitometry examination is its ability to predict fracture risk, and the most reliable way to evaluate and compare the alternative techniques is through prospective studies of incident fractures *(27)*. Figure 2 illustrates how data from a fracture study are analysed to quantify the relationship between BMD and fracture risk. When the study subjects are divided into quartiles on the basis of their baseline BMD measurements, an inverse relationship is found between fracture risk and BMD. To describe this relationship the BMD figures are converted into *Z*-scores. *Z*-scores are similar to *T*-scores except that instead of comparing the patient's measured BMD with the mean and SD for young

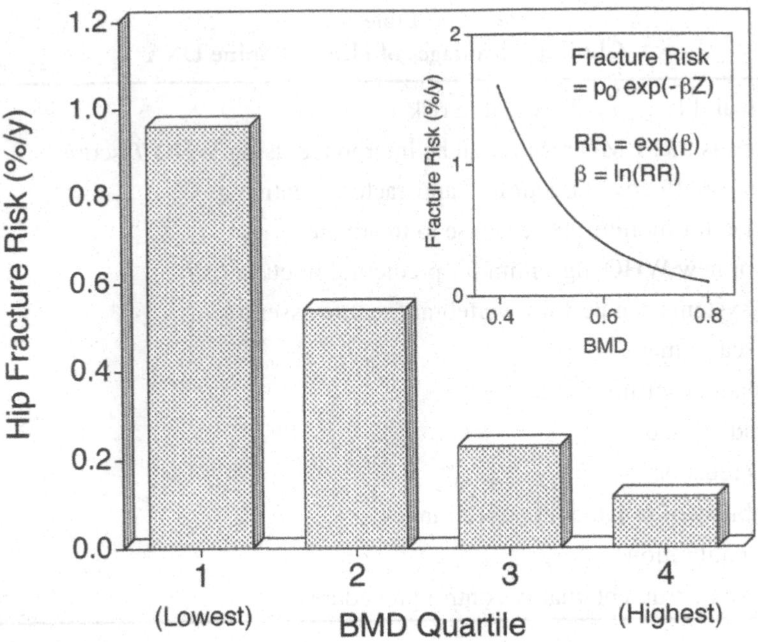

Fig. 2. Incidence of hip fracture risk by bone mineral density (BMD) quartile for femoral neck BMD. Data are taken from the 2-year follow-up of the Study of Osteoporotic Fractures (SOF) *(41)*. Inset diagram: data from fracture studies are fitted using a gradient-of-risk model, in which the fracture risk varies exponentially with Z-score with gradient β. Results are expressed in terms of the relative risk (RR), the increased risk of fracture for each unit decrease in Z-score. The value of RR is found from β using the exponential function (RR $=\exp(\beta)$). Alternatively, the gradient of risk is found by taking the natural logarithm of RR ($\beta = \ln(\text{RR})$).

adults, it is compared instead with the mean BMD and SD for healthy normal subjects matched for age, gender, and ethnic group:

$$\text{Z-score} = \frac{\text{Measured BMD} - \text{Age-matched mean BMD}}{\text{Age matched population SD}} \tag{2}$$

Data from fracture studies are fitted using a gradient-of-risk model in which the fracture risk increases exponentially with decreasing Z-score (Fig. 2, inset). Results are usually expressed in terms of the relative risk (RR), which is defined as the increased risk of fracture for each unit decrease in Z-score.

The larger the value of RR (or equivalently, the steeper the gradient-of-risk β in Fig. 2), the more effective the technique at discriminating between patients who will suffer a fracture in the future and those who will not. To understand the reason for this, consider a large group of subjects chosen randomly from the general population. For such a group the distribution of Z-score values approximates to a Gaussian curve (Fig. 3A). The distribution of Z-score values for the group of patients who will at some future date experience an osteoporotic fracture is found by multiplying the Gaussian curve representing the general population by the gradient-of-risk curve shown in the inset to Fig. 2. When this is done the distribution of Z-score values for the fracture population is found to be a second Gaussian

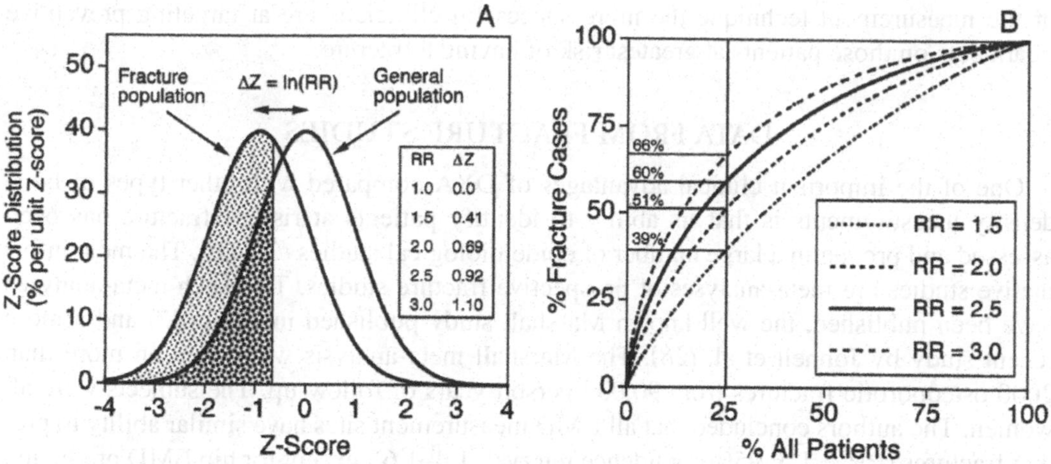

Fig. 3. (**A**) Distribution of *Z*-score values in a fracture population compared with the age-matched general population. The curve for the general population is a bell-shaped curve symmetrically distributed around its peak at $Z = 0$. The corresponding curve for the population of patients who will suffer an osteoporotic fracture is a similar bell-shaped curve that is offset from the general population by a *Z*-score difference of $\Delta Z = \ln(\mathrm{RR})$, where RR = relative risk. The inset table lists values of RR and ΔZ. (**B**) Plot of the receiver operating characteristic (ROC) curves obtained by evaluating the areas under the two bell-shaped curves shown in (**A**) up to an arbitrarily chosen *Z*-score threshold and plotting the two areas against each other for different values of the relative risk (RR). The ROC curve shows the percentage of fracture cases that fall below the bone mineral density (BMD) threshold (*shaded area* under the fracture population curve in (**A**)) plotted against the percentage of subjects in the general population who fall below the same threshold (*shaded area* under the general population curve in (**A**)). It therefore shows the true positive fraction (those patients who sustain a fracture and were correctly identified as being at risk) against the false-positive fraction (those patients identified as being at risk but who never actually have a fracture). The larger the value of RR the wider the separation of the two curves in (A) and the more effective BMD measurements are at discriminating the patients who will have a fracture. For example, if patients in the lowest quartile of BMD are identified for treatment, then for RR values of 1.5, 2.0, 2.5, and 3.0 this group will include 39, 51, 60 and 66%, respectively, of all patients who will suffer a fracture.

curve with the same SD as the first but with its peak offset to the left by an amount ΔZ equal to the gradient-of-risk β (or equivalently to the natural logarithm of RR) ($\Delta Z = \beta = \ln(\mathrm{RR})$) (Fig. 3A) *(39)*.

To understand the importance of selecting a technique with a high RR value, consider choosing some arbitrary *Z*-score value in Fig. 3A as the threshold for making decisions about patients' treatment (for example, this might be the *Z*-score value equivalent to a *T*-score of –2.5). The areas under the two curves can be evaluated to find the percentages of patients in the fracture population and the general population with BMD values below the chosen threshold. As the threshold is varied and the two percentages plotted against each other we obtain a receiver operating characteristic (ROC) curve (Fig. 3B) in which the percentage of true positives (those patients who will suffer a fracture in the future and were correctly identified to be at risk) is plotted against the percentage of false positives (those patients identified to be at risk but who never have a fracture). Figure 3B is fundamental to understanding the clinical value of any type of bone density measurement used to identify and treat patients at risk of fracture. It shows that the larger the RR value of the measurement technique the more successful clinicians are at targeting preventive treatments on those patients at greatest risk of having a fracture.

DATA FROM FRACTURE STUDIES

One of the important clinical advantages of DXA compared with other types of bone density measurements is that its ability to identify patients at risk of fracture has been assessed and proven in a large number of epidemiological studies *(27–29)*. The most informative studies are meta-analyses of prospective fracture studies. Two such meta-analyses have been published, the well-known Marshall study published in 1996 *(27)* and a more recent study by Johnell et al. *(28)*. The Marshall meta-analysis was based on more than 2000 osteoporotic fractures from 90,000 person-years of follow-up. The subjects were all women. The authors concluded that all BMD measurement sites have similar ability to predict fractures (RR = 1.5; 95% confidence interval: 1.4–1.6), except for hip BMD predicting hip fractures (RR = 2.6; 95% CI: 2.0–3.5) (Fig. 4) and spine BMD predicting vertebral fractures (RR = 2.3; 95% CI: 1.9–2.8). The authors concluded that hip and spine BMD

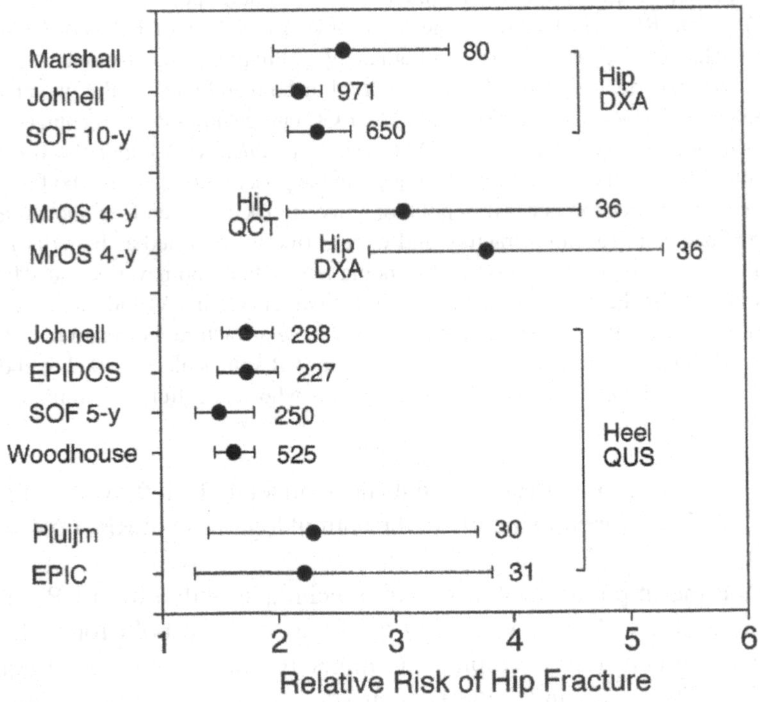

Fig. 4. Values of the relative risk (RR) (defined as the increased risk of fracture for a 1 standard deviation decease in bone mineral density) for hip fracture for (1) hip DXA measurements (Marshall meta-analysis *(27)*, Johnell meta-analysis *(28)*, Study of Osteoporotic Fractures (SOF) 10-year study *(29)*); (2) QCT and DXA hip BMD measurements (MrOS study *(43)*); (3) heel QUS measurements (Johnell meta-analysis *(28)*, EPIDOS study *(51)*, SOF 5-year study *(42)*, Woodhouse meta-analysis *(47)*, Amsterdam study *(46)*, and EPIC study *(50)*). The errors bars show the 95% confidence intervals. The number beside each data point shows the number of hip fractures in the study. The graph illustrates the importance of having a large number of fractures in order to reduce the error bars and allow a meaningful comparison between different bone densitometry techniques.

were the best measurements for predicting hip and spine fractures, respectively. A limitation of the Marshall study was that these latter conclusions were based on a relatively small number of fracture cases (80 hip fractures and 98 vertebral fractures, respectively).

The Johnell meta-analysis examined the relationship between hip fracture and hip BMD based on data from 12 different fracture studies from Australia, Canada, Europe, and Japan including both men and women *(28)*. There were data on 971 hip fractures from a total of 168,000 person-years of follow-up. As would be expected given the much larger number of hip fractures, the statistical errors are considerably reduced and consequently the results are more informative. When corrected to the population SD of the female reference range of the Third National Health and Nutrition Examination Survey (NHANES III) *(40)*, the RR figure for men and women combined was 2.21 (95% CI: 2.03–2.41) (Fig. 4). There was no significant difference between men and women (women: RR = 2.18; 95% CI: 1.99–2.39; men: RR = 2.28; 95% CI: 1.81–2.87). Interestingly the relative risk figures decreased progressively with increasing age varying from RR = 3.68 (95% CI: 2.61–5.19) at age 50 to RR = 1.93 (95% CI: 1.76–2.10) at age 85. Relative risk figures for hip fracture did not vary significantly with the length of follow-up (0–10 years) or baseline Z-score ($-4 < Z < +4$).

Among individual fracture studies, perhaps the most informative is the Study of Osteoporotic Fractures (SOF), a study of 9704 white US women aged 65 and over who had baseline measurements of hip, spine, forearm, and heel BMD when the study commenced in the late 1980 s *(29)*. One of the strengths of the SOF study is the large number of recorded fracture cases, with the recently published 10-year follow-up including over 650 hip fractures and 2900 fractures at all sites. A second important strength is that the baseline measurements included a variety of bone densitometry sites including DXA of the hip and spine, peripheral absorptiometry of the forearm and heel, and QUS of the heel. A large number of fracture cases are essential for achieving adequate statistical power if meaningful comparisons are to be made between different bone density techniques. This is illustrated in Fig. 4, which shows RR values for hip fracture from various studies with their 95% confidence intervals and the number of fractures recorded in the study. As the SOF study has progressed the results have consistently confirmed the ability of hip BMD measurements to predict hip fracture risk with an RR value of around 2.5 *(29,41,42)*. The 10-year follow-up data confirm the association between BMD and fracture risk with high statistical reliability for many types of fracture and show that the prediction of hip fracture risk from a hip BMD measurement has the largest RR value and is the most effective single type of DXA examination (Fig. 5) *(29)*.

In comparison to DXA, until recently there were no prospective studies of QCT and fracture risk. However, the first results of a prospective study of QCT and hip fracture risk from the Osteoporotic Fractures in Men (MrOS) study were recently announced *(43)*. The MrOS study enrolled 5995 white men aged 65 and over from six US centres. As well as baseline DXA scans, 3357 men had spine and hip QCT scans. The first results based on 36 hip fracture cases recorded after an average follow-up period of 4.4 years show comparable RR values for femoral neck BMD measured by QCT or DXA (Fig. 4). As can be seen, because of the small number of fracture cases so far recorded the statistical errors are still too large to make any meaningful comparison between QCT and DXA.

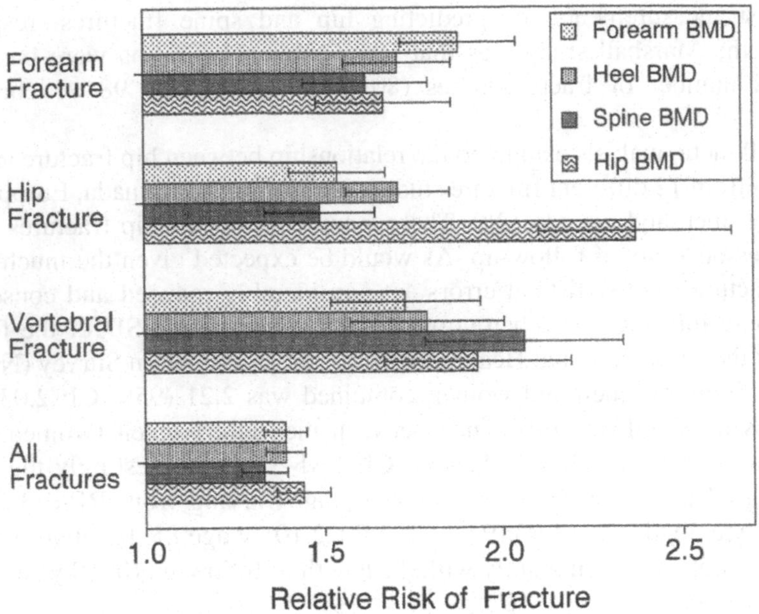

Fig. 5. Values of the relative risk (RR) (defined as the increased risk of fracture for a 1 standard deviation decrease in bone mineral density (BMD)) for fractures at different skeletal sites (wrist, hip, spine, and any fracture) for BMD measurements made at four different sites (forearm, heel, spine, and femoral neck). The errors bars show the 95% confidence intervals. Data are taken from the 10-year follow-up of the Study of Osteoporotic Fractures (SOF) study population *(29)*. In the SOF data the largest value of RR is for the prediction of hip fracture risk from a hip BMD measurement (RR = 2.4). From the ROC curves shown in Fig. 3B this means that the clinically most effective DXA scan measurement is to use hip BMD to predict hip fracture risk.

In contrast with QCT, there are a large number of published studies of QUS and fracture risk *(44–52)*. The Johnell meta-analysis includes QUS data from two cohorts (EPIDOS and Sheffield) with a total of 288 hip fractures *(28)*. RR values were 1.74 (95% CI: 1.53–1.97) for broadband ultrasonic attenuation (BUA) and 1.50 (95% CI: 1.31–1.70) for speed of sound (SOS). These and some other data for QUS are plotted in Fig. 4. Comparison of the various results plotted in Fig. 4 illustrates the importance of having studies with a large number of recorded fracture cases in order to reduce the error bars and allow a meaningful comparison between different techniques.

APPROPRIATE TARGETING OF ANTIFRACTURE TREATMENTS

Another of the clinical advantages of hip and spine BMD scans are their proven ability to identify patients who will respond successfully to treatments for preventing fractures. Table 4 lists the principal clinical trials of the pharmaceutical agents proven to prevent vertebral and/or non-vertebral fractures *(11–20)*. It is notable that all the trials listed enrolled patients on the basis of study entry criteria that included a DXA scan *T*-score at the hip or spine demonstrating either osteoporosis or severe osteopenia. In a number of these trials the data analysis showed that treatment was effective only in those subjects with a hip or spine *T*-score of –2.5 or less *(12,14,15,20)*. These findings have created difficulty in selecting

Table 4
Fracture Prevention Studies that Have Selected Subjects Using Hip and Spine DXA

Class of agent	*Name of drug*	*Study name*	T-*score thresholds for patient enrolment*[a]
Bisphosphonate	Alendronate	FIT 1 *(11)*	Femoral neck *T*-score < –1.5[b]
		FIT 2 *(12)*	Femoral neck *T*-score < –1.5
	Risedronate	VERT NA *(13)*	Spine *T*-score < –2[b]
		HIP *(14)*	Femoral neck *T*-score < –3.2[c]
	Ibandronate	BONE *(15)*	Spine *T*-score in range –2 to –5[b]
	Zolendronate	HORIZON *(16)*	Femoral neck *T*-score < –2.5[b]
Selective oestrogen receptor modulator	Raloxifene	MORE *(17)*	Spine or Fem neck *T*-score < –1.8[b]
Parathyroid hormone	PTH (1–34)	Neer study *(18)*	Spine or Fem neck *T*-score < –1[b]
Strontium	Strontium ranelate	SOTI *(19)*	Spine *T*-score < –1.9[b]
		TROPOS *(20)*	Femoral neck *T*-score < –2.2

[a] *T*-score thresholds are those calculated using the NHANES III reference range for the hip *(40)* and the Hologic reference range for spine BMD.
[b] Study entry criteria also included previous vertebral fracture.
[c] Study entry criteria also included clinical risk factors.

patients for treatment using techniques other than hip or spine DXA because of the poor correlation between different techniques and the lack of evidence that patients selected using other techniques will respond to treatment *(53)*.

VERTEBRAL FRACTURE ASSESSMENT

One important outcome of the recent trials of new treatments for osteoporosis has been the recognition of the importance of a previous vertebral fracture as a risk factor for future fractures that is independent of BMD *(54,55)*. Trial subjects with a previous vertebral fracture were five times more likely to have a further fracture than those without *(54)*. Other epidemiological studies confirm that patients with a prevalent vertebral fracture are at substantially greater risk of a future fracture than patients without a prevalent fracture *(56)*. Conventionally, the diagnosis of vertebral fracture is made from the semi-quantitative assessment of lateral X-ray films of the lumbar and thoracic spine *(57)*. However, many modern DXA systems are designed to acquire fast, high-resolution lateral images of the spine that can provide equivalent information, a technique referred to as vertebral fracture assessment (VFA). ISCD has published guidelines on the clinical indications for a VFA study and the method for defining and reporting vertebral fractures on a VFA study *(26)*.

Advantages of VFA studies using DXA equipment include the low radiation dose compared with X-ray films, and the ability to combine an assessment for vertebral fracture and a BMD measurement at a single patient visit *(58,59)*. Although the spatial resolution of the DXA images is poorer than a conventional radiograph, a normal scan image has been shown to be a highly reliable method of excluding the presence of vertebral fractures *(58)*.

AVAILABILITY OF RELIABLE REFERENCE RANGES

Over the last 10 years the interpretation of DXA scans has been guided by the WHO *T*-score definition of osteoporosis (Table 1). However, if scan results are to be interpreted reliably care is necessary in the choice of reference data for the calculation of *T*-scores. For consistency, ISCD recommends the use of the NHANES III reference database *(40)* for *T*-score derivation in the hip *(26)*. This recommendation was made following the publication of a study comparing the spine and hip *T*-score results obtained on the two principal brands of DXA scanner (manufactured by GE-Lunar and Hologic) and calculated using the manufacturers' reference ranges *(60)*. Although good agreement was found for spine *T*-scores measured on the two manufacturers' systems, a systematic difference of almost one *T*-score unit was found between the hip *T*-scores. The discrepancy was resolved by all the manufacturers agreeing to use the NHANES III hip reference range *(61)*, which is based on measurements of over 14,000 randomly selected men and women from across the whole of the United States. Comparison of reference ranges from different manufacturers for the same BMD site can show surprising large differences in the plots of mean *T*-score against age due to factors that include the use of inappropriate populations, different conventions for deriving the reference curve from the data, and insufficient numbers of subjects *(62)*. When the principal DXA manufacturers adopted the NHANES III hip BMD reference range with its large, randomly selected population this was an important factor in improving confidence in the interpretation of scan results.

INTERPRETATION OF T-SCORES USING THE WHO CRITERIA

As explained above, one of the important clinical advantages of DXA is the widespread consensus that spine, hip, and forearm BMD measurements should be interpreted using the WHO *T*-score definition of osteoporosis (Table 1). However, the WHO definition should not be applied to QCT or QUS measurements or pDXA results at sites other than the 33% radius *(26)*. The reason why this rule is so important can be understood from Fig. 6. When the reference ranges for different types of bone density measurement are plotted as graphs of mean *T*-score against age the curves obtained are found to be very different for different techniques. For example, the curve for spine QCT decreases rapidly with age and crosses the WHO threshold of $T = -2.5$ at age 60 (Fig. 6). This means that if QCT measurements were interpreted using the WHO definition 50% of 60-year-old women would be diagnosed with osteoporosis. In contrast, for some types of heel pDXA and QUS measurements the curve decreases so slowly with age that patients need to be age 100 before 50% of them have osteoporosis. For spine, femoral neck, and 33% radius DXA measurements the three curves decrease in a similar manner crossing the $T = -2.5$ threshold at age 75. It is clear that

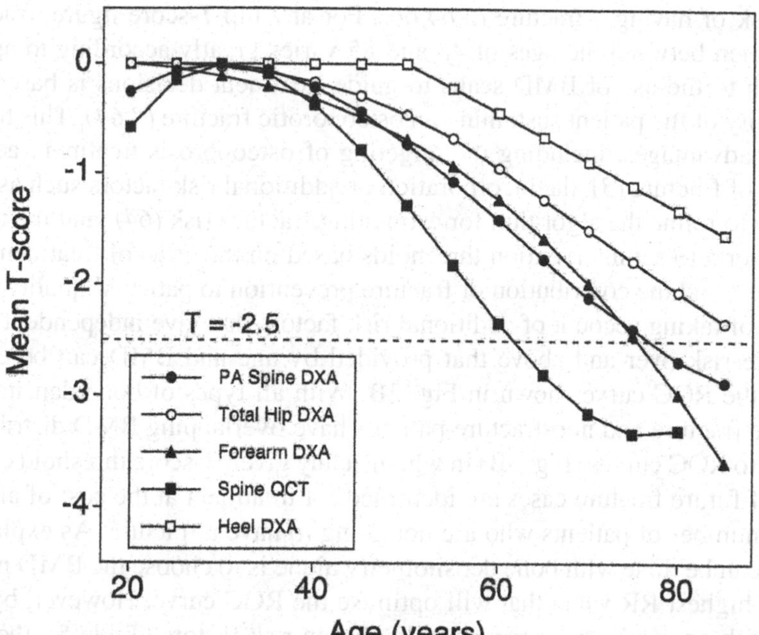

Fig. 6. Age-related decline in mean *T*-scores at different bone mineral density sites for healthy white female subjects. The hip DXA data are taken from the National Health and Nutrition Examination Survey (NHANES III) study *(40,61)*. The DXA normative data for the lumbar spine (L1–L4) and forearm (total forearm region) were obtained from the Hologic manufacturer's reference ranges. Heel data are for the GE-Lunar PIXI pDXA device. Spinal QCT is that used by the Image Analysis reference system. *Filled circles*: lumbar spine; *Open circles*: total hip; *Triangles*: total forearm; *Filled squares*: QCT spine; *Open squares*: Heel.

if care is not taken in applying the WHO criteria appropriately then cases of osteoporosis may be either seriously underdiagnosed or overdiagnosed depending on the measurement technique *(37)*. In principle, measurements other than spine and hip DXA can be used with appropriate device-specific thresholds to identify a group of patients with high peripheral BMD that are unlikely to be at risk, and another group with low BMD and who can be treated for osteoporosis. Patients with intermediate peripheral BMD results can be referred for a central DXA examination for a definitive diagnosis. However, the clinical application of this triage algorithm requires the availability of adequate information about the device-specific thresholds *(62)*.

THE NEW WHO FRACTURE RISK ALGORITHM

Views on the best way of using the information from DXA scans to advise patients about the use of antifracture treatment continue to evolve *(3,63–65)*. As emphasised above, the clinical value of a BMD examination lies in the information it provides about fracture risk. An important limitation of the WHO *T*-score approach to making decisions about patient treatment is that age as well as BMD is an important factor in determining the patient's short-term risk of having a fracture *(3,64,66)*. For any hip *T*-score figure, fracture risk in men and women between the ages of 45 and 85 varies greatly according to age *(3,66)*. A new approach to the use of BMD scans to guide treatment decisions is based on the 10-year probability of the patient sustaining an osteoporotic fracture *(3,64)*. This has a number of important advantages, including the targeting of osteoporosis treatment according the patient's risk of fracture *(3)*, the incorporation of additional risk factors such as a history of prior fracture to refine the algorithm for estimating fracture risk *(64)*, and the use of health economic criteria to set intervention thresholds based on the costs of treatment, savings to health services, and the contribution of fracture prevention to patients' quality of life *(63)*.

The value of taking account of additional risk factors that give independent information about fracture risk over and above that provided by age and BMD can be explained by reference to the ROC curve shown in Fig. 3B. With all types of bone densitometry measurement, the fracture and non-fracture patients have overlapping BMD distributions (Fig. 3A), leading to ROC curves (Fig. 3B) in which at any given *T*-score threshold only a certain percentage of future fracture cases are identified for treatment at the cost of also having to treat a large number of patients who are not going to have a fracture. As explained above, the best that can be done with bone densitometry alone is to choose the BMD measurement site with the highest RR value that will optimise the ROC curve. However, by combining BMD data with age and other appropriately chosen risk factors (Table 5), the ROC curve can be further improved so that treatments are better targeted on the patients at highest risk.

Table 5
Clinical Risk Factors Included in WHO Fracture Algorithm *(64)*

Age
Low body mass index
Prior fracture after age 50
Parental history of hip fracture
Current smoking habit
Current or past use of systemic corticosteroids
Alcohol intake > 2 U daily
Rheumatoid arthritis

The new WHO fracture risk algorithm is based on a series of meta-analyses of data from 12 independent fracture studies from North America, Europe, Asia, and Australia *(67–72)*. The DXA scan information required is femoral neck BMD. Because of the need to build the correct parameters into the statistical model, including the interdependence of the various risk factors, there is a specific requirement that the BMD information is provided by a hip DXA scan. The reliance on BMD information from a single skeletal site raises the important question of whether fracture risk prediction is improved by combining BMD measurements from more than one site. A meta-analysis of spine and femoral neck BMD data showed that use of the lowest *T*-score did not improve the ROC curve *(73)*. This finding is perhaps surprising, but mathematical analysis provides the reason: although hip and spine BMD measurements are quite poorly correlated ($r = 0.5$–0.7), even this degree of correlation is too high for a second BMD site to provide significant additional information about fracture risk *(74)*. A further point that follows from the WHO fracture risk algorithm is that not all patients necessarily require a DXA scan *(75)*. For some the use of age, fracture history, and the other risk factors are sufficient to place them in either the high-risk group requiring antifracture treatment or the low-risk group who can be reassured that their likelihood of having a fracture is small. Thus in future a triage approach could be adopted for BMD scanning in which the fracture risk algorithm is used to select those patients for a DXA examination in whom BMD information is most likely to contribute to their management.

Another advantage of the new WHO algorithm is that it enables fracture risk thresholds for intervention to be established based on economic criteria that can be adjusted for practice in different countries *(76,77)*. A series of health economic analyses have examined the rationale for fracture prevention and the cost-effectiveness of different osteoporosis treatments *(78–82)*. These analyses show that, taking account of all types of fracture, the cost-effective intervention thresholds correspond to *T*-score values between –2 and –3 over a range of ages from 50 to 80 *(63,64)*. At the present time it is unclear how quickly the new fracture risk approach will become the new paradigm for the management of osteoporosis.

MONITORING RESPONSE TO TREATMENT

Verifying response to treatment using follow-up DXA scans is widely believed to have a beneficial role in encouraging patients to continue taking their medication, and also in identifying non-responders who may benefit from a different treatment regimen. DXA has a number of advantages as a technique for monitoring patients' response, of which one of the most important is the good precision of the measurements. Precision is usually expressed in terms of the coefficient of variation (CV) which is typically around 1–1.5% for spine and total hip BMD and 2–2.5% for femoral neck BMD *(83)*. DXA scanners have good long-term precision because among other reasons their calibration is extremely stable and there are effective instrument quality control procedures provided by manufacturers to detect any long-term drifts (Table 3). A second requirement for effective patient monitoring is a BMD measurement site that shows a large response to treatment. The best DXA site for follow-up measurements is the spine because the treatment changes are usually largest and the precision error is as good or better than that at most other sites *(84–85)*.

CONCLUSIONS

As a technique for performing bone densitometry, hip and spine DXA examinations have a number of important clinical advantages including compatibility with the WHO *T*-score definition of osteoporosis, their proven effectiveness at predicting fracture risk, proven effectiveness for targeting of antifracture treatment, effectiveness at monitoring patients' response to treatment, and compatibility with the new WHO fracture risk algorithm. Other advantages include the stable calibration of hip and spine DXA scanners, the good precision of the measurements, and the availability of reliable reference ranges. Their future clinical use is likely to be guided by the new paradigm of basing patient treatment on individual fracture risk. It is likely in the future that most decisions about treatment will be based on a hip BMD examination while spine BMD examinations will be performed for treatment monitoring.

REFERENCES

1. Cummings SR, Melton LJ. Epidemiology and outcomes of osteoporotic fractures. Lancet 2002;359: 1761–1767.
2. Bone health and osteoporosis: a report of the Surgeon General. Issued October 2004. Available online at www.surgeongeneral.gov/library/bonehealth.
3. Kanis JA, Black D, Cooper C, et al. A new approach to the development of assessment guidelines for osteoporosis. Osteoporos Int 2002;13:527–536.
4. Ray NF, Chan JK, Thamer M, Melton LJ. Medical expenditures for the treatment of osteoporotic fractures in the United States in 1995: report from the National Osteoporosis Foundation. J Bone Miner Res 1997:12:24–35.
5. Melton LJ, Gabriel SE, Crowson CS, Tostesen ANA, Johnell O, Kanis JA. Cost-equivalence of different osteoporotic fractures. Osteoporos Int 2003;14:383–388.
6. Cooper C, Atkinson EJ, Jacobsen SJ, O'Fallon M, Melton LJ. Population based study of survival after osteoporotic fractures. Am J Epidemiol 1993;137:1001–1005.
7. Centre JR, Nguyen TV, Schneider D, Sambrook PN, Eisman JA. Mortality after all major types of osteoporotic fractures in men and women: an observational study. Lancet 1999;353:878–882.
8. Genant HK, Engelke K, Fuerst T, et al. Noninvasive assessment of bone mineral and structure: state of the art. J Bone Miner Res 1996;11:707–730.
9. Storm T, Thamsborg G, Steiniche T, Genant HK, Sorensen OH. Effect of intermittent cyclical etidronate therapy on bone mass and fracture rate in women with postmenopausal osteoporosis. N Engl J Med 1990;322:1265–1271.
10. WHO. Assessment of fracture risk and its application to screening for postmenopausal osteoporosis: technical report series 843. Geneva: WHO, 1994.
11. Black DM, Cummings SR, Karpf DB, et al. Randomised trial of the effect of alendronate on risk of fracture in women with existing vertebral fractures. Lancet 1996;348:1535–1541.
12. Cummings SR, Black DM, Thompson DE, et al. Effect of alendronate on risk of fracture in women with low bone density but without vertebral fractures: results from the Fracture Intervention Trial. JAMA 1998;280:2077–2082.
13. Harris ST, Watts NB, Genant HK, et al. Effects of risedronate treatment on vertebral and non-vertebral fractures in women with postmenopausal osteoporosis. JAMA 1999;282:1344–1352.
14. McClung MR, Geusens P, Miller PD, et al. Effect of risedronate treatment on hip fracture risk in elderly women. N Engl J Med 2001;344:333–340.
15. Chesnut CH, Skag A, Christiansen C, et al. Effects of oral ibandronate administered daily or intermittently on fracture risk in postmenopausal osteoporosis. J Bone Miner Res 2004;19:1241–1249.
16. Black DM, Boonen S, Cauley J, et al. Effect of once-yearly infusion of zolendronic acid 5 mg on spine and hip fracture reduction in postmenopausal women with osteoporosis: the HORIZON pivotal fracture trial. J Bone Miner Res 2006;21(Suppl 1):S16.
17. Ettinger B, Black DM, Mitlak BH, et al. Reduction of vertebral fracture risk in postmenopausal women with osteoporosis treated with raloxifene: results from a 3-year randomised clinical trial. JAMA 1999;282:637–645.
18. Neer RM, Arnaud CD, Zanchetta JR, et al. Effect of recombinant human parathyroid hormone (1–34) fragment on spine and non-spine fractures and bone mineral density in postmenopausal osteoporosis. N Engl J Med 2001;344:1434–1441.
19. Meunier PJ, Roux C, Seeman E, et al. The effects of strontium ranelate on the risk of vertebral fracture in women with postmenopausal osteoporosis. N Engl J Med 2004;350:459–468.
20. Reginster JY, Seeman E, De Vernejoul MC, et al. Strontium ranelate reduces the risk of nonvertebral fractures in postmenopausal women with osteoporosis: TROPOS study. J Clin Endocrinol Metab 2005;90:2816–2822.
21. Seeman E, Vellas B, Benhamou C, et al. Strontium ranelate reduces the risk of vertebral and nonvertebral fractures in women eighty years of age and older. J Bone Miner Res 2006;21:1113–1120.
22. Kanis JA, Delmas P, Burckhardt P, Cooper C, Torgerson D, On behalf of the European Foundation for Osteoporosis and Bone Disease. Guidelines for diagnosis and treatment of osteoporosis. Osteoporos Int 1997;7:390–406.

23. Anon. Osteoporosis: review of the evidence for prevention, diagnosis, and treatment and cost-effectiveness analysis. Osteoporos Int 1998;8(Suppl 4):S7–S80.
24. Genant HK, Cooper C, Poor G, et al. Interim report and recommendations of the World Health Organization task-force for osteoporosis. Osteoporos Int 1999;10:259–264.
25. Kanis JA, Gluer CC, For the Committee of Scientific Advisors, International Osteoporosis Foundation. An update on the diagnosis and assessment of osteoporosis with densitometry. Osteoporos Int 2000;11: 192–202.
26. Official positions of the International Society for Clinical Densitometry: updated 2005. Available online at www.iscd.org/visitors/positions/official.cfm.
27. Marshall D, Johnell O, Wedel H. Meta-analysis of how well measures of bone mineral density predict occurrence of osteoporotic fractures. BMJ 1996;312:1254–1259.
28. Johnell O, Kanis JA, Oden A, et al. Predictive value of BMD for hip and other fractures. J Bone Miner Res 2005;20:1185–1194.
29. Stone KL, Seeley DG, Lui L-Y, et al. BMD at multiple sites and risk of fracture of multiple types: long-term results from the Study of Osteoporotic Fractures. J Bone Miner Res 2003;18:1947–1954.
30. Eastell R. Treatment of postmenopausal osteoporosis. N Engl J Med 1998;338:736–746.
31. Gluer C-C. Monitoring skeletal change by radiological techniques. J Bone Miner Res 1999;14: 1952–1962.
32. Fogeman I, Blake GM. Different approaches to bone densitometry. J Nucl Med 2000;41:2015–2025.
33. Guglielmi G, Lang TF. Quantitative computed tomography. Semin Musculoskelet Radiol 2002;6: 219–227.
34. Lang TF, Guglielmi G, Van Kuijk C, De Serio A, Cammisa M, Genant HK. Measurement of vertebral bone mineral density at the spine and proximal femur by volumetric quantitative computed tomograph and dual-energy X-ray absorptiometry in elderly women with and without vertebral fractures. Bone 2002;30: 247–250.
35. Blake GM, Fogelman I. Clinical use of instruments that measure peripheral bone mass. Curr Opin Endocrinol Diab 2002;9:502–511.
36. Stewart A, Reid DM. Quantitative ultrasound in osteoporosis. Semin Musculoskelet Radiol 2002;6: 229–232.
37. Lu Y, Genant HK, Shepherd J, et al. Classification of osteoporosis based on bone mineral densities. J Bone Miner Res 2001;16:901–910.
38. Faulkner KG, Von Stetton E, Miller P. Discordance in patient classification using T-scores. J Clin Densitom 1999;2:343–350.
39. Blake GM, Fogelman I. Peripheral or central densitometry: does it matter which technique we use? J Clin Densitom 2001;4:83–96.
40. Looker AC, Wahner HW, Dunn WL, et al. Updated data on proximal femur bone mineral levels of US adults. Osteoporos Int 1998;8:468–489.
41. Cummings SR, Black DM, Nevitt MC, et al. Bone density at various sites for prediction of hip fractures. Lancet 1993;341:72–75.
42. Black DM, Palermo L, Bauer D. How well does bone mass predict long-term risk of hip fracture? Osteoporosis Int 2000;11(Suppl 2):S59.
43. Orwoll ES, Marshall LM, Chan BK, et al. Measures of hip structure are important determinants of hip fracture risk independent of BMD. J Bone Miner Res 2006;20(Suppl 1):S35.
44. Hans D, Dargent-Molina P, Schott AM, et al. Ultrasonographic heel measurements to predict hip fracture in elderly women: the EPIDOS prospective study. Lancet 1996;348:511–514.
45. Bauer DC, Gluer C-C, Cauley JA, et al. Broadband ultrasonic attenuation predicts fractures strongly and independently of densitometry in older women. Arch Intern Med 1997;157:629–634.
46. Pluijm SMF, Graafmans WC, Bouter LM, Lips P. Ultrasound measurements for the prediction of osteoporotic fractures in elderly people. Osteoporos Int 1999;9:550–556.
47. Woodhouse A, Black DM. BMD at various sites for the prediction of hip fracture: a meta-analysis. J Bone Miner Res 2000;15(Suppl 2):S145.
48. Bauer DC, Palermo L, Black DM, Hillier TA, Cauley JA. A prospective study of dry calcaneal quantitative ultrasound and fracture risk in older women: the Study of Osteoporotic Fractures. J Bone Miner Res 2001;16(Suppl 1):S166.

49. Miller PD, Siris ES, Barrett-Connor E, et al. Prediction of fracture risk in postmenopausal white women with peripheral bone densitometry: evidence from the National Osteoporosis Risk Assessment. J Bone Miner Res 2002;17:2222–2230.
51. Hans D, Schott A-M, Duboeuf F, Durosier C, Meunier PJ. Does follow-up duration influence the ultrasound and DXA prediction of hip fracture? The EPIDOS prospective study. Bone 2004;35:357–363.
52. Durosier C, Hans D, Kreig M-A, Schott A-M. Prediction and discrimination of osteoporotic hip fracture in postmenopausal women. J Clin Densitom 2006;9:475–495.
53. Barr RJ, Adebajo A, Fraser WD, et al. Can peripheral DXA measurements be used to predict fractures in elderly women living in the community? Osteoporos Int 2005;16:1177–1183.
54. Delmas PD. How does antiresorptive therapy decrease the risk of fracture in women with osteoporosis? Bone 2000:27;1–3.
55. Lindsay R, Silverman SL, Cooper C, et al. Risk of new vertebral fracture in the year following a fracture. JAMA 2001;285:320–323.
56. Melton L, Atkinson EJ, Cooper C, O'Fallon WM, Riggs BL. Vertebral fractures predict subsequent fractures. Osteoporos Int 1999;10:214–221.
57. Genant HK, Wu CY, van Kuijk C, Nevitt MC. Vertebral fracture assessment using a semiquantitative technique. J Bone Miner Res 1993;8:1137–1148.
58. Rea JA, Li J, Blake GM, et al. Visual assessment of vertebral deformity by X-ray absorptiometry: a highly predictive method to exclude vertebral deformity. Osteoporos Int 2000;11:660–668.
59. Rea JA, Chen MB, Li J, et al. Morphometric X-ray absorptiometry and morphometric radiography of the spine: a comparison of prevalent vertebral deformity identification. J Bone Miner Res 2000;15:564–574.
60. Faulkner KG, Roberts LA, McClung MR. Discrepancies in normative data between Lunar and Hologic DXA systems. Osteoporosis Int 1996;6:432–436.
61. Hanson J. Standardization of femur BMD. J Bone Miner Res 1997;12:1316–1317.
62. Blake GM, Chinn DJ, Steel SA, et al. A list of device specific thresholds for the clinical interpretation of peripheral X-ray absorptiometry examinations. Osteoporos Int 2005;16:2149–2156.
63. Kanis JA. Diagnosis of osteoporosis and assessment of fracture risk. Lancet 2002;359:1929–1936.
64. Kanis JA, Borgstrom F, De Laet C, et al. Assessment of fracture risk. Osteoporos Int 2005;16:581–589.
65. De Laet C, Oden A, Johansson H, Johnell O, Jonsson B, Kanis JA. The impact of the use of multiple risk factors for fracture on case-finding strategies: a mathematical approach. Osteoporos Int 2005;16:313–318.
66. Kanis JA, Johnell O, Oden A, Dawson A, De Laet C, Jonsson B. Ten year probabilities of osteoporotic fractures according to BMD and diagnostic thresholds. Osteoporos Int 2001;12:989–995.
67. Kanis JA, Johnell O, De Laet C, et al. A meta-analysis of previous fracture and subsequent fracture risk. Bone 2004;35:375–382.
68. Kanis JA, Johansson H, Oden A, et al. A meta-analysis of prior corticosteroid use and fracture risk. J Bone Miner Res 2004;19:893–899.
69. Kanis JA, Johansson H, Oden A, et al. A family history of fracture and fracture risk: a meta-analysis. Bone 2004;35:1029–1037.
70. Kanis JA, Johnell O, Oden A, et al. Smoking and fracture risk: a meta-analysis. Osteoporos Int 2005;16:155–162.
71. Kanis JA, Johansson H, Johnell O, et al. Alcohol intake as a risk factor for fracture. Osteoporos Int 2005;16:737–742.
72. De Laet C, Kanis JA, Oden A, et al. Body mass index as a predictor of fracture risk: a meta-analysis. Osteoporos Int 2005;16:1330–1338.
73. Kanis JA, Johnell O, Oden A, et al. The use of multiple sites for the diagnosis of osteoporosis. Osteoporos Int 2006;17:527–534.
74. Blake GM, Patel R, Knapp KM, Fogelman I. Does the combination of two BMD measurements improve fracture discrimination? J Bone Miner Res 2003;18:1955–1963.
75. Johansson H, Oden A, Johnell O, et al. Optimisation of BMD measurements to identify high risk groups for treatment – a test analysis. J Bone Miner Res 2004;19:906–913.
76. Kanis JA, Oden A, Johnell O, Jonsson B, De Laet C, Dawson A. The burden of osteoporotic fractures: a method of setting intervention thresholds. Osteoporos Int 2001;12:417–427.
77. Borgstrom F, Johnell O, Kanis JA, et al. At what hip fracture risk is it cost effective to treat? International intervention thresholds for the treatment of osteoporosis. Osteoporos Int 2006;17: 1459–1471.

78. Kanis JA, Borgstrom F, Zethraeus N, Johnell O, Oden A, Jonsson B. Intervention thresholds for osteoporosis in the UK. Bone 2005;36:22–32.
79. Zethraeus N, Borgstrom F, Strom O, Kanis JA. Cost-effectiveness of the treatment and prevention of osteoporosis – a review of the literature and a reference model. Osteoporos Int 2007;18:9–23.
80. Kanis JA, Borgstrom F, Johnell O, Oden A, Sykes D, Jonsson B. 2005 Cost-effectiveness of raloxifene in the UK: an economic evaluation based on the MORE study. Osteoporos Int 16:15–25.
81. Borgstrom F, Carisson A, Sintonen H, et al. Cost-effectiveness of risedronate in the treatment of osteoporosis: an international perspective. Osteoporos Int 2006;17:996–1007.
82. Borgstrom F, Jonsson B, Strom O, Kanis JA. An economic evaluation of strontium ranelate in the treatment of osteoporosis in a Swedish setting based on the results of the SOTI and TROPOS trials. Osteoporos Int 2006;17:1781–1793.
83. Patel R, Blake GM, Rymer J, Fogelman I. Long-term precision of DXA scanning assessed over seven years in forty postmenopausal women. Osteoporos Int 2000;11;68–75.
84. Faulkner KG. Bone densitometry: choosing the proper site to measure. J Clin Densitom 1998;1:279–285.
85. Blake GM, Herd RJM, Fogelman I. A longitudinal study of supine lateral DXA of the lumbar spine: a comparison with posteroanterior spine, hip and total body DXA. Osteoporos Int 1996;6:462–470.

5 Biochemical Markers of Bone Turnover – Basic Biochemistry and Variability

Markus J. Seibel and Christian Meier

CONTENTS

SUMMARY

Disorders of bone and mineral metabolism are frequent and constitute an important part of everyday clinical practice. Consequently, there is a need for effective measures to be used in the screening, diagnosis, and follow-up of such pathologies. Together with clinical and imaging techniques, biochemical markers of bone metabolism and other laboratory tests offer useful assistance in the assessment and differential diagnosis of metabolic bone disease. In recent years, the isolation and characterization of cellular and extracellular components of the skeletal matrix have resulted in the development of molecular markers that are considered to reflect either bone formation or bone resorption. These biochemical indices are non-invasive, comparatively inexpensive and, when applied and interpreted correctly, helpful tools in the assessment of metabolic bone disease. The following chapter provides an overview of the basic biochemistry of "bone markers" and sources of their non-specific variability. The clinical use of these markers in osteoporosis will be reviewed in Chapter 6.

Key Words: Bone metabolism, phosphatase, osteocalcin, propeptide, cross-links, sialoprotein, collagen, osteoblast, osteoclast, bone formation, bone resorption, variability

From: *Contemporary Endocrinology: Osteoporosis: Pathophysiology and Clinical Management*
Edited by: R. A. Adler, DOI 10.1007/978-1-59745-459-9_5,

BIOCHEMISTRY OF MARKERS OF BONE TURNOVER

Bone is a metabolically active tissue that undergoes continuous remodeling by two counteracting processes, namely bone formation and bone resorption. These processes rely on the activity of osteoclasts (resorption), osteoblasts (formation), and osteocytes (maintenance). Under normal conditions, bone resorption and formation are tightly coupled to each other, so that the amount of bone removed is always equal to the amount of bone newly formed. This balance is achieved and regulated through the action of various systemic hormones (e.g., parathyroid hormone, vitamin D, other steroid hormones) and local mediators (e.g., cytokines, growth factors). In contrast, somatic growth, aging, metabolic bone diseases, states of increased or decreased mobility, therapeutic interventions, and many other conditions are characterized by more or less pronounced imbalances in bone turnover. The results of such uncoupling in bone turnover are often changes in bone structure, strength, and mass. While bone structure and strength are difficult to measure in vivo, bone mass can be assessed by densitometric techniques. In contrast to these rather static measures, however, molecular markers of bone metabolism are helpful tools to detect the dynamics of the metabolic imbalance itself *(1,2)*.

Although the currently available markers of bone turnover include both enzymes and non-enzymatic peptides derived from cellular and non-cellular compartments of bone, they are usually classified according to the metabolic process they are considered to reflect. Most biochemical indices of bone resorption are related to collagen breakdown products such as hydroxyproline or the various collagen cross-links and telopeptides. Other markers of bone resorption include non-collagenous matrix proteins such as bone sialoprotein, or osteoclast-specific enzymes like tartrate-resistant acid phosphatase or cathepsin K. In contrast, markers of bone formation are either by-products of collagen neosynthesis (e.g., propeptides of type I collagen) or osteoblast-related proteins such as osteocalcin and alkaline phosphatase. For clinical purposes, therefore, markers of bone formation are distinguished from indices of bone resorption (Table 1, Fig. 1). This distinction, however, is not as sharp as it may appear. For example, some marker components reflect, at least in part, both bone formation and bone resorption (e.g., hydroxyproline, certain osteocalcin fragments). Furthermore, most of the molecules used as markers of bone turnover are also present in tissues other than bone, and non-skeletal processes may therefore influence their circulating or urinary levels. Finally, changes in markers of bone turnover are not disease specific but reflect, as an integral measure, alterations in the metabolism of the entire skeletal envelope independently of the underlying cause. Hence, results of bone marker measurements should always be interpreted against the background of their basic science and the clinical picture.

The following section summarizes commonly used biochemical markers of bone formation and bone resorption.

MARKERS OF BONE FORMATION

Bone formation markers are products of active osteoblasts expressed during different phases of osteoblast development. They are considered to reflect different aspects of osteoblast function and of bone formation. All markers of bone formation are measured in serum or plasma.

Table 1
Markers of Bone Turnover

Marker	*Tissue of origin*	*Specimen*	*Analytical method*	*Remarks*
Markers of bone formation				
Bone-specific alkaline phosphatase (BAP)	Bone	Serum	Electrophoresis, precipitation, IRMA, EIA	Specific product of osteoblasts. Some assays show up to 20% cross-reactivity with liver isoenzyme (LAP)
Osteocalcin (OC)	Bone, platelets	Serum	RIA, IRMA, ELISA	Specific product of osteoblasts; many immunoreactive forms in blood; some may be derived from bone resorption
C-terminal propeptide of type I procollagen (PICP)	Bone, soft tissue, skin	Serum	RIA, ELISA	Specific product of proliferating osteoblasts and fibroblasts
N-terminal propeptide of type I procollagen (PINP)	Bone, soft tissue, skin	Serum	RIA, ELISA	Specific product of proliferating osteoblast and fibroblasts; partly incorporated into bone extracellular matrix
Markers of bone resorption				
Collagen-related markers				
Hydroxyproline, total and dialyzable (Hyp)	Bone, cartilage, soft tissue, skin	Urine	Colorimetry, HPLC	Present in all fibrillar collagens and partly collagenous proteins, including C1q and elastin. Present in newly synthesized and mature collagen, i.e., both collagen synthesis and tissue breakdown contribute to urinary hydroxyproline

(*Continued*)

Table 1
(continued)

Marker	*Tissue of origin*	*Specimen*	*Analytical method*	*Remarks*
Hydroxylysine-glycosides	Bone, soft tissue, skin, serum complement	Urine (serum)	HPLC, ELISA	Hydroxylysine in collagen is glycosylated to varying degrees, depending on tissue type. Glycosylgalactosyl-OHLys in high proportion in collagens of soft tissues, and C1q; Galyctosyl-OHLys in high proportion in skeletal collagens
Pyridinoline (PYD)	Bone, cartilage, tendon, blood vessels	Urine, serum	HPLC, ELISA	Collagens, with highest concentrations in cartilage and bone; absent from skin; present in mature collagen only
Deoxypyridinoline (DPD)	Bone, dentin	Urine, serum	HPLC, ELISA	Collagens, with highest concentration in bone; absent from cartilage or skin; present in mature collagen only
Carboxy-terminal cross-linked telopeptide of type I collagen (ICTP, CTX-MMP)	Bone, skin	Serum	RIA	Collagen type I, with highest contribution probably from bone; may be derived from newly synthesized collagen
Carboxy-terminal cross-linked telopeptide of type I collagen (CTX-I)	All tissues containing type I collagen	Urine: α or β; serum: α α or ββ	ELISA, RIA	Collagen type I, with highest contribution probably from bone. Isomerization of aspartyl to β-aspartyl occurs with ageing of collagen molecule

Amino-terminal cross-linked telopeptide of type I collagen (NTX-I)	All tissues containing type I collagen	Urine, serum	ELISA, CLIA, RIA	Collagen type I, with highest contribution from bone
Collagen I alpha 1 helicoidal peptide (HELP)	All tissues containing type I collagen	Urine	ELISA	Degradation fragment derived from the helical part of type I collagen (α1 chain, AA 620–633). Correlates highly with other markers of collagen degradation, no specific advantage or difference in regard to clinical outcomes
Non-collagenous proteins				
Bone sialoprotein (BSP)	Bone, dentin, hypertrophic cartilage	Serum	RIA, ELISA	Acidic, phosphorylated glycoprotein, synthesized by osteoblasts and osteoclastic-like cells, laid down in bone extracellular matrix. Appears to be associated with osteoclast function
Osteocalcin fragments (ufOC, U-Mid-OC, U-LongOC)	Bone	Urine	ELISA	Certain age-modified OC fragments are released during osteoclastic bone resorption and may be considered an index of bone resorption

(*Continued*)

Table 1
(continued)

Marker	*Tissue of origin*	*Specimen*	*Analytical method*	*Remarks*
Osteoclast enzymes				
Tartrate-resistant acid phosphatase (TRAcP)	Bone, blood	Plasma, serum	Colorimetry, RIA, ELISA	Six isoenzymes found in human tissues (osteoclasts, platelets, erythrocytes). Band 5b predominant in bone (osteoclasts). Enzyme identified in both the ruffled border of the osteoclast membrane and the secretions in the resorptive space
Cathepsins (e.g., K, L)	K: primarily in osteoclasts; L: macrophage, Osteoclasts	Plasma, serum	ELISA	Cathepsin K, cysteine protease, plays an essential role in osteoclast-mediated bone matrix degradation by cleaving helical and telopeptide regions of collagen type I. Cathepsin K and L cleave the loop domain of TRACP and activate the latent enzyme. Cathepsin L has a similar function in macrophages. Tests for measurement of Cathepsins in blood are presently under evaluation

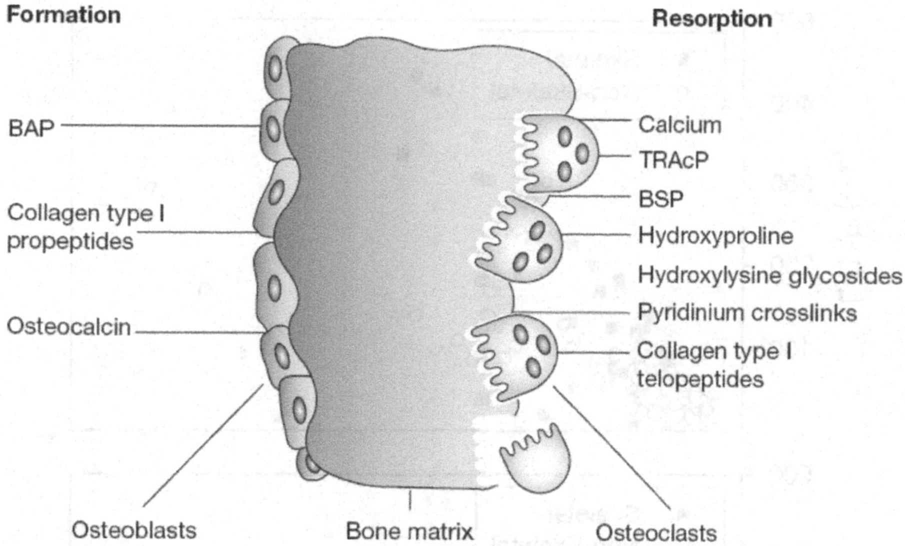

Fig. 1. Biochemical markers of bone remodeling.

Alkaline phosphatase (ALP) is a ubiquitous, membrane-bound tetrameric enzyme attached to glycosyl-phosphatidylinositol moieties located on the outer cell surface *(3)*. The precise function of the enzyme is yet unknown *(4)*, but it obviously plays an important role in osteoid formation and mineralization. The total AP serum pool (TAP) consists of several dimeric isoforms, which originate from various tissues: liver, bone, intestine, spleen, kidney, and placenta. In addition, certain tumors may express macromolecular forms of AP (e.g., "Nagao AP") *(5,6)*.

The physiological isoforms of AP are coded by four gene loci, including three tissue-specific and one non-tissue-specific gene on chromosome 1. The latter encodes for the most abundant isoforms, namely bone, liver, and kidney AP. The differences between these non-specifically encoded isoenzymes are solely due to post-translational modifications in the carbohydrate moiety *(7)*. In adults with normal liver function, approximately 50% of the total AP activity in serum is derived from the liver, whereas 50% arises from bone *(8)*. In children and adolescents the bone-specific isoenzyme predominates (up to 90%) because of skeletal growth *(9,10)*.

Many techniques have been developed to differentiate between the two main isoforms of circulating AP, including heat denaturation, electrophoresis, precipitation, selective inhibition and, more recently, immunoassays *(11–15)*. In healthy adults, most methods show a good correlation between bone-specific and total AP (Fig. 2). The newer immunoassays allow simple and rapid quantitation of either enzyme activity or enzyme mass. However, like all of the other techniques, even these assays show a certain degree of cross-reactivity between bone and liver AP (15–20%). Therefore, in subjects with high liver AP, results of bone AP measurements may be artificially high, leading to false-positive results *(7,16,17)*.

Serum total AP is the most widely used marker of bone metabolism due to the wide availability of inexpensive and simple methods. Once liver disease is ruled out, serum levels of total AP provide a good impression of the extent of new bone formation and osteoblast

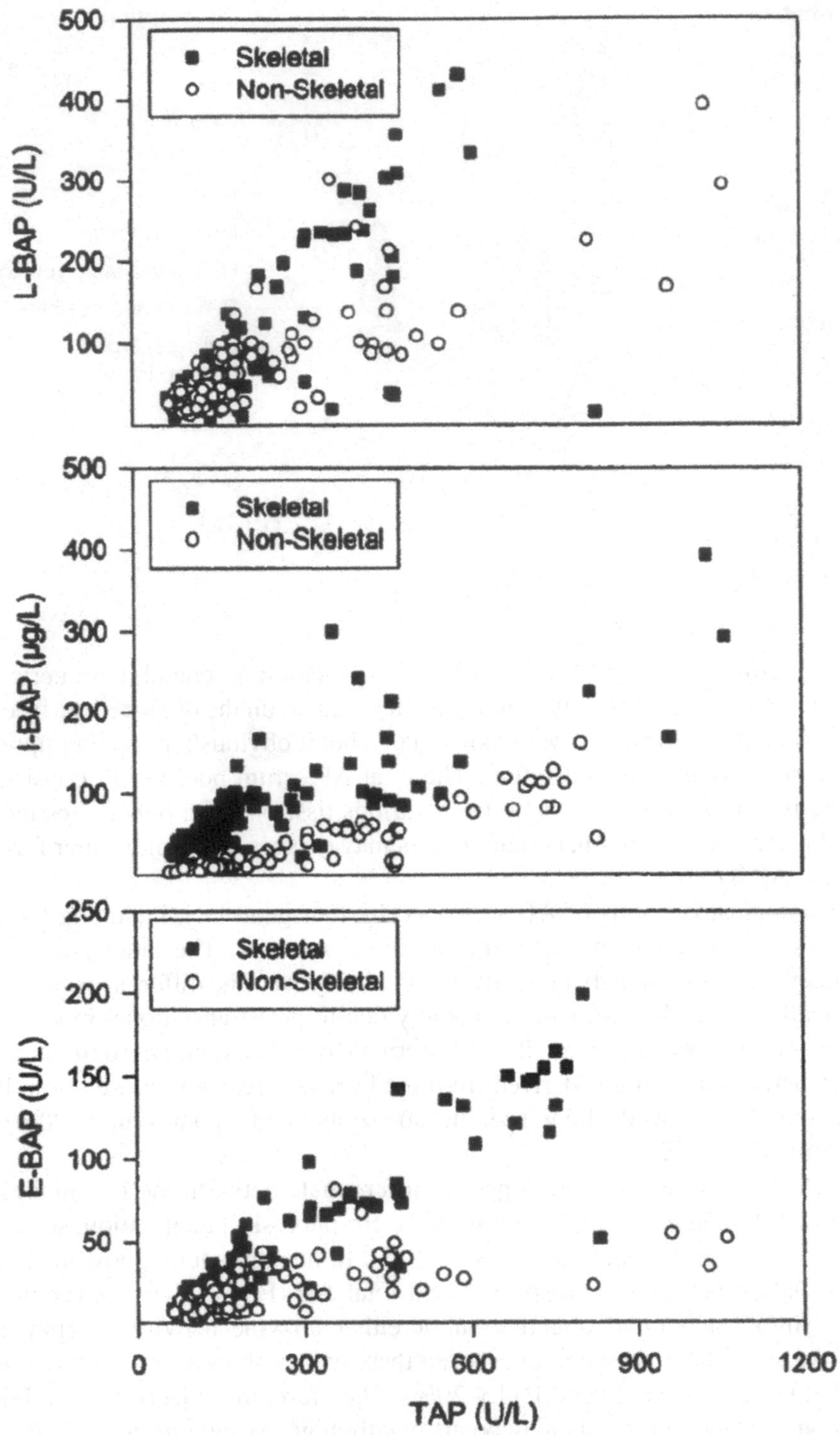
Skeletal
Non-Skeletal
L-BAP (U/L)
500
400
300
200
100
Skeletal
Non-Skeletal
I-BAP (µg/L)
500
400
300
200
100
Skeletal
Non-Skeletal
E-BAP (U/L)
250
200
150
100
50
0
300
600
900
1200
TAP (U/L)

Fig. 2.

activity *(18,19)*. From a clinical perspective, however, detection of the bone-specific AP (BAP) isoenzyme is increasingly preferred because of its higher specificity *(8,20,21)*.

Osteocalcin (OC) is a 5.8 kDa, hydroxyapatite-binding protein exclusively synthesized by osteoblast, odontoblasts, and hypertrophic chondrocytes *(22–24)*. One of the major characteristics of OC are three vitamin K-dependent, gamma-carboxyglutamic acid (Gla) residues, which are responsible for the calcium binding properties of the protein *(25)*. At its carboxy-terminus, OC can also interact with other proteins, including cell surface receptors. These functions predispose OC as a molecule active in the organization of the extracellular matrix. Earlier research has suggested that OC is involved in the process of osteoid mineralization, as the protein is expressed mainly during this phase of bone formation. However, although OC is now known for more than 20 years, its precise function has yet to be determined. More recently, new light has been cast on this issue through the development of an osteocalcin knockout mouse model. Unexpectedly, these animals have increased cortical and trabecular thickness, and their bones seem mechanically more stable than those of the wild type *(26)*. Although the knockout model awaits further characterization, it seems that OC is involved in the bone remodeling process and may act via a negative feedback mechanism.

OC is considered as a specific marker of osteoblast function *(27)*. It is estimated that, directly after its release from osteoblasts, the largest part of the newly synthesized protein is incorporated into the extracellular bone matrix where it constitutes approximately 15% of the non-collagenous protein fraction. A smaller fraction is released into the circulation where it can be detected by immunoassays *(28–34)*. Serum levels of immunoreactive OC have been shown to correlate well with the bone formation rate as assessed by histomorphometry *(35)*. However, the peptide is readily subject to rapid degradation in serum, so that both intact peptides and OC fragments of various sizes coexist in the circulation *(36–38)*. Furthermore, since OC is incorporated into the bone matrix, some investigators have suggested that OC fragments may be released even during bone resorption. This may be particularly true for some smaller N-terminal fragments of OC, which are found in individuals with high bone turnover *(39–41)*. The ensuing heterogeneity of OC fragments in serum results in considerable limitations in the clinical application of this a priori highly specific marker. Thus, the various assays used to measure OC in serum detect fragments of various sizes and usually, epitope specificity and antibody cross-reactivity of the assays are ill defined. In practice, different immunoassays have routinely yielded such varying results in measurements that they are incomparable *(42–44)*.

Two-site immunoassays, utilizing antibodies detecting different parts of the OC molecule, have been introduced that detect the intact 1–49 OC molecule. However, only one-third of the total OC serum pool represents intact OC, and due to the instability of

Fig. 2. (continued) Correlation between serum total and bone-specific alkaline phosphatase. Patients with non-skeletal disease had chronic hepatic failure, chronic obstructive pulmonary disease, or chronic renal failure. Patients with skeletal disease had Paget's disease of bone, primary or secondary hyperparathyroidism, or metastatic bone disease. TAP, total alkaline phosphatase; L-BAP, bone alkaline phosphatase measured by lectin precipitation assay; I-BAP, bone alkaline phosphatase measured by immunoradiometric assay (IRMA); E-BAP, bone alkaline phosphatase measured by enzyme-linked immunosorbant assay (ELISA) (From Woitge et al. *(17)* with permission).

OC in serum, rapid loss of immunoreactivity is seen with these assays when samples are being left alone for more than 1 h at room temperature. To circumvent this problem, newer assays measure the largest degradation product of OC, the 1–43 (N-terminal/mid-molecule) fragment. This fragment, which represents one-third of the circulating OC pool, is a result of proteolytic degradation of the intact molecule and may in part be generated by active osteoblasts. Although little is known about the function of the N-terminal fragment, its measurement eliminates in part the problem of pre-analytical instability *(44,45)*. However, quick processing of the blood sample after drawing is essential for most assays since a loss of reactivity is noted within a few hours at room temperature. The same applies to sera subjected to multiple thawing, or prolonged storage at temperatures above –25°C.

The *procollagen type I propeptides* are derived from collagen type I, the most abundant form of collagen found in bone *(46)*. However, type I collagen is also present in other tissues such as skin, dentin, cornea, vessels, fibrocartilage, and tendons. In bone, collagen is synthesized by osteoblasts in the form of pre-procollagen. These precursor molecules are characterized by short-terminal extension peptides: the amino (N-) terminal propeptide (PINP) and the carboxy (C-) terminal propeptide (PICP) *(47)* (Fig. 3). After secretion into the extracellular space, the globular trimeric propeptides are enzymatically cleaved *(48)* and liberated into the circulation. PICP has a Mw of 115 kDa, is stabilized by disulfide bonds, is cleared by liver endothelial cells via the mannose receptor and therefore has a short serum half-life of 6–8 min *(49,50)*. PINP has a Mw of only 70 kDa, is rich in proline and hydroxyproline, and is eliminated from the circulation by liver endothelial cells by a scavenger receptor. Since both PICP and PINP are generated from newly synthesized collagen in a stoichiometric fashion, the propeptides are considered quantitative measures of newly formed type I collagen. Although type I collagen propeptides may also arise from other sources, most of the non-skeletal tissues exhibit a slower turnover than bone and contribute very little to the circulating propeptide pool.

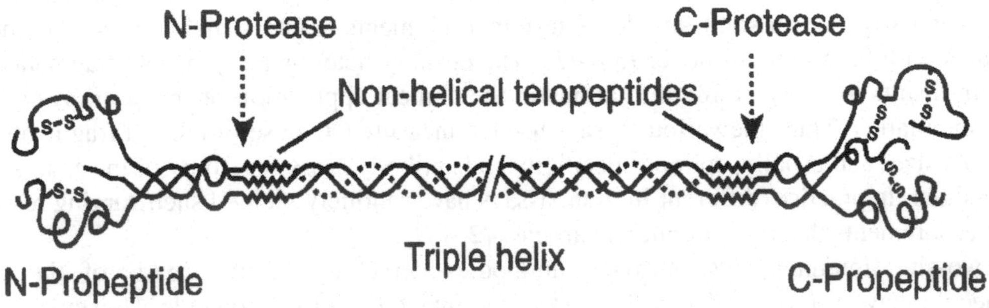

Fig. 3. Schematic representation of the collagen type I molecule. The carboxy- and amino-terminal propeptides are cleaved by specific propeptidases and are partly released into the circulation (Figure courtesy of Dr. Simon Robins, Aberdeen).

Both propeptides are currently measured by specific immunoassays *(51,52)*. Different studies have shown good correlations between serum PICP levels and the rate of bone formation *(53,54)*. While the clinical relevance of PICP in the evaluation of metabolic bone diseases is still viewed with skepticism *(55,56)*, serum PINP appears to be of greater diagnostic validity. From a practical point of view, the thermostability of the propeptides is an advantage in that extended transport and storage times are well tolerated without significant loss of signal. The propeptides share these properties with most of the parameters of collagen metabolism (e.g., cross-links, ICTP, NTx, CTx, hydroxyproline; vide infra).

MARKERS OF BONE RESORPTION

Except for tartrate-resistant acid phosphatase, the majority of bone resorption markers are degradation products of bone collagen (Fig. 4). Only recently, non-collagenous proteins, such as bone sialoprotein, and osteoclast-derived enzymes, such as cathepsin K and L, have been investigated as markers of bone turnover.

Hydroxyproline (OHP) is formed intracellularly from the post-translational hydroxylation of proline and constitutes 12–14% of the total amino acid content of mature collagen. About 90% of the OHP liberated during the degradation of bone collagen is primarily metabolized in the liver *(57)*. Subsequently, it is excreted in the urine where it may be detected either as a free or as a peptide-bound hydroxyproline by colorimetric or HPLC methods *(58,59)*. Urinary OHP is usually considered an index of bone resorption. However, it should be noted that significant amounts of urinary OHP are derived from the degradation of newly synthesized collagens *(60)*. In addition, hydroxyproline can be found in other tissues such as the skin *(61)* and, moreover, liberated from the metabolism of elastin and C1q *(62)*. Urinary hydroxyproline is therefore considered an unspecific index of collagen turnover and, consequently, has been largely replaced by more specific techniques.

The *hydroxylysine-glycosides* arise during the posttranslational phase of collagen synthesis and occur in two forms, glycosyl-galactosyl-hydroxylysine (GGHL) and galactosyl-hydroxylysine (GHL) *(63)* (Fig. 4). Both components are released into the circulation during collagen degradation and may be measured in urine by HPLC after appropriate derivatization *(64)*. The intrinsic advantage of hydroxylysine over that of hydroxyproline is that the glycosylated forms are not metabolized and are not influenced by dietary components *(63,64)*. Moreover, GGHL is present in skin and C1q, while GHL is more specific for bone. Thus the ratio of GGHL/GHL may allow for the recognition of existent tissue specificity. Although the hydroxylysines have potential as markers of bone resorption *(65–67)*, their major disadvantage is presently the absence of a convenient immunoassay format.

The *3-hydroxypyridinium cross-links of collagen, pyridinoline (PYD) and deoxypyridinoline* (DPD) are formed during the extracellular maturation of fibrillar collagens. As trifunctional cross-links, they bridge several collagen peptides and mechanically stabilize the collagen molecule *(68–70)* (Fig. 4). During bone resorption, cross-linked collagens are proteolytically broken down and the cross-link components are released into the circulation and the urine *(71–73)*. The measurement of hydroxypyridinium cross-links is not influenced by the degradation of newly synthesized collagens and their levels strictly reflect the degradation of mature, i.e., cross-linked collagens. In addition, the urinary excretion of pyridinium cross-links is independent of dietary sources since neither PYD nor DPD are taken up from food *(74)*. Finally, the two hydroxypyridinium components show a high specificity for skeletal tissues. While PYD is found in cartilage, bone, ligaments and vessels, DPD is almost exclusively found in bone and dentin. Neither derivative is present in the collagen of skin or in other sources such as C1q or elastin *(62,75,76)*. Since bone has a much higher turnover than cartilage, ligaments, vessels or tendons, the amounts of

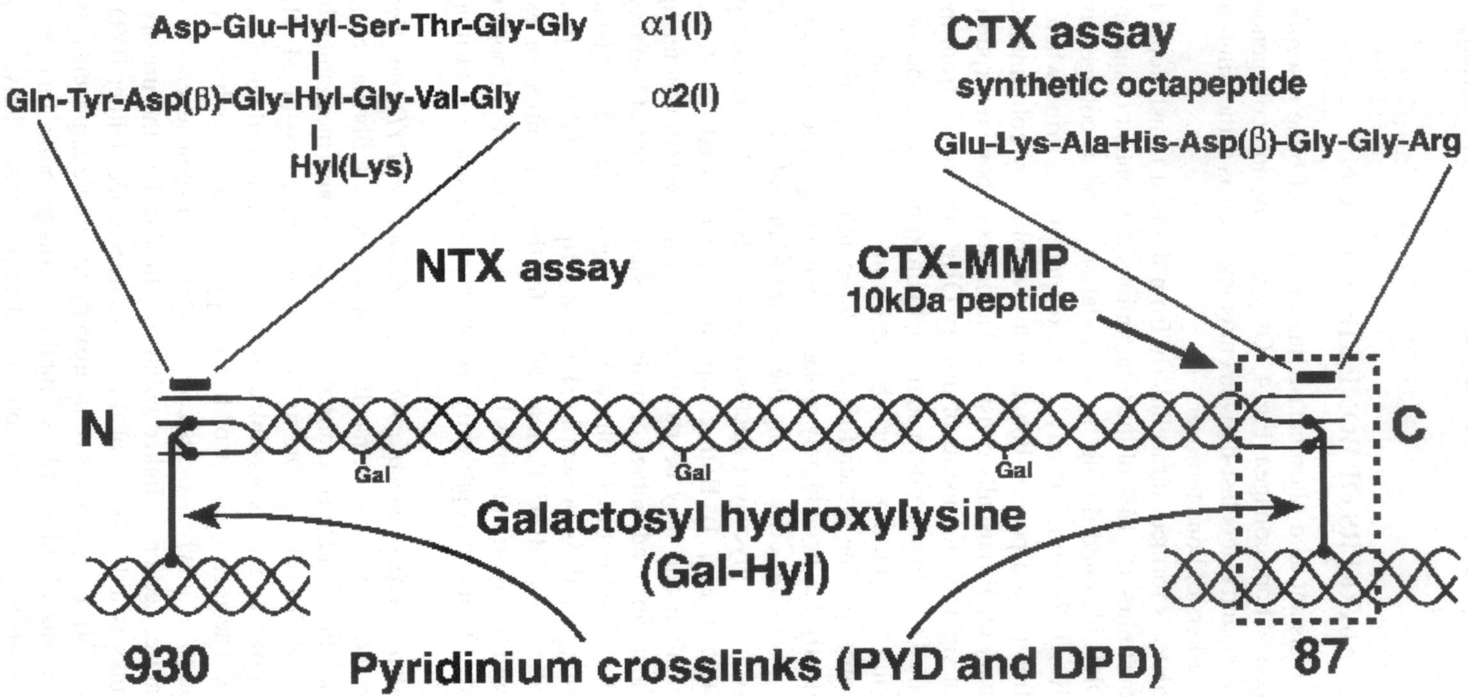

Fig. 4. Molecular basis of currently used markers of type I collagen-related degradation. For more details, see text and Table 1 (Figure courtesy Dr. Simon Robins, Aberdeen).

PYD and DPD in serum or urine are mainly derived from the skeleton. Thus, the pyridinium cross-links are currently viewed the best indices for assessing bone resorption *(77–79)*.

Initially, PYD and DPD were quantified in urine by reverse-phase ion-paired HPLC technique, combined with a pre-fractionation step using cellulose partition chromatography, and hydrolysis of urine samples to convert all cross-links into the peptide free forms *(76,80–82)*. Today, automated techniques for the measurement in urine and serum are available. Analysis of urine by HPLC without initial hydrolysis showed that 40–50% of the cross-links were present in peptide-free form *(83)*. Although the amounts of free and peptide-bound cross-links seem to vary with bone pathologies, today direct immunoassays for *free* and peptide-bound cross-links are widely used. Under normal conditions, these assays have been shown to produce results similar to those provided by the traditional HPLC technique *(84–86)*.

The *cross-linked telopeptides of type I collagen* are derived from specific regions of the collagen type I molecule, namely the amino-terminal (NTP) and the carboxy-terminal (CTP) telopeptide (Fig. 4).

The first collagen telopeptide assay was a RIA for the carboxy-terminal type I collagen telopeptide (ICTP) in serum *(87)*. The respective antibodies were raised against a cross-link-containing collagen peptide (Mw 8.5 kDa) isolated from human bone. The antigenic determinant requires a trivalent cross-link, including two phenylalanine-rich domains of the telopeptide region of the alpha-1 chain of type I collagen. Divalently and non-cross-linked peptides do not react with the antibody, nor do peptides isolated from skin. Despite the fact that the initial peptide contained pyridinoline, the assay also detected other cross-link forms such as deoxypyridinoline or pyrrole cross-links. The ICTP assay appears to be sensitive for pathological bone resorption as seen in multiple myeloma, metastatic bone disease, and other degradation processes involving hasty breakdown of skeletal and non-skeletal type I collagen *(88)*.

Another group of immunoassays involves the carboxy-terminal telopeptide of type I collagen, abbreviated CTX-I *(89)* (Fig. 4). Employing a polyclonal antiserum against a synthetic octapeptide containing the cross-linking site, a first ELISA (termed β-CTX) recognized the C-terminal type I collagen telopeptide containing an isoaspartyl (=β-aspartyl) peptide bond in its L-enantiomeric form *(90)*. The β-L-aspartyl is considered to result mainly from the aging of extracellular proteins. Only one peptide strand is necessary for immunoreactivity. Meanwhile, a monoclonal-based RIA for the non-isomerized octapeptide (EKAH-αD-GGR) in urine has been developed ("α-CTX") *(91)*. Simultaneous measurement of both forms may be used to calculate the ratio of α-CTX/β-CTX as an index of bone turnover. This ratio has been shown to be elevated in the urine of patients with untreated Paget's disease of bone, where rapid bone formation and resorption result in an increase of α-CTx (non-isomerized octapeptide) *(92)*.

Further to isomerization, many proteins are also subjected to racemization of certain residues. Both processes are considered an effect of aging, as the extent of racemization and isomerization increases with the time elapsed since synthesis of the protein. Additionally, antibodies directed against the D-aspartic acid residues in the CTX molecule have been described *(93)*. Thus, immunoassays are now existing for all four possible isomers of the CTX molecule: the native α-L form, the β-isomerized isoaspartyl peptide (βL), and the respective racemized forms α-D and β-D. The differential use of these assays may possibly provide information on the age-dependent changes of collagen in health and disease *(94)*, although the clinical relevance is questionable.

More recently, sandwich ELISAs for the measurement of ββ-CTX and αα-CTX in serum have been developed, and both assays have been shown to reflect bone resorption in a number of different pathologies *(95)*. Serum and urinary CTX values are highly correlated ($r = 0.86$) suggesting that the antigen is similar in both analytical media.

Yet another peptide assay measures the cross-linked N-terminal telopeptide of type I collagen. This assay (termed NTX assay) utilizes a monoclonal antibody raised against an epitope on the alpha-2 chain of type I collagen. *(96)* (Fig. 4). However, the antibody seems to react with several cross-linking components, and the presence of a pyridinium cross-link is not essential for reactivity. As a matter of fact, digests of skin collagen exhibited similar reactivity with the NTX assay as skeletal extracts *(97)*. Both the monoclonal antibody and the assay format are identical for the urine and the serum-based assays. Expectedly, both assays show good correlation, and the analyte seems to be stable at room temperature and during up to three freeze-thaw cycles *(98)*.

Bone sialoprotein (BSP) is a phosphorylated glycoprotein with an apparent Mw of 70–80 kDa, which accounts for 5–10% of the non-collagenous matrix of bone *(99,100)*. The protein has been shown to be a major synthetic product of active osteoblasts and odontoblasts, but was also found in osteoclast-like and malignant cell lines. Consequently, BSP or its mRNA is detected mainly in mineralized tissue such as bone, dentin, and at the interface of calcifying cartilage *(101–103)*. Intact BSP contains an Arg-Gly-Asp (RGD) integrin recognition sequence, improves the attachment of osteoblasts and osteoclasts to plastic surfaces *(104)*, binds preferentially to the α2 chain of collagen, nucleates hydroxyapatite crystal formation in vitro *(105)*, and appears to enhance osteoclast-mediated bone resorption *(104)*. The protein is therefore considered to play an important role in cell–matrix adhesion processes and in the supramolecular organization of the extracellular matrix of mineralized tissues.

Others and we have developed immunoassays for the measurement of bone sialoprotein in serum *(106,107)*. So far, all of these assays are based upon polyclonal antisera, and little is known about the specific nature of the respective epitopes. Antibodies do not cross-react with non-collagenous proteins such as osteonectin, fibronectin, or osteocalcin *(107)*. In serum, the majority of BSP is bound to factor H, a major regulator of the alternate complement pathway, which is found at 0.5 mg/ml in serum. Although this phenomenon is of unknown physiological relevance, BSP/factor H-binding studies suggest that current immunoassays do detect only a fraction of bioavailable BSP in serum *(108)*. Based upon clinical data and the rapid reduction of serum BSP levels following intravenous bisphosphonate treatment, it is assumed that serum BSP reflects processes mainly related to bone resorption *(109)*.

Tartrate-resistant acid phosphatase (TRAP) belongs to the family of ubiquitously occurring acid phosphatases, of which at least five different isoforms are known. These isoforms are expressed by different tissues and cells such as prostate, bone, spleen, platelets, erythrocytes, and macrophages. All acid phosphatases are inhibited by L(+)-tartrate, except band 5, which was therefore termed tartrate-resistant acid phosphatase (TRAP). Of the latter, two subforms, 5a and 5b, are known, and recent research has shown that TRAP-5b is characteristic of osteoclasts *(110)*. The origin of TRAP-5a is unknown, but may be expressed by macrophages. The two isoforms 5a and 5b are different in that 5a contains sialic acid, whereas 5b does not. So far, most assays for the measurement of TRAP in blood were colorimetric and detected both isoforms without differentiating between bands 5a and 5b. More recently, specific immunoassays for TRAP 5b have been described and clinical results indicate that this marker may be useful to assess osteoclast activity *(111,112)*. The antibodies for these assays were raised against material isolated from the spleen of a patient with hairy cell leukemia *(113)* or against TRAP 5b isolated from human cord plasma *(114)*. For the conventional TRAP assays, care should be taken after phlebotomy to stabilize the enzyme since TRAP loses more than 20% of its activity per hour at room temperature. This can be prevented by the addition of citrate buffer to the sample *(115)*.

Cathepsin K is a member of the cysteine protease family that, unlike other cathepsins, has the unique ability to cleave both helical and telopeptide regions of collagen I *(116,117)*. Its clinical relevance was appreciated with the discovery that pycnodysostosis, an autosomal recessive disease characterized by osteopetrosis, was the result of mutations in the cathepsin K gene *(118)*. This clinical phenotype has been confirmed in cathepsin K null mice showing dysfunctional matrix digestion *(119,120)*. Immunocytochemical studies have shown that cathepsin K is located intracellularly in vesicles, granules, and vacuoles throughout the cytoplasm of osteoclasts and that it is secreted into bone resorption lacunae for extracellular collagen degradation *(121)*. Recently, a new enzyme-linked immunoassay for measurements of cathepsin K in serum has been developed. Due to the fact that cathepsin K is expressed and secreted by osteoclasts during active bone resorption, cathepsin K, and specifically its circulating form, may be a useful and specific biochemical marker of osteoclastic activity.

VARIABILITY

Most bone turnover markers exhibit significant within-subject variability. This poses a major problem in the practical use of bone markers: Whenever a change in a bone marker level is observed in an individual patient (e.g., following an invention), this change must be interpreted against the background of the respective marker's variability. Therefore, knowledge of the sources of variability and the strategies used to cope with "background noise" are essential for the meaningful interpretation of bone markers.

In general, non-specific variability comprises both pre-analytical (i.e., mostly subject related; CV_{PA}) and analytical (i.e., mostly assay related; CV_A) factors. Total variability is considered the sum of pre-analytical and analytical variation and defined as $CV_T^2 = CV_{PA}^2 + CV_A^2$. The ideal marker and assay are characterized by (i) excellent analytical performance (i.e., high precision and accuracy) and (ii) minimal and predictable pre-analytical variability. Unfortunately, no method in clinical chemistry completely meets all of these criteria. Indeed, most of the currently available assays for biochemical markers of bone turnover are characterized by substantial pre-analytical variability. The relevant pre-analytical factors affecting marker variability are summarized in Table 2.

A number of factors need to be taken into account when employing serial measurements of biochemical markers to determine changes in bone turnover. To minimize some of the limitations linked to pre-analytical and analytical variability, standardized sampling and sample handling are mandatory to obtain reliable results.

Table 2
Sources of Pre-analytical Variability

- Technical sources
  - Specimen and mode of sample collection
  - Specimen handling and storage
  - Thermodegradation
  - Photolysis
  - Timing of sample collection (see also diurnal variation)
  - Between laboratory variation
  - Biological (subject-related) sources
  - Age
    - Puberty, somatic growth, menopausal transition, menopause, aging, frailty
  - Gender
  - Ethnicity
  - Recent fractures (up to 1 year)
  - Pregnancy/lactation
  - Drugs
    - Anti-resorptive agent (e.g., HRT, bisphosphonates, SERMs, strontium, OPG)
    - Anabolic agents (e.g., anabolic steroids, PTH, PTHrP, strontium)
    - Glucocorticosteroids
    - Anticonvulsants
    - GnRH agonists
    - Oral Contraception
  - Non-skeletal disease
    - Diabetes
    - Thyroid disease
    - Renal impairment (GFR < 20 ml/min/1.73 m^2)
    - Liver disease
    - Systemic inflammatory disease (IBD, RA, COPD, etc.)
    - Degenerative joint disease
  - Immobility/loss of gravity (bed rest, space flight)
  - Diet
  - Exercise
  - Temporal variability
  - Diurnal (circadian)
  - Menstrual
  - Seasonal

TECHNICAL SOURCES OF VARIABILITY

In addition to parameters of assay performance (Figs. 5 and 6), factors such as the choice of sample (i.e., serum vs. urine), mode of sample collection (e.g., 24-h collection vs. first or second morning void), the appropriate preparation of the patient (e.g., pre-sampling diet/fasting/exercise before phlebotomy), the correct handling, processing, and storage of specimens should always be considered. This is important as these technical sources of variability are controllable and hence modifiable. For the purpose of practical use, some technical aspects of variability shall be discussed in more detail (Table 2).

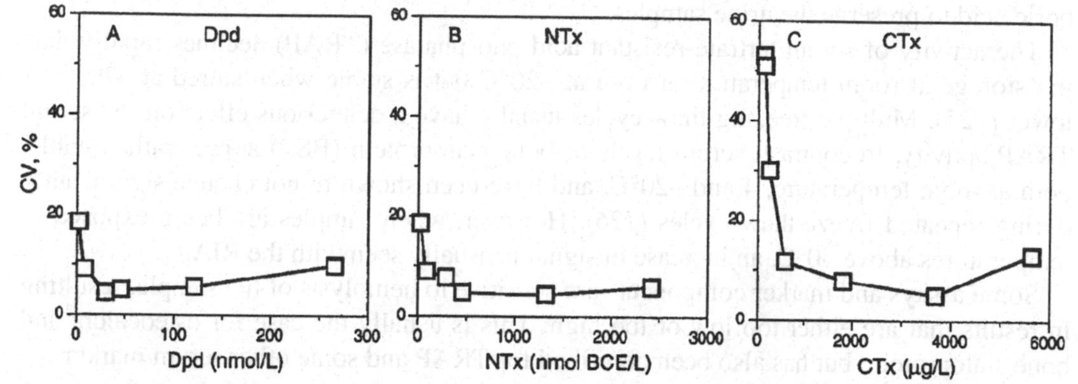

Fig. 5. Intra-assay precision profiles for three immunoassays measuring type I collagen degradation products in urine. (A) Deooxypyridinoline (DPD), (B) amino-terminal cross-linked telopeptide (NTX), and (C) carboxy-terminal octapeptide (CTX) (From Ju et al. *(197)* with permission).

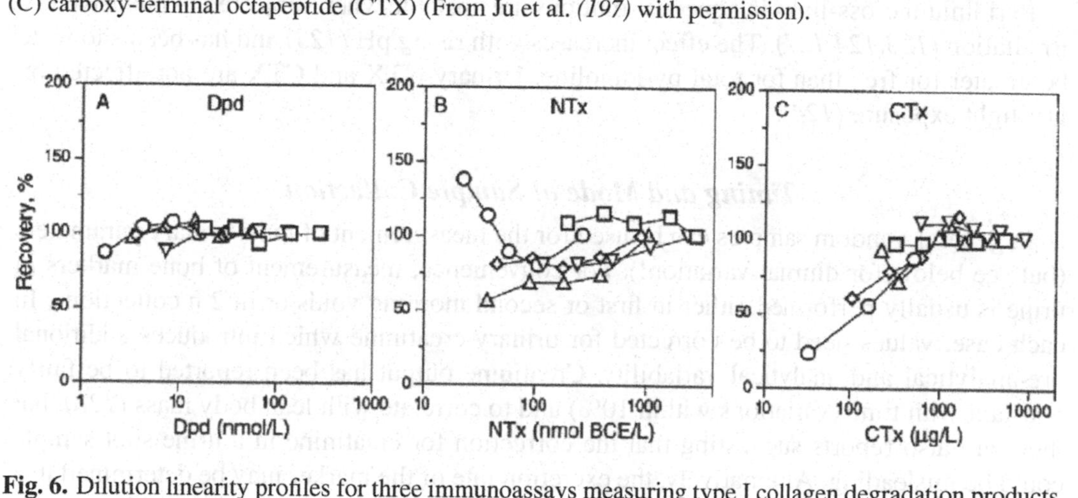

Fig. 6. Dilution linearity profiles for three immunoassays measuring type I collagen degradation products in urine ($n = 4$). (A) Deoxypyridinoline (DPD), (B) amino-terminal cross-linked telopeptide (NTX), and (C) carboxy-terminal octapeptide (CTX)(From Ju et al. *(197)* with permission).

Thermodegradation

Some bone markers are sensitive to ambient conditions such as temperature. Thermodegradation should always be a concern with assays directed against the intact OC(1–49) molecule. Rapid enzymatic cleavage of the peptide into smaller fragments will lead to significant signal losses if the serum sample is kept at room temperature for more than 1–2 h. Adding protease inhibitors will delay, but by no means prevent this process *(122)*. Both the free and the conjugated forms of PYD and DPD have been shown to be stable in urine samples kept at room temperature for several weeks. Several reports show that pyridinium cross-links can be stored at –20°C for years and that repeated freeze-thaw cycles of urine samples have no effect on the concentrations of PYD and DPD *(123)*. Similar stability has been reported for the urinary N-terminal (NTX) and C-terminal (CTX) collagen type I telopeptides, while C-terminal telopeptide in serum (ICTP) loses up to 12% of the signal when stored at room temperature for 5 days *(124)*. The stability of glycosylated hydroxylysine residues has not been fully characterized yet, but it may be necessary to add boric acid to preserve the urine samples.

The activity of serum tartrate-resistant acid phosphatase (TRAP) declines rapidly during storage at room temperature or even at –20°C but is stable when stored at –70°C or lower *(125)*. Multiple freezing-thaw cycles usually have a deleterious effect on the serum TRAP activity. In contrast, serum levels of bone sialoprotein (BSP) appear rather stable, both at room temperature, 4 and –20°C, and have been shown to not change significantly during repeated freeze-thaw cycles *(126)*. However, when samples are being exposed to temperatures above 30°C, an increase in signal is usually seen with the RIA.

Some assays and marker components are sensitive to hemolysis of the sample, resulting in results that are either too low or too high. This is usually the case for osteocalcin and bone sialoprotein, but has also been described for TRAP and some other serum markers.

Photolysis

Pyridinium cross-links in aqueous solutions are unstable when subjected to intensive UV irradiation *(123,124,127)*. The effect increases with rising pH *(123)* and has been shown to be greater for free than for total pyridinoline. Urinary NTX and CTX are not affected by UV light exposure *(124)*.

Timing and Mode of Sample Collection

In general, random samples can be used for the measurement of most urinary parameters (but see below for diurnal variation!). For convenience, measurement of bone markers in urine is usually performed either in first or second morning voids or in 2 h collections. In each case, values need to be corrected for urinary creatinine which introduces additional pre-analytical and analytical variability. Creatinine output has been reported to be fairly constant with time (variations within 10%) and to correlate with lean body mass *(128)*, but there are also reports suggesting that the correction for creatinine in a urine spot sample could be misleading. Alternatively, the excretion rate of the marker may be determined in a 24-h urine collection. However, these collections are subject to inevitable inaccuracies due to collection errors. With most markers, similar results are obtained from either 24-h, 2-h, or spot urine (FMV, SMV) collections.

It is long known that bone turnover and thus bone markers show significant diurnal variations, with highest values in the early morning hours and lowest values during the afternoon and evening *(129)*. Most studies report daily amplitudes of 15–30% *(130–135)*, although the most pronounced diurnal changes have been communicated for CTX *(136)* (Fig. 7). It should be borne in mind that the slope of diurnal changes is steepest during the morning hours, which is usually the time at which urine samples are collected. This is true for both

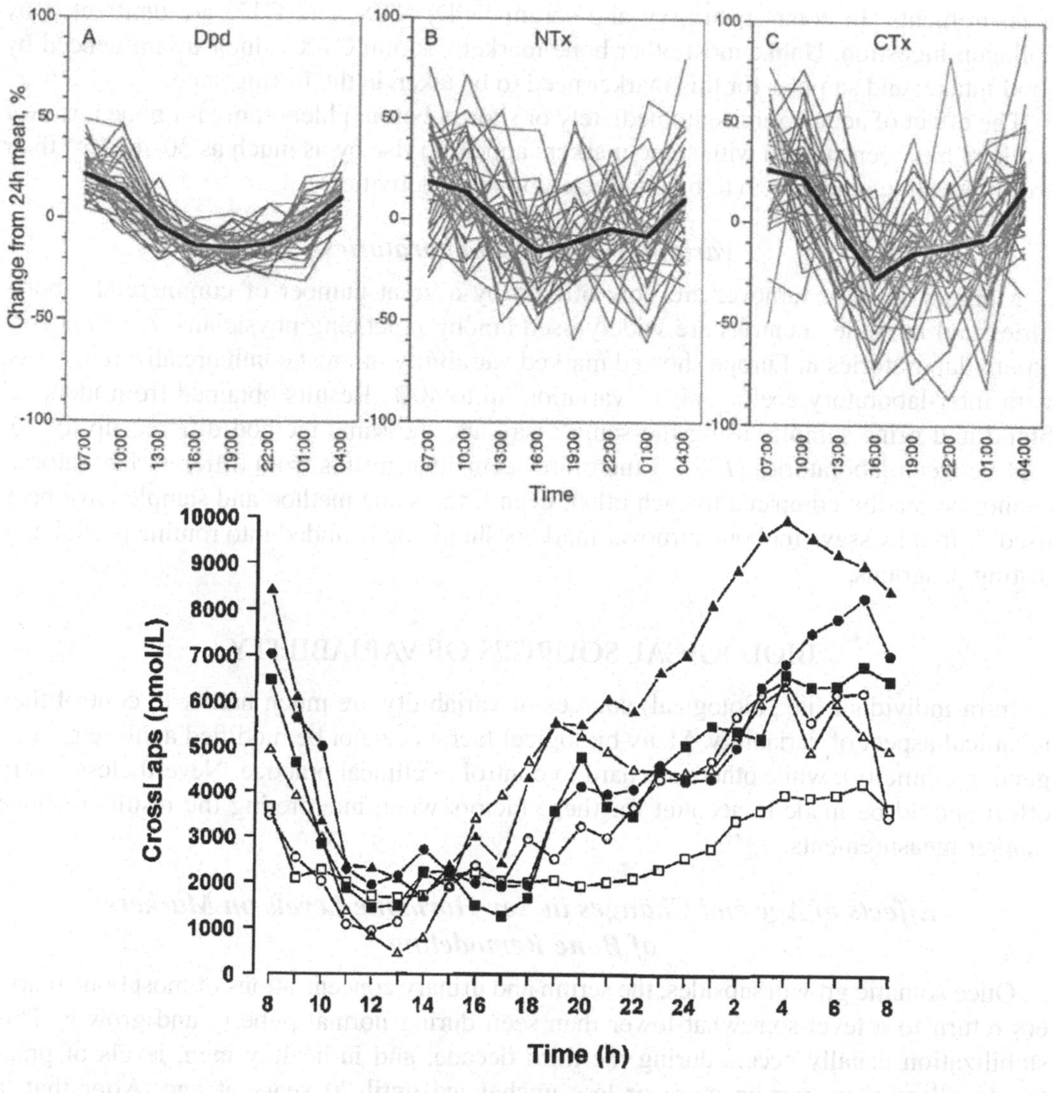

Fig. 7. Diurnal variation. (A–C) Comparison of three immunoassays measuring type I collagen degradation products in urine. (A) Deoxypyridinoline (DPD), (B) amino-terminal cross-linked telopeptide (NTX), and (C) carboxy-terminal octapeptide (CTX). All values are creatinine corrected. The thick line represents the mean, while thin lines are individual subjects (From Ju et al. *(197)* with permission). (D) Diurnal variation in serum CTX levels in six healthy male volunteers. On an average, the peak value was 66% higher and the nadir was 60% lower than the calculated daily mean (From Wichers et al. *(136)* with permission).

urinary and serum markers. Controlling the timing of sample collection is therefore a "bare necessity" for all types of markers (see also further below).

In addition, the effects of diet and food intake need to be considered with certain markers. For example, the ingestion of hydroxyproline-rich foods, such as meat or gelatine, will markedly affect measurements of OHP in urine *(137)*. It is therefore necessary to instruct patients to keep a collagen-free diet for at least 24 h before collecting their urine for OHP measurements. In contrast, urinary and serum DPD, NTX, and CTX are unaffected by collagen ingestion. Unlike most other bone markers, serum CTX values are influenced by food intake, and samples for this marker need to be taken in the fasting state.

The effect of acute exercise immediately or shortly before phlebotomy for bone turnover markers has been studied with some markers appear to rise by as much as 30–40% of their baseline value, others seem to be unaffected by these activities.

Variation Between Laboratories

Markers of bone turnover are now offered by a great number of commercial laboratories and in some countries are widely used among practicing physicians. A recent trial among laboratories in Europe showed marked variability of most commercialized test kits, with inter-laboratory coefficients of variation up to 40%. Results obtained from identical blood and urine samples using the same assay and the same method differed up to 5.6-fold between laboratories *(138)*. It therefore seems that results from different laboratories cannot be readily compared to each other, even if the same method and sample have been used. Immunoassays for bone turnover markers should be included into routine proficiency testing programs.

BIOLOGICAL SOURCES OF VARIABILITY

Intra-individual (i.e., biological) sources of variability are much harder to control than technical aspect of variability. Many biological factors cannot be modified at all (e.g., age, gender, ethnicity), while others are hard to control in clinical practice. Nevertheless, every effort should be made to account for these factors when interpreting the results of bone marker measurements.

Effects of Age and Changes in Sex Hormone Levels on Markers of Bone Remodeling

Once somatic growth subsides, the serum and urinary concentrations of most bone markers return to a level somewhat lower than seen during normal puberty and growth. This stabilization usually occurs during the third decade, and in healthy men, levels of practically all markers remain more or less unchanged until 70 years of age. After that, a slight increase is usually seen in formation markers such as serum BAP or OC, and most resorption markers *(139–142)*.

Menopause is associated with a substantial acceleration in bone turnover, which is mirrored by a 50–100% increase in both bone formation and bone resorption markers *(139,142–151)* (Fig. 8). In early postmenopausal women, this increase in bone turnover may be attenuated by calcium supplementation *(152)*. Long-term treatment of women with estrogen was shown to reduce resorption markers such as DPD and NTx to premenopausal levels and to correct secondary hyperparathyroidism *(153,154)*. A prospective study covering the perimenopausal transition in healthy women suggests that changes in bone turnover start during late pre-menopause with a decrease in bone formation, which only later is followed by a rise in bone resorption *(155)*. It is now widely accepted that the accelerated rate of bone loss seen after the menopause is mainly due to an uncoupling in bone turnover and an increase in bone resorption. Studies employing specific bone markers indicate that bone turnover continues to be increased (and to be associated with bone loss) even during

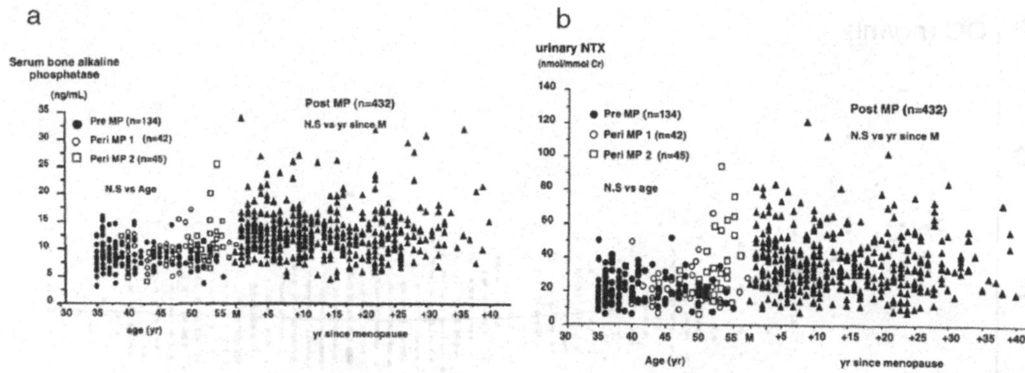

Fig. 8. Age-related changes in (**A**) bone-specific alkaline phosphatase and (**B**) urinary collagen type I amino-terminal cross-linked telopeptide (NTX). Pre, premenopausal women; peri MP 1, early perimenopausal women; peri MP 2, late perimenopausal women; post MP, postmenopausal women; M, menopause (From Garnero et al. *(156)* with permission).

late menopause *(156)*. In some postmenopausal women *(157)*, but particularly in the very elderly *(158,159)*, this increase in bone turnover is often, but not always, found to due to vitamin D and/or calcium deficiency and secondary hyperparathyroidism.

In men, the pattern of age-dependent change in bone markers is quite different from that observed in women. Markers of bone formation and resorption are high in men aged 20–30 years which corresponds to the late phase of formation of peak bone mass. Thereafter they decrease reaching their lowest levels between 50 and 60 years *(160–163)* (Fig. 9).

While there is general agreement on the age-related changes of bone turnover in adult men between 20 and 60 years of age, data on bone turnover rates in men over the age of 60 years are largely discordant. Based on recent cross-sectional studies, concentrations of bone formation markers remained unchanged *(163)*, decreased *(160,164)*, or increased *(161,165,166)* with age in men over 60 years. Most studies evaluating age-related changes in bone resorption markers observed an increase in serum and urinary indices *(160,161,163,166,167)*. However, this was not confirmed in other population-based studies showing no change in resorption indices with age *(162,168)*. A careful analysis of the published data provides clues that may help to explain some of these discrepancies. Differences in studies investigating age-dependent changes in bone formation and resorption may be related to diverse population characteristics and sample size, to the use of marker assays with different specificities, to age-related changes in renal and hepatic function, and lastly to the inclusion of men with osteoporosis.

As some biochemical markers of bone turnover are cleared via the kidney (i.e., OC, collagen telopeptides), age-associated decrease in glomerular filtration rate may affect urinary and, to a larger extent, serum marker concentrations. In case of decreased renal function, urinary excretion of bone resorption markers expressed as 24-h output may be falsely decreased. Conversely, levels of markers corrected by urinary creatinine can be falsely increased because of decreased creatinine filtration and decreased muscle mass *(169–171)*.

Both static and dynamic histomorphometric studies suggest that bone formation decreases with age in healthy men. In contrast, osteoclast function remains largely constant with age. Consequently, decreased bone formation seems to be the principal factor in

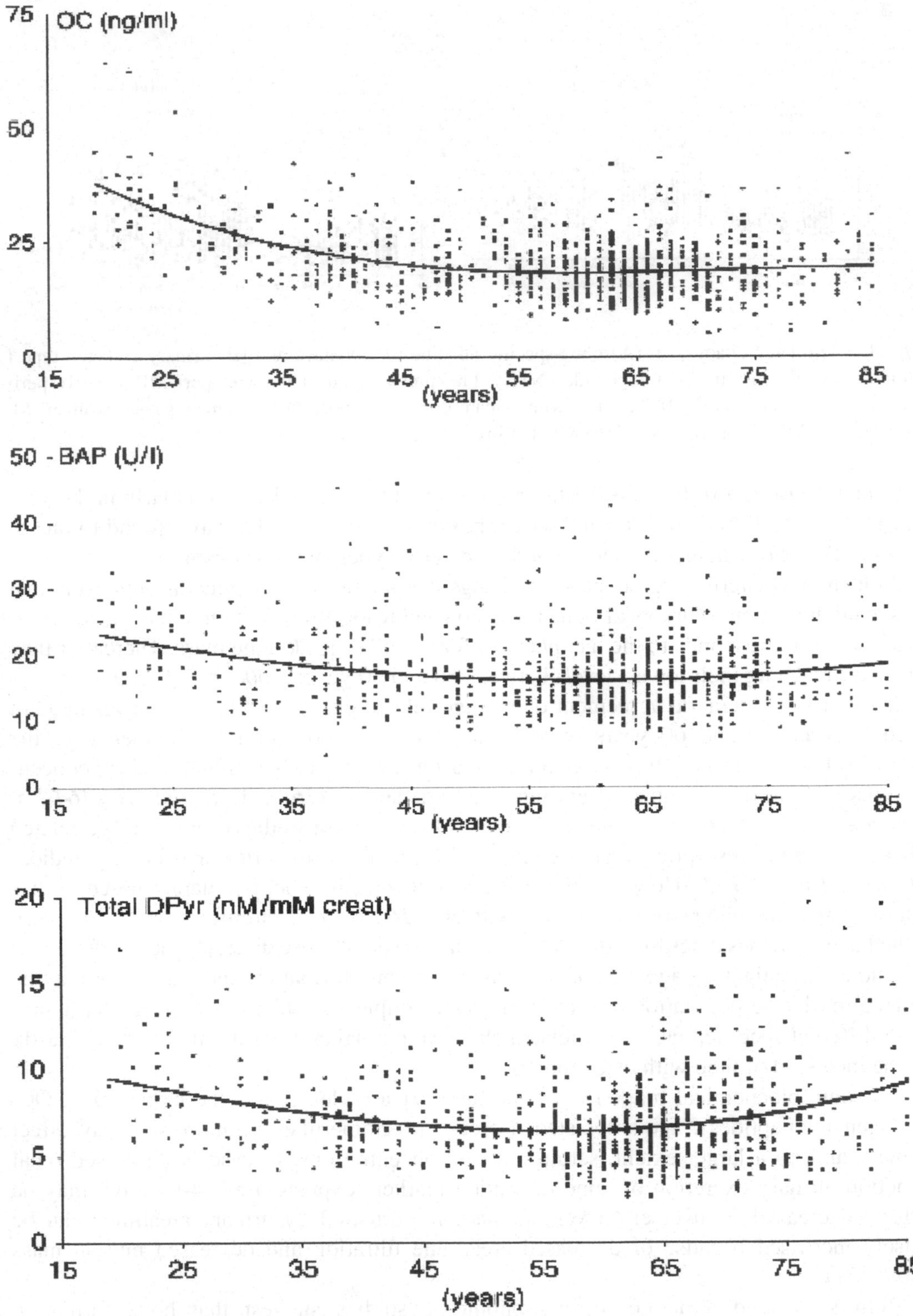

Fig. 9. Age-related changes of biochemical markers of bone formation and resorption in men. **(A)** Serum osteocalcin, **(B)** serum bone-specific alkaline phosphatase, and **(C)** 24-h urinary excretion of deoxypyridinoline (From Szulc et al. *(170)* with permission).

bone loss in men *(172,173)*. In the cohort of healthy men studied by Clarke et al. *(173)*, specific markers of bone resorption (urinary DPD) did not change with age, confirming the histomorphometric findings that osteoclast function is preserved with increasing age in these men. These results are in contrast to some of the previously mentioned cross-sectional studies reporting an age-dependent increase in serum and urinary indices of bone resorption *(160–163,166,167,170–172)*. As mentioned before, differences in population characteristics may, at least in part, explain these inconsistencies. Furthermore, men with idiopathic osteoporosis are histomorphometrically characterized by increased bone resorption with an increase in eroded surfaces up to 90% when compared with age-matched controls *(174)*. Hence, the observed increase in biochemical markers of bone resorption in population-based studies might also be due to the heterogeneity of men investigated including men with osteoporosis.

Taken together it remains controversial to what extent biochemical markers of bone resorption change as a function of age in men over 60 years. Observational studies investigating age-dependent changes in bone marker levels indicate that in elderly men there seems to be an imbalance in bone turnover with increased bone resorption and stable bone formation after the age of 60. As biochemical markers have been shown to be negatively correlated with BMD *(161,170)*, this imbalance in bone turnover may, at least in part, be responsible for the age-related bone loss in men. However, confounding factors such as population characteristics, specificity of bone marker, as well as estimates of renal and liver function have to be taken into account when evaluating age-dependent changes in bone turnover.

Effects of Diurnal Variation on Bone Marker Measurements

Diurnal variation appears not to be affected by age, menopause, physical activity, or season. Although in postmenopausal women bone turnover is higher than in premenopausal women, the circadian variation is similar for both pre- and postmenopausal women and, thus, is not influenced by sex hormones *(175–177)*. The etiology of diurnal variations is unknown. Several hormones, such as parathyroid hormone, growth hormone, or cortisol show diurnal changes and may therefore be involved in the generation of diurnal changes in bone metabolism *(178)*. Independent of this, there is wide agreement that controlling the time of sampling is crucial in order to obtain clinically relevant information from bone markers. Most biochemical markers show significant diurnal variations, with highest values in the early morning hours and lowest values during the afternoon and at night. This has been well documented for most urinary markers *(129)* and amplitudes usually vary between 20 and 30% (Fig. 7). Serum markers usually show less pronounced changes during the day than urine-based indices. However, largely discrepant results have been reported for serum CTX. Wichers et al. *(136)* reported daily amplitudes of serum CTX of up to 66%, while others describe smaller changes (Fig. 7D).

Effect of Low-Frequency Biological Rhythms on Bone Marker Measurements

Intra-individually, biochemical markers of bone turnover not only vary within a single day but in most cases also between consecutive days. This phenomenon is called between-day or day-to-day variability and is apparently due to genuine variations in marker levels and not to analytical imprecision. In general, serum markers show less day-to-day variability than markers of bone turnover measured in urine *(179)*. The day-to-day variation in the urinary excretion of PYD and DPD, measured by HPLC and corrected for creatinine, ranges between 16 and 26% *(180)*. Similar results have been reported for free pyridinoline by EIA (7–25%), for the N-terminal collagen type I telopeptide (NTX, 13–35%), for the C-terminal collagen type I telopeptide (CTX, 12–35%), and for tartrate-resistant acid phosphatase (TRAP, 10–12%) *(179,181)*. Day-to-day variability adds considerably to the total variation of biochemical markers of bone turnover and unlike diurnal variations, day-to-day variability cannot be controlled.

Bone turnover varies with the menstrual cycle with an overall amplitude of approximately 10–20% *(182,183)*. There is evidence to support the suggestion that bone formation is higher during the luteal than the follicular phase *(182)*, whereas bone resorption is higher during the mid-follicular, late-follicular, and early luteal phase *(184)*. Cyclical changes in bone turnover have also been reported in postmenopausal women treated with sequential estrogen/gestagen regimens, showing decreases during estrogen treatment and increases during gestagen treatment *(185)*. In premenopausal women with metabolic bone disease, menstrual variability should be taken into account, and the timing for sampling is probably best during the first 3–7 days of the menstrual cycle.

Bone turnover and its regulation seem to vary with seasonal changes. Some studies have shown that serum 25-OH vitamin D and urinary calcium are higher in summer than in winter and that parathyroid hormone levels show inverse changes *(186,187)*. More recently, seasonal changes were also described for markers of bone metabolism, with a 20–30% lower turnover rate in summer than in winter *(188)*. The increase in bone turnover during the winter period may be due, at least in part, to subclinical vitamin D deficiency.

Effects of Somatic Growth

During early childhood and then again during the pubertal growth spurt, biochemical markers of bone turnover are significantly higher than during adulthood *(189)*. In girls, peak bone marker levels are observed approximately 2 years earlier than in boys, and estradiol seems to be the major determinant of the increase in bone turnover. In men between 20 and 30 years of age, bone turnover markers are usually higher than in women of the same age bracket. After the age of 50, most bone turnover markers tend to increase with further ageing, but less in men than in women. In the latter, the age-related increase in bone turnover is more pronounced due to the menopause, when both bone resorption and formation increase by about 50–100% *(190,191)*.

Other Biological Sources of Variability

A number of non-skeletal diseases have been shown to strongly affect bone turnover markers. These conditions mostly relate to impairments in the clearance and/or metabolism of the components measured. Thus, even moderate impairment of renal function (GFR 50 ml/min) has been shown to have significant effects on the serum levels of osteocalcin *(192)*, of bone sialoprotein *(109)*, and of the collagen type I telopeptides (NTX, CTX) *(193)*.

In summary, numerous factors influence bone turnover, but there are even more sources of variability that need to be taken into account when measuring biochemical markers of bone turnover. To minimize some of the limitations linked to pre-analytical and analytical variability, standardized sampling and sample handling are mandatory to obtain reliable results. Controllable factors such as the mode of sample collection, samples handling and storage, diurnal and menstrual rhythms, pre-sampling exercise, and pre-sampling diet should be taken care of wherever possible. Laboratories are encouraged to establish their own reference ranges and to use gender- and age-specific reference intervals. In order to further reduce variability, standardization of bone marker assays and routine proficiency testing programs are strongly recommended.

HOW TO DEAL WITH VARIABILITY

If bone markers vary so much, how can we ever use them in our patients? Admittedly, most data on the use of bone markers have been generated in large populations or controlled clinical trials, which may not be representative of a routine clinical setting. However, bone markers can well be used in individual patients if methods are used that account for potential sources of variability and thus integrate the inherent limitations of bone markers measurements.

The Concept of Least Significant Change

Numerous biological factors affect bone turnover and therefore bone marker levels (Table 2). As a rule, markers showing large changes in response to disease processes or interventions also show substantial degrees of biological variability. In the clinical setting, variability of bone markers should be of particular concern when it comes to serial measurements, for example, during therapeutic monitoring. Often, a moderate reduction in a bone resorption marker is believed to be the effect of anti-resorptive treatment, when it really should be attributed to non-specific variability. However, a true ("significant") response to either BMD or bone turnover can only be assumed, when within a single individual the change in signal is greater than the imprecision of the measurement. This change is called the "least significant change" (LSC). The LSC can be defined for various levels of confidence (e.g., 80 or 95%) and by large depends on the short- and long-term within subject variability (CV) of a given marker. The CV of bone formation markers is lower than that of most bone resorption markers, and so is their LSC. Thus, for formation markers, a change >25% should under regular circumstances be considered significant, while for most bone resorption markers (serum and urine) the LSC is around 60–80%.

Another phenomenon to be considered when interpreting any serial measurement is the regression to the mean (RTM). This effect is independent of biological variability and relates to the changes in extreme baseline values.

The pronounced variability and heterogeneity of bone markers makes it difficult to determine precise thresholds or cutoffs for practical use in individual patients. In clinical medicine, two interrelated approaches are often used to assess the clinical significance of a change. These include a comparison of the actual difference to a predefined cutoff, and a comparison of the measured value to a predefined range.

The first method defines certain cutoff levels that a change in a marker must exceed to be considered "clinically significant." Some models apply the LSC or similar statistical approaches to define a priori cutoffs *(194)*. Other models have used the placebo and treatment groups of large RCTs and calculated the fracture incidence according to the change in a marker above or below a certain cutoff. For example, using data from the fracture intervention trial, Bauer et al. demonstrated that alendronate-treated women with a reduction in serum BALP of 30% or more at 1 year had fewer hip and non-spine (but not vertebral) fractures than alendronate-treated women with a 1 year change in serum BALP of less than

30%. However, when compared to the *placebo* group, there was no difference in the incidence of vertebral fractures between the alendronate-treated groups (>30 vs. <30% change at 1 year). In this instance, therefore, setting a 30% cutoff helped to define – a posteriori – a valid response to alendronate treatment for non-spine and hip fractures, but appears to be useless for vertebral fractures *(195)*.

Another widely used method to assess therapy-induced changes in laboratory parameters is to compare the actual marker level to a predefined range (similar to the *T*- and *Z*-score approach in bone mineral density). In most instances, this range will be the "reference" or "normal" range, which may or may not be standardized between methods and/or laboratories. In the bone field, most people would agree that patients with accelerated bone turnover are likely to benefit from anti-resorptive treatment if their bone markers return to the respective "normal," i.e., premenopausal range. Such a "normalization" would be considered a valid response, while changes that do not lead to a return of the marker into the reference range would be labeled as an invalid response. Furthermore, a reduction of the marker below the reference range could be indicative of overtreatment.

A recent paper by Sambrook et al. illustrates the usefulness of this approach. In a double-masked and double placebo-controlled study, the authors compared the effects of alendronate 70 mg once weekly with raloxifene 60 mg daily on markers of bone turnover in 487 postmenopausal women with low bone mineral density *(196)*. Both anti-resorptive agents reduced serum osteocalcin and urinary NTX-I levels after 1 year of treatment, but the effect was more pronounced for alendronate. Large RCTs have shown that both alendronate and raloxifene reduce fracture risk in women with low bone mineral density. It is therefore interesting to note that in the head-to-head trial by Sambrook et al. *(196)*, both alendronate and raloxifene returned bone markers into their respective reference ranges.

The problem with this method is that the reference ranges for most markers have not been well defined. Also, a reduction into the "normal" range can only be achieved if the pre-treatment values are abnormally high, which is the case in less than 50% of patients with osteoporosis. Clearly, the approach is also invalid for anabolic treatments, which increase both bone formation and resorption. Finally, standardization of most assays is presently insufficient to provide a basis for a wider application of such a reference-based approach *(138)*.

REFERENCES

1. Lian JB, Stein GS. The cells of bone. In: Seibel MJ, Robins SP, Bilezikian JP, eds. Dynamics of bone and cartilage metabolism, 2nd ed. San Diego: Academic Press, 2006:221–258.
2. Rizzoli R, Bonjour JP. Physiology of calcium and phosphate homeostasis. In: Seibel MJ, Robins SP, Bilezikian JP, eds. Dynamics of bone and cartilage metabolism, 2nd ed. San Diego: Academic Press, 2006:345–360.
3. Stinson RA, Hamilton BA. Human liver plasma membranes contain an enzyme activity that removes membrane anchor from alkaline phosphatase and converts it to a plasma-like form. Clin Biochem 1994;27:49–55.
4. Harris H. The human alkaline phosphatases: what we know and what we don't know. Clin Chim Acta 1989;186:133–150.
5. Crofton PS. Biochemistry of alkaline phosphatase isoenzymes. CRC Crit Rev Clin Lab Sci 1982:16; 161–194.
6. Koyama I, Miura M, Matsuzaki H, Sakagishi Y, Komoda T. Sugar-chain heterogeneity of human alkaline phosphatases: differences between normal and tumor-associated isoenzymes. Am J Dis Child 1985;139:736–740.

7. Langlois MR, Delanghe JR, Kaufman JM, et al. Posttranslational heterogeneity of bone alkaline phosphatase in metabolic bone disease. Eur J Cli Chem Clin Biochem 1994;32:675–680.
8. Green S, Antiss CL, Fishman WH. Automated differential isoenzyme analysis. II. The fractionation of serum alkaline phosphatase into liver, intestinal, and other components. Enzymologia 1971;41:9–26.
9. Van Hoof VO, Holyaerts MF, Geryl H, Van Mullem M, Lepoutre LG, De Broe ME. Age and sex distribution of alkaline phosphatase isoenzymes by agarose electrophoresis. Clin Chem 1990;36:875–878.
10. Magnusson P, Larsson L, Magnusson M, Davie MW, Sharp CA. Isoforms of bone alkaline phosphatase: characterization and origin in human trabecular and cortical bone. J Bone Miner Res 1999;14: 1926–1933.
11. Hill CS, Wolfert RL. The preparation of monoclonal antibodies which react preferentially with human bone alkaline phosphatase and not liver alkaline phosphatase. Clin Chem Acta 1989;186:315–320.
12. Rosalki SB, Foo AY. Two new methods for separating and quantifying bone and liver alkaline phosphatase isoenzymes in plasma. Clin Chem 1984;30:1182–1186.
13. Rosalki SB, Foo AY. Lectin affinity electrophoresis of alkaline phosphatase for the differentiation of bone hepatobiliary disease. Electrophoresis 1987;10:604–611.
14. Crofton PM. Wheat-germ lectin affinity electrophoresis for alkaline phosphatase isoforms in children: age-dependent reference ranges and changes in liver and bone disease. Clin Chem 1992;38:663–670.
15. Gomez B Jr, Ardakani S, Ju J, et al. Monoclonal antibody assay for measuring bone-specific alkaline phosphatase activity in serum. Clin Chem 1995;41:1560–1566.
16. Martin M, Van Hoof V, Couttenye M, Prove, A, Blokx P. Analytical and clinical evaluation of a method to quantify bone alkaline phosphatase, a marker of osteoblastic activity. Anticancer Res 1997;17: 3167–3170.
17. Woitge H, Seibel MJ, Ziegler R. Comparison of total and bone-specific alkaline phosphatase in patients with nonskeletal disorders or metabolic bone disease. Clin Chem 1996;42:1796–1804.
18. Van Straalen JP, Sanders E, Prummel MF, Sanders GTB. Bone alkaline phosphatase as indicator of bone formation. Clin Chim Acta 1991;201:27–34.
19. Alpers DH, Goodwin CL, Young GP. Quantitation of human intestinal and liver/bone alkaline phosphatase in serum by rocket electroimmunoassay. Analyt Biochem 1984;140:129–137.
20. Farley JR, Chesnut CH III, Baylink DJ. Improved method for quantitative determination in serum of alkaline phosphatase of skeletal origin. Clin Chem 1981;27:2002–2007.
21. Gorman L, Statland BE. Clinical usefulness of alkaline phosphatase isoenzyme determinations. Clin Biochem 1977;10:171–174.
22. Gallop PM, Lian JB, Hauschka PV. Carboxylated calcium-binding proteins and vitamin K. New Eng J Med 1980;302:1460–1466.
23. Hauschka PV, Lian JB, Cole DE, Gundberg C. Osteocalcin and matrix Gla protein: vitamin K-dependent proteins in bone. Physiol Rev 1989;69:990–1047.
24. Gundberg CM, Nishimoto SK. Vitamin K dependent proteins of bone and cartilage. In: Seibel MJ, Robins SP, Bilezikian JP, eds. Dynamics of bone and cartilage metabolism, 2nd ed. San Diego: Academic Press, 2006:55–70.
25. Price PA. Vitamin K-dependent proteins. In: Cohn DV, ed. Calcium regulation and bone metabolism: basic and clinical aspects. Amsterdam: Elsevier Science, 1987:419–425.
26. Ducy P, Desbois C, Boycem B, et al. Increased bone formation in osteocalcin-deficient mice. Nature 1996;382:448–452.
27. Brown JP, Delmas PD, Malaval L, et al. Serum bone Gla-protein: a specific marker for bone formation in postmenopausal osteoporosis. Lancet 1984;1:1091–1093.
28. Bouillon R, Vanderschueren D, Van Herck E, et al. Homologous radioimmunoassay of human osteocalcin. Clin Chem 1992;38:2055–2060.
29. Delmas PD, Stenner D, Wahner HW, et al. Increase in serum bone gamma-carboxyglutamic acid protein with aging in women. J Clin Invest 1983;71:1316–1321.
30. Gundberg CM, Wilson PS, Gallop PM, Parfitt AM. Determination of osteocalcin in human serum: results with two kits compared with those by a well-characterized assay. Clin Chem 1985;31:1720–1723.
31. Taylor AK, Linkhart SG, Mohan S, Baylink DJ. Development of a new radioimmunoassay for human osteocalcin: evidence for a midmolecule epitope. Metabolism 1988;37:872–877.
32. Monaghan DA, Power MJ, Fottrell PF. Sandwich enzyme immunoassay of osteocalcin in serum with use of an antibody against human osteocalcin. Clin Chem 1993;39:942–947.

33. Parviainen M, Kuronen I, Kokko H, Lakaniemi M, Savolainen K, Mononen I. Two-site enzyme immunoassay for measuring intact human osteocalcin in serum. J Bone Min Res 1994;9:347–354.
34. Chen JT, Hosoda K, Hasumi K, Ogata E, Shiraki M. Serum N-terminal osteocalcin is a good indicator for estimating responders to hormone replacement therapy in postmenopausal women. J Bone Min Res 1996;11:1784–1792.
35. Delmas PD, Malaval L, Arlot M, et al. Serum bone-Gla-protein compared to bone histomorphometry in endocrine diseases. Bone 1985;6:339–341.
36. Fournier B, Gineyts E, Delmas PD. Evidence that free gamma carboxyglutamic acid circulates in serum. Clin Chim Acta 1989;182:173–182.
37. Taylor AK, Linkhart S, Mohan S, et al. Multiple osteocalcin fragments in human urine and serum as detected by a midmolecule osteocalcin radioimmunoassay. J Clin Endocrinol Metab 1990;70:467–472.
38. Baumgrass R, Williamson MK, Price PA. Identification of peptide fragments generated by digestion of bovine and human osteocalcin with the lysosomal proteinases cathepsin B, D, L, H, and S. J Bone Min Res 1997;12:447–455.
39. Gorai L, Hosoda K, Taguchi Y, et al. A heterogeneity in serum osteocalcin N-terminal fragments in Paget's disease: comparison with other biochemical indices in pre- and post-menopause. J Bone Min Res 1997;12(S1):T678.
40. Page AE, Hayman AR, Andersson LMB, Chambers TJ, Warburton MJ. Degradation of bone matrix proteins by osteoclast cathepsins. Internat J Biochem 1993;25:545–550.
41. Delmas PD, Christiansen C, Mann KG, Price PA. Bone gla protein (osteocalcin) assay standardization report. J Bone Min Res 1990;5:5–10.
42. Masters PW, Jones RG, Purves DA, Cooper EH, Cooney JM. Commercial assays for serum osteocalcin give clinically discordant result Clin Chem 1994;40:358–363.
43. Diego ED, Guerrero R, de la Piedra C. Six osteocalcin assays compared. Clin Chem 1994;40:2071–2077.
44. Liu SH, Yang RS, al-Shaikh R, Lane JM. Collagen in tendon, ligament, and bone healing. A current review. Clin Orthop 1995;318:265–278.
45. Dumon JC, Wantier H, Mathieu JJ, Body JJ. Technical and clinical validation of a new immunoradiometric assay for human osteocalcin. Eur J Endocrinol 1996;135:231–237.
46. Liu SH, Yang RS, al-Shaikh R, Lane JM. Collagen in tendon, ligament, and bone healing. A current review. Clin Orthop 1995;318:265–278.
47. Merry AH, Harwood R, Wooley DE, Grant ME, Jackson DS. Identification and partial characterization of the non-collagenous amino- and carboxy-terminal extension peptides of cartilage procollagen. Biochem Biophys Res Commun 1976;71:83–90.
48. Fessler LI, Morris NP, Fessler JH. Procollagen: biological scission of amino and carboxy extension peptides. Proc Nat Acad Sci USA 1975;72:4905–4909.
49. Olsen BR, Guzman NA, Engel J, Condit C, Aase S. Purification and characterization of a peptide from the carboxy-terminal region of chick tendon procollagen type I. Biochemistry 1977;16:3030–3036.
50. Smedsrod B, Melkko J, Risteli L, Risteli J. Circulating C-terminal propeptide of type I procollagen is cleared mainly via the mannose receptor in liver endothelial cells. Biochem J 1990;271:345–350.
51. Taubman MB, Goldberg B, Sherr C. Radioimmunoassay for human procollagen. Science 1974;186:1115–1117.
52. Melkko J, Niemi S, Risteli L, Risteli J. Radioimmunoassay of the carboxyterminal propeptide of human type I procollagen. Clin Chem 1990;36:1328–1332.
53. Eriksen EF, Charles P, Meisen F, et al. Serum markers of type 1 collagen formation and degradation in metabolic bone disease: correlation with bone histomorphometry. J Bone Min Res 1993;8:127–132.
54. Hassager C, Jensen LT, Johansen JS, et al. The carboxy-terminal propeptide of type 1 procollagen in serum as a marker of bone formation: the effect of nandrolone decanoate and female sex hormones. Metabolism 1991;40:205–208.
55. Ebeling PR, Peterson JM, Riggs BL. Utility of type I procollagen propeptide assays for assessing abnormalities in metabolic bone diseases. J Bone Min Res 1992;7:1243–1250.
56. Charles P, Mosekilde L, Risteli L, et al. Assessment of bone remodeling using biochemical indicators of type I collagen synthesis and degradation: relation to calcium kinetics. Bone Miner 1994;24:81–94.
57. Lowry M, Hall D, Brosnan J. Hydroxyproline metabolism by the rat kidney: distribution of renal enzymes of hydroxyproline catabolism and renal conversion of hydroxyproline to glycine and serine. Metabolism 1985;34:955–961.

58. Kivirikko KI. Urinary excretion of hydroxyproline in health and disease. Int Rev Connect Tissue Res 1970;5:93–163.
59. Krane SM, Kantrowitz FG, Byrne M, Pinnell SR, Singer FR. Urinary excretion of hydroxylysine and its glycosides as an index of collagen degradation. J Clin Invest 1977;59:819–827.
60. Smith R. Collagen and disorders of bone. Clin Sci 1980;59:215–223.
61. Prockop DJ, Kivirikko KI, Tuderman L, Guzman NA. The biosynthesis of collagen and its disorders. New Engl J Med 1979;301:13–23.
62. Robins SP. Turnover of collagen and its precursors. In: Viidik A, Vuust J, eds. Biology of collagen. Academic Press: New York, 1980:135–151.
63. Cunningham LW, Ford JD, Segrest JP. The isolation of identical hydroxylysyl glycosides from hydroxylates of soluble collagen and from human urine. J Biol Chem 1967;242:2570–2571.
64. Moro L, Modricki C, Stagni N, et al. High performance liquid chromatography analysis of urinary hydroxylysine glycosides as indicators of collagen turnover. Analyst 1984;109:1621–1628.
65. Moro L, Noris-Suarez K, Michalsky M, Romanello M, de Bernard B. The glycosides of hydroxylysine are final products of collagen degradation in humans. Biochim Biophys Acta 1993;1156:288–290.
66. Segrest JP, Cunningham LW. Variations in human urinary O-hydroxylysyl glycoside levels and their relationship to collagen metabolism. J Clin Invest 1970;49:1497–1509.
67. Bettica P, Moro L, Robins SP, et al. The comparative performance of urinary bone resorption markers: galactosyl hydroxylysine, pyridinium crosslinks, hydroxyproline. Clin Chem 1992;38:2313–2318.
68. Fujimoto D, Moriguchi T, Ishida T, Hayashi H. The structure of pyridinoline, a collagen crosslink. Biochem Biophys Res Commun 1978;84:52–57.
69. Robins SP. Fibrillogenesis and maturation of collagens. In: Seibel MJ, Robins SP, Bilezikian JP, eds. Dynamics of bone and cartilage metabolism, 2nd ed. San Diego: Academic Press, 2006:41–54.
70. von der Mark K. Structure and Biosynthesis of Collagens. In: Seibel M, Robins S, Bilezikian J, eds. Dynamics of bone and cartilage metabolism, 2nd ed. San Diego: Academic Press, 2006:3–40.
71. Gunja-Smith Z, Boucek RJ. Collagen crosslink components in human urine. Biochem J 1981;197: 759–762.
72. Delmas PD, Schlemmer A, Gineyts E, et al. Urinary excretion of pyridinoline crosslinks correlates with bone turnover measured on iliac crest biopsy in patients with vertebral osteoporosis. J Bone Min Res 1991;6:639–644.
73. Eastell R, Colwell A, Hampton L, Reeve J. Biochemical markers of bone resorption compared with estimates of bone resorption from radiotracer kinetic studies in osteoporosis. J Bone Miner Res 1997;12:59–65.
74. Colwell A, Russell R, Eastell R. Factors affecting the assay of urinary 3-hydroxy pyridinium crosslinks of collagen as markers of bone resorption. Eur J Clin Invest 1993;23:341–349.
75. Boucek RJ, Noble NL, Gunja-Smith Z, Butler WT. The Marfan syndrome: a deficiency in chemically stable collagen crosslinking. New Engl J Med 1981;305:988–991.
76. Eyre DR, Dickson IR, Van Ness KP. Collagen crosslinking in human bone and articular cartilage. Biochem J 1988;252:495–500.
77. Seibel MJ, Robins SP, Bilezikian JP. Urinary pyridinium crosslinks of collagen: specific markers of bone resorption in metabolic bone disease. Trends Endocrinol Metab 1992;3:263–270.
78. Kraenzlin EM, Seibel MJ. Measurement of biochemical markers of bone resorption. In: Seibel MJ, Robins SP, Bilezikian JP, eds. Dynamics of bone and cartilage metabolism, 2nd ed. San Diego: Academic Press, 2006:541–565.
79. Brixen K, Eriksen EF. Validation of local and systemic markers of bone turnover. In: Seibel MJ, Robins SP, Bilezikian JP, eds. Dynamics of bone and cartilage metabolism, 2nd ed. San Diego: Academic Press, 2006:583–594.
80. Black D, Duncan A, Robins SP. Quantitative analysis of the pyridinium crosslinks of collagen in urine using ion-paired reversed-phase high-performance liquid chromatography. Anal Biochem 1988;169: 197–203.
81. Pratt DA, Daniloff Y, Duncan A, Robins SP. Automated analysis of the pyridinium crosslinks of collagen in tissue and urine using solid-phase extraction and reversed-phase high-performance liquid chromatography. Anal Biochem 1992;207:168–175.
82. James IT, Perrett D. Automated on-line solid-phase extraction and high-performance liquid chromatographic analysis of total and free pyridinium crosslinks in serum. J Chromatogr 1998;79:159–166.

83. Robins SP, Duncan A, Riggs BL. Direct measurement of free hydroxy-pyridinium crosslinks of collagen in urine as new markers of bone resorption in osteoporosis. In: Christiansen C, Overgaard K, eds. Osteoporosis 1990. Copenhagen: Osteopress, 1990:465–468.
84. Seyedin SM, Kung VT, Daniloff YN, et al. Immunoassay for urinary pyridinoline: the new marker of bone resorption. J Bone Miner Res 1993;8:635–641.
85. Robins SP, Woitge H, Hesley R, Ju J, Seyedin S, Seibel MJ. Direct, enzyme-linked immunoassay for urinary deoxypyridinoline as a specific marker for measuring bone resorption. J Bone Miner Res 1994;9:1643–1649.
86. Delmas PD, Gineyts E, Bertholin A, Garnero P, Marchand F. Immunoassay of urinary pyridinoline crosslink excretion in normal adults and in Paget's disease. J Bone Min Res 1993;8:643–648.
87. Ristell J, Niemi S, Elomaa I, Risteli L. Bone resorption assay based on a peptide liberated during type I collagen degradation. J Bone Min Res 1991;6:S251,A670
88. Risteli J, Risteli L. Products of bone collagen metabolism. In: Seibel M, Robins S, Bilezikian J, eds. Dynamics of bone and cartilage metabolism, 2nd ed. San Diego: Academic Press, 2006:391–406.
89. Bonde MQP, Fledelius C, Riis BJ, Christiansen C. Immunoassay for quantifying type I degradation products in urine evaluated. Clin Chem 1994;40:2022–2025.
90. Fledelius C, Johnsen AH, Cloos PAC, Bonde M, Qvist P. Characterization of urinary degradation products derived from type I collagen. Identification of a beta-isomerized Asp-Gly sequence within the C-terminal telopeptide (alpha1) region. J Biol Chem 1997;272:9755–9763.
91. Bonde M, Fledelius C, Qvist P, Christiansen C. Coated-tube radioimmunoassay for C-telopeptides of type I collagen to assess bone resorption. Clin Chem 1996;42:1639–1644.
92. Garnero P, Fledelius C, Gineyts E, et al. Decreased beta-isomerization of the C-terminal telopeptide of type I collagen alpha 1 chain in Paget's disease of bone. J Bone Miner Res 1997;12:1407–1415.
93. Cloos PAC, Fledelius C. Two new bone resorption assays measuring racemized protein fragments: measurement of age-modified peptides to mssess bone quality. Bone 1998;23(Suppl):T114.
94. Cloos PAC, Fledelius C, Ovist P, Garnero P. Biological clocks of bone aging: racemization and isomerization, potential tools to assess bone turnover. Bone 1998;23(Suppl):F440.
95. Leeming J, Koizumi M, Byrjalsen I, et al. The relative use of eight collagenous and noncollagenous markers for diagnosis of skeletal metastases in breast, prostate, or lung cancer patients. Cancer Epidemiol Biomarkers Prev 2006;15:32–38.
96. Hanson DA, Weis MA, Bollen AM, Maslan SL, Singer FR, Eyre DR. A specific immunoassay for monitoring human bone resorption: quantitation of type I collagen cross-linked N-telopeptides in urine. J Bone Miner Res 1992;7:1251–1258.
97. Robins SP. Collagen crosslinks in metabolic bone disease. Acta Orthop Scand Suppl 1995;266:171–175.
98. Woitge HW, Oberwittler H, Farahmand I, et al. Novel serum markers of bone resorption. J Bone Mineral Res 1999;14:792–801.
99. Fisher LW, Whitson SW, Avioli LW, Termine JD. Matrix sialoprotein of developing bone. J Biol Chem. 1983;258:12723–12727.
100. Oldberg Å, Franzen A, Heinegard D. Isolation and characterization of two sialoproteins present only in bone. Biochem J. 1985;232:715–724.
101. Chen J, Shapiro HS, Wrana JL, Reimers S, Heersche J, Sodek J. Localization of bone sialoprotein (BSP) expression to sites of mineral tissue formation in fetal rat tissue by in situ hybridization. Matrix 1991;11:133–143.
102. Bianco P, Fisher LW, Young MF, Termine JD, Robey PG. Expression of bone sialoprotein (BSP) in developing human tissues. Calcif Tissue Int 1991;49(6):421–426.
103. Bellahcene A, Castronovo V. Expression of bone matrix proteins in human breast cancer: potential roles in microcalcification formation and in the genesis of bone metastases. Bull Cancer 1997;84:17–24.
104. Ross FP, Chappel J, Alvarez JI, et al. Interactions between the bone matrix proteins osteopontin and bone sialoprotein and the osteoclast integrin $\alpha_V \beta_3$ potentiate bone resorption. J Biol Chem 1993;268: 9901–9907.
105. Hunter GK, Goldberg HA. Modulation of crystal formation by bone phosphoproteins: role of glutamic acid-rich sequences in the nucleation of hydroxyapatite by bone sialoprotein. Biochem J 1994;302: 175–179.
106. Saxne T, Zunino L, Heinegard D. Increased release of bone sialoprotein into synovial fluid reflects tissue destruction in rheumatoid arthritis. Arthritis Rheum 1995;38:82–90.

107. Karmatschek M, Woitge HW, Armbruster FP, Ziegler R, Seibel MJ. Improved purification of human bone sialoprotein and development of a homologous radioimmunoassay. Clin Chem 1997;43:2076–2082.
108. Fedarko NS, Fohr B, Robey PG, Young MF, Fisher LW. Factor H binding to bone sialoprotein and osteopontin enables tumor cell evasion from complement-mediated attack. J Biol Chem 2000;275(22): 16666–16672.
109. Seibel MJ, Woitge HW, Pecherstorfer M, et al. Serum immunoreactive bone sialoprotein as a new marker of bone turnover in metabolic and malignant bone disease. J Clin Endocrinol Metab 1996;81:3289–3294.
110. Minkin C. Bone acid phosphatase: tartrate-resistant acid phosphatase as a marker of osteoclast function. Calcif Tissue Int 1982;34:285–290.
111. Halleen JM, Karp M, Viloma S, Laaksonen P, Hellman J, Kakonen SM, Stepan JJ, et al. Two-site immunoassays for osteoclastic tartrate-resistant acid phosphatase based on characterization of six monoclonal antibodies. J Bone Miner Res 1999;14:464–469.
112. Halleen JM, Alatalo SL, Suominen H, Cheng S, Janckila AJ, Vaananen HK. Tartrate-resistant acid phosphatase 5b: a novel serum marker of bone resorption. J Bone Miner Res 2000;15:1337–1345.
113. Kraenzlin ME, Lau KH, Liang L, et al. Development of an immunoassay for human serum osteoclastic tartrate-resistant acid phosphatase. J Clin Endocrinol Metab 1990;71:442–451.
114. Cheung C, Panesar N, Haines C, Masarei J, Swaminathan R. Immunoassay of a tartrate-resistant acid phosphatase in serum. Clin Chem 1995;41:679–686.
115. Bais R, Edwards JB. An optimized continuous-monitoring procedure for semiautomated determination of serum acid phosphatase activity. Clin Chem 1976;22:2025–2028.
116. Kafienah W, Bromme D, Buttle DJ, Croucher LJ, Hollander AP. Human cathepsin K cleaves native type I and II collagens at the N-terminal end of the triple helix. Biochem J 1998;331:727–732.
117. Li Z, Yasuda Y, Li W, Bogyo M, Katz N, Gordon RE, Fields GB, Bromme D. Regulation of collagenase activities of human cathepsins by glycosaminoglycans. J Biol Chem 2004;279:5470–5479.
118. Gelb BD, Shi GP, Chapman HA, Desnick RJ. Pycnodysostosis, a lysosomal disease caused by cathepsin K deficiency. Science 1996;273:1236–1238.
119. Saftig P, Hunziker E, Wehmeyer O, Jones S, Boyde A, Rommerskirch W, Moritz JD, Schu P, von Figura K. Impaired osteoclastic bone resorption leads to osteopetrosis in cathepsin-K-deficient mice. Proc Natl Acad Sci USA 1998;95:13453–13458.
120. Gowen M, Lazner F, Dodds R, Kapadia R, Feild J, Tavaria M, Bertoncello I, Drake F, Zavarselk S, Tellis I, Hertzog P, Debouck C, Kola I. Cathepsin K knockout mice develop osteopetrosis due to a deficit in matrix degradation but not demineralization. J Bone Miner Res 1999;14:1654–1663.
121. Goto T, Yamaza T, Tanaka T. Cathepsins in the osteoclast. J Electron Microsc 2003;52:551–558.
122. Lang M, Seibel MJ, Zipf A, Ziegler R. Influence of a new protease inhibitor on the stability of osteocalcin in serum. Clin Lab 1996;42:5–10.
123. Colwell A, Hamer A, Blumsohn A, Eastell R. To determine the effects of ultraviolet light, natural light and ionizing radiation on pyridinium cross-links in bone and urine using high-performance liquid chromatography. Eur J Clin Invest 1996;26:1107–1114.
124. Blumsohn A, Colwell A, Naylor KE, Eastell R. Effect of light and gamma-irradiation on pyridinolines and telopeptides of type I collagen in urine. Clin Chem 1995;41:1195–1197.
125. Bais R, Edwards JB. An optimized continuous-monitoring procedure for semiautomated determination of serum acid phosphatase activity. Clin Chem 1976;22:2025–2028.
126. Karmatschek M, Woitge HW, Armbruster FP, Ziegler R, Seibel MJ. Improved purification of human bone sialoprotein and development of a homologous radioimmunoassay. Clin Chem 1997;43:2076–2082.
127. Walne AJ, James IT, Perret D. The stability of pyridinium crosslinks in urine and serum. Clin Chem Acta 1995;240:95–97.
128. Heymsfield SB, Artega C, McManus BS, Smith J, Moffitt S. Measurements of muscle mass in humans: valaidity of the 24 hour urinary creatinine method. Am J Clin Nutr 1983;37:478–494.
129. Mautalen CA. Circadian rhythm of urinary total and free hydroxyproline excretion and its relation to creatinine excretion. J Lab Clin Med 1970;75:11–18.
130. Eastell R, Calvo MS, Burritt MF, Offord KP, Russell, RGG, Riggs, BL. Abnormalities in circadian patterns of bone resorption and renal calcium conservation in type I osteoporosis. J Clin Endocrinol Metab 1992;74:487–494.
131. Greenspan SL, Dresner-Pollak R, Parker RA, London D, Ferguson L. Diurnal variation of bone mineral turnover in elderly men and women. Calcif Tissue Int 1997;60:419–423.

132. Li Y, Woitge W, Kissling C, et al. Biological variability of serum immunoractive bone sialoprotein. Clin Lab 1998;44:553–555.
133. Jensen JB, Kollerup G, Sorensen A, Sorensen OH. Intraindividual variability of bone markers in the urine. Scand J Clin Lab Invest 1997;57:29–34.
134. Sarno M, Powell H, Tjersland G, Schoendorfer D, et al. A collection method and high-sensitivity enzyme immunoassay for sweat pyridinoline and deoxypyridinoline crosslinks. Clin Chem 1999;45: 1501–1509.
135. Schlemmer A, Hassager C. Acute fasting diminishes the circadian rhythm of biochemical markers of bone resorption. Eur J Endocrinol 1999;140:332–337.
136. Wichers M, Schmidt E, Bidlingmaier F, Klingmüller D. Diurnal rhythm of crosslaps in human serum. Clin Chem 1999;45:1858–1860.
137. Lang M, Haag P, Schmidt-Gayk H, Seibel MJ, Ziegler R. Influence of ambient storage conditions and of diet on the measurement of biochemical markers of bone turnover. Calcif Tissue Int 1995;56:497
138. Seibel MJ, Lang M, Geilenkeuser WJ. Interlaboratory variation of biochemical markers of bone turnover. Clin Chem 2001;47:1443–1450.
139. Beardsworth LJ, Eyre DR, Dickson IR. Changes with age in the urinary excretion of lysyl- and hydroxylysylpyridinoline, two new markers of bone collagen turnover. J Bone Miner Res 1990;5:671.
140. Eastell R, Simmons PS, Colwell A, et al. Nyctohemeral changes in bone turnover assessed by serum bone Gla-protein concentration and urinary deoxypyridinoline excretion: effects of growth and ageing. Clin Sci 1992;83:375–382.
141. Robins SP, Woitge H, Hesley R, Ju J, Seyedin S, Seibel MJ. Direct, enzyme-linked immunoassay for urinary deoxypyridinoline as a specific marker for measuring bone resorption. J Bone Miner Res 1994;9:1643–1649.
142. Seibel M, Woitge H, Scheidt NC, et al. Urinary hydroxypyridinium crosslinks of collagen in population-based screening for overt vertebral osteoporosis: results of a pilot study. J Bone Miner Res 1994;9: 1433–1440.
143. Cantatore F, Carrozzo M, Magli D, D'Amore M, Pipitone V. Serum osteocalcin levels in normal humans of different sex and age. Panminerva Med 1988;30:23–25.
144. Catherwood B, Marcus R, Madvig P, Cheung A. Determinants of bone gamma-carboxyglutamic acid-containing protein in plasma of healthy aging subjects. Bone 1985;6:9–13.
145. Eastell R, Calvo MS, Burritt MF, Offord KP, Russell RGG, Riggs BL. Abnormalities in circadian patterns of bone resorption and renal calcium conservation in type I osteoporosis. J Clin Endocrinol Metab 1992;74:487–494.
146. Epstein S, McClintock R, Bryce G, Poser J, Johnston CC Jr, Hui S. Differences in serum bone gla protein with age and sex. Lancet 1984;11:307–310.
147. Galli M, Caniggia M. Osteocalcin in normal adult humans of different sex and age. Horm Metab Res 1984;17:165–166.
148. Garnero P, Delmas PD. Assessment of the serum levels of bone alkaline phosphatase with a new immunoradiometric assay in patients with metabolic bone disease. J Clin Endocrinol Metab 1993;77:1046–1053.
149. Hassager C, Risteli J, Risteli L, Christiansen C. Effect of the menopause and hormone replacement therapy on the carboxy-terminal pyridinoline cross-linked telopeptide of type I collagen. Osteoporos Int 1994;4:349–352.
150. Midtby M, Magnus JH, Joakimsen RM. The tromso study: a population-based study on the variation in bone formation markers with age, gender, anthropometry and season in both men and women. Osteoporos Int 2001;12:835–843.
151. Sgherzi M, Fabbri G, Bonati M, et al. Episodic changes of serume procollagen type I carboxy-terminal propeptide levels in fertile and postmenopausal women. Gynecol Obstet Invest 1994;38:60–64.
152. Cleghorn DB, O'Loughlin PD, Schroeder BJ, Nordin BE. An open, crossover trial of calcium-fortified milk in prevention of early postmenopausal bone loss. Med J Aust 2001;175:242–245.
153. McKane W, Khosla S, Risteli J, Robins S, Muhs J, Riggs B. Role of estrogen deficiency in pathogenesis of secondary hyperparathyroidism and increased bone resorption in elderly women. Proc Assoc Am Physicians 1997;109:174–180.
154. Prestwood K, Pilbeam C, Burleson J, et al. The short-term effects of conjugated estrogen on bone turnover in older women. J Clin Endocrinol Metab 1994;79:366–371.

155. Seifert-Klauss V, Mueller JE, Luppa P, et al. Bone metabolism during the perimenopausal transition: a prospective study. Maturitas 2002;41:23–33.
156. Garnero P, Sornay-Rendu E, Chapuy M-C, Delmas PD. Increased bone turnover in late postmenopausal women is a major determinant of osteoporosis. J Bone Miner Res 1996;11:337–349.
157. Mezquita-Raya P, Munoz-Torres M, Luna JD, et al. Relation between vitamin D insufficiency, bone density, and bone metabolism in healthy postmenopausal women. J Bone Miner Res 2001;16:1408–1415.
158. Harris SS, Soteriades E, Dawson-Hughes B. Secondary hyperparathyroidism and bone turnover in elderly blacks and whites. J Clin Endocrinol Metab 2001;86:3801–3804.
159. Sambrook PN, Chen JS, March LM, Cameron ID, Cumming RG, Lord SR, Schwarz J, Seibel MJ. Serum parathyroid hormone is associated with increased mortality independent of 25-hydroxy vitamin d status, bone mass, and renal function in the frail and very old: a cohort study. J Clin Endocrinol Metab 2004;89:5477–5481.
160. Wishart JM, Need AG, Horowitz M, Morris HA, Nordin BE. Effect of age on bone density and bone turnover in men. Clin Endocrinol (Oxf) 1995;42:141–146.
161. Khosla S, Melton LJ III, Atkinson EJ, O'Fallon WM, Klee GG, Riggs BL. Relationship of serum sex steroid levels and bone turnover markers with bone mineral density in men and women: a key role for bioavailable estrogen. J Clin Endocrinol Metab 1998;83:2266–2274.
162. Orwoll ES, Bell NH, Nanes MS, Flessland KA, Pettinger MB, Mallinak NJ, Cain DF. Collagen N-telopeptide excretion in men: the effects of age and intrasubject variability. J Clin Endocrinol Metab 1998;83:3930–3935.
163. Fatayerji D, Eastell R. Age-related changes in bone turnover in men. J Bone Miner Res 1999;14: 1203–1210.
164. Tsai KS, Pan WH, Hsu SH, Cheng WC, Chen CK, Chieng PU, Yang RS, Twu ST. Sexual differences in bone markers and bone mineral density of normal Chinese. Calcif Tissue Int 1996;59:454–460.
165. Garnero P, Delmas PD. Assessment of the serum levels of bone alkaline phosphatase with a new immunoradiometric assay in patients with metabolic bone disease. J Clin Endocrinol Metab 1993;77: 1046–1053.
166. Gallagher JC, Kinyamu HK, Fowler SE, Dawson-Hughes B, Dalsky GP, Sherman SS. Calciotropic hormones and bone markers in the elderly. J Bone Miner Res 1998;13:475–482.
167. Clarke BL, Ebeling PR, Jones JD, Wahner HW, O'Fallon WM, Riggs BL, Fitzpatrick LA. Predictors of bone mineral density in aging healthy men varies by skeletal site. Calcif Tissue Int 2002;70:137–145.
168. Sone T, Miyake M, Takeda N, Fukunaga M. Urinary excretion of type I collagen crosslinked N-telopeptides in healthy Japanese adults: age- and sex-related changes and reference limits. Bone 1995;17:335–339.
169. Szulc P, Delmas PD. Biochemical markers of bone turnover in men. Calcif Tissue Int 2001;69:229–234.
170. Szulc P, Garnero P, Munoz F, Marchand F, Delmas PD. Cross-sectional evaluation of bone metabolism in men. J Bone Miner Res 2001;16:1642–1650.
171. Szulc P, Munoz F, Claustrat B, Garnero P, Marchand F, Duboeuf F, Delmas PD. Bioavailable estradiol may be an important determinant of osteoporosis in men: the MINOS study. J Clin Endocrinol Metab 2001;86:192–199.
172. Aaron JE, Makins NB, Sagreiya K. The microanatomy of trabecular bone loss in normal aging men and women. Clin Orthop 1987:215;260–271.
173. Clarke BL, Ebeling PR, Jones JD, Wahner HW, O'Fallon WM, Riggs BL, Fitzpatrick LA. Changes in quantitative bone histomorphometry in aging healthy men. J Clin Endocrinol Metab 1996;81:2264–2270.
174. Chavassieux P, Meunier PJ. Histomorphometric approach of bone loss in men. Calcif Tissue Int 2001;69:209–213.
175. Schlemmer A, Hassager C, Jensen SB, Christiansen C. Marked diurnal variation in urinary excretion of pyridinium cross-links in premenopausal women. J Clin Endocrinol Metab 1992;74:476–480.
176. Schlemmer A, Hassager C, Pedersen B, Christiansen C. Posture, age, menopause, and osteopenia do not influence the circadian variation in the urinary excretion of pyridinium crosslinks. J Bone Miner Res 1994;9:1883–1888.
177. Eastell R, Simmons PS, Assiri AM, Burritt MF, Russel RGG, Riggs BL. Nyctohemeral changes in bone turnover assessed by serum bone gla-protein concentration and urinary deoxypyridinoline excretion: effect of growth and aging. Clin Sci 1992;83:375–382.

178. Nielsen HK, Laurberg P, Brixen K, Mosekilde L. Relations between diurnal variations in serum osteocalcin, cortisol, parathyroid hormone, and ionized calcium in normal individuals. Acta Endocrinol (Copenh) 1991;124:391–398.
179. Popp-Snijders C, Lips P, Netelenbos JC. Intra-individual variation in bone resorption markers in urine. Ann Clin Biochem 1996;33:347–348.
180. McLaren AM, Isdale AH, Whitings PH, Bird HA, Robins SP. Physiological variations in the urinary excretion of pyridinium crosslinks of collagen. Br J Rheumatol 1993;32:307–312.
181. Blumsohn A, Hannon RA, al-Dehaimi AW, Eastell R. Short-term intraindividual variability of markers of bone turnover in healthy adults. J Bone Miner Res 1994;9(Suppl 1):S153.
182. Nielsen HK, Brixen K, Bouillon R, Mosekilde L. Changes in biochemical markers of osteoblastic activity during the menstrual cycle. J Clin Endocrinol Metab 1990;70:1431–1437.
183. Schlemmer A, Hassager C, Risteli J, Risteli L, Jensen SB, Christiansen C. Possible variation in bone resorption during the normal menstrual cycle. Acta Endocrinol (Copenh) 1993;129:388–392.
184. Gorai I, Chaki O, Nakayama M, Minaguchi H. Urinary biochemical markers for bone resorption during the menstrual cycle. Calcif Tissue Int 1995;57:100–104.
185. Christiansen C, Riis BJ, Nilas L, Rodbro P, Deftos L. Uncoupling of bone formation and resorption by combined estrogen and progestagen therapy in postmenopausal osteoporosis. Lancet 1985;2(8459): 800–801.
186. Scharla S, Scheidt-Nave C, Leidig G, Seibel MJ, Ziegler R. Lower serum 25-hydroxyvitamin D is associated with increased bone resorption markers and lower bone density at the proximal femur in normal females: a population-based study. Exp Clin Endocrinol Diab 1996;104:289–292.
187. Morgan DB, Rivlin RS, Davis R. Seasonal changes in the urinary excretion of calcium. Am J Clin Nutr 1972;25:652–654.
188. Woitge H, Scheidt-Nave C, Kissling C, Leidig G, Meyer K, Grauer A, Scharla S, Ziegler R, Seibel MJ. Seasonal variation of biochemical indices of bone turnover: results of a population based study. J Clin Endocrinol Metab 1998;83:68–75.
189. Stepan JJ, Tesarova A, Havranek T, Jodl J, Normankova J, Pacovsky V. Age and sex dependency of the biochemical indices of bone remodeling. Clin Chem Acta 1985;151:273–283.
190. Eastell R, Delmas PD, Hodgson SF, Eriksen EF, Mann KG, Riggs BL. Bone formation rate in older normal women: concurrent assessment with bone histomorphometry, calcium kinetics, and biochemical markers. J Clin Endocrinol Metab 1988;67:741–748.
191. Kelly PJ, Pocock NA, Sambrook PN, Eisman JA. Age and menopause-related changes in indices of bone turnover. J Clin Endocrinol Metab 1989;69:1160–1165.
192. Gundberg CM, Hanning R, Liu A, Zlotkin S, Balfe J, Cole D. Clearance of osteocalcin by peritoneal dialysis in children with end-stage renal disease. Pediatr Res 1987;21:296–300.
193. Woitge HW, Oberwittler H, Farahmand I, Lang M, Ziegler R, Seibel MJ. New serum assays for bone resorption. Results of a cross-sectional study. J Bone Miner Res 1999;14:792–801
194. Delmas PD. Markers of bone turnover for monitoring treatment of osteoporosis with antiresorptive drugs. Osteoporos Int 2000;11(Suppl 6):S66–S76.
195. Bauer DC, Black DM, Garnero P, Hochberg M, Ott S, Orloff J, Thompson DE, Ewing SK, Delmas PD. Change in bone turnover and hip, non-spine, and vertebral fracture in alendronate-treated women: the fracture intervention trial. J Bone Miner Res 2004;19:1250–1258.
196. Sambrook PN, Geusens P, Ribot C, Solimano JA, Ferrer-Barriendos J, Gaines K, Verbruggen N, Melton ME. Alendronate produces greater effects than raloxifene on bone density and bone turnover in postmenopausal women with low bone density: results of EFFECT (efficacy of fosamax versus evista comparison trial). Int J Intern Med 2004;255:503–511
197. Ju HSJ, Leung S, Brown B, Stringer MA, Leigh S, Scherrer C, Shepard K, Jenkins D, Knudsen J, Cannon R. Comparison of analytical performance and biological variability of three bone resorption assays. Clin Chem 1997;43:1570–1576.

6 Biochemical Markers of Bone Turnover – Clinical Aspects

Christian Meier, Markus J. Seibel, and Marius E. Kraenzlin

CONTENTS

Key Words: Bone turnover marker, monitoring, antiresorptive treatment, bone loss, fracture risk, compliance

From: *Contemporary Endocrinology: Osteoporosis: Pathophysiology and Clinical Management*
Edited by: R. A. Adler, DOI 10.1007/978-1-59745-459-9_6,

SUMMARY

The long-term result of imbalances in bone turnover (i.e., osteoblastic bone formation and osteoclastic bone resorption) is a change in bone mass, strength, and structure, and ultimately may lead to osteoporosis and fragility fractures. In recent years, considerable progress has been made in the isolation and characterization of cellular and extracellular components of the skeletal matrix, which in turn have facilitated the development of biochemical markers that specifically reflect either bone formation or bone resorption. These biochemical indices are non-invasive, comparatively inexpensive, and, when applied and interpreted correctly, helpful tools in the diagnostic and therapeutic assessment of metabolic bone disease. In clinical practice, bone turnover markers have been shown to predict the risk for fractures, independent from BMD. Furthermore, bone markers may be useful for monitoring anti-osteoporotic treatment in order to evaluate treatment efficacy and patients' compliance. In contrast, however, bone markers cannot be used for diagnosis of osteoporosis. The following chapter will give an overview on these clinical aspects of bone turnover markers; the basic biochemistry of bone markers and sources of their non-specific variability are reviewed in Chapter 5.

BONE TURNOVER MARKERS AND PREDICTION OF BONE LOSS

Induced by estrogen deficiency, bone turnover increases rapidly after menopause, and this increase in bone turnover persists long after the menopause, up to 40 years *(1)*. In general bone loss at the spine in the immediate menopausal period is approximately 1% per year; however, as many as one-third of postmenopausal women lose bone at a rate exceeding 1% per year. Cross-sectional data suggest that a sustained increase in bone turnover is associated with a faster and greater bone loss. It has been more difficult to confirm this relationship in longitudinal studies as the amount of bone loss is in the same order of magnitude as the precision error of BMD measurement *(2,3)*. A strong relationship between baseline bone turnover markers and the rate of bone loss has only been demonstrated in a study measuring BMD at the radius, a precise site with small maximal CV *(4)*. In a cohort of 305 postmenopausal women (aged 50–88 years) who had annual forearm BMD measurements over 4 years markers of both bone resorption (S-CTX, U-NTX) and bone formation (OC, PINP) were found to be positively correlated with the rate of bone loss. Furthermore, women with baseline levels of bone markers above the premenopausal range had a rate of bone loss four- to sixfold higher than women with a lower turnover *(4)*.

The clinical utility of bone turnover markers to predict subsequent bone loss in an individual woman seems uncertain. This is illustrated by a study evaluating the association between bone markers and bone loss at the hip in elderly postmenopausal women (aged 73–89 years) *(5)*. Higher levels of bone turnover markers were associated with somewhat faster hip bone loss; however, the predictive value of these markers for bone loss in an individual patient was limited. Nevertheless there is some evidence indicating that biochemical markers can detect "rapid losers" and can predict those women most likely to respond to antiresorptive therapy, i.e., hormone replacement therapy *(6,7)*. Increased bone turnover markers therefore can be regarded as a risk factor for rapid bone loss in postmenopausal women.

In men, the pattern of age-dependent change in bone markers is quite different from that observed in women. While there is general agreement on the age-related changes of bone turnover in adult men between 20 and 60 years of age, data on bone turnover rates in men over the age of 60 years are discordant. Observational studies investigating age-dependent changes in bone marker levels indicate that there seems to be an imbalance in bone turnover with increased bone resorption and stable bone formation after the age of 60 *(8)*. As biochemical markers have been shown to be negatively correlated with BMD *(9,10)*, this imbalance in bone turnover may, at least in part, be responsible for the age-related bone loss in men. However, in elderly men, age-dependent bone loss (as measured by BMD) is less pronounced than in postmenopausal women *(11,12)*, and the association between bone turnover markers and change in BMD remains weak or mostly absent *(13–15)*. Hence, the contribution of bone markers to the prediction of bone loss in elderly men is of limited clinical value.

BONE TURNOVER MARKERS AND PREDICTION OF FRACTURE RISK

Early detection of patients at risk for fractures is the basis for preventive and therapeutic strategies in the management of osteoporosis. A lot of effort has gone into the identification of predictors of osteoporotic fracture risk. Several prospective epidemiological studies in postmenopausal women demonstrated a strong association between BMD and the risk of hip, spine, and forearm fractures. However, up to half of patients with incident fractures have baseline BMD assessed by DXA above the diagnostic threshold of osteoporosis defined as a *T*-score of –2.5 SD or more below the average value of young healthy women *(16–18)*. Importantly, there is increasing evidence that the decision to use pharmacological intervention for prevention of fracture should be based on the fracture probability rather than only on the presence of osteoporosis as defined by BMD *(19,20)*. There is thus need for improvement in the identification of patients at risk for fracture.

Bone strength and fracture risk not only depend on bone mass but also on morphology, the architecture, remodeling of bone, as well as on qualitative properties of bone matrix *(19,21)*. More recently, it has become evident that accelerated bone turnover also is associated with a higher risk of osteoporotic fracture, independent of age, disability and bone mass in women at the menopause and in elderly women, and more recently also for men. In these studies, patients with low bone mineral density and/or high bone turnover were shown to be at the highest risk for osteoporotic fractures.

In postmenopausal women, five prospective studies (EPIDOS, Rotterdam, OFELY, HOS, and Malmö) demonstrated a significant relationship between baseline levels of bone resorption markers (U-CTX, S-CTX, U-DPD, TRAP5b) and subsequent fracture risk *(1,22–26)*. After adjustments for BMD, an increase of these markers above the premenopausal range was associated with a twofold increase in risk for hip, vertebral and non-vertebral fractures, over a follow-up period of 1.8–5 years. Importantly, the prediction of fracture risk is independent of BMD measurements, indicating that accelerated bone resorption deteriorates bone strength beyond a given bone mass. This suggests that a combined approach, with BMD and indices of bone turnover, could improve fracture prediction in postmenopausal women. In fact, Garnero et al. *(23)* showed that in women who had low hip BMD and an increase in U-CTX, the relative risk of hip fracture increased by 4.2 (95% CI, 1.9–9.3), whereas the risk increased by 2.3 if they had high U-CTX (95% CI, 1.3–4.2) and by 2.8

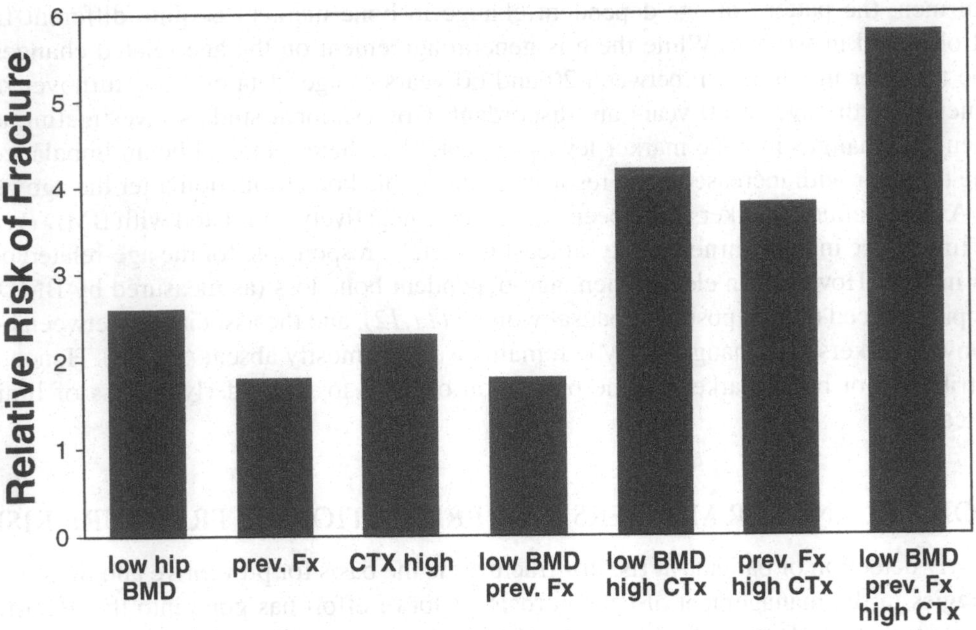

Fig. 1. Combination of different independent predictors to identify women with the highest risk of fracture. Low hip BMD was defined as values at 2.5 SD or below the mean of young adults. High urinary CTX corresponds to values in the highest quartile. RRs are adjusted for age and physical activity. From: Garnero et al. with permission *(23)*.

(95% CI, 1.4–5.6) if they had low BMD (Fig. 1). Calculating the absolute risk such as the 10-year probability of fracture based on two prospective studies (EPIDOS and OFELY), it was found that combining clinical risk factors (i.e., previous fracture), BMD and bone turnover, results in a 10-year probability of hip fracture that was about 70–100% higher than that associated with low BMD alone *(27)* (Fig. 2). Thus there is evidence that patients with low bone mineral density and high bone turnover are at high risk for osteoporotic fractures.

In contrast to bone resorption markers data on the association between bone formation markers and fracture risk are conflicting. In the French cohort study of elderly women (EPIDOS) no significant relationship between OC and BAP and the risk of hip fracture could be demonstrated during a 2-year follow-up, whereas in younger healthy postmenopausal women (OFELY, HOS) a significant relationship between increased BAP levels and risk of vertebral as well as non-vertebral fracture was found *(22–24)*. Difference in study populations, sampling conditions, fracture types, and the duration of follow-up may in part explain the contradictory results. In this context it is noteworthy that in the OFELY study (initial follow-up 5 years) a reassessment was performed after a median of 9 years follow-up and a significant positive association between baseline bone formation markers and the risk of fracture was confirmed *(2,18)*.

In a recent study including 151 elderly men (aged over 60) followed prospectively over 6.3 years, high bone resorption (as assessed by serum ICTP) was associated with increased

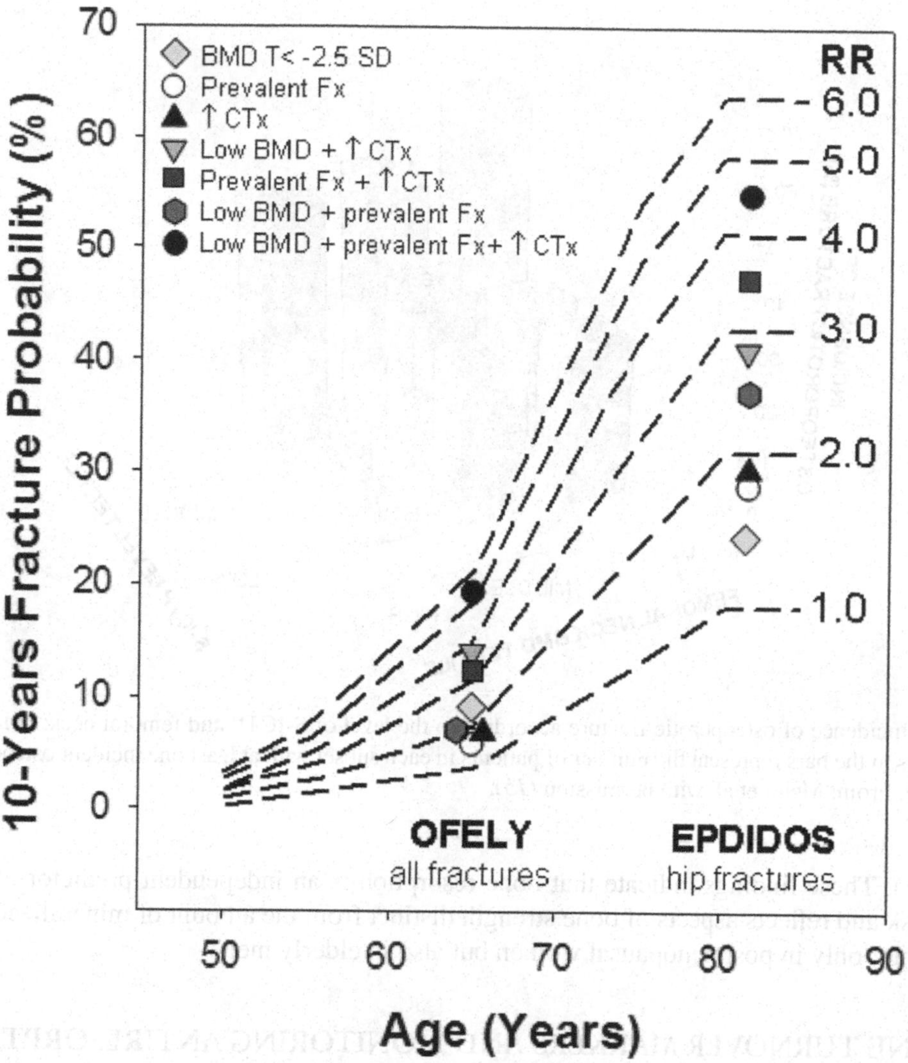

Fig. 2. Combination of clinical risk factors, bone mineral density, and bone turnover measurements to identify women with the highest risk of fracture. The figure shows the 10-year probability of hip fracture according to age and relative risk. The symbols show the effect of risk factors on fracture probability derived from women aged 65 (OFELY study) and 80 (EPIDOS study). The data from the OFELY study are derived from information of all fractures. Low hip BMD was defined as values at 2.5 SD or below the mean of young adults. High urinary CTX corresponds to values above the upper limit of premenopausal women (mean+2SD). From: Johnell et al. with permission *(27)*.

risk of osteoporotic fracture, independent of BMD *(15)*. For each increase in ICTP concentrations by 1 SD, overall fracture probability increased by 40%. The association was significant for hip fractures (RR 1.7; 95% CI; 1.2–2.6) and vertebral fractures (RR 2.1; 95% CI; 1.3–3.3). Men with ICTP levels in the highest quartile had a 2.8-fold increased risk of incident fractures compared to men with ICTP levels in the lowest quartile. In addition, fracture incidence was about 10 times higher in men with low BMD combined with a high bone resorption rate compared to men with high BMD and lower values of ICTP

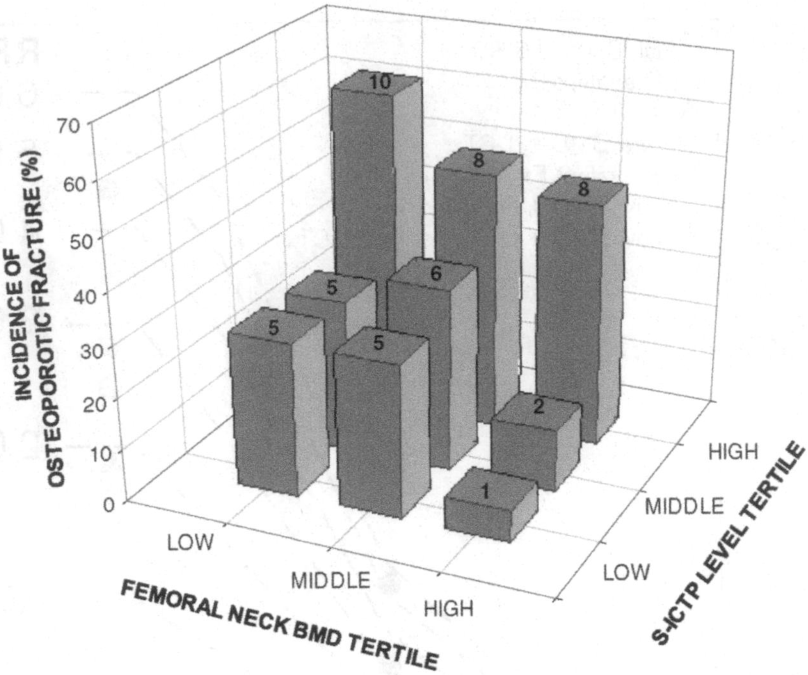

Fig. 3. Incidence of osteoporotic fracture according to the level of S-ICTP and femoral neck BMD. The numbers in the bars represent the number of patients in each subset with at least one incident osteoporotic fracture. From: Meier et al. with permission *(15)*.

(Fig. 3). These findings indicate that bone resorption is an independent predictor of fracture risk and reflects aspects of bone strength distinct from the amount of mineralized bone tissue not only in postmenopausal women but also in elderly men.

BONE TURNOVER MARKERS AND MONITORING ANTIRESORPTIVE TREATMENT

A major domain for the clinical use of biochemical bone markers is the monitoring of osteoporosis therapy. This application includes keeping an eye on both therapeutic efficacy (i.e., the prediction of the therapeutic response in regard to changes in BMD and reduction in fracture risk) and patient compliance. The ultimate goal in treating patients with osteoporosis is to reduce their fracture risk. However, the short-term incidence of osteoporotic fractures is low, and the absence of fracture during treatment does not necessarily mean that the treatment is effective. Thus monitoring the effect of treatment by fracture incidence alone would be inadequate for most practical purposes. Consequently, serial measurements of changes in BMD as a surrogate marker of therapeutic efficacy are currently the standard approach to monitor osteoporosis therapy. However, changes in BMD occur slowly and significant therapeutic effects are usually not detectable before several years of treatment *(28–30)*. In contrast, biochemical markers of bone turnover change much faster than BMD in response to therapeutic interventions and therefore may be used for monitoring antiresorptive treatment efficacy and treatment adherence.

EFFECT OF ANTIRESORPTIVE TREATMENT ON BONE TURNOVER MARKERS

Most antiresorptive agents induce a profound decrease in bone turnover with maximal suppression of bone resorption markers within 1–6 months of treatment, and a somewhat delayed decrease in bone formation markers. The magnitude of suppression in bone markers appears to depend on the dose and potency of the drug chosen as well as the marker used *(31,32)*.

Estrogen deficiency is associated with a significant increase in bone remodeling as reflected by a 50–100% increase in both bone formation and bone resorption markers *(33–37)*. Many studies, including large randomized placebo-controlled trials evaluating the effect of estrogen replacement therapy on bone turnover, have consistently demonstrated that hormone replacement therapy can reverse these changes by decreasing markers of bone turnover into the premenopausal range. Irrespective of the route of administration, a rapid and sustained decrease in bone resorption markers is observed during the initial weeks of HRT, reaching a plateau within 3–6 months. Due to the normal coupling of bone resorption and formation processes, bone formation markers usually follow with a short delay *(6,7,38–60)*. After discontinuation of HRT, markers of bone resorption and, at a later stage, markers of bone formation return to postmenopausal (i.e., elevated) levels *(52,56,61)*.

As shown in early postmenopausal women treated with conjugated estrogens (0.625 mg/day), urinary NTX levels significantly decrease by 23% as early as 2 weeks after starting replacement therapy. After 3 months, urinary NTX levels decreased by 39% *(48)*, whereas urinary DPD concentrations showed a less pronounced effect with a mean decrease of 20% *(6)*. Comparable antiresorptive effects have been observed for formulations using alternate routes of administration, including transdermal *(42,49,59)*, percutaneous *(38)*, and intranasal *(55,60)* estrogen applications.

With both conjugated estrogens (CEE) *(57)* and transdermal 17β-estradiol *(62)*, a dose-dependent suppressive effect on bone resorption markers has been observed in early postmenopausal women. Lindsay et al. *(57)* report on significant reductions in urinary NTX levels after 24 months of treatment with either 0.625 or 0.3 mg CEE daily. However, the reduction in urinary NTX levels was significantly smaller for women taking CEE at 0.3 mg/d (34%) as compared to women on 0.625 mg/d (55%). In older postmenopausal women, however, the response of biochemical markers of bone turnover was similar for lower or higher estrogen doses *(53,56,58)* indicating that lower than usual doses of estrogen may equally reduce bone resorption and, thereby prevent bone loss in older postmenopausal women.

Raloxifene is a selective estrogen receptor modulator (SERM) with estrogen agonistic effects on the skeleton. Studies in different cohorts including early menopausal *(63)*, late postmenopausal *(64–66)*, as well as older, institutionalized women *(67)* demonstrate that raloxifene induces a sustained decrease in markers of bone resorption and formation, reaching a plateau after 6–12 months of treatment. Delmas et al. *(63)* reported significant reductions in urinary CTX by 34%, BAP by 23%, and OC by 15% after 24 months of continuous treatment with raloxifene 60 mg/d. Two recent studies comparing the effects of raloxifene and estrogen treatment on bone turnover suggest that raloxifene results in a less pronounced reduction in bone markers *(68,69)*.

Treatment of postmenopausal women, and of men, with bisphosphonates such as alendronate *(3,70–78)*, risedronate *(79–83)*, ibandronate *(84–89)*, pamidronate *(90)*, and zoledronate *(91)* results in suppression of bone turnover. As with HRT, bone resorption markers decrease earlier than markers of bone formation, consistent with a direct effect of bisphosphonates on osteoclasts. Several studies have shown that the absolute amount of metabolic suppression achieved by any bisphosphonate depends on the dose, the way of administration, and the biochemical marker chosen. Independent of these factors, the effects of bisphosphonates on bone turnover seem more pronounced than those of either HRT *(92,93)* or raloxifene *(94)* (Fig. 4).

Most studies would suggest that the suppressive effect of bisphosphonates on bone turnover is "largest" when measured by telopeptides of type I collagen (NTX, CTX), and that less pronounced effects are observed when using urinary DPD and PYD as resorption markers. Furthermore, treatment with intravenous bisphosphonates leads to a reduction in resorption markers as early as 12–72 h after the injection *(90,95,96)*, while oral bisphosphonates act much slower. For example, postmenopausal women treated with oral alendronate had a 58% decrease in urinary NTX levels after 4 weeks of treatment *(74)*, and achieved the maximal response after 6–12 months of treatment. At this point in time, mean reductions were 50–80% for urinary NTX, 35–50% for urinary CTX, 20–50% for total DPD and PYD, and 20–25% for free DPD and PYD *(3,70–72,74,78,94)*. When looking at these numbers, one should not forget that a numerical result alone has little value if not viewed against the background of that marker's non-specific variability. As a rule of thumb, markers showing a pronounced response (signal) to bisphosphonate therapy also exhibit the greatest degree of non-specific variability (noise). Calculating the respective signal-to-noise ratios for the various markers can be helpful in distinguishing between spurious and true differences in the magnitude of response.

Due to the coupling of bone resorption and bone formation, markers of bone formation decrease in parallel to markers of bone resorption, but with a delay of several weeks to months. In postmenopausal women treated with alendronate, a decrease in serum OC by 30–50%, BAP by 35–45%, and PICP by 35–40% has been reported *(70,71,74,78)*.

Several recent studies investigated the effect of combined treatments on bone mass and bone turnover, comparing HRT alone with combinations of HRT with either alendronate *(92,97)* or risedronate *(98)*. Elderly postmenopausal women treated with HRT plus alendronate had a more pronounced decrease in bone turnover than women on HRT alone. Although a significantly greater decrease in bone turnover markers was seen in the combined bisphosphonate-HRT groups, the differences between the various treatment groups were small and, hence, of uncertain clinical significance when it comes to differences in the change of BMD or fracture risk.

Upon cessation of most bisphosphonates given for 2 or 3 years, indices of bone turnover increase to attain pre-treatment values within 3–12 months *(97,99)*. However, following a group of postmenopausal women treated with the highest doses of oral ibandronate, Ravn et al. *(86)* observed that serum OC and BALP values remained reduced at 12 months after discontinuation of treatment. Similar data were reported for both bone formation and bone resorption markers after a single dose of zoledronate *(91)*, indicating that high-dose bisphosphonate regimens may induce long-term suppression of bone turnover. Bone et al. *(100)* showed that after 5 years of alendronate treatment, NTX levels rise about 20–25% in the first year and then are maintained at the new reduced level for the next 4 years.

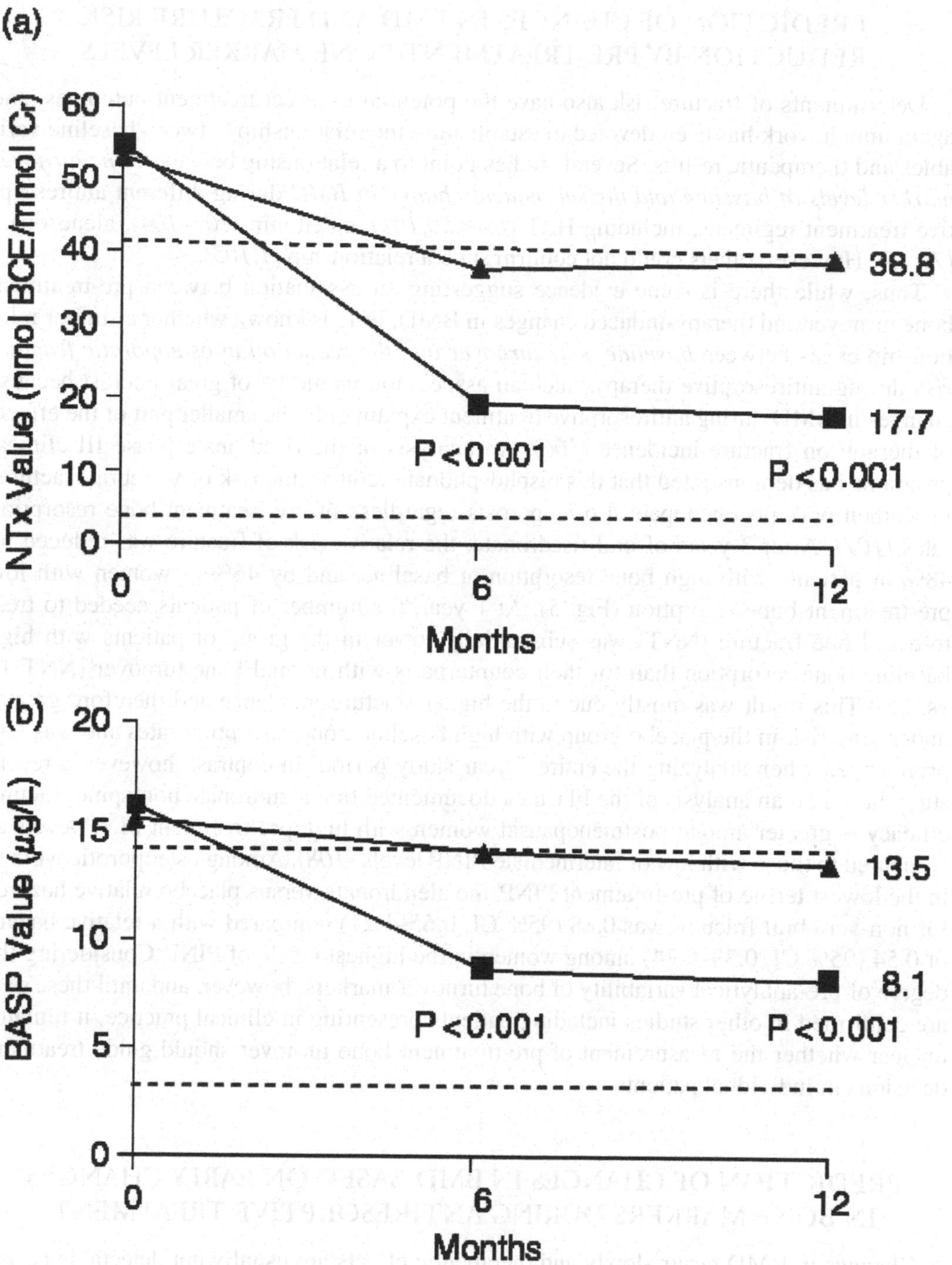

Fig. 4. Change in bone turnover markers during treatment with alendronate 70 mg once weekly (■) and raloxifene 60 mg daily (▲) for 12 months. **(a)** Urinary N-telopeptide of type I collagen (NTX) absolute values, **(b)** serum bone-specific alkaline phosphatase (BSAP) absolute values. Apparently, the effects of alendronate on both markers are more pronounced than those of raloxifene. However, both antiresorptive agents reduce both bone markers into their respective reference range (area between *dashed lines*). From: Sambrook et al. with permission *(94)*.

PREDICTION OF CHANGES IN BMD AND FRACTURE RISK REDUCTION BY PRE-TREATMENT BONE MARKER LEVELS

Determinants of fracture risk also have the potential to affect treatment outcomes, and again, much work has been devoted to establishing the relationship between baseline variables and therapeutic results. Several studies point to a relationship between *bone turnover marker levels at baseline and the subsequent change in BMD* during different antiresorptive treatment regimens, including HRT *(6,48,50,101)*, calcitonin *(102–104)*, alendronate *(72,75)*. However, others could not confirm such a relationship *(1,105)*.

Thus, while there is some evidence suggesting an association between pre-treatment bone turnover and therapy-induced changes in BMD, little is known whether a similar relationship exists between *baseline bone turnover and the reduction in osteoporotic fracture risk* during antiresorptive therapy. Such an association would be of great interest because changes in BMD during antiresorptive treatment explain only the smaller part of the effects of therapy on fracture incidence *(106)*. An analysis of the risedronate phase III clinical programs has demonstrated that this bisphosphonate reduces the risk of vertebral fractures in women with postmenopausal osteoporosis regardless of pre-treatment bone resorption rates *(107)*. After 3 years of oral risedronate, the relative risk of fracture was reduced by 48% in patients with high bone resorption at baseline, and by 46% in women with low pre-treatment bone resorption (Fig. 5). At 1 year, the number of patients needed to treat to avoid one fracture (NNT) was substantially lower in the group of patients with high baseline bone resorption than for their counterparts with normal bone turnover (NNT 15 vs. 25). This result was mostly due to the higher fracture incidence and therefore greater underlying risk in the placebo group with high baseline bone resorption rates and was less pronounced when analyzing the entire 3-year study period. In contrast, however, a recent study based on an analysis of the FIT data documented that alendronate non-spine fracture efficacy is greater among postmenopausal women with high pre-treatment PINP levels as compared to those with low or intermediate PINP levels *(108)*. Among osteoporotic women in the lowest tertile of pre-treatment PINP, the alendronate versus placebo relative hazards for non-vertebral fracture was 0.88 (95% CI, 0.65–1.21) compared with a relative hazard of 0.54 (95% CI, 0.39–0.74) among women in the highest tertile of PINP. Considering the degree of pre-analytical variability of bone turnover markers, however, and until these data are confirmed in other studies including patients presenting in clinical practice, it remains unclear whether the measurement of pre-treatment bone turnover should guide treatment decisions in individual patients.

PREDICTION OF CHANGES IN BMD BASED ON EARLY CHANGES IN BONE MARKERS DURING ANTIRESORPTIVE TREATMENT

Changes in BMD occur slowly and therapeutic effects are usually not detectable before several years of treatment. This is partly due to the disadvantageous short-term signal-to-noise ratio of most BMD measurements. Within a year of treatment, comparatively small changes in bone density (2–4%) are contrasted by relatively high precision errors (1–3%), which renders BMD measurements unreliable for short-term assessment of antiresorptive treatment efficacy *(109)*. Owing to their significant biological variability, biochemical markers of bone turnover also exhibit a high degree of imprecision and a signal-to-noise

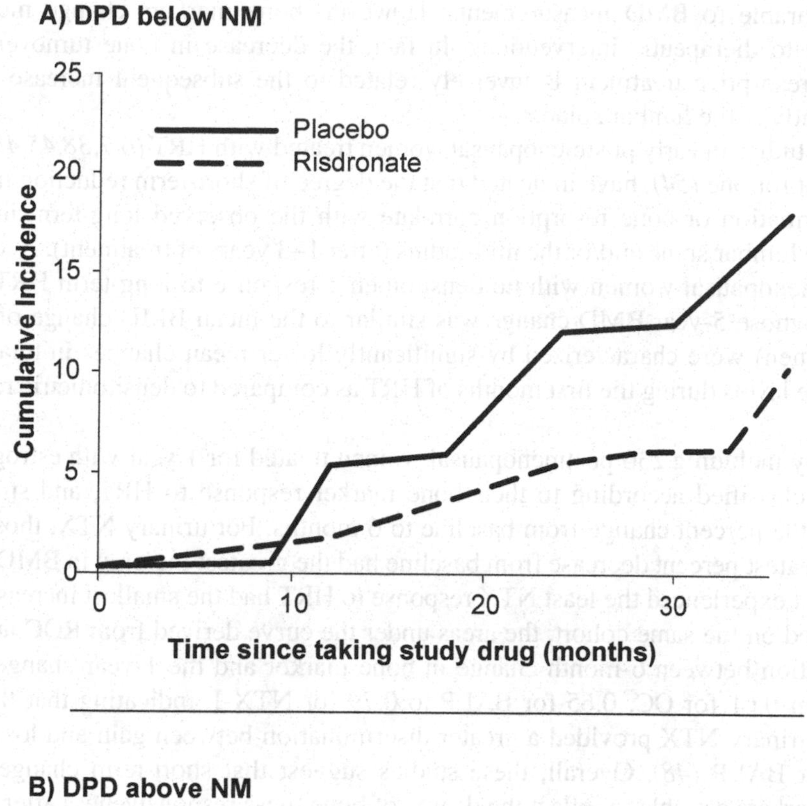

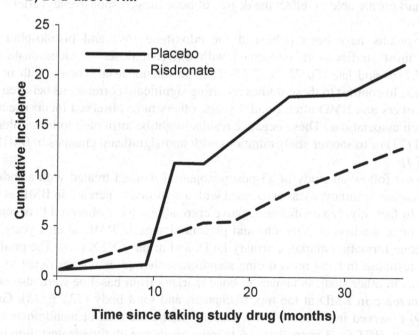

Fig. 5. Cumulative incidence of new vertebral fractures by bone resorption status (urinary DPD). **(A)** Below normative mean (NM). **(B)** Above normative mean (NM). The *dotted lines* represent risedronate-treated patients, whereas the *solid lines* represent patients receiving placebo. From: Seibel et al. with permission *(107)*.

ratio comparable to BMD measurements. However, bone markers change much faster in response to therapeutic interventions. In fact, the decrease in bone turnover markers during antiresorptive treatment is inversely related to the subsequent increase in BMD, predominantly at the lumbar spine.

Several studies in early postmenopausal women treated with HRT *(6,7,38,45,48,50,110–114)*, except for one *(54)*, have indicated that the degree of short-term reduction in markers of bone formation or bone resorption correlate with the observed long-term increase in BMD at the lumbar spine and/or the mid-radius (after 1–3 years of treatment). Accordingly, early postmenopausal women with no densitometric response to long-term HRT (defined as women whose 5-year BMD change was similar to the mean BMD change of placebo-treated women) were characterized by significantly lower mean changes in total alkaline phosphatase levels during the first months of HRT as compared to densitometric responders *(113)*.

In a study including 236 postmenopausal women treated for 1 year with estrogens, subjects were classified according to their bone marker response to HRT, and stratified by quartile of the percent change from baseline to 6 months. For urinary NTX, those women with the greatest percent decrease from baseline had the greatest increase in BMD, whereas subjects that experienced the least NTX response to HRT had the smallest increase in spine BMD. Based on the same cohort, the areas under the curve derived from ROC analyses of the association between 6-month change in bone marker and the 1-year change in BMD ranged from 0.61 for OC, 0.65 for BALP to 0.79 for NTX-I, indicating that the percent change in urinary NTX provided a greater discrimination between gain and loss of BMD than OC or BALP *(48)*. Overall, these studies suggest that short-term changes in bone turnover markers are able to reflect the degree of bone mass responsiveness after 1–3 years of HRT.

Similar results have been published for raloxifene *(69)* and bisphosphonates. Of the latter, most studies were performed with different doses of alendronate in early *(73,78,115,116)* and late *(70,72,76,77,117,118)* postmenopausal women with or without osteoporosis. In contrast to these studies reporting significant correlations between changes in bone markers and BMD after 1 and 4 years, others have observed inconsistent *(71)* or no *(74)* such associations. These negative results might be attributed to lower alendronate doses used *(71)* or to shorter study durations with non-significant changes in BMD (after 6 months) *(74)*.

In a 2-year follow-up study in 85 postmenopausal women treated with alendronate, a marked decrease in turnover was associated with a significant increase in BMD at the lumbar spine. In fact, highly significant negative correlations were observed between percent change in bone markers at 3 months and percent change in BMD after 2 years of treatment for bone formation markers, urinary DPD, and urinary NTX *(70)*. The prediction of long-term response in bone mass during alendronate therapy is not restricted to the lumbar spine, as in other studies changes in bone markers from baseline were also correlated with the increase in BMD at the hip, trochanter, and total body *(72,73,118)*. Greenspan et al. *(119)* observed in a double-blind, placebo-controlled trial of alendronate treatment combined with HRT for 3 years that at 6 months, women with the greatest drop in urinary NTX (66% or greater) had the largest gain in BMD at all sites compared with patients who had smaller decreases in NTX (Fig. 6). Furthermore, Garnero et al. *(76)* showed that both the absolute serum BALP level and the percent change in BALP at 6 months of treatment

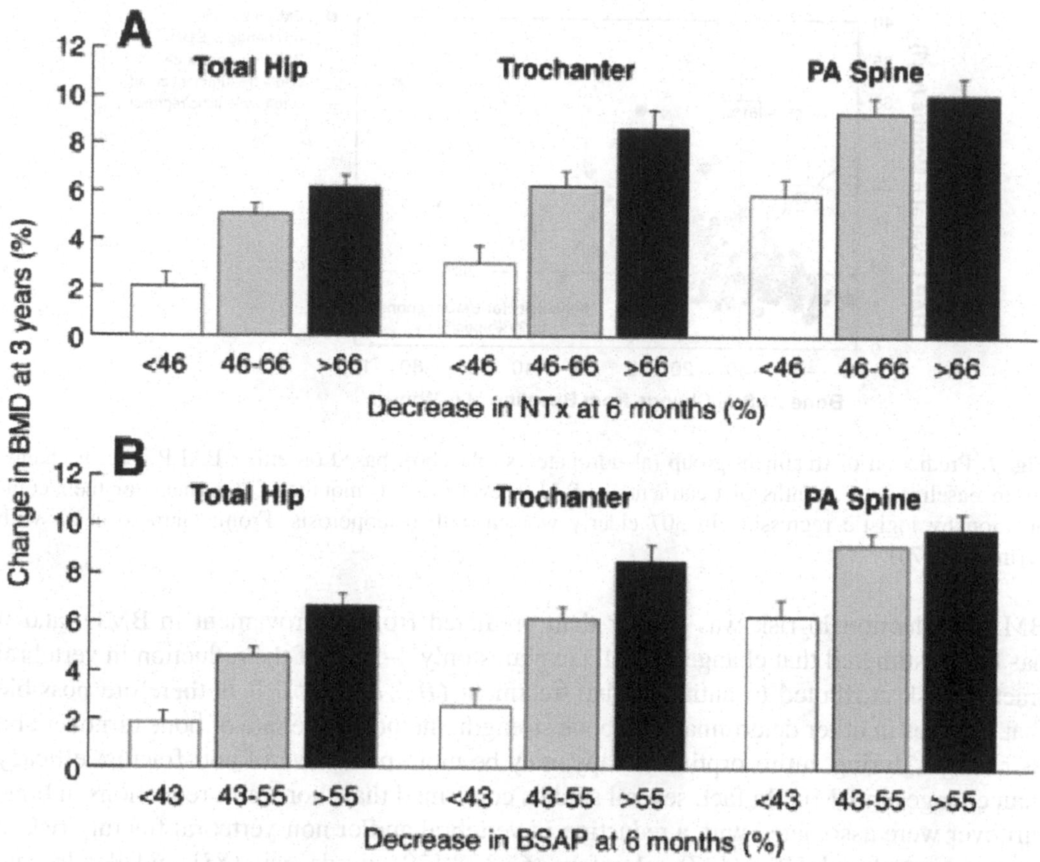

Fig. 6. Percent changes in BMD at the total hip, trochanter, and posteroanterior (PA) spine after 3 years of active treatment (alendronate, HRT, or combination therapy), grouped by percent decreases in (**A**) urinary NTX and (**B**) serum BAP levels at 6 months. From: Greenspan et al. with permission *(119)*.

are independent predictors of BMD gain (defined as an increase in spine BMD of at least 3% after 2 years). Based on these data it could be stated that in order to define treatment responsiveness, assessment of the relative change from baseline at 3–6 months may be imprecise to identify BMD responders. The combination of the absolute bone marker level at 6 months (as an estimate of the current bone turnover rate) and the change from baseline (as a measure of treatment efficacy) may improve the prediction of changes in BMD *(76)* (Fig. 7). Further validation of such models using different bone markers is required before they can be safely applied to clinical practice.

PREDICTION OF FRACTURE RISK REDUCTION BASED ON EARLY CHANGES IN BONE MARKERS DURING ANTIRESORPTIVE TREATMENT

Although several randomized trials have found that antiresorptive agents improve BMD and reduce the risk of fractures *(64,80,120–124)*, recent studies have evidenced that the observed reduction in fracture risk is only partly explained by the observed changes in

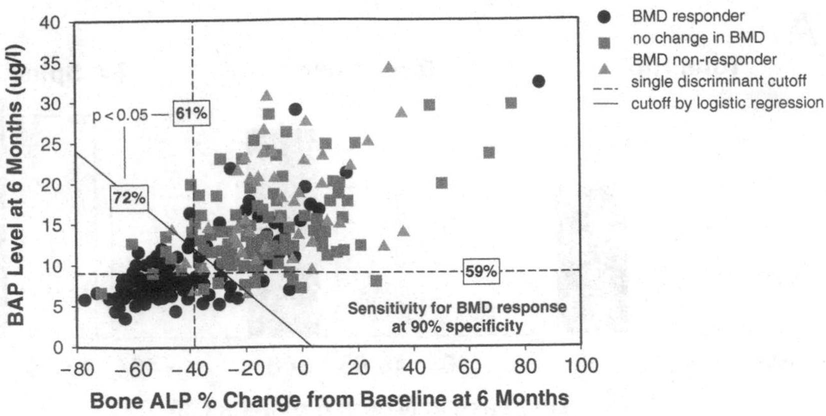

Fig. 7. Prediction of treatment group (alendronate vs. placebo), based on either BALP percent change (from baseline to 6 months of treatment) or BALP level (after 6 months of treatment) or their combination by logistic regression in 307 elderly women with osteoporosis. From: Garnero et al. with permission *(76)*.

BMD. Reduction in risk was greater than predicted from improvement in BMD, and it has been estimated that change in BMD explains only 4–28% of the reduction in vertebral fracture risk attributed to antiresorptive treatment *(106,125,126)*. It is therefore possible that changes in other determinants of bone strength, including the rate of bone turnover and its changes during antiresorptive therapy, may be more predictive of anti-fracture efficacy than changes in BMD. In fact, several studies confirmed that short-term reductions in bone turnover were associated with a reduction in vertebral and/or non-vertebral fracture risk in women treated with HRT *(127)*, raloxifene *(66,128,129)*, risedronate *(83)*, and alendronate *(130)*.

Bjarnason et al. *(128)* studied the relationship between changes in bone turnover markers and vertebral fracture risk after 3 years of raloxifene treatment in postmenopausal women. Decreases in serum levels of OC and BAP after 1 year of treatment were significantly associated with a decreased risk of new vertebral fractures after 3 years. Importantly, these relationships remained after adjustment for baseline vertebral fracture status and BMD. Two subsequent analyses including postmenopausal women with osteoporosis from the same cohort (MORE trial) extended and confirmed these results showing that both 1-year percentage changes in serum PINP *(66)* and OC *(129)* are able to predict the reduction in vertebral fracture risk after 3 years of treatment.

Recently, two studies have been published investigating the change in bone turnover markers and fracture risk in bisphosphonate treated postmenopausal women *(83,130)*. Using data from the VERT studies including postmenopausal women with at least one vertebral fracture, Eastell et al. *(83)* found that reductions in urinary CTX (by 60%) and NTX (by 51%) at 3–6 months of risedronate treatment were significantly associated with the reduction in vertebral and non-vertebral fracture risk after 3 years. The change in bone resorption markers explained more than 50% of the risedronate-related fracture risk reduction for both, vertebral and non-vertebral fractures.

Bauer et al. *(130)* reported that in alendronate-treated women, greater reductions in bone turnover were associated with fewer osteoporotic fractures. In their study, each SD reduction in the change in serum BAP at 1 year was associated with fewer spine (HR, 0.74; 95% CI; 0.63 –0.87), non-spine (0.89; 95% CI; 0.78–1.00), and hip fractures (0.61; 95% CI; 0.46–0.78). Furthermore, alendronate-treated women with at least a 30% reduction in serum BALP had a lower risk of non-spine (0.72; 95% CI; 0.55–0.92) and hip fractures (0.26; 95% CI; 0.08–0.83) relative to those with reductions < 30% (Fig. 8).

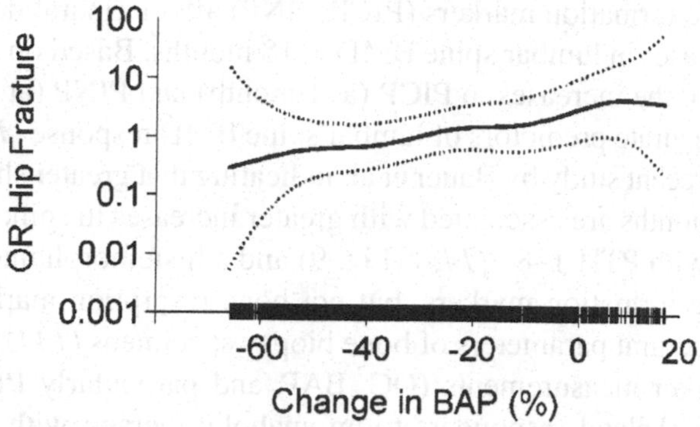

Fig. 8. One-year change in bone ALP and hip fracture risk among alendroante-treated women. Percent change in bone ALP and predicted risk (log OR) of hip fracture (*solid line*) and 95% CI (*dotted lines*) from logistic regression model. Individual data points represented on the *x* axis. Departure from linearity *p* value 0.33. From: Bauer et al. with permission *(130)*.

These data suggest that increased bone turnover is an important determinant of fracture susceptibility and early reductions in bone turnover during antiresorptive treatment in fact reduces fracture risk beyond changes in BMD.

BONE TURNOVER MARKERS AND MONITORING ANABOLIC THERAPY

Recently anabolic agents from the parathyroid hormone family have become available as a new advance in the treatment of osteoporosis. Both, the aminoterminal fragment of human PTH [PTH 1–34; teriparatide] *(131–134)* and the full-length molecule PTH 1–84,*135–137* stimulate new bone formation on bone surfaces by preferentially stimulating osteoblastic activity over osteoclastic activity in both, postmenopausal women and men. The anabolic effects of PTH are resulting in increased bone mass, bone turnover, and bone strength, and importantly improved microarchitectural qualities of bone beyond the effects known from bisphosphonates.

Similar to the antiresorptive agents, it can be assumed that the therapeutic effects of PTH are based on its actions to influence bone turnover. Several randomized studies have demonstrated that bone formation markers (TAP, OC, PINP) increase early after teriparatide therapy has been initiated, with a delayed but substantial increase in bone resorption markers (S-CTX, S-NTX) *(135,138–140)*. The difference in time course between the initial stimulation of bone formation and the subsequent stimulation of bone resorption has given rise to the concept of the "anabolic window," a period of time when the anabolic actions of PTH are maximal and allow for a substantial gain in bone mass before bone remodeling is stimulated *(141)*. Based on changes in bone turnover marker levels (as well as changes in

BMD) it is suggested, however, that the concurrent use of bisphosphonates may reduce the anabolic properties of PTH most likely due to the dominating effects of the antiresorptive drug on bone dynamics *(133,134,136)*.

Similar as for antiresorptive drugs, it can be questioned whether short-term changes in bone turnover markers can be used to monitor the effect of PTH on BMD or fracture risk reduction. Indeed, Chen et al. have shown that in postmenopausal women with osteoporosis, early changes in bone formation markers (PICP, PINP) after teriparatide administration are associated with increases in lumbar spine BMD at 18 months. Based on ROC analysis it has been shown that both, the increases in PICP (at 1 month) and PINP (at 3 months) were the most sensitive and accurate predictors of lumbar spine BMD response *(142)*. These findings were confirmed in a recent study by Bauer et al. indicating that greater short-term changes in PINP levels after 3 months are associated with greater increases in spine and hip BMD after 1 year of treatment with PTH 1–84 *(143)* (Fig. 9) and a histomorphometric study showing that changes in bone formation markers, but not bone resorption markers, are associated with increases in structural parameters of bone biopsy specimens *(144)*. These data suggest that serial bone marker measurements (OC, BAP, and particularly PINP) could become useful in identifying skeletal responders to an anabolic therapy with PTH, especially as the two- to fourfold increase in bone formation marker above baseline exceeds the least significant change of the measurement.

For clinical practice a strategy based on PINP measurements at baseline and after 1–3 months of PTH therapy has been proposed *(145)*. Positive PINP responses (defined as increases > 10 μg/L) were observed in 77–97% of teriparatide- and in 6% of placebo-treated patients after 3 months of study drug. Patients with PINP increases < 10 μg/L therefore should be assessed for adherence, PTH administration and storage techniques, and for the presence of medical conditions that might limit their therapeutic response. In patient without these issues, repeat bone marker measurement in another 3 months by which time one would expect clear changes to be detectable seems prudent. Data assessing the relationship between changes in bone markers and fracture risk are not available yet. On the other hand it is interesting to note that in postmenopausal women with osteoporosis increases in BMD account only for approximately one-third of the vertebral fracture risk reduction seen with teriparatide *(146)*. The majority of the risk reduction, however, results from improvements in non-BMD determinants of bone strength, which might include changes in bone markers. Nevertheless, teriparatide-mediated relative fracture risk reduction was independent of pre-treatment bone marker levels (BAP, PINP, U-NTX, U-DPD) *(147)* indicating that anabolic treatment with PTH might offer clinical benefit to patients irrespective of baseline bone turnover.

MONITORING PATIENT COMPLIANCE USING BONE MARKERS

Compliance with long-term treatment, such as for osteoporosis, is usually poor *(148,149)*. Several studies reported that up to 50% of postmenopausal women were not adherent to their treatment after 1–5 years of antiresorptive therapy *(150–156)*. Poor adherence to medication has an adverse effect on outcome with non-adherent patients exhibiting smaller BMD gains, and a significantly greater risk of fracture *(157,158)*. Hence, monitoring patients on antiresorptive medication is an eminent part of patient management in order to improve adherence and persistence to therapy, and ultimately treatment effectiveness.

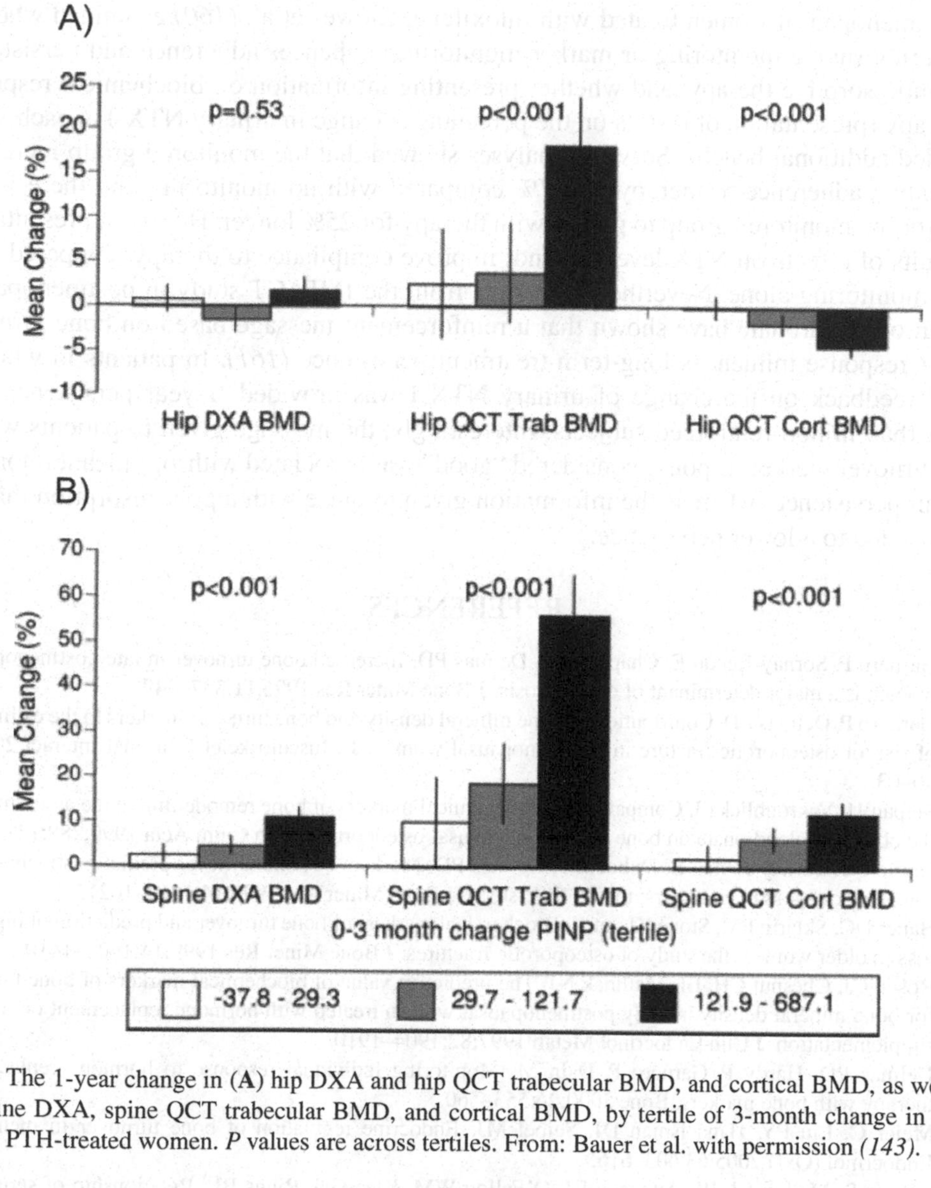

Fig. 9. The 1-year change in **(A)** hip DXA and hip QCT trabecular BMD, and cortical BMD, as well as, **(B)** spine DXA, spine QCT trabecular BMD, and cortical BMD, by tertile of 3-month change in PINP among PTH-treated women. *P* values are across tertiles. From: Bauer et al. with permission *(143)*.

Biochemical markers of bone turnover have been advocated to facilitate follow-up of patients receiving antiresorptive treatments for osteoporosis. As bone turnover markers, in particular indices of bone resorption, decrease rapidly after initiation of treatment within 3–6 months, they might represent useful surrogate markers for monitoring patient compliance.

Using a decision analysis model, Chapurlat et al. *(159)* compared two strategies of follow-up: (a) treatment of a woman without specific monitoring and (b) treatment of this woman with measurement of a serum marker of bone resorption after 3 months of treatment, with change of treatment if response to treatment as assessed by this marker was not satisfactory. It has been suggested that the approach of monitoring osteoporotic women with measurements of bone markers early during treatment course may increase effectiveness of treatment with greater quality-adjusted life years than no follow-up. In a recent study in

75 postmenopausal women treated with raloxifene, Clowes et al. *(160)* examined whether monitoring (nurse monitoring or marker monitoring) enhances adherence and persistence with antiresorptive therapy, and whether presenting information on biochemical response to therapy (presentation of results on the percentage change in urinary NTX-I at each visit) provided additional benefit. Survival analyses showed that the monitored group increased cumulative adherence to therapy by 57% compared with no monitoring and there was a trend for the monitored group to persist with therapy for 25% longer. However, presentation of results of effects on NTX levels did not improve compliance to therapy compared with nurse monitoring alone. Nevertheless, results from the IMPACT study in postmenopausal women on risedronate have shown that a reinforcement message based on bone turnover marker response influences long-term treatment persistence *(161)*. In patients in whom a verbal feedback on the change of urinary NTX-I was provided, 1-year persistence was higher than in non-reinforced subjects. Interestingly, the message given to patients with a bone turnover marker response considered "good" was associated with significant improvement in persistence, whereas the information given to those with a poor resorption marker response led to a lower persistence.

REFERENCES

1. Garnero P, Sornay-Rendu E, Chapuy MC, Delmas PD. Increased bone turnover in late postmenopausal women is a major determinant of osteoporosis. J Bone Miner Res 1996;11:337–349.
2. Garnero P, Delmas PD. Contribution of bone mineral density and bone turnover markers to the estimation of risk of osteoporotic fracture in postmenopausal women. J Musculoskelet Neuronal Interact 2004;4: 50–63.
3. Stepan JJ, Vokrouhlicka J. Comparison of biochemical markers of bone remodelling in the assessment of the effects of alendronate on bone in postmenopausal osteoporosis. Clin Chim Acta 1999;288:121–135.
4. Garnero P, Sornay-Rendu E, Duboeuf F, Delmas PD. Markers of bone turnover predict postmenopausal forearm bone loss over 4 years: the OFELY study. J Bone Miner Res 1999;14:1614–1621.
5. Bauer DC, Sklarin PM, Stone KL, et al. Biochemical markers of bone turnover and prediction of hip bone loss in older women: the study of osteoporotic fractures. J Bone Miner Res 1999;14:1404–1410.
6. Rosen CJ, Chesnut CH, III, Mallinak NJ. The predictive value of biochemical markers of bone turnover for bone mineral density in early postmenopausal women treated with hormone replacement or calcium supplementation. J Clin Endocrinol Metab 1997;82:1904–1910.
7. Delmas PD, Hardy P, Garnero P, Dain M. Monitoring individual response to hormone replacement therapy with bone markers. Bone 2000;26:553–560.
8. Meier C, Liu PY, Handelsman DJ, Seibel MJ. Endocrine regulation of bone turnover in men. Clin Endocrinol (Oxf) 2005;63:603–616.
9. Khosla S, Melton LJ, III, Atkinson EJ, O'Fallon WM, Klee GG, Riggs BL. Relationship of serum sex steroid levels and bone turnover markers with bone mineral density in men and women: a key role for bioavailable estrogen. J Clin Endocrinol Metab 1998;83:2266–2274.
10. Szulc P, Garnero P, Munoz F, Marchand F, Delmas PD. Cross-sectional evaluation of bone metabolism in men. J Bone Miner Res 2001;16:1642–1650.
11. Nguyen TV, Sambrook PN, Eisman JA. Bone loss, physical activity, and weight change in elderly women: the Dubbo Osteoporosis Epidemiology Study. J Bone Miner Res 1998;13:1458–1467.
12. Ensrud KE, Palermo L, Black DM, et al. Hip and calcaneal bone loss increase with advancing age: longitudinal results from the study of osteoporotic fractures. J Bone Miner Res 1995;10:1778–1787.
13. Yoshimura N, Hashimoto T, Sakata K, Morioka S, Kasamatsu T, Cooper C. Biochemical markers of bone turnover and bone loss at the lumbar spine and femoral neck: the Taiji study. Calcif Tissue Int 1999;65:198–202.
14. Chandani AK, Scariano JK, Glew RH, Clemens JD, Garry PJ, Baumgartner RN. Bone mineral density and serum levels of aminoterminal propeptides and cross-linked N-telopeptides of type I collagen in elderly men. Bone 2000;26:513–518.

15. Meier C, Nguyen TV, Center JR, Seibel MJ, Eisman JA. Bone resorption and osteoporotic fractures in elderly men: The Dubbo Osteoporosis Epidemiology Study. J Bone Miner Res 2005;20:579–587.
16. Siris ES, Miller PD, Barrett-Connor E, et al. Identification and fracture outcomes of undiagnosed low bone mineral density in postmenopausal women: results from the National Osteoporosis Risk Assessment. JAMA 2001;286:2815–2822.
17. Schuit SC, van der Klift M, Weel AE, et al. Fracture incidence and association with bone mineral density in elderly men and women: the Rotterdam Study. Bone 2004;34:195–202.
18. Sornay-Rendu E, Munoz F, Garnero P, Duboeuf F, Delmas PD. Identification of osteopenic women at high risk of fracture: the OFELY study. J Bone Miner Res 2005;20:1813–1819.
19. Kanis JA, Borgstrom F, De Laet C, et al. Assessment of fracture risk. Osteoporos Int 2005;16:581–589.
20. Kanis JA. Diagnosis of osteoporosis and assessment of fracture risk. Lancet 2002;359:1929–1936.
21. Seeman E. Pathogenesis of bone fragility in women and men. Lancet 2002;359:1841–1850.
22. Garnero P, Hausherr E, Chapuy MC, et al. Markers of bone resorption predict hip fracture in elderly women: the EPIDOS Prospective Study. J Bone Miner Res 1996;11:1531–1538.
23. Garnero P, Sornay-Rendu E, Claustrat B, Delmas PD. Biochemical markers of bone turnover, endogenous hormones and the risk of fractures in postmenopausal women: the OFELY study. J Bone Miner Res 2000;15:1526–1536.
24. Ross PD, Kress BC, Parson RE, Wasnich RD, Armour KA, Mizrahi IA. Serum bone alkaline phosphatase and calcaneus bone density predict fractures: a prospective study. Osteoporos Int 2000;11:76–82.
25. van Daele PL, Seibel MJ, Burger H, et al. Case-control analysis of bone resorption markers, disability, and hip fracture risk: the Rotterdam study. BMJ 1996;312:482–483.
26. Gerdhem P, Ivaska KK, Alatalo SL, et al. Biochemical markers of bone metabolism and prediction of fracture in elderly women. J Bone Miner Res 2004;19:386–393.
27. Johnell O, Oden A, De Laet C, Garnero P, Delmas PD, Kanis JA. Biochemical indices of bone turnover and the assessment of fracture probability. Osteoporos Int 2002;13:523–526.
28. Delmas PD. Markers of bone turnover for monitoring treatment of osteoporosis with antiresorptive drugs. Osteoporos Int 2000;11(Suppl 6):S66–S76.
29. Bonnick SL, Shulman L. Monitoring osteoporosis therapy: bone mineral density, bone turnover markers, or both? Am J Med 2006;119:S25–S31.
30. Roux C, Garnero P, Thomas T, Sabatier JP, Orcel P, Audran M. Recommendations for monitoring antiresorptive therapies in postmenopausal osteoporosis. Joint Bone Spine 2005;72:26–31.
31. Meier C, Nguyen TV, Seibel MJ. Monitoring of antiresorptive therapy. In: Seibel MJ, Robins S, Bilezikian JP, eds. Dynamics of bone and cartilage metabolism. San Diego: Academic Press, 2006:649–669.
32. Kraenzlin EM, Seibel MJ. Measurement of biochemical markers of bone resorption. In: Seibel MJ, Robins S, Bilezikian JP, eds. Dynamics of bone and cartilage metabolism. San Diego: Academic Press, 2006:541–564.
33. Epstein S, Poser J, McClintock R, Johnston CC, Jr., Bryce G, Hui S. Differences in serum bone GLA protein with age and sex. Lancet 1984;1:307–310.
34. Beardsworth LJ, Eyre DR, Dickson IR. Changes with age in the urinary excretion of lysyl- and hydroxylysylpyridinoline, two new markers of bone collagen turnover. J Bone Miner Res 1990;5:671–676.
35. Garnero P, Delmas PD. Assessment of the serum levels of bone alkaline phosphatase with a new immunoradiometric assay in patients with metabolic bone disease. J Clin Endocrinol Metab 1993;77:1046–1053.
36. Seibel MJ, Woitge H, Scheidt-Nave C, et al. Urinary hydroxypyridinium crosslinks of collagen in population-based screening for overt vertebral osteoporosis: results of a pilot study. J Bone Miner Res 1994;9:1433–1440.
37. Hassager C, Risteli J, Risteli L, Christiansen C. Effect of the menopause and hormone replacement therapy on the carboxy-terminal pyridinoline cross-linked telopeptide of type I collagen. Osteoporos Int 1994;4:349–352.
38. Johansen JS, Riis BJ, Delmas PD, Christiansen C. Plasma BGP: an indicator of spontaneous bone loss and of the effect of oestrogen treatment in postmenopausal women. Eur J Clin Invest 1988;18:191–195.
39. Stepan JJ, Pospichal J, Schreiber V, et al. The application of plasma tartrate-resistant acid phosphatase to assess changes in bone resorption in response to artificial menopause and its treatment with estrogen or norethisterone. Calcif Tissue Int 1989;45:273–280.
40. Uebelhart D, Schlemmer A, Johansen JS, Gineyts E, Christiansen C, Delmas PD. Effect of menopause and hormone replacement therapy on the urinary excretion of pyridinium cross-links. J Clin Endocrinol Metab 1991;72:367–373.

41. Hasling C, Eriksen EF, Melkko J, et al. Effects of a combined estrogen-gestagen regimen on serum levels of the carboxy-terminal propeptide of human type I procollagen in osteoporosis. J Bone Miner Res 1991;6:1295–1300.
42. Reginster JY, Christiansen C, Dequinze B, et al. Effect of transdermal 17 beta-estradiol and oral conjugated equine estrogens on biochemical parameters of bone resorption in natural menopause. Calcif Tissue Int 1993;53:13–16.
43. Prestwood KM, Pilbeam CC, Burleson JA, et al. The short-term effects of conjugated estrogen on bone turnover in older women. J Clin Endocrinol Metab 1994;79:366–371.
44. Cicinelli E, Galantino P, Pepe V, et al. Bone metabolism changes after transdermal estradiol dose reduction during estrogen replacement therapy: a 1-year prospective study. Maturitas 1994;19:133–139.
45. Riis BJ, Overgaard K, Christiansen C. Biochemical markers of bone turnover to monitor the bone response to postmenopausal hormone replacement therapy. Osteoporos Int 1995;5:276–280.
46. Bonde M, Qvist P, Fledelius C, Riis BJ, Christiansen C. Applications of an enzyme immunoassay for a new marker of bone resorption (CrossLaps): follow-up on hormone replacement therapy and osteoporosis risk assessment. J Clin Endocrinol Metab 1995;80:864–868.
47. Raisz LG, Wiita B, Artis A, et al. Comparison of the effects of estrogen alone and estrogen plus androgen on biochemical markers of bone formation and resorption in postmenopausal women. J Clin Endocrinol Metab 1996;81:37–43.
48. Chesnut CH III, Bell NH, Clark GS, et al. Hormone replacement therapy in postmenopausal women: urinary N-telopeptide of type I collagen monitors therapeutic effect and predicts response of bone mineral density. Am J Med 1997;102:29–37.
49. Hannon R, Blumsohn A, Naylor K, Eastell R. Response of biochemical markers of bone turnover to hormone replacement therapy: impact of biological variability. J Bone Miner Res 1998;13:1124–1133.
50. Hesley RP, Shepard KA, Jenkins DK, Riggs BL. Monitoring estrogen replacement therapy and identifying rapid bone losers with an immunoassay for deoxypyridinoline. Osteoporos Int 1998;8:159–164.
51. Cooper C, Stakkestad JA, Radowicki S, et al. Matrix delivery transdermal 17beta-estradiol for the prevention of bone loss in postmenopausal women. The International Study Group. Osteoporos Int 1999;9:358–366.
52. Prestwood KM, Thompson DL, Kenny AM, Seibel MJ, Pilbeam CC, Raisz LG. Low dose estrogen and calcium have an additive effect on bone resorption in older women. J Clin Endocrinol Metab 1999;84:179–183.
53. Recker RR, Davies KM, Dowd RM, Heaney RP. The effect of low-dose continuous estrogen and progesterone therapy with calcium and vitamin D on bone in elderly women. A randomized, controlled trial. Ann Intern Med 1999;130:897–904.
54. Marcus R, Holloway L, Wells B, et al. The relationship of biochemical markers of bone turnover to bone density changes in postmenopausal women: results from the Postmenopausal Estrogen/Progestin Interventions (PEPI) trial. J Bone Miner Res 1999;14:1583–1595.
55. Garnero P, Tsouderos Y, Marton I, Pelissier C, Varin C, Delmas PD. Effects of intranasal 17beta-estradiol on bone turnover and serum insulin-like growth factor I in postmenopausal women. J Clin Endocrinol Metab 1999;84:2390–2397.
56. Prestwood KM, Kenny AM, Unson C, Kulldorff M. The effect of low dose micronized 17ss-estradiol on bone turnover, sex hormone levels, and side effects in older women: a randomized, double blind, placebo-controlled study. J Clin Endocrinol Metab 2000;85:4462–4469.
57. Lindsay R, Gallagher JC, Kleerekoper M, Pickar JH. Effect of lower doses of conjugated equine estrogens with and without medroxyprogesterone acetate on bone in early postmenopausal women. JAMA 2002;287:2668–2676.
58. Prestwood KM, Kenny AM, Kleppinger A, Kulldorff M. Ultralow-dose micronized 17beta-estradiol and bone density and bone metabolism in older women: a randomized controlled trial. JAMA 2003;290: 1042–1048.
59. Valimaki MJ, Laitinen KA, Tahtela RK, Hirvonen EJ, Risteli JP. The effects of transdermal estrogen therapy on bone mass and turnover in early postmenopausal smokers: a prospective, controlled study. Am J Obstet Gynecol 2003;189:1213–1220.
60. Nielsen TF, Ravn P, Bagger YZ, Warming L, Christiansen C. Pulsed estrogen therapy in prevention of postmenopausal osteoporosis. A 2-year randomized, double blind, placebo-controlled study. Osteoporos Int 2004;15:168–174.

61. Gallagher JC, Rapuri PB, Haynatzki G, Detter JR. Effect of discontinuation of estrogen, calcitriol, and the combination of both on bone density and bone markers. J Clin Endocrinol Metab 2002;87:4914–4923.
62. Delmas PD, Pornel B, Felsenberg D, et al. A dose-ranging trial of a matrix transdermal 17beta-estradiol for the prevention of bone loss in early postmenopausal women. International Study Group. Bone 1999;24:517–523.
63. Delmas PD, Bjarnason NH, Mitlak BH, et al. Effects of raloxifene on bone mineral density, serum cholesterol concentrations, and uterine endometrium in postmenopausal women. N Engl J Med 1997;337:1641–1647.
64. Ettinger B, Black DM, Mitlak BH, et al. Reduction of vertebral fracture risk in postmenopausal women with osteoporosis treated with raloxifene: results from a 3-year randomized clinical trial. Multiple Outcomes of Raloxifene Evaluation (MORE) Investigators. JAMA 1999;282:637–645.
65. Morii H, Ohashi Y, Taketani Y, et al. Effect of raloxifene on bone mineral density and biochemical markers of bone turnover in Japanese postmenopausal women with osteoporosis: results from a randomized placebo-controlled trial. Osteoporos Int 2003;14:793–800.
66. Reginster JY, Sarkar S, Zegels B, et al. Reduction in PINP, a marker of bone metabolism, with raloxifene treatment and its relationship with vertebral fracture risk. Bone 2004;34:344–351.
67. Hansdottir H, Franzson L, Prestwood K, Sigurdsson G. The effect of raloxifene on markers of bone turnover in older women living in long-term care facilities. J Am Geriatr Soc 2004;52:779–783.
68. Prestwood KM, Gunness M, Muchmore DB, Lu Y, Wong M, Raisz LG. A comparison of the effects of raloxifene and estrogen on bone in postmenopausal women. J Clin Endocrinol Metab 2000;85: 2197–2202.
69. Reid IR, Eastell R, Fogelman I, et al. A comparison of the effects of raloxifene and conjugated equine estrogen on bone and lipids in healthy postmenopausal women. Arch Intern Med 2004;164:871–879.
70. Garnero P, Shih WJ, Gineyts E, Karpf DB, Delmas PD. Comparison of new biochemical markers of bone turnover in late postmenopausal osteoporotic women in response to alendronate treatment. J Clin Endocrinol Metab 1994;79:1693–1700.
71. Bone HG, Downs RW, Jr., Tucci JR, et al. Dose-response relationships for alendronate treatment in osteoporotic elderly women. Alendronate Elderly Osteoporosis Study Centers. J Clin Endocrinol Metab 1997;82:265–274.
72. Greenspan SL, Parker RA, Ferguson L, Rosen HN, Maitland-Ramsey L, Karpf DB. Early changes in biochemical markers of bone turnover predict the long-term response to alendronate therapy in representative elderly women: a randomized clinical trial. J Bone Miner Res 1998;13:1431–1438.
73. Ravn P, Hosking D, Thompson D, et al. Monitoring of alendronate treatment and prediction of effect on bone mass by biochemical markers in the early postmenopausal intervention cohort study. J Clin Endocrinol Metab 1999;84:2363–2368.
74. Braga de Castro Machado A, Hannon R, Eastell R. Monitoring alendronate therapy for osteoporosis. J Bone Miner Res 1999;14:602–608.
75. Gonnelli S, Cepollaro C, Pondrelli C, et al. Bone turnover and the response to alendronate treatment in postmenopausal osteoporosis. Calcif Tissue Int 1999;65:359–364.
76. Garnero P, Darte C, Delmas PD. A model to monitor the efficacy of alendronate treatment in women with osteoporosis using a biochemical marker of bone turnover. Bone 1999;24:603–609.
77. Greenspan SL, Rosen HN, Parker RA. Early changes in serum N-telopeptide and C-telopeptide cross-linked collagen type 1 predict long-term response to alendronate therapy in elderly women. J Clin Endocrinol Metab 2000;85:3537–3540.
78. Ravn P, Thompson DE, Ross PD, Christiansen C. Biochemical markers for prediction of 4-year response in bone mass during bisphosphonate treatment for prevention of postmenopausal osteoporosis. Bone 2003;33:150–158.
79. Mortensen L, Charles P, Bekker PJ, Digennaro J, Johnston CC, Jr. Risedronate increases bone mass in an early postmenopausal population: two years of treatment plus one year of follow-up. J Clin Endocrinol Metab 1998;83:396–402.
80. Harris ST, Watts NB, Genant HK, et al. Effects of risedronate treatment on vertebral and nonvertebral fractures in women with postmenopausal osteoporosis: a randomized controlled trial. Vertebral Efficacy With Risedronate Therapy (VERT) Study Group. JAMA 1999;282:1344–1352.
81. Raisz L, Smith JA, Trahiotis M, et al. Short-term risedronate treatment in postmenopausal women: effects on biochemical markers of bone turnover. Osteoporos Int 2000;11:615–620.

82. Brown JP, Kendler DL, McClung MR, et al. The efficacy and tolerability of risedronate once a week for the treatment of postmenopausal osteoporosis. Calcif Tissue Int 2002;71:103–111.
83. Eastell R, Barton I, Hannon RA, Chines A, Garnero P, Delmas PD. Relationship of early changes in bone resorption to the reduction in fracture risk with risedronate. J Bone Miner Res 2003;18:1051–1056.
84. Ravn P, Clemmesen B, Riis BJ, Christiansen C. The effect on bone mass and bone markers of different doses of ibandronate: a new bisphosphonate for prevention and treatment of postmenopausal osteoporosis: a 1-year, randomized, double-blind, placebo-controlled dose-finding study. Bone 1996;19:527–533.
85. Thiebaud D, Burckhardt P, Kriegbaum H, et al. Three monthly intravenous injections of ibandronate in the treatment of postmenopausal osteoporosis. Am J Med 1997;103:298–307.
86. Ravn P, Christensen JO, Baumann M, Clemmesen B. Changes in biochemical markers and bone mass after withdrawal of ibandronate treatment: prediction of bone mass changes during treatment. Bone 1998;22:559–564.
87. Cooper C, Emkey RD, McDonald RH, et al. Efficacy and safety of oral weekly ibandronate in the treatment of postmenopausal osteoporosis. J Clin Endocrinol Metab 2003;88:4609–4615.
88. Christiansen C, Tanko LB, Warming L, et al. Dose dependent effects on bone resorption and formation of intermittently administered intravenous ibandronate. Osteoporos Int 2003;14:609–613.
89. Miller PD, McClung MR, Macovei L, et al. Monthly oral ibandronate therapy in postmenopausal osteoporosis: 1-year results from the MOBILE study. J Bone Miner Res 2005;20:1315–1322.
90. Garnero P, Gineyts E, Arbault P, Christiansen C, Delmas PD. Different effects of bisphosphonate and estrogen therapy on free and peptide-bound bone cross-links excretion. J Bone Miner Res 1995;10: 641–649.
91. Reid IR, Brown JP, Burckhardt P, et al. Intravenous zoledronic acid in postmenopausal women with low bone mineral density. N Engl J Med 2002;346:653–661.
92. Evio S, Tiitinen A, Laitinen K, Ylikorkala O, Valimaki MJ. Effects of alendronate and hormone replacement therapy, alone and in combination, on bone mass and markers of bone turnover in elderly women with osteoporosis. J Clin Endocrinol Metab 2004;89:626–631.
93. Johnell O, Scheele WH, Lu Y, Reginster JY, Need AG, Seeman E. Additive effects of raloxifene and alendronate on bone density and biochemical markers of bone remodeling in postmenopausal women with osteoporosis. J Clin Endocrinol Metab 2002;87:985–992.
94. Sambrook PN, Geusens P, Ribot C, et al. Alendronate produces greater effects than raloxifene on bone density and bone turnover in postmenopausal women with low bone density: results of EFFECT (Efficacy of FOSAMAX versus EVISTA Comparison Trial) International. J Intern Med 2004;255:503–511.
95. Pedrazzoni M, Alfano FS, Gatti C, et al. Acute effects of bisphosphonates on new and traditional markers of bone resorption. Calcif Tissue Int 1995;57:25–29.
96. Seibel MJ, Woitge HW, Pecherstorfer M, et al. Serum immunoreactive bone sialoprotein as a new marker of bone turnover in metabolic and malignant bone disease. J Clin Endocrinol Metab 1996;81:3289–3294.
97. Greenspan SL, Emkey RD, Bone HG, et al. Significant differential effects of alendronate, estrogen, or combination therapy on the rate of bone loss after discontinuation of treatment of postmenopausal osteoporosis. A randomized, double-blind, placebo-controlled trial. Ann Intern Med 2002;137:875–883.
98. Harris ST, Eriksen EF, Davidson M, et al. Effect of combined risedronate and hormone replacement therapies on bone mineral density in postmenopausal women. J Clin Endocrinol Metab 2001;86: 1890–1897.
99. Rossini M, Gatti D, Zamberlan N, Braga V, Dorizzi R, Adami S. Long-term effects of a treatment course with oral alendronate of postmenopausal osteoporosis. J Bone Miner Res 1994;9:1833–1837.
100. Bone HG, Hosking D, Devogelaer JP, et al. Ten years' experience with alendronate for osteoporosis in postmenopausal women. N Engl J Med 2004;350:1189–1199.
101. Gonnelli S, Cepollaro C, Pondrelli C, Martini S, Monaco R, Gennari C. The usefulness of bone turnover in predicting the response to transdermal estrogen therapy in postmenopausal osteoporosis. J Bone Miner Res 1997;12:624–631.
102. Civitelli R, Gonnelli S, Zacchei F, et al. Bone turnover in postmenopausal osteoporosis. Effect of calcitonin treatment. J Clin Invest 1988;82:1268–1274.
103. Overgaard K, Hansen MA, Nielsen VA, Riis BJ, Christiansen C. Discontinuous calcitonin treatment of established osteoporosis – effects of withdrawal of treatment. Am J Med 1990;89:1–6.
104. Nielsen NM, von der Recke P, Hansen MA, Overgaard K, Christiansen C. Estimation of the effect of salmon calcitonin in established osteoporosis by biochemical bone markers. Calcif Tissue Int 1994;55: 8–11.

105. Stevenson JC, Hillard TC, Lees B, Whitcroft SI, Ellerington MC, Whitehead MI. Postmenopausal bone loss: does HRT always work? Int J Fertil Menopausal Stud 1993;38 Suppl 2:88–91.
106. Cummings SR, Karpf DB, Harris F, et al. Improvement in spine bone density and reduction in risk of vertebral fractures during treatment with antiresorptive drugs. Am J Med 2002;112:281–289.
107. Seibel MJ, Naganathan V, Barton I, Grauer A. Relationship between pretreatment bone resorption and vertebral fracture incidence in postmenopausal osteoporotic women treated with risedronate. J Bone Miner Res 2004;19:323–329.
108. Bauer DC, Garnero P, Hochberg MC, et al. Pretreatment levels of bone turnover and the antifracture efficacy of alendronate: the fracture intervention trial. J Bone Miner Res 2006;21:292–299.
109. Seibel MJ. Biochemical markers of bone remodeling. Endocrinol Metab Clin North Am 2003;32:83–113, vi–vii.
110. Filipponi P, Pedetti M, Fedeli L, et al. Cyclical clodronate is effective in preventing postmenopausal bone loss: a comparative study with transcutaneous hormone replacement therapy. J Bone Miner Res 1995;10:697–703.
111. Dresner-Pollak R, Mayer M, Hochner-Celiniker D. The decrease in serum bone-specific alkaline phosphatase predicts bone mineral density response to hormone replacement therapy in early postmenopausal women. Calcif Tissue Int 2000;66:104–107.
112. Bjarnason NH, Christiansen C. Early response in biochemical markers predicts long-term response in bone mass during hormone replacement therapy in early postmenopausal women. Bone 2000;26: 561–569.
113. Komulainen M, Kroger H, Tuppurainen MT, Heikkinen AM, Honkanen R, Saarikoski S. Identification of early postmenopausal women with no bone response to HRT: results of a five-year clinical trial. Osteoporos Int 2000;11:211–218.
114. Fall PM, Kennedy D, Smith JA, Seibel MJ, Raisz LG. Comparison of serum and urine assays for biochemical markers of bone resorption in postmenopausal women with and without hormone replacement therapy and in men. Osteoporos Int 2000;11:481–485.
115. Ravn P, Clemmesen B, Christiansen C. Biochemical markers can predict the response in bone mass during alendronate treatment in early postmenopausal women. Alendronate Osteoporosis Prevention Study Group. Bone 1999;24:237–244.
116. Fink E, Cormier C, Steinmetz P, Kindermans C, Le Bouc Y, Souberbielle JC. Differences in the capacity of several biochemical bone markers to assess high bone turnover in early menopause and response to alendronate therapy. Osteoporos Int 2000;11:295–303.
117. Bone HG, Greenspan SL, McKeever C, et al. Alendronate and estrogen effects in postmenopausal women with low bone mineral density. Alendronate/Estrogen Study Group. J Clin Endocrinol Metab 2000;85:720–726.
118. Watts NB, Jenkins DK, Visor JM, Casal DC, Geusens P. Comparison of bone and total alkaline phosphatase and bone mineral density in postmenopausal osteoporotic women treated with alendronate. Osteoporos Int 2001;12:279–288.
119. Greenspan SL, Resnick NM, Parker RA. Early changes in biochemical markers of bone turnover are associated with long-term changes in bone mineral density in elderly women on alendronate, hormone replacement therapy, or combination therapy: a three-year, double-blind, placebo-controlled, randomized clinical trial. J Clin Endocrinol Metab 2005;90:2762–2767.
120. Storm T, Thamsborg G, Steiniche T, Genant HK, Sorensen OH. Effect of intermittent cyclical etidronate therapy on bone mass and fracture rate in women with postmenopausal osteoporosis. N Engl J Med 1990;322:1265–1271.
121. Overgaard K, Hansen MA, Jensen SB, Christiansen C. Effect of salcatonin given intranasally on bone mass and fracture rates in established osteoporosis: a dose-response study. BMJ 1992;305:556–561.
122. Lufkin EG, Wahner HW, O'Fallon WM, et al. Treatment of postmenopausal osteoporosis with transdermal estrogen. Ann Intern Med 1992;117:1–9.
123. Liberman UA, Weiss SR, Broll J, et al. Effect of oral alendronate on bone mineral density and the incidence of fractures in postmenopausal osteoporosis. The Alendronate Phase III Osteoporosis Treatment Study Group. N Engl J Med 1995;333:1437–1443.
124. Cummings SR, Black DM, Thompson DE, et al. Effect of alendronate on risk of fracture in women with low bone density but without vertebral fractures: results from the Fracture Intervention Trial. JAMA 1998;280:2077–2082.

125. Sarkar S, Mitlak BH, Wong M, Stock JL, Black DM, Harper KD. Relationships between bone mineral density and incident vertebral fracture risk with raloxifene therapy. J Bone Miner Res 2002;17:1–10.
126. Li Z, Meredith MP. Exploring the relationship between surrogates and clinical outcomes: analysis of individual patient data vs. meta-regression on group-level summary statistics. J Biopharm Stat 2003;13:777–792.
127. Riggs BL, Melton LJ III, O'Fallon WM. Drug therapy for vertebral fractures in osteoporosis: evidence that decreases in bone turnover and increases in bone mass both determine antifracture efficacy. Bone 1996;18:197S–201S.
128. Bjarnason NH, Sarkar S, Duong T, Mitlak B, Delmas PD, Christiansen C. Six and twelve month changes in bone turnover are related to reduction in vertebral fracture risk during 3 years of raloxifene treatment in postmenopausal osteoporosis. Osteoporos Int 2001;12:922–930.
129. Sarkar S, Reginster JY, Crans GG, Diez-Perez A, Pinette KV, Delmas PD. Relationship between changes in biochemical markers of bone turnover and BMD to predict vertebral fracture risk. J Bone Miner Res 2004;19:394–401.
130. Bauer DC, Black DM, Garnero P, et al. Change in bone turnover and hip, non-spine, and vertebral fracture in alendronate-treated women: the fracture intervention trial. J Bone Miner Res 2004;19:1250–1258.
131. Neer RM, Arnaud CD, Zanchetta JR, et al. Effect of parathyroid hormone (1–34) on fractures and bone mineral density in postmenopausal women with osteoporosis. N Engl J Med 2001;344:1434–1441.
132. Jiang Y, Zhao JJ, Mitlak BH, Wang O, Genant HK, Eriksen EF. Recombinant human parathyroid hormone (1–34) [teriparatide] improves both cortical and cancellous bone structure. J Bone Miner Res 2003;18:1932–1941.
133. Finkelstein JS, Hayes A, Hunzelman JL, Wyland JJ, Lee H, Neer RM. The effects of parathyroid hormone, alendronate, or both in men with osteoporosis. N Engl J Med 2003;349:1216–1226.
134. Finkelstein JS, Leder BZ, Burnett SA, et al. Effects of teriparatide, alendronate, or both on bone turnover in osteoporotic men. J Clin Endocrinol Metab 2006;91:2882–2887.
135. Orwoll ES, Scheele WH, Paul S, et al. The effect of teriparatide [human parathyroid hormone (1–34)] therapy on bone density in men with osteoporosis. J Bone Miner Res 2003;18:9–17.
136. Black DM, Greenspan SL, Ensrud KE, et al. The effects of parathyroid hormone and alendronate alone or in combination in postmenopausal osteoporosis. N Engl J Med 2003;349:1207–1215.
137. Black DM, Bilezikian JP, Ensrud KE, et al. One year of alendronate after one year of parathyroid hormone (1–84) for osteoporosis. N Engl J Med 2005;353:555–565.
138. Lindsay R, Nieves J, Formica C, et al. Randomised controlled study of effect of parathyroid hormone on vertebral-bone mass and fracture incidence among postmenopausal women on oestrogen with osteoporosis. Lancet 1997;350:550–555.
139. Kurland ES, Cosman F, McMahon DJ, Rosen CJ, Lindsay R, Bilezikian JP. Parathyroid hormone as a therapy for idiopathic osteoporosis in men: effects on bone mineral density and bone markers. J Clin Endocrinol Metab 2000;85:3069–3076.
140. Rittmaster RS, Bolognese M, Ettinger MP, et al. Enhancement of bone mass in osteoporotic women with parathyroid hormone followed by alendronate. J Clin Endocrinol Metab 2000;85:2129–2134.
141. Bilezikian JP, Rubin MR. Monitoring anabolic treatment. In: Seibel MJ, Robins S, Bilezikian JP, eds. Dynamics of bone and cartilage metabolism. San Diego: Academic Press, 2006:629–647.
142. Chen P, Satterwhite JH, Licata AA, et al. Early changes in biochemical markers of bone formation predict BMD response to teriparatide in postmenopausal women with osteoporosis. J Bone Miner Res 2005;20:962–970.
143. Bauer DC, Garnero P, Bilezikian JP, et al. Short-term changes in bone turnover markers and bone mineral density response to parathyroid hormone in postmenopausal women with osteoporosis. J Clin Endocrinol Metab 2006;91:1370–1375.
144. Dobnig H, Sipos A, Jiang Y, et al. Early changes in biochemical markers of bone formation correlate with improvements in bone structure during teriparatide therapy. J Clin Endocrinol Metab 2005;90:3970–3977.
145. Eastell R, Krege JH, Chen P, Glass EV, Reginster JY. Development of an algorithm for using PINP to monitor treatment of patients with teriparatide. Curr Med Res Opin 2006;22:61–66.
146. Chen P, Miller PD, Delmas PD, Misurski DA, Krege JH. Change in lumbar spine BMD and vertebral fracture risk reduction in teriparatide-treated postmenopausal women with osteoporosis. J Bone Miner Res 2006;21:1785–1790.

147. Delmas PD, Licata AA, Reginster JY, et al. Fracture risk reduction during treatment with teriparatide is independent of pretreatment bone turnover. Bone 2006;39:237–243.
148. McCombs JS, Thiebaud P, McLaughlin-Miley C, Shi J. Compliance with drug therapies for the treatment and prevention of osteoporosis. Maturitas 2004;48:271–287.
149. Yood RA, Emani S, Reed JI, Lewis BE, Charpentier M, Lydick E. Compliance with pharmacologic therapy for osteoporosis. Osteoporos Int 2003;14:965–968.
150. Marwick C. Hormone combination treats women's bone loss. JAMA 1994;272:1487.
151. Cano A. Compliance to hormone replacement therapy in menopausal women controlled in a third level academic centre. Maturitas 1994;20:91–99.
152. Faulkner DL, Young C, Hutchins D, McCollam JS. Patient noncompliance with hormone replacement therapy: a nationwide estimate using a large prescription claims database. Menopause 1998;5:226–229.
153. Kotzan JA, Martin BC, Wade WE. Persistence with estrogen therapy in a postmenopausal Medicaid population. Pharmacotherapy 1999;19:363–369.
154. Kayser J, Ettinger B, Pressman A. Postmenopausal hormonal support: discontinuation of raloxifene versus estrogen. Menopause 2001;8:328–332.
155. Tosteson AN, Grove MR, Hammond CS, et al. Early discontinuation of treatment for osteoporosis. Am J Med 2003;115:209–216.
156. Cramer JA, Amonkar MM, Hebborn A, Altman R. Compliance and persistence with bisphosphonate dosing regimens among women with postmenopausal osteoporosis. Curr Med Res Opin 2005;21:1453–1460.
157. Caro JJ, Ishak KJ, Huybrechts KF, Raggio G, Naujoks C. The impact of compliance with osteoporosis therapy on fracture rates in actual practice. Osteoporos Int 2004;15:1003–1008.
158. Reginster JY, Rabenda V, Neuprez A. Adherence, patient preference and dosing frequency: understanding the relationship. Bone 2006;38:S2–S6.
159. Chapurlat RD, Cummings SR. Does follow-up of osteoporotic women treated with antiresorptive therapies improve effectiveness? Osteoporos Int 2002;13:738–744.
160. Clowes JA, Peel NF, Eastell R. The impact of monitoring on adherence and persistence with antiresorptive treatment for postmenopausal osteoporosis: a randomized controlled trial. J Clin Endocrinol Metab 2004;89:1117–1123.
161. Delmas PD, Vrijens B, Roux C, et al. A reinforcement message based on bone turnover marker response influences long-term persistence with risedronate in osteoporosis: The IMPACT Study. J Bone Miner Res 2003;18:S374.

7 Biomechanics of Bone

Jacqueline H. Cole and Marjolein C.H. van der Meulen

CONTENTS

SUMMARY

The ability to bear loads is a critical function of the skeleton, in addition to its metabolic and physiological roles. Load-bearing ability depends on both the applied loads and the structural properties of the loaded bone. When the loads exceed the structural properties, fracture will occur. Because the nature of the applied loads can be difficult to predict, the greatest potential impact on minimizing fracture risk is through targeted interventions and therapies to improve bone strength. The strength and fracture resistance of the skeleton depend primarily on the mass, morphology/architecture, and material properties of bone tissue. Although each of these attributes has been examined independently in both cortical and cancellous bone, no single measurement can fully characterize the structural integrity of bone or reliably predict the occurrence of a fracture. In addition, factors such as aging, trauma, and disease affect the tissue properties and can compromise bone strength. While bone mass and, more recently, morphology have been widely examined in vivo, to date these measures do not fully explain variations in bone mechanical properties observed experimentally in vitro. Healthy bone tissue exhibits spatial and temporal variations in tissue-level material properties that are altered by aging and disease. Characterizing bone material properties, whether at the tissue level or at the chemical composition level of the mineral and matrix constituents, may improve the ability to predict structural competence and fracture risk reliably.

From: *Contemporary Endocrinology: Osteoporosis: Pathophysiology and Clinical Management*
Edited by: R. A. Adler, DOI 10.1007/978-1-59745-459-9_7,

Key Words: Biomechanics, bone strength, failure load, osteoporotic fracture, bone stiffness, bone quality, bone mass, bone density, architecture, material properties

BONE STRENGTH AND FRACTURE

In addition to metabolic and physiologic roles, the ability to bear functional loads is a critical function of the skeletal system. Individuals constantly impose dynamic mechanical stimuli on their bones during daily activities. Throughout much of life the skeleton performs as expected, successfully supporting the loads applied during normal function. Whole bone strength, or the resistance of a bone to fracture, is generally not a consideration for a healthy skeleton subjected to such loading conditions. However, with trauma, aging, and disease, the ability of the skeleton to perform its structural function can become compromised. With trauma, loading may exceed the load-bearing capacity of the skeleton, either healthy or otherwise, and produce fracture. Aging and many skeletal diseases reduce bone strength, thereby producing skeletal failure even under normal or non-traumatic loading conditions. Fractures result not only in individual morbidity and mortality but also in high healthcare and societal costs *(45,63,85)*. Therefore, an understanding of the factors that contribute to bone strength is critical to the prevention and treatment of skeletal fractures.

Failure of any load-bearing structure can stem from a single traumatic overload or from the accumulation of damage with repetitive loading. Here we will focus on the former: what determines whether a given load applied to a bone will result in fracture? The interaction between applied loading and the ability of a bone to bear the applied loads can be summarized in a term called *factor of risk (56)*. The factor of risk is the ratio of the load applied to a bone divided by the load required to produce fracture (Fig. 1). If the applied load exceeds the failure load of the bone of interest, then the factor of risk is greater than one and fracture will occur. To predict fracture accurately, characteristics of the applied load such as the manner and location of its application must be considered. In addition, the failure load for a particular skeletal site or bone must be sufficiently defined, since it

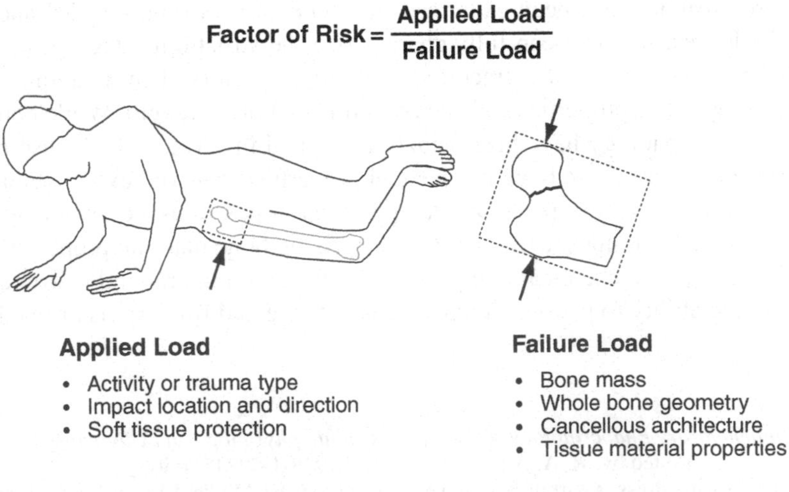
Factor of Risk = Applied Load / Failure Load
Applied Load
• Activity or trauma type
• Impact location and direction
• Soft tissue protection
Failure Load
• Bone mass
• Whole bone geometry
• Cancellous architecture
• Tissue material properties

Fig. 1. Factor of Risk proposed by Hayes is the ratio of the applied loads to the structural strength of the whole bone at the skeletal site of interest. When the applied load exceeds the failure load (Factor of risk > 1) then failure is predicted.

is influenced by characteristics of the constituent material and the material's distribution and structural arrangement *(131)*. The ability of the skeleton to resist fracture under applied loading varies with aging and disease, primarily through changes in these constituents of bone failure load and bone strength. Our focus here will be on the determinants of whole bone strength and factors that affect whole bone behavior when loaded.

The mechanical performance of bone governs skeletal function and is strongly shaped by the in vivo loading experienced by the skeleton. Bone tissue is exquisitely mechanosensitive, and the cell populations associated with bone respond to mechanical stimuli by altering turnover to increase or decrease the amount of tissue present, which in turn alters both the architecture and material properties *(43,130)*. Therefore, as we consider the effects of loading on the failure of bone tissue, we must remember that the structure of a given bone represents the integration of the loading history experienced throughout the individual's lifetime *(25)*. Skeletal mechanobiology is detailed in Chapter 8 (Judex and Rubin).

FACTORS CONTRIBUTING TO WHOLE BONE STRENGTH

The response of the skeleton to applied loads is similar to that of any other load-bearing structure, with the exception that man-made structures are not metabolically active and are unable to heal themselves. In vivo, activities such as walking and stair climbing produce complex loading states that are combinations of the individual loading modes studied in the laboratory in vitro *(15,69)*. Loading in the laboratory can be applied axially (tension or compression), in bending, or in torsion to a whole bone such as a femur or vertebra. Different structural characteristics will be measured for different loading modes.

When a force is applied to a whole bone, deformation is produced throughout the structure (Fig. 2). When the load is examined as a function of the deformation, the resulting curve has several distinct characteristics: an initial linear or *elastic* region, a nonlinear region with

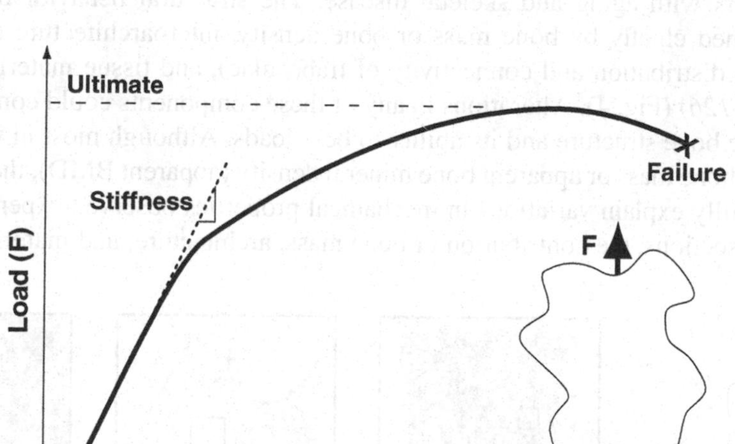

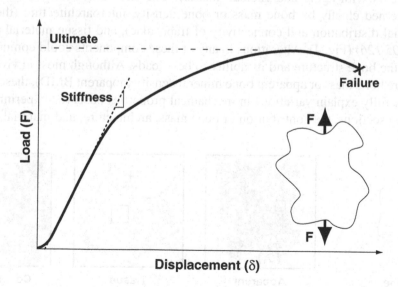

Fig. 2. Load-displacement behavior for a structural test such as a whole bone. The structural stiffness is determined from the initial linear region. The structural strength is the load required to fail the whole bone. These parameters depend on the loading mode (tension, compression, bending or torsion).

a maximum defined as the ultimate point, and a failure point that indicates the level at which the bone fractures and can no longer withstand the applied load. Applied loads that fall within the initial linear range can be resisted without permanently deforming the bone or causing failure. The two most critical measures obtained from the load-displacement data are the structural stiffness and strength. The stiffness of a whole bone is the resistance to deformation for a given applied load and is the slope of the linear portion of the load-displacement curve. For a whole bone, the structural strength is the load required to fail the whole bone and is usually defined as the load at the ultimate point. Different loading modes, such as compression, bending, and torsion, will produce different strengths and stiffnesses, and these values will be a function of the properties of the bone tissue, how much tissue is present, and where the tissue is located. For example, the failure strength of a vertebral body will be different when loaded in compression than in bending. Stiffness and strength are distinct parameters, but are often correlated. Other parameters of interest may include the yield point (the transition between the linear and nonlinear regions) and energy absorbed to failure (the area under the entire load-displacement curve). The forces and deformations of the whole bone also create internal forces and deformations within the bone tissue that are known as stresses and strains.

Whole bone behavior can also be viewed as depending on the behavior of the constituent tissues, cortical and cancellous bone. In bending of a whole bone, for example, the behavior is dominated by cortical bone geometry and material properties. Cortical and cancellous bone are both complex structures in their own right; their behavior depends on similar factors as those for whole bone strength and is also be discussed below. The continuum properties of these bulk tissues is referred to as the *apparent* level here, which is a level above the tissue material properties and is distinct from the whole bone structural behavior (Fig. 3). The porous structure of cancellous bone and its location in vertebral bodies and the ends of long bones lend it importance in the distribution of joint contact forces during daily activities but also make the tissue more susceptible to the surface-focused resorption that occurs with aging and skeletal disease. The structural behavior of cancellous bone is governed chiefly by bone mass or bone density, microarchitecture (the geometric and spatial distribution and connectivity of trabeculae), and tissue material properties *(27,49,81,105,126)* (Fig. 4). Alterations in any of these components could compromise the integrity of the bone structure and its ability to bear loads. Although most in vivo imaging tools measure bone mass or apparent bone mineral density (apparent BMD), these measures alone do not fully explain variations in mechanical properties observed experimentally. In the following sections, the contribution of bone mass, architecture, and material properties

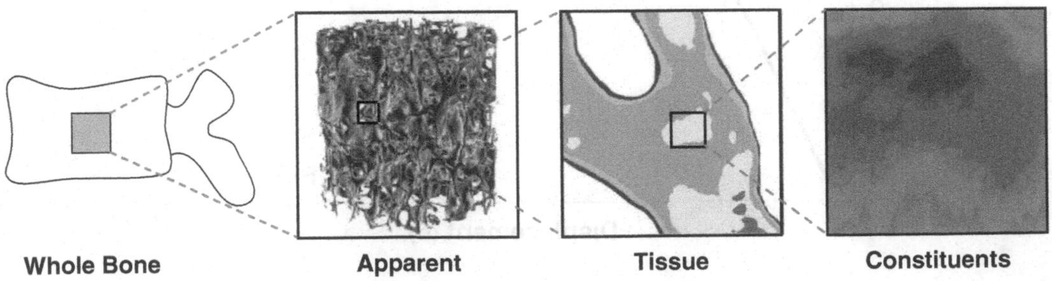

Fig. 3. Definition of levels of consideration for bone: Whole bone structure to apparent level structure (cortical or cancellous bone) to tissue materials to constituents.

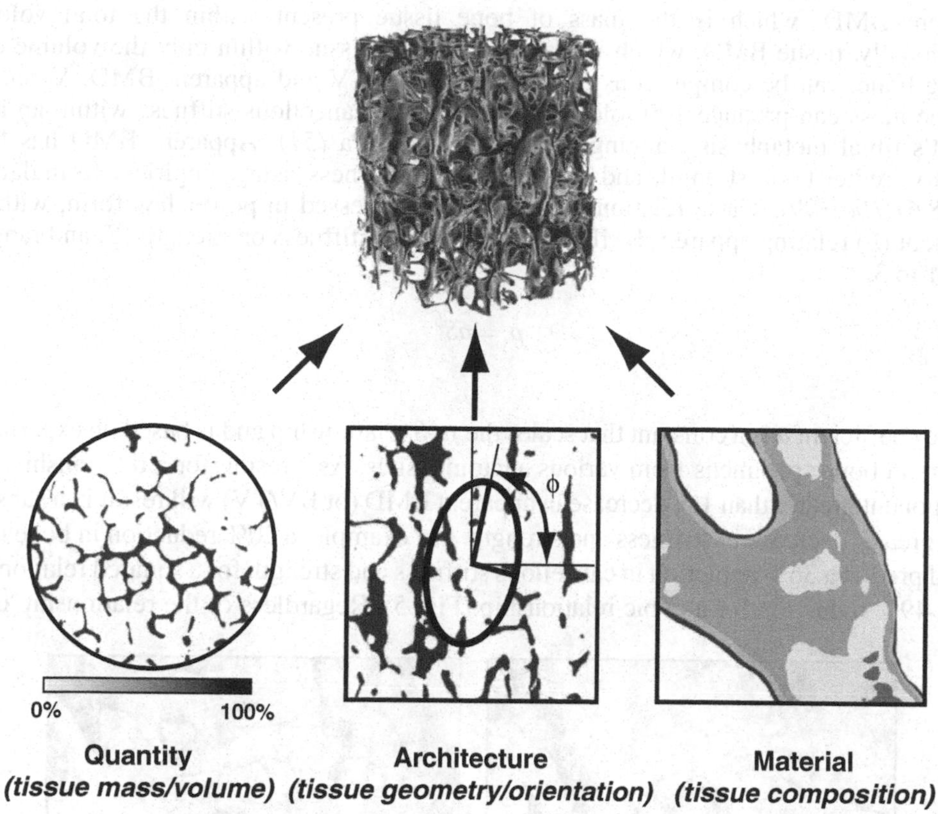

Fig. 4. Determinants of cancellous apparent bone strength include how much tissue is present (quantity), where the tissue is located (architecture), and the properties of the tissue (material).

to the structural behavior of cancellous bone will be described, as well as the clinical and laboratory tools used to characterize them. The role of bone quantity (bone mass) has been studied most extensively. The effect of architecture on structural performance is less well-characterized, and the role of tissue material properties still requires more investigation.

BONE MASS

The most-studied determinant of bone structural behavior is the amount of tissue present, the bone mass. When a long bone is loaded during daily activities in vivo, the loading is primarily bending and compression, and the dense cortical bone tissue of the diaphysis bears the highest loads and deformations. At the ends of a long bone, the cancellous bone tissue distributes the loads from the joint surface and transfers this load to the cortex. In cortical bone, the amount of bone is represented by geometric measures such as the cross-sectional area. In cancellous bone, which consists of an intricate network of trabeculae, the measurement of bone mass cannot be performed based on geometry and has been examined instead by analyzing small volumes of tissue.

Cancellous bone mass is typically measured either by bone volume fraction (BV/TV), which is the volume of bone tissue present within the total volume of interest, or by apparent BMD, which is the mass of bone tissue present within the total volume. Additionally, tissue BMD, which is the mass of bone tissue within only the volume containing bone, can be computed as the product of BV/TV and apparent BMD. Variations in bone mass can produce 100-fold differences in the cancellous stiffness within an individual's tibial metaphysis, ranging from 4 to 433 MPa *(51)*. Apparent BMD has been used to predict bone strength and apparent tissue stiffness using empirical formulations *(27,48,61,106,109)*. These relationships are often expressed in power law form, with the exponent (b) relating apparent BMD (ρ) to cancellous stiffness or strength (S) and ranging from 1 to 3:

$$\rho = aS^b$$

The coefficient a is a constant that scales the ρ–S relationship and is based on experimental data in bone specimens from various anatomic sites. As a result, for a relationship with an exponent greater than 1, a decrease in apparent BMD (or BV/TV) will result in a substantially greater decrease in stiffness and strength. For example, a 20% reduction in bone mass would predict a 36% reduction in cancellous stiffness and strength for a squared relationship and a 49% reduction for a cubic relationship (Fig. 5). Regardless of the relationship used,

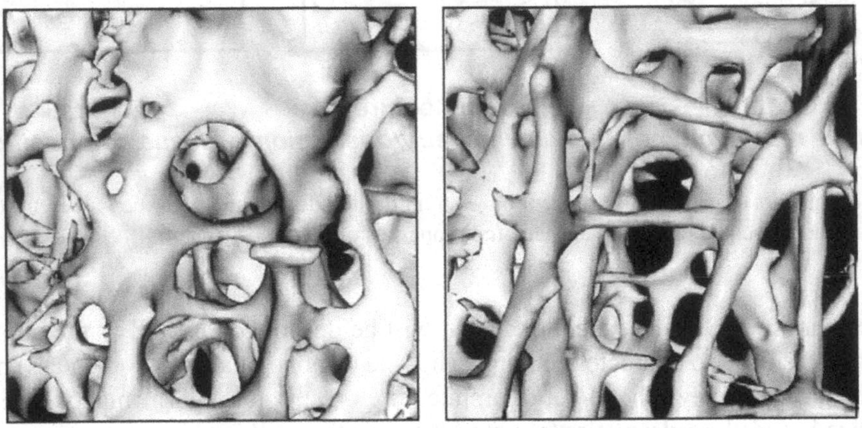

Normal	**Osteoporotic**
74 year old female	92 year old female
T-score = –0.8	T-score = –2.6
BV/TV = 12.7%	BV/TV = 10.0% (–21% vs Normal)
Tb.Th = 117 μm	Tb.Th = 90 μm
Modulus, E = 844 MPa	Modulus, E = 470 MPa (–44%)
Strength, σ_u = 3.5 MPa	Strength, σ_u = 2.1 MPa (–40%)

Fig. 5. MicroCT images of two cancellous cores taken from the center of the L2 vertebra of two different females. Measured T-score, bone volume fraction (BV/TV), trabecular thickness (Tb.Th), and apparent modulus and strength indicated. Percent differences indicated for the osteoporotic female relative to the normal female. For the 21% loss of bone mass, a squared power law relationship would predict a 38% reduction in mechanical properties, and a cubic power law would predict a 51% reduction, both of which are comparable to the 40–44% reductions found experimentally.

apparent BMD and BV/TV obtained experimentally or from microcomputed tomography (microCT) can explain 60–85% of the variability in compressive apparent stiffness and strength for human cancellous bone *(66,68,74,75,89)*. Although bone mass measurements generally have a high explanatory power for bone mechanical properties, these surrogate measures only capture one aspect of bone strength and cannot capture differences in how this mass is distributed. While mass is critical to bone integrity, additional factors are clearly needed to distinguish between individuals who do or do not fracture.

BONE SIZE AND ARCHITECTURE

The size and distribution of cross-sectional geometry strongly influences the resistance to fracture for cortical bone under any loading condition. If the tissue material properties are assumed to be constant, geometric parameters (such as the periosteal diameter, cross-sectional area, cross-sectional moment of inertia, and a geometric indicator of failure strength called the section modulus) all influence the whole bone structural behavior *(80)*. For bones loaded in bending, the cross-sectional moment of inertia (I) is a geometric measure of the distribution of bone about a central or *neutral* plane. It is a measure of the bone's resistance to bending and deflection and is computed as follows for a hollow circular cross-section *(59)*:

$$I = \frac{\pi}{4}(R_p^4 - R_e^4)$$

where R_p is the periosteal radius and R_e is the endosteal radius, computed about the neutral plane.

For bones loaded in torsion, the polar moment of inertia (J) is the distribution about the longitudinal or *neutral* axis and represents the bone's resistance to angular deflection or twist. It is computed as follows for a hollow circular cross-section *(59)*:

$$J = \frac{\pi}{2}(R_p^4 - R_e^4) = 2I$$

The section modulus (Z) represents a whole bone's resistance to bending or torsional loads and is computed as follows for a hollow circular cross-section:

$$Z_{\text{Torsion}} = \frac{J}{R_p} = \frac{\pi}{2R_p}(R_p^4 - F_e^4) = 2Z_{\text{Bending}}$$

For a long bone loaded in bending, as seen in the proximal femur, both the size and geometric distribution of bone relative to the loading axis contribute to the whole bone's resistance to applied loads and thus to fracture. Assuming a circular cross section, a hollow bone with the same periosteal diameter as a solid bone, and with cortical thickness equal to 20% of the periosteal diameter, will have a 25% smaller cortical area but only a 6% lower section modulus, which is proportional to the bending failure strength (Fig. 6). On the other hand, a hollow bone with the same cortical thickness as the previous hollow bone but with the same cortical area of the solid bone will have a 70% larger section modulus (and, hence, structural strength) for only a 25% increase in the periosteal diameter as compared to the solid bone. Therefore, even small changes in overall bone size can compensate for losses in bone strength when the remaining bone is redistributed with reference to the neutral plane or axis.

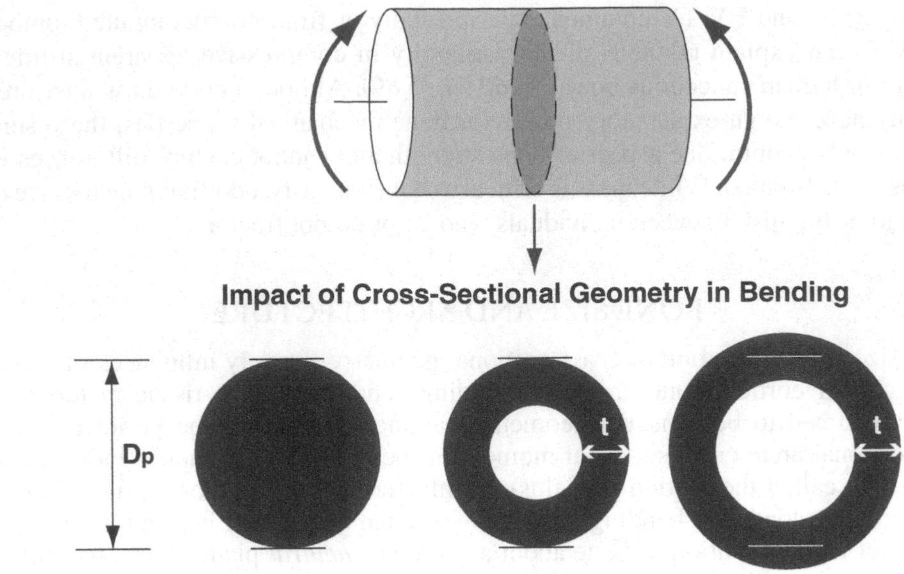

Periosteal Diameter (D_p)	100%	100%	125%
Cortical Area (A)	100%	75%	100%
Section Modulus (Z)	100%	94%	170%

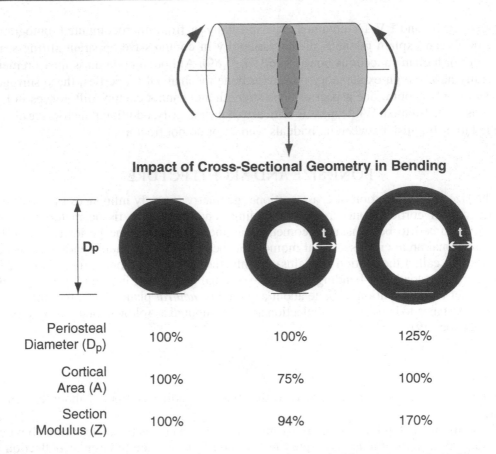

Fig. 6. Variations in the size and distribution of bone mass in a cortical bone cross section influence the section modulus, which is proportional to the bending failure strength of the whole bone. The resorption of bone on the endosteal surface or the apposition of bone on the periosteal surface may change the cortical thickness (*t*) or the distribution of bone about the loading axis, thereby altering the ability of the bone to resist fracture. For example, compared to the reference bone (left), a bone of the same girth but with less material (middle) will be slightly weaker, but a bone with the same amount of material distributed further away from the neutral axis of the bone will be much stronger.

Similarly for cancellous bone, the size and spatial arrangement of trabeculae that make up the cancellous microarchitecture also play a key role in the structural competence of bone. As early as the mid-19th century, increased fracture incidence was observed in older patients with thinning bone *(31)*. Two different sites of cancellous bone with similar apparent BMD can vary substantially in their strength and stiffness due to differences in tissue architecture *(47,128)*. In addition, the architecture of cancellous bone often has a preferred orientation, creating substantially different modulus and strength values when bone from a given location is loaded in different directions, a characteristic called material anisotropy. In human vertebrae, for example, the primary trabecular orientation is superior–inferior, corresponding to the strongest direction when loaded *(93)*. The strength of cancellous bone loaded along the superior–inferior direction of the spine is nearly twice as strong as when loaded in the anterior–posterior or medial–lateral directions *(47)*. Therefore, characterizing the cancellous bone structure is important for understanding the relationship between architecture and mechanical properties.

Similar to bone mass measures, architecture parameters have also been experimentally correlated with elastic mechanical properties *(32,50,52,64,99,132)*. Independent of apparent BMD, bone regions with different architectures exhibited variable elastic mechanical properties that differed by over 50% *(128)*. Based on studies using two-dimensional serial sectioning techniques, trabecular orientation and connectivity correlated with cancellous bone strength *(52,104,126)*. In sheep femoral bone assessed with microCT, architecture indices explained 10–70% of the variation in compressive strength *(88)*. A study using static histomorphometry indicated that similar architecture–strength correlations also hold true in human vertebral bone *(125)*.

BONE TISSUE MATERIAL PROPERTIES

The material properties of bone are the properties of the constituent material, referred to here as the tissue-level behavior (Fig. 3). Both cortical and cancellous tissues are formed by surface-based processes that develop lamellar tissue. These tissues are believed to be similar, so apparent differences between cortical and cancellous bone result from differences in mass and architecture. Material characteristics are independent of bone size and shape and are measured on small, homogeneous tissue samples. Similar to a whole bone test, a bone materials test examines deformation in response to an applied load for the small, standardized tissue samples, and this response differs depending on the direction or mode of loading. The samples can be loaded perpendicular to the face of the material to determine the tensile and compressive properties or parallel to the face to find the shear properties. From these material tests, bone material properties are computed by normalizing the resulting load-displacement parameters by geometric measures representing the sample size and shape. For example, applied load is converted to tissue stress and displacement converted to tissue strain, as described below.

Tissue stress is defined as the ratio of the applied load (tension, compression, or shear) to the sample cross-sectional area (Fig. 7). For a tissue sample tested in tension or compression, the tissue stress is defined as the applied load divided by the cross-sectional area perpendicular to that load (i.e., the area of the sample face on which the load acts). For a tissue sample tested in shear, the applied load is parallel to the surface and again normalized by the area the force acts across. Bone tissue strain is measured as the amount of deformation in the direction of loading normalized by the initial sample dimension. Tensile or compressive loads produce stretched or compacted displacements, respectively, along the direction of the applied load. The resulting strain is computed as the ratio of the change in length to initial length. Shear loads create distortions in the sample by inducing the sample surfaces on which the loads are applied to slide with respect to each other. For shear strain, the distortion ratio is related to the change in angle (Fig. 7).

The properties used to characterize bone material include the failure or ultimate stress, failure strain, modulus of elasticity (i.e., material stiffness), and toughness (Fig. 8). The ultimate stress represents the strength of bone tissue and is generally defined as the maximum stress on the stress–strain curve. The failure strain is the strain corresponding to the

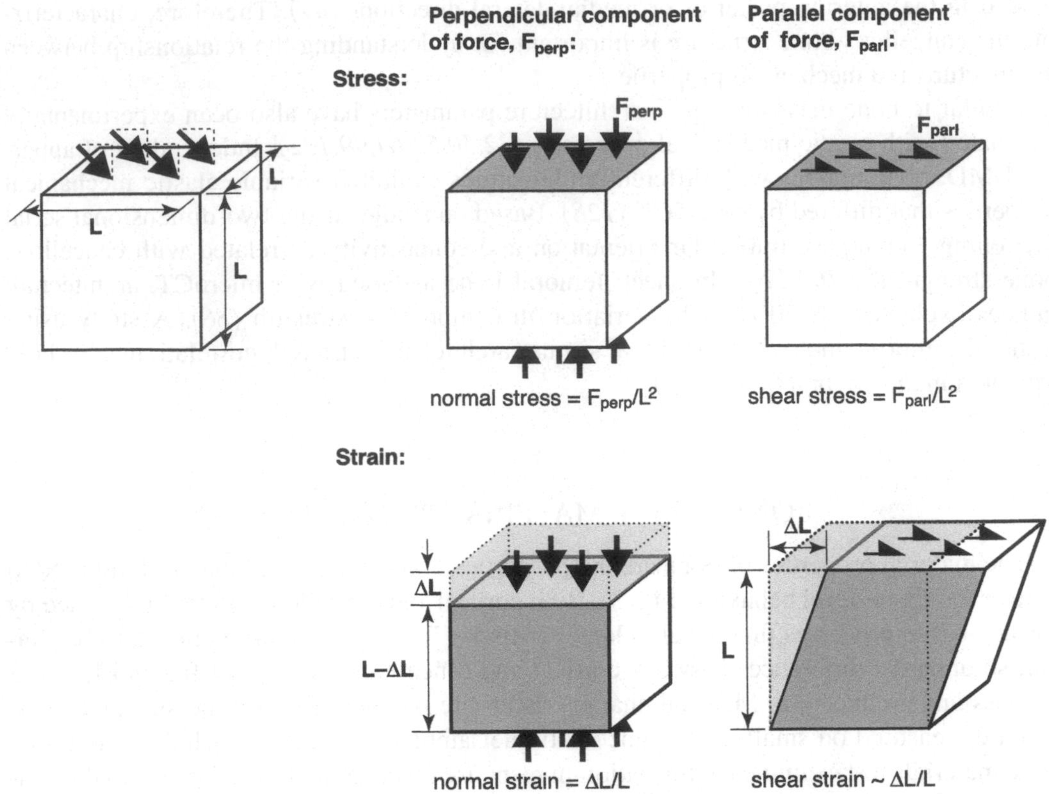

Fig. 7. Material stresses (local tissue forces) and strains (local tissue deformations) for bone tissue samples loaded in compression and shear. The applied loading is decomposed into the component perpendicular (compression) and parallel (shear) to the cube face. The face for which the stress or strain is calculated is shaded. For strain, the original, undeformed volume is shaded.

ultimate stress, and modulus of elasticity, or tissue stiffness, is the slope of the linear portion of the curve. Bone toughness is a measure of the ability of the bone material to absorb energy without fracture and is calculated as the area under the stress–strain curve.

As explained earlier, this material behavior is characteristic of a single load applied to failure. However, bones continually experience cyclic loading in vivo during normal activities. In fact, such loading is more common than single increasing loads to failure *(24)*. Cyclic loading of material at levels below the failure strength is known as fatigue. In bone, fatigue loading produces microscale damage in the tissue, known as microdamage. Microdamage changes the tissue properties and thus may alter the ability of the whole bone to withstand loads and avoid fracture.

Bone is a composite tissue comprised of an organic matrix made mostly of collagen that is reinforced by inorganic mineral crystals. The characteristics of these organic and inorganic constituents, as well as their interaction with each other, determine the tissue material properties of bone, properties that at least partially define the popular term *bone quality*. To date, little is known about the individual and collective contributions of the collagen matrix and mineral constituents to bone quality and bone strength. Indeed, the strength of

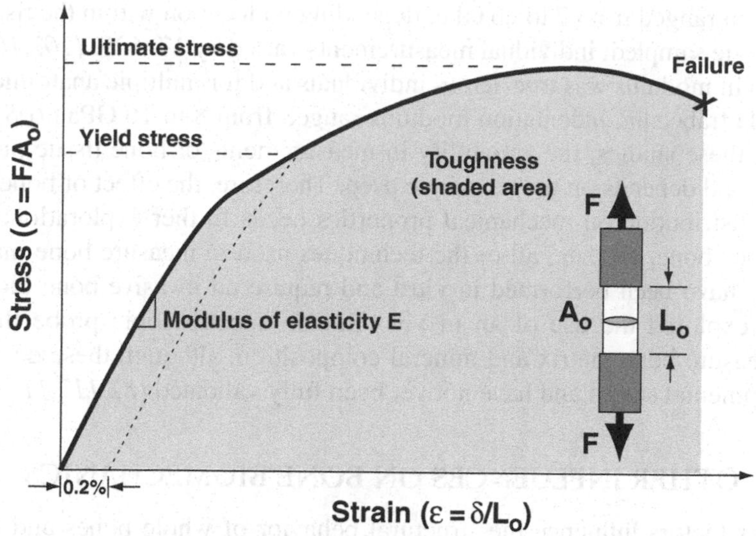

Fig. 8. Stress–strain behavior for a materials test. These measurements are independent of specimen size and shape but do depend on the loading mode (tension, compression, bending, or shear). The modulus of elasticity is determined from the initial linear region; yield is the transition from linear to nonlinear behavior; toughness is the shaded area.

the composite bone tissue is greater than that of other materials composed primarily of only one of the constituents, such as collagen-rich tendon or mineral samples of calcium phosphate *(37)*. Studies of radiation in human bone and allograft specimens revealed that collagen damage compromises the toughness but not the stiffness of bone tissue *(38,53)*. In addition, numerous studies have shown a clear relationship between bone mineral content and material stiffness or strength *(22,35,36,79)*. These results suggest that the collagen and mineral phases of bone tissue contribute differently to its material behavior.

Characterizing the molecular structure of bone tissue is important for examining the relative contributions of the matrix and mineral constituents to the overall material behavior. Important compositional measures of bone matrix include collagen content, maturity, and orientation, as well as the molecular structure of various matrix proteins that aid in mineral crystal formation, binding, and maturation (e.g., osteopontin, osteocalcin, and bone sialoprotein). Important measures for bone mineral include the apatitic crystal size, orientation, and structure, as well as the degree of ion substitution, particularly the substitution of carbonate in the phosphate binding site, within the lattice or on the surface of the mineral crystals. These structural and compositional measures can be quantified using classic techniques such as gravimetry or more sophisticated techniques such as X-ray diffraction, backscattered electron imaging, and infrared (IR), Raman, and nuclear magnetic resonance (NMR) spectroscopies.

Healthy bone tissue properties show substantial variation both spatially *(19,78,98)* and temporally *(54,55)* even for a given site and species. Materials testing techniques used to examine tissue properties include microbeam testing and nanoindentation. Using microbeam testing, the trabecular tissue modulus ranged from 3.8 to 20.7 GPa and varied depending on the loading mode *(28,71,106)*. The mean tissue modulus assessed by nanoindentation ranged from 7 to 26 GPa, depending on location within the tissue and type of lamellar tissue sampled; individual measurements varied by 17–62% *(107,108,127,136)*. This variation in modulus was true across individuals and for multiple anatomic sites. Even within a single trabecula, indentation modulus ranged from 8 to 16 GPa *(108)*. As clearly evidenced by these studies, the variability in measurements of bone tissue properties can be quite large and depends on the technique used. Therefore, the effect of bone tissue composition and distribution on mechanical properties needs further exploration, particularly for a cancellous bone. To date, all of the techniques used to measure bone material properties directly have been performed in vitro and require an invasive bone biopsy. Recent studies have explored the use of an in vivo Raman spectroscopic probe that can non-invasively measure bone matrix and mineral composition, although these devices are still in the developmental stages and have not yet been fully validated *(82,117,118)*.

OTHER INFLUENCES ON BONE BIOMECHANICS

Many other factors influence the structural behavior of whole bones and the apparent behavior of cancellous tissue, including age, sex and disease. These influences alter bone mass, architecture, and tissue properties, all of which govern the mechanical performance of whole bones and cancellous bone tissue. For example, with aging, the compressive modulus of vertebral cancellous bone decreases 17% per decade *(95)*. Osteoporosis and aging are tightly coupled in women, and osteoporosis may in fact be the natural outcome of the aging process.

Aging

The factors described above (i.e., bone mass, geometry/architecture, and material properties) vary independently with age. Age-related degradation of bone mass and architecture can seriously compromise bone integrity. Bone mass decreases with age after peak bone mass has been attained in both men and women *(1,10,41,73,76,133)*, but especially in women due to peri-menopausal bone loss. By age 80, BMD at the common fracture sites of the spine, hip, and forearm decreases by 13–18% in men *(122)* and 15–54% in women *(3,5,8,110)*, thereby increasing the likelihood for developing osteoporosis *(62,113,114)*. As the life expectancy of the general population continues to increase, age-related declines will result in even lower bone mass, and the total incidence of skeletal fractures will rise, unless diagnosis and treatment of skeletal deficiencies can be significantly improved *(84,97)*.

While our understanding of the relationship between tissue composition and material behavior is limited, substantial progress has been made recently in characterizing tissue composition and variation with age. For example, osteons of cortical bone and individual trabeculae of iliac crest biopsies demonstrate spatially varying mineral crystallinity and collagen cross-linking by Fourier transform infrared microscopy *(103)*. The most crystalline (mature) bone mineral is located at the center of trabeculae, and newly deposited mineral is less crystalline than older mineral. Changes in mineral-to-matrix ratio and mineral maturity are documented with age and disease *(20,70,100,102,123)*. Femoral heads from patients with hip fractures undergoing total hip arthroplasty demonstrated a significantly increased mineral-to-matrix ratio compared to femoral heads of patients without fractures, suggesting that compositional changes may precede failure *(83)*. The critical question is how these compositional changes relate to tissue and whole bone mechanical behavior. The results to date are contradictory, making them difficult to interpret. For example, reductions in whole bone stiffness correlate with increasing mineral-to-matrix ratio and mineral maturity *(4)*. In contrast, the mineral-to-matrix ratio has recently been correlated with the locally measured compressive modulus of both cortical and cancellous tissue *(23)*.

Sex Effects

Given the relatively higher incidence of fragility fractures in women, understanding the sex-related differences in bone mass, architecture, and material properties with aging is critical for improved diagnosis and treatment of osteoporosis. For both sexes, volume fraction in human cancellous bone declines steadily throughout life *(2,40,92,124)*, as does ash density *(94,95)*. However, histomorphometry studies indicated that sex appeared to have minimal or no impact on this relationship *(2,16,44,92,124,134)*. Although ash density and volume fraction may change similarly with age for both sexes, thereby changing bone mechanical performance, the mechanisms of bone loss seem to be different and are at least partially related to sex-specific changes in the cancellous architecture. Regardless of sex, mean trabecular thickness as measured with traditional histomorphometry techniques decreased with age for vertebral bone *(40,60,92,124)*. For men, decreased bone volume resulted more from progressive thinning of trabeculae while maintaining the trabecular network, but for women, bone volume reductions resulted mainly from a loss of trabeculae (and consequently an increase in trabecular separation) while the thickness of the remaining trabeculae was maintained *(2)*.

Interestingly, these sex-specific changes in architecture with age alter the modulus and strength of cancellous bone very differently. When a 10% reduction in bone density was modeled in human vertebral cancellous bone, uniform thinning of trabeculae only reduced the bone strength by 20%, while the random removal of entire trabeculae reduced strength by 70%, and a reduction in both thickness and number reduced strength by 77% *(120)*. Even when normal bone density was restored by increasing the thickness of trabeculae to compensate for the bone loss, a strength deficit of 63% remained, which may help explain the higher fracture incidence observed clinically in women.

Disease

Although bone is a living tissue that adapts to its mechanical environment, disruptions in bone metabolism by diseases such as osteoporosis, osteogenesis imperfecta, and cystic fibrosis can seriously compromise structural integrity and the ability of bone to bear loads. Osteoporosis is a skeletal condition marked by reduced bone mass and a deteriorated architecture, which reduces bone strength and increases the likelihood of fracture *(1,129)*. At 50 years of age, white women have a 40% lifetime risk, and white men have a 13% lifetime risk, of sustaining an osteoporotic fracture at the spine, hip, or forearm *(34,86)*. By 2010, the prevalence of osteoporosis and low bone mass are expected to increase by 20%, thereby increasing fracture rates *(97)*. Osteoporosis is often asymptomatic prior to fracture, thus making prediction and possible prevention difficult.

In addition to reducing bone mass, osteoporosis also detrimentally affects the other contributors to bone strength, architecture, and material properties. Osteoporotic patients that sustain a vertebral fracture experience more trabecular thinning at the spine and iliac crest than normal, non-fractured aging subjects, resulting in a lower trabecular density, loss of trabecular connectivity, and the disappearance of load-bearing trabecular struts *(67,101)*. This architectural disruption from osteoporosis is sometimes accompanied by a compensatory increase in the trabecular thickness *(67)*, although this adaptive mechanism does not necessarily prevent fracture. Similarly at the proximal femur, female patients with hip fractures had a lower bone volume fraction, trabecular number, and connectivity than normal cadaveric controls, and the orientation of the trabecular structure was more aligned with the primary direction of loading, a characteristic known as *anisotropy (29)*. The architectural deficits in subjects with osteoporotic fractures were accompanied by reduced bone material stiffness and strength. In addition, bone biopsies of fracture patients revealed changes in tissue composition with osteoporosis, with fracture patients having a lower mineral content, higher crystallinity, and higher collagen maturity than age-matched controls *(46,102)*.

Often referred to as brittle bone disease, osteogenesis imperfecta (OI) literally means *imperfect bone formation* and is a group of hereditary genetic disorders that primarily affect bone and lead to increased bone fragility. OI results from mutations in the genes that encode for type I collagen *(30)*. Therefore, most patients with clinical OI (i.e., types I–IV) experience abnormalities in type I collagen, the primary component of the bone tissue matrix, which may alter the normal mineralization process. Bone strength is compromised in patients with OI, as evidenced by the degradation in bone mass and material properties. Cortical bone in the femora of adult mice with a moderate-to-severe phenotype of OI (*oim/oim*) was significantly weaker than in wild-type mice, and the bone tissue was less compliant and resistant to fracture, as evidenced by reduced moment of inertia, ultimate load, stiffness, energy to failure, ultimate stress, and toughness and increased brittleness *(87)*. In this mouse model, the mineral-to-matrix ratio was increased, likely due to a lower matrix collagen content *(24)*. In children and adults with OI types I–IV, bone mineral content and bone size were substantially reduced by 1.6–5.2 standard deviations as compared to normal controls *(72,77)*. Matrix collagen defects will adversely affect bone mineral formation and likely compromise bone tissue properties.

Cystic fibrosis (CF) is another inherited disease whose name refers to the typical tissue scarring and cyst formation that occur in the pancreas. CF is characterized by a genetic mutation that impairs the mobility of chloride ions across the cell membrane of epithelial cells, which disrupts the osmotic regulation necessary to produce normal fluid and mucus coatings inside the lungs, pancreas, and other organs. The coatings become abnormally thick and obstruct digestive and respiratory passageways, thereby inhibiting enzyme production important for nutrient absorption and resulting in breathing difficulties and chronic lung infections. Low bone mass is common among children and adults with cystic fibrosis. When compared to sex-matched or age- and sex-matched controls, children and adults with CF had an average BMD that was 1–3 standard deviations lower at the spine and femoral neck *(6,7,9,17,18,39,57,119)*. Although, CF patients were generally one standard deviation shorter than their age- and sex-matched controls *(11)*, size-corrected mineral status as assessed by bone mineral apparent density (BMAD) was still significantly reduced *(9)*. In a mouse model of CF, histomorphometry revealed bone geometry and architecture deficits in both cortical and trabecular bone, with significantly reduced cortical thickness, trabecular thickness, and trabecular number in the distal femur when compared with normal littermates *(42)*. In addition, the CF-related osteopenia is likely driven by a bone modeling/remodeling imbalance characterized by accelerated bone resorption (i.e., an increase in the number and activity of osteoclasts) without sufficient increases in bone formation (i.e., an increase in the osteoblast surface and mineral apposition rate) *(11,42)*. The reduced bone mass and other aspects of the disease, including nutritional deficiencies, pancreatic insufficiencies, and reduced activity and exercise, all contribute to the increased risk for fragility fractures in patients with CF. Although data on fracture prevalence with CF are limited, studies have reported a history of skeletal fractures in 25–50% of children and young adult patients *(7,58)*. Vertebral and rib fractures can be especially detrimental, resulting in height loss and kyphosis, as well as exacerbated pulmonary symptoms. Therefore, the accurate evaluation of bone strength using surrogate predictions from routine clinical and laboratory assessment tools is essential, as is understanding the determinants of bone mechanical behavior.

BONE STRENGTH PREDICTIONS FROM IN VIVO MEASUREMENTS

Clinical imaging techniques are routinely used to assess bone mass and external geometry, although cancellous architecture and tissue material properties cannot be measured non-invasively at present. Several analytical techniques can be used to extract structural properties from subject-specific clinical data with varying degrees of simplifying assumptions. These structural properties can then be used to predict the strength and fracture risk of skeletal sites that commonly fracture. The analytical approaches include structural analyses of densitometric data based on assumed geometric models, and engineering beam theory and finite element (FE) analyses based on CT data. The strength of these methods is that a mechanically meaningful mechanism can be determined to compare the structural performance of bones from different individuals, rather than representing the complex structure with a single bone density value. Clinical validation of these approaches is needed to examine whether they represent appropriate metrics of bone fragility and correlate with fracture risk.

Bone mass is most commonly assessed in vivo using dual-energy X-ray absorptiometry (DXA), which evaluates the inorganic mineral phase of bone with minimal radiation exposure to patients. DXA scans can be performed for large regions, such as the lumbar spine, proximal femur, forearm, or even the whole body, thereby providing a non-invasive global measure of bone mass. However, DXA-based BMD alone cannot account for differences in mineral distribution and bone structure, and only partially discriminates individuals who will fracture from those who will not *(112,116)*. This is not surprising: DXA scans are two-dimensional and provide projected areal measurements of bone mineral density, which integrate geometric and material contributions to BMD and create a size bias that overestimates the volumetric mineral density for larger individuals *(26)*. Because the resolution of DXA is relatively low (on the order of 1 mm), cortical bone tissue cannot be distinguished from cancellous tissue, architectural features of cancellous bone (on the order of 0.1 mm) cannot be captured, and the mineral distribution within the bone tissue cannot be measured. Because unmineralized tissues do not inherently attenuate X-rays, DXA scans cannot evaluate the organic phase of bone or the soft tissues surrounding bone. DXA-based BMD correlates well with in vitro vertebral failure load in compression *(90)*. The attenuation profile obtained from DXA can be used to determine geometric properties, including cross-sectional area and polar moment of inertia about a plane perpendicular to the scan direction, assuming that these measures are defined solely by the mineral phase

(14,80,96,135). If structural changes in whole bone properties are assumed to arise only from geometric changes and not from alterations in tissue properties, then DXA-derived parameters can also be used to predict structural performance. This method has been applied extensively to the femoral neck and midshaft *(12–14,91)* and the distal radius *(96)*. Calculating the structural behavior with this method requires assumptions to determine the underlying geometry, mineral distribution and density, and relative cortical and cancellous fractions; therefore, the application of this technique may be most appropriate for cortical sites.

Quantitative computed tomography (QCT) is a true three-dimensional method based on X-ray imaging that overcomes many of the limitations of DXA, though with a higher radiation exposure for the patient. For bone, QCT images reflect the spatial distribution of mineral, with the degree of attenuation (CT number, in Hounsfield units) directly proportional to the mineral content. The resolution of this technique is typically better in the scan plane (~0.5 mm) than axially between slices (~1 mm). Therefore, QCT cannot capture cancellous architecture but rather measures apparent BMD for the voxel volume. In contrast to DXA, QCT can distinguish cortical and cancellous tissue and measures both external geometry and tissue BMD, which can be related to apparent stiffness.

Using engineering beam theory and more complex FE models, QCT data have been used to examine the structural performance of sites where fractures occur clinically *(21,33,65,111,121)*. The axial and bending rigidity can be calculated from a QCT data slice based on composite beam theory. This approach uses the true external geometry of the bone or bone segment, and incorporates the spatial variation in material properties based on the spatial distribution of the apparent-level tissue density. Model-based estimates of bone rigidity correlated better with experimental data than did BMD-based structural measures *(23)*. This straightforward approach has been applied to the spine, femoral neck, and distal radius *(21,23,116)*. To date, population-based analyses have been performed to compare the mechanical competence of bone across ages and between sexes. Next, these methods need to be applied to the prediction of individual fracture risk. In tumor patients with skeletal lesions, this approach was substantially more accurate for predicting fracture risk than radiographic methods were *(126)*.

Finite element models of the vertebra and femoral neck take this QCT-based approach further and provide the opportunity to include the full bone geometry, distribution of apparent properties, and more complex loading conditions in a fully three-dimensional analysis *(37,69)*. As in the two-dimensional analysis, the bone geometry is modeled with high fidelity from the scan data, and apparent-level material properties can be included based on the CT-measured density. In contrast to the stiffness determined from the two-dimensional analyses, FE models can predict both stiffness and strength when nonlinear analyses are performed. When FE models are compared to in vitro testing data, the correlations between the strength predicted by the models and the failure strength measured in the experiments are high and stronger than those with BMD from DXA or QCT *(23,33,37,71)*. In the spine, the emphasis of FE models has been on the vertebral body, omitting the posterior elements and facet joints and modeling purely compressive loading without including discs, muscles, and ligaments. Comparisons with QCT-based rigidity for predicting compressive strength have shown both better *(37)* and equivalent *(22,23)* results. FE models clearly have the potential to mechanistically elucidate skeletal structural performance and improve our ability to predict skeletal fragility *(69)*. For this to be realized, FE models must be validated with established clinical metrics and fracture risk and perhaps also improved to include better modeling of in vivo loading conditions.

In summary, current clinical tools that assess fracture risk based primarily on bone mass and geometry do not reliably predict whether or not a patient will fracture. Based on the concepts of bone mechanics and laboratory studies presented here, we see that the structure and properties of bones are complex and depend on many factors. Future techniques should combine information regarding an individual's bone mass, architecture, and tissue material properties to provide a more precise measurement of bone strength and susceptibility to fracture, regardless of age, sex, or the presence of skeletal diseases (and perhaps even more so because of these). A combined imaging–modeling approach can include all of these factors, and recent laboratory studies using this type of analysis have produced promising results, although the clinical implementation of such a technique is still on the horizon.

REFERENCES

1. None. Bone density reference data. In: Favus MJ, ed. Primer on the metabolic bone diseases and disorders of mineral metabolism. Philadelphia: Lippincott Williams & Wilkins, 1996:483.
2. Aaron JE, Makins NB, Sagreiya K. The microanatomy of trabecular bone loss in normal aging men and women. Clin Orthop Relat Res 1987;215:260–271.
3. Ahlborg HG, Johnell O, Turner CH, Rannevik G, Karlsson MK. Bone loss and bone size after menopause. N Engl J Med 2003;349(4):327–334.
4. Akkus O, Adar F, Schaffler MB. Age-related changes in physicochemical properties of mineral crystals are related to impaired mechanical function of cortical bone. Bone 2004;34(3):443–453.
5. Aloia JF, Vaswani A, Mikhail M, Badshah M, Flaster E. Cancellous bone of the spine is greater in black women. Calcif Tissue Int 1999;65(1):29–33.
6. Aris RM, Neuringer IP, Weiner MA, Egan TM, Ontjes D. Severe osteoporosis before and after lung transplantation. Chest 1996;109(5):1176–1183.
7. Aris RM, Renner JB, Winders AD, Buell HE, Riggs DB, Lester GE, Ontjes DA. Increased rate of fractures and severe kyphosis: sequelae of living into adulthood with cystic fibrosis. Ann Intern Med 1998;128(3):186–193.
8. Arlot ME, Sornay-Rendu E, Garnero P, Vey-Marty B, Delmas PD. Apparent pre- and postmenopausal bone loss evaluated by DXA at different skeletal sites in women: the OFELY cohort. J Bone Miner Res 1997;12(4):683–690.
9. Bachrach LK, Loutit CW, Moss RB. Osteopenia in adults with cystic fibrosis. Am J Med 1994;96(1): 27–34.
10. Barden H. Bone mineral density of the spine and femur in normal U.S. white females. J Bone Miner Res 1997;12(Suppl. 1):S248.
11. Baroncelli GI, De Luca F, Magazzu G, Arrigo T, Sferlazzas C, Catena C, Bertelloni S, Saggese G. Bone demineralization in cystic fibrosis: evidence of imbalance between bone formation and degradation. Pediatr Res 1997;41(3):397–403.
12. Beck TJ, Oreskovic TL, Stone KL, Ruff CB, Ensrud K, Nevitt MC, Genant HK, Cummings SR. Structural adaptation to changing skeletal load in the progression toward hip fragility: the study of osteoporotic fractures. J Bone Miner Res 2001;16(6):1108–1119.
13. Beck TJ, Ruff CB, Scott WW, Jr, Plato CC, Tobin JD, Quan CA. Sex differences in geometry of the femoral neck with aging: a structural analysis of bone mineral data. Calcif Tissue Int 1992;50:24–29.
14. Beck TJ, Ruff CB, Warden KE, Scott WWJ, Rao GU. Predicting femoral neck strength from bone mineral data. A structural approach. Invest Radiol 1990;25:6–18.
15. Bergmann G, Graichen F, Rohlmann A. Hip joint loading during walking and running, measured in two patients. J Biomech 1993;26(8):969–990.
16. Bergot C, Laval-Jeantet AM, Preteux F, Meunier A. Measurement of anisotropic vertebral trabecular bone loss during aging by quantitative image analysis. Calcif Tissue Int 1988;43(3):143–149.

17. Bhudhikanok GS, Lim J, Marcus R, Harkins A, Moss RB, Bachrach LK. Correlates of osteopenia in patients with cystic fibrosis. Pediatrics 1996;97(1):103–111.
18. Bhudhikanok GS, Wang MC, Eckert K, Matkin C, Marcus R, Bachrach LK. Differences in bone mineral in young Asian and Caucasian Americans may reflect differences in bone size. J Bone Miner Res 1996;11(10):1545–1556.
19. Bonucci E, Ballanti P, Della Rocca C, Milani S, Lo Cascio V, Imbimbo B. Technical variability of bone histomorphometric measurements. Bone Miner 1990;11(2):177–186.
20. Boskey AL, Dicarlo E, Paschalis E, West P, Mendelsohn R. Comparison of mineral quality and quantity in iliac crest biopsies from high- and low-turnover osteoporosis: an FT-IR microspectroscopic investigation. Osteoporos Int 2005;16:2031–2038.
21. Bouxsein ML, Melton LJ, III, Riggs BL, Muller J, Atkinson EJ, Oberg AL, Robb RA, Camp JJ, Rouleau PA, McCollough CH, Khosla S. Age- and sex-specific differences in the factor of risk for vertebral fracture: a population-based study using QCT. J Bone Miner Res 2006;21(9):1475–1482.
22. Buckley JM, Cheng L, Loo K, Slyfield C, Xu Z. Quantitative computed tomography-based predictions of vertebral strength in anterior bending. Spine 2007;32(9):1019–1027.
23. Buckley JM, Loo K, Motherway J. Comparison of quantitative computed tomography-based measures in predicting vertebral compressive strength. Bone 2007;40(3):767–774.
24. Burr DB, Forwood MR, Fyhrie DP, Martin RB, Schaffler MB, Turner CH. Bone microdamage and skeletal fragility in osteoporotic and stress fractures. J Bone Miner Res 1997;12(1):6–15.
25. Burstein AH, Zika JM, Heiple K, Klein L. Contribution of collagen and mineral to the elastic–plastic properties of bone. J Bone Joint Surg (Am) 1975;57(7):956–961.
26. Busa B, Miller LM, Rubin CT, Qin YX, Judex S. Rapid establishment of chemical and mechanical properties during lamellar bone formation. Calcif Tissue Int 2005;77(6):386–394.
27. Camacho NP, Landis WJ, Boskey AL. Mineral changes in a mouse model of osteogenesis imperfecta detected by Fourier transform infrared microscopy. Connect Tissue Res 1996;35(1–4): 259–265.
28. Carter DR. Mechanical loading history and skeletal biology. J Biomech 1987;20:1095–1109.
29. Carter DR, Bouxsein ML, Marcus R. New approaches for interpreting projected bone densitometry data. J Bone Miner Res 1992;7(2):137–145.
30. Carter DR, Hayes WC. The compressive behavior of bone as a two-phase porous structure. J Bone Joint Surg Am 1977;59-A:954–962.
31. Choi K, Kuhn JL, Ciarelli MJ, Goldstein SA. The elastic moduli of human subchondral, trabecular, and cortical bone tissue and the size-dependency of cortical bone modulus. J Biomech 1990;23(11): 1103–1113.
32. Ciarelli TE, Fyhrie DP, Schaffler MB, Goldstein SA. Variations in three-dimensional cancellous bone architecture of the proximal femur in female hip fractures and in controls. J Bone Miner Res 2000;15(1):32–40.
33. Cody DD, Hou FJ, Divine GW, Fyhrie DP. Femoral structure and stiffness in patients with femoral neck fracture. J Orthop Res 2000;18(3):443–448.
34. Cole WG. Osteogenesis imperfecta. Baillieres Clin Endocrinol Metab 1988;2(1):243–265.
35. Cooper A. A treatise on dislocations and fractures of the joints. London: Longman, Hurst, Rees, Orme, and Brown, 1842.
36. Cowin SC. The relationship between the elasticity tensor and the fabric tensor. Mech Mater 1985;4: 137–147.
37. Crawford RP, Cann CE, Keaveny TM. Finite element models predict in vitro vertebral body compressive strength better than quantitative computed tomography. Bone 2003;33(4):744–750.
38. Cummings SR, Melton LJ. Epidemiology and outcomes of osteoporotic fractures. Lancet 2002;359(9319):1761–1767.
39. Currey JD. The effect of porosity and mineral content on the Young's modulus of elasticity of compact bone. J Biomech 1988;21(2):131–139.
40. Currey JD. What determines the bending strength of compact bone? J Exp Biol 1999;202(Pt 18): 2495–2503.
41. Currey JD. Role of collagen and other organics in the mechanical properties of bone. Osteoporos Int 2003;14(Suppl 5):S29-S36.

42. Currey JD, Foreman J, Laketic I, Mitchell J, Pegg DE, Reilly GC. Effects of ionizing radiation on the mechanical properties of human bone. J Orthop Res 1997;15(1):111–117.
43. De Schepper J, Smitz J, Dab I, Piepsz A, Jonckheer M, Bergmann P. Low serum bone gamma-carboxyglutamic acid protein concentrations in patients with cystic fibrosis: correlation with hormonal parameters and bone mineral density. Horm Res 1993 39(5–6):197–201.
44. Dempster DW, Ferguson-Pell MW, Mellish RW, Cochran GV, Xie F, Fey C, Horbert W, Parisien M, Lindsay R. Relationships between bone structure in the iliac crest and bone structure and strength in the lumbar spine. Osteoporos Int 1993;3(2):90–96.
45. Diaz Curiel M, Carrasco de la Peña JL, Honorato Perez J, Perez Cano R, Rapado A, Ruiz Martinez I. Study of bone mineral density in lumbar spine and femoral neck in a Spanish population. Multicentre Research Project on Osteoporosis. Osteoporos Int 1997;7(1):59–64.
46. Dif F, Marty C, Baudoin C, de Vernejoul MC, Levi G. Severe osteopenia in CFTR-null mice. Bone 2004;35(3):595–603.
47. Duncan RL, Turner CH. Mechanotransduction and the functional response of bone to mechanical strain. Calcif Tissue Int 1995;57(5):344–358.
48. Dunnill MS, Anderson JA, Whitehead R. Quantitative histological studies on age changes in bone. J Pathol Bacteriol 1967;94(2):275–291.
49. Gabriel SE, Tosteson AN, Leibson CL, Crowson CS, Pond GR, Hammond CS, Melton LJ III. Direct medical costs attributable to osteoporotic fractures. Osteoporos Int 2002;13(4): 323–330.
50. Gadeleta SJ, Boskey AL, Paschalis E, Carlson C, Menschik F, Baldini T, Peterson M, Rimnac CM. A physical, chemical, and mechanical study of lumbar vertebrae from normal, ovariectomized, and nandrolone decanoate-treated cynomolgus monkeys (Macaca fascicularis). Bone 2000;27(4): 541–550.
51. Galante J, Rostoker W, Ray RD. Physical properties of trabecular bone. Calcif Tissue Res 1970;5: 236–246.
52. Gibson LJ. The mechanical behavior of cancellous bone. J Biomech 1985;18:317–328.
53. Goldstein SA. The mechanical properties of trabecular bone: dependence on anatomic location and function. J Biomech 1987;20(11–12):1055–1061.
54. Goldstein SA, Goulet R, McCubbrey D. Measurement and significance of three-dimensional architecture to the mechanical integrity of trabecular bone. Calcif Tissue Int 1993;53:S127–32; discussion S132–133.
55. Goldstein SA, Wilson DL, Sonstegard DA, Matthews LS. The mechanical properties of human tibial trabecular bone as a function of metaphyseal location. J Biomech 1983;16(12):965–969.
56. Goulet RW, Goldstein SA, Ciarelli MJ, Kuhn JL, Brown MB, Feldkamp LA. The relationship between the structural and orthogonal compressive properties of trabecular bone. J Biomech 1994;27(4): 375–389.
57. Hamer AJ, Stockley I, Elson RA. Changes in allograft bone irradiated at different temperatures. J Bone Joint Surg Br 1999;81(2):342–344.
58. Handschin RG, Stern WB. Crystallographic and chemical analysis of human bone apatite (Crista Iliaca). Clin Rheumatol 1994;13(Suppl 1):75–90.
59. Handschin RG, Stern WB. X-ray diffraction studies on the lattice perfection of human bone apatite (Crista iliaca). Bone 1995;16(4 Suppl):355S–363S.
60. Hayes WC, Piazza SJ, Zysset PK. Biomechanics of fracture risk prediction of the hip and spine by quantitative computed tomography. Radiol Clin North Am 1991;29(1):1–18.
61. Henderson RC, Madsen CD. Bone density in children and adolescents with cystic fibrosis. J Pediatr 1996;128(1):28–34.
62. Henderson RC, Specter BB. Kyphosis and fractures in children and young adults with cystic fibrosis. J Pediatr 1994;125(2):208–212.
63. Hibbeler RC. Mechanics of materials. Upper Saddle River, New Jersey: Prentice Hall, 1997.
64. Hildebrand T, Laib A, Müller R, Dequeker J, Rüegsegger P. Direct three-dimensional morphometric analysis of human cancellous bone: microstructural data from spine, femur, iliac crest, and calcaneus. J Bone Miner Res 1999;14(7):1167–1174.
65. Hodgskinson R, Currey JD. Young's modulus, density and material properties in cancellous bone over a large density range. J Mater Sci Mater Med 1992;3(377–381)

66. Hui SL, Slemenda CW, Johnston CC, Jr. Age and bone mass as predictors of fracture in a prospective study. J Clin Invest 1988;81(6):1804–1809.
67. Johnell O. The socioeconomic burden of fractures: today and in the 21st century. Am J Med 1997;103(2A):20S–25S; discussion 25S–26S.
68. Kabel J, Odgaard A, van Rietbergen B, Huiskes R. Connectivity and the elastic properties of cancellous bone. Bone 1999;24(2):115–120.
69. Keaveny TM, Donley DW, Hoffmann PF, Mitlak BH, Glass EV, San Martin JA. Effects of teriparatide and alendronate on vertebral strength as assessed by finite element modeling of QCT scans in women with osteoporosis. J Bone Miner Res 2007;22(1):149–157.
70. Keaveny TM, Pinilla TP, Crawford RP, Kopperdahl DL, Lou A. Systematic and random errors in compression testing of trabecular bone. J Orthop Res 1997;15(1):101–110.
71. Keyak JH, Kaneko TS, Tehranzadeh J, Skinner HB. Predicting proximal femoral strength using structural engineering models. Clin Orthop Relat Res 2005;(437):219–228.
72. Kleerekoper M, Villanueva AR, Stanciu J, Rao DS, Parfitt AM. The role of three-dimensional trabecular microstructure in the pathogenesis of vertebral compression fractures. Calcif Tissue Int 1985;37(6): 594–597.
73. Kopperdahl DL, Keaveny TM. Yield strain behavior of trabecular bone. J Biomech 1998;31(7):601–608.
74. Kotzar GM, Davy DT, Goldberg VM, Heiple KG, Berilla J, Heiple KG, Jr., Brown RH, Burstein AH. Telemeterized in vivo hip joint force data: a report on two patients after total hip surgery. J Orthop Res 1991;9(5):621–633.
75. Kozloff KM, Carden A, Bergwitz C, Forlino A, Uveges TE, Morris MD, Marini JC, Goldstein SA. Brittle IV mouse model for osteogenesis imperfecta IV demonstrates postpubertal adaptations to improve whole bone strength. J Bone Miner Res 2004;19(4):614–622.
76. Kuhn JL, Goldstein SA, Choi K, London M, Feldkamp LA, Matthews LS. Comparison of the trabecular and cortical tissue moduli from human iliac crests. J Orthop Res 1989;7(6):876–884.
77. Kurtz D, Morrish K, Shapiro J. Vertebral bone mineral content in osteogenesis imperfecta. Calcif Tissue Int 1985;37(1):14–18.
78. Lehmann R, Wapniarz M, Randerath O, Kvasnicka HM, John W, Reincke M, Kutnar S, Klein K, Allolio B. Dual-energy X-ray absorptiometry at the lumbar spine in German men and women: a cross-sectional study. Calcif Tissue Int 1995;56(5):350–354.
79. Linde F, Gøthgen CB, Hvid I, Pongsoipetch B. Mechanical properties of trabecular bone by a non-destructive compression testing approach. Eng Med 1988;17(1):23–29.
80. Linde F, Hvid I, Pongsoipetch B. Energy absorptive properties of human trabecular bone specimens during axial compression. J Orthop Res 1989;7(3):432–439.
81. Löfman O, Larsson L, Ross I, Toss G, Berglund K. Bone mineral density in normal Swedish women. Bone 1997;20(2):167–174.
82. Lund AM, Molgaard C, Muller J, Skovby F. Bone mineral content and collagen defects in osteogenesis imperfecta. Acta Paediatr 1999;88(10):1083–1088.
83. Malluche HH, Meyer W, Sherman D, Massry SG. Quantitative bone histology in 84 normal American subjects. Micromorphometric analysis and evaluation of variance in iliac bone. Calcif Tissue Int 1982;34(5):449–455.
84. Martin RB, Boardman DL. The effects of collagen fiber orientation, porosity, density, mineralization on bovine cortical bone bending properties. J Biomech 1993;26(9):1047–1054.
85. Martin RB, Burr DB. Non-invasive measurement of long bone cross-sectional moment of inertia by photon absorptiometry. J Biomech 1984;17(3):195–201.
86. Martin RB, Burr DB, Sharkey NA. Skeletal tissue mechanics. New York: Springer, 1998.
87. Matousek P, Draper ER, Goodship AE, Clark IP, Ronayne KL, Parker AW. Noninvasive Raman spectroscopy of human tissue in vivo. Appl Spectrosc 2006;60(7):758–763.
88. McCreadie BR, Morris MD, Chen TC, Sudhaker Rao D, Finney WF, Widjaja E, Goldstein SA. Bone tissue compositional differences in women with and without osteoporotic fracture. Bone 2006;39(6): 1190–1195.
89. Melton LJ III. Hip fractures: a worldwide problem today and tomorrow. Bone 1993;14:S1–8.
90. Melton LJ III. Who has osteoporosis? A conflict between clinical and public health perspectives. J Bone Miner Res 2000;15(12):2309–2314.

91. Melton LJ, 3rd, Chrischilles EA, Cooper C, Lane AW, Riggs BL. Perspective. How many women have osteoporosis? J Bone Miner Res 1992;7(9):1005–1010.
92. Misof BM, Roschger P, Baldini T, Raggio CL, Zraick V, Root L, Boskey AL, Klaushofer K, Fratzl P, Camacho NP. Differential effects of alendronate treatment on bone from growing osteogenesis imperfecta and wild-type mouse. Bone 2005;36(1):150–158.
93. Mittra E, Rubin C, Qin YX. Interrelationship of trabecular mechanical and microstructural properties in sheep trabecular bone. J Biomech 2005;38(6):1229–1237.
94. Morgan EF, Bayraktar HH, Keaveny TM. Trabecular bone modulus-density relationships depend on anatomic site. J Biomech 2003;36(7):897–904.
95. Moro M, Hecker AT, Bouxsein ML, Myers ER. Failure load of thoracic vertebrae correlates with lumbar bone mineral density measured by DXA. Calcif Tissue Int 1995;56(3):206–209.
96. Moro M, van der Meulen MC, Kiratli BJ, Marcus R, Bachrach LK, Carter DR. Body mass is the primary determinant of midfemoral bone acquisition during adolescent growth. Bone 1996;19(5):519–526.
97. Mosekilde L. Sex differences in age-related loss of vertebral trabecular bone mass and structure – biomechanical consequences. Bone 1989;10:425–432.
98. Mosekilde L. Consequences of the remodelling process for vertebral trabecular bone structure: a scanning electron microscopy study (uncoupling of unloaded structures). Bone Miner 1990;10(1):13–35.
99. Mosekilde L, Mosekilde L. Sex differences in age-related changes in vertebral body size, density and biomechanical competence in normal individuals. Bone 1990;11:67–73.
100. Mosekilde L, Mosekilde L, Danielsen CC. Biomechanical competence of vertebral trabecular bone in relation to ash density and age in normal individuals. Bone 1987;8(2):79–85.
101. Myers ER, Hecker AT, Rooks DS, Hipp JA, Hayes WC. Geometric variables from DXA of the radius predict forearm fracture load in vitro. Calcif Tissue Int 1993;52(3):199–204.
102. National Osteoporosis Foundation. America's bone health: the state of osteoporosis and low bone mass in our nation. Washington D.C.: National Osteoporosis Foundation, 2002.
103. Ninomiya JT, Tracy RP, Calore JD, Gendreau MA, Kelm RJ, Mann KG. Heterogeneity of human bone. J Bone Miner Res 1990;5(9):933–938.
104. Odgaard A, Kabel J, van Rietbergen B, Dalstra M, Huiskes R. Fabric and elastic principal directions of cancellous bone are closely related. J Biomech 1997;30(5):487–495.
105. Ou-Yang H, Paschalis EP, Mayo WE, Boskey AL, Mendelsohn R. Infrared microscopic imaging of bone: spatial distribution of CO3(2-). J Bone Miner Res 2001;16(5):893–900.
106. Parfitt AM, Mathews CH, Villanueva AR, Kleerekoper M, Frame B, Rao DS. Relationships between surface, volume, thickness of iliac trabecular bone in aging and in osteoporosis. Implications for the microanatomic and cellular mechanisms of bone loss. J Clin Invest 1983;72(4):1396–1409.
107. Paschalis EP, Betts F, DiCarlo E, Mendelsohn R, Boskey AL. FTIR microspectroscopic analysis of human iliac crest biopsies from untreated osteoporotic bone. Calcif Tissue Int 1997;61(6):487–492.
108. Paschalis EP, Betts F, DiCarlo E, Mendelsohn R, Boskey AL. FTIR microspectroscopic analysis of normal human cortical and trabecular bone. Calcif Tissue Int 1997;61(6):480–486.
109. Pugh JW, Rose RM, Radin EL. A structural model for the mechanical behavior of trabecular bone. J Biomech 1973;6(6):657–670.
110. Raux P, Townsend PR, Miegel R, Rose RM, Radin EL. Trabecular architecture of the human patella. J Biomech 1975;8(1):1–7.
111. Rho JY, Ashman RB, Turner CH. Young's modulus of trabecular and cortical bone material: ultrasonic and microtensile measurements. J Biomech 1993;26(2):111–119.
112. Rho JY, Roy ME II, Tsui TY, Pharr GM. Elastic properties of microstructural components of human bone tissue as measured by nanoindentation. J Biomed Mater Res 1999;45(1):48–54.
113. Rho JY, Tsui TY, Pharr GM. Elastic properties of human cortical and trabecular lamellar bone measured by nanoindentation. Biomaterials 1997;18(20):1325–1330.
114. Rice JC, Cowin SC, Bowman JA. On the dependence of the elasticity and strength of cancellous bone on apparent density. J Biomech 1988;21(2):155–168.
115. Riggs BL, Khosla S, Melton LJ III. Sex steroids and the construction and conservation of the adult skeleton. Endocr Rev 2002;23(3):279–302.
116. Riggs BL, Melton LJ, 3rd, Robb RA, Camp JJ, Atkinson EJ, Oberg AL, Rouleau PA, McCollough CH, Khosla S, Bouxsein ML. Population-based analysis of the relationship of whole bone strength indices

and fall-related loads to age- and sex-specific patterns of hip and wrist fractures. J Bone Miner Res 2006;21(2):315–323.
117. Riggs BL, Wahner HW, Seeman E, Offord KP, Dunn WL, Mazess RB, Johnson KA, Melton LJ III. Changes in bone mineral density of the proximal femur and spine with aging. Differences between the postmenopausal and senile osteoporosis syndromes. J Clin Invest 1982;70(4):716–723.
118. Ross PD, Davis JW, Epstein RS, Wasnich RD. Pre-existing fractures and bone mass predict vertebral fracture incidence in women. Ann Intern Med 1991;114(11):919–923.
119. Ross PD, Davis JW, Vogel JM, Wasnich RD. A critical review of bone mass and the risk of fractures in osteoporosis. Calcif Tissue Int 1990;46(3):149–161.
120. Schuit SC, van der Klift M, Weel AE, de Laet CE, Burger H, Seeman E, Hofman A, Uitterlinden AG, van Leeuwen JP, Pols HA. Fracture incidence and association with bone mineral density in elderly men and women: the Rotterdam Study. Bone 2004;34(1):195–202.
121. Schulmerich MV, Dooley KA, Vanasse TM, Goldstein SA, Morris MD. Subsurface and transcutaneous Raman spectroscopy and mapping using concentric illumination rings and collection with a circular fiber-optic array. Appl Spectrosc 2007;61(7):671–678.
122. Schulmerich MV, Finney WF, Fredricks RA, Morris MD. Subsurface Raman spectroscopy and mapping using a globally illuminated non-confocal fiber-optic array probe in the presence of Raman photon migration. Appl Spectrosc 2006;60(2):109–114.
123. Shane E, Silverberg SJ, Donovan D, Papadopoulos A, Staron RB, Addesso V, Jorgesen B, McGregor C, Schulman L. Osteoporosis in lung transplantation candidates with end-stage pulmonary disease. Am J Med 1996;101(3):262–269.
124. Silva MJ, Gibson LJ. Modeling the mechanical behavior of vertebral trabecular bone: effects of age-related changes in microstructure. Bone 1997;21(2):191–199.
125. Silva MJ, Keaveny TM, Hayes WC. Computed tomography-based finite element analysis predicts failure loads and fracture patterns for vertebral sections. J Orthop Res 1998;16(3):300–308.
126. Snyder BD, Hauser-Kara DA, Hipp JA, Zurakowski D, Hecht AC, Gebhardt MC. Predicting fracture through benign skeletal lesions with quantitative computed tomography. J Bone Joint Surg Am 2006;88(1):55–70.
127. Szulc P, Munoz F, Duboeuf F, Marchand F, Delmas PD. Bone mineral density predicts osteoporotic fractures in elderly men: the MINOS study. Osteoporos Int 2005;16(10):1184–1192.
128. Tarnowski CP, Ignelzi MA, Jr., Morris MD. Mineralization of developing mouse calvaria as revealed by Raman microspectroscopy. J Bone Miner Res 2002;17(6):1118–1126.
129. Thomsen JS, Ebbesen EN, Mosekilde L. A new method of comprehensive static histomorphometry applied on human lumbar vertebral cancellous bone. Bone 2000;27(1):129–138.
130. Thomsen JS, Ebbesen EN, Mosekilde L. Predicting human vertebral bone strength by vertebral static histomorphometry. Bone 2002;30(3):502–508.
131. Townsend PR, Raux P, Rose RM, Miegel RE, Radin EL. The distribution and anisotropy of the stiffness of cancellous bone in the human patella. J Biomech 1975;8(6):363–367.
132. Turner CH, Rho J, Takano Y, Tsui TY, Pharr GM. The elastic properties of trabecular and cortical bone tissues are similar: results from two microscopic measurement techniques. J Biomech 1999;32(4):437–441.
133. Ulrich D, Hildebrand T, van Rietbergen B, Müller R, Rüegsegger P. The quality of trabecular bone evaluated with micro-computed tomography, FEA and mechanical testing. Stud Health Technol Inform 1997;40:97–112.
134. U.S. Department of Health and Human Services, Office of the Surgeon General. Bone Health and Osteoporosis: A Report of the Surgeon General. Rockville, MD 2004.
135. van der Meulen MC, Huiskes R. Why mechanobiology? A survey article. J Biomech 2002;35(4):401–414.
136. van der Meulen MC, Jepsen KJ, Mikić B. Understanding bone strength: size isn't everything. Bone 2001;29(2):101–104.
137. van Rietbergen B, Majumdar S, Pistoia W, Newitt DC, Kothari M, Laib A, Rüegsegger P. Assessment of cancellous bone mechanical properties from micro-FE models based on micro-CT, pQCT and MR images. Technol Health Care 1998;6(5–6):413–420.

138. Vega E, Bagur A, Mautalen CA. Densidad mineral âosea en mujeres osteoporâoticas y normales de Buenos Aires. Medicina 1993;53(3):211–216.
139. Weaver JK, Chalmers J. Cancellous bone: its strength and changes with aging and an evaluation of some methods for measuring its mineral content. J Bone Joint Surg Am 1966;48(2):289–298.
140. Yoshikawa T, Turner CH, Peacock M, Slemenda CW, Weaver CM, Teegarden D, Markwardt P, Burr DB. Geometric structure of the femoral neck measured using dual-energy x-ray absorptiometry [published erratum appears in J Bone Miner Res 1995 Mar;10(3):510]. J Bone Miner Res 1994;9(7):1053–1064.
141. Zysset PK, Guo XE, Hoffler CE, Moore KE, Goldstein SA. Elastic modulus and hardness of cortical and trabecular bone lamellae measured by nanoindentation in the human femur. J Biomech 1999;32(10):1005–1012.

8 Mechanical Influences on Bone Mass and Morphology

Stefan Judex and Clinton Rubin

CONTENTS

SUMMARY

While the ability of exercise to favorably influence bone mass and strength has been established long ago, the challenge becomes to determine which specific components of the loading milieu are anabolic and anti-resorptive to bone tissue and how to translate this information to the clinic. Loading parameters such as force magnitude, loading duration, or loading frequency all have a critical impact on altering the levels of bone formation and resorption and may interact with each other to define the skeletal outcome of any applied loading regime. Recent advances in understanding which components of bone's mechanical milieu are osteogenic have allowed the development of biomechanical prophylaxes against bone loss, including the anabolic potential of extremely low-level, high-frequency mechanical signals, an example of a non-drug intervention for the prevention of bone loss. Studies such as these, while preliminary, emphasize that signals need not be large to be effective and that there may be ways of stimulating the skeleton mechanically without necessarily requiring an individual to exercise.

Key Words: Mechanical influences, bone mass, morphology, bone morphology, exercise, Wolff's Law, physical activity, osteocytes, osteoblasts, osteoclasts, mechanical environment

From: *Contemporary Endocrinology: Osteoporosis: Pathophysiology and Clinical Management*
Edited by: R. A. Adler, DOI 10.1007/978-1-59745-459-9_8,

CLINICAL EVIDENCE OF MECHANICAL INFLUENCES ON BONE MORPHOLOGY

Introduction

There is strong agreement that exercise is a critical deterrent to osteoporosis, a goal achieved through bone tissue's sensitivity to its mechanical loading environment. While mounting evidence from clinical and animal studies demonstrates these functional stimuli to be potent growth factors to the skeleton, the challenge becomes to determine which specific components of the loading milieu are anabolic (and anti-resorptive) to bone tissue, and how to translate this information to the clinic where physical interventions might be tuned to most efficiently and effectively harness the skeleton's responsiveness to mechanical signals.

In 1638, the first connection between mechanical forces and skeletal architecture was proposed by Galileo Galilei, where he emphasized that *. . .nature cannot grow a tree nor construct an animal beyond a certain size, while retaining the proportions and employing the materials which suffice in the case of the smaller structure* (*1*). Clearly, for the skeleton to succeed as animals get larger and put greater demands on the tissue, bone morphology must compensate to effectively survive these new challenges. Two centuries later, several investigators including Julius Wolff theorized that the interdependence of skeletal form and mechanical stress (force per unit area) followed a specific (but as of yet undetermined) set of mathematical rules, which could be used to anticipate bone's response to new functional and pathologic demands, an interrelationship now referred to as "Wolff's Law" (*2–4*). Under the tenets of this law, an increase in the level of physical activity would cause an increase in bone mass (e.g., exercise) and reduced physical activity would stimulate bone loss (e.g., bedrest, spaceflight). While these early observations were made primarily from pathologic architecture, their importance in bringing to light the adaptive capacity of bone cannot be underestimated.

A host of human-based studies have worked toward quantifying the effects of general and specific exercise regimens on bone mass and morphology, taking into account interdependent variables such as gender, age, and nutritional status of the individuals. While some studies have provided encouraging results, the large majority of data have been equivocal, perhaps as much a reflection of our limited understanding of which specific components of the mechanical signal are perceived as osteogenic by the resident bone cells populations (e.g., osteocytes, osteoblasts, and osteoclasts), and which are irrelevant byproducts of loading, thus confusing our efforts to design the "optimal exercise intervention." For the design of such an idealized exercise intervention (e.g., least amount of physical exertion for the greatest gain in skeletal strength), many critical questions have to be addressed, such as should the exercise protocol incorporate large loads or could they be small if they are applied rapidly? How long does an individual have to exercise to maximize benefits? Are the attributes of mechanical loading accumulated or is there a threshold that is past in which additional challenges no longer are perceived as regulatory influences to the skeleton? Can exercises be designed to stimulate bone formation at skeletal sites most prone to fracture or is the response systemic? Ideally, by identifying critical aspects of bone's loading environment, it is hoped that specific exercise interventions or devices which induce regulatory mechanical signals can be developed to prevent the bone loss which leads to osteoporosis.

Here, we briefly overview exercise effects on bone (please see the companion chapter by Beck and colleagues for an in-depth review), define the functional mechanical environment of bone, and demonstrate that the ability of physical signals to influence bone morphology is strongly dependent on the character of the signal. It is with this improved understanding of which components of bone's mechanical milieu are osteogenic that has allowed the development of biomechanical prophylaxes against bone loss, including the anabolic potential of extremely low-level, high-frequency mechanical signals, an example of a non-drug intervention for the prevention of bone loss. Studies such as these, while preliminary, emphasize that signals need not be large to be effective, and that there may be ways of stimulating the skeleton mechanically without necessarily requiring an individual to exercise.

Can Exercise Increase Bone Mass?

Cross-sectional studies in humans reveal that bone morphology can change markedly in response to long-term exercise. One of the most definitive examples can be found in professional tennis players, where the cortical wall thickness of humeri in the "playing arm" can be up to 45% larger in the male and 30% larger in the female compared to humeri in the arm which simply throws the ball into the air (*5*). Similar evidence of bone hypertrophy has been reported in a range of athletes and locations, such as the feet of classical ballet dancers (*6*). Other cross-sectional studies have related a variety of different kinds of physical activities to increased bone mass including soccer, weightlifting, speed skating, squash, dancing/gymnastics, and a generally higher level of physical activity (*7–10*). Self-selection bias, however, cannot be discounted in cross-sectional comparative studies and results from longitudinal prospective studies may provide more reliable information on how bone responds to exercise. Further, the specific aspect of the sport which is relevant to bone is difficult to define: is it because the athletes practice for so long each day and for so many years (duration)? That their exercise regimens are so strenuous (intensity)? Or does the humeral hypertrophy in these tennis players arise because the Roger Federers and Venus Williams of the world hit the ball so fast (rate)? Surely, it is some interdependence of variables such as duration, intensity, and rate, yet broad-spectrum human trials make it difficult to tease apart specific contributions of each component.

Only very few prospectively designed exercise trials indicate that exercise can rapidly and effectively produce large increases in bone mass. Even considering the increases in bone mineral density (BMD) that result from the intense training regimen demanded during army training (*11*), it is unclear whether this was an adaptation of the skeletal system or the early pathological stages of a stress fracture reaction. In premenarchal girls, a high-impact strength building regimen significantly increased BMD over a 10-month period in particular at the femoral neck where the increase in exercisers was 12.0% compared to 1.7% in controls. Unfortunately, the large majority of longitudinal studies have found only modest (*12–16*) if not negligible (*17–20*) increases in bone mass. For instance, in a 12-month trial, young adult females unilaterally performed high-resistance strength training (*18*). The training significantly increased muscle strength but bone mass was unaffected by the exercise intervention.

When results from cross-sectional and prospective exercise studies are stratified for the different exercise interventions used (e.g., gymnastics, running, or swimming), the results only hint that certain types of exercise are more effective than others in stimulating bone formation or inhibiting resorption. Some studies suggest that high-load, high-impact exercises using few repetitions are superior to those exercises using low loads and high repetitions (*21–23*). Swimming, as an example of a low-load high-repetition exercise, has often failed to demonstrate significant skeletal benefits (*23,24*). Nevertheless, some reports indicate that aerobic exercise (including swimming) is also capable of eliciting an adaptive response in bone (*25–28*), while a few strength exercise regimens failed to increase BMD (*20,29*). Comparative studies often find only modest differences among different modes of exercise and the largest differences are frequently observed between those who exercise and controls (*14,25,28*).

Constraints in Clinical Studies

Numerous clinical exercise studies have attempted to relate adaptive changes in bone to specific aspects of a particular exercise regimen including exercise mode (e.g., running, swimming, weightlifting), intensity (e.g., percent of maximal heart rate), duration, and frequency (number of times per month, week, day). Unfortunately, none of these parameters has been successfully correlated to exercise-related changes in bone formation or resorption, but is this necessarily evidence that mechanical factors are ineffective in influencing bone mass and morphology? To a certain extent, this inability to demonstrate a robust correlation may be a result of a failure to fully characterize and evaluate the local mechanical milieu engendered by the specific exercise protocol. Further, bone adaptation is site-specific and focal in nature at both the organ and the tissue level and, therefore, can only weakly relate to parameters that are systemic to the entire skeleton such as exercise mode or intensity. At the organ level, bone adaptation is site-specific because only those bones that are subjected to changes in relevant mechanical stimuli respond with adaptive changes. This is particularly obvious in tennis and squash players who display significant bone hypertrophy in the playing extremity but not in the contralateral arm. Similarly, in a longitudinal prospective study of postmenopausal women, unilateral strength exercise increased BMD in the mechanically stressed arm while the contralateral arm was unaffected (*30*). And of course, there are the inevitable human factors which are difficult and/or impossible to control, including genetics, gender, body habitus and nutrition, and that critical – but evasive – parameter called compliance.

When considering bone's adaptive response to mechanical signals, it is important to consider what happens at the level of the tissue, and that not all bone cells will respond equally to any given exercise-related stimulus, as some surfaces change their osteoblastic or osteoclastic activity while other surfaces remain unchanged. An example for these focal changes within a bone is a study in which adult roosters were exercised on a treadmill for 3 weeks while a second group of roosters served as sedentary controls (*31*). High-speed running for 9 min/day activated previously quiescent periosteal middiaphyseal surfaces in the tarsometatarsus of exercised roosters, while no periosteal activity was observed in control roosters. The periosteal activation measured in exercisers occurred primarily at the medial and antero-lateral aspects of the middiaphysis while activation at anterior and posterior surfaces was minimal. The total percentage of activated surface in exercises was only 23% of the entire periosteal surface. While the bone structure may be accommodating to the new load challenges, it is apparently being done with only very subtle changes in morphology.

The focal nature of bone's adaptation to mechanical stimuli prompts the question whether the assays used to evaluate potential skeletal benefits in clinical studies are sensitive enough to detect site-specific changes and, further, whether alterations in bone mineral density accurately reflect the structural result of bone's adaptive response to exercise. The most common technique for evaluating bone's response in clinical setting is dual energy

X-ray absorptiometry (DXA). DXA is easy to use, non-invasive, and quantifies bone mineral content, BMC, in grams (g). A potential limitation of DXA, however, is that it provides only a two-dimensional "apparent density" of bone mineral density, BMD (g/cm^2), by normalizing BMC to the scanned area. As such, BMD would not be highly sensitive to focal, highly selective changes in bone quantity and/or quality.

The incomplete correction for size causes DXA to underestimate true bone mineral density in people with small bones and to overestimate bone mineral density in people with large bones (*32*). Further, DXA cannot differentiate between changes in the quantity of a bone from those changes related to the quality of a bone. In a general sense, bone quality is an index of the structural efficiency of the extracellular matrix (e.g., the architectural alignment and/or interconnectedness of trabecular bone, the degree of mineralization of the inorganic matrix, the organization and integrity of the collagen). Neglecting bone quality poses a critical limitation for the assessment of bone integrity as bone is a complex structure which mechanical function cannot be explained just by its mass. Fluoride treatment, for instance, evokes large increases in BMD at certain doses, yet has the potential to compromise the structural integrity of the bone due to a reduction of the strength of the mineralized (compressive) component of the bone tissue (*33*). Consequently, the addition of only a small amount of new bone that is well mineralized and deposited at a mechanically relevant site may well have a markedly more beneficial impact than the addition of a large amount of bone that is mechanically inferior. DXA, however, may fail to detect these focal changes in bone quality, particularly if they are subtle.

The difficulty of quantifying specific aspects of bone's mechanical environment during exercise in humans as well as the limited ability to quantify beneficial effects of exercise on the human skeleton are two of the reasons that many investigators have turned to animal studies to study bone's adaptive response to new functional challenges. Using animals, bone's mechanical loading environment can be more comprehensively quantified and controlled, and variables such as genetics, gender, nutrition, and compliance can be better accounted for. Further, several assays are available to determine changes in bone quantity and quality at the organ, as well as tissue (e.g., micro-computed tomography, static and dynamic histomorphometry, mechanical determination of stiffness and strength), cell and molecular-level responses can be evaluated. Overall, these assays can help to identify site-specific and focal changes in bone formation/resorption and distinguish between altered bone quality and bone quantity. They are also instrumental in identifying the cells that are the responders (e.g., osteoblasts, osteocytes) as well as the molecules that regulate the response, as a function of time and space. Taken together, such an interdisciplinary, hierarchical approach will help to define the relation of specific components of bone's mechanical milieu to changes in bone quantity and quality, thus enabling the identification of distinct aspects of the functional loading environment that play a critical role in bone adaptation.

BONE'S MECHANICAL ENVIRONMENT

The inability of parameters such as exercise mode or intensity to predict adaptive changes in bone quantity or quality emphasizes the need to more closely evaluate specific candidate parameters in terms of their role in influencing mechanically mediated bone modeling and remodeling. Toward this end, the mechanical environment that bone is subject to during functional load bearing has been characterized to gain insights into the structural demands that are placed onto the skeleton. In contrast to the notion that bone is purely loaded under compression, these experiments have definitively demonstrated that the long bones of the appendicular skeleton are also subject to a complex combination of forces and moments produced by torsion and bending even during relatively simple activities such as steady-state locomotion.

These forces and moments applied to a bone generate a mechanical state in the bone matrix which is quantified by spatial and temporal measures. Mechanical *strain* (ε) is the most common measure to quantify deformations in the bone matrix and is expressed as a change in length (ΔL) normalized to the original length (L) of any given specimen ($\varepsilon = \Delta L/L$) (Fig. 1a). Thus, strain is a dimensionless measure, and given the exceedingly small strains that arise in bone under load, is most commonly expressed in microstrain (10^{-6} strain). Thus, 1% deformation, which would occur in a meter stick (100 cm) being loaded such that it deformed to 99 cm, would indicate that the ruler is subject to 1.0% ε (strain), or its nomenclature equivalents of 0.01 $\varepsilon = 10{,}000 \times 10^{-6}$ strain $= 10{,}000$ $\mu\varepsilon$ (μstrain).

Strains can be divided into normal and shear strains with normal strains producing volumetric changes and shear strains producing geometric angular changes (Fig. 1b). Spatial *strain gradients* give information about how strain magnitude changes across a volume of tissue, and it is easy to imagine the resulting fluid flow within the bone matrix arising. These gradients can be calculated for different directions within the bone matrix (e.g., circumferential, radial, longitudinal). *Strain rate* takes the temporal component of mechanical loading into account and is used to describe how quickly strain changes within a given time; the larger the strain rate the quicker the load (or moment) applied to the bone. *Strain frequency* gives information about how many strain events occur within a certain time frame, most typically considered in terms of cycles per second. One Hertz = 1 Hz = one cycle per second. Alternating electrical current in the United States is delivered at 60 cycles per second or 60 Hz.

The magnitude of these parameters can be determined during functional activities when strain gages are surgically implanted onto bone's surface. While these gages only record deformation from the specific sites that they are attached to, mechanical models such as beam theory can be used to extrapolate measured deformations to other sites within the bone. This approach works well for cortical bone because of its accessibility to strain gages but is exceedingly difficult for trabecular bone where sophisticated finite element models with numerous loading assumptions are needed to estimate bone's strain state. In cortical bone, strain gages have been used to quantify activity-related bone strains in a great variety of species including humans (*34,35*), dogs (*36,37*), primates (*38,39*), roosters (*31,40*), horses (*41,42*), sheep (*43*), and rats (*44*). From these strain gage data, there are a number of critical observations to be made regarding the structural demands made on the skeleton.

Vigorous physical activity induces similar peak strains in the 2000–3000 $\mu\varepsilon$ (microstrain) range (*45–47*). This indicates that bone loading and architecture is finely tuned to achieve a safety factor of 2–3 with respect to the level of bone strain at which permanent deformation (damage) is induced. Whether measured in a galloping horse (metacarpal), running human (tibia), flying goose (humerus), trotting sheep (femur), or chewing macaque (mandible), this "dynamic strain similarity" suggests that skeletal morphology is adjusted in such a way that functional activity elicits a very specific (and perhaps beneficial) level of strain to the bone tissue (*48*). This similarity in peak strain magnitudes also supports a

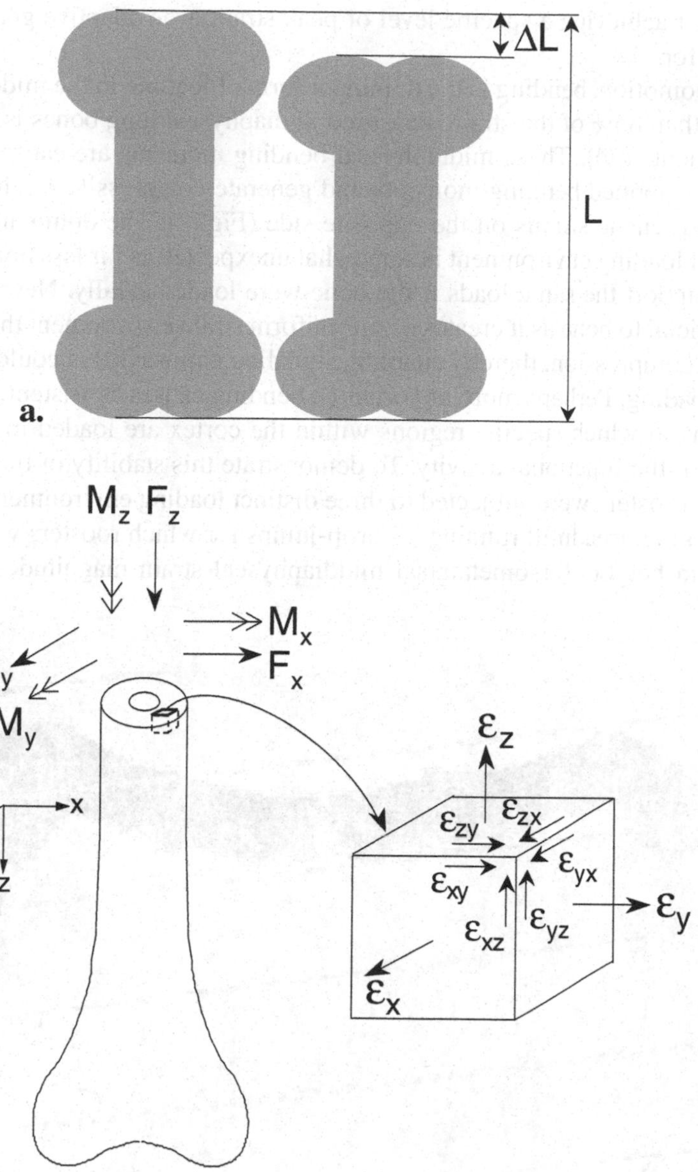

Fig. 1. (**a**) Illustration of the calculation of strain. Assuming that the original length of the bone is "L" and the bone is compressed by "ΔL," then strain is determined as the ratio of deformation ΔL to the original length L. Thus, strain represents a normalized deformation and is dimensionless. (**b**) Functional load environment acting on a middiaphyseal section of a long bone consisting of bending moments (M_x, M_y), a torsional moment (M_z), shear forces (F_x, F_y), and an axial force (F_z). Many functional activities induce diaphysial strains that are generated primarily by moments. Diaphysial moments are influenced by joint and muscular forces and moments as well as by the degree of bone curvature. (**b**) Although strain as illustrated in (**a**) is a conceptually simple parameter when measured in only one direction, it is critical to realize that functional activities produce a complex state of strain in any given cube within the bone structure. This strain state can be characterized by normal strains (ε_{xx}, ε_{yy}, ε_{zz}) acting perpendicular to the faces of the cube which compress or elongate the cube. Shear strains (ε_{xy}, ε_{xz}, ε_{yz}, etc.) that are primarily produced by shear forces and torsional moments cause an angular change in cube geometry.

hypothesis that achieving a specific level of peak strain is an adaptive goal that bone as an organ strives for.

During locomotion, bending is the dominant form of loading in the middiaphysis of limb bones; more than 85% of the strain measured in diaphyseal long bones is accounted for by bending moments (*46*). These mididphyseal bending moments are caused by bone curvature as well as applied bending moments and generate compressive strains on one side of the cortex and tensile strains on the opposite side (Fig. 2). The dominance of bending in the functional loading environment is somewhat unexpected as far less bone mass would be required to support the same loads if the bone were loaded axially. Nevertheless, bending may be beneficial to bone as it creates a non-uniform strain environment that is more diverse than uniform compression, thereby enabling signaling pathways that could not be generated by uniform loading. Perhaps more importantly, bending causes consistent, predictable loading conditions in which specific regions within the cortex are loaded in a similar fashion independent of the functional activity. To demonstrate this stability of the functional strain environment, roosters were subjected to three distinct loading environments engendered by treadmill walking, treadmill running, or drop-jumps for which roosters were released from a 50 to 60 cm height. Tarsometatarsal middiaphyseal strain magnitudes and distribution

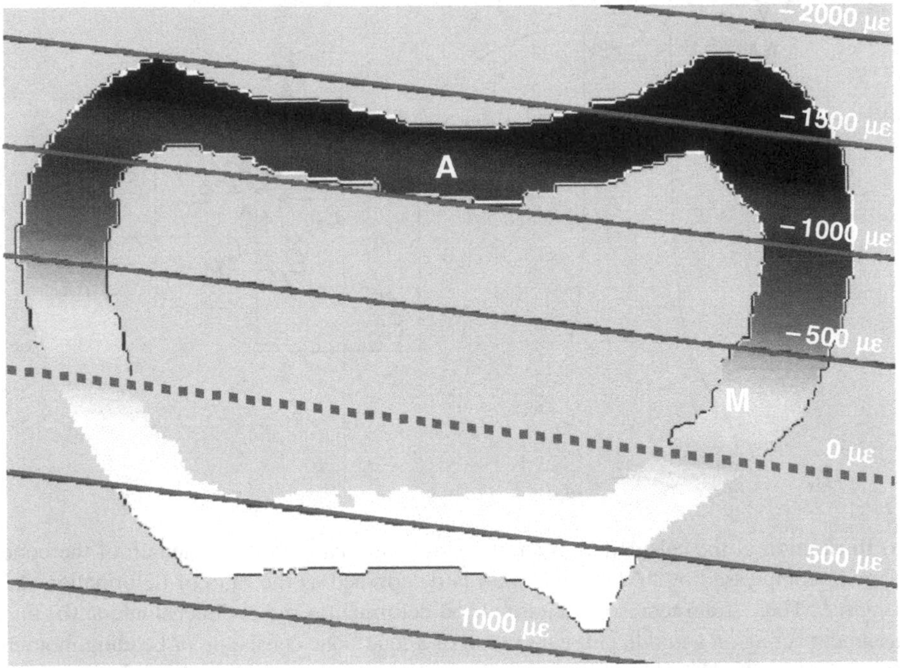

Fig. 2. Distribution of longitudinal normal strain superimposed upon a middiaphyseal tarsometatarsal section in a rooster running at a treadmill speed of 1.7 m/s. Bending moments generated regions of large compressive strains (~1500–1800 με) at the anterior cartex (*shaded dark*) and regions of large tensile strains (~500–800 με) at the posterior cortex (*white*). The neutral axis (zero strain) is dotted with strain isopleths running parallel to it. This distribution was determined during mid-stance phase when peak strains were induced but the manner of loading (i.e., position of the neutral axis) did not change throughout stance phase or with changes in exercise mode (see also Fig. 3). A, anterior; M, medial.

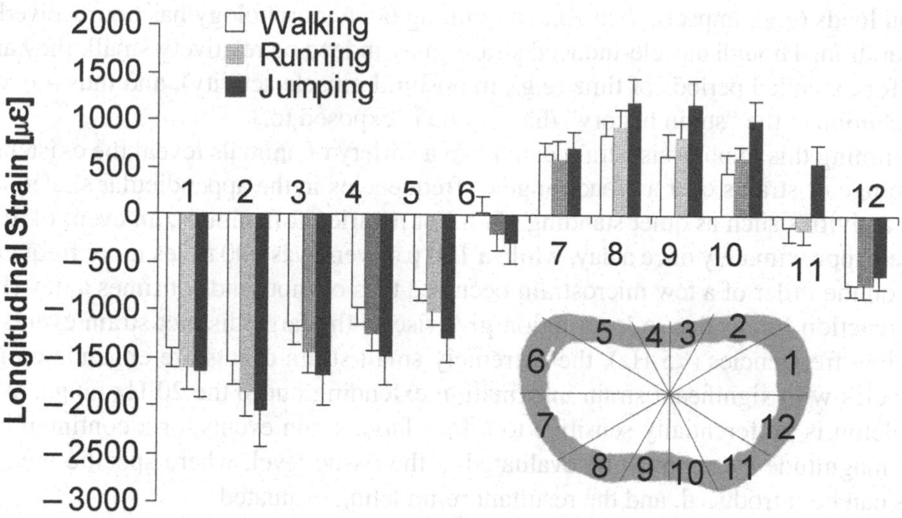

Fig. 3. Peak longitudinal strain determined in each of 12 sectors subdividing a middiaphyseal section when growing roosters were subjected to either slow walking, high-speed running, or drop jumps. Peak strains increased from walking to running and jumping, yet the relative distribution across the middiaphysis was similar for the three activities, indicating an extremely stable strain environement independent of exercise mode. Numbers along the abscissa refer to the sector sumbers in the inset (mean ± SE).

were determined via strain gages and linear beam theory (*49*). We found that peak compressive strains produced by these three activities increased from –1570 µε for walking to –1870 µε for running and –2070 µε for jumping. Despite this increase in peak strains, the relative distribution of strain across the middiaphysis remained remarkably stable across the three activities (Fig. 3).

With bending causing tension on one surface and compression on another, the transition between these two areas creates a region of the cortex which experiences very low peak strain magnitudes. Even though this neutral axis is far removed from the area of the cortex subject to the peak strains, somehow tissue is retained in this low-magnitude strain state. A conceivable mechanism to save bone from resorbing in this region could be differential coupling of bone cells to the matrix with cells in low strain regions being tightly coupled and cells from peak strain regions being more loosely coupled to the matrix. In this way, the cells have "tuned" themselves to the mechanical strain environment, a means of functional adaptation at the level of the cell. Certainly, it is clear that bone cannot be presumed to be solely a compressive element, and strain cannot be presumed to be uniform across the cortex.

Recognizing that bone is first a biologic tissue and second a mechanical structure, it is important to consider the biologic implications associated with physical stimuli. Indeed, tissue viability may depend on aspects of the mechanical environment which may not be at all rooted in maximal strain events. Alternatively, bone adaptation may depend on some camouflaged subset of the mechanical milieu, for example, the mechanical strains induced by muscle. While the symbiotic relationship between muscle and bone is inherently obvious, only seldom is it explicitly considered in the context of one defining the other (*50*). As muscle contraction imposes far smaller strains on the skeleton than that caused by ground reaction loads (e.g., impact), their role in defining bone morphology has not received much consideration. Though muscle-induced strains may indeed be relatively small, they are sustained for extended periods of time (e.g., in postural muscle activity), and thus – over time – may dominate the "strain history" that a bone is exposed to.

Examining this hypothesis, strain data from a variety of animals reveal the existence of a broad range of strains over a broad range of frequencies in the appendicular skeleton, even during activities such as quiet standing (*51*). For a variety of animals, an event of 1000 με occurred approximately once a day, while a 100 με event was 100 times more frequent, and events on the order of a few microstrain occurred tens of thousands of times a day (Fig. 4). While reaction forces due to locomotion give rise to the large distinct strain events (1000 με) at low frequencies (<5 Hz), the extremely small strain events are engendered at high frequencies with significant strain information extending out to the 20 Hz range. Whether the skeleton is preferentially sensitive to a few, large strain events, or a continual barrage of low-magnitude events must be evaluated at the tissue level, where specific mechanical signals can be introduced, and the resultant remodeling evaluated.

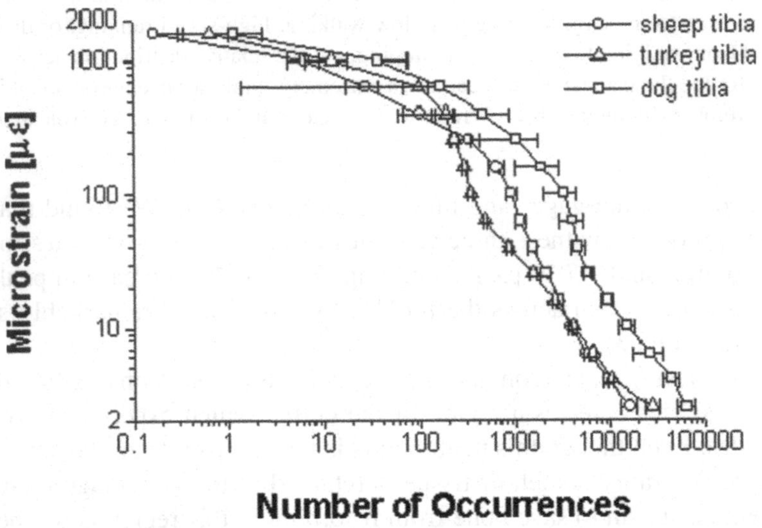

Fig. 4. Strain events measured in a sheep, turkey, and dog tibia over a 24 h period. Large strain events approaching 2000 με were exceedingly rare and the total number of strain events occurring during the 24 h period (strain history) were dominated by strain events that were very small in magnitude (2–10 με) but high in frequency (>5 Hz). Thus, the strain magnitude of an event decreased with its number of occurrences. From Fritton et al. (*51*).

In summary, it is clear that the skeletal organ is subject to a wide range of mechanical signals, from low- to high-frequency strains, normal and shear strains, compressive and tensile strains. It is also clear that the cells on and within the mineralized matrix are subject not only to mechanical parameters such as strain but also derivatives of tissue deformation such as fluid flow and electrokinetic currents, parameters which may represent an important physiologic pathway in mediating an adaptive response. This accentuates the importance of studying the adaptation of bone to (exercise-induced) mechanical stimuli at its tissue level.

WHAT MECHANICAL PARAMETERS INFLUENCE BONE ADAPTATION?

The design of exercise protocols that can effectively stimulate bone growth or inhibit resorption requires the identification of specific mechanical parameters that can achieve this goal. For instance, if strain magnitude (i.e., deformation of the matrix) was identified as the single most important parameter, then large loads should be imposed. If, on the other hand, strain rate was identified as more influential in defining skeletal morphology (e.g., the increase rate of fluid flow that arises with higher rates of loading), then exercise interventions could apply loads that need not necessarily be high in magnitude but are applied rapidly. Similarly, determining that only a few cycles are necessary to saturate the response may allow interventions that are of minimal duration. Or, if a change in the distribution of bone strain (as defined by bending) is required, then complex exercises creating diverse loading conditions would be called for. Relating specific aspects of bone's mechanical milieu to an adaptive response is a critical step toward efficient biomechanical interventions and has led to the development of models in which the applied mechanical milieu can be quantified at bone's tissue level.

Models that have been used to investigate bone's adaptive response to its mechanical environment include overloads by osteotomies (*52*), vigorous exercise (*53*), or exogenous loading models in which external forces are applied to the bone. Physical exercise represents a physiological means of enhanced mechanical loading, but a disadvantage of exercise models is the limited exercise repertoire of most laboratory animals making it difficult to generate and control distinct mechanical milieus. Exogenous loading models such as the functionally isolated avian ulna (*54*), the axially loaded rat ulna (*55*), or the rat tibia placed in a four-point bending apparatus (*56*) allow the generation of controllable mechanical environments but a disadvantage of some these models is that the morphological response may be confounded by injury caused by the means of load application (*55*).

Since Wolff's treatise (Wolff's Law) (*3*) which stated that physical laws govern the modeling and remodeling processes in bone, researchers' attention has focused primarily on strain magnitude as the dominant determinant of bone mass and morphology. Other parameters have received only limited attention. Isolating the effect of a single mechanical parameter is not trivial due to the interdependence of many of the parameters. Changing strain magnitude while maintaining a constant loading frequency, for example, may result in a concomitant change in strain rate (Fig. 5). Despite these difficulties, several mechanical parameters have emerged from controlled experimental studies that related the mechanical environment to induced morphological changes.

Strain Magnitude

When holding strain frequency and number of loading events constant, longitudinal normal strain magnitude (strain in the direction of bone's longitudinal axis) is highly related to the osteogenic response (*55,57,58*). In other words, the larger the maximal deformation that is generated in the bone, the larger the overall response of the bone. Strains applied at 1 Hz that do not reach a certain magnitude are permissive to bone loss. This relationship was first demonstrated in the functionally isolated turkey ulna preparation to which strains in the range of 500–4000 $\mu\varepsilon$ were applied for 100 cycles per day. In this model, the ulna of adult male turkeys is functionally isolated by proximal and distal epiphyseal osteotomies, leaving the entire diaphyseal shaft undisturbed. The only stimuli applied to the diaphysis

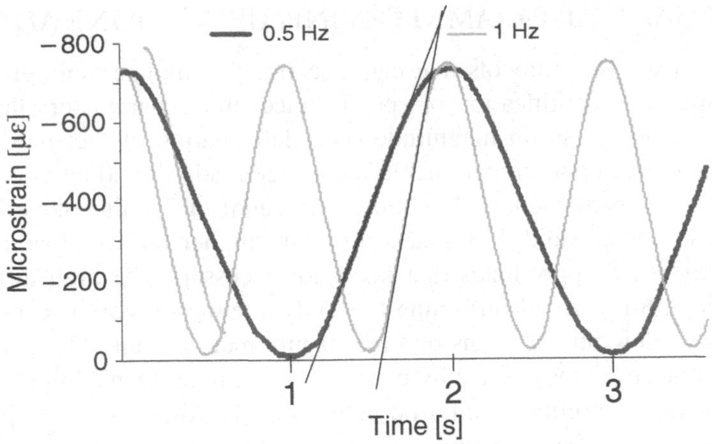

Fig. 5. Recording from a strain gage attached to the ventral surface of the turkey ulna subjected to either a 0.5 or 1 Hz load. Both frequencies cause longitudinal normal strains of about 700 με in compression at this strain gage, but strain rate, the change in strain magnitude over time, is affected by the altered frequency. The 1 Hz signals induce peak strain rates that are twice as large (2200 με/s) as the peak strain rates induced by the 0.5 Hz signal (1100 με/s) as shown by the different tangents of the sine waves.

are the mechanical regimen prescribed by the investigators, with no aberrant biophysical signals entering the preparation. In this model, strains smaller than 1000 με caused bone loss with strains larger than 1000 με leading to new bone formation in a dose-dependent relationship (Fig. 6a).

The question as to how much strain in bone has to be generated to obtain an osteogenic effect is dependent upon the interrelationship between strain magnitude, strain rate, and strain frequency. While in the previously described isolated turkey ulna preparation, 100 loading cycles per day at 1 Hz inducing 1000 με prevented bone loss from occurring, this threshold can be reduced to 700 με when 600 loading cycles are applied at 1 Hz, to 270 με when 36,000 loading cycles are applied at 60 Hz, or to 100 με when 108,000 loading cycles are applied at 30 Hz (*59*) (Fig. 6b). This demonstrates that the search for a particular strain (loading) threshold has to take other mechanical parameters into account as well and that this relationship can be exploited to design safer exercise regimens using smaller loads.

The complete strain state of the bone tissue (strain tensor) of the functional regimen is very complex but it can be described in general terms by two predominant components, normal strains and shear strains. While only normal strains were considered in previous studies investigating the relation between strain and new bone formation, it is essential to know which specific component of this strain actually influences the metabolism of the osteocyte, osteoblast, or osteoclast to retain bone homeostasis, initiate modeling, or turn on remodeling.

This goal of investigating the osteogenic effects of different aspects of the strain tensor has been approached using the turkey ulna model of disuse osteopenia, in which the modeling and remodeling response was quantified following 4 weeks of either axial or torsional loading or disuse (*60*). Each of the two load groups was subject to peak principal strains of 1000 με (predominately normal strain in the axial case and shear strain when subject to torsion). Of the three distinct groups, only disuse caused a significant change in gross

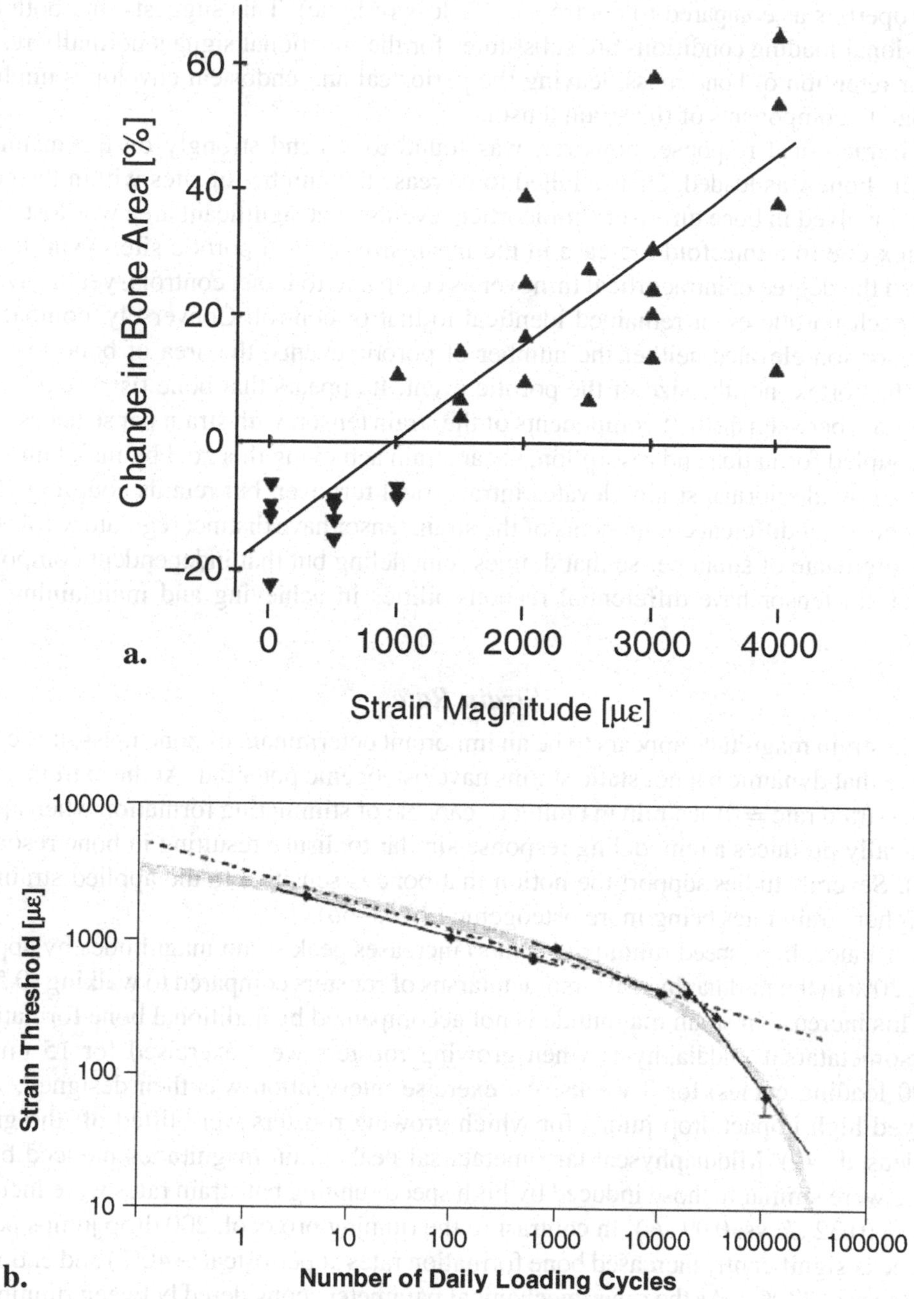

Fig. 6. (**a**) Relation between strain magnitude and changes in bone morphology when 100 cycles per day were applied at 1 Hz. Peak strain magnitudes engendered in the diaphyseal turkey ulna of about 1000 με retained bone mass. Strain magnitudes below this threshold caused bone resorption and strain magnitudes above 1000 με were osteogenic in a dose-dependent relationship. Adapted from Rubin and Lanyon (*58*). (**b**) Empiral evidence compiled from several studies suggesting that the strain threshold at which bone mass is maintained (*gray line*) can be lowered when the number of daily loading cycles is increased; either 4 cycles of 2000 με at 0.5 Hz, 100 cycles of 1000 με at 1 Hz, or 108,000 cycles of 100 με at 30 Hz provide the same information with respect to the maintenance of bone tissue. Adapted from Qin et al. (*59*).

areal properties as compared to controls (13% loss of bone). This suggests that both axial and torsional loading conditions are substitutes for the functional signals normally responsible for retention of bone mass, leaving the periosteal and endosteal envelopes unphased by disparate components of the strain tensor.

The intracortical response, however, was found to depend strongly on the manner in which the bone was loaded. Disuse failed to increase the number of sites within the cortex actively involved in bone turnover (intracortical events), yet significant area was lost within the cortex due to a threefold increase in the mean size of each porotic site. Axial loading increased the degree of intracortical turnover as compared to intact controls, yet the average size of each porotic event remained identical to that of control. Conversely, compared to control, torsion elevated neither the number of porotic events, the area of bone lost from within the cortex, nor the size of the porotic event. It appears that bone tissue can readily differentiate between distinct components of the strain tensor, with strain per se necessary to retain coupled formation and resorption, shear strain achieving this goal by maintaining the status quo, while normal strain elevates intracortical turnover, but retains coupling. These data suggest that different components of the strain tensor have distinct regulatory roles. It is not the aggregate of strain per se that defines remodeling but that independent components of the strain tensor have differential responsibilities in achieving and maintaining bone mass.

Strain Rate

While strain magnitude appears to be an important determinant of bone mass, it is critical to realize that dynamic but not static strains have osteogenic potential. At the extreme, static loading (strain rate = 0) at strain magnitudes capable of stimulating formation when applied dynamically produces a remodeling response similar to disuse resulting in bone resorption (*61,62*). Several studies support the notion that bone is sensitive to the applied strain rate, with higher strain rates being more osteogenic (*49,63–66*).

For instance, high speed running (1.7 m/s) increases peak strain magnitudes by approximately 20% in the middiaphyseal tarsometatarsus of roosters compared to walking (0.5 m/s) (53). This increase in strain magnitude is not accompanied by additional bone formation in the tarsometatarsal middiaphysis when growing roosters were exercised for 15 min/day (~2600 loading cycles) for 8 weeks. An exercise intervention was then designed, which employed high impact drop jumps for which growing roosters were lifted off the ground and released (*49*). Middiaphyseal tarsometatarsal peak strain magnitudes induced by this exercise were similar to those induced by high speed running but strain rates were increased by 260% (0.32 ε/s vs. 0.09 ε/s). In contrast to the running protocol, 200 drop jumps per day for 3 weeks significantly increased bone formation rates at periosteal (+40%) and endocortical surfaces (+370%). As the other mechanical parameters considered between running and drop-jumping, the differential osteogenic effect associated with these two exercise protocols could be attributed directly to the large difference in generated strain rates. Site-specific analyses within the middiaphyseal cortex revealed that drop-jumping deposited additional bone preferentially in those regions that were subjected to the largest strain rates. This further emphasized bone's sensitivity to high strain rates.

Extrapolated for the design of exercise interventions, these results imply that loads should be applied rapidly. Although exercise studies have been unable to identify a specific exercise intervention that is most effective in producing beneficial skeletal effects, a trend has emerged with high-impact exercise being more efficient than low impact exercises in terms of stimulating new bone formation. This trend may support the notion that high strain rates have a critical impact on bone morphology as high-impact exercises have been assumed to induce high strain rates. Unfortunately, bone strain rates have rarely been measured in humans and the occurrence of high strain rates in presumably high impact sports such as gymnastics or volleyball still has to be verified.

Cycle Number

A threshold behavior exists for the number of loading cycles. The full response can be triggered after only a limited number of loading cycles (*54,67*). In the functionally isolated turkey ulna preparation, a loading regime inducing peak strains of approximately 2000 $\mu\varepsilon$ maintained bone mass with only four cycles a day. When the cycle number was increased, this particular loading regime stimulated new bone formation. Thirty-six load cycles saturated the osteogenic response, with as many as 1800 cycles being not more effective than 36 cycles.(*54*) The notion that a finite number of loading cycles employing large loads may increase BMD or inhibit bone loss is supported by exercise studies involving weight lifters (*7,13*). It is critical to realize, though, that the saturation threshold to cycle number is influenced by other mechanical parameters including strain magnitude (as described in the Strain Magnitude section).

Strain Distribution

While a relation between peak strain magnitude generated in a bone and the resulting adaptive response has been proposed, bone also appears to be sensitive to how the strains are distributed across a bone section. Simply imposing a strain distribution that produces similar peak strain magnitudes as habitual loading conditions – but at different locations within the section (i.e., rotating the strain distribution) – may initiate new bone formation (*68*). Thus, unusual strain events (strain errors) have been suggested to drive bone adaptation. Running, for instance, may not be the osteogenically optimal exercise partly because it may generate strain distributions that are very similar to strain distributions induced by normal walking (Fig. 4) (*31*). Interestingly, sports that involve many a great variety of changes in loading directions such as soccer or badminton have been suggested to possess a higher osteogenic capacity although it has not been confirmed that these changes in loading directions actually cause altered bone strain distributions.

Strain Gradients

Parameters such as peak strain magnitude or strain rate were primarily tested at the organ level. In other words, the region of the bone that was studied in response to a given mechanical stimulus was large (e.g., the middiaphysis of a long bone) and encompassed a large range of strain magnitudes. For instance, applying peak strain magnitudes of 2500 $\mu\varepsilon$ in bending may produce 2500 $\mu\varepsilon$ in compression on one side of the middiaphyseal cortex, 2000 $\mu\varepsilon$ in tension on the other cortex, and very low strains at the midline between these cortices. Rather than simply considering the peak magnitude of the stimulus and averaging the morphological response across a section, one could investigate whether new bone is actually deposited in those regions where the applied stimulus is the largest (i.e., the distribution of a mechanical parameter can be correlated with the distribution of bone's response). If such a site-specific relationship exists, then the knowledge of this specific osteogenic component may provide information about a mechanism by which bone cells perceive their mechanical environment. Further, if a particular mechanical parameter is capable of consistently predicting the specific sites of bone formation in different models, then exercise interventions could be designed that deposit bone at sites where additional structural strength is required.

This issue was addressed in an exercise study in which young adult rooster were ran on treadmill for 9 min/day (~1500 gait cycles) for 3 weeks (*31*). Strain gages were attached to the tarsometatarsus to determine the distribution of candidate mechanical parameters across a middiaphyseal section. Periosteal activation (as measured by histomorphometry) and mechanical parameters, such as strain magnitude, strain rate, and strain gradients, were quantified in twelve 30° sectors of a transverse section, thus enabling a site-specific correlation with each other (Fig. 7). The brief daily running regime activated periosteal surfaces but the amount of periosteal mineralizing surfaces per sector was only weakly associated with strain magnitude ($R^2 = 0.24$, negative correlation). In contrast, circumferential strain gradients (changes in strain magnitude across a volume of tissue) correlated strongly ($R^2 = 0.63$) with the sites of periosteal activation (Fig. 7), consistent with results from an external loading model (*69*). Generally, circumferential strain gradients are largest where strains (deformations) are the smallest. While it is counterintuitive from a structural (engineering) perspective that new bone formation is activated at sites subjected to low strains rather than large strains, physiologically, it is important to point out that strain gradients are proportional to fluid flow in bone (*70*), a byproduct of strain which has been implicated to play an important role in mechanotransduction in bone. The result that the distribution of

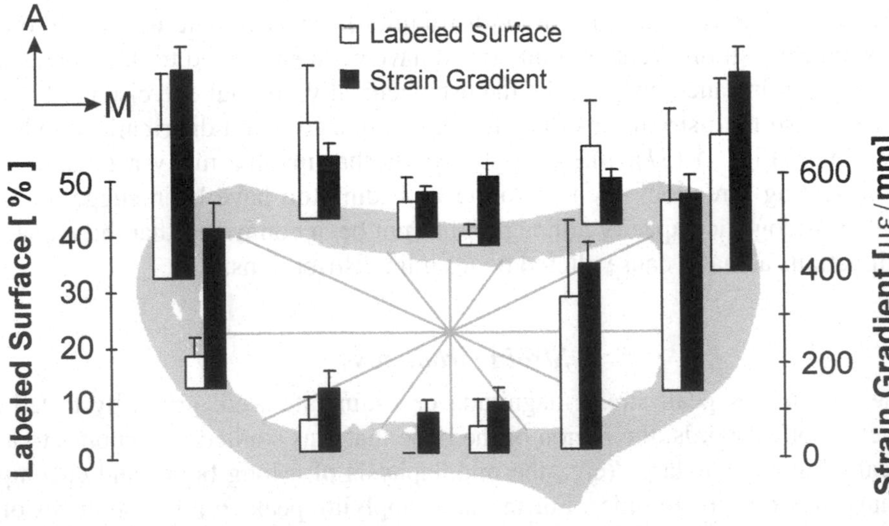

Fig. 7. Distribution of circumferential strain gradients and percentage of periosteal labeled surface per sector superimposed on a middiaphyseal TMT cross section (Mean ± SE). Sectors with the largest strain gradients correlated highly ($R^2 = 0.63$) with the sectors that exhibited the largest regions of bone forming surfaces (mean ± SE). From Judex et al. (*31*).

strain magnitude was poorly related to the specific sites of bone formation may also imply that bone is possibly not sensitive to strain magnitude per se but rather to a parameter or combination of parameters that is only indirectly related to strain magnitude such as strain gradients.

Further, as exercise-related new bone accretion is linked to specific sites within a bone, the structural enhancement of bone could be maximized if the deposition of new tissue could be directed toward sites that are at greatest risk to fracture. If strain gradients can be confirmed as consistent predictors of the specific sites of bone formation, then exercise protocols could be designed in which the sites of very low strains (large circumferential gradients) are aligned with those sites within the bone that would most efficiently enhance the structural strength of the tissue.

Strain Frequency

A common theme of the mechanical parameters described above is that only peak events are considered (e.g., peak strain magnitude, peak strain rate). From this, one could conclude that mechanical modulation of bone physiology depends on large signals to have any morphologic impact. However, the weak correlation of new bone formation with exercise intensity or with the specific sites of peak strain magnitudes suggests that other factors may also be relevant for defining bone mass and morphology.

As indicated in the Strain Magnitude section, a nonlinear interdependence between cycle number, strain frequency, and strain magnitude was observed in the functionally isolated turkey ulna preparation. When loaded at 1 Hz, peak strains larger than 700 με are necessary to maintain bone mass. This loading threshold can be reduced to 400 με at 30 Hz and to 70 με at 30 Hz (*59*). The ability to reduce this strain threshold is most likely influenced by the increased frequency at which loading occurred. The concept that high-frequency but low-magnitude strains can be beneficial to bone quantity as well as quality is supported by host of studies. Whole-body vibrations applied at 1 g (1 g = Earth's gravitational field), 25 Hz for 12 h/day to rats increased the modulus of elasticity and the micro-hardness of cortical bone harvested from the femur (*71*). Even vibrations applied at less than 0.5 g have been shown to promote anabolic activity (*72,73*), decrease catabolic activity (*74*), and increase bone quantity (*75*) and quality (*76*).

Considering that high-frequency mechanical stimuli can stimulate bone formation, it is important to consider whether their presence is critical for maintaining bone formation. To address this question, female, 6 months old Sprague–Dawley rats were subjected to tail-suspension, removing mechanical loading from the hind limbs (*77*). It was hypothesized that the exposure of a bone to high-frequency but low-magnitude mechanical stimuli may prevent the decline in bone formation during disuse. First, the extent to which hind limb unloading induced bone loss was assessed. It was then determined whether a mechanical signal consisting of high-frequency whole-body vibration at 90 Hz (0.25 g) for 10 min/day can return altered bone formation rates to normal in hind limb unloaded animals. The ability of this high-frequency mechanical stimulus to rescue the bone phenotype was compared to control rats, as well as to rats subjected to tail suspension interrupted by weight bearing for 10 min/day. At the end of the 28 days protocol, hind limb suspension significantly decreased trabecular bone formation rates by 92% compared to controls. Hind limb suspension interrupted by 10 min of weight-bearing per day failed to negate bone loss. In contrast, when high-frequency low-magnitude mechanical stimulation was used

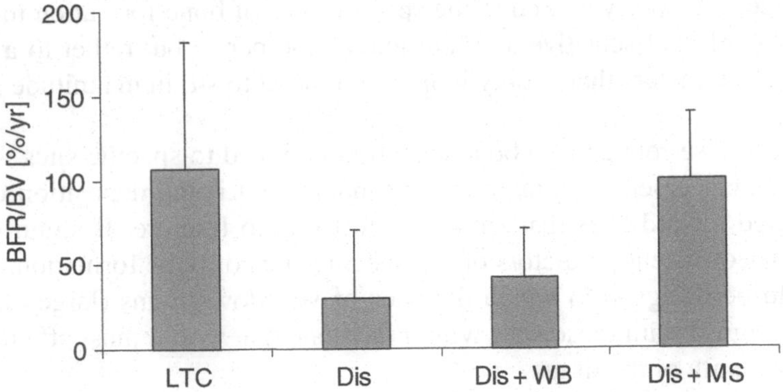

Fig. 8. Tibial trabecular bone formation rates (BFR/BV, mean ± SD) of age-matched controls (LTC) and after 28 days of hindlimb suspension-related disuse (Dis), disuse interrupted by 10 min/day of weight bearing (Dis + WB), and disuse interrupted by 10 min/day of high-frequency low-magnitude mechanical stimulation (Dis + MS). Adapted from Rubin et al. (*77*).

for 10 min/day to combat disuse, the impact of the intervention served to normalize the response back to control values (Fig. 8). This demonstrates the capability of extremely low-level vibration to inhibit the decline in bone formation rates associated with hind limb disuse. Clinically, these data are encouraging as this safe biomechanical intervention effectively prevented disuse-related osteopenia from occurring, even when the bone was subjected to 23 h and 50 min/day of this strong stimulus for resorption. Based on these observations, high-frequency, low-magnitude, mechanical strains effectively served as a "surrogate" for musculoskeletal forces and, thus, may represent a countermeasure to the osteopenia which parallels disuse.

Longer term animal studies (1 year) have shown that such low-magnitude, high-frequency loading, inducing cortical strains of 5 $\mu\varepsilon$ can increase cancellous bone volume fraction (*72*), thicken trabeculae (*75*), increase trabecular number (*78*), and enhance bone stiffness and strength (*76*). Considering that these high-frequency strains are far below (<1/1000th) those which may cause damage to bone tissue, they are unique in that they may represent the basis of a mechanical intervention which would serve as a non-pharmacologic prophylaxis for osteoporosis.

These data demonstrate that signals need not be large to be influential, and that the signals need not be long in duration to be effective. This "other than peak" perspective is employed in several biologic systems which perceive and respond to exogenous stimuli, such as vision, hearing, and touch. In considering the mechanically mediated control of bone remodeling, there is little argument that biophysical stimuli are potent determinants of skeletal morphology but too much may only damage the system. To identify the criteria by which these processes are controlled, it is necessary to look beyond the material consequences of a structure subject to load and consider the biologic benefit of a viable tissue subject to functional levels of strain. Indeed, in a "complete" departure from the interaction of bone strain and cell responses, it has even been proposed that mechanical signals are sensed by bone cells through a factor independent of matrix strain, such that acceleration itself represents an efficient means of delivering mechanical signals to a cell yet requires no deformation of the matrix whatsoever (*79*).

Summary

This overview on the relative influence of specific mechanical parameters on skeletal adaptation emphasizes both the complexity of functional loading environment and the potency of mechanical signals to stimulate formation and inhibit resorption of bone tissue. Clearly, the ability to "explain" bone adaptation through a single parameter (e.g., magnitude, rate, frequency, duration) further emphasizes how little we actually know of the key regulatory parameters or the cellular and molecular means which control the response (*80*). Further, even given bone's sensitivity to mechanical loading, the relative importance of these physical signals is certain to change relative to factors such as gender, age, and hormonal status.

EXAMPLE FOR A SAFE CLINICAL APPLICATION OF BIOPHYSICAL STIMULI

Transmission of Low-Level Mechanical Stimuli to the Skeleton

While a biophysical approach contrasts sharply with pharmaceutical strategies for the treatment of osteoporosis, in essence, the structural success of the skeleton is a product of bone tissue's ability to adapt to this constant barrage of mechanically based signals. As outlined earlier, animal work has led us to the hypothesis that high-frequency but low-magnitude mechanical stimuli can influence bone formation and resorption. Considering that these signals are so low, they could clinically be used to inhibit or reverse osteopenia. Certainly, low-level biophysical signals would be simpler and safer to impose into the skeletal system than large stimuli that are typically associated with exercise regimens.

As a first step, the feasibility of transmitting these low-level mechanical stimuli to the human skeleton was examined. The nature of the weight-supporting skeleton facilitates the transmission of mechanical energy into bone tissue in a relatively direct manner. That the weight-bearing skeleton certainly subjects the skeleton to strain, a dynamic strain on the skeleton can presumably be induced by perturbing its effective gravity. The modulation of g-force can be accomplished by placing the standing human on a platform which is made to oscillate at a specific frequency and acceleration (*81*). The strains arising from dynamic alterations in g-force would be transferred into the skeleton along a normal trajectory, ensuring that the stimulus is concentrated at those sites with greatest weight-bearing responsibility (e.g., femoral neck), yet weak at sites not subject to resisting gravity (e.g., cranium). While conceptually simple, it must be demonstrated that ground-based accelerations are indeed transmitted through the bones and joints of the lower appendicular skeleton; little is known of transmissibility of ground-based vibration at frequencies above 12 Hz (*82*). To establish the relationship between acceleration at the plate surface and transmission of acceleration through the appendicular and axial skeleton, accelerations were measured from the femur and spine of the human standing on a vibrating platform. Force transmission to these bones was determined using accelerometers mounted on Steinman pins transcutaneously imbedded in the spinous process of L3 and the greater trochanter of the right femur of six volunteers (*81*). To determine damping as a function of posture, data were also collected from subjects while standing with bent knees.

Negligible loss of acceleration was observed in the femur and spine up to frequencies of 30 Hz but transmissibility fell off by as much as 60% when the frequency approached

40 Hz. Further, when the subject was asked to stand with bent knees, transmissibility fell to below 20% at the femur and spine. Presumably, this is due – at least in part – to the uncoupling of the body segments, such that they are no longer working efficiently as a fixed, stiff system. More importantly, these measurements confirm the ability of the standing adult skeleton to transmit a substantial fraction of ground accelerations to regions of the weight-bearing skeleton most susceptible to osteopenic bone loss.

Using Low-Level Mechanical Signals in the Clinic

Three human trials have been completed, each independently evaluating the potential of high-frequency, low-magnitude mechanical loading for use in the clinic as a means of influencing bone mass and morphology in the human. In the first, 62 post-menopausal women were randomized into in a double-blind, placebo-controlled pilot study (*83*). Thirty-two women underwent mechanical loading for two 10-min periods per day, through floor-mounted devices that produced a 0.2 g mechanical stimulus at 30 Hz (TX). Thirty-two women received placebo devices (PL). Evaluating those in the highest quartile of compliance (86% compliant), PL lost 2.13% in the femoral neck over the year, while TX was associated with a gain of 0.04%, reflecting a 2.17% relative benefit of treatment ($p=0.06$). In this quartile, the spine of lighter women (<65 kg) exhibited a relative benefit of TX of 3.35% greater BMD ($p=0.009$); and for the mean compliance group a 2.73% benefit was measured ($p=0.02$).

In a parallel study, 20 children with cerebral palsy (4–19 years) were randomized into TX (0.3 g, 90 Hz, 10 min/day) and PL (*84*). Over the 6-month trial, the mean change in tibial vTBMD in children who stood on placebo devices vTBMD decreased by –9.45 mg/ml (–11.9%), while children who stood on active devices increased by 6.27 mg/ml (+6.3%), reflecting a net benefit of treatment of +15.72 mg/ml (17.7%; $p=0.003$). At the spine, the net benefit of treatment as compared to placebo was not significant, at +6.72 mg/ml ($p=0.14$). Overall compliance was 44% of the 10 min/day period (4.4 min/day), implying that the anabolic response could be achieved with very short duration stimuli – a phenomenon also observed in animal experiments (*54*), and suggesting that the biologic response was "triggered," rather than accumulated.

Finally, a 12-month trial was conducted in 48 young women (15–20 years) with half of the subjects subject to brief (10 min/day), low-level whole-body vibration (30 Hz, 0.3 g) each day, with the remaining women served as controls (*85*). CT scans performed at baseline and the end of study was used to establish changes in muscle and bone mass in weight-bearing regions of the skeleton. Using an intention to treat (ITT) analysis, cancellous bone in the lumbar vertebrae and cortical bone in the femoral midshaft of the experimental group increased by 2.1% ($p=0.025$) and 3.4% ($p<0.001$), respectively, as compared to 0.1% ($p=0.74$) and 1.1% ($p=0.14$) in controls. Increases in cancellous and cortical bone were 2.0% ($p=0.06$) and 2.3% ($p=0.04$) greater, respectively, in the experimental group when compared with controls. Cross-sectional area of paraspinous musculature was 4.9% greater ($p=0.002$) in the experimental group vs. controls. When a per-protocol (PP) analysis was performed, gains in both muscle and bone were strongly correlated to a threshold in compliance, where the benefit of the mechanical intervention as compared to controls was realized once the device was used for at least 2 min/day ($n=18$), as reflected by a 3.9% increase in cancellous bone of the spine ($p=0.007$), 2.9% increase in cortical bone of the femur ($p = 0.009$), and 7.2% increase in musculature of the spine ($p = 0.001$), as compared to controls plus the low compliers ($n = 30$).

Evidence in the animal and human indicates that brief exposure to low-magnitude, high-frequency mechanical signals can benefit bone quantity and quality, and perhaps a benefit to the musculoskeletal "system," including muscle. Such a biomechanical intervention is self-targeting, endogenous to bone tissue, and auto-regulated, and provides insight toward a unique, non-pharmacologic intervention for osteoporosis.

SUMMARY AND OUTLOOK

The critical role that biophysical stimuli are playing in achieving and maintaining a structurally appropriate bone mass is clear. It is also clear that bone is capable of responding to exercise-induced mechanical stimuli by improving its quality and quantity or by preventing resorption from occurring. Although many exercise regimens have been ineffective in producing any morphological changes, bone cells should not be accused of being unresponsive to mechanical stimuli. Rather, exercise regimens will have to be designed that target specific skeletal sites with just the right amount and aspect of the complex mechanical environment generated by exercise. To enable the formulation of these exercise interventions, the mechanisms by which bone senses mechanical stimuli have to be explored at the organ, tissue, and molecular level.

The often used trial-and-error approach to finding an osteogenically optimal exercise program is highly inefficient. Instead of attempting to associate specific physical activities to altered BMD, mechanical milieus induced by these activities should be estimated, which then can be correlated with changes (of lack of them) in bone morphology. It is also critical to employ alternative clinical assays to DXA that are capable of detecting focal changes in bone mass and that can delineate both changes in bone quality as well as changes in bone quantity. At the same time, specific mechanical parameters derived from carefully controlled animal studies should be incorporated into the design of exercise protocols and tested. Current data from studies examining the ability of specific components of the mechanical milieu to stimulate bone formation indicate that osteogenic mechanical stimuli neither have to be large in magnitude nor do they have to be applied over a long duration, important prerequisites for the design of clinically successful exercise interventions. Ultimately, exercise protocols will also have to take the systemic state of the patient into account (e.g., growing vs. young adult vs. aging, hormonal and nutritional status), as it is unlikely that one universally applicable exercise regimen will provide maximal efficacy to the skeleton in all phases of life.

In summary, exercise may represent a unique means to improve bone quality as well as inhibit resorption. This represents an idealized strategy because the strain generated by exercise is native to the bone tissue and incorporates all aspects of the remodeling cycle, an attribute that is not inherent to systemic, pharmaceutical interventions. Given the great deal that has been learned about bone since the days of Galileo and Wolff, it should not be surprising to anyone to expect that we have much more to understand about bone adaptation, and much more to learn about how to apply this information in the clinic, to stem diseases such as osteoporosis. While the controversy around which mechanical signal is most important in regulating bone is certain to continue, it is also certain the scientific, engineering, and clinical disciplines will continue to agree that mechanical factors are critical to establishing and retaining bone mass and morphology.

ACKNOWLEDGMENTS

This work has been supported, in part, by grants from NIH, the Whitaker Foundation, Juvent, Inc., NASA, NSF, NSBRI, and the Coulter Foundation.

REFERENCES

1. Galileo G. Discorsi e dimonstrazioni matematiche, intorno a due nuove scienze attentanti alla meccanica ed a muovementi localli. Madison WI: University of Wisconsin Press, 1638.
2. Roux W. Beiträge zur Morphologie der funktionellen Anpassung. 3. Beschreibung und Erläuterung einer knöchernen Kniegelenksankylose. Archiv für Anatomie, Physiologie und wissenschaftliche Medizin, 1885120–158.
3. Wolff J. Das Gesetz der Transformation der Knochen (The Law of Bone Remodeling). Berlin, Verlag von August Hirschwald, 1892.
4. Wyman J. On the cancellated structure of some of the bones of the human body. Memoirs Boston Soc Nat Hist 1857;4:125–140.
5. Haapasalo H, Kannus P, Sievanen H, Heinonen A, Oja P, Vuori I. Long-term unilateral loading and bone mineral density and content in female squash players. Calcif Tissue Int 1994;54(4):249–255.
6. Kravitz SR, Fink KL, Huber S, Bohanske L, Cicilioni S. Osseous changes in the second ray of classical ballet dancers. J Am Podiatr Med Assoc 1985;75(7):346–348.
7. Hamdy RC, Anderson JS, Whalen KE, Harvill LM. Regional differences in bone density of young men involved in different exercises. Med Sci Sports Exerc 1994;26(7):884–888.
8. Heinonen A, Oja P, Kannus P, et al. Bone mineral density in female athletes representing sports with different loading characteristics of the skeleton. Bone 1995;17(3):197–203.
9. Snow-Harter C, Whalen R, Myburgh K, Arnaud S, Marcus R. Bone mineral density, muscle strength, and recreational exercise in men. J Bone Miner Res 1992;7(11):1291–1296.
10. Wittich A, Mautalen CA, Oliveri MB, Bagur A, Somoza F, Rotemberg E. Professional football (soccer) players have a markedly greater skeletal mineral content, density and size than age- and BMI-matched controls. Calcif Tissue Int 1998;63(2):112–117.
11. Leichter I, Simkin A, Margulies JY, et al. Gain in mass density of bone following strenuous physical activity. J Orthop Res 1989;7(1):86–90.
12. Dornemann TM, McMurray RG, Renner JB, Anderson JJ. Effects of high-intensity resistance exercise on bone mineral density and muscle strength of 40–50-year-old women. J Sports Med Phys Fitness 1997;37(4):246–251.
13. Nelson ME, Fiatarone MA, Morganti CM, Trice I, Greenberg RA, Evans WJ. Effects of high-intensity strength training on multiple risk factors for osteoporotic fractures. A randomized controlled trial. JAMA 1994;272(24):1909–1914.
14. Bennell KL, Malcolm SA, Khan KM, et al. Bone mass and bone turnover in power athletes, endurance athletes, and controls: a 12-month longitudinal study. Bone 1997;20(5):477–484.
15. Friedlander AL, Genant HK, Sadowsky S, Byl NN, Gluer CC. A two-year program of aerobics and weight training enhances bone mineral density of young women. J Bone Miner Res 1995;10(4):574–585.
16. Pruitt LA, Jackson RD, Bartels RL, Lehnhard HJ. Weight-training effects on bone mineral density in early postmenopausal women. J Bone Miner Res 1992;7(2):179–185.
17. Gleeson PB, Protas EJ, LeBlanc AD, Schneider VS, Evans HJ. Effects of weight lifting on bone mineral density in premenopausal women. J Bone Miner Res 1990;5(2):153–158.
18. Heinonen A, Sievanen H, Kannus P, Oja P, Vuori I. Effects of unilateral strength training and detraining on bone mineral mass and estimated mechanical characteristics of the upper limb bones in young women. J Bone Miner Res 1996;11(4):490–501.
19. Pruitt LA, Taaffe DR, Marcus R. Effects of a one-year high-intensity versus low-intensity resistance training program on bone mineral density in older women. J Bone Miner Res 1995;10(11): 1788–1795.
20. Vuori I, Heinonen A, Sievanen H, Kannus P, Pasanen M, Oja P. Effects of unilateral strength training and detraining on bone mineral density and content in young women: a study of mechanical loading and deloading on human bones. Calcif Tissue Int 1994;55(1):59–67.

21. McKay HA, MacLean L, Petit M, et al. "Bounce at the Bell": a novel program of short bouts of exercise improves proximal femur bone mass in early pubertal children. Br J Sports Med 2005;39(8):521–526.
22. Robinson TL, Snow-Harter C, Taaffe DR, Gillis D, Shaw J, Marcus R. Gymnasts exhibit higher bone mass than runners despite similar prevalence of amenorrhea and oligomenorrhea. J Bone Miner Res 1995;10(1):26–35.
23. Taaffe DR, Snow-Harter C, Connolly DA, Robinson TL, Brown MD, Marcus R. Differential effects of swimming versus weight-bearing activity on bone mineral status of eumenorrheic athletes. J Bone Miner Res 1995;10(4):586–593.
24. Fehling PC, Alekel L, Clasey J, Rector A, Stillman RJ. A comparison of bone mineral densities among female athletes in impact loading and active loading sports. Bone 1995;17(3):205–210.
25. Grove KA, Londeree BR. Bone density in postmenopausal women: high impact vs low impact exercise. Med Sci Sports Exerc 1992;24(11):1190–1194.
26. Heinonen A, Oja P, Sievanen H, Pasanen M, Vuori I. Effect of two training regimens on bone mineral density in healthy perimenopausal women: a randomized controlled trial. J Bone Miner Res 1998;13(3):483–490.
27. Orwoll ES, Ferar J, Oviatt SK, McClung MR, Huntington K. The relationship of swimming exercise to bone mass in men and women. Arch Intern Med 1989;149(10):2197–2200.
28. Snow-Harter C, Bouxsein ML, Lewis BT, Carter DR, Marcus R. Effects of resistance and endurance exercise on bone mineral status of young women: a randomized exercise intervention trial. J Bone Miner Res 1992;7(7):761–769.
29. Rockwell JC, Sorensen AM, Baker S, et al. Weight training decreases vertebral bone density in premenopausal women: a prospective study. J Clin Endocrinol Metab 1990;71(4):988–993.
30. Kerr D, Morton A, Dick I, Prince R. Exercise effects on bone mass in postmenopausal women are site-specific and load-dependent. J Bone Miner Res 1996;11(2):218–225.
31. Judex S, Gross TS, Zernicke RF. Strain gradients correlate with sites of exercise-induced bone-forming surfaces in the adult skeleton. J Bone Miner Res 1997;12(10):1737–1745.
32. Carter DR, Bouxsein ML, Marcus R. New approaches for interpreting projected bone densitometry data. J Bone Miner Res 1992;7(2):137–145.
33. Riggs BL, Hodgson SF, O'Fallon WM, et al. Effect of fluoride treatment on the fracture rate in postmenopausal women with osteoporosis. N Engl J Med 1990;322(12):802–809.
34. Burr DB, Milgrom C, Fyhrie D, et al. In vivo measurement of human tibial strains during vigorous activity. Bone 1996;18(5):405–410.
35. Lanyon LE, Hampson WG, Goodship AE, Shah JS. Bone deformation recorded in vivo from strain gauges attached to the human tibial shaft. Acta Orthop Scand 1975;46(2):256–268.
36. Burr DB, Schaffler MB, Yang KH, et al. The effects of altered strain environments on bone tissue kinetics. Bone 1989;10(3):215–221.
37. Szivek JA, Johnson EM, Magee FP, Emmanual J, Poser R, Koeneman JB. Bone remodeling and in vivo strain analysis of intact and implanted greyhound proximal femora. J Invest Surg 1994;7(3): 213–233.
38. Demes B, Qin YX, Stern JT, Jr, Larson SG, Rubin CT. Patterns of strain in the macaque tibia during functional activity. Am J Phys Anthropol 2001;116(4):257–265.
39. Swartz SM, Bertram JE, Biewener AA. Telemetered in vivo strain analysis of locomotor mechanics of brachiating gibbons. Nature 1989;342(6247):270–272.
40. Biewener AA, Bertram JE. Skeletal strain patterns in relation to exercise training during growth. J Exp Biol 1993;185:51–69.
41. Biewener AA, Thomason J, Goodship A, Lanyon LE. Bone stress in the horse forelimb during locomotion at different gaits: a comparison of two experimental methods. J Biomech 1983;16(8):565–576.
42. Gross TS, McLeod KJ, Rubin CT. Characterizing bone strain distributions in vivo using three triple rosette strain gages. J Biomech 1992;25(9):1081–1087.
43. Lanyon LE. Strain in sheep lumbar vertebrae recorded during life. Acta Orthop Scand 1971;42(1): 102–112.
44. Keller TS, Spengler DM. Regulation of bone stress and strain in the immature and mature rat femur. J Biomech 1989;22(11–12):1115–1127.
45. Biewener AA, Taylor CR. Bone strain: a determinant of gait and speed? J Exp Biol 1986;123:383–400.

46. Rubin CT, Lanyon LE. Limb mechanics as a function of speed and gait: a study of functional strains in the radius and tibia of horse and dog. J Exp Biol 1982;101:187–211.
47. Rubin CT, Lanyon LE. Dynamic strain similarity in vertebrates; an alternative to allometric limb bone scaling. J Theor Biol 1984;107(2):321–327.
48. Rubin CT, McLeod KJ, Bain SD. Functional strains and cortical bone adaptation: epigenetic assurance of skeletal integrity. J Biomech 1990;23(Suppl 1):43–54.
49. Judex S, Zernicke RF. High-impact exercise and growing bone: relation between high strain rates and enhanced bone formation. J Appl Physiol 2000;88(6):2183–2191.
50. Adams DJ, Spirt AA, Brown TD, Fritton SP, Rubin CT, Brand RA. Testing the daily stress stimulus theory of bone adaptation with natural and experimentally controlled strain histories. J Biomech 1997;30(7): 671–678.
51. Fritton SP, McLeod KJ, Rubin CT. Quantifying the strain history of bone: spatial uniformity and self-similarity of low-magnitude strains. J Biomech 2000;33(3):317–325.
52. Lanyon LE, Goodship AE, Pye CJ, MacFie JH. Mechanically adaptive bone remodelling. J Biomech 1982;15(3):141–154.
53. Judex S, Zernicke RF. Does the mechanical milieu associated with high-speed running lead to adaptive changes in diaphyseal growing bone? Bone 2000;26(2):153–159.
54. Rubin CT, Lanyon LE. Regulation of bone formation by applied dynamic loads. J Bone Joint Surg (Am) 1984;66(3):397–402.
55. Torrance AG, Mosley JR, Suswillo RF, Lanyon LE. Noninvasive loading of the rat ulna in vivo induces a strain-related modeling response uncomplicated by trauma or periostal pressure. Calcif Tissue Int 1994;54(3):241–247.
56. Turner CH, Akhter MP, Raab DM, Kimmel DB, Recker RR. A noninvasive, in vivo model for studying strain adaptive bone modeling. Bone 1991;12(2):73–79.
57. Mosley JR, March BM, Lynch J, Lanyon LE. Strain magnitude related changes in whole bone architecture in growing rats. Bone 1997;20(3):191–198.
58. Rubin CT, Lanyon LE. Regulation of bone mass by mechanical strain magnitude. Calcif Tissue Int 1985;37(4):411–417.
59. Qin YX, Rubin CT, McLeod KJ. Nonlinear dependence of loading intensity and cycle number in the maintenance of bone mass and morphology. J Orthop Res 1998;16(4):482–489.
60. Rubin C, Gross T, Qin YX, Fritton S, Guilak F, McLeod K. Differentiation of the bone-tissue remodeling response to axial and torsional loading in the turkey ulna. J Bone Joint Surg Am 1996;78(10):1523–1533.
61. Hert J, Liskova M, Landa J. Reaction of bone to mechanical stimuli. 1. Continuous and intermittent loading of tibia in rabbit. Folia Morphol (Praha) 1971;19(3):290–300.
62. Lanyon LE, Rubin CT. Static vs dynamic loads as an influence on bone remodelling. J Biomech 1984;17(12):897–905.
63. Mosley JR, Lanyon LE. Strain rate as a controlling influence on adaptive modeling in response to dynamic loading of the ulna in growing male rats. Bone 1998;23(4):313–318.
64. O'Connor JA, Lanyon LE, MacFie H. The influence of strain rate on adaptive bone remodelling. J Biomech 1982;15(10):767–781.
65. Turner CH, Owan I, Takano Y. Mechanotransduction in bone: role of strain rate. Am J Physiol 1995;269 (3 Pt 1):E438–E442.
66. Lamothe JM, Hamilton NH, Zernicke RF. Strain rate influences periosteal adaptation in mature bone. Med Eng Phys 2005;27(4):277–284.
67. Stanford CM, Morcuende JA, Brand RA. Proliferative and phenotypic responses of bone-like cells to mechanical deformation. J Orthop Res 1995;13(5):664–670.
68. Rubin CT, Lanyon LE. Kappa Delta Award paper. Osteoregulatory nature of mechanical stimuli: function as a determinant for adaptive remodeling in bone. J Orthop Res 1987;5(2):300–310.
69. Gross TS, Edwards JL, McLeod KJ, Rubin CT. Strain gradients correlate with sites of periosteal bone formation. J Bone Miner Res 1997;12(6):982–988.
70. Beck BR, Qin YX, McLeod KJ, Otter MW. On the relationship between streaming potential and strain in an in vivo bone preparation. Calcif Tissue Int 2002;71(4):335–343.
71. Jankovich JP. The effects of mechanical vibration on bone development in the rat. Journal of Biomechanics 1972;5(3):241–250.

72. Rubin C, Turner AS, Bain S, Mallinckrodt C, McLeod K. Anabolism: low mechanical signals strengthen long bones. Nature 2001;412(6847):603–604.
73. Judex S, Donahue LR, Rubin C. Genetic predisposition to low bone mass is paralleled by an enhanced sensitivity to signals anabolic to the skeleton. FASEB J. 2002;16(10):1280–1282.
74. Xie L, Jacobson JM, Choi ES, et al. Low-level mechanical vibrations can influence bone resorption and bone formation in the growing skeleton. Bone 2006;39(5):1059–1066.
75. Rubin C, Turner AS, Muller R, et al. Quantity and quality of trabecular bone in the femur are enhanced by a strongly anabolic, noninvasive mechanical intervention. J Bone Miner Res 2002;17(2):349–357.
76. Judex S, Boyd S, Qin YX, et al. Adaptations of trabecular bone to low magnitude vibrations result in more uniform stress and strain under load. Ann Biomed Eng 2003;31(1):12–20.
77. Rubin C, Xu G, Judex S. The anabolic activity of bone tissue, suppressed by disuse, is normalized by brief exposure to extremely low-magnitude mechanical stimuli. FASEB J. 2001;15(12):2225–2229.
78. Rubin C, Turner AS, Mallinckrodt C, Jerome C, McLeod K, Bain S. Mechanical strain, induced noninvasively in the high-frequency domain, is anabolic to cancellous bone, but not cortical bone. Bone 2002;30(3):445–452.
79. Garman R, Gaudette G, Donahue LR, Rubin C, Judex S. Low-level accelerations applied in the absence of weight bearing can enhance trabecular bone formation. J Orthop Res 2007;25:732–740.
80. Rubin J, Rubin C, Jacobs CR. Molecular pathways mediating mechanical signaling in bone. Gene 2006;367:1–16.
81. Huang RP, Rubin CT, McLeod KJ. Changes in postural muscle dynamics as a function of age. J Gerontol A Biol Sci Med Sci 1999;54(8):B352–B357.
82. Fritton JC, Rubin CT, Qin YX, McLeod KJ. Whole-body vibration in the skeleton: development of a resonance-based testing device. Ann Biomed Eng 1997;25(5):831–839.
83. Rubin C, Recker R, Cullen D, Ryaby J, McCabe J, McLeod K. Prevention of postmenopausal bone loss by a low-magnitude, high-frequency mechanical stimuli: a clinical trial assessing compliance, efficacy, and safety. J Bone Miner Res 2004;19(3):343–351.
84. Ward K, Alsop C, Caulton J, Rubin C, Adams J, Mughal Z. Low magnitude mechanical loading is osteogenic in children with disabling conditions. J Bone Miner Res 2004;19(3):360–369.
85. Gilsanz V, Wren TA, Sanchez M, Dorey F, Judex S, Rubin C. Low-level, high-frequency mechanical signals enhance musculoskeletal development of young women with low BMD. J Bone Miner Res 2006;21(9):1464–1474.

9 Exercise in the Prevention of Osteoporosis-Related Fractures

Belinda R. Beck, PhD
and Kerri M. Winters-Stone, PhD

Contents

Summary

The prevention of osteoporotic fracture by exercise intervention requires a two-pronged approach, that is, the maximization of bone strength and the minimization of falls. The former is most effectively addressed before peak bone mass has been attained, so that the latter is the primary option for the older, osteoporotic individual. Intense animal and human research activity over the last 20 years has generated a wealth of data that has led to recommendations for exercise prescriptions to both enhance bone strength and minimize risk of falling. Whether those exercise protocols will be shown to effectively reduce actual fracture incidence requires the analysis of longer term data than is currently available.

Key Words: Exercise, osteoporosis, bone mass, hip fracture, bone strength, physical activity

From: *Contemporary Endocrinology: Osteoporosis: Pathophysiology and Clinical Management*
Edited by: R. A. Adler, DOI 10.1007/978-1-59745-459-9_9,

INTRODUCTION

The utility of exercise in preventing osteoporosis-related fractures is a topic of considerable interest and research effort. It is well known that skeletal unloading, such as occurs following spinal cord injury, prolonged bed rest, limb immobilization, and microgravity, precipitates generalized skeletal loss, particularly in bones that bear weight under normal conditions *(1–6)*, and that losses may not be entirely regained with return to normal weight bearing *(7)*. By contrast, the effect of additional loading (exercise) on the skeleton is both variable and only modestly understood. The bone response to exercise varies as a function of skeletal age, diet, reproductive hormone status, and nature of the activity.

In humans, the practical goal of an exercise intervention is not merely to increase bone mass, but to reduce the incidence of fracture. The etiology of osteoporotic fractures includes both low bone mass and falls. Falls account for over 90% of hip fractures and over 50% of vertebral fractures. Thus, developing exercise interventions that serve to improve bone mass *and* prevent falls is necessary to reduce the risk of fracture.

This chapter provides a discussion of exercise as a strategy to reduce the factor of risk (a predictor of fracture risk), in order to maximize skeletal health and prevent osteoporosis-related fractures. We summarize the literature specific to promoting bone health across the life span with critical reference to study design. Guidelines for prescribing exercise to reduce the factor of risk are proposed and directions for future research are identified.

FACTOR OF RISK

The factor of risk, based on engineering principles, is defined as the ratio between the applied load and the fracture load ($\phi =$ applied load/fracture load). If the applied load is greater than the fracture load, then fracture is probable. If the applied load is less than the fracture load, fracture is unlikely. In a 70-year-old individual with average hip bone mass, the factor of risk of hip fracture ranges from 1.25 to 3.0 for a fall from standing height *(8–10)*.

Exercise is a potentially powerful strategy to reduce the risk of hip fracture by altering both the numerator and the denominator of the factor of risk. It can affect the numerator in two ways. First, by eliminating falls, the numerator becomes zero and fracture becomes highly unlikely. Second, by improving lower extremity neuromuscular function, exercise can reduce applied load at the hip by lowering the energy of a fall to the side. To raise the denominator, exercise can increase bone mass and reduce skeletal fragility, thus increasing the force required to fracture.

Given the strong relationship between a bone mass surrogate (DXA-derived bone mineral density – BMD) and failure load, increasing BMD is an important strategy for reducing fractures *(11–13)*. Bone strength is also strongly influenced by its geometric proportions. Small increases in cross-sectional area, width, and moment of inertia convey disproportionately large improvements in the resistance of long bones to bending *(14)*. Effecting changes in cross-sectional geometry is, therefore, an important strategy to reducing the factor of risk. Recent advances in the non-invasive measurement of bone geometry have improved measurement validity and reliability of techniques such as QCT *(15)*, pQCT *(16–22)*, quantitative ultrasound *(23)*, and MRI *(24)*, with commensurate improvement in our understanding of exercise effects.

EXERCISE STUDY DESIGN

The influence of study design and implementation on the ability to interpret research findings is particularly relevant when examining the effect of exercise on bone. In general, cross-sectional data reveal that physically active individuals have superior bone mass than those who are less active. An important limitation of cross-sectional data, however, is that of self-selection bias. That is, individuals who select a specific type of exercise may have predisposing skeletal attributes that influence the initial choice to participate and the ability to successfully continue the activity, without injury. For example, while power lifters have higher than average bone mass, the ability to succeed in a sport that entails repetitive lifting of very heavy weights depends on an inherently strong skeleton from the outset. This predisposition will largely account for the larger bones observed in power lifters in comparison with non-weight lifting individuals. Another limitation of most cross-sectional exercise studies is the use of standard physical activity questionnaires (PAQs). Most PAQs are designed to measure energy expenditure and do not assess the magnitude of forces applied to the skeleton during an activity. Attempts to relate bone mass to total energy expenditure introduce validity error and, as a consequence, the likelihood of drawing inappropriate conclusions. As in most forms of clinical research, randomized, controlled, intervention trials (RCTs) are the most valid method to examining the effects of exercise on bone.

In the following chapter, we have chosen to emphasize observations derived from exercise RCTs with bone as the primary outcome measure. Cross-sectional observations are included where appropriate to illustrate consistency in experimental findings or when RCT data are absent or equivocal.

GENERAL PRINCIPLES OF EFFECTIVE BONE LOADING

Principles of Exercise Training

Drinkwater *(25)* emphasized the need to incorporate the following five principles of exercise training into the design of exercise interventions for bone health: specificity, overload, reversibility, initial values, and diminishing returns. While the principles are clearly interrelated, independent consideration will assist in the development of customized programs of training for bone.

SPECIFICITY

According to the principle of specificity, an exercise protocol should be designed to load a target bone. For example, lower body resistance and impact exercise will improve bone mass at the hip, but not the spine. Only when upper body resistance exercise is added will spine bone mass increase *(26)*. Similarly, lower extremity impact activities that prevent bone loss at the hip do not influence bone mass at the forearm *(27)*.

OVERLOAD

Exercise must overload bone in order to stimulate it. That is, loads experienced at the skeleton must be either sufficiently different from or greater in intensity than normal daily loading to stimulate adaptive accretion *(28)*. Lack of attention to overload is a frequent shortcoming of published intervention studies, and one that is particularly challenging to address given the difficulty of directly measuring loads experienced at skeletal sites during exercise. Existing techniques are highly invasive and impractical for many sites.

Although not definitive, it is possible to make inferences from studies examining high- versus low-intensity loading to illustrate the principle of overload. For example, high-intensity strength training (>80% of one repetition maximum) more effectively increases spine and hip bone mass than low- or moderate-intensity strength training *(29,30)*. Similarly, weight squatted over the course of a 1-year progressive strength training program positively predicted change in trochanteric BMD *(31)*. Recently, the relationship between exercise intensity measured by accelerometry and hip bone mass was reported for a cohort of premenopausal women over the course of a year *(32)*. It was found that physical activities that induced accelerations exceeding 3.6 g were positively related to bone mass at the hip, suggesting that an exercise intensity threshold may exist. Advances in technology that will improve our ability to directly measure bone strain during exercise will facilitate quantification of the overload principle.

Reversibility

When exercise is an adaptive stimulus, reversibility is demonstrable. That is, cessation of an activity reverses exercise-induced bone accretion. It is possible that the principle of reversibility applies only to mature adult bone *(33–35)* rather than to the growing skeleton. Recent data indicate that gains achieved from increased mechanical loading during growth are maintained in the medium long term *(36)*, but longer term data are yet to be reported. Cross-sectional adult data are supportive of a bone maintenance effect from childhood loading, as individuals who exercised before or during puberty have significantly higher bone mass in adulthood than those who were less active *(37)*. These data are, however, subject to the previously mentioned self-selection bias.

Initial Values

The principle of initial values refers to the concept that responses from bone are greatest in individuals with lower than average bone mass. For example, premenopausal women with the lowest initial bone mass demonstrated the greatest improvement at the hip to 12 months of impact plus resistance training *(26)*. Interventions targeting postmenopausal cohorts with low bone mass have observed exercise-induced gains in spine and/or hip bone mass that are over twice as high *(38,39)* as reported gains in similar cohorts with average bone mass *(29,30,33,40–42)*.

The initial values effect is likely to reflect the principle of overload, as smaller lighter bones will experience greater strain than larger heavier ones exposed to the same load. When loading is extremely high (>10 body weights), skeletal improvements are observed regardless of initial values *(43)*, suggesting that even very robust skeletons will be overloaded at such high-load intensities.

Diminishing Returns

The principle of diminishing returns is evident when a ceiling effect in bone adaptation is observed after a period of same or like loading. Diminishing returns are similarly related to the principles of initial values and overload, as bone will be strained less by the same load once mass and geometric adaptations to an exercise stimulus have taken place. Indeed, it is the *raison d'être* of the adaptive response to mechanical loading.

Characteristics of Bone Response to Exercise Loading

Important factors that distinguish the exercise response of the skeletal system from other body systems are as follows: (1) changes are typically small (1–5%), (2) the time required to elicit a measurable response is considerable, (3) overload is required from the outset, (4) older bone is less responsive than younger bone, and (5) exercise-induced improvements in bone strength can occur in the absence of BMD change via geometric adaptation.

Whereas both the neuromuscular and cardiovascular systems typically respond to a training stimulus within 4–6 weeks, bone requires at least 6 months to initiate measurable adaptation, that is, complete a full remodeling cycle and achieve a modicum of mineralization in new osteoid.

In contrast with the soft tissue systems that require progressive loading increments to prevent injury, it is increasingly clear that bone does not require such a graduated approach *(44,45)*. In fact, as described above, substantial overload is critical to stimulate a response from bone. Depending upon the age and health status of the individual, however, progressive incremental loading may be necessary to allow neuromuscular adaptation and prevent non-bone injury.

Although there are some data to the contrary *(46)*, it is thought that bone age will influence the skeletal response to exercise *(47)*. Not only does younger human bone appear to respond more vigorously to a similar activity than older bone *(45)*, but a younger individual can withstand higher load magnitudes than an older person. Thus, it is likely that exercise prescription to strengthen bone or reduce bone loss in the elderly requires some creativity.

Substantial gains in the resistance of a long bone to bending and fracture can be achieved by the strategic addition of even small amounts of new bone around the circumference of the shaft *(48)*. While changes in bone mass are not always observed following exercise intervention, measurement of the cross-sectional geometry of a long bone before and after an intervention may reveal these subtle but critical structural improvements.

Important Load Parameters

From studies in animals, bone responds preferentially to certain forms of mechanical loading. It has long been known that, when other factors remain constant, high-magnitude loads that induce relatively large bone strains (deformations) are more osteogenic than low *(49)*. As the frequency (cycles per second) of loading increases, however, the magnitude of the load required to stimulate an adaptive response from bone declines *(50)*. Strain rate (the speed at which a bone deforms under load) is also a highly influential adaptive stimulus *(51)*. And finally, strain gradient, or the pattern of strain experienced across a loaded bone, is known to direct the location of bone remodeling *(52)*.

EXERCISE STUDIES ACROSS THE LIFE SPAN

Exercise and Peak Bone Mass

The NIH Consensus Conference on Osteoporosis *(53)* reported that optimizing peak bone mass should be a primary strategy to prevent osteoporosis.

Children, Exercise, and Bone – Cross-Sectional Observations

Studies of children and adolescents of various races/ethnicities generally support significant associations between physical activity and total body, hip, spine, and forearm bone mass *(54–62)*. Evidence is accumulating to suggest that exercise confers the greatest long-term benefit when initiated in the prepubertal years *(37,63)*; however, the data are not consistent.

Prepubertal gymnasts have greater bone mass at weight-bearing sites than controls, an effect that strengthens as years of training increases *(57,58,64)*. Compared with less-active children, highly active children have a greater rate of bone mineral accumulation for the two peripubertal years during which bone is most rapidly accruing (12.5 years for girls and 14.1 years for boys) *(62)*. Bailey and colleagues noted that this greater accrual translated into 9 and 17% higher total body bone mineral content 1 year after peak bone mineral content velocity for active boys and girls, respectively. Slemenda et al. *(65)*, however, found no relationship between physical activity and bone mass in peripubertal children. They suggested that exercise exerts an influence on bone mass before puberty, but that during puberty other factors, such as estrogen, become more influential on bone acquisition. By contrast, Haapasalo et al. *(66)* reported that the differences in spine bone mass of athletic and control children were greatest at the peripubertal years Tanner stages IV and V (average ages 13.5 and 15.5, respectively). The lack of consistency in reports likely reflects the inability of cross-sectional study design to control for the myriad of variables that influence skeletal status in growing children.

Variations in skeletal response to different activities reflect the different loading patterns of each sport and exemplify the principle of specificity *(61,67)*. The effect is elegantly demonstrated by a comparison between limbs. Dominant limbs have greater bone mass than non-dominant limbs *(68)*, and athletes loading their dominant limbs preferentially while exercising develop even greater bilateral disparity *(69,70)*. Differences in bone mass between playing and non-playing arms in female squash and tennis players are about two times greater if participation in the sport begins prior to or during menarche than after puberty *(37)*, although some have observed that the effect does not become evident until the adolescent growth spurt or Tanner stage III (mean age 12.6 years) *(66)*.

In general then, the data from the majority of cross-sectional studies would suggest that exercise benefits to the skeleton are site specific and best achieved when exercise is performed before puberty and/or during the peripubertal years.

Pediatric Exercise Intervention Findings

The influence of exercise intervention on growing bone has become a focus of intense research interest in recent years.

Infants In a study of premature infants, five repetitions of range of motion, gentle compression, flexion, and extension exercises five times a week induced greater acquisition of bone mass at 4 weeks in exercised babies than in controls *(71)*. A similar protocol initiated at 1 week of age prevented typical postnatal loss of tibial speed of sound (a marker of bone strength) in very low birth weight infants *(72)*. Others have observed, however, that calcium intake exerts a greater influence on bone mineral accrual than 18 months of either gross or fine motor activity in 6-month-old infants *(73)*.

Preschoolers The only intervention to target bone health in preschoolers assessed the material and structural response of bone of children randomized to gross motor activities compared with fine motor activities 30 min/day, 5 days/week for 12 months *(74)*. Within each group children were also supplemented with calcium (1000 mg/day) or placebo. Exercise alone increased tibial periosteal and endosteal circumferences, but exercise plus calcium improved leg bone mass, cortical thickness, and cortical area of the distal tibia most markedly (Fig. 1). While the differences in periosteal circumference remained between the groups 12 months after cessation of the intervention, the investigators reported that persistently higher activity levels among those in the gross motor activity group may have accounted for the disparity *(75)*.

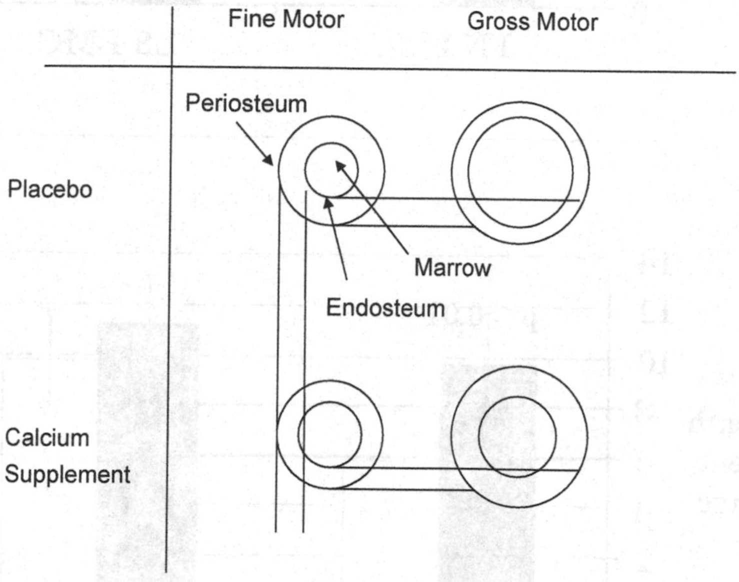

Fig. 1. Diagrammatic representation of the effects of 1 year fine motor or gross motor activities and calcium supplementation on the cross section of the 20% distal tibial shaft by pQCT in young children (not to scale). Reproduced from Specker and Binkley *(74)* with permission of the American Society for Bone and Mineral Research.

Pre-puberty In a randomized study of 89 prepubescent boys and girls (mean age = 7.1 years), jumping 100 times, 3 days/week at ground reaction forces of 8 times body weight, increased femoral neck and lumbar spine bone mass 4.5 and 3.1%, respectively, in comparison with controls *(76)*. The effect was maintained 7 months after detraining *(36)*, suggesting the program may have augmented peak bone mass (Fig. 2). Geometric changes have also been observed in response to exercise training in this age group. Femoral mid-shaft cortical thickness increased in prepubertal boys after 8 months of weight-bearing activity *(77)*. Similarly, 2 years participation in a school-based, high-impact, weight-bearing exercise program that supplemented regular physical education enhanced structural properties of the femoral neck in prepubescent boys (mean age 10.2 years) compared to controls *(78)*. A mere 10 min of jumping activity twice weekly for 9 months improved both femoral neck

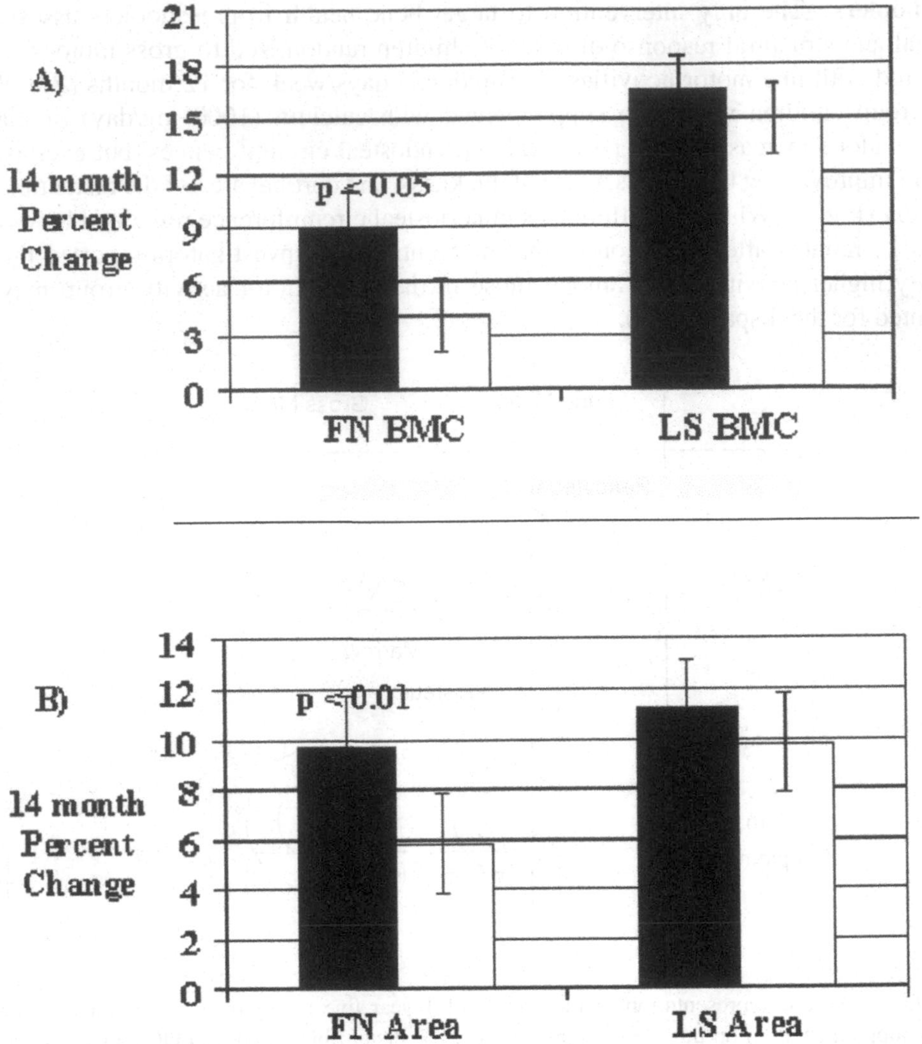

Fig. 2. (**A**) Fourteen-month changes (exercise intervention plus detraining) in femoral neck BMC were significantly greater ($p < 0.05$) in jumpers ($n = 37$, black bar) than controls ($n = 37$, white bar). No significant differences were observed between groups for lumbar spine BMC. (**B**) Fourteen-month changes (exercise intervention plus detraining) in femoral neck area were significantly greater ($p < 0.01$) in jumpers ($n = 37$, black bar) than controls ($n = 37$, white bar). No significant differences were observed between groups for lumbar spine area. Values reported as percent change (%), mean ± SEM. Reprinted from Fuchs and Snow *(36)*. Copyright (2002) with permission from Elsevier.

geometry and spine bone mass compared with controls in a healthy cohort of peripubertal boys and girls (mean age = 13.7 years) *(78a)*.

Favorable responses to bone loading exercise that included resistance and/or jump training, have also been observed for both prepubescent *(79–81)* and early pubertal girls *(79,82,83)*. MacKelvie et al. *(84)*, however, did not observe the improvements at the hip and spine in prepubertal girls that were observed in early pubertal girls in response to brief high-impact exercise.

Postpuberty Few exercise interventions have been completed with acutely postpubertal adolescents. Following 8 months of plyometric and jumping exercise in an adolescent female cohort (mean age = 14.2 years, approximately 2 years past menarche), no significant difference between intervention or control groups was observed at any bone site, with the exception of an increase in trochanteric bone mineral content in the exercisers *(85)*. Because the trial was not randomized and controls were highly active, it was unclear whether the lack of response was due to the high level of activity in controls or if adolescent bone does not respond as dramatically to increased loading as prepubertal bone. Another trial reported that 15 months of resistance training produced a significant increase in femoral neck bone mass in adolescent girls (roughly 2.5 years postmenarche), despite major challenges with subject compliance *(86)*. A study comparing the effects of twice weekly step aerobics for 9 months in pre- versus postmenarcheal girls reported bone mass and geometric parameters of bone strength increased at the spine and hip for premenarcheal girls only *(87)*.

Thus, in support of cross-sectional findings, data from intervention trials suggest exercise has a very positive effect on bone mass and geometry in children. The consensus suggests the effect is most marked in the years just prior to or during early puberty. It remains to be seen if those benefits translate to a reduced risk of osteoporosis and/or fracture in later life. Only large, very long-term follow-up investigations can determine if such an objective will be realized.

Exercise and Bone Mass in Adults

Although the response of the adult skeleton to exercise has been studied extensively, the considerable logistical challenges and methodological inconsistency associated with exercise trials may account for the diversity of findings. Randomization is particularly difficult, as adults who volunteer for an exercise study do not wish to be allocated to a control group. Innumerable studies are casualties to poor compliance, given the necessarily protracted duration of interventions, and poor acceptance of exercise by those who often need it most. Furthermore, there are relatively few studies of men due to the common misperception that osteoporosis is a disease unique to women.

ADULTS, EXERCISE, AND BONE – CROSS-SECTIONAL OBSERVATIONS

Observational data indicate that adults engaged in weight-bearing exercise at intensities of >60% of aerobic capacity have consistently greater bone mass than non-exercisers or those exercising at low aerobic intensities. These differences have been observed in the whole body *(88–96)*, spine, proximal femur *(56,88–91,93,95–104)*, pelvis *(90,94)*, distal femur *(105)*, tibia *(88,90,102,106,107)*, humerus *(90)*, calcaneus *(108,109)*, and forearm *(102)*. Broadband ultrasound attenuation and speed of sound transmission in the calcaneus are similarly higher in runners than controls *(93)*. Consistent with the principle of specificity, high bone mass is typically observed local to the loaded bone(s) *(94,110–112)*.

Certain activities do not sufficiently overload the skeleton to cause an adaptive response *(113)*. Athletes participating in moderate- to high-intensity impact activities such as running, jumping, and power lifting have greater bone mass than those performing low-intensity or non-weight-bearing activities *(92,104,114,115)*. By contrast, individuals who participate in non-weight-bearing activities such as swimming have similar bone mass to non-exercisers *(105,116)*, although some data to the contrary exist for men *(117)*. Muscle forces on the skeleton during elite-level swimming training do not appear to offset the substantially reduced daily weight-bearing activity associated with long periods of time spent in a weight-supported environment (water).

In non-exercising adults, as in children, the dominant arm exhibits greater total and cortical bone mass than the non-dominant arm *(68,118)* and side-to-side differences are exaggerated when the dominant limb is chronically overloaded *(69,70,98,105)*. Some have found the difference is accounted for by increased periosteal area and cortical thickness rather than bone mass *(118)*, while others have observed both expanded diaphyseal diameters and increased bone mass in the dominant limb of athletes. Dalen et al. *(69)* observed a 27% difference in cortical cross-sectional area between left and right humeri of tennis players compared to a non-significant 5% difference in controls. Krahl et al. *(119)* observed differences in diameter *and* length of playing arm ulnae of tennis players compared to the contralateral arms. The second metacarpals of playing hands were also wider and longer than those of the contralateral hands, whereas no differences were observed between limbs of controls. The latter somewhat isolated observations suggest that exercise may potentiate long bone growth in length, a curious finding with implications for overall height. That side dominance is not evident in athletes who load both limbs equally in the course of their training (rowers and triathletes) *(120)* attests to the principle of site specificity.

Although data exist to question the role of exercise in the prevention of age-related bone loss *(121)*, there is no denying that active people who have exercised for many years, generally have higher bone mass than less-active people *(58,91,97,122–126)*. Unfortunately, while bone loss may be reduced by lifelong exercise, it may bear little or no relationship to the incidence of fractures. For example, Greendale and colleagues *(125)* reported a significant linear trend in older men between both lifetime and current exercise and hip bone mass, but found no relationship between osteoporotic fracture rate and exercise history. The paradox could be related to other risk factors for falling and the lack of a persistent neuromuscular benefit from early life exercise.

Exercise Interventions in Young and Mature Premenopausal Women

Randomized, controlled trials confirm that exercise training programs enhance the bone mass of young women in a site-specific manner. Both resistance and weight-bearing endurance exercise programs increase spine, hip, and calcaneal bone mass of young adult women *(45,127–131)*. However, in contrast to the developing skeleton, the principle of reversibility applies, that is, osteogenic loading must be sustained in order to maintain bone gains. For example, increases in trochanteric and femoral neck BMD observed after 12 months of resistance plus jump exercise declined to baseline values after only 6 months of detraining in premenopausal women *(132)* (Fig. 3). Two-year observations of college gymnasts indicate that bone at the hip, spine, and whole body consistently increased over the training seasons and decreased in the off-season *(133)* (Fig. 4). By contrast, the relatively lower magnitude loading associated with field hockey playing was not sufficient to stimulate seasonal changes in a similar cohort *(134)*.

Based on an awareness of the importance of load magnitude and rate for bone stimulation, researchers have frequently employed impact loading (jumping) as an exercise intervention. While load magnitude is similar for jogging and jumping (2–5 times body

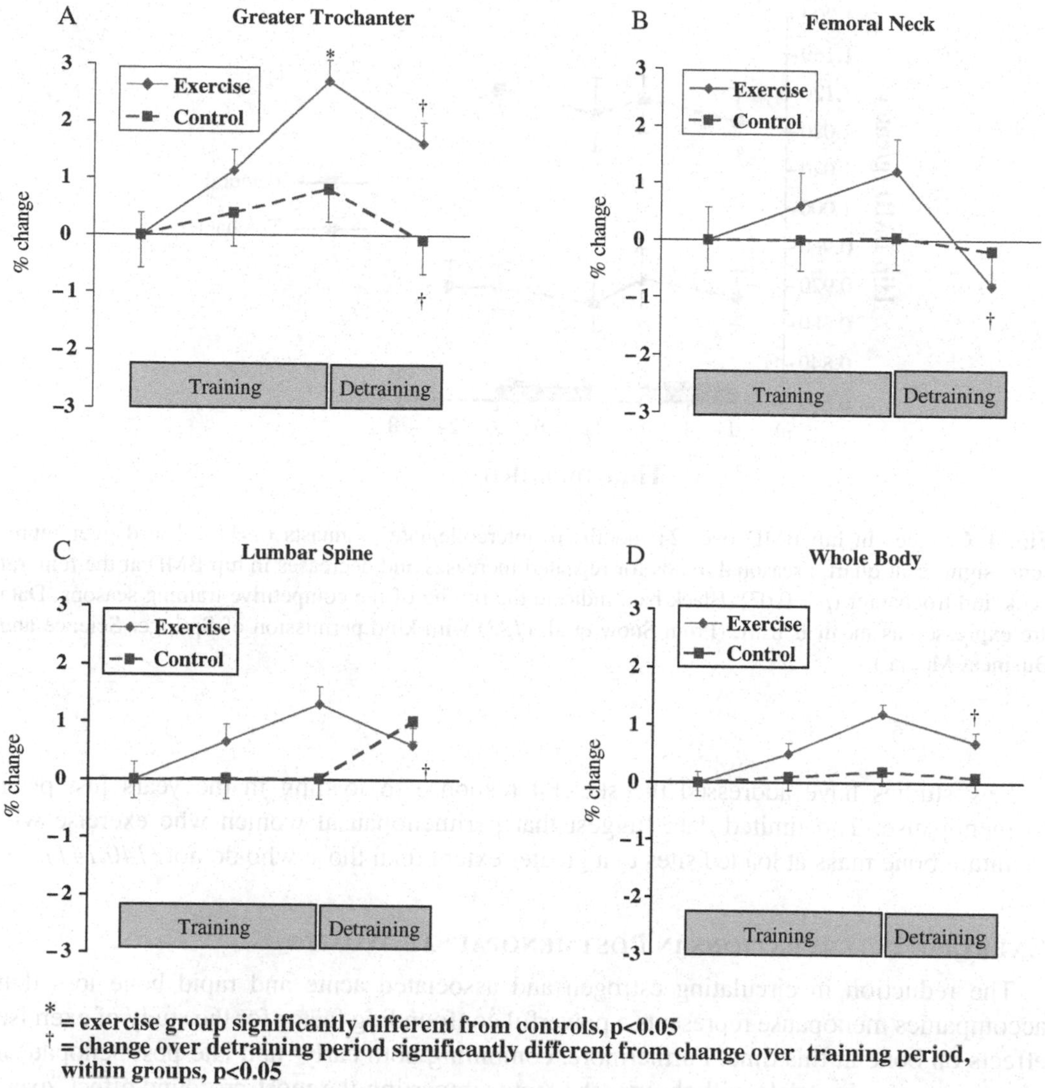

Fig. 3. Percent changes in BMD across training and detraining periods (mean ± SEM) at the (**A**) greater trochanter, (**B**) femoral neck, (**C**) lumbar spine, and (**D**) whole body. Reproduced from Winters and Snow *(34)* with permission of the American Society for Bone and Mineral Research.

weight), the loading rate for jogging is roughly 75 body weights/s while jumping is approximately 300 body weights/s. Commensurately, jumping has consistently been shown to increase femoral and sometimes lumbar spine bone mass in premenopausal women *(34,45,127,135–137)*. Curiously, the number of reported impacts performed per session in the studies describing a bone effect ranges from a low of 10 *(135)* to a high of 100 *(138,139)*. Direct comparisons among studies to evaluate a dose–response of bone to jump number are thus clouded by variance between training protocols, varying age of participants, and the lack of accurate information with respect to total impact exposure (other aerobic activity).

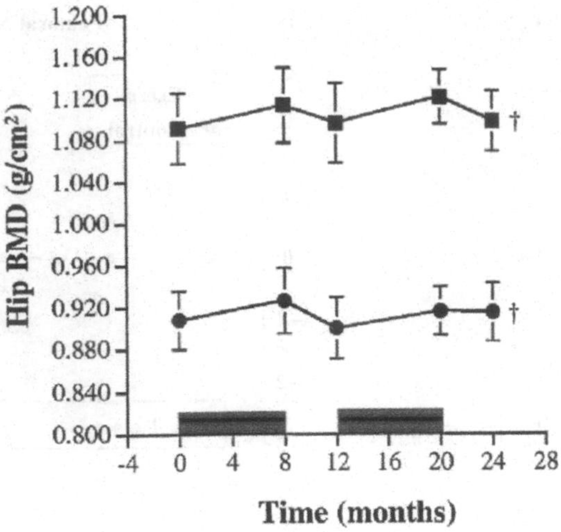

Fig. 4. Changes in hip BMD over 24 months in intercollegiate gymnasts ($n = 8$). The dagger represents significant quartic seasonal trends for repeated increases and decreases in hip BMD at the femoral neck and trochanter ($p = 0.03$). Black bars indicate the timing of the competitive training seasons. Data are expressed as mean ± SEM. (From Snow et al. *(133)* with kind permission of Springer Science and Business Media.)

Few studies have addressed the skeletal response to loading in the years just prior to menopause. The limited data suggest that perimenopausal women who exercise will maintain bone mass at loaded sites to a greater extent than those who do not *(140,141)*.

EXERCISE INTERVENTIONS IN POSTMENOPAUSAL WOMEN

The reduction in circulating estrogen and associated acute and rapid bone loss that accompanies menopause represents a powerful confounding factor for the study of exercise effects on bone at this time. Furthermore, combining both early- and late-postmenopausal women in exercise trials will obscure the factor imparting the most profound effect, exercise or estrogen. Even those investigations specifically targeting estrogen-deplete early postmenopausal women have reported inconsistent findings with respect to the ability of exercise to prevent bone loss at all sites. Resistance training effectively maintained only spine bone mass in some cases *(142,143)* and only trochanteric bone mass in others *(30)*. A rare finding that walking prevented hip bone loss, an effect that was enhanced by isoflavone intake, was recently reported in a cohort of early postmenopausal Japanese women *(144)*. High-intensity resistance training was as effective as hormone therapy in preventing bone loss at the spine and was more effective than no hormone therapy in attenuating bone loss at the spine in women an average of 2 years postmenopause *(145)*. A 4-year progressive strength training program found exercise frequency to be significantly positively associated with changes in bone mass at the hip and spine in women an average of 6 years postmenopause regardless of hormone therapy status *(146)*.

Resistance training programs of 9–24 months duration in estrogen-deplete late-postmenopausal women are generally associated with an increase or maintenance of bone mass compared to losses in controls at the whole body *(41)*, lumbar spine *(41,42,142, 147 – 149)*, proximal femur *(29,42,148,149)*, calcaneus *(149)*, and radius *(29)*, although not without exception *(150–152)*. A recent meta-analysis of high-intensity resistance training and postmenopausal bone loss concluded that high-intensity resistance training confers a significant positive effect on spine bone mass but that findings are highly heterogeneous at the femoral neck *(153)*. Significant changes at the hip were observed only in trials that recruited subjects not taking hormone therapy. Exercise effects were augmented with calcium supplementation and in women with low initial values. The authors also remarked on the poor methodological quality of studies, that non-randomized trials report markedly greater treatment effects than randomized, and that reporting bias toward studies finding positive bone outcomes was evident.

The most clinically relevant sites are primarily comprised of trabecular bone, thus cortical bone is often ignored in research trials. As long bone fractures indeed occur at cortical sites in osteoporotic individuals, an observation that both resistance and agility training increased cortical bone density in elderly osteopenic women is of clinical relevance *(154)*. Although substantial changes in femoral neck bone mass were not observed, tibial shaft bone strength index was maintained to a greater extent in elderly women performing 1 year of resistance and balance-jumping training than in controls *(155)*.

Weight-bearing aerobic or impact exercise interventions of 7–30 months duration are also generally associated with increases or maintenance of bone mass compared to losses in control subjects at the whole body *(41,156)*, lumbar spine *(33,40,143,156,157)*, proximal femur *(41,156,158)*, radius *(157)*, and calcaneus *(159,160)*.

As for other groups discussed previously, lower intensity activities typically do not promote bone gain or reduce loss in postmenopausal women. A 12-month, 5 days/week, 45-min moderate-intensity aerobic exercise intervention did not provide sufficient overload to the skeletons of obese postmenopausal women to improve bone mass *(161)*. Similarly, 12 months of unloaded exercise in waist-deep water did not prevent spine bone loss or improve femoral bone mass in osteoporotic women, despite changes in other functional fitness parameters *(162)*. It is generally agreed that walking alone is not an effective strategy for osteoporosis prevention in postmenopausal women *(163)*. Exceptions include the above-mentioned Japanese study and a report by Hatori et al. *(40)* who found that 7 months of walking 3 days/week at walking speeds equivalent to those reached in race walking (>4.5 mph) increased lumbar spine bone mass in postmenopausal women. The increased muscular forces associated with arm movements required for walking at high speeds combined with lower initial bone mass values might explain these isolated positive responses.

Unfortunately, high magnitude loading is not appropriate for individuals with osteoporosis whose bones would likely fracture under such loads. It has been observed, however, that lower magnitude loading may be osteogenic if applied at high enough rate and/or frequency (roughly 30 Hz). While the active application of loads at frequencies higher than 2–3 Hz is not physically feasible for most, whole body vibration (WBV) devices have been developed that can apply passive, low-magnitude loads at osteogenic frequencies. Preliminary findings of the effectiveness of WBV to enhance bone strength are encouraging *(164–168)*; however, as WBV is primarily a passive rather than active stimulus, it cannot strictly be considered exercise and will not be discussed further (see Chapter 8).

The length of participation in weight-bearing exercise may be an important consideration for exercise programming in older adults. For example, although no change in femoral neck bone mass was observed in postmenopausal women following 9 months of jump plus resistance exercise wearing weighted vests *(169)*, 5 years of participation in the program prevented bone loss of more than 4% at the hip *(35)* (Fig. 5). It is possible that the delayed response is a function of mineralization, a process known to continue long after new bone tissue (osteoid) has been secreted by osteoblasts.

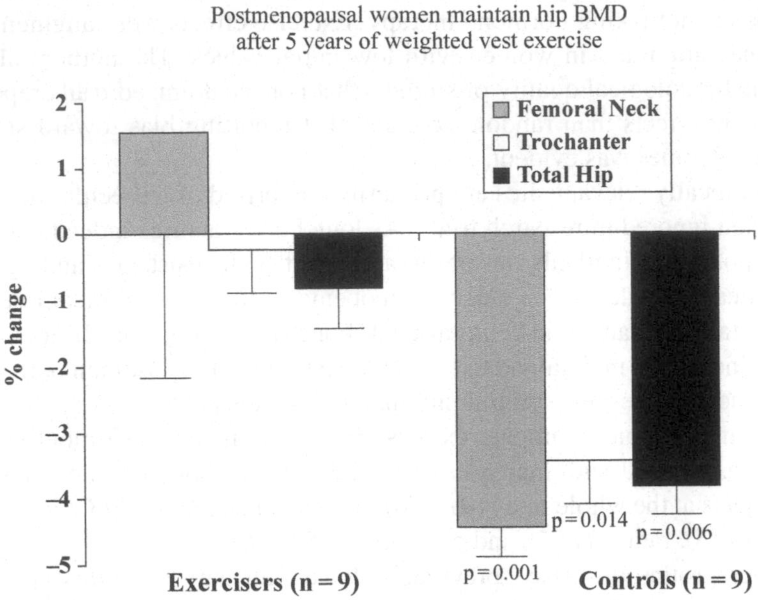

Fig. 5. Percent changes in BMD at the femoral neck, trochanter, and total hip in exercisers and controls after 5 years. Changes for exercisers were 1.54 ± 2.37% (CI = –3.9 to 7.0%) at the femoral neck, –0.24 ± 1.02% (CI = –2.6 to 2.1%) at the trochanter, and –0.82 ± 1.04% (CI = –3.2 to 1.6%) at the total hip, whereas controls decreased 4.43 ± 0.93% (CI = –6.6 to –2.3%) at the femoral neck, 3.43 ± 1.09% (CI = –5.9 to –0.92%) at the trochanter, and 3.80 ± 1.03 (CI = –6.2 to –1.4%) at the total hip. Decreases in controls are significantly different from zero (unpaired *t*-tests). Data are presented as means ± SEM. From Snow et al. *(35)*, Copyright © The Gerontological Society of America. Reproduced by permission of the publisher.

Given the importance of site specificity, it is not surprising that weight-bearing exercise does not increase forearm bone mass in postmenopausal women *(41,137)*. In fact, some have suggested that upper body bone mass may suffer at the expense of lower body bone mass in female runners *(170)*. For those at risk of Colles (distal forearm) fractures, however, it is encouraging to observe that upper extremity loading of high rate and magnitude, stimulated higher forearm bone density in osteoporotic, postmenopausal women after only 5 months *(171,172)*.

Hormone Therapy and Exercise As hormone therapy (HT) has been a common treatment for postmenopausal symptoms and side effects in the past, the efficacy of exercise in comparison to and in combination with HT has been examined. In some reports, exercise enhanced the bone maintenance effect of HT. Resistance exercise has been shown to significantly increase spine, hip, total body, and radial mid-shaft bone mass in menopausal women who were estrogen-replaced compared to maintenance effects observed in estrogen-replaced, non-exercising controls *(173,174)*. Similarly, the interaction of HT and 9 months of weight-bearing exercise (walking, jogging, stairs) resulted in greater increases in total body and lumbar spine bone mass in 60–72-year-old postmenopausal women than exercise or HT alone *(175)*.

By contrast, other studies report no interaction between exercise and HT. For example, a 3 h/week program of resistance exercise plus walking or running for 1 year did not enhance the positive effect of estrogen supplementation on lumbar vertebral or femoral neck bone mass in postmenopausal women *(176)*. Similar results were observed at the lumbar spine and hip in early postmenopausal women on HT, despite a positive effect of 3 h/week exercise on bone mass in a placebo group *(177)*. In these studies, a longer intervention period and higher load magnitudes may have been necessary for more positive outcomes. Somewhat perplexingly, given the usual site-specific effect of bone loading, Judge et al. observed changes in total hip bone mass in postmenopausal women on long-term hormone therapy regardless of randomization status to either upper body-only or lower body-only resistance training *(178)*. The investigators concluded that any kind of moderate resistance exercise in the presence of hormone therapy conferred a generalized positive effect at the hip.

Exercise Interventions in Young Adult Men

Although there have been few longitudinal studies in this cohort, the response of the male skeleton to exercise appears to be similar to that of same-aged women.

Basic military training has served as an opportune model to observe the effect of brief, high-intensity, multi-mode, physical training interventions. After 14 weeks of basic training, male army recruits have been observed to improve calcaneal strength *(179)* and increase leg bone mass by around 12%; those with the lowest initial values gaining the greatest amount *(106,180)*. Recruits who temporarily stopped training due to stress fracture also gained bone mass, but to a lesser degree (5%). Curiously, 10% of the same recruits lost bone mass. The latter effect may have been a function of either incomplete remodeling owing to the short observation period or abnormal remodeling due to fatigue and inadequate rest intervals.

The influence of training intensity on bone response becomes evident when findings from military trials are compared with those of recreational athletes. By contrast to recruits, men aged 25–52 failed to gain bone at the spine, humerus, femur, calcaneus, or forearm following 3 months of either walking (3 km, 5 days/week) or running (5 km, 3 days/week) *(114)*. The disparity of findings likely reflects the novelty of loading and higher load magnitudes experienced during basic training and the youth of the army recruits. The only other young male exercise intervention to have been reported involved 9 months of marathon training. The investigators observed significantly higher calcaneal bone mass in the runners than in non-runners, with a positive association between average distance run and percent change in bone mass *(159)*.

A 7.8-year longitudinal study of young Caucasian men (mean age = 17 years) measured change in bone mass over time according to change in level of activity *(181)*. The investigators reported those men who stayed active gained bone mass, those who ceased activity lost bone mass at the hip, but remained significantly higher than controls at final follow-up. The study is an illustration of the ability of exercise to potentiate male peak bone mass even in the very final stages of skeletal growth.

Exercise Interventions in Older Adult Men

There are even fewer reports of exercise interventions with older men. From a combined male and female trial, Welsh and Rutherford *(156)* reported a significant increase in trochanteric bone mass in six men aged 50–73 years who performed 12 months of step and jumping exercise. More recently, the effects of 6 months of either a high-intensity, standing, free-weight program or a moderate-intensity, seated, resistance training program on bone mass were examined in older men and women *(30)*. High-intensity training increased lumbar spine BMD by 2% in the men (mean age = 54.6 years), whereas moderate-intensity training produced no change. Increased bone mass was observed at the greater trochanter regardless of training intensity.

Summary of Exercise Effects Across the Life Span

Evidence from exercise interventions longer than 6 months indicates that activities of high magnitude and rate of loading improve bone mass and geometry in children and adults of both sexes. While gains may be maintained if achieved during the growing years, adults will likely lose new bone if exercise is discontinued. Effective activities include jumping and high-intensity weight training. Although walking and other low-intensity exercises are unlikely to be substantially osteogenic, a lifetime of walking appears to be beneficial to the skeleton.

CALCIUM AND EXERCISE

The permissive action of calcium in enhancing the effect of exercise on bone mass is somewhat controversial. In a review of 17 trials, Specker *(182)* concluded that an intake of 1000 mg/day of calcium is necessary in order to observe a skeletal response to exercise. Specifically, the evidence suggests that the combination of calcium supplementation and exercise is more effective for a bone response in children *(74,183,184)*, adolescents *(185)*, and postmenopausal women than calcium supplementation alone *(33,39,186)*.

By contrast to the positive reports, a recent cross-sectional study of 422 women found that even though high levels of physical activity and calcium intake were associated with a higher total body bone mass than low activity levels and low calcium intake, there was no significant interaction between exercise and calcium *(95)*. Furthermore, 2 years of combined aerobics and weight training increased bone mass in young women, but calcium supplementation neither enhanced the exercise benefit nor improved bone mass in the absence of exercise *(128)*.

Although exercise likely provides a greater stimulus to bone than does calcium, at least in older children and adults, adequate calcium intake is recommended, particularly in children, to provide the building blocks for exercise-induce gains in bone mass.

HORMONE RESPONSE TO ITENSE EXERCISE

Women

Exercise-associated amenorrhea occurs in some premenopausal women who train at high exercise intensities. While low body fat was once thought to precipitate exercise-associated amenorrhea, it is now thought that reduced energy availability disrupts the hypothalamic–pituitary–thyroid axis *(187)* and ultimately circulating reproductive hormones. The effect of reduced energy availability on bone resorption and formation markers is well documented *(188)*. The reduction in estrogen provides the link between exercise-associated amenorrhea and bone loss *(113,189,190)*. The Female Athlete Triad describes the combined conditions of excessive dietary restraint, reproductive hormone disturbance, and bone loss in female athletes.

The question of whether the Triad should be considered a pathological or even psychopathological condition has recently become contentious *(191–193)*. What is generally accepted is that in all but cases of extreme (high-magnitude) loading, the positive effect of exercise on bone cannot offset the negative effects of inadequate energy availability during high-intensity, high-volume exercise training. To illustrate, gymnasts load their skeletons at very high magnitudes and rates, and thus, despite a high prevalence of menstrual disturbance, have bone mass well above normal *(194)*. Long distance runners, on the other hand, who load their skeletons at much lower rates, are not protected from amenorrhea-related bone loss. Although there are individual differences, the loss of bone mass in amenorrheic distance runners increases their risk of stress fracture and premature osteoporosis compared with their eumenorrheic running counterparts *(195)*. Loucks et al. *(196)* suggest that exercise-associated amenorrhea may be prevented or reversed by increasing energy consumption, without alterations in training.

There is some suggestion that oral contraceptives (OC) may offset bone loss in athletes with menstrual dysfunction, but there are insufficient data to fully corroborate the effect *(197)*. Keen and Drinkwater *(198)* reported that initiating OC use approximately 8 years after the onset of athletic oligo- or amenorrhea did not improve bone mass, concluding that intervention should begin at the onset of dysfunction in order to prevent significant loss. The effect of OCs, alone or in combination with exercise, on bone strength indices is, however, poorly understood. In fact, for women aged 18–31 years, exercise alone and OCs alone depressed normal age-related increases in femoral neck mass and size, although the combination of exercise and OC was slightly less detrimental *(199)*. It is likely that a complex interaction of factors yet to be identified will account for these puzzling findings.

Men

Intense training is not associated with commensurately severe alterations in reproductive hormones in men. Male athletes exercising at a range of intensities have serum concentrations of testosterone that lie within the normal range *(107,108,120,200,201)* including adolescents *(202)*. In some athletes, however, a degree of subtle hormonal perturbation can occur. Smith and Rutherford *(120)* reported that, although in the normal range, serum total testosterone was significantly lower in triathletes than controls, but not rowers. Further, total serum testosterone, non-sex hormone binding globulin (SHBG)-bound testosterone, and free testosterone concentrations in men running more than 64 km/week was 83, 69.5, and 68.1% that of controls, respectively *(203)*. Others have similarly observed that resting and free testosterone concentrations of trained athletes are 68.8 and 72.6% that of controls *(204)*. Age may influence the effect as elderly endurance athletes have significantly greater levels of SHBG than controls whereas younger athletes demonstrate no differences compared to controls *(108,205)*.

Whether hormones potentiate the effect of exercise on bone in men is relatively unexamined. Suominen and Rahkila *(108)* reported a negative correlation between bone mass and SHBG in older endurance athletes but no relationship of bone mass with testosterone. Further, the addition of self-administered anabolic steroids (testosterone: 193.75 ± 147.82 mg/week) to high-intensity body building training does not stimulate greater osteoblastic activity or bone formation than exercise alone *(206)*. Four months of progressive resistance exercise training 4 days/week, with or without growth hormone supplementation, did not significantly increase whole body, spine, or proximal femur bone mass in elderly men (mean age = 67) with normal bone mass *(207)*. Similarly, the addition of recombinant human growth hormone to 6 months of resistance exercise training induced no change in bone mass of older men *(208,209)*.

OSTEOPOROTIC FRACTURE AND FALLS

Fracture and Exercise

Exercise studies that include fractures as an outcome measure are difficult and expensive to conduct. Very long-term follow-up of interventions is required and many men and women at risk for fracture due to poor bone health are on pharmacological therapy that can mask the effect of exercise. In general, the literature supports a protective effect of physical activity on the risk of fracture, especially at the hip *(210–213)*. Specifically, the Study of Osteoporotic Fractures, a large, prospective, community-based, observational study of healthy, older, Caucasian women, reported that moderately to vigorously active women had significantly fewer hip and vertebral fractures compared to inactive women *(210)*. Similarly, data from the Nurse's Health Study showed that moderate levels of activity, including walking, were associated with a significantly lower risk of hip fracture in postmenopausal women *(214)*. Two studies that tracked fractures over a prolonged period of exercise *(215)* or over a follow-up period after completion of an exercise intervention *(216)* suggest a protective effect of exercise against fracture. The incidence of vertebral fractures was lower (1.6%) 8 years after a 2-year back extension exercise program compared to controls (4.3%) *(216)*. Original exercisers had better back extension strength at follow-up and a 2.7 lower relative risk of vertebral compression fracture than controls.

Falls and Exercise

Falls are the cause of almost 90% of all hip fractures *(217–219)*. As previously indicated, exercise can affect both the numerator and the denominator of the factor of risk. Discussion thus far has focused on exercise as a means of altering the denominator of the factor of risk, that is, on increasing fracture load by improving parameters of bone strength. However, exercise can also reduce the numerator either by preventing a fall entirely or by lowering the applied load of falls through improved neuromuscular responses.

Risk factors for falls are numerous, and some can be modified by exercise. Lateral instability, muscle weakness of the lower extremities, and poor gait have been found to independently predict hip fracture and falls *(220–223)*. Impaired balance is similarly related to incidence of vertebral fracture *(224)*. In the Study of Osteoporotic Fractures in Men (MrOS), men in the upper quartile of leg power and grip strength had an 18–24% lower risk of falls compared to men in the lowest quartile *(225)*. Since exercise promotes and maintains muscle strength, balance, and mobility, it is an intuitive strategy for reducing osteoporosis-related fractures *(226,227)*. In fact, muscle strengthening and balance training have been shown to reduce extraskeletal risk factors for hip fracture in elderly men and women *(228,229)* and overall risk of falling by as much as 75% *(229,230)*. That vibration superimposed on muscle training exercise augments the strengthening effect *(231)* suggests whole body vibration may be a preventative strategy with dual (anti-fall and bone-building) benefits (see Chapter 8).

A 30-month randomized controlled trial of high-impact exercise in 160 elderly women with low bone mass reported a lower incidence of fall-related fractures among exercisers compared to controls, despite minimal effects on hip bone mass *(215)*. Improvements in neuromuscular function resulting from low-intensity exercise, including water-based exercise *(155,232,233)*, while not osteogenic, may likewise be efficacious for fall and fracture prevention.

Exercise interventions with falls and injurious falls as primary outcomes are limited but tend to support the role of exercise as a preventative strategy. Data from the FICSIT trials (Frailty and Injuries: Cooperative Studies of Intervention Techniques) indicate that activities that are most beneficial for reducing incidence of falls include those that result in muscle strength gains and dynamic balance improvements *(234)*. However, Lord et al. *(235)* reported improvements in strength and balance in elderly women but no change in incidence of falls after 12 months of exercise that included resistance and a similar null effect on falls after an individualized prevention program that included exercise *(236)*. Yet other trials by the same group reported a reduction in falls among the elderly who participated in group exercise in both community-dwelling *(237)* and retirement home *(238)* settings. Campbell et al. *(239)* found that a multifactorial exercise intervention involving muscle building plus walking exercise reduced injurious and non-injurious falls by 40% in elderly women. The study required home visits by physical therapists; and it is not known which component of the program, muscle building, walking, or the two combined, was most potent for reducing falls.

Sadly, the fall-reducing benefit of exercise may not extend to the very frail elderly *(240–243)* despite improvements in fall risk factors and physical function *(240,242)*. Trends toward lower falls among exercisers, however, were apparent in studies of longer duration *(242,243)*, suggesting that a longer period of adaptation may be required to detect protective effects in this population.

RECOMMENDATIONS: EXERCISE PRESCRIPTION

The Osteogenic Index – An Exercise Algorithm Derived from Animal Data

Charles Turner *(244,245)* has translated the findings of a generation of basic animal research into a theory for practical exercise application. With Alex Robling, he developed the Osteogenic Index (OI), a method to predict the effectiveness of an exercise regime to improve parameters of bone strength based on the known response of bone cells and tissue to certain types of loading *(245)*. The OI requires dynamic (cyclical) loading and accounts for load magnitude, rate, and frequency *(29,41,131,246–248)*. They note that animal bone tissue becomes desensitized to prolonged loading stimuli and, in fact, loses the majority of its mechanosensitivity after 20 loading cycles *(49,249)*. Adding rest periods between bouts of loading markedly improves the bone response to a cyclical stimulus *(250)*. Thus, they propose that a regime of frequent, short, intense bouts of exercise should be most beneficial to bone.

The validity of the Osteogenic Index for human application remains to be tested. Preliminary evidence suggests the human response may vary in subtle ways, such as the importance of cycle number. For example, while 300 jump repetitions per week for 7 months produced positive effects at the hip and spine in prepubescent children, reducing the jump number to 150 failed to reproduce the effect *(251)*. Collective findings of jumping studies in premenopausal women, however, support the OI theory as even low numbers of weekly jumps can produce a bone response with little added benefit from additional impacts *(44,135,138,139)*. Recently, it was reported that women who performed the greatest amount of impact activity, measured by accelerometry, above a threshold level of intensity had significantly greater improvements in hip BMD compared to women who performed lower amounts of activity *(252)*. These data suggest that the cycle number may be an important determinant of bone responsiveness to impact activity, but that the effect may follow more of a threshold rather than dose–response pattern.

ACSM Position Stand – Recommendations Based on Human Data

Based on the best evidence to date, recently the American College of Sports Medicine published a Position Stand for Physical Activity and Bone Health *(253)* with the following recommendations. Children should engage in 10–20 min (split into two sessions if possible) of high-intensity activities that include jumping-type activities at least three times a week. Adults should engage in 30–60 min of a combination of weight-bearing endurance of moderate to high intensity, jumping 3–5 times per week, and resistance exercises targeting all major muscle groups 2–3 times per week. Prolonged immobilization and bed rest should be avoided at all costs, given the very negative effect of unloading on bone mass and the limited ability to fully regain losses with remobilization.

While high-magnitude (impact) activities are recommended for increasing bone mass of the younger, more robust skeleton, they are not recommended for those with advanced osteoporosis. In the frail elderly population, particular care must be taken to maintain a balance between safety and efficacy because the exercise intervention itself (through increasing activity levels) presents not only the possibility of skeletal and neuromuscular benefit but also an increased risk of fracture. Osteoporotic individuals, with or without a history of vertebral compression fractures, should not engage in jumping activities or deep forward trunk flexion exercises such as rowing, toe touching, and full situps. Through a combination of dynamic force analyses at the hip and spine and ex vivo measurements in cadaveric bone, it is possible to determine the factor of risk for most of the exercise activities that might be used in exercise studies in the elderly. Understanding and maintaining a safe value of the factor of risk for a specific exercise program is crucial. Until such understanding is achieved, caution is warranted in the use of overload concepts in the frail elderly. Before initiating a program of high intensity, elderly individuals should consider a bone density evaluation and perhaps an image of the spine. Any individual undertaking a new program should begin slowly with careful attention to exercise form and appropriate progressions. Exercises that produce severe joint pain or muscle soreness of more than 3 days should be discontinued until exercise of lower intensity can be tolerated.

FUTURE RESEARCH

The large body of research data notwithstanding, in fact it remains impossible to say without reservation that exercise will reduce the likelihood of fracturing. As Karlsson *(254)* has stated, much of the research has been "hypothesis generating" rather than "hypothesis testing" – a consequence of the confounding challenges associated with exercise RCTs and the protracted nature of follow-up required to compare real fracture rates between exercise and control groups. Indeed, while much has been achieved in our understanding of the use of exercise for the prevention of age-related fractures, many questions and challenges remain. For instance we know little about the relative importance of mechanical, endocrine, and genetic factors and how these interact to potentiate or blunt the exercise response in bone over the life span. How these mechanisms relate to the temporal sequence of the bone remodeling cycle is also unclear.

It is likely that the complex interplay of genetics, nutrition, hormone status, and even a degree of central control *(255)* accounts for much that remains unexplained about the bone response to exercise. That mechanical loading cannot entirely prevent spinal cord injury-related bone loss *(6)* is testament to the presence of influences yet to be explained.

Thus, while the power law model incorporating load magnitude and number of repetitions of Whalen and colleagues *(256)* and the Osteogenic Index of Turner and Robling *(257)* have moved us forward in our ability to design and test exercise regimes for bone health, a definitive exercise prescription remains elusive. The challenge remains to identify a means by which optimal overload can be determined in order to safely stimulate a positive bone response. The complex interplay of dose (load magnitude and rate), cycle number, and duration must be elucidated in human models. Only then can we customize exercise prescription for bone with confidence.

Finally, it is important to consider the issue of compliance. The commitment to regular exercise of any kind, much less the relatively specific form required to effect change in bone, is known to be challenging for the vast majority of individuals. Compliance even with study protocols, when volunteers often have access to state-of-the-art facilities and personnel to encourage and support their efforts, is routinely disappointing. For example, compliance of a mere 17.8% was reported for an 18-month, home-based, exercise program for the prevention of postmenopausal osteoporosis, primarily due to lack of motivation *(258)*. Few maintain a lifelong exercise routine, and those who do are unlikely to vary their regime the extent required to stimulate ongoing bone adaptation. In reality, the greatest challenge for bone physiologists may not be the identification of the optimal exercise program, but the engagement of the community to utilize the knowledge. In this respect, the health of the skeletal system shares commonality with the cardiovascular and neuromuscular systems.

CONCLUSIONS

Regular physical activity has the potential to reduce the risk of osteoporosis and fragility fractures by (1) optimizing peak bone mass, (2) consolidating or maintaining adult bone, and (3) reducing the risk and incidence of falls. As each strategy is age specific, the exercise prescription for the prevention of osteoporosis-related fractures will differ across the life span.

Exercise will only affect bones that are loaded during the activity. Bone requires substantial overload for prolonged durations for positive adaptations to be stimulated. With the possible exception of the pediatric population, bone gains will likely be lost if a stimulatory exercise is discontinued. Individuals with the weakest bones can expect the greatest improvements from initiating exercise. Exercise is most efficacious when accompanied by adequate calcium consumption.

Exercises that are most or least likely to substantially alter bone mass and prevent falls can be identified with relative certainty. Development of individualized and population-specific exercise prescription across the life span is more challenging. Issues such as determining actual bone strain exposure during activity, optimal dose–response, safety, and the interaction of exercise with pharmacologic agents remain opportunities for future research. It will be important to determine the degree to which exercise-invoked improvements in bone strength and falls prevention will translate to a reduction in the incidence of fracture.

REFERENCES

1. Krolner B, Toft B. Vertebral bone loss: an unheeded side effect of therapeutic bed rest. Clin Sci (Lond) 1983;64:537–540.
2. Donaldson CL, Hulley SB, Vogel JM, Hattner RS, Bayers JH, McMillan DE. Effect of prolonged bed rest on bone mineral. Metabolism 1970;19:1071–1084.
3. Tilton FE, Degioanni JJ, Schneider VS. Long-term follow-up of Skylab bone demineralization. Aviat Space Environ Med 1980;51:1209–1213.
4. Leblanc AD, Schneider VS, Evans HJ, Engelbretson DA, Krebs JM. Bone mineral loss and recovery after 17 weeks of bed rest. J Bone Miner Res 1990;5:843–850.
5. NASA. The effects of space travel on the musculoskeletal system, 1992.
6. Jiang SD, Dai LY, Jiang LS. Osteoporosis after spinal cord injury. Osteoporos Int 2006;17:180–192.
7. Lang TF, Leblanc AD, Evans HJ, Lu Y. Adaptation of the proximal femur to skeletal reloading after long-duration spaceflight. J Bone Miner Res 2006;21:1224–1230.
8. Courtney AC, Wachtel EF, Myers ER, Hayes WC. Effects of loading rate on strength of the proximal femur. Calcif Tissue Int 1994;55:53–58.
9. Courtney AC, Wachtel EF, Myers ER, Hayes WC. Age-related reductions in the strength of the femur tested in a fall-loading configuration. J Bone Joint Surg Am 1995;77:387–395.
10. Hayes WC, Myers ER, Robinovitch SN, Van Den Kroonenberg A, Courtney AC, McMahon TA. Etiology and prevention of age-related hip fractures. Bone 1996;18:77S–86S.
11. Moro M, Hecker AT, Bouxsein ML, Myers ER. Failure load of thoracic vertebrae correlates with lumbar bone mineral density measured by DXA. Calcif Tissue Int 1995;56:206–209.
12. Myers ER, Hecker AT, Rooks DS, Hayes WC. Correlations of the failure load of the femur with densitometric and geometric properties from QDR. Transactions of the 38th Annual Meeting of the Orthopaedic Research Society 1992:115.
13. Myers ER, Sebeny EA, Hecker AT, et al. Correlations between photon absorption properties and failure load of the distal radius in vitro. Calcif Tissue Int 1991;49:292–297.
14. Seeman E, Delmas PD. Bone quality-the material and structural basis of bone strength and fragility. N Engl J Med 2006;354:2250–2261.
15. Marshall LM, Lang TF, Lambert LC, Zmuda JM, Ensrud KE, Orwoll ES. Dimensions and volumetric BMD of the proximal femur and their relation to age among older U.S. men. J Bone Miner Res 2006;21:1197–1206.
16. Ashe MC, Khan KM, Kontulainen SA, et al. Accuracy of pQCT for evaluating the aged human radius: an ashing, histomorphometry and failure load investigation. Osteoporos Int 2006;17:1241–1251.

17. Brodt MD, Pelz GB, Taniguchi J, Silva MJ. Accuracy of peripheral quantitative computed tomography (pQCT) for assessing area and density of mouse cortical bone. Calcif Tissue Int 2003;73: 411–418.
18. DiLeo C, Tarolo GL, Bagni B, et al. Peripheral quantitative Computed Tomography (PQCT) in the evaluation of bone geometry, biomechanics and mineral density in postmenopausal women. Radiol Med (Torino) 2002;103:233–241.
19. Jiang Y, Zhao J, Augat P, et al. Trabecular bone mineral and calculated structure of human bone specimens scanned by peripheral quantitative computed tomography: relation to biomechanical properties. J Bone Miner Res 1998;13:1783–1790.
20. Moisio KC, Podolskaya G, Bamhart B, Berzins A, Sumner DR. pQCT provides better prediction of canine femur breaking load than does DXA. J Musculoskelet Neuronal Interact 2003;3:240–245.
21. Siu WS, Qin L, Leung KS. pQCT bone strength index may serve as a better predictor than bone mineral density for long bone breaking strength. J Bone Miner Metab 2003;21:316–322.
22. Wosje KS, Binkley TL, Specker BL. Comparison of bone parameters by dual-energy X-ray absorptiometry and peripheral quantitative computed tomography in Hutterite vs. non-Hutterite women aged 35–60 years. Bone 2001;29(2):192–197.
23. Sakata S, Barkmann R, Lochmuller EM, Heller M, Gluer CC. Assessing bone status beyoned BMD: evaluation of bone geometry and porosity by quantitative ultrasound of human finger phalanges. J Bone Miner Res 2004;19:924–930.
24. Hong J, Hipp JA, Mulkern RV, Jaramillo D, Snyder BD. Magnetic resonance imaging measurements of bone density and cross-sectional geometry. Calcif Tissue Int 2000;66:74–78.
25. Drinkwater BL. 1994 C. H. McCloy Research Lecture: does physical activity play a role in preventing osteoporosis? Res Q Exerc Sport 1994;65:197–206.
26. Winters-Stone KM, Snow CM. Musculoskeletal response to exercise is greatest in women with low initial values. Med Sci Sports Exerc 2003;35:1691–1696.
27. Korpelainen R, Keinanen-Kiukaanniemi S, Heikkinen J, Vaananen K, Korpelainen J. Effect of impact exercise on bone mineral density in elderly women with low BMD: a population-based randomized controlled 30-month intervention. Osteoporos Int 2006;17:109–118.
28. Carter DR. Mechanical loading histories and cortical bone remodeling. Calcif Tissue Int 1984;36:S 19–S24.
29. Kerr D, Morton A, Dick I, Prince R. Exercise effects on bone mass in postmenopausal women are site-specific and load-dependent. J Bone Miner Res 1996;11:218–225.
30. Maddalozzo GF, Snow CM. High intensity resistance training: effects on bone in older men and women. Calcif Tissue Int 2000;66:399–404.
31. Cussler EC, Lohman TG, Going SB, et al. Weight lifted in strength training predicts bone change in postmenopausal women. Med Sci Sports Exerc 2003;35:10–17.
32. Jamsa T, Vainionpaa A, Korpelainen R, Vihriala E, Leppaluoto J. Effect of daily physical activity on proximal femur. Clin Biomech (Bristol, Avon) 2006;21:1–7.
33. Dalsky GP, Stocke KS, Ehsani AA, Slatopolsky E, Lee WC, Birge SJ, Jr. Weight-bearing exercise training and lumbar bone mineral content in postmenopausal women. Ann Intern Med 1988;108:824–828.
34. Winters KM, Snow CM. Detraining reverses positive effects of exercise on the musculoskeletal system in premenopausal women. J Bone Miner Res. 2000;15:2495–2503.
35. Snow CM, Shaw JM, Winters KM, Witzke KA. Long-term exercise using weighted vests prevents hip. J Gerontol Med Sci 2000;55A(9):M489–M491.
36. Fuchs R, Snow C. Gains in hip bone mass from 7 months of high-impact jumping are maintained after 7 months of detraining. J Pediatr 2002;141:357–362.
37. Kannus P, Haapasalo H, Sankelo M, et al. Effect of starting age of physical activity on bone mass in the dominant arm of tennis and squash players. Ann Intern Med 1995;123:27–31.
38. Chien MY, Wu YT, Hsu AT, Yang RS, Lai JS. Efficacy of a 24-week aerobic exercise program for osteopenic postmenopausal women. Calcif Tissue Int 2000;67:443–448.
39. Iwamoto J, Takeda T, Otani T, Yabe Y. Effect of increased physical activity on bone mineral density in postmenopausal osteoporotic women. Keio J Med 1998;47:157–161.
40. Hatori M, Hasegawa A, Adachi H, et al. The effects of walking at the anaerobic threshold level on vertebral bone loss in postmenopausal women. Calcif Tissue Int 1993;52:411–414.

41. Kohrt WM, Ehsani AA, Birge SJ, Jr. Effects of exercise involving predominantly either joint-reaction or ground-reaction forces on bone mineral density in older women. J Bone Miner Res 1997;12:1253–1261.
42. Nelson ME, Fiatarone MA, Morganti CM, Trice I, Greenberg RA, Evans WJ. Effects of high-intensity strength training on multiple risk factors for osteoporotic fractures. A randomized controlled trial. JAMA 1994;272:1909–1914.
43. Taaffe DR, Robinson TL, Snow CM, Marcus R. High-impact exercise promotes bone gain in well-trained female athletes. J Bone Miner Res 1997;12:255–260.
44. Bassey EJ, Ramsdale SJ. Increase in femoral bone density in young women following high-impact exercise. Osteoporos Int 1994;4:72–75.
45. Bassey EJ, Rothwell MC, Littlewood JJ, Pye DW. Pre- and postmenopausal women have different bone mineral density responses to the same high-impact exercise [see comments]. J Bone Miner Res 1998;13:1805–1813.
46. Raab DM, Smith EL, Crenshaw TD, Thomas DP. Bone mechanical properties after exercise training in young and old rats. J Appl Physiol 1990;68:130–134.
47. Rubin CT, Bain SD, McLeod KJ. Suppression of the osteogenic response in the aging skeleton. Calcif Tissue Int 1992;50:306–313.
48. Robling AG, Hinant FM, Burr DB, Turner CH. Improved bone structure and strength after long-term mechanical loading is greatest if loading is separated into short bouts. J Bone Miner Res 2002;17: 1545–1554.
49. Rubin CT, Lanyon LE. Regulation of bone formation by applied dynamic loads. J Bone Joint Surg 1984;66:397–402.
50. Rubin CT, McLeod KJ. Promotion of bony ingrowth by frequency-specific, low-amplitude mechanical strain. Clin Orthop Relat Res 1994:165–174.
51. O'Connor JA, Lanyon LE, MacFie H. The influence of strain rate on adaptive bone remodelling. J Biomech 1982;15:767–781.
52. Gross TS, Edwards JL, McLeod KJ, Rubin CT. Strain gradients correlate with sites of periosteal bone formation. J Bone Miner Res 1997;12:982–988.
53. Osteoporosis prevention, diagnosis, and therapy. JAMA 2001;285:785–795.
54. Welten DC, Kemper HCG, Post GB, et al. Weight-bearing activity during youth is a more important factor for peak bone mass than calcium intake. J Bone Miner Res 1994;9:1089–1096.
55. Boot AM, de Ridder MAJ, Pols HAP, Krenning EP, de Muinck Keizer-Schrama SMPF. Bone mineral density in children and adolescents: relation to puberty, calcium intake, and physical activity. J Clin Endocrinol Metab 1997;82:57–62.
56. Duppe H, Gardsell P, Johnell O, Nilsson BE, Ringsberg K. Bone mineral density, muscle strength and physical activity. A population-based study of 332 subjects aged 15–42 years. Acta Orthop Scan 1997;68:97–103.
57. Courteix D, Lespessailles E, Peres SL, Obert P, Germain P, Benhamou CL. Effect of physical training on bone mineral density in prepubertal girls: a comparative study between impact-loading and non-impact-loading sports. Osteoporos Int 1998;8:152–158.
58. Bass S, Pearce G, Bradney M, et al. Exercise before puberty may confer residual benefits in bone density in adulthood: studies in active prepubertal and retired female gymnasts. J Bone Miner Res 1998;13: 500–507.
59. Grimston SK, Willows ND, Hanley DA. Mechanical loading regime and its relationship to bone mineral density in children. Med Sci Sports Exerc 1993;25:1203–1210.
60. Gunnes M, Lehmann EH. Physical activity and dietary constituents as predictors of forearm cortical and trabecular bone gain in healthy children and adolescents: a prospective study. Acta Paediatr 1996;85: 19–25.
61. Tsai SC, Kao CH, Wang SJ. Comparison of bone mineral density between athletic and non-athletic Chinese male adolescents. Kaohsiung J Med Sci 1996;12:573–580.
62. Bailey DA, McKay HA, Mirwald RL, Crocker PR, Faulkner RA. A six-year longitudinal study of the relationship of physical activity to bone mineral accrual in growing children: The University of Saskatchewan Bone Mineral Accrual Study. J Bone Miner Res 1999;14:1672–1679.
63. Khan KM, Bennell KL, Hopper JL, et al. Self-reported ballet classes undertaken at age 10–12 years and hip bone mineral density in later life. Osteoporos Int 1998;8:165–173.

64. Daly RM, Rich PA, Klein R, Bass S. Effects of high-impact exercise on ultrasonic and biochemical indices of skeletal status: A prospective study in young male gymnasts [In Process Citation]. J Bone Miner Res 1999;14:1222–1230.
65. Slemenda CW, Reister TK, Hui SL, Miller JZ, Christian JC, Johnston CC, Jr. Influences on skeletal mineralization in children and adolescents: evidence for varying effects of sexual maturation and physical activity. J Pediatr 1994;125:201–207.
66. Haapasalo H, Kannus P, Sievanen H, et al. Effect of long-term unilateral activity on bone mineral density of female junior tennis players. J Bone Miner Res 1998;13:310–319.
67. Nordstrom P, Nordstrom G, Thorsen K, Lorentzon R. Local bone mineral density, muscle strength, and exercise in adolescent boys: a comparitive study of two groups with different muscle strength and exercise levels. Calcif Tissue Int 1996;58:402–408.
68. Rico H, Revilla M, Cardenas JL, et al. Influence of weight and seasonal changes and radiogrammetry and bone densitometry. Calcif Tissue Int 1994;54:385–388.
69. Dalen N, Laftman P, Ohlsen H, Stromberg L. The effect of athletic activity on the bone mass in human diaphyseal bone. Orthopedics 1985;8:1139–1141.
70. Haapasalo H, Sievanen H, Kannus P, Heinenon A, Oja P, Vuori I. Dimensions and estimated mechanical characteristics of the humerus after long-term tennis loading. J Bone Miner Res 1996;11:864–872.
71. Moyer-Mileur L, Luetkemeier M, Boomer L, Chan GM. Effect of physical activity on bone mineralization in premature infants. J Pediatr 1995;127:620–625.
72. Litmanovitz I, Dolfin T, Friedland O, et al. Early physical activity intervention prevents decrease of bone strength in very low birth weight infants. Pediatrics 2003;112:15–19.
73. Specker BL, Mulligan L, Ho M. Longitudinal study of calcium intake, physical activity, and bone mineral content in infants 6–18 months of age. J Bone Miner Res 1999;14:569–576.
74. Specker B, Binkley T. Randomized trial of physical activity and calcium supplementation on bone mineral content in 3- to 5-year-old children. J Bone Miner Res 2003;18:885–892.
75. Specker B, Binkley T, Fahrenwald N. Increased periosteal circumference remains present 12 months after an exercise intervention in preschool children. Bone 2004;35:1383–1388.
76. Fuchs R, Bauer J, Snow C. Jumping improves hip and lumbar spine bone mass in prepubescent children: a randomized controlled trial. J Bone Miner Res 2001;16:148–156.
77. Bradney M, Pearce G, Naughton G, et al. Moderate exercise during growth in prepubertal boys: changes in bone mass, size, volumetric density, and bone strength: a controlled prospective study [see comments]. J Bone Miner Res 1998;13:1814–1821.
78. MacKelvie KJ, Petit MA, Khan KM, Beck TJ, McKay HA. Bone mass and structure are enhanced following a 2-year randomized controlled trial of exercise in prepubertal boys. Bone 2004;34:755–764.
78a. Weeks BK, Young CM, and Beck BR. Eight months of regular in-school jumping improves indices of bone strength in adolescent boys and girls: Results of the POWER PE study. Journal of Bone and Mineral Research, 2008;23(7):1002–1011.
79. Johannsen N, Binkley T, Englert V, Neiderauer G, Specker B. Bone response to jumping is site-specific in children: a randomized trial. Bone 2003;33:533–539.
80. McKay HA, Petit MA, Schutz RW, Prior JC, Barr SI, Khan KM. Augmented trochanteric bone mineral density after modified physical education classes: a randomized school-based exercise intervention study in prepubescent and early pubescent children. J Pediatr 2000;136:156–162.
81. Morris FL, Naughton GA, Gibbs JL, Carlson JS, Wark JD. Prospective ten-month exercise intervention in premenarcheal girls: positive effects on bone and lean mass. J Bone Miner Res 1997;12:1453–1462.
82. MacKelvie KJ, Khan KM, Petit MA, Janssen PA, McKay HA. A school-based exercise intervention elicits substantial bone health benefits: a 2-year randomized controlled trial in girls. Pediatrics 2003;112:e447.
83. Petit MA, McKay HA, MacKelvie KJ, Heinonen A, Khan KM, Beck TJ. A randomized school-based jumping intervention confers site and maturity-specific benefits on bone structural properties in girls: a hip structural analysis study. J Bone Miner Res 2002;17:363–372.
84. Mackelvie KJ, McKay HA, Khan KM, Crocker PR. A school-based exercise intervention augments bone mineral accrual in early pubertal girls. J Pediatr 2001;139:501–508.
85. Witzke KA, Snow CM. Effects of plyometric jump training on bone mass in adolescent girls. Med Sci Sports Exerc 2000;32:1051–1057.
86. Nichols DL, Sanborn CF, Love AM. Resistance training and bone mineral density in adolescent females. J Pediatr 2001;139:494–500.

87. Heinonen A, Sievanen H, Kannus P, Oja P, Pasanen M, Vuori I. High-impact exercise and bones of growing girls: a 9-month controlled trial. Osteoporos Int 2000;11:1010–1017.
88. Snow-Harter C, Whalen R, Myburgh K, Arnaud S, Marcus R. Bone mineral density, muscle strength, and recreational exercise in men. J Bone Miner Res 1992;7:1291–1296.
89. Madsen KL, Adams WC, Van Loan MD. Effects of physical activity, body weight and composition, and muscular strength on bone density in young women. Med Sci Sports Exerc 1998;30:114–120.
90. Pettersson U, Nordstrom P, Lorentzon R. A comparison of bone mineral density and muscle strength in young male adults with different exercise level. Calcif Tissue Int 1999;64:490–498.
91. Karlsson MK, Hasserius R, Obrant KJ. Bone mineral density in athletes during and after career: A comparison between loaded and unloaded skeletal regions. Calcif Tissue Int 1996;59:245–248.
92. Bennell KL, Malcolm SA, Khan KM, et al. Bone mass and bone turnover in power athletes, endurance athletes, and controls: a 12-month longitudinal study. Bone 1997;20:477–484.
93. Brahm H, Strom H, Piehl-Aulin K, Mallmin H, Ljunghall S. Bone metabolism in endurance trained athletes: a comparison to population-based controls based on DXA, SXA, quantitative ultrasound, and biochemical markers. Calcif Tissue Int 1997;61:448–454.
94. Wittich A, Mautalen CA, Oliveri MB, Bagur A, Somoza F, Rotemberg E. Professional football (soccer) players have a markedly greater skeletal mineral content, density and size than age- and BMI-matched controls. Calcif Tissue Int 1998;63:112–117.
95. Uusi-Rasi K, Sievanen H, Vuori I, Pasanen M, Heinonen A, Oja P. Associations of physical activity and calcium intake with bone mass and size in healthy women at different ages. J Bone Miner Res 1998;13:133–142.
96. Tsuzuku S, Ikegami Y, Yabe K. Effects of high-intensity resistance training on bone mineral density in young male powerlifters. Calcif Tissue Int 1998;63:283–286.
97. Sone T, Miyake M, Takeda N, Tomomitsu T, Otsuka N, Fukunaga M. Influence of exercise and degenerative vertebral changes on BMD: a cross-sectional study in Japanese men. Gerontology 1996;42:57–66.
98. Calbet JA, Moysi JS, Dorado C, Rodriguez LP. Bone mineral content and density in professional tennis players. Calcif Tissue Int 1998;62:491–496.
99. Block JE, Friedlander AL, Brooks GA, Steiger P, Stubbs HA, Genant HK. Determinants of bone density among athletes engaged in weight-bearing and non-weight-bearing activity. J Appl Physiol 1989;67:1100–1105.
100. Block JE, Genant HK, Black D. Greater vertebral bone mineral mass in exercising young men. West J Med 1986;145:39–42.
101. Colletti LA, Edwards J, Gordon L, Shary J, Bell NH. The effects of muscle-building exercise on bone mineral density of the radius, spine, and hip in young men. Calcif Tissue Int 1989;45:12–14.
102. Karlsson MK, Johnell O, Obrant KJ. Bone mineral density in weight lifters. Calcif Tissue Int 1993;52:212–215.
103. Mayoux-Benhamou MA, Leyge JF, Roux C, Revel M. Cross-sectional study of weight-bearing activity on proximal femur bone mineral density. Calcif Tissue Int 1999;64:179–183.
104. Need AG, Wishard JM, Scopacasa F, Horowitz M, Morris HA, Nordin BE. Effect of physical activity on femoral bone density on men. Br Med J 1995;310:6993:1501–1502.
105. Nilsson BE, Westlin NE. Bone density in athletes. Clin Orthop Relat Res 1971;77:179–182.
106. Leichter I, Simkin A, Margulies JY, et al. Gain in mass density of bone following strenuous physical activity. J Orthop Res 1989;7:86–90.
107. MacDougall JD, Webber CE, Martin J, et al. Relationship among running mileage, bone density, and serum testosterone in male runners. J Appl Physiol 1992;73:1165–1170.
108. Suominen H, Rahkila P. Bone mineral density of the calcaneus in 70- to 80-yr-old male athletes and a population sample. Med Sci Sports Exerc 1991;23:1227–1233.
109. Hutchinson TM, Whalen RT, Cleet TM, Vogel JM, Arnaud SB. Factors in daily physical activity related to calcaneal mineral density in men. Med Sci Sports Exerc 1995;27:745–750.
110. Hamdy RC, Anderson JS, Whalen KE, Harvill LM. Regional differences in bone density of young men involved in different exercises. Med Sci Sports Exerc 1994;26:884–888.
111. Aloia JF, Cohn SH, Babu T, Abesamis C, Kalici N, Ellis K. Skeletal mass and body composition in marathon runners. Metabolism 1978;27:1793–1796.
112. Flodgren G, Hedelin R, Henriksson-Larsen K. Bone mineral density in flatwater sprint kayakers. Calcif Tissue Int 1999;64:374–379.

113. Myburgh KH, Charette S, Zhou L, Steele CR, Arnaud S, Marcus R. Influence of recreational activity and muscle strength on ulnar bending stiffness in men. Med Sci Sports Exerc 1993;25:592–596.
114. Dalen N, Olsson KE. Bone mineral content and physical activity. Acta Orthop Scand 1974;45:170–174.
115. Michel BA, Bloch DA, Fries JF. Weight-bearing exercise, overexercise, and lumbar bone density over age 50 years. Arch Int Med 1989;149:2325–2329.
116. Taaffe DR, Snow-Harter C, Connolly DA, Robinson TL, Brown MD, Marcus R. Differential effects of swimming versus weight-bearing activity on bone mineral status on eumenorrheic athletes. J Bone Miner Res 1995;10:586–593.
117. Orwoll ES, Ferar J, Ovaitt SK, McClung MR, Huntington K. The relationship of swimming exercise to bone mass in men and women. Arch Int Med 1989;149:2197–2200.
118. Ashizawa N, Nonaka K, Michikami S, et al. Tomographical description of tennis-loaded radius: reciprocal relation between bone size and volumetric BMD. J Appl Physiol 1999;86:1347–1351.
119. Krahl H, Michaelis U, Pieper H-G, Quack G, Montag M. Stimulation of bone growth through sports. A radiologic investigation of the upper extremities in professional tennis players. Am J Sports Med 1994;22:751–757.
120. Smith R, Rutherford OM. Spine and total body bone mineral density and serum testosterone levels in male athletes. Eur J Appl Physiol 1993;67:330–334.
121. Ryan AS, Elahi D. Loss of bone mineral density in women athletes during aging. Calcif Tissue Int 1998;63:287–292.
122. Karlsson MK, Johnell O, Obrant KJ. Is bone mineral density advantage maintained long-term in previous weight lifters? Calcif Tissue Int 1995;57:325–328.
123. Glynn NW, Meilahn EN, Charron M, Anderson SJ, Kuller LH, Cauley JA. Determinants of bone mineral density in older men. J Bone Miner Res. 1995;10:1769–1777.
124. Pollock ML, Mengelkoch LJ, Graves JE, et al. Twenty-year follow-up of aerobic power and body composition of older track athletes. J Appl Physiol 1997;82:1508–1516.
125. Greendale GA, Barrett-Connor E, Edelstein S, Ingles S, Haile R. Lifetime leisure exercise and osteoporosis. The Rancho Bernardo study. Am J Epidemiol 1995;141:951–959.
126. Ulrich CM, Georgiou CC, Gillis DE, Snow CM. Lifetime physical activity is associated with bone mineral density in premenopausal women. J Womens Health 1999;8:365–375.
127. Bassey E, Ramsdale S. Increase in femoral bone mineral density in young women following high impact exercise. Osteoporos Int 1994;4:72–75.
128. Friedlander AL, Genant HK, Sadowsky S, Byl NN, Gluer CC. A two-year program of aerobics and weight-training enhances BMD of young women. J Bone Miner Res 1995;10:574.
129. Heinonen A, Sievanen H, Kannus P, Oja P, Vuori I. Effects of unilateral strength training and detraining on bone mineral mass and estimated mechanical characteristics of the upper limb bones in young women. J Bone Miner Res 1996;11:490–501.
130. Lohman T, Going S, Pamenter R, et al. Effects of resistance training on regional and total bone mineral density in premenopausal women: a randomized prospective study. J Bone Miner Res 1995;10:1015.
131. Snow-Harter C, Bouxsein M, Lewis BT, Carter DR, Marcus R. Effects of resistance and endurance exercise on bone mineral status of young women: A randomized exercise intervention trial. J Bone Miner Res 1992;7:761–769.
132. Winters KM, Snow CM. Detraining reverses positive effects of exercise on the musculoskeletal system in premenopausal women. J Bone Miner Res 2000;15:2495–2503.
133. Snow CM, Williams DP, LaRiviere J, Fuchs RK, Robinson TL. Bone gains and losses follow seasonal training and detraining in gymnasts. Calcif Tissue Int 2001;69:7–12.
134. Beck BR, Doecke JD. Seasonal bone mass of college and senior female field hockey players. J Sports Med Phys Fitness 2005;45:347–354.
135. Kato T, Terashima T, Yamashita T, Hatanaka Y, Honda A, Umemura Y. Effect of low-repetition jump training on bone mineral density in young women. J Appl Physiol 2006;100:839–843.
136. Vainionpaa A, Korpelainen R, Leppaluoto J, Jamsa T. Effects of high-impact exercise on bone mineral density: a randomized controlled trial in premenopausal women. Osteoporos Int 2005;16:191–197.
137. Heinonen A, Kannus P, Sievanen H, et al. Randomised controlled trial of effect of high-impact exercise on selected risk factors for osteoporotic fractures [see comments]. Lancet 1996;348:1343–1347.
138. Heinonen A, Kannus P, Sievanen H, et al. Randomised controlled trial of effect of high-impact exercise on selected risk factors for osteoporotic fractures. Lancet 1996;348:1343–1347.

139. Winters KM, Snow CM. Detraining reverses positive effects of exercise on the musculoskeletal system in premenopausal women. J. Bone Miner Res 2000;15:2495–2503.
140. Dornemann TM, McMurray RG, Renner JB, Anderson JJ. Effects of high-intensity resistance exercise on bone mineral density and muscle strength of 40–50-year-old women. J Sports Med Phys Fitness 1997;37:246–251.
141. Heinonen A, Oja P, Sievanen H, Pasanen M, Vuori I. Effect of two training regimens on bone mineral density in healthy perimenopausal women: A randomized controlled trial. J Bone Miner Res 1998;13:483–490.
142. Pruitt LA, Jackson RD, Bartells RL, Lehnhard HJ. Weight-training effects on bone mineral density in early postmenopausal women. J Bone Miner Res 1992;7:179–185.
143. Grove KA, Londeree BR. Bone density in postmenopausal women: high impact vs low impact exercise. Med Sci Sports Exerc 1992;24:1190–1194.
144. Wu J, Oka J, Tabata I, et al. Effects of isoflavone and exercise on BMD and fat mass in postmenopausal Japanese women: a 1-year randomized placebo-controlled trial. J Bone Miner Res 2006;21:780–789.
145. Maddalozzo G, Maddalozzo GF, Widrick JJ, Cardinal BJ, Winters-Stone KM, Hoffman MA, Snow CM. The effects of hormone replacement therapy and resistance training on spine bone mineral density in early postmenopausal women. Bone 2007;40(5):1244–1251.
146. Cussler EC, Going SB, Houtkooper LB, et al. Exercise frequency and calcium intake predict 4-year bone changes in postmenopausal women. Osteoporos Int 2005;16:2129–2141.
147. Revel M, Mayoux-Benhamou MA, Rabourdin JP, Bagheri F, Roux C. One-year psoas training can prevent lumbar bone loss in postmenopausal women: a randomized controlled trial. Calcif Tissue Int 1993;53:307–311.
148. Smidt GL, Lin SY, O′Dwyer KD, Blanpied PR. The effect of high-intensity trunk exercise on bone mineral density of postmenopausal women. Spine 1992;17:280–285.
149. Engelke K, Kemmler W, Lauber D, Beeskow C, Pintag R, Kalender WA. Exercise maintains bone density at spine and hip EFOPS: a 3-year longitudinal study in early postmenopausal women. Osteoporos Int 2006;17:133–142.
150. Pruitt LA, Taaffe DR, Marcus R. Effects of a one-year high-intensity versus low-intensity resistance training program on bone mineral density in older women. J Bone Miner Res 1995;10:1788–1795.
151. Sinaki M, Wahner HW, Offord KP, Hodgson SF. Efficacy of nonloading exercises in prevention of vertebral bone loss in postmenopausal women: a controlled trial. Mayo Clin Proc 1989;64:762–769.
152. Bassey EJ, Ramsdale SJ. Weight-bearing exercise and ground reaction forces: A 12-month randomized controlled trial of effects on bone mineral density in healthy postmenopausal women. Bone 1995;16: 469–476.
153. Martyn-St James M, Carroll S. High-intensity resistance training and postmenopausal bone loss: a meta-analysis. Osteoporos Int 2006;17:1225–1240.
154. Liu-Ambrose TY, Khan KM, Eng JJ, Heinonen A, McKay HA. Both resistance and agility training increase cortical bone density in 75- to 85-year-old women with low bone mass: a 6-month randomized controlled trial. J Clin Densitom 2004;7:390–398.
155. Karinkanta S, Heinonen A, Sievanen H, et al. A multi-component exercise regimen to prevent functional decline and bone fragility in home-dwelling elderly women: randomized, controlled trial. Osteoporos Int 2006.
156. Welsh L, Rutherford OM. Hip bone mineral density is improved by high-impact aerobic exercise in postmenopausal women and men over 50 years. Eur J Appl Physiol Occup Physiol 1996;74:511–517.
157. Krolner B, Toft B, Nielsen SP, Tondevold E. Physical exercise as prophylaxis against involutional vertebral bone loss: a controlled trial. Clinical Science 1983;64:541–546.
158. Vainionpaa A, Korpelainen R, Sievanen H, Vihriala E, Leppaluoto J, Jamsa T. Effect of impact exercise and its intensity on bone geometry at weight-bearing tibia and femur. Bone 2006.
159. Williams JA, Wagner J, Wasnich R, Heilbrun L. The effect of long-distance running upon appendicular bone mineral content. Med Sci Sports Exerc 1984;16:223–227.
160. Rundgren A, Aniansson A, Ljungberg P, Wetterqvist H. Effects of a training programme for elderly people on mineral content of the heel bone. Arch Gerontol Geriatr 1984;3:243–248.
161. Chubak J, Ulrich CM, Tworoger SS, et al. Effect of exercise on bone mineral density and lean mass in postmenopausal women. Med Sci Sports Exerc 2006;38:1236–1244.

162. Bravo G, Gauthier P, Roy PM, Payette H, Gaulin P. A weight-bearing, water-based exercise program for osteopenic women: its impact on bone, functional fitness, and well-being. Arch Phys Med Rehabil 1997;78:1375–1380.
163. Cavanaugh DJ, Cann CE. Brisk walking does not stop bone loss in postmenopausal women. Bone 1988;9:201–204.
164. Gilsanz V, Wren TA, Sanchez M, Dorey F, Judex S, Rubin C. Low-level, high-frequency mechanical signals enhance musculoskeletal development of young women with low BMD. J Bone Miner Res 2006;21:1464–1474.
165. Johnell O, Eisman J. Whole lotta shakin′ goin′ on. J Bone Miner Res 2004;19:1205–1207.
166. Rubin C, Recker R, Cullen D, Ryaby J, McCabe J, McLeod K. Prevention of postmenopausal bone loss by a low-magnitude, high-frequency mechanical stimuli: a clinical trial assessing compliance, efficacy, and safety. J Bone Miner Res 2004;19:343–351.
167. Verschueren SM, Roelants M, Delecluse C, Swinnen S, Vanderschueren D, Boonen S. Effect of 6-month whole body vibration training on hip density, muscle strength, and postural control in postmenopausal women: a randomized controlled pilot study. J Bone Miner Res 2004;19:352–359.
168. Beck BR, Kent K, Holloway L, Marcus R. Novel, high frequency, low strain, mechanical loading for premenopausal women with low bone mass: early findings. J Bone Miner Metab 2006;24(6):505–507.
169. Shaw JM, Snow CM. Weighted vest exercise improves indices of fall risk in older women. J Gerontol A Biol Sci Med Sci 1998;53:M53–M58.
170. Nevill AM, Burrows M, Holder RL, Bird S, Simpson D. Does lower-body BMD develop at the expense of upper-body BMD in female runners? Med Sci Sports Exerc 2003;35:1733–1739.
171. Simkin A, Ayalon J, Leichter I. Increased trabecular bone density due to bone-loading exercises in postmenopausal osteoporotic women. Calcif Tissue Int 1987;40:59–63.
172. Ayalon J, Simkin A, Leichter I, Raifmann S. Dynamic bone loading exercises for postmenopausal women: effect on the density of the distal radius. Arch Phys Med Rehabil 1987;68:280–283.
173. Notelovitz M, Martin D, Tesar R, et al. Estrogen therapy and variable-resistance weight training increase bone mineral in surgically menopausal women. J Bone Miner Res 1991;6:583–590.
174. Going S, Lohman T, Houtkooper L, et al. Effects of exercise on bone mineral density in calcium-replete postmenopausal women with and without hormone replacement therapy. Osteoporos Int 2003;14: 637–643.
175. Kohrt WM, Ehsani AA, Birge SJ, Jr. HRT preserves increases in bone mineral density and reductions in body fat after a supervised exercise program. J Appl Physiol 1998;84:1506–1512.
176. Heikkinen J, Kurttila-Matero E, Kyllonen E, Vuori J, Takala T, Vaananen HK. Moderate exercise does not enhance the positive effect of estrogen on bone mineral density in postmenopausal women. Calcif Tissue Int 1991;49:S83–S84.
177. Heikkinen J, Kyllonen E, Kurttila-Matero E, et al. HRT and exercise: effects on bone density, muscle strength and lipid metabolism. A placebo controlled 2-year prospective trial on two estrogen-progestin regimens in healthy postmenopausal women. Maturitas 1997;26:139–149.
178. Judge JO, Kleppinger A, Kenny A, Smith JA, Biskup B, Marcella G. Home-based resistance training improves femoral bone mineral density in women on hormone therapy. Osteoporos Int 2005;16:1096–1108.
179. Valimaki VV, Loyttyniemi E, Valimaki MJ. Quantitative ultrasound variables of the heel in Finnish men aged 18–20 yr: predictors, relationship to bone mineral content, and changes during military service. Osteoporos Int 2006;17:1763–1771.
180. Margulies JY, Simkin A, Leichter I, et al. Effect of intense physical activity on the bone-mineral content in the lower limbs of young adults. J Bone Joint Surg 1986;68:1090–1093.
181. Nordstrom A, Olsson T, Nordstrom P. Sustained benefits from previous physical activity on bone mineral density in males. J Clin Endocrinol Metab 2006;91:2600–2604.
182. Specker BL. Evidence for an interaction between calcium intake and physical activity on changes in bone mineral density. J Bone Miner Res 1996;11:1539–1544.
183. Courteix D, Jaffre C, Lespessailles E, Benhamou L. Cumulative effects of calcium supplementation and physical activity on bone accretion in premenarchal children: a double-blind randomised placebo-controlled trial. Int J Sports Med 2005;26:332–338.

184. Iuliano-Burns S, Saxon L, Naughton G, Gibbons K, Bass SL. Regional specificity of exercise and calcium during skeletal growth in girls: a randomized controlled trial. J Bone Miner Res 2003;18:156–162.
185. Stear SJ, Prentice A, Jones SC, Cole TJ. Effect of a calcium and exercise intervention on the bone mineral status of 16–18-y-old adolescent girls. Am J Clin Nutr 2003;77:985–992.
186. Prince R, Devine A, Dick I, et al. The effects of calcium supplementation (milk powder or tablets) and exercise on bone density in postmenopausal women. J Bone Miner Res 1995;10:1068–1075.
187. Loucks AB, Laughlin GA, Mortola JF, Girton L, Nelson JC, Yen SS. Hypothalamic-pituitary-thyroidal function in eumenorrheic and amenorrheic athletes. J Clin Endocrinol Metab 1992;75:514–518.
188. Ihle R, Loucks AB. Dose-response relationships between energy availability and bone turnover in young exercising women. J Bone Miner Res 2004;19:1231–1240.
189. Tomten SE, Falch JA, Birkeland KI, Hemmersbach P, Hostmark AT. Bone mineral density and menstrual irregularities. A comparative study on cortical and trabecular bone structures in runners with alleged normal eating behavior. Int J Sports Med 1998;19:92–97.
190. Zanker CL, Cooke CB. Energy balance, bone turnover, and skeletal health in physically active individuals. Med Sci Sports Exerc 2004;36:1372–1381.
191. Loucks AB, Stachenfeld NS, DiPietro L. The female athlete triad: do female athletes need to take special care to avoid low energy availability? Med Sci Sports Exerc 2006;38:1694–1700.
192. Loucks AB. Refutation of "the myth of the female athlete triad". Br J Sports Med 2007;41:55–57; author reply 57–58.
193. DiPietro L, Stachenfeld NS. The myth of the female athlete triad. Br J Sports Med 2006;40:490–493.
194. Robinson TL, Snow-Harter C, Taaffe DR, Gillis D, Shaw J, Marcus R. Gymnasts exhibit higher bone mass than runners despite similar prevalence of amenorrhea and oligomenorrhea. J Bone Miner Res 1995;10:26–35.
195. Constantini NW, Warren MP. Special problems of the female athlete. Baillieres Clin Rheumatol 1994;8:199–219.
196. Loucks AB, Heath EM. Induction of low-T3 syndrome in exercising women occurs at a threshold of energy availability. Am J Physiol 1994;266:R817–R823.
197. Hartard M, Bottermann P, Bartenstein P, Jeschke D, Schwaiger M. Effects on bone mineral density of low-dosed oral contraceptives compared to and combined with physical activity. Contraception 1997;55: 87–90.
198. Keen AD, Drinkwater BL. Irreversible bone loss in former amenorrheic athletes [editorial]. Osteoporos Int 1997;7:311–315.
199. Burr DB, Yoshikawa T, Teegarden D, et al. Exercise and oral contraceptive use suppress the normal age-related increase in bone mass and strength of the femoral neck in women 18–31 years of age. Bone 2000;27:855–863.
200. MacConnie SE, Barkan A, Lampman RM, Schork MA, Beitins IZ. Decreased hypothalmic gonadotrophin-releasing hormone secretion in male marathon runners. N Eng J Med 1986;315: 411–417.
201. Hetland ML, Haarbo J, Christiansen C. Low bone mass and high bone turnover in male long distance runners. J Clin Endocrinol Metab 1993;77:770–775.
202. Rowland TW, Morris AH, Kelleher JF, Haag BL, Reiter EO. Serum testosterone response to training in adolescent runners. Am J Dis Child 1987;141:881–883.
203. Wheeler GD, Wall SR, Belcastro AN, Cumming DC. Reduced serum testosterone and prolactin levels in male distance runners. Journal of the American Medical Association 1984;252:514–516.
204. Hackney AC, Sinning WE, Bruot BC. Reproductive hormonal profiles of endurance-trained and untrained males. Med Sci Sports Exerc 1988;20:60–65.
205. Cooper CS, Taaffe DR, Guido D, Packer E, Holloway L, Marcus R. Relationship of chronic endurance exercise to the somatotropic and sex hormone status of older men. Eur J Endocrinol 1998;138: 517–523.
206. Fiore CE, Cottini E, Fargetta C, di Salvio G, Foti R, Raspagliesi M. The effects of muscle-building execise on forearm bone mineral content and osteoblast activity in drug-free and anabolic steroids self-administering young men. Bone Miner 1991;13:77–83.
207. Yarasheski KE, Campbell JA, Kohrt WM. Effect of resistance exercise and growth hormone on bone density in older men. Clin Endocrinol 1997;47:223–229.

208. Taaffe DR, Pruitt L, Riem J, et al. Effect of recombinant human growth hormone on the muscle strength response to resistance exercise in elderly men. J Clin Endocrinol Metab 1994;79:1361–1366.
209. Taaffe DR, Jin IH, Vu TH, Hoffman AR, Marcus R. Lack of effect of recombinant growth hormone (GH) on muscle morphology and GH-insulin-like growth factor expression in resistance-trained elderly men. J Clin Endocrinol Metab 1996;81:421–425.
210. Gregg EW, Cauley JA, Seeley DG, Ensrud KE, Bauer DC. Physical activity and osteoporotic fracture risk in older women. Study of Osteoporotic Fractures Research Group [see comments]. Ann Intern Med 1998;129:81–88.
211. Jaglal SB, Kreiger N, Darlington G. Past and recent physical activity and risk of hip fracture. Am J Epidemiol 1993;138:107–118.
212. Jaglal SB, Kreiger N, Darlington GA. Lifetime occupational physical activity and risk of hip fracture in women. Ann Epidemiol 1995;5:321–324.
213. Schwartz AV, Kelsey JL, Sidney S, Grisso JA. Characteristics of falls and risk of hip fracture in elderly men. Osteoporos Int 1998;8:240–246.
214. Feskanich D, Willett W, Colditz G. Walking and leisure-time activity and risk of hip fracture in postmenopausal women. JAMA 2002;288:2300–2306.
215. Korpelainen R, Korpelainen J, Heikkinen J, Vaananen K, Keinanen-Kiukaanniemi S. Lifelong risk factors for osteoporosis and fractures in elderly women with low body mass index – a population-based study. Bone 2006;39:385–391.
216. Sinaki M, Lynn SG. Reducing the risk of falls through proprioceptive dynamic posture training in osteoporotic women with kyphotic posturing: a randomized pilot study. Am J Phys Med Rehabil 2002;81:241–246.
217. Cummings SR, Melton LJ. Epidemiology and outcomes of osteoporotic fractures. Lancet 2002;359:1761–1767.
218. Norton R, Campbell AJ, Lee-Joe T, Robinson E, Butler M. Circumstances of falls resulting in hip fractures among older people. J Am Geriatr Soc 1997;45:1108–1112.
219. Cummings SR, Black DM, Nevitt MC, et al. Appendicular bone density and age predict hip fracture in women. The Study of Osteoporotic Fractures Research Group [see comments]. JAMA 1990;263: 665–668.
220. Whipple RH, Wolfson LI, Amerman PM. The relationship of knee and ankle weakness to falls in nursing home residents: an isokinetic study. J Am Geriatr Soc 1987;35:13–20.
221. Aniansson A, Zetterberg C, Hedberg M, Henriksson KG. Impaired muscle function with aging. A background factor in the incidence of fractures of the proximal end of the femur. Clin Orthop 1984:193–201.
222. Dargent-Molina P, Favier F, Grandjean H, et al. Fall-related factors and risk of hip fracture: the EPIDOS prospective study. [published erratum appears in Lancet 1996 Aug 10;348(9024):416]. Lancet 1996;348:145–149.
223. Maki BE, Holliday PJ, Topper AK. A prospective study of postural balance and risk of falling in an ambulatory and independent elderly population. J Gerontol 1994;49:M72–M84.
224. Greig AM, Bennell KL, Briggs AM, Wark JD, Hodges PW. Balance impairment is related to vertebral fracture rather than thoracic kyphosis in individuals with osteoporosis. Osteoporos Int 2006.
225. Chan B, Marshall L, Winters K, Faulkner K, Schwartz A, Orwoll E. Incident falls and physical activity and physical performance among older men: The osteoporotic fractures in men (MrOS) study. Am J Epidemiol. 2007;165(6):696–703.
226. Drinkwater BL. Exercise in the prevention of osteoporosis. Osteoporos Int 1993;3:169–171.
227. Allen SH. Exercise considerations for postmenopausal women with osteoporosis. Arthritis Care Res 1994;7:205–214.
228. Korpelainen R, Keinanen-Kiukaanniemi S, Heikkinen J, Vaananen K, Korpelainen J. Effect of exercise on extraskeletal risk factors for hip fractures in elderly women with low BMD: a population-based randomized controlled trial. J Bone Miner Res 2006;21:772–779.
229. Madureira MM, Takayama L, Gallinaro AL, Caparbo VF, Costa RA, Pereira RM. Balance training program is highly effective in improving functional status and reducing the risk of falls in elderly women with osteoporosis: a randomized controlled trial. Osteoporos Int 2006.
230. Robertson MC, Campbell AJ, Gardner MM, Devlin N. Preventing injuries in older people by preventing falls: a meta-analysis of individual-level data. J Am Geriatr Soc 2002;50:905–911.

231. Mileva KN, Naleem AA, Biswas SK, Marwood S, Bowtell JL. Acute effects of a vibration-like stimulus during knee extension exercise. Med Sci Sports Exerc 2006;38:1317–1328.
232. Englund U, Littbrand H, Sondell A, Pettersson U, Bucht G. A 1-year combined weight-bearing training program is beneficial for bone mineral density and neuromuscular function in older women. Osteoporos Int 2005;16:1117–1123.
233. Devereux K, Robertson D, Briffa NK. Effects of a water-based program on women 65 years and over: a randomised controlled trial. Aust J Physiother 2005;51:102–108.
234. Wolfson L, Judge J, Whipple R, King M. Strength is a major factor in balance, gait, and the occurrence of falls. J Gerontol A Biol Sci Med Sci 1995;50:64–67.
235. Lord SR, Ward JA, Williams P, Strudwick M. The effect of a 12-month exercise trial on balance, strength, and falls in older women: a randomized controlled trial. J Am Geriatr Soc 1995;43:1198–1206.
236. Lord SR, Tiedemann A, Chapman K, et al. The effect of an individualized fall prevention program on fall risk and falls in older people: a randomized, controlled trial. J Am Geriatr Soc 2005;53:1296–1304.
237. Barnett A, Smith B, Lord SR, Williams M, Baumand A. Community-based group exercise improves balance and reduces falls in at-risk older people: a randomised controlled trial. Age Ageing 2003;32: 407–414.
238. Lord SR, Castell S, Corcoran J, et al. The effect of group exercise on physical functioning and falls in frail older people living in retirement villages: a randomized, controlled trial. J Am Geriatr Soc 2003;51:1685–1692.
239. Campbell AJ, Robertson MC, Gardner MM, Norton RN, Tilyard MW, Buchner DM. Randomised controlled trial of a general practice programme of home based exercise to prevent falls in elderly women. BMJ 1997;315:1065–1069.
240. Jensen J, Nyberg L, Rosendahl E, Gustafson Y, Lundin-Olsson L. Effects of a fall prevention program including exercise on mobility and falls in frail older people living in residential care facilities. Aging Clin Exp Res 2004;16:283–292.
241. Latham NK, Anderson CS, Lee A, Bennett DA, Moseley A, Cameron ID. A randomized, controlled trial of quadriceps resistance exercise and vitamin D in frail older people: the Frailty Interventions Trial in Elderly Subjects (FITNESS). J Am Geriatr Soc 2003;51:291–299.
242. Shimada H, Obuchi S, Furuna T, Suzuki T. New intervention program for preventing falls among frail elderly people: the effects of perturbed walking exercise using a bilateral separated treadmill. Am J Phys Med Rehabil 2004;83:493–499.
243. Wolf SL, Barnhart HX, Kutner NG, McNeely E, Coogler C, Xu T. Selected as the best paper in the 1990s: Reducing frailty and falls in older persons: an investigation of tai chi and computerized balance training. J Am Geriatr Soc 2003;51:1794–1803.
244. Turner CH. Three rules for bone adaptation to mechanical stimuli. Bone 1998;23:399–407.
245. Turner CH, Robling AG. Designing exercise regimens to increase bone strength. Exerc Sport Sci Rev 2003;31:45–50.
246. Hsieh YF, Turner CH. Effects of loading frequency on mechanically induced bone formation. J Bone Miner Res 2001;16:918–924.
247. Rockwell JC, Sorensen AM, Baker S, et al. Weight training decreases vertebral bone density in premenopausal women: a prospective study. J Clin Endocrinol Metab 1990;71:988–993.
248. Nelson ME, Fisher EC, Dilmanian FA, Dallal GE, Evans WJ. A 1-y walking program and increased dietary calcium in postmenopausal women: effects on bone. Am J Clin Nutr 1991;53:1304–1311.
249. Umemura Y, Ishiko T, Yamauchi T, Kurono M, Mashiko S. Five jumps per day increase bone mass and breaking force in rats. J Bone Miner Res 1997;12:1480–1485.
250. Robling AG, Burr DB, Turner CH. Recovery periods restore mechanosensitivity to dynamically loaded bone. J Exp Biol 2001;204:3389–3399.
251. Fuchs RK, Williams DP, Snow C. Response of growing bones to a jumping protocol of reduced repetitions: a randomized controlled trial, 23rd Annual Meeting of the American Society for Bone and Mineral Research, Phoenix, AR, J Bone Miner Res.2001;16(Suppl 1).
252. Vainionpaa A KR, Vihriala E, Rinta-Paavola A, Leppaluoto J, Jamsa T. Intensity of exercise is associated with bone density change in premenopausal women. Osteoporos Int 2006;17:455–463.
253. Kohrt WM, Bloomfield SA, Little KD, Nelson ME, Yingling VR. American College of Sports Medicine Position Stand: physical activity and bone health. Med Sci Sports Exerc 2004;36:1985–1996.

254. Karlsson M. Does exercise reduce the burden of fractures? A review. Acta Orthop Scand 2002;73: 691–705.
255. Strotmeyer ES, Cauley JA, Schwartz AV, et al. Reduced peripheral nerve function is related to lower hip BMD and calcaneal QUS in older white and black adults: the Health, Aging, and Body Composition Study. J Bone Miner Res 2006;21:1803–1810.
256. Whalen RT, Carter DR, Steele CR. Influence of physical activity on the regulation of bone density. J Biomech 1988;21:825–837.
257. Turner C, Robling A. Designing exercise regimens to increase bone strength. Exercise and Sport Sciences Reviews 2003;331:45–50.
258. Mayoux-Benhamou MA, Roux C, Perraud A, Fermanian J, Rahali-Kachlouf H, Revel M. Predictors of compliance with a home-based exercise program added to usual medical care in preventing post-menopausal osteoporosis: an 18-month prospective study. Osteoporos Int 2005;16:325–331.

10 The Physiology and Cell Biology of Calcium Transport in Relation to the Development of Osteoporosis

Richard L. Prince, MD

Contents

Key Words: Calcium transport, calcium homeostasis, organ level regulation, extracellular calcium balance

INTRODUCTION TO THE PHYSIOLOGY AND CELL BIOLOGY OF CALCIUM HOMEOSTASIS

This chapter will review the physiological and cell biological basis of the effects of hormonal agents on transmembrane calcium transport and their consequent effects on bone biology. In the short term, extracellular calcium balance is far more important to the survival of the individual than total body calcium. The vital role that calcium plays as a second messenger in cell signaling processes highlights its importance in a wide range of cellular activities and its fundamental importance to the sustenance of health. In addition to this central role in the functioning of all cells, calcium also has a specific role in the conduction

From: *Contemporary Endocrinology: Osteoporosis: Pathophysiology and Clinical Management*
Edited by: R. A. Adler, DOI 10.1007/978-1-59745-459-9_10,

of action potentials along nerves and in the coupling of excitation and contraction in striated and cardiac muscle. Since the skeleton contains most of the total body calcium (1–2 kg), it is this compartment that compensates for any reduction in extracellular calcium and does so at the expense of bone mineral.

Consequently, it is the tension between the requirements of separate body compartments that sets the scene for the importance of calcium nutrition in the prevention and treatment of many of the causes of osteoporosis. In light of these issues, the principal focus of this chapter will be the mechanisms regulating extracellular calcium levels and how these affect bone structure and function resulting in osteoporosis.

Calcium deficiency as a cause of loss of skeletal structures has been recognized for years *(1)*. However, the complexity and efficiency of the systems, defending both extracellular calcium and the mechanical aspects of the skeleton, have led to a lack of understanding of the important role that deficient calcium nutrition plays in the development of various causes of osteoporosis, in particular following gonadal failure. This chapter sets out to review the mechanisms controlling calcium in the various body compartments and how these interact to protect the skeleton from damage due to a low dietary calcium and how these fail under the influence of gonadal hormone deficiency, intestinal and renal disorders.

Overview of Organ Level Regulation of Calcium Homeostasis

At the tissue level, the principal organs involved in extracellular calcium homeostasis are bone, gut, and kidney, as it is these structures that regulate the principal flow of calcium into or out of the extracellular space (Fig. 1). It is critically important to realize that calcium is continually cycling in and out of the bloodstream bathing these organs. In the kidney 98% of the dialyzed calcium filtered at the glomerulus is reabsorbed, approximating 150 mmol/day. In the bone, it can be calculated that 5–10 mmol/day of calcium cycles into and out of the skeleton. In the bowel, calcium is secreted into the lumen as part of the secretions from the exocrine pancreas, bile, and intestinal enterocyte amounting to about 4 mmol/day. Food contributes about 20 mmol of calcium to intestinal calcium. Approximately 7.0 mmol of calcium is absorbed and reabsorbed in the gut per day. Thus, calcium is in a state of continuous flux into and out of these principal organs involved in extracellular calcium homeostasis. Similarly, calcium is continually moving in and out of all the cells of the body. Thus the critical issue in the control of this system is to regulate the relative activity of the various organs and cells in order to maintain a constant internal cellular environment.

Overview of Cell Level Regulation of Calcium Homeostasis

A detailed understanding of cell biology is required in order to understand the principal mechanisms involved in transmembrane calcium transportation *(2)*. One of the unifying concepts that will be addressed in this chapter is the similarity between the calcium transport mechanisms in the kidney distal tubule, small intestinal epithelium, and bone cells. These calcium transport mechanisms exist in all three areas to contend with the changing need of the whole organism in order to adapt to times of calcium deprivation as competently as at times of calcium sufficiency.

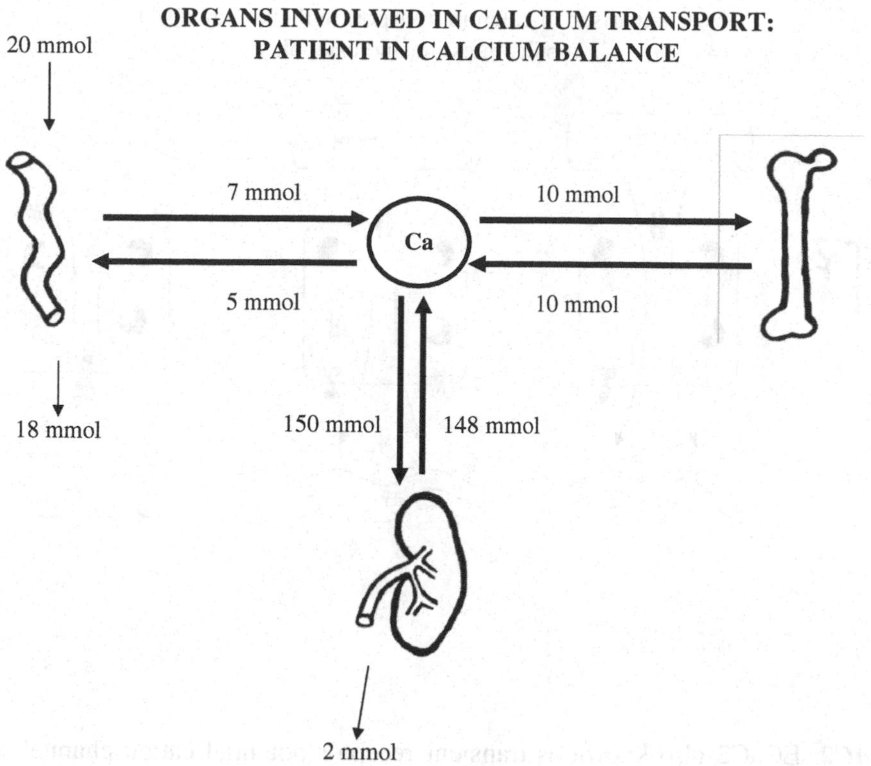

Fig. 1.

Cellular Proteins Involved in Calcium Transport

The transcellular, diffusional-active transport of calcium reabsorption in the kidney and intestine involves three separate components at the subcellular level (Fig. 2).

First, calcium enters the cell across the apical plasma membrane mediated through discrete calcium channels *(3)* characterized at the gene, mRNA, and protein levels as epithelial calcium channel one (ECaC1) *(4)* and two (ECaC2) *(5)*. Second, the presence of two intracellular calcium-binding proteins, appropriately termed calbindin proteins, are thought to expedite transcellular calcium movement and prompt delivery to the opposing, basolateral membrane *(6)*. Lastly, calcium efflux at the basolateral membrane occurs via two active transport mechanisms on the basolateral membrane to subserve this purpose: the plasma membrane calcium ATPase (PMCA) *(7)* and the Na^+/Ca^{2+} (NCX) exchanger *(8)*.

ECaCs

ECaC1. The epithelial calcium channel is an 83 kDa 729 amino acid protein localized to the apical membrane of enterocytes and distal tubule cells *(4)*. There are a variety of alternate names for this protein including transient receptor potential cation channel, subfamily V, member 5 (TrpV5); osm-9-like TRP channel 3 (OTRPC3); and calcium transport protein 2 (CaT2).

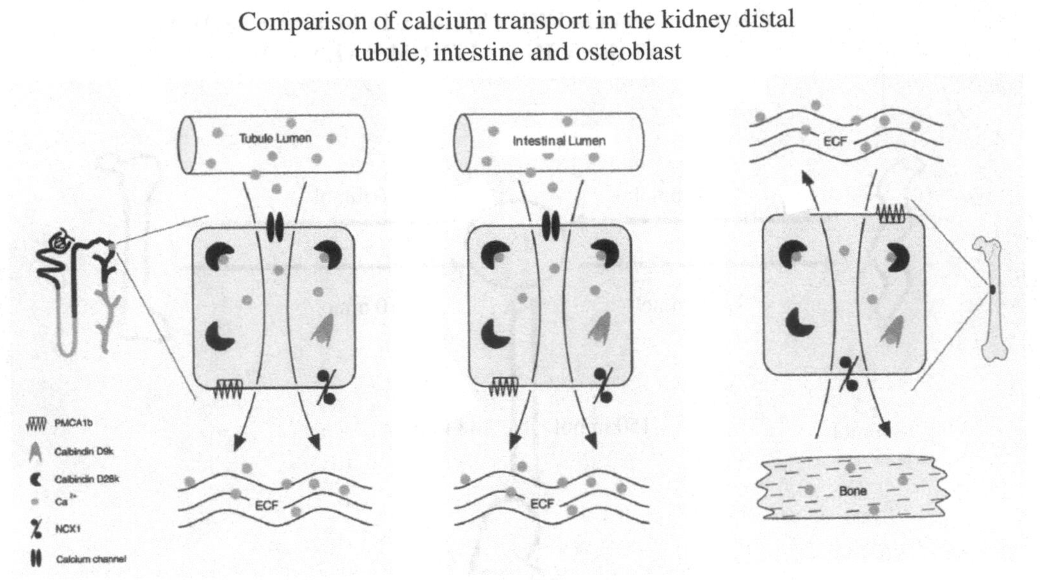

Fig. 2.

ECaC2. ECaC2 also known as transient receptor potential cation channel, subfamily V, member 6 (TrpV6) and calcium transport protein 1 (CaT1) has 727 amino acids *(5)*. Both are found on chromosome 7. The proteins contain six transmembrane domains with the putative calcium transport region occurring between transmembrane domains five and six. Both combine in tetramers to facilitate calcium transport and both bind calbindins and possibly calmodulin *(9)*. In the rat, ECaC1 is expressed at higher concentration in the kidney while ECaC2 is more highly expressed in the intestine; however not only is there evidence of co-expression in the same cell, but also evidence that they may be co-expressed in the same calcium channel structure *(10)*.

CALBINDINS

Calbindin-D$_{28K}$. It is a 28 kDa cytoplasmic protein of approximately 261 amino acid residues. It is a member of the EF-hand helix-loop-helix protein family that binds calcium with high affinity. Each molecule has six high-affinity calcium-binding sites although only four are active *(11)*. The distribution of calbindin-D$_{28K}$ has been shown to be widespread in mammalian tissue. In addition to classical transport tissue including the distal convoluted tubule and collecting duct of the kidney, the intestinal enterocyte in some species, and the osteoblast, calbindin-D$_{28K}$ expression has also been found in neurons, in pancreatic islet cells, and in testes.

Calbindin-D$_{9K}$. It is another high-affinity calcium-binding protein containing two EF-hand structures. It has little sequence homology with calbindin-D$_{28K}$, consisting of about 79 amino acid residues and two high-affinity calcium-binding sites *(11)*. The tissue distribution of calbindin-D$_{9K}$ has similarities to that of calbindin-D$_{28K}$ except that it is more highly expressed in the intestine than calbindin-D$_{28K}$.

PMCAs

At least four different genes code for the pump (PMCA1-4), and post-transcriptional modification of each primary gene transcript produces distinct isoforms which create an even greater diversity of functional consequences *(12,13)*. PMCAs are members of the P-type ATPase family, are calmodulin dependent, and form phosphorylated intermediates. Calmodulin affinity chromatography was the first method utilized to separate and purify PMCA *(13)*. The PMCAs consists of a single 130–140kDa polypeptide chain with around 75% identical amino acids recognized between each isoform. The amino acid residues which are near identical or similar between each isoform are not scattered throughout the polypeptide chain but are restricted to several highly conserved regions within the protein *(14)*. The site of ATP binding and the site of phosphorylation represent two of these highly conserved regions.

NCXs

The Na^+/Ca^{2+} (NCX) exchanger *(8)* has three isoforms. It is a secondary active transport protein which uses the electrochemical gradient produced by sodium ATPase activity to move calcium across the basolateral membrane *(15)*. Although NCX is particularly abundant in cells that handle large fluxes of calcium across their membranes such as contractile and neuronal cells, in the regulation of calcium transport across the kidney and intestine only NCX1 has been identified. It is a 970 amino acid protein with a primary structure that contains 11 transmembrane spanning regions and a large cytoplasmic loop between transmembrane segments 6 and 7. The orientation of NCX is determined by the predominance of two inwardly directed electrochemical gradients generated by plasma membrane sodium and calcium pumps.

Regulation of Calcium Transport

PTH and Vitamin D

In light of the fact that three organs are intimately involved in extracellular calcium regulation, it is clear that endocrine regulation plays a leading role in coordinating responses to calcium excess or deficiency. Two hormones, PTH and calcitriol, play a major role in regulating extracellular calcium concentrations on a minute-to-minute basis (Fig. 3). For example, if the dietary calcium intake is reduced, the coordinated action of PTH and calcitriol causes increased absorption of calcium from the bowel, urine, and bone compartments to correct the extracellular deficit *(16)*.

By feedback regulation between themselves, they influence the relative levels of the two hormones and work in a coordinated way to influence the movement of calcium across membranes in the bowel, kidney, or bone to maintain the calcium concentrations in the extracellular compartment. Parathyroid hormone (PTH) is regulated by the concentration of calcium in the extracellular fluid via a G protein-linked calcium receptor in the membrane of parathyroid hormone cells and proximal tubule cells of the kidney, the calcium-sensing receptor *(17)*, and thus may play the lead sensing and activation role in correcting calcium deficits.

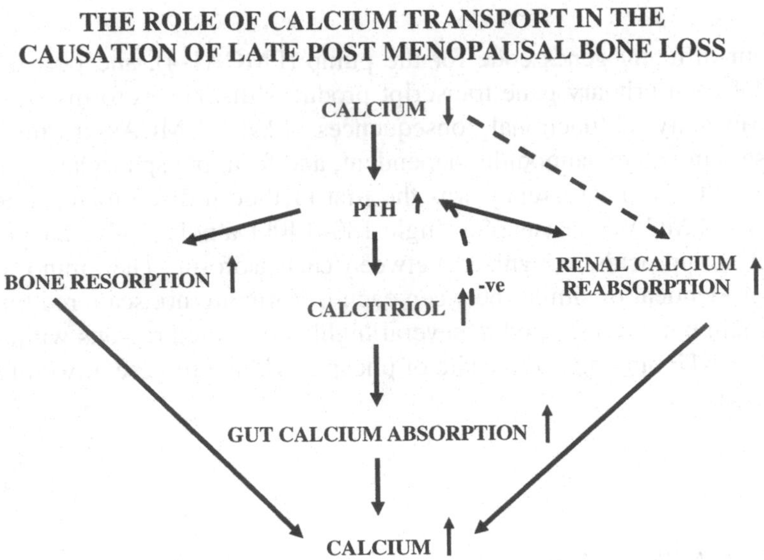

Fig. 3.

Gonadal Hormones

Estrogen deficiency plays a central role in the development of postmenopausal osteoporosis and also has an important role in male osteoporosis *(18)*, and there is a prima facie case for the involvement of estrogen in the regulation of calcium transport across membranes either directly or indirectly. As indicated in the previous paragraphs there is evidence that estrogen is important in determining the rate of flux of calcium into and out of the bone, kidney tubule, and bowel lumen and thus can indirectly determine circulating concentrations of PTH and calcitriol *(19)*.

The role of estrogen deficiency appears to be involved in the release of calcium from specific skeletal sites, particularly those with trabecular bone. It is possible that the physiological connection between estrogen deficiency and skeletal calcium mobilization relates to supply of calcium for lactation *(20)*. Parallels with avian species are appropriate in that medullary bone formation, a prominent source of calcium supply for the eggshell, is thought to be dependent on estrogen for its development .

In light of evidence that estrogen deficiency is a critical determinant of male osteoporosis, it is likely that similar factors may be operating in the male *(18)*.

Calcium

Calcium itself has been shown to regulate calcium transport in the kidney and osteoclast via a short-loop feedback system involving the calcium-sensing receptor (CaSR) located along the renal tubule and on the surface of the mature osteoclast. Mutations within the CaSR are of course the genetic basis for familial hypocalciuric hypercalcemia (FHH). In addition CaSR is the primary regulatory protein controlling PTH production in the parathyroid gland *(21)*.

Relevance to Osteoporosis

Abnormal calcium transport plays a role in the etiology of a variety of causes of osteoporosis including estrogen and testosterone deficiency, vitamin D deficiency, intestinal malabsorption, and hypercalciuria-related osteoporosis. These disorders are usually more serious in the presence of genetically determined low-peak bone mass which may occasionally affect the calcium homeostatic system. For example, there are data to implicate variation in the vitamin D receptor gene leading to reduced intestinal calcium absorption and possibly a predisposition to osteoporosis *(22)*.

THE ROLE OF THE KIDNEY IN EXTRACELLULAR CALCIUM BALANCE

Physiology of Calcium Handling in the Nephron

The kidneys filter approximately 100–200 mmol of calcium per 24 h of which about 98% is reabsorbed. Because of the high rate at which calcium is cycling across the renal tubular membrane, it is possible for subtle variations in the rate of reabsorption to have profound effects on the extracellular calcium balance. Approximately 70% of calcium reabsorption occurs in the proximal tubule *(23)* and is largely passive, voltage-dependent, and associated with active reabsorption of sodium, glucose, and other solutes.

There is evidence that three dietary constituents influence renal calcium excretion. These are sodium chloride, protein, and food acid. The overall effect on skeletal calcium depends on the ability of the intestine to increase calcium absorption and thus maintain calcium balance without requiring increased bone resorption. Sodium competes with calcium for reabsorption in the proximal and distal tubule as demonstrated by the association between sodium excretion and calcium excretion *(24)*. These data seem specific for sodium chloride as other sodium salts, such as bicarbonate or citrate, do not increase renal calcium excretion *(25,26)*. In a 2-year, prospective, epidemiological study of the effects of sodium intake on bone mass in elderly postmenopausal women, higher sodium intake was associated with a greater degree of bone loss *(27)*. In the same cohort, high calcium intake prevented bone loss and the interaction of both minerals predicted the change in bone mass better than either alone.

Dietary protein intake increases renal calcium excretion *(28,29)*. The protein effect may increase glomerular filtration rate; however, the effect appears to be related to excretion of fixed organic acid as a result of protein metabolism of sulfur-containing amino acids, in particular. Certainly the effect can be reversed by increasing alkali intake at the same time *(30)*. In population studies of the effects of dietary intake in renal calculi, there was no excess risk of protein intakes over 76 g/day compared to intakes under 42 g/day *(31)*. In old age there is evidence that a protein supplement will improve bone density and clinical outcomes after hip fracture *(32)*. In postmenopausal women there is a positive association between protein intake and IGF1 levels *(33)* and protein intake and bone mass *(34)*.

The effect of alkali to reduce renal calcium excretion is well described and has been attributed to effects on bone resorption and renal calcium excretion *(35,36)*. The primary effect is uncertain and indeed it is likely that effects on both bone and kidney may be linked as a method of buffering excess food acid.

Cell Biology of Renal Epithelial Transport

The specific mechanism of transcellular calcium transport in the kidney distal tubule involves the ECaC, the calbindins, and PMCA and NCX.

ECaC1

An apical influx channel in the distal kidney tubule (ECaC1) has been characterized, although it is unknown whether this channel is hormonally regulated *(4)*.

Calbindin D_{28K} and Calbindin D_{9K}

Two other calcium transporters exist within the cytosol of the epithelial cells lining the distal kidney tubule and were named according to their cellular mass as calbindin D_{28K} and calbindin D_{9K} *(37)*. While hypercalciuria develops in the calbindin D_{28K} knockout mouse, circulating serum calcium levels are maintained due to the fact that both D_{28K} and D_{9K} play a role in renal calcium transport *(38)*. Chronic metabolic acidosis has also been noted to increase calbindin D_{28K} expression in rat kidney distal tubule *(39)*.

NCX1

NCX is expressed on the basolateral membrane of the kidney distal tubule (40–42). Stimulation of the Na^+–H^+ antiporter in the distal kidney tubule by calbindin D_{28K}, which reduces intracellular sodium and may consequently increase calcium transport, highlights one mechanism that may explain how calbindin D_{28K} may influence NCX1 activity in this cell *(43)*.

PMCA

PMCA is expressed on the basolateral membrane of the kidney distal tubule in conjunction with NCX *(37,42)*. The availability of isogene-specific antibodies to PMCA confirmed results of earlier immunohistochemical studies with the detection of PMCA1 and PMCA4 but not PMCA2 and PMCA3 isogenes in human kidney crude plasma membranes using polyclonal antibodies specific for each of the four isogenes of PMCA *(44)*. This finding was verified using crude microsomal preparations from human kidney and monoclonal antibodies to PMCA1, PMCA4a, and PMCA4b *(45)*. Thus, all four transport proteins probably act in a coordinated fashion to regulate calcium excretion in the distal kidney tubule.

Regulation of Renal Calcium Transport

It is clear that the kidney is a vital part of the regulation of extracellular calcium in humans. However, the exact mechanisms whereby this occurs have proved difficult to characterize because of the complexity of the interacting systems. It has of course been essential to undertake most of the work in non-primate species. In view of the species variation, it is difficult to categorically extend the data to humans. Finally, the nutritional and hormonal status pertaining to the experimental situation is not always specified, again making extrapolation difficult.

CALCITRIOL

ECaC 1 and 2, PMCA1b, calbindin D_{28K}, and calbindin D_{9K} are all upregulated by calcitriol *(46)*. Vitamin D deficiency has no effect on NCX1 activity indicating that this transporter is unlikely to be regulated by vitamin D *(47)*. While several isoforms of PMCA exist within the kidney, only one isoform (PMCA1b) appears to be hormonally responsive. PMCA1b is regulated by calcitriol in rabbit and bovine distal kidney tubule cells (48–50), and it is probably this effect that accounts for the increased calcium reabsorption demonstrable in calcitriol-treated vitamin D-deficient rabbits *(47)*.

The mechanism for activation of PMCA probably involves calbindin D_{28K} and calbindin D_{9K}, both of which are upregulated by calcitriol in the chick *(51)*, rat *(52)*, and mouse *(53)*, probably by transcriptional regulation *(54)*.

PTH

Regulation by parathyroid hormone (PTH) and cAMP occurs predominantly in the distal tubule *(55)*. Within the kidney distal tubule, NCX1 has been shown to be the primary mechanism by which PTH modulates renal calcium reabsorption *(56)*. Phospholipase D and protein kinase C are involved in PTH-induced calcium reabsorption in the distal kidney tubule *(57)*.

ESTROGEN

Estrogen increases calbindin D_{28K} expression in rat kidney indicating a possible common mechanism of hormonal regulation in the kidney *(58)*. Recent studies in our laboratory have shown that distal kidney tubule PMCA is also directly regulated by estrogen and testosterone in vitro *(59)*. In postmenopausal women the effect size of estrogen on renal calcium excretion is similar to PTH *(60)*. A recent review discusses these issues in relation to renal physiology *(61)*.

CALCIUM

Renal calcium handling is regulated by the CaSR within various locations along the renal tubule *(62,63)*. Paracellular and transcellular calcium transport in the cortical ascending limb is regulated by the extracellular ionized calcium concentration that acts via the CaSR *(64)*.

THE ROLE OF THE INTESTINE IN EXTRACELLULAR CALCIUM BALANCE

The Physiology of Calcium Handling in the Intestine

In the adult human, 40–90% of the calcium consumed each day is excreted in feces and 10–60% is absorbed by the intestine. Three processes determine the overall role of the intestine in calcium balance. These are dietary calcium consumption, intestinal secretions containing calcium, and intestinal calcium absorption. It is not sufficiently recognized that calcium is entering the bowel not only from dietary consumption but also from pancreatic, bile, and enterocyte secretions into the intestine. The secreted calcium from these latter sources, which is not reabsorbed, is entitled the endogenous fecal calcium. It is important to note that under conditions of low calcium intake, it is possible to excrete more calcium in the feces from pancreatic, bile, and enterocyte secretions than is consumed in the diet. Further, it is claimed that the magnitude of the endogenous fecal calcium is equivalent to the urine calcium in perimenopausal women *(65)*. Under these circumstances the individual will be in negative calcium balance in the bowel compartment. Net calcium absorption is the difference between the net amount of calcium consumed and the amount excreted as fecal calcium excretion. True calcium absorption takes into account the amount of calcium secreted into the intestine.

There are several known determinants of intestinal calcium secretion. In women these include dietary phosphate intake *(66)* and oophorectomy in rats *(67)*. However, the exact site of the action of these determinants or indeed the direct effects of calcitropic hormones on intestinal calcium secretion is unknown.

Gut calcium absorption is determined first by the intraluminal concentration of calcium achieved at various points in the bowel and second by gut wall factors determining absorption efficiency, including the vitamin D status. The actual site of calcium absorption in the bowel varies depending on the magnitude of the calcium load in the food and on its rate of transit through the bowel. In general, 95% of calcium absorption occurs in the small bowel. Duodenal absorption, although having the highest rate of active absorption, is not the most important site for calcium absorption on a quantitative basis, except at very low calcium intakes. This is because the time that calcium resides within the duodenum is relatively short.

Intestinal Factors Affecting Intestinal Calcium Absorption

Lactose

In normal subjects lactose increases calcium absorption from 22 to 36% *(68)*. However, in patients with lactose intolerance, lactose will itself induce a reduction in calcium absorption of about 5% *(68)*. This may be due to the osmotic effects of the lactose reducing the effective concentration of calcium within the bowel *(69)*. The connection between lactose intolerance and osteoporotic fracture would appear to be due to a reduced calcium intake associated with avoidance of milk products *(70,71)*.

Fiber

High-fiber diets have been recommended for various benefits on the bowel and cardiovascular system. Studies that have examined the effects of these diets on calcium consumption have not found any significant deleterious effects, at least from moderate consumption of fiber-containing foods *(72)*. However, at high-fiber intakes, calcium retention is reduced from 25 to 19% *(73)*.

Achlorhydria

It has been shown that in achlorhydric individuals the absorption of calcium when administered as calcium carbonate is less than when administered as calcium citrate. This differential absorption is abolished if the calcium is taken with food *(74)*. Certainly, in terms of preventing bone loss, calcium lactate gluconate has identical effects to milk powder that contains the same amount of calcium *(75,76)*.

Mechanisms of Intestinal Calcium Absorption

The absorption of calcium occurs by transcellular and paracellular mechanisms. In general, the paracellular route is considered to be unregulated, although there is some evidence that vitamin D can stimulate the non-saturable phase of calcium transport *(77,78)*. The driving force behind the paracellular route of calcium uptake is thought to be mediated by the concentration gradient and solvent drag. Paracellular movement of calcium takes place throughout the length of the intestine and may account for two-thirds of calcium flux in the rat intestine. In the human, passive paracellular absorption appears to have an absorption efficiency of about 15%. Thus, at high dietary intakes, it may be possible to supply sufficient calcium to maintain extracellular homeostasis from this source. Paracellular movement favors absorption in the duodenum, with paracellular calcium secretion occurring in the jejunum and ileum indicating that net calcium absorption is determined by transcellular mechanisms as well as the net difference between paracellular absorption and secretion *(78,79)*. There are two mechanisms of transcellular transport: active transport and transcellular vesicular transport termed transcaltachia *(80)*.

Cell Biology of Intestinal Epithelial Transport

As in the kidney active transport in the enterocyte involves ECaCs, calbindins, NCX1, and PMCA

ECaC

In contrast to the kidney it appears that in mammals in the bowel ECaC2 (CaT1) mRNA is expressed at higher concentrations than ECaC1 transcript *(81)*. The ECaC1 null allele mouse hyperabsorbs calcium from the intestine suggesting that ECaC1 is not an essential component of this physiological activity *(82)*.

Calbindin

In the human calbindin D_{9K} but not calbindin D_{28K} is expressed within the proximal small intestine and exhibits a similar expression profile as PMCA1b *(83)*.

NCX1

NCX1 activity has been shown in the intestine in both rats *(84)* and humans *(85)*.

PMCA

A careful study of rat and human enterocytes has shown that PMCA1 is the predominant transcript especially in the duodenum *(86)*. However, at least in the rat, PMCA1b activity declines with age *(87)*. Both NCX1 and PMCA1 activities have been reported in human small bowel enterocyte preparations *(85)*. In the Hildman study *(84)* which utilized basolateral membrane preparations, PMCA1b had the predominant calcium translocation activity compared to NCX1, suggesting that PMCA1b is the more important mechanism for translocation of calcium in the intestine.

Regulation of Intestinal Calcium Transport

PTH has no direct effect on intestinal calcium transport. It does of course have a potent regulatory effect on the renal production of calcitriol which itself has a potent feedback inhibitory effect on PTH synthesis.

CALCITRIOL

Transcellular calcium transport is stimulated by calcitriol, thus there is evidence that calcitriol stimulates all three proteins involved in calcium transport in the intestine.

ECaC1 and 2 are both regulated by calcitriol in the rat *(46)*. Support for calcitriol control of ECaC2 in the male human duodenum but not in female elderly human duodenum has been published *(88)*. Clearly these findings raise the possibility that circulating estrogen levels may play a role in ECaC2 expression in females.

Calbindin D_{9K} expression correlates with serum calcitriol in animals *(89)* and humans *(90)*. Post-transcriptional reduction in degradation of calbindin D_{9K} appears to be quantitatively more important than transcriptional regulation in the rat *(91)*. There is also evidence that transcription may be reduced with aging in the rat *(89)*. PMCA1b activity and mRNA expression are stimulated by calcitriol in the rat *(87)*.

A rapid stimulation of calcium transport (transcaltachia) by a non-genomic action of calcitriol has been described *(92)*. In this process calcium uptake into lysosomes at the apical membrane is stimulated, with subsequent delivery to the basolateral membrane and a time course in the order of 30 min at least in the chicken *(93)*.

GONADAL HORMONES

Studies in animals confirm that estrogen increases duodenal calcium transport, independent of any effect on serum calcitriol *(94)*. The genes involved in this action have now been characterized and include the expected candidates. However the principal effect was on ECaC2 mRNA expression *(95)* with no effect on VDR expression.

These data support calcium absorption studies in women that show a reduction in calcium absorption at menopause *(96,97)* corrected by estrogen *(98)*.

CALCIUM

Although the calcium-sensing receptor has been reported to be present in the rat intestine *(99)*, its role on calcium homeostasis is uncertain. Interestingly, evidence that feeding with calcium can induce a short-term increase in calbindin D_{9K} has been presented *(100)*.

ROLE OF BONE IN EXTRACELLULAR CALCIUM BALANCE

Although it is universally agreed that the skeleton plays a vital role in extracellular calcium homeostasis, the exact mechanisms underlying this role remain controversial. There are two concepts that are not necessarily in opposition. First, some consider that calcium exit from and entry into the skeleton occurs across the bone extracellular fluid surfaces, perhaps mediated by physicochemical forces, a bone membrane, and/or bone-lining cells in contact with bone. Second and more widely accepted, calcium transport out of and into the bone via the cells involved in the basic multicellular unit, the osteoclast and osteoblast, is considered to be the principal method by which calcium exits or enters the skeleton.

The next problem is that unlike the intestine and kidney where it is absorption of calcium into the extracellular space that is considered to be regulated, in bone there is clearly two-way traffic of calcium into and out of the bone.

The Physiology of Calcium Transport Across Bone Surfaces

The concept that the mechanism by which bone plays a role in extracellular calcium homeostasis related to a physicochemical balance between bone and extracellular fluid (ECF) was developed in the 1950s. It suggests that bone surfaces, without the intervention of lining cells, play a direct regulatory role in calcium homeostasis by virtue of the solubility product balance between bone and ECF *(101)*. The problem that bone was observed to be a very large sink for calcium with a much lower solubility product than ECF was countered by an argument that osteonectin and osteocalcin covering the bone could maintain the supersaturation of the ECF in relation to calcium and provide a "buffering" capacity for calcium at the bone surface *(102)*.

Physiology of Calcium Transport Across Osteoblast/Lining Cells

The bone membrane model in which bone-lining cells play a role in calcium regulation is based on histological and ultrastructural evidence for the presence of a bone-lining cell layer made up of cells which probably arise from the osteoblast cell lineage *(103,104)*. As a result of tracer calcium-45 studies combined with histological studies, this layer is postulated to play a role in the maintenance of extracellular calcium homeostasis and could be modified by hormonal regulators involved in extracellular calcium homeostasis, including PTH and calcitonin (103,105,106). The lining cell concept has also been tied in with the physicochemical concept such that the surface area of the bone available for regulation of extracellular calcium is controlled by the amount of surface covered by cells *(107)*.

The Physiology of Calcium Transport in the Basic Multicellular Unit

Bone structure can be divided into two types: trabecular and cortical bone. Each of these structures undergoes remodeling in which osteoclast-mediated bone resorption is followed by osteoblast-mediated bone formation. The combination of the osteoclast-induced Howship's lacunae and the consequent osteoblast-mediated bone formation to refill the resorption pit comprises the two components that define the basic multicellular unit (BMU). The physiological rationale for the need for constant remodeling relates to removal of stress fractures *(108)* in old bone and is also one of the physiological bases for the maintenance of extracellular calcium homeostasis.

Calcium re-entry into the skeleton occurs at the time of new bone formation by plump osteoblasts associated with the BMU. The mechanism of extracellular calcification in the newly formed osteoid is still uncertain but may require the transport of calcium into the area to allow the formation of hydroxyapatite during the mineralization lag time. Thus calcium transport in the BMU consists of two major components: calcium transport out of the bone under the influence of osteoclastic bone resorption and calcium transport into the bone across the osteoblast to allow for the deposition of hydroxyapatite on the collagen molecule.

The BMU may itself have a localized environment in light of data that a vascular space enclosed by a syncytium of osteoblast-like cells has been observed microscopically in relation to the BMU such that it may form a closed system *(109,110)*.

Cell biology of Calcium Transport in Bone – Osteoclasts and Osteoblasts

OSTEOCLASTS

The mechanism of osteoclast-mediated bone resorption is dependent on developing a low pH in the sub-osteoclastic lacuna to allow dissolution of the hydroxyapatite. This is undertaken by forming hydrogen ions under the action of carbonic anhydrase type II in the cytoplasm and pumping them into the sealed sub-osteoclastic lacuna *(111,112)*. Transport of organic and inorganic bone breakdown products to the extracellular fluid occurs by vesicular transcytosis across the cell from the sealed bone resorption pit *(113)*. However it appears that such vesicular transcytosis may not be the physiological basis for the transport of calcium *(114)*, raising the possibility that the osteoclast uses similar molecular machinery as other calcium transport cells.

In a series of elegant experiments, the proteins associated with transcellular calcium transport in the intestine and kidney (ECaC1, calbindin D_{9K} and D_{28K}, NCX1, and PMCA1b) have been shown to be present in human and mouse osteoclasts *(115)*. NCX transcripts have also been found within the plasma membrane of mouse osteoclasts both on the bone and ECF surfaces, providing a potential pathway for transcellular cytoplasmic transport *(116)*. PMCA has been localized within the chick osteoclast principally on the ECF surface where it may play a role on pumping calcium out of the cell *(117)*.

OSTEOBLAST/LINING CELLS

Review of most of the studies of osteoblast-like cells shows that it is difficult to differentiate cells forming bone in the multicellular unit from those active on bone surfaces without prior resorption or indeed quiescent lining cells. It is now clear that four proteins involved in calcium transport, NCX1, PMCA1b, calbindin D_{9K}, and calbindin D_{28K}, are expressed within the osteoblast, consistent with the notion that the osteoblast plays a direct role in calcium transport in bone. Interestingly, to date ECaC1 has not been found in osteoblast-like cells.

These data provide possible mechanisms for the role of the osteoblast or osteoblast-like cells in calcium transport into and out of the skeleton to support calcification of osteoid or to provide calcium for the extracellular compartment, including control of the life cycle of the cells by an effect on apoptosis. The role of the osteoblast in calcium homeostasis may be independent of the role that the osteoblast plays in the maintenance of skeletal integrity or in bone remodeling.

Calbindin D_{28K} and Calbindin D_{9K}. These have been identified in rat osteoblasts *(118)*. The role of these molecules remains unclear with evidence that a primary role may be to suppress apoptosis of osteoblasts or as a calcium buffer rather than in calcium transport *(119)*.

PMCA1b. It is expressed on the apical plasma membrane of osteoblast-like cells *(117,120)*, in contrast to the intestine and kidney distal tubule where it is expressed on the basolateral membrane.

NCX1. It is localized to the basolateral membrane of the avian osteoblast *(121,122)*. Inhibition of NCX1 has been shown to impair mineralization of bone formed by cultured primary osteoblasts suggesting an important role for this protein in this process *(122)*.

Regulation of Bone Cell Activity in Relation to Extracellular Calcium Homeostasis

Although a large number of factors influence the activity of osteoclasts and osteoblasts and thus may influence the calcium transport into and out of the skeleton, the main ones are PTH, calcitriol, and estrogen. These work together to optimize both the mechanical and extracellular calcium homeostasis of the skeleton during normal and reproductive life. The mechanisms surrounding the action of these hormones on bone cells are still the subject of a huge research effort involving the study of the production, activity, and longevity of the cells of the bone. There is also evidence of a short-loop regulatory effect of extracellular calcium on bone cell activity.

The complexities of the regulation of the overall balance between osteoclast-mediated release of calcium from bone and osteoblast-mediated uptake of calcium into bone in the BMU in relation to maintenance of extracellular calcium homeostasis have not been elucidated *(123)*. The complexities will be considerable, as there are likely to be site-specific effects modulating the overall balance between bone and calcium accretion and dissolution. These site-specific effects will include mechanical effects and the presence of microdamage.

Osteoclasts

Physiological evidence in favor of the importance of osteoclastic activity in calcium homeostasis relates to the action of bisphosphonates which are considered to reduce osteoclast activity rather than alter the physicochemical balance between bone and extracellular fluid. In osteoporosis, osteomalacia, and Paget's disease, bisphosphonates may induce either marked hypocalcemia or secondary hyperparathyroidism (124–126). Calcitonin also plays a direct role in reducing osteoclast activity. However, the importance of this hormone in extracellular calcium homeostasis in humans is uncertain, nor does it play a role in the development of osteoporosis *(127)*.

PTH and Calcitriol. In light of the fact that neither PTH/PTHrP nor vitamin D receptors have been found in mature osteoclasts, it is unlikely that these regulators directly influence osteoclast activity but rather influence the supply of new active osteoclasts to resorption sites. There is a considerable literature on this issue which is covered in other chapters.

One of the potential weaknesses of the concept that the early effect of PTH to increase plasma calcium depends on increasing osteoclastic bone resorption relates to evidence that injected PTH has a demonstrable effect to increase plasma calcium within 4 h *(128)*. If the osteoclast is to play a role in this effect, differentiation of osteoclast precursors into mature bone resorbing osteoclasts would have to occur in this time frame.

Estrogen. In epidemiological terms estrogen deficiency is clearly the most potent factor associated with net transport of calcium out of the skeleton *(19)*. This is considered to occur as a result of an increase in the activation frequency of initiation of BMUs with a consequent increase in osteoclast activity compared to osteoblast activity *(129)*. As with PTH/PTHRP and vitamin D receptors, the evidence that estrogen receptors are found on mature human osteoclasts is controversial *(130)*.

Calcium. There is evidence that osteoclast activity is directly inhibited by high extracellular calcium concentrations, perhaps by inducing apoptosis *(131)*. There are at least two putative mechanisms whereby osteoclast activity could be regulated by calcium. There is some evidence for direct regulation of osteoclast resorptive activity via a membrane ryanodine receptor *(132)*. There is also evidence for mRNA expression for the classical calcium-sensing receptor present in the parathyroid and kidney in mature osteoclasts and osteoclast precursors *(133,134)*. This may allow extracellular calcium sensing by the osteoclast, which may regulate the differentiation and apoptosis of osteoclasts *(135)*.

In conclusion apart from a possible direct effect of ECF calcium on osteoclast-mediated resorption of bone calcium, the various calcitropic hormones are considered to have their effects by control of osteoclast differentiation or apoptosis.

OSTEOBLASTS

PTH and Calcitriol. Human osteoblasts have receptors for calcitriol and PTH. Calcitriol upregulates calbindin D_{28K} protein expression in chick bone and human osteoblasts *(136,137)*, which may play a role in the mineralization of matrix. The effect of calcitriol on PMCA1b has been recently studied in osteoblast-like cells (ROS 17/2.8) and in accord with the kidney distal tubule and intestinal enterocyte, PMCA1b is upregulated by calcitriol *(49,50)*. These effects are consistent with the concept that calcitriol acts to increase the calcium supply to the basolateral side of the osteoblast, which is in contact with the calcifying bone matrix. Nevertheless, bone mineralization can occur in the absence of vitamin D or calcitriol as shown by experiments in 1-hydroxylase or vitamin D receptor knockout animals rescued with a high intake of calcium *(138)*.

Finally, calcitriol and PTH have been reported to downregulate NCX1 expression *(139)*, which may indicate a mechanism for a negative effect on bone mineralization consistent with an effect of both agents to maintain extracellular calcium under certain circumstances (see also Chapter 21).

Estrogen. Human osteoblasts have receptors for estrogen *(130)*. The role of estrogen in relation to the osteoblast has been shown to increase activity and possibly number of osteoblasts and thus to increase bone formation, particularly in the medullary area of the metaphysis *(140,141)* via estrogen receptor alpha *(142)* (see also Chapter 14).

INTEGRATION OF CALCIUM HOMEOSTASIS

In summarizing the data discussed so far, several issues are worthy of more detailed consideration. The similarities in the regulation of calcium transport mechanisms (viz. ECaC1, calbindin D_{28K}, calbindin D_{9K}, PMCA1b, and NCX1) in the kidney, intestine, and bone and evidence that these are regulated by similar hormonal factors suggests that current concepts of regulation of calcium homeostasis by PTH and calcitriol are correct. However, detailed understanding of the effect of endocrine regulators on each part of the Ca^{2+} transport system and how this relates to the optimization of calcium availability in the ECF and bone is still unclear.

Catabolic Effects of PTH and Calcitriol

Interestingly, the localization of PMCA1 on the basolateral or apical membrane differs among organs. In the intestine and kidney it is on the basolateral membrane facing the ECF, while in the osteoclast and osteoblast it is on the apical membrane again facing the ECF. Thus this transporter is ideally located to maintain ECF calcium when stimulated by either PTH or calcitriol or both. These two hormones have the most urgent role in calcium homeostasis to maintain ECF calcium. The role of NCX1 is a little more complicated because in the intestine and kidney, it plays an important role in increasing ECF calcium where it is stimulated by both PTH and calcitriol. In the osteoblast, however, it is located on the bone matrix side of the cell, where its role in calcium transport is unclear.

Anabolic Effects of PTH and Calcitriol

It is clear from much cell, animal, and human data that both hormones play a role in skeletal regeneration. Defining mechanisms whereby PTH and calcitriol may have both a destructive and an anabolic effect on the skeleton has proven difficult. However, at a conceptual level there is a way in which these two aspects of calcium regulatory hormone action could be harmonized.

One of the principal roles of the BMU may be to allow for the possibility of regeneration of bone calcium lost during periods of low calcium intake at the precise site of prior bone resorption. The mechanism for this is the recognized linkage of bone formation to osteoclastic bone resorption within the BMU. Because calcium is cycling in and out of the skeleton on a continuous basis, if the individual is in calcium balance the amount of bone removed by osteoclastic bone resorption will be matched by the amount of bone replaced by osteoblastic bone formation. However, during episodes of calcium deprivation, there is a temporary imbalance in which bone resorption exceeds formation, thus releasing calcium into the circulation *(143)*. During high calcium intakes, the bone hydroxyapatite deficit is replaced by a relative increase in mineralized bone deposition. This constitutes an elegant mechanism for smoothing out the intermittent demands on the skeleton for calcium during periods of dietary calcium deficiency without seriously impairing the mechanical function of the bone. This is because bone is replaced exactly at the site it has been removed from ready to be available for the next episode of calcium deficiency.

ESTROGENS AND ANDROGENS

Although it is clear that estrogens and androgens do not play a regulatory role in the maintenance of extracellular calcium, they clearly play a major role in the development and maintenance of skeletal mass to allow effective reproduction. An essential part of this is supply of calcium to mineralizing sites during bone growth and regeneration. In addition, reduction in estrogen levels during lactation subserves an increase in the formation and survival of osteoclasts while reducing its anabolic effect on osteoblasts to increase the supply of bone calcium for lactation (see Chapters 14 and 16).

CALCIUM

In addition to the calcium regulatory factors outlined above, calcium itself is an important regulator of ECF calcium both via effects on PTH secretion and via effects on the kidney and osteoclast as outlined above. Thus there is a second line of defense of ECF calcium as demonstrated by the fact that low ECF calcium in hypoparathyroidism is compatible with life. Presumably, the kidney and osteoclast CaSRs play a role in the defense of ECF under these circumstances.

CALCIUM PHYSIOLOGY AND THE CAUSATION OF BONE DISEASE

Osteoporosis or Osteomalacia

There is still disagreement about the effects of calcium deprivation on the skeletal structure. Irrespective of the cause of calcium deficiency, an unresolved question is whether calcium deficiency produces osteoporosis, that is, "too little bone in the bone" but of normal appearance under light microscopy or osteomalacia, that is, a delay in osteoid mineralization that may give the appearance of excessive uncalcified osteoid protein. There are clear data that in the growing skeleton, calcium deficiency alone without the additional effects of vitamin D deficiency can result in osteomalacia *(144)*. In the adult skeleton, because the size of the "bone bank" of calcium is larger and the fact that there is an internal redistribution of bone calcium from areas of less biomechanical importance under the influence of relative secondary hyperparathyroidism *(145)*, calcium deficiency usually results in less bone within the bone. This internal economy of the skeleton is a critically important part of the defense of extracellular calcium and bone structure in the face of calcium deficiency. In this process calcium is resorbed from certain areas, in particular, the endocortical area to be made available for defense of more critical mechanical structures.

Many causes of bone loss resulting in such a damaged skeletal structure are associated with a negative whole body calcium balance although whether this is a primary or secondary effect has been surprisingly controversial. If the primary cause of the bone loss is due to mechanisms originating in the skeleton itself, then improvement in extracellular calcium balance may only result in hypercalcemia. Thus treatment with calcium is only of value where a reduction in calcium absorption in the intestine and reabsorption in the kidney is a cause of bone loss rather than a result of bone loss.

Intestinal and Renal Disorders of Calcium Transport Resulting in Bone Disorders

Malabsorptive Disorders. It is commonly present with bone or calcium disorders usually osteoporosis as diagnosed by bone mineral density (BMD) testing. It is important to remember that BMD testing actually measures calcified bone so that if the results are low this could be due to too little bone in the bone, osteoporosis, or reduced mineralization of the bone, osteomalacia.

One of the best characterized of these disorders is celiac disease which is often not diagnosed until quite advanced because of the relatively subtle symptoms associated with the disorder. In this disorder secondary hyperparathyroidism with appendicular skeleton osteoporosis is typical *(146)*. The pathogenesis is of disordered intestinal calcium absorption resulting in parathyroid overactivity to maintain extracellular calcium homeostasis. This results in increased renal calcium reabsorption via the ECaC1, calbindin, and NCX1 in the distal tubule. In bone increased osteoclast recruitment to areas of low biomechanical importance, the endocortical surfaces of long bones, occurs which then entrains increased release of bone calcium.

Hypercalciuria. It is a complex disorder *(147)* but has been related to low bone mass in men and women *(148)*. Sodium-induced increases in urine calcium have also been associated with low bone mass in postmenopausal women (27) corrected in part by increased dietary calcium. No clear biochemical mechanism for the association between high urine calcium and low bone mass has been elucidated. Nevertheless, it would be reasonable to consider that hypercalciuria can result in a negative calcium balance which may not be compensated for by a sufficient increase in intestinal calcium absorption to protect the skeleton against bone loss.

Age-Related Osteoporosis in Women

There is now good evidence that the bone loss occurring in women after the age of 65 is due to defects in intestinal calcium absorption and renal calcium reabsorption resulting in increased resorption of bone calcium as a result of estrogen deficiency. It can partly be corrected by calcium supplementation and vitamin D.

An outline of the physiological interactions important in the development of negative calcium balance in aging is shown in Fig. 4. In essence, osteoporosis in these women could be regarded as a bi-hormonal deficiency disorder in which the importance of estrogen deficiency is most marked close to the menopause and in which vitamin D deficiency becomes more important as renal function declines with age. The combined effects result in relative secondary hyperparathyroidism inducing bone resorption and osteoporosis (19).

The principal causes of the decreased absorption of calcium with aging *(149,150)* are the effects of decreased calcitriol and estrogen on the gut. In addition, there may be an intrinsic age-related defect in the gut wall. The principal cause of the decreased reabsorption

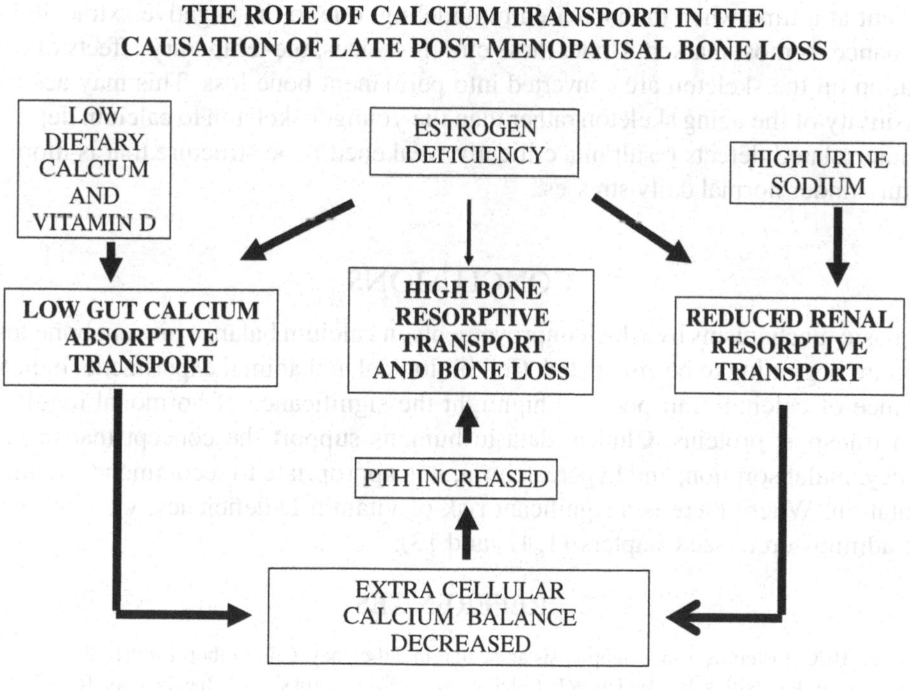

Fig. 4.

of calcium in the kidney is due to estrogen deficiency (19). The combined problem of reduced intestinal calcium absorption and decreased renal calcium reabsorption results in a negative extracellular calcium balance that results in increased bone resorption to maintain the calcium concentration by an increase in PTH (151–153). The increased bone resorption results in trabecular plate perforation and endocortical bone resorption.

Dietary Factors

A low calcium intake exacerbates the intestinal calcium absorptive defect and a high salt intake exacerbates the renal calcium loss. Vitamin D deficiency due to lack of sunlight exposure and poor dietary intake will also exacerbate the calcitriol deficiency and impair gut calcium absorption. The data from randomized controlled trials of calcium supplementation and vitamin D have supported this concept, with studies showing a reduction in bone loss with increased calcium intake at all skeletal sites at which the bone density was measured. The data from clinical trials of increased calcium intake on fracture rates have been variable largely due to variable compliance with the supplements; however, those with good compliance have shown beneficial effects of calcium (145) and calcium and vitamin D (154) (see also Chapter 11).

Osteoblast Defect

An important defect in age-related osteoporosis is the defect in osteoblastic bone formation that occurs with aging. In age-related osteoporosis, in addition to the potential for relative extracellular calcium deficiency causing increased bone resorption and consequent formation, there is also evidence for a specific age-related defect in bone formation associated with osteoblast senescence *(129,155)*. Thus the bone formation function of the BMU is deficient at a time when the increased remodeling, due to the negative extracellular calcium balance, is most marked. Under these circumstances, the temporary effects of calcium deprivation on the skeleton are converted into permanent bone loss. This may account for the sensitivity of the aging skeleton rather than the younger skeleton to calcium deprivation. These interrelated defects result in a critically weakened bone structure that is more likely to fracture under normal daily stresses.

CONCLUSIONS

The basic mechanisms by which improvements in calcium balance prevent bone loss and fracture are beginning to be elucidated. Cell biological and animal experiments indicate the importance of calcium transport and highlight the significance of hormonal regulation of calcium transport proteins. Clinical data in humans support the concept that in gonadal deficiency, malabsorption, and hypercalciuria, it is appropriate to recommend calcium supplementation. Where there is a significant risk of vitamin D deficiency, vitamin D should also be administered (see Chapters 11, 12, and 13).

REFERENCES

1. Nordin BEC. Osteomalacia, osteoporosis and calcium deficiency. Clin Orthop 1960;17:235–258.
2. Hoenderop JG, Nilius B, Bindels RJ. Calcium absorption across epithelia. Physiol Rev 2005;85(1): 373–422.

3. Hofmann F, Biel M, Flockerzi V. Molecular basis for Ca2+ channel diversity. Annu Rev Neurosci 1994;17:399–418.
4. Hoenderop JG, van der Kemp AW, Hartog A, van de Graaf SF, van Os CH, Willems PH, Bindels RJ. Molecular identification of the apical Ca2+ channel in 1, 25-dihydroxyvitamin D3-responsive epithelia. J Biol Chem 1999;274(13):8375–8378.
5. Fatalities and injuries from falls among older adults – United States, 1993–2003 and 2001–2005. MMWR Morb Mortal Wkly Rep 2006; 55 (45): 1221–1224.
6. Christakos S, Gill R, Lee S, Li H. Molecular aspects of the calbindins. J Nutr 1992;122(3 Suppl):678–682.
7. Carafoli E, Garcia-Martin E, Guerini D. The plasma membrane calcium pump: recent developments and future perspectives. Experientia 1996;52(12):1091–1100.
8. Dominguez JH, Juhaszova M, Feister HA. The renal sodium-calcium exchanger. J Lab Clin Med 1992;119(6):640–649.
9. Lambers TT, Weidema AF, Nilius B, Hoenderop JG, Bindels RJ. Regulation of the mouse epithelial Ca2(+) channel TRPV6 by the Ca(2+)-sensor calmodulin. J Biol Chem 2004;279(28):28855–28861.
10. Hoenderop JG, Voets T, Hoefs S, Weidema F, Prenen J, Nilius B, Bindels RJ. Homo- and heterotetrameric architecture of the epithelial Ca2+ channels TRPV5 and TRPV6. EMBO J 2003;22(4):776–785.
11. Christakos S, Gabrielides C, Rhoten WB. Vitamin D-dependent calcium binding proteins: chemistry, distribution, functional considerations, and molecular biology. Endocr Rev 1989;10(1):3–26.
12. Strehler EE, Zacharias DA. Role of alternative splicing in generating isoform diversity among plasma membrane calcium pumps. Physiol Rev 2001;81(1):21–50.
13. Niggli V, Penniston JT, Carafoli E. Purification of the (Ca2+-Mg2+)-ATPase from human erythrocyte membranes using a calmodulin affinity column. J Biol Chem 1979;254(20):9955–9958.
14. Carafoli E. Biogenesis: plasma membrane calcium ATPase:15 years of work on the purified enzyme. FASEB J 1994;8(13):993–1002.
15. Blaustein MP, Lederer WJ. Sodium/calcium exchange: its physiological implications. Physiol Rev 1999;79(3):763–854.
16. Prince RL, Dick I, Garcia-Webb P, Retallack RW. The effects of the menopause on calcitriol and parathyroid hormone: responses to a low dietary calcium stress test. J Clin Endocrinol Metab 1990;70(4):1119–1123.
17. Brown EM, MacLeod RJ. Extracellular calcium sensing and extracellular calcium signaling. Physiol Rev 2001;81(1):239–297.
18. Riggs BL, Khosla S, Melton LJ III. Sex steroids and the construction and conservation of the adult skeleton. Endocr Rev 2002;23(3):279–302.
19. Prince RL. Counterpoint: estrogen effects on calcitropic hormones and calcium homeostasis. Endocr Rev 1994;15(3):301–309.
20. Kalkwarf HJ, Specker BL, Bianchi DC, Ranz J, Ho M. The effect of calcium supplementation on bone density during lactation and after weaning. N Engl J Med 1997;337(8):523–528.
21. Thakker RV. Diseases associated with the extracellular calcium-sensing receptor. Cell Calcium 2004;35(3):275–282.
22. Dawson Hughes B, Harris SS, Finneran S. Calcium absorption on high and low calcium intakes in relation to Vitamin D receptor genotype. J Clin Endocrinol Metab 1995;80:3657–3661.
23. Suki WN. Calcium transport in the nephron. Am J Physiol 1979;237(1):F1–F6.
24. Massey LK, Whiting SJ. Dietary salt, urinary calcium, and bone loss. J Bone Miner Res 1996;11: 731–736.
25. Sakhaee K, Nicar M, Hill K, Pak CY. Contrasting effects of potassium citrate and sodium citrate therapies on urinary chemistries and crystallization of stone-forming salts. Kidney Int 1983;24(3):348–352.
26. Lemann J Jr, Gray RW, Pleuss JA. Potassium bicarbonate, but not sodium bicarbonate, reduces urinary calcium excretion and improves calcium balance in healthy men. Kidney Int 1989;35(2):688–695.
27. Devine A, Criddle RA, Dick IM, Kerr DA, Prince RL. A longitudinal study of the effect of sodium and calcium intakes on regional bone density in postmenopausal women. Am J Clin Nutr 1995;62(4): 740–745.
28. Hegsted MS, Schuette SA, Zemel MB, Linkswiler HM. Urinary calcium and calcium balance in young men as affected by level of protein and phosphorus intake. J Nutr 1981;111: 553–562.

29. Schuette SA, Hegsted M, Zemel MB, Linkswiler HM. Renal acid, urinary cyclic AMP, and hydroxyproline excretion as affected by level of protein, sulfur amino acid, and phosphorus intake. J Nutr 1981;111:2106–2116.
30. Lutz J. Calcium balance and acid-base status of women as affected by increased protein intake and by sodium bicarbonate ingestion. Am J Clin Nutr 1984;39(2):281–288.
31. Curhan GC, Willett WC, Rimm EB, Stampfer MJ. A prospective study of dietary calcium and other nutrients and the risk of symptomatic kidney stones [see comments]. N Engl J Med 1993;328(12): 833–838.
32. Schurch MA, Rizzoli R, Slosman D, Vadas L, Vergnaud P, Bonjour JP. Protein supplements increase serum insulin-like growth factor-I levels and attenuate proximal femur bone loss in patients with recent hip fracture. A randomized, double-blind, placebo-controlled trial. Ann Intern Med 1998;128(10): 801–809.
33. Devine A, Rosen C, Mohan S, Baylink DJ, Prince RL. Effects of zinc and other nutritional factors on insulin-like growth factor 1 and insulin-like growth factor binding proteins in postmenopausal women. Am J Clin Nutr 1998;68:200–206.
34. Devine A, Dick IM, Islam AF, Dhaliwal SS, Prince RL. Protein consumption is an important predictor of lower limb bone mass in elderly women. Am J Clin Nutr 2005;81(6):1423–1428.
35. Barzel US. The skeleton as an ion exchange system: implications for the role of acid-base imbalance in the genesis of osteoporosis. J Bone Miner Res 1995;10(10):1431–1436.
36. Sebastian A, Harris ST, Ottaway JH, Todd KM, Morris RC Jr. Improved mineral balance and skeletal metabolism in postmenopausal women treated with potassium bicarbonate. N Engl J Med 1994;330(25):1776–1781.
37. Borke JL, Minami J, Verma AK, Penniston JT, Kumar R. Co-localization of erythrocyte Ca++-Mg++ ATPase and vitamin D-dependent 28-kDa-calcium binding protein. Kidney Int 1988;34(2): 262–267.
38. Zheng W, Xie Y, Li G, Kong J, Feng JQ, Li YC. Critical role of calbindin-D28k in calcium homeostasis revealed by mice lacking both vitamin D receptor and calbindin-D28k. J Biol Chem 2004;279(50): 52406–52413.
39. Rizzo M, Capasso G, Bleich M, Pica A, Grimaldi D, Bindels RJ, Greger R. Effect of chronic metabolic acidosis on calbindin expression along the rat distal tubule. J Am Soc Nephrol 2000;11(2):203–210.
40. Bourdeau JE, Taylor AN, Iacopino AM. Immunocytochemical localization of sodium-calcium exchanger in canine nephron. J Am Soc Nephrol 1993;4(1):105–110.
41. Reilly RF, Shugrue CA, Lattanzi D, Biemesderfer D. Immunolocalization of the Na+/Ca2+ exchanger in rabbit kidney. Am J Physiol 1993;265(2 Pt 2):F327–F332.
42. Magyar CE, White KE, Rojas R, Apodaca G, Friedman PA. Plasma membrane Ca2+-ATPase and NCX1 Na+/Ca2+ exchanger expression in distal convoluted tubule cells. Am J Physiol Renal Physiol 2002;283(1):F29–F40.
43. Brunette MG, Leclerc M, Huo TL, Porta A, Christakos S. Effect of calbindin D 28K on sodium transport by the luminal membrane of the rabbit nephron. Mol Cell Endocrinol 1999;152(1–2):161–168.
44. Stauffer TP, Guerini D, Carafoli E. Tissue distribution of the four gene products of the plasma membrane Ca2+ pump. A study using specific antibodies. J Biol Chem 1995;270(20):12184–12190.
45. Caride AJ, Filoteo AG, Enyedi A, Verma AK, Penniston JT. Detection of isoform 4 of the plasma membrane calcium pump in human tissues by using isoform-specific monoclonal antibodies. Biochem J 1996;316(Pt 1):353–359.
46. Song Y, Peng X, Porta A, Takanaga H, Peng JB, Hediger MA, Fleet JC, Christakos S. Calcium transporter 1 and epithelial calcium channel messenger ribonucleic acid are differentially regulated by 1,25 dihydroxyvitamin D3 in the intestine and kidney of mice. Endocrinology 2003;144(9): 3885–3894.
47. Bouhtiauy I, Lajeunesse D, Brunette MG. Effect of vitamin D depletion on calcium transport by the luminal and basolateral membranes of the proximal and distal nephrons. Endocrinology 1993;132(1): 115–120.
48. Bindels RJ, Hartog A, Timmermans J, Van Os CH. Active Ca2+ transport in primary cultures of rabbit kidney CCD: stimulation by 1,25-dihydroxyvitamin D3 and PTH. Am J Physiol 1991;261(5 Pt 2): F799–F807.

49. Glendenning P, Ratajczak T, Dick IM, Prince RL. Calcitriol upregulates expression and activity of the 1b isoform of the plasma membrane calcium pump in immortalized distal kidney tubular cells. Arch Biochem Biophys 2000;380(1):126–132.
50. Glendenning P, Ratajczak T, Prince RL, Garamszegi N, Strehler EE. The promoter region of the human PMCA1 gene mediates transcriptional downregulation by 1,25-dihydroxyvitamin D(3). Biochem Biophys Res Commun 2000;277(3):722–728.
51. Hall AK, Norman AW. Regulation of calbindin-D28K gene expression by 1,25-dihydroxyvitamin D3 in chick kidney. J Bone Miner Res 1990;5(4):325–330.
52. Huang YC, Christakos S. Modulation of rat calbindin-D28 gene expression by 1,25-dihydroxyvitamin D3 and dietary alteration. Mol Endocrinol 1988;2(10):928–935.
53. Li H, Christakos S. Differential regulation by 1,25-dihydroxyvitamin D3 of calbindin-D9k and calbindin-D28k gene expression in mouse kidney. Endocrinology 1991;128(6):2844–2852.
54. Gill RK, Christakos S. Identification of sequence elements in mouse calbindin-D28k gene that confer 1,25-dihydroxyvitamin D3- and butyrate-inducible responses. Proc Natl Acad Sci USA 1993;90(7): 2984–2988.
55. Costanzo LS, Windhager EE, Ellison DH. Calcium and sodium transport by the distal convoluted tubule of the rat. 1978. J Am Soc Nephrol 2000;11(8):1562–1580.
56. Bouhtiauy I, LaJeunesse D, Brunette MG. The mechanism of parathyroid hormone action on calcium reabsorption by the distal tube. Endocrinology 1991;128(1):251–258.
57. Friedman PA, Gesek FA, Morley P, Whitfield JF, Willick GE. Cell-specific signaling and structure-activity relations of parathyroid hormone analogs in mouse kidney cells. Endocrinology 1999;140(1):301–309.
58. Criddle RA, Zheng MH, Dick IM, Callus B, Prince RL. Estrogen responsiveness of renal calbindin-D28k gene expression in rat kidney. J Cell Biochem 1997;65(3):340–348.
59. Dick IM, Liu J, Glendenning P, Prince RL. Estrogen and androgen regulation of plasma membrane calcium pump activity in immortalized distal tubule kidney cells. Mol Cell Endocrinol 2003;212(1–2): 11–18.
60. Dick IM, Devine A, Beilby J, Prince RL. Effects of endogenous estrogen on renal calcium and phosphate handling in elderly women. Am J Physiol Endocrinol Metab 2005;288(2):E430–E435.
61. Lambers TT, Bindels RJ, Hoenderop JG. Coordinated control of renal Ca2+ handling. Kidney Int 2006;69(4):650–654.
62. Riccardi D, Hall AE, Chattopadhyay N, Xu JZ, Brown EM, Hebert SC. Localization of the extracellular Ca2+/polyvalent cation-sensing protein in rat kidney. Am J Physiol 1998;274(3 Pt 2):F611–F622.
63. Aida K, Koishi S, Tawata M, Onaya T. Molecular cloning of a putative Ca(2+)-sensing receptor cDNA from human kidney. Biochem Biophys Res Commun 1995;214(2):524–529.
64. Motoyama HI, Friedman PA. Calcium-sensing receptor regulation of PTH-dependent calcium absorption by mouse cortical ascending limbs. Am J Physiol Renal Physiol 2002;283(3):F399–F406.
65. Heaney RP, Recker RR, Saville PD. Menopausal changes in calcium balance performance. J Lab Clin Med 1978;92(6):953–963.
66. Davies KM, Rafferty K, Heaney RP. Determinants of endogenous calcium entry into the gut. Am J Clin Nutr 2004;80(4):919–923.
67. Draper CR, Dick IM, Prince RL. The effect of estrogen deficiency on calcium balance in mature rats. Calcif Tissue Int 1999;64(4):325–328.
68. Cochet B, Jung A, Griessen M, Bartholdi P, Schaller P, Donath A. Effects of lactose on intestinal calcium absorption in normal and lactase-deficient subjects. Gastroenterology 1983;84(5 Pt 1):935–940.
69. Sheikh MS, Schiller LR, Fordtran JS. In vivo intestinal absorption of calcium in humans. Miner Electrolyte Metab 1990;16(2–3):130–146.
70. Jackson KA, Savaiano DA. Lactose maldigestion, calcium intake and osteoporosis in African-, Asian-, and Hispanic-Americans. J Am Coll Nutr 2001;20(2):198S–207S.
71. Honkanen R, Kroger H, Alhava E, Turpeinen P, Tuppurainen M, Saarikoski S. Lactose intolerance associated with fractures of weight-bearing bones in Finnish women aged 38–57 years. Bone 1997;21(6):473–477.
72. Wisker E, Nagel R, Tanudjaja TK, Feldheim W. Calcium, magnesium, zinc, and iron balances in young women: effects of a low-phytate barley-fiber concentrate. Am J Clin Nutr 1991;54(3): 553–559.

73. Knox TA, Kassarjian Z, Dawson-Hughes B, Golner BB, Dallal GE, Arora S, Russell RM. Calcium absorption in elderly subjects on high- and low-fiber diets: effect of gastric acidity. Am J Clin Nutr 1991;53(6):1480–1486.
74. Recker RR. Calcium absorption and achlorhydria. N Engl J Med 1985;313(2):70–73.
75. Prince R, Devine A, Dick I, Criddle A, Kerr D, Kent N, Price R, Randell A. The effects of calcium supplementation (milk powder or tablets) and exercise on bone density in postmenopausal women. J Bone Miner Res 1995;10(7):1068–1075.
76. Devine A, Dick IM, Heal SJ, Criddle RA, Prince RL. A 4-year follow-up study of the effects of calcium supplementation on bone density in elderly postmenopausal women. Osteoporosis Int 1997;7:23–28.
77. Wasserman RH, Kallfelz FA. Vitamin D3 and unidirectional calcium fluxes across the rachitic chick duodenum. Am J Physiol 1962;203:221–224.
78. Karbach U. Paracellular calcium transport across the small intestine. J Nutr 1992;122(3 Suppl):672–677.
79. Karbach U. Segmental heterogeneity of cellular and paracellular calcium transport across the rat duodenum and jejunum. Gastroenterology 1991;100(1):47–58.
80. Norman AW. Minireview: vitamin D receptor: new assignments for an already busy receptor. Endocrinology 2006;147(12):5542–5548.
81. van Abel M, Hoenderop JG, van der Kemp AW, van Leeuwen JP, Bindels RJ. Regulation of the epithelial Ca2+ channels in small intestine as studied by quantitative mRNA detection. Am J Physiol Gastrointest Liver Physiol 2003;285(1):G78–G85.
82. Hoenderop JG, van Leeuwen JP, van der Eerden BC, Kersten FF, van der Kemp AW, Merillat AM, Waarsing JH, Rossier BC, Vallon V, Hummler E, Bindels RJ. Renal Ca2+ wasting, hyperabsorption, and reduced bone thickness in mice lacking TRPV5. J Clin Invest 2003;112(12):1906–1914.
83. Barley NF, Prathalingam SR, Zhi P, Legon S, Howard A, Walters JR. Factors involved in the duodenal expression of the human calbindin-D9k gene. Biochem J 1999;341 (Pt 3):491–500.
84. Hildmann B, Schmidt A, Murer H. Ca++-transport across basal-lateral plasma membranes from rat small intestinal epithelial cells. J Membr Biol 1982;65(1–2):55–62.
85. Kikuchi K, Kikuchi T, Ghishan FK. Characterization of calcium transport by basolateral membrane vesicles of human small intestine. Am J Physiol 1988;255(4 Pt 1):G482–G489.
86. Howard A, Legon S, Walters JR. Human and rat intestinal plasma membrane calcium pump isoforms. Am J Physiol 1993;265(5 Pt 1):G917–G925.
87. Armbrecht HJ, Boltz MA, Wongsurawat N. Expression of plasma membrane calcium pump mRNA in rat intestine: effect of age and 1,25-dihydroxyvitamin D. Biochim Biophys Acta 1994;1195(1):110–114.
88. Walters JR, Balesaria S, Chavele KM, Taylor V, Berry JL, Khair U, Barley NF, van Heel DA, Field J, Hayat JO, Bhattacharjee A, Jeffery R, Poulsom R. Calcium channel TRPV6 expression in human duodenum: different relationships to the vitamin D system and aging in men and women. J Bone Miner Res 2006;21(11):1770–1777.
89. Armbrecht HJ, Boltz MA, Christakos S, Bruns ME. Capacity of 1,25-dihydroxyvitamin D to stimulate expression of calbindin D changes with age in the rat. Arch Biochem Biophys 1998;352(2): 159–164.
90. Staun M, Boesby S, Daugaard H, Jarnum S. Calcium-binding protein in human duodenal biopsies. Calcif Tissue Int 1988;42(4):205–209.
91. Dupret JM, Brun P, Perret C, Lomri N, Thomasset M, Cuisinier-Gleizes P. Transcriptional and post-transcriptional regulation of vitamin D-dependent calcium-binding protein gene expression in the rat duodenum by 1,25-dihydroxycholecalciferol. J Biol Chem 1987;262(34):16553–16557.
92. Nemere I, Norman AW. Transcaltachia, vesicular calcium transport, and microtubule-associated calbindin-D28K: emerging views of 1,25-dihydroxyvitamin D3-mediated intestinal calcium absorption. Miner Electrolyte Metab 1990;16(2-3):109–114.
93. Nemere I. Vesicular calcium transport in chick intestine. J Nutr 1992;122(3 Suppl):657–661.
94. Colin EM, Van Den Bemd GJ, Van Aken M, Christakos S, De Jonge HR, Deluca HF, Prahl JM, Birkenhager JC, Buurman CJ, Pols HA, Van Leeuwen JP. Evidence for involvement of 17beta-estradiol in intestinal calcium absorption independent of 1,25-dihydroxyvitamin D3 level in the Rat. J Bone Miner Res 1999;14(1):57–64.
95. Van Cromphaut SJ, Rummens K, Stockmans I, Van Herck E, Dijcks FA, Ederveen AG, Carmeliet P, Verhaeghe J, Bouillon R, Carmeliet G. Intestinal calcium transporter genes are upregulated by

estrogens and the reproductive cycle through vitamin D receptor-independent mechanisms. J Bone Miner Res 2003;18(10):1725–1736.
96. Heaney RP, Recker RR, Saville PD. Menopausal changes in calcium balance performance. J Lab Clin Med 1978;92(6):953–963.
97. Heaney RP, Recker RR, Stegman MR, Moy AJ. Calcium absorption in women: Relationships to calcium intake, estrogen status, and age. J Bone Miner Res 1989;4(4):469–475.
98. Gennari C, Agnusdei D, Nardi P, Civitelli R. Estrogen preserves a normal intestinal responsiveness to 1,25-dihydroxyvitamin D3 in oophorectomized women. J Clin Endocrinol Metab 1990;71(5):1288–1293.
99. Chattopadhyay N, Cheng I, Rogers K, Riccardi D, Hall A, Diaz R, Hebert SC, Soybel DI, Brown EM. Identification and localization of extracellular Ca(2+)-sensing receptor in rat intestine. Am J Physiol 1998;274(1 Pt 1):G122–G130.
100. Lemay J, Demers C, Hendy GN, Gascon-Barre M. Oral calcium transiently increases calbindin9k gene expression in adult rat duodena. Calcif Tissue Int 1997;60(1):43–47.
101. Talmage RV, Talmage DW. Calcium homeostasis: solving the solubility problem. J Musculoskelet Neuronal Interact 2006;6(4):402–407.
102. Neuman WF, Neuman MW, Diamond AG, Menanteau J, Gibbons WS. Blood:bone disequilibrium. VI. Studies of the solubility characteristics of brushite: apatite mixtures and their stabilization by noncollagenous proteins of bone. Calcif Tissue Int 1982;34(2):149–157.
103. Matthews JL, Wiel CV, Talmage RV. Bone lining cells and the bone fluid compartment, an ultrastructural study. Adv Exp Med Biol 1978;103:451–458.
104. Miller SC, Jee WS. The bone lining cell: a distinct phenotype? Calcif Tissue Int 1987;41(1):1–5.
105. Norimatsu H, Wiel CJ, Talmage RV. Electron microscopic study of the effects of calcitonin on bone cells and their extracellular milieu. Clin Orthop Relat Res 1979;(139):250–258.
106. Norimatsu H, Yamamoto T, Ozawa H, Talmage RV. Changes in calcium phosphate on bone surfaces and in lining cells after the administration of parathyroid hormone or calcitonin. Clin Orthop Relat Res 1982;(164):271–278.
107. Bronner F, Stein WD. Calcium homeostasis - an old problem revisited. J Nutr 1995;125(7 Suppl):1987S–1995S.
108. Burr DB, Forwood MR, Fyhrie DP, Martin RB, Schaffler MB, Turner CH. Bone microdamage and skeletal fragility in osteoporotic and stress fractures. J Bone Miner Res 1997;12(1):6–15.
109. Hauge EM, Qvesel D, Eriksen EF, Mosekilde L, Melsen F. Cancellous bone remodeling occurs in specialized compartments lined by cells expressing osteoblastic markers. J Bone Miner Res 2001;16(9):1575–1582.
110. Eriksen EF, Eghbali-Fatourechi GZ, Khosla S. Remodeling and vascular spaces in bone. J Bone Miner Res 2007;22(1):1–6.
111. Gay CV, Mueller WJ. Carbonic anhydrase and osteoclasts: localization by labeled inhibitor autoradiography. Science 1974;183(123):432–434.
112. Riihonen R, Supuran CT, Parkkila S, Pastorekova S, Vaananen HK, Laitala-Leinonen T. Membrane-bound carbonic anhydrases in osteoclasts. Bone 2007;40(4):1021–1031.
113. Salo J, Lehenkari P, Mulari M, Metsikko K, Vaananen HK. Removal of osteoclast bone resorption products by transcytosis. Science 1997;276(5310):270–273.
114. Berger CE, Rathod H, Gillespie JI, Horrocks BR, Datta HK. Scanning electrochemical microscopy at the surface of bone-resorbing osteoclasts: evidence for steady-state disposal and intracellular functional compartmentalization of calcium. J Bone Miner Res 2001;16(11):2092–2102.
115. van der Eerden BC, Hoenderop JG, de Vries TJ, Schoenmaker T, Buurman CJ, Uitterlinden AG, Pols HA, Bindels RJ, van Leeuwen JP. The epithelial Ca2+ channel TRPV5 is essential for proper osteoclastic bone resorption. Proc Natl Acad Sci USA 2005;102(48):17507–17512.
116. Li JP, Kajiya H, Okamoto F, Nakao A, Iwamoto T, Okabe K. Three Na+/Ca2+ exchanger (NCX) variants are expressed in mouse osteoclasts and mediate calcium transport during bone resorption. Endocrinology 2007;148(5):2116–2125.
117. Akisaka T, Yamamoto T, Gay CV. Ultracytochemical investigation of calcium-activated adenosine triphosphatase (Ca++-ATPase) in chick tibia. J Bone Miner Res 1988;3(1):19–25.

118. Berdal A, Hotton D, Saffar JL, Thomasset M, Nanci A. Calbindin-D9k and calbindin-D28k expression in rat mineralized tissues in vivo. J Bone Miner Res 1996;11(6):768–779.
119. Bellido T, Huening M, Raval-Pandya M, Manolagas SC, Christakos S. Calbindin-D28k is expressed in osteoblastic cells and suppresses their apoptosis by inhibiting caspase-3 activity. J Biol Chem 2000;275(34):26328–26332.
120. Shen V, Hruska K, Avioli LV. Characterization of a (Ca2+ + Mg2+)-ATPase system in the osteoblast plasma membrane. Bone 1988;9(5):325–329.
121. Stains JP, Gay CV. Asymmetric distribution of functional sodium-calcium exchanger in primary osteoblasts. J Bone Miner Res 1998;13(12):1862–1869.
122. Stains JP, Gay CV. Inhibition of Na+/Ca2+ exchange with KB-R7943 or bepridil diminished mineral deposition by osteoblasts. J Bone Miner Res 2001;16(8):1434–1443.
123. Suda T, Udagawa N, Nakamura I, Miyaura C, Takahashi N. Modulation of osteoclast differentiation by local factors. Bone 1995;17(2 Suppl):87S–91S.
124. Devlin RD, Retallack RW, Fenton AJ, Grill V, Gutteridge DH, Kent GN, Prince RL, Worth GK. Long-term elevation of 1,25-dihydroxyvitamin D after short-term intravenous administration of pamidronate (aminohydroxypropylidene bisphosphonate, APD) in Paget's disease of bone. J Bone Miner Res 1994;9(1):81–85.
125. Vasikaran SD. Bisphosphonates: an overview with special reference to alendronate. Ann Clin Biochem 2001;38(Pt 6):608–623.
126. Rosen CJ, Brown S. Severe hypocalcemia after intravenous bisphosphonate therapy in occult vitamin D deficiency. N Engl J Med 2003;348(15):1503–1504.
127. Prince RL, Dick IM, Price RI. Plasma calcitonin levels are not lower than normal in osteoporotic women. J Clin Endocrinol Metab 1989;68(3):684–687.
128. Winer KK, Yanovski JA, Sarani B, Cutler GB Jr. A randomized, cross-over trial of once-daily versus twice-daily parathyroid hormone 1-34 in treatment of hypoparathyroidism. J Clin Endocrinol Metab 1998;83(10):3480–3486.
129. Eriksen EF, Hodgson SF, Eastell R, Cedel SL, O' Fallon WM, Riggs BL. Cancellous bone remodeling in type I (postmenopausal) osteoporosis: quantitative assessment of rates of formation, resorption, and bone loss at tissue and cellular levels. J Bone Miner Res 1990;5(4):311–319.
130. Kusec V, Virdi AS, Prince R, Triffitt JT. Localization of estrogen receptor-alpha in human and rabbit skeletal tissues. J Clin Endocrinol Metab 1998;83(7):2421–2428.
131. Lorget F, Kamel S, Mentaverri R, Wattel A, Naassila M, Maamer M, Brazier M. High extracellular calcium concentrations directly stimulate osteoclast apoptosis. Biochem Biophys Res Commun 2000;268(3):899–903.
132. Zaidi M, Moonga BS, Adebanjo OA. Novel mechanisms of calcium handling by the osteoclast: A review-hypothesis. Proc Assoc Am Physicians 1999;111(4):319–327.
133. Kameda T, Mano H, Yamada Y, Takai H, Amizuka N, Kobori M, Izumi N, Kawashima H, Ozawa H, Ikeda K, Kameda A, Hakeda Y, Kumegawa M. Calcium-sensing receptor in mature osteoclasts, which are bone resorbing cells. Biochem Biophys Res Commun 1998;245(2): 419–422.
134. Kanatani M, Sugimoto T, Kanzawa M, Yano S, Chihara K. High extracellular calcium inhibits osteoclast-like cell formation by directly acting on the calcium-sensing receptor existing in osteoclast precursor cells. Biochem Biophys Res Commun 1999;261(1):144–148.
135. Mentaverri R, Yano S, Chattopadhyay N, Petit L, Kifor O, Kamel S, Terwilliger EF, Brazier M, Brown EM. The calcium sensing receptor is directly involved in both osteoclast differentiation and apoptosis. FASEB J 2006;20(14):2562–2564.
136. Christakos S, Norman AW. Vitamin D3-induced calcium binding protein in bone tissue. Science 1978;202(4363):70–71.
137. Faucheux C, Bareille R, Amedee J. Synthesis of calbindin-D28K during mineralization in human bone marrow stromal cells. Biochem J 1998;333(Pt 3):817–823.
138. Panda DK, Miao D, Bolivar I, Li J, Huo R, Hendy GN, Goltzman D. Inactivation of the 25-hydroxyvitamin D 1alpha-hydroxylase and vitamin D receptor demonstrates independent and interdependent effects of calcium and vitamin D on skeletal and mineral homeostasis. J Biol Chem 2004;279(16):16754–16766.

139. Krieger NS. Parathyroid hormone, prostaglandin E2, and 1,25-dihydroxyvitamin D3 decrease the level of Na+-Ca2+ exchange protein in osteoblastic cells. Calcif Tissue Int 1997;60(5): 473–478.
140. Chow J, Tobias JH, Colston KW, Chambers TJ. Estrogen maintains trabecular bone volume in rats not only by suppression of bone resorption but also by stimulation of bone formation. J Clin Invest 1992;89(1):74–78.
141. Tobias JH, Chow J, Colston KW, Chambers TJ. High concentrations of 17 beta-estradiol stimulate trabecular bone formation in adult female rats. Endocrinology 1991;128(1):408–412.
142. McDougall KE, Perry MJ, Gibson RL, Bright JM, Colley SM, Hodgin JB, Smithies O, Tobias JH. Estrogen-induced osteogenesis in intact female mice lacking ERbeta. Am J Physiol Endocrinol Metab 2002;283(4):E817–E823.
143. Horowitz M, Need AG, Philcox JC, Nordin BE. Effect of calcium supplementation on urinary hydroxyproline in osteoporotic postmenopausal women. Am J Clin Nutr 1984;39(6): 857–859.
144. Thacher TD, Fischer PR, Pettifor JM, Lawson JO, Isichei CO, Reading JC, Chan GM. A comparison of calcium, vitamin D, or both for nutritional rickets in Nigerian children. N Engl J Med 1999;341(8): 563–568.
145. Prince RL, Devine A, Dhaliwal SS, Dick IM. Effects of calcium supplementation on clinical fracture and bone structure: results of a 5-year, double-blind, placebo-controlled trial in elderly women. Arch Intern Med 2006;166(8):869–875.
146. Selby PL, Davies M, Adams JE, Mawer EB. Bone loss in celiac disease is related to secondary hyperparathyroidism. J Bone Miner Res 1999;14(4):652–657.
147. Giannini S, Nobile M, Sella S, Dalle Carbonare L. Bone disease in primary hypercalciuria. Crit Rev Clin Lab Sci 2005;42(3):229–248.
148. Asplin JR, Donahue S, Kinder J, Coe FL. Urine calcium excretion predicts bone loss in idiopathic hypercalciuria. Kidney Int 2006;70(8):1463–1467.
149. Gallagher JC, Riggs BL, Eisman J, Hamstra A, Arnaud SB, DeLuca HF. Intestinal calcium absorption and serum vitamin D metabolites in normal subjects and osteoporotic patients. J Clin Invest 1979;64:729736.
150. Devine A, Prince RL, Kerr DA, Dick IM, Criddle RA, Kent GN, Price RI, Webb PG. Correlates of intestinal calcium absorption in women 10 years past the menopause. Calcif Tissue Int 1993;52(5): 358–360.
151. Wiske PS, Epstein S, Bell NH, Queener SF, Edmondson J, Johnston CC. Increases in immunoreactive parathyroid hormone with age. N Engl J Med 1979;300(25):1419–1421.
152. Insogna KL, Lewis AM, Lipinski CB, Baran DT. Effect of age on serum immunoreactive parathyroid hormone and its biological effects. J Clin Endocrinol Metab 1981;53(5):1072–1075.
153. Prince RL, Dick I, Devine A, Price RI, Gutteridge DH, Kerr D, Criddle A, Garcia-Webb P, St John A. The effects of menopause and age on calcitropic hormones: a cross-sectional study of 655 healthy women aged 35 to 90. J Bone Miner Res 1995;10(6):835–842.
154. Chapuy MC, Arlot ME, Delmas PD, Meunier PJ. Effect of calcium and cholecalciferol treatment for three years on hip fractures in elderly women. Br Med J 1994;308:1081–1082.
155. Parfitt AM, Villanueva AR, Foldes J, Rao DS. Relations between histologic indices of bone formation: implications for the pathogenesis of spinal osteoporosis. J Bone Miner Res 1995;10(3):466–473.

11 Calcium, Bone, and Life

Robert P. Heaney, MD

CONTENTS

SUMMARY

Calcium is a divalent mineral cation that functions as an intracellular messenger in virtually all life forms. In multicellular organisms it functions also as an integrator tying body systems together, and in land-living vertebrates it provides the principal mineral component of the endoskeleton (bone). Calcium cannot be synthesized and must be ingested, first to build an adult skeleton and then to maintain it. Because calcium was abundant in the terrestrial vertebrate diet, humans, like most mammals, did not develop mechanisms to absorb or retain calcium efficiently, and human physiology is optimized to defend against calcium excess rather than calcium deficiency. Unfortunately, modern diets have low calcium densities, and for that reason contemporary humans face the threat of calcium deficiency. Since calcium is regularly lost from the body through skin and excreta, it must be replaced with ingested calcium. If not, the body tears down units of bone in order to scavenge their calcium. This is the context in which calcium functions in bone health.

This chapter describes the details of the operation of the calcium economy and sets forth calcium intake requirements, the factors that influence them, and calcium sources, both from foods and from supplements.

Key Words: Bone, calcium, biosphere, complexation, life, oxygen atoms, glutamic acid, aspartic acid, peptide backbone

From: *Contemporary Endocrinology: Osteoporosis: Pathophysiology and Clinical Management*
Edited by: R. A. Adler, DOI 10.1007/978-1-59745-459-9_11,

CALCIUM AND THE ORIGINS OF LIFE ON EARTH

Calcium in the Biosphere

Calcium is the fifth most abundant element in the biosphere (after iron, aluminum, silicon, and oxygen). It is the stuff of limestone and marble, coral and pearls, seashells and eggshells, antlers, and bones. Because calcium salts exhibit intermediate solubility, calcium is found both in solid form (rocks) and in solution. It was probably present in abundance in the watery environment in which life first appeared. Today, seawater contains approximately 10 mmol calcium per liter (approximately eight times higher than the calcium concentration in the extracellular water of higher vertebrates). Even fresh waters, if they support an abundant biota, typically contain calcium at concentrations of 1–2 mmol. In most soils, calcium exists as an exchangeable cation in the soil colloids. It is taken up by plants, whose parts typically contain from 0.1 to as much as 8.0% calcium. Generally, calcium concentrations are highest in the leaves, lower in the stems and roots, and lowest in the seeds.

Calcium–Protein Complexation and Life

Evolving life developed an intimate association with calcium, which is used both in the operation of the most fundamental cell processes and for the coordination of the myriads of cells and tissues that go to make up a complex organism. The calcium ion [Ca^{2+}] has an ionic radius of 0.99 Å and is able to form coordination bonds with up to 12 oxygen atoms *(1)*. The combination of these two features makes calcium nearly unique among all cations in its ability to fit neatly into the folds of the peptide chain. By binding with the oxygen atoms of glutamic and aspartic acid residues projecting off of the peptide backbone, calcium stiffens the protein molecule and fixes its tertiary structure. Magnesium and strontium, which are chemically similar to calcium in the test tube, have different ionic radii and do not bond so well with protein. Lead and cadmium ions, by contrast, substitute quite well for calcium. In fact, lead binds to various calcium-binding proteins with greater avidity than does calcium itself. (This property is probably a principal basis for lead toxicity.)

Binding of calcium to various cell proteins results in activation of their unique functions *(2)*. These proteins range from those involved with cell movement and muscle contraction to, for example, nerve transmission, glandular secretion, and cell division. In most of these situations, calcium acts both as a signal transmitter from the outside of the cell to the inside and as an activator of the functional proteins within. In fact, ionized calcium is the most common signal transmitter in all of biology, operating in cells from bacteria all the way up to the highly specialized tissues in the higher mammals.

Intracellular Calcium and Its Regulation

If all of the functional proteins of a cell were fully activated by calcium at the same time, the cell would rapidly self-destruct. For that reason, cells must keep free calcium ion concentrations in the cytosol at extremely low levels, typically on the order of 0.1 μmol. This is 10,000-fold lower than the concentration of calcium ion ([Ca^{2+}]) in the extracellular water outside of the cell. Cells maintain this concentration gradient by a combination of mechanisms: (a) a cell membrane with limited calcium permeability; (b) ion pumps which move calcium rapidly out of the cytosol, either to the outside of the cell or into storage vesicles within the cell; and (c) a series of specialized proteins in the storage vesicles that have no catalytic function in their own right, but which serve only to bind (and hence sequester) large quantities of calcium. Low cytosolic [Ca^{2+}] ensures that the various functional proteins will remain dormant until the cell activates certain of them; and it does this simply by letting [Ca^{2+}] rise in critical cytosolic compartments.

CALCIUM IN THE HUMAN BODY

In land-living mammals, calcium accounts for 2–4% of gross body weight. A 60 kg adult human female typically contains about 1000–1200 g (25–30 mol) of calcium in her body. More than 99% of that total is in the bones and teeth. About 1 g is in the plasma and extracellular fluid (ECF) bathing the cells and 6–8 g in the tissues themselves (mostly sequestered in calcium storage vesicles inside of cells).

In the circulating blood, calcium concentration is typically 2.25–2.5 mmol. About 40–45% of this quantity is bound to plasma proteins, about 8–10% is complexed with ions such as citrate, and about 45–50% is dissociated as free ions. In the ECF outside of the blood vessels, total calcium concentration is on the order of 1.25 mmol/L. It is the ionic calcium concentration ([Ca^{2+}]) in the ECF which the cells perceive and which is tightly regulated by the parathyroid, calcitonin, and vitamin D hormonal control systems (see below).

ECF [Ca^{2+}] is one of nature's great physiological constants, extending across the vertebrate phylum (at least in healthy individuals of the species concerned). When elevations of serum calcium occur in different physiological situations (such as during egg laying in reptiles and birds), the elevation is always in the protein-bound fraction, not in the ionized calcium concentration.

The ECF calcium serves two major groups of functions. It is the source of the calcium that pours into the cells of many tissues at the point of their activation, thereby triggering the specific cascade that produces tissue-specific cellular responses. Here, concentration is critically important, and clinicians have long recognized that hyper- and hypocalcemia are each associated with neuromuscular symptoms such as hypo- and hypertonia, conduction defects on electrocardiograms, and overt clinical symptoms such as constipation or muscular spasms and rigidity.

Calcium Traffic

The second role of ECF calcium lies in the fact that its ions constitute the multidirectional calcium "traffic," i.e., calcium entering the circulation through absorption of dietary calcium or resorption of bone calcium, and calcium leaving the blood in the process of bone mineralization, or through excretory or cutaneous losses. Both sets of processes are closely integrated in many complex ways, one of the more obvious of which is the fact that the physiological apparatus regulating ECF [Ca^{2+}] also affects the fluxes in and out of the extracellular fluid.

Figure 1 depicts the calcium traffic entering and leaving the extracellular fluid in a healthy adult and includes typical values for transfer rates. It is necessary to stress, however, that the indicated values of these transfer rates are highly interdependent. The individual processes will be considered briefly in the paragraphs that follow, but their

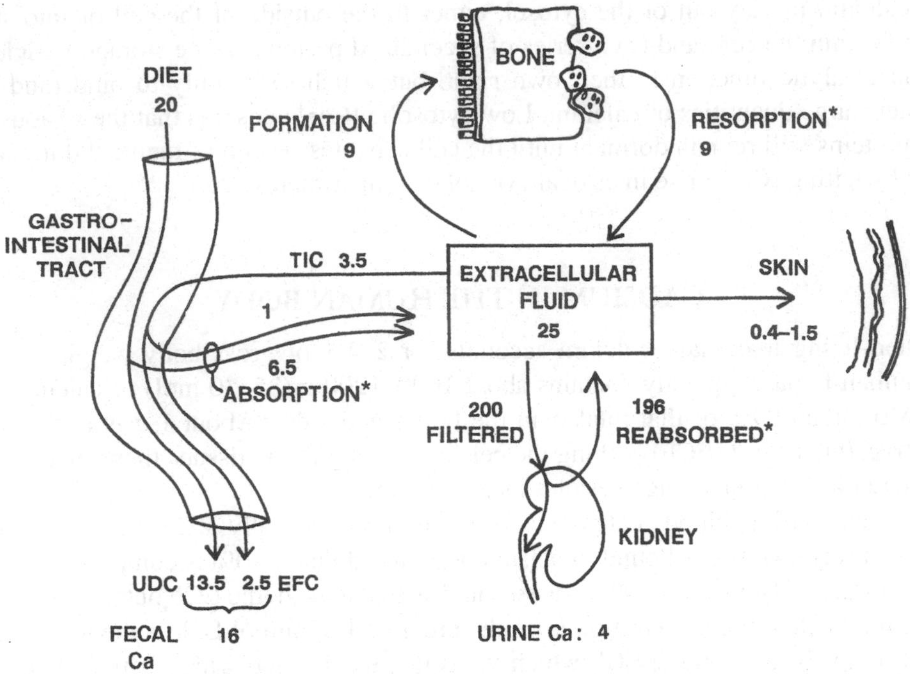

Fig. 1. Principal routes of calcium entry into and exit from the extracelluar fluid of an adult human. Rates are given in mmol/day and represent typical values. (TIC is total intestinal calcium from endogenous sources, UDC is unabsorbed dietary calcium, and EFC is endogenous fecal calcium (to convert mmol to mg, multiply by 40). (Copyright Robert P. Heaney, 1996. Used with permission.)

interrelationships can be briefly summarized with an example. When absorptive input from the diet falls, bony resorption rises to offset the absorptive shortfall. This effect is produced by an increased secretion of parathyroid hormone. The immediate consequences are maintenance of the extracellular [Ca^{2+}] and an offsetting reduction (however small) of the bony reserves of calcium. The *totality* of the traffic changes little, while the various routes of entry and exit are adjusted up or down.

Similarly, vigorous physical exercise leads to sweat losses that can be 10–20 times the level of resting losses shown in Fig. 1 *(3)*. Also, various nutrient–nutrient interactions may alter either calcium absorption efficiency or obligatory urinary calcium losses. Protein, for example, can increase urinary calcium by about 0.025 mmol for every 1 g of protein ingested *(4,5)*, and sodium (in the form of sodium chloride) regularly increases urinary calcium by about 1 mmol per 100 mmol salt *(6,7)* (see "Nutrient–Nutrient Interactions"). These nutrient influences, together with great variability in food choices and hence dietary calcium intake, constitute unregulated stresses on the system, i.e., they are perturbations to which the control mechanisms (and the fluxes in Fig. 1) must respond. For all such stresses, bone resorption is regulated up or down to compensate for the altered inputs or outputs.

The examples just cited represent influences that, if not countered, would result in a lowering of ECF [Ca^{2+}]. But the opposite stress, i.e., a trend toward hypercalcemia, can be equally important and/or threatening. This half of the regulatory control environment is relatively uncommonly encountered in adult human physiology, largely because contemporary diets are low in calcium and hypercalcemic stresses, accordingly, are uncommon. However, animals with naturally high calcium intakes, subjected to thyroparathyroidectomy but given thyroid replacement (i.e., deprived only of PTH and calcitonin), tend to exhibit not so much *hypo*calcemia as wildly fluctuating levels of ECF calcium, sometimes low, sometimes high, depending almost totally on absorptive inputs from the gut which, in the absence of PTH and CT, cannot be damped.

These examples are intended simply to illustrate the "push–pull" character of the regulatory system and the way it responds to unregulated inputs.

Dystrophic Calcification

With advancing age humans commonly accumulate calcium deposits in various damaged tissues, such as atherosclerotic plaques in arteries, healed granulomas, and other scars left by disease or injury, and often in the rib cartilages as well. These deposits are called dystrophic calcification and rarely amount to more than a few grams of calcium. These deposits are not caused by diet calcium but by local injury, coupled with the tendency of many proteins to bind calcium. So long as ECF [Ca^{2+}] remains normal, calcification in tissues other than bones and teeth is a sign of tissue damage and cell death, not of calcium excess.

Bone as the Nutrient Reserve for Calcium

Aside from its obvious structural role, the skeleton is an important reservoir of calcium which serves to maintain plasma calcium concentrations. For the most part it does this principally by adjusting the balance between bone formation and bone resorption. An excess of the latter releases calcium into the blood, and an excess of the former soaks up calcium from the blood.

Additionally, this process of formation and resorption is what constitutes bone structural modeling and remodeling. Bone replacement, or turnover, continues throughout life, renewing skeletal tissue on average every 10–12 years. Bone-resorbing osteoclasts begin the remodeling process by attaching onto a bone surface, sealing it from the rest of the ECF; they then extrude packets of citric, lactic, and carbonic acids to dissolve bone mineral and proteolytic enzymes to digest organic matrix. Later bone-forming osteoblasts synthesize new bone to replace bone previously resorbed.

Formation and resorption are coupled both systemically and locally, and when resorption is high, formation is generally high as well. But the coupling is not perfect. Bone formation exceeds resorption during growth, and resorption exceeds formation during development of osteoporosis or in the face of ongoing dietary shortage of calcium. It is important to stress that calcium cannot be withdrawn from (or added to) bone per se; instead calcium is scavenged from the tearing down of structural bony units. Thus, reduction in skeletal calcium reserves involves reduction in bone mass.

THE CALCIUM ECONOMY OF THE HUMAN ORGANISM: INPUTS, OUTPUTS, AND THEIR CONTROLS

Control Mechanisms

The concentration of calcium in the ECF is maintained by a combination of adjustments to the inputs and outputs in Fig. 1 and, perhaps more importantly, by controlling the level of the renal calcium threshold. This latter function, though very well established, is commonly underappreciated. Since the threshold is the point at which blood calcium begins to spill into the urine, it is clear that raising that point is a first line defense against renal calcium loss. Parathyroid hormone (PTH) is the principal regulator of the renal calcium threshold. The importance of the threshold in the regulation of ECF [Ca^{2+}] is clearly evidenced in the common clinical experience of the difficulty of elevating serum calcium in patients with hypoparathyroidism, even with sometimes heroic inputs of calcium into the system.

The physiological effects of PTH are complex and are diagrammed schematically in Fig. 2. These hormonal actions, in approximately the order in which they occur, can be described briefly as follows: (1) decreased renal tubular reabsorption of serum inorganic phosphate (P_i) with a corresponding decrease in serum P_i; (2) increased resorptive efficiency of osteoclasts already working on bone surfaces; (3) increased renal 1-α-hydroxylation of circulating 25(OH)-vitamin D to produce the hormonally most active form of vitamin D; (4) increased renal tubular reabsorption of calcium; and (5) activation of new bone remodeling loci. These effects interact and reinforce one another in important ways, indicated by the connections between the loops of Fig. 2. For example, the reduced ECF P_i caused by the immediate fall in tubular reabsorption of phosphate is a potent stimulus to the synthesis of $1,25(OH)_2D$, and it also increases the resorptive efficiency of osteoclasts already in place and working in bone. $1,25(OH)_2D$ directly increases intestinal absorption of both ingested calcium and the endogenous calcium contained in the digestive secretions. It is also necessary for the full expression of PTH effects in bone, particularly the maturation of cells in the myelomonocytic line that produce new osteoclasts.

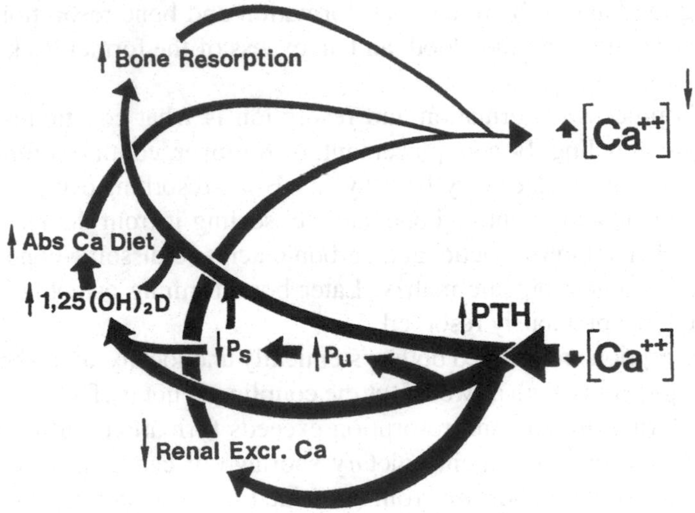

Fig. 2. Schematic depiction of the three-arm control loop regulating ECF [Ca^{++}], showing specifically the response to a drop in [Ca^{++}]. (P_s is serum inorganic phosphorus and P_u is urinary phosphorus clearance.) [Adapted from Arnaud *(8)*. Copyright Robert P. Heaney, 1981. Used with permission.]

The three arms of Fig. 2 make graphic the fact that the system uses three independent end-organs to regulate ECF [Ca^{2+}]; their actions are to reduce losses through the kidneys, to improve utilization of dietary calcium, and to draw down calcium from the bony reserves. The aggregate effect of all of them, as Fig. 2 indicates, is to prevent or reverse a fall in ECF [Ca^{2+}]. It is important, also, to understand that the three arms respond independently of one another. Thus, resistance of bone resorption to PTH leads to higher PTH secretion, which drives the other two control arms harder. Ethnic, menopausal, and treatment-related differences in the operation of the system are all based in differential responsiveness of the three arms of this control system (see "Quantitative Operation of the System").

While hypocalcemia is a much more common risk in adults than is hypercalcemia, in infants and small children both deviations are a threat. The principal defense against hypercalcemia is release of calcitonin by the *C* cells of the thyroid gland. Calcitonin (CT) is a peptide hormone with binding sites in the kidney, bone, and central nervous system. Absorption of calcium from an 8-oz feeding in a 6-month-old infant dumps up to 3.75 mmol (150 mg) calcium into the ECF. This is enough, given the small size of the ECF compartment at that age (1.5–2 L), to produce near fatal hypercalcemia if other adjustments are not made. What happens is that CT is released, in part in response to the rise in serum calcium concentration, but even before that, in response to gut hormones signaling the digestive activity that will lead to absorption. This burst of CT very rapidly blocks osteoclastic resorption, thus stopping bony release of calcium. Later, when absorption falls, CT levels also fall and osteoclastic resorption resumes.

By contrast, CT has little significance in adults because adult calcium absorption is less efficient to begin with, and the ECF is vastly larger. As a result, transient absorptive calcemia from a high calcium intake raises the ECF [Ca^{2+}] by only a few percentage points (up to ~1% for each 100 mg ingested at typical intakes).

Endogenous Fecal Calcium Loss

Calcium is contained in all of the digestive secretions, as well as in the mucosal cells themselves (which turn over about every 5 days). Together these sources account for entry of endogenous calcium into the gut amounting to about 0.05 mmol (2 mg)/kg/day or in a typical middle-aged woman, about 3.5 mmol (140 mg)/day *(9)*. Because absorption efficiency for calcium is low (see below), and because some of the digestive juice calcium enters the lumen downstream of the sites of most active absorption, most of this endogenous calcium ends up in the feces and is generally designated "endogenous fecal calcium (EFCa)." The quantity entering the gut is not regulated by the hormones otherwise controlling the calcium economy, and the principal known influences on calcium entry into the gut are phosphorus intake *(9)* and mucosal mass. EFCa, in turn, is inversely related to absorption efficiency (and hence to calcium intake). It constitutes one of the unregulated drains on the calcium economy to which the control system must react. EFCa is measurable only by isotopic tracer methods and hence cannot be assessed clinically. Nevertheless, when it is measured, it is found to account for a somewhat greater share of the variability in total body calcium balance than does actual oral calcium intake.

Urinary Loss

Calcium losses in the urine are dependent on filtered load except during adolescence. During this period of rapid growth, at calcium intakes typically ingested, most of the absorbed calcium is diverted to bone growth and little spills into the urine.

Machinery for calcium transport, most extensively studied in intestinal epithelial cells, is also present in the nephrons of the kidney, but it is not known to what extent it is functional there. The process is calcium load dependent, stimulated by PTH and $1{,}25(OH)_2D$, and has a microvillar myosin I–calmodulin complex that could serve as a calcium transporter *(10)*. Active transport occurs in the distal convoluted tubule against a concentration gradient. Renal calcium clearance is increased when PTH concentration in blood is low, thereby protecting against hypercalcemia when bone resorption is high for reasons other than homeostatic. Tubular reabsorption is determined to some extent by Na^+ excretion (see "Nutrient–Nutrient Interactions"). For every 100 mmol of sodium excreted, approximately 0.5–1.5 mmol of calcium is pulled out with it in the urine *(6,7)*.

Urine calcium rises with absorbed calcium intake, but the relationship is loose and depends strongly on the circulating level of PTH at the time. The alimentary rise is partly due to the small increase in blood calcium following absorption of ingested calcium, with a corresponding increase in the filtered load of calcium. Available data from healthy adults indicate that urinary calcium rises on dietary intake with a slope of about +0.045, meaning that, for every 10 mmol (400 mg) rise in intake, urine calcium rises by about 0.45 mmol (18 mg). But there is much variability about this average figure and the range of normal is accordingly very broad. Table 1 sets forth observed ranges in healthy estrogen-replete and estrogen-deprived adult women, both as absolute values and as weight-adjusted values. The latter can be applied to men since the difference in urine calcium between the sexes is due principally to the generally greater body weight of men.

Table 1
Distribution of 24-h Urinary Calcium Values in Normal Middle-Aged Women[a]

Percentile	*mmol (mg)/day*	*mmol (mg)/kg/day*
Estrogen-replete		
97.5	6.3 (252)	0.104 (4.15)
95.0	5.4 (215)	0.093 (3.72)
90.0	4.9 (197)	0.081 (3.23)
50.0	2.9 (116)	0.046 (1.86)
10.0	1.5 (62)	0.024 (0.99)
5.0	1.3 (53)	0.021 (0.83)
2.5	1.1 (44)	0.017 (0.67)
Estrogen-deprived		
97.5	7.6 (303)	0.126 (5.05)
95.0	6.6 (264)	0.107 (4.27)
90.0	5.6 (225)	0.091 (3.66)
50.0	3.3 (134)	0.054 (2.15)
10.0	2.0 (81)	0.028 (1.12)
5.0	1.4 (55)	0.020 (0.80)
2.5	0.9 (38)	0.014 (0.56)

[a]Reproduced from Ref. *(11)*.

Illustrative of the dependence of urine calcium on the settings of the calcium economy is the fact that the sum of endogenous fecal and urinary losses has a smaller coefficient of variation than does either route alone *(11)*. In other words, as EFCa rises, urine calcium tends to fall, and vice versa, reflecting, in this instance, reciprocal renal conservation in the face of varying digestive juice losses.

Cutaneous Loss

Calcium is contained in all cells and organs such as the intestinal mucosa, which turns over approximately every 5 days, thereby constituting a loss to the body of the calcium those cells contain. The same is true with epidermis and skin appendages (hair and nails), all of which contain some calcium. This shedding thereby produces a steady calcium drain on the system. It is the sum total of these cell-related cutaneous calcium losses which is represented in Fig. 1 by the rough estimate of 0.4–1.5 mmol/day. Sweat losses, not included in that figure, have not been extensively studied, but such data as are available indicate that heavy physical exercise in a hot environment can increase sweat calcium losses to levels as high as 5–10 mmol (200–400 mg)/day. In one study of athletes, these losses were sufficient to produce a measurable decrease in bone mineral density (i.e., a detectable reduction of the nutrient calcium reserve) across a playing season, despite the relatively high dietary calcium intakes typical of varsity athletes *(3)*. Calcium supplementation in the same athletes prevented this seasonal, exercise-related bone loss. This instance probably represents an extreme situation, but it illustrates nicely the function of bone as the body's nutrient calcium reserve, and also a point to be discussed further in the following section that, given relatively inefficient dietary extraction of calcium, there are limits to how much calcium the organism can get from food to offset unregulated losses.

Intestinal Calcium Absorption

Intestinal calcium absorption occurs by two pathways *(12–14)*: (1) transcellular, saturable (active) transfer that involves a vitamin D-dependent calcium-binding protein, calbindin; and (2) paracellular, a nonsaturable (diffusional) transfer that is to some extent a linear function of the calcium content of the chyme.

Active absorption is more efficient in the duodenum and proximal jejunum where calbindin is present in highest concentration. However, total absorption is probably greatest in the ileum where the residence time is longer. Absorption from the colon accounts for about 5% of the total amount absorbed in normal individuals but may be larger in patients with small bowel resections and in individuals in whom colonic bacteria break down dietary calcium complexes.

The main regulator of transport across the epithelial cell against an energy gradient is $1{,}25(OH)_2D$, which controls the synthesis of calbindin by DNA transcription after binding of the hormone with receptors in the mucosal cell. Calbindin operates by complexing Ca^{2+} on the surface of the cell, then internalizing the ions via endocytic vesicles that probably fuse with lysosomes. After release of the bound calcium in the acidic lysosomal interior, the calbindin returns to the cell surface and the Ca^{2+} ions exit the cell through the basolateral membrane *(12)*. Calbindin serves both as a Ca^{2+} translocator and a cytosolic Ca^{2+} buffer. Relative Ca^{2+} binding capacities across the enterocyte are brush border = 1, calbindin = 4, and the ATP-dependent Ca^{2+} pump = 10, a gradient that ensures unidirectional transfer of Ca^{2+} *(13)*.

In the paracellular pathway, calcium movement occurs not through the cell interior but through the junctions that bind one cell to another, i.e., *around* the cells. Theoretically, this can be in both directions, but normally the predominant direction is from lumen into blood. Rate of transfer depends on calcium load and tightness of the junctions. Water probably carries calcium through the junctions by solvent drag *(14)*. Calcium usually is freed from complexes in the diet during digestion and is released in a soluble and probably ionized form for absorption. However, low molecular weight complexes, such as calcium oxalate and calcium carbonate, can be absorbed, though weakly, as non-dissociated compounds *(15)*.

The relationship between calcium intake and absorption fraction is shown in Fig. 3. At lower calcium intakes, the active component contributes importantly to absorbed calcium. As calcium intake increases, the active component becomes saturated and vitamin D-mediated synthesis of calbindin drops. Thus an increasing proportion of calcium is absorbed by passive diffusion. The figure illustrates that, across most of the intake range, the adaptive component is rather small. This partly explains the inefficiency of human ability to compensate for a fall in calcium intake.

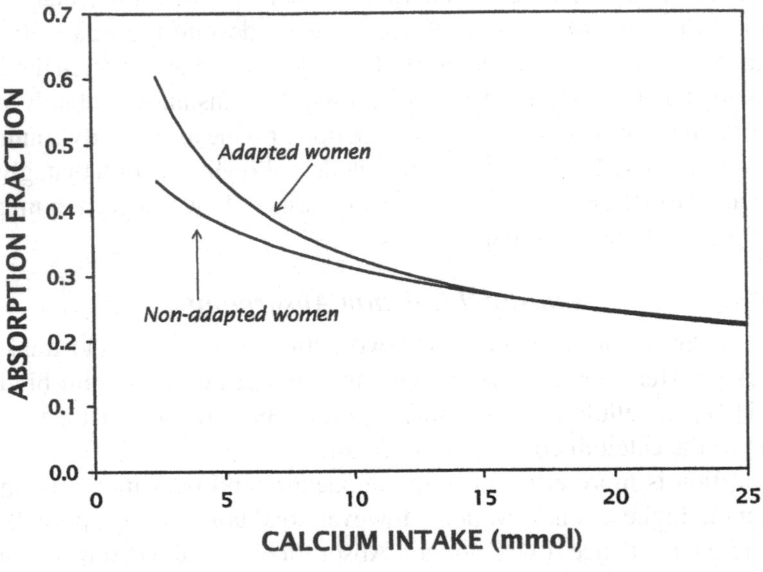

Fig. 3. Relationship between calcium intake and absorption fraction in women studied on their usual calcium intakes (adapted) and in women tested with no prior exposure to the test load (non-adapted). (Copyright Robert P. Heaney, 1999. Used with permission.)

Various host factors affect calcium absorption efficiency. Vitamin D status, intestinal transit time, mucosal mass, and stage of life are the best established. In infancy, absorption is dominated by paracellular diffusion. For that reason, the vitamin D status of the mother has little effect on calcium absorption in young breast-fed infants. Both active and passive calcium transport are increased during pregnancy and lactation. Calbindin and plasma $1,25(OH)_2D$ and PTH levels increase during pregnancy. From midlife on, absorption fraction declines from a premenopausal value of ~0.30, by about 0.002 per year, with an additional 0.02 decrease at menopause *(16)*. Thus, from age 45 to 65, absorption fraction declines by 0.06, or a decrease of ~20%.

It has long been recognized that calcium absorption efficiency increases as the size of the ingested load falls. This relationship has two components, an effect of load itself and variation in vitamin D-mediated active absorption. Within individuals, absorptive efficiency generally varies approximately inversely with the logarithm of intake, but the *absolute* quantity of calcium absorbed increases non-linearly with intake *(17,18)*. However, only 20% of the variation in calcium absorption can be accounted for by differences in intake. Individuals seem to have preset absorptive efficiencies, some high, others low.

The generally recognized inverse relationship between intake and absorption fraction has often been uncritically assumed to mean that the body can fully adapt to reduced intake. However, extensive studies in which absorption has been measured by isotopic tracer methods show very clearly that, while fractional absorption does rise (see, for example, Fig. 3), the rise is far short of what would be needed to maintain constant mass transfer across the intestinal mucosa. Figure 4 illustrates this point with one such set of data. The regression line through the data in Fig. 4 is for a simple linear model, and more detailed investigations of the low intake end of the curve indicate that the rise is initially steeper, reflecting the active transport response to low intake discussed above. The slope of the line in Fig. 4 is +0.158, meaning that 15.8% of ingested calcium is absorbed, overall. If analysis is confined to intakes at the high end of the range, the slope drops to about +0.12. This means that the body absorbs ~12% of any additional amount of calcium that may be ingested. At all intakes, the distribution of absorption values is broad, as the spread of the data in Fig. 4 demonstrates.

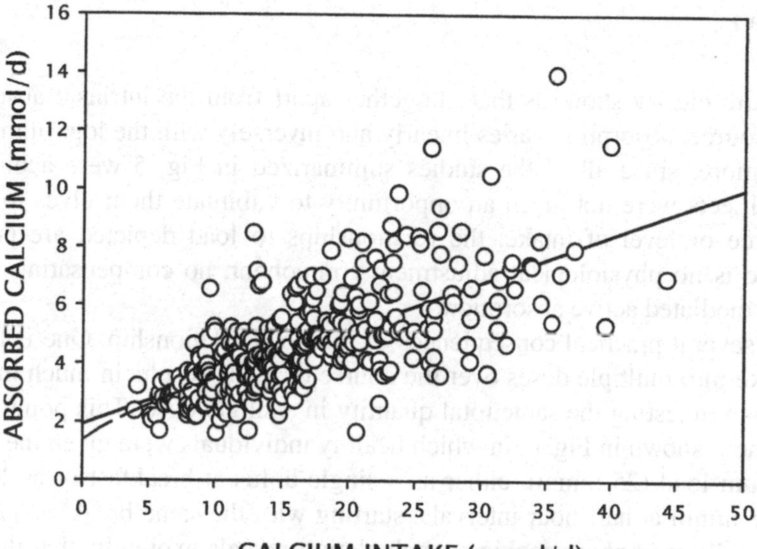

Fig. 4. Absorbed calcium plotted as a function of intake in 332 studies in middle-aged healthy women studied on their usual calcium intakes. (Copyright Robert P. Heaney, 2001. Used with permission.)

The relationship of absorption both to load size and to source is illustrated in Fig. 5, which summarizes the data from three groups of sources: milk calcium (the principal dietary source of calcium in the industrialized nations), calcium carbonate (the principal calcium salt used in calcium supplements in North America), and finally calcium oxalate.

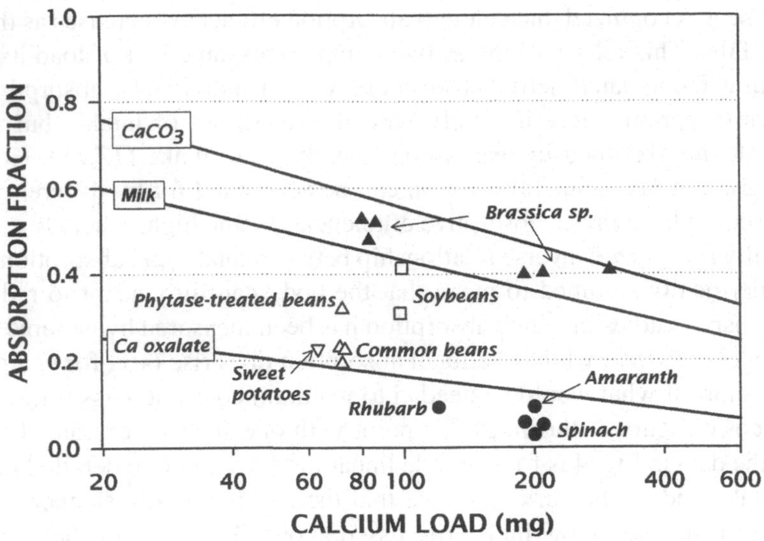

Fig. 5. Regression lines fitted to fractional absorption values at various load sizes for three families of calcium sources. Topmost is the line for plain calcium carbonate. Next is the line for milk calcium. The lowest is the line for calcium oxalate and the high oxalate vegetables (e.g., spinach and rhubarb). For all three groups there is an inverse linear relationship with the logarithm of load size, i.e., at low load sizes, a larger fraction of the load is absorbed than at high loads. Mean fractional absorption values for various other food sources are plotted for their respective intake loads. (Copyright Robert P. Heaney, 2001. Used with permission.)

What the figure clearly shows is that altogether apart from the intrinsic absorbability of the calcium source, absorption varies linearly and inversely with the logarithm of the load size. Furthermore, since all of the studies summarized in Fig. 5 were acute studies, in which the subjects were not given an opportunity to habituate themselves to a particular calcium source or level of intake, the relationships to load depicted are purely physical, i.e., there is no physiological adjustment component, no compensating alteration of $1,25(OH)_2D$-mediated active absorption.

There are several practical consequences of this load relationship. One is that dividing calcium intake into multiple doses over the course of a day results in much more efficient absorption than ingesting the same total quantity in a single dose. This point is illustrated in an experiment shown in Fig. 6, in which healthy individuals were given the same tracer-labeled calcium load (25 mmol), either as a single bolus at breakfast or as 17 individual doses of 1.47 mmol at half-hour intervals, starting with the same breakfast *(19)*. Figure 6 shows graphically, and pharmacokinetic calculation reveals explicitly, that the area under the curve (AUC_{∞}) for the divided-dose regimen was nearly twice that for the single-dose regimen. A consequence relates to the interpretation of published studies in which calcium supplements were used. Even if the aggregate daily doses were the same in two studies, when the dosing regimens are different, the effective delivered dose will be predictably different as well.

It is worth noting in passing that the primitive human diet, which would have been relatively calcium rich in most of its constituents, would more closely have approximated the continuous dosing regimen. Hence, not only would the primitive calcium intake have been

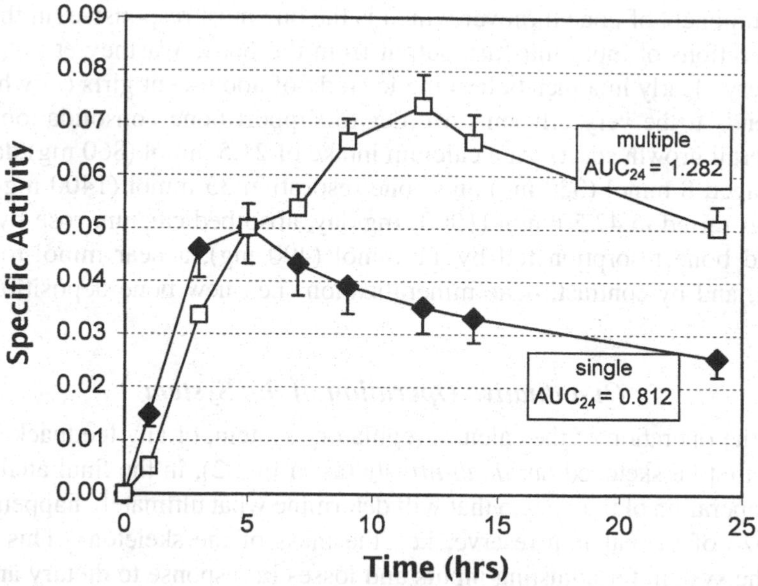

Fig. 6. Time course through 24 h for the mean specific activity values for two calcium dosing regimens. In the first (labeled "single"), 1000 mg Ca (25 mmol) was ingested as a single bolus at breakfast, and in the second (labeled "multiple"), the same total load was ingested in 17 equally spaced doses of 1.5 mmol (59 mg) each, ingested at 0.5 h intervals. (Copyright Robert P. Heaney, 2000. Used with permission.)

higher than we currently experience, but its pattern of ingestion would have likely delivered calcium into the body more efficiently than modern humans generally manage.

Bone Calcium Turnover

As the numbers in Fig. 1 suggest, the turnover of bone, in the process of bone modeling and remodeling, accounts for roughly half of the total turnover of the ECF in a typical healthy adult. (This proportion is substantially higher during growth.) A single cubic centimeter of bone contains ~10 mmol calcium, equivalent to ~40% of the total calcium in the entire ECF of an adult. Essentially all of that bone calcium is locked away in intimate association with the collagen fibers of the bone matrix, and it can be released into the blood only by physically tearing down a unit of bone through osteoclastic resorption. Similarly, calcium deposition in bone occurs as a result of another cellular activity, the osteoblastic deposition of collagen matrix and its subsequent alteration to create crystal nuclei suitable for aggregating calcium and phosphate as hydroxyapatite. Both processes are cell mediated. However, with mineral deposition, the timing of the mineral entry lags several days behind the cell's deposition and activation of the matrix. Nucleated bone matrix creates a mineral drain, or debt, which is paid by extracting mineral from blood flowing past the new bone-forming site. Thus, stopping osteoblastic bone formation will not stop the mineralization of the last several days' accumulation of deposited matrix.

Since hormonal control mechanisms, whether endocrine or paracrine, act only through functioning cells, it follows that mineral deposition in bone is not *acutely* controllable, as is mineral removal. By contrast, both PTH and calcitonin, and their attendant mechanisms can act very promptly to alter osteoclastic resorption. That is why, as noted earlier, it is the resorptive component of bone turnover which is the one most responsive, in the scheme of Fig. 2, to alterations of input into and output from the body. Wastney et al. *(20)* demonstrated this very clearly in a metabolic-kinetic study of adolescent girls (in whom calcium absorption tends to be very efficient in order to support bone consolidation during and after the pubertal growth spurt). At a calcium intake of 21.5 mmol (860 mg)/day, absorbed calcium averaged 8 mmol (320 mg) and bone resorption 35 mmol (1400 mg)/day. When the intake was raised to 47.5 mmol (1900) mg/day, absorbed calcium rose by 11.6 mmol (464 mg) and bone resorption fell by 11 mmol (490 mg), a near mmol-for-mmol offset. However, and by contrast, bone mineralization (i.e., new bone deposition) remained unchanged.

Quantitative Operation of the System

Although the operation of the calcium regulatory system, or any feedback loop for that matter, must first be sketched out *qualitatively* (as in Fig. 2), in the final analysis it is the *quantitative* operation of the system that will determine what ultimately happens (for example, to the size of the calcium reserve, i.e., the mass of the skeleton). This *quantitative* working of the system for adjusting inputs and losses in response to dietary and other perturbations is often ignored. For example, it is commonly, if erroneously, assumed that, because intestinal calcium absorption efficiency varies inversely with intake, the body can fully compensate for declines in intake or increases in excretory loss. But quantitative analysis of the system (as well as data such as those assembled in Fig. 4) shows the fallacy of that assumption (see below). In the face of reduced intake, ECF [Ca^{2+}] tends to fall and the prior rate of absorption of food calcium no longer suffices. The result is an increase in PTH secretion, which produces the three end-organ effects described in Fig. 2, i.e., more bone resorption, improved renal conservation, and increased calcium absorption efficiency. In brief, all the three control loops are called upon to offset a shortfall caused by just one of them. The net effect with respect to total bone mass depends both on the relationship between the sensitivity of the individual effector organs and on their capacity to provide the needed calcium *(21)*. *Sensitivity* of the effectors is genetically and hormonally determined, whereas *capacity* to respond is largely determined by unregulated factors outside the control loop, such as the calcium content of the diet and factors that influence obligatory loss.

If for some reason the response of one or the other of these effectors is blunted, PTH rises further, forcing more response from the other two effectors. Conversely, if one effector (such as bone) becomes highly responsive to PTH, the hormone level rises to a lesser extent because the needed calcium is readily supplied from the nearly limitless skeletal reserves. As a result, less improvement in external calcium utilization ensues. Similarly, if the gut is unresponsive or the diet is so low in calcium that its capacity to yield the needed amount is exceeded, then PTH secretion rises further and bone is driven to meet the needs of the ECF [Ca^{2+}]. The two key insights here are (1) it is ECF [Ca^{2+}] that is being regulated, not bone mass and (2) the dose–response relationships for the three effector systems are independent of one another.

Examples of different patterns of effector responsiveness abound. Thus, American blacks (and probably African blacks as well) have a bony resorptive apparatus relatively resistant to PTH *(22–24)*. As a result, they develop and maintain a higher bone mass than do Caucasians and Orientals, despite an often poor diet. As predicted from the foregoing,

African-Americans exhibit higher PTH and calcitriol levels but lower levels of bone remodeling. In brief, they utilize and conserve diet calcium more efficiently than Caucasians. Somewhat the opposite situation occurs in all women at normal menopause. Because estrogen appears to decrease bony responsiveness to PTH, estrogen loss at menopause increases the skeletal response to PTH. This is a part of the explanation for the increase in recommended calcium intake after menopause *(25,26)*. Obese individuals also increase their bone mass as they gain weight *(27)*, and they lose less bone at menopause *(28)*. Like blacks, they have high circulating PTH levels and (presumably) a relatively resistant bone remodeling apparatus.

Age-Related Changes in Operation of the Control System

Important changes occur in these quantitative settings of the system with age, as well as in unregulated forces acting on the system. An example of the latter is the fall in calcium intake among women in the United States from early adolescence to the end of life. In NHANES-III, median calcium intake was 685 mg (~17 mmol) in early adolescence, 640 mg (~16 mmol) in the twenties, and 557 mg (~14 mmol) at menopause *(29)*. At the same time, absorption efficiency also falls with age.[1] Peripubertal girls absorb calcium with about 45% greater efficiency for the same intake than do perimenopausal women *(30)*. As already noted, from age 45 to age 60, absorption fraction drops by about 0.06 *(16)*. In concrete terms, if a 45-year-old woman absorbed a standard load at an efficiency of 30%, the same woman, at age 65 and deprived of estrogen, would absorb at an efficiency of 24% or about a 20% worsening in absorptive performance.

To complicate the situation further, renal calcium clearance rises at menopause *(31)*, an effect seen most clearly with low calcium intakes, when urinary calcium for the same intake will typically be as much as 36% higher than premenopause *(11)*. Vitamin D status declines with age as well *(32,33)*, partly because of decreases in solar exposure, cutaneous vitamin D synthetic efficiency, and milk consumption. In Europe, where solar vitamin D synthesis is low for reasons of latitude and climate and milk is generally not fortified, serum 25(OH)D concentration drops from over 100 nmol/l (40 ng/ml) in young adults to under 40 nmol/l (16 ng/ml) in individuals over age 70 years.

Not surprisingly, serum PTH rises with age as a consequence of this aggregate of age-related changes. The 24-h-integrated PTH is 70% higher in healthy 65-year-old US women consuming diets containing 800 mg calcium per day than in third-decade women on the same diets *(34)*. That this difference is due to insufficient absorptive input is shown by the fact that the difference can be completely obliterated by increasing calcium intake *(34)*.

Two Examples of System Operation

As stressed in the foregoing, it is a quantity that is being optimized (i.e., ECF [Ca^{2+}]); this is accomplished by the algebraic sum of various quantitative inputs and outputs. Two

[1] A part of this absorptive decline is due to estrogen deficiency, which both decreases renal 1-α-hydroxytation of 25(OH)D and appears to have a small effect on the intestinal mucosa. A further part may be due to decrease in mucosal mass, which, in animals varies with food intake.

examples will serve to illustrate further the importance of attending to quantities. One examines the contrast between calcium handling at menarche and menopause just described, and the second describes the response of the system at any given age to a fixed increase in obligatory loss.

Menarche and Menopause

True trabecular bone density increases by about 15% across menarche *(35)* and about the same quantum of bone is lost across menopause *(36)*. Curiously, administration of estrogen to women more than 3 years postmenopausal has generally failed to reproduce the pubertal increase in BMD, and it has been customary to say, in recent years, that apart from whatever remodeling transient estrogen (or hormone) replacement therapy (ERT/HRT) may produce in postmenopausal women *(37)*, the principal effect of ERT/HRT on bone is to stabilize bone mass, rather than to cause restoration of what had been lost. But this conclusion was drawn without attending to the quantitative aspects of the age-related changes in the calcium economy, summarized in the foregoing.

Table 2 assembles published data for median calcium intake and mean data for absorption efficiency and endogenous fecal calcium loss and shows very clearly how quantitative changes occurring in the 40 years from menarche to menopause account for the rather different performance of the two age groups. In brief (and despite an intake less than recommended), a peripubertal girl is able to achieve net absorption of 174 mg (4.3 mmol) calcium from the median diet of her age cohort, whereas an early menopausal woman extracts only about 40% as much from hers. The drop in intake amounts to about 19%, but the fall in net absorption is 61%. As Table 2 shows, this is the resultant of lower intake, lower absorption efficiency, and higher digestive juice calcium losses. Given the level of total body obligatory losses at midlife, this absorbed quantity is simply not sufficient to support an estrogen-stimulated increase in BMD. As would be predicted from this understanding, higher calcium intakes permit estrogen to produce in postmenopausal women bony increases closer to those seen at puberty *(38)* (see also "Calcium as Co-therapy").

Table 2
Net Calcium Absorption at Menarche and Menopause

	Menarche	*Menopause*
Ca intake[a]	685 mg/day (17.1 mmol/day)	557 mg/day (14 mmol/day)
Ca absorption efficiency[b]	35.2%	30.5%
Endogenous fecal Ca[c]	67 mg/day (1.7 mmol/day)	102 mg/day (2.5 mmol/day)
Net Ca absorption	174 mg/day (4.3 mmol/day)	68 mg/day (1.7 mmol/day)

[a]NHANES-III median values *(29)*.
[b]Heaney et al. *(16)*; O'Brien et al. *(30)*; values adjusted for intake.
[c]Heaney et al. *(9)*.

RESPONSE TO AUGMENTED LOSSES

As already noted, it is commonly (and uncritically) considered that the absorptive apparatus is able to compensate either for a change in intake or a change in excretory loss. However, quantitative considerations make it clear that this depends entirely on the level of calcium in the diet. Thus, an individual increasing his/her sodium intake by an amount equivalent to a single daily serving of a fast food, fried chicken meal experiences an increase in urinary calcium of about 1 mmol (40 mg)/day. Without compensating adjustments in input to the ECF, [Ca^{2+}] would drop. PTH, of course, would rise, and with it, synthesis of 1,25(OH)$_2$D, resulting ultimately in better extraction of calcium from the diet.

Published data allow rough estimation that a calcium drain of this magnitude produces an increase in 1,25(OH)$_2$D of about 6–7 pmol/l *(39)*, and dose–response measurements for 1,25(OH)$_2$D indicate that this stimulus would increase calcium absorption fraction by about 0.02–0.03 *(40)*. An increase in extraction of that magnitude from a 50 mmol (2000 mg) diet yields 1–1.5 mmol (40–60 mg) of extra calcium, more than enough to offset the increased urinary loss, whereas from a 5 mmol (200 mg) diet, the same absorptive increase yields less than 0.1 mmol (4 mg).[2] Thus, on a high-calcium diet, the body easily compensates for varying drains; both bone and ECF [Ca^{2+}] are protected. But on a low-calcium diet, although the ECF [Ca^{2+}] is protected, bone is not. Why does serum 1,25(OH)$_2$D not rise more on a low-calcium diet? Simply because the 1-α-hydroxylation step is responding to PTH. Bone calcium meets much (or most) of the ECF need, and PTH secretion is regulated by ECF [Ca^{2+}], not by bone mass.

In brief, as the body adjusts to varying demands, the portion of the demand met by bone will be determined both by factors influencing bony responsiveness and by the level of diet calcium, the principal component of the system that is not regulated. However, it must also be stressed that, although an adequate calcium intake is a necessary condition for bone building and for adaptation to varying calcium demands, it is not by itself sufficient. Calcium alone will not stop estrogen-deficiency bone loss nor disuse bone loss (because neither is due to calcium deficiency). But by the same token, recovery from immobilization or restoration of bone lost because of hormone deficiency will not be possible without an adequate supply of the raw materials needed to build bone substance.

THE CALCIUM REQUIREMENT

Calcium requirements for bone health are not uniform throughout life, first because of differences in skeletal growth rate and then because of age-related changes in absorption and excretion. In adults the calcium requirement is the amount of calcium that must be ingested to replace losses through urine, feces, and skin. During growth, pregnancy, and lactation, the requirement must also provide the calcium needed for skeletal augmentation, fetal development, and milk production. Calcium is a threshold nutrient. Above a certain intake, at each life stage, calcium retention reaches an age-specific plateau above which little or no further increase in calcium retention occurs. The ingested excess is

[2] This is partly because extraction efficiency is already relatively high on low intakes, and there is less calcium still unabsorbed on which the mucosa can work to extract additional calcium.

simply excreted. Threshold intakes for achieving maximal calcium retention at each life stage were used to set the 1997 dietary reference intakes for calcium *(26)*.

Recommendations by various national policy groups for calcium intake across the life span are given in Table 3, and their background is discussed briefly in the following sections.

Table 3
Various Estimates of the Calcium Requirement in Women[a]

Age	*1989 RDA[b]*	*NIH[c]*	*1997 DRI (AI)[d]*
1–5	800	800	500/800
6–10	800	800–1200	800/1300
11–24	1200	1200–1500	1300/1000
Pregnancy/lactation	1200	1200–1500	1000
24–50/65	800	1000	1000/1200
65–	800	1500	1200

[a]All values are given in milligrams, as this is how the respective bodies reported their recommendations. To convert to SI units, divide the values in the table by 40.

[b]Ref. *(41)*.

[c]Recommendations for women as proposed by the Consensus Development Conference on Optimal Calcium Intake *(25)*

[d]"AI" refers to "Adequate Intake" *(26)*, a value which, in this context, is equivalent to an average requirement. The corresponding RDA could be 20–30% higher, i.e., 1000 in children, 1600 in adolescents, 1200 in adults upto age 50, 1200 during pregnancy and lactation, and 1450 in those over age 50. The presence of two values in this column reflects the fact that the age categories for the DRIs overlapped those of the NIH.

Childhood and Adolescence

Net calcium accretion continues from birth through the late twenties. Rate of growth slows from the infancy high to about age 8 and then increases rapidly again. Maximal accretion occurs during the pubertal growth spurt, which occurs for most girls between the ages of 12 and 14 years and for boys, between 14 and 16 years. The intake required for mean maximal calcium retention in adolescents is 32.5–40 mmol (1300–1600 mg)/day *(42)*. Between the ages of 9 and 17, approximately 45% of the adult skeleton is acquired. Although not a linear process, this represents an average gain in bone mass of about 7–8%/year.

Several calcium or dairy supplementation trials have been conducted in children. They all demonstrate that calcium intake can positively influence bone accumulation *(43–47)*. As would be expected for any nutrient ingested basally in suboptimal amounts and then supplemented, the additional gain in bone mass during supplementation often wanes when intake drops *(48)*. This fact is sometimes used to argue that calcium augmentation is of little value, but this is to attribute magical properties to calcium. All nutrients must be ingested more or less continually to ensure adequacy of nutrition.

Milk-avoiding children have lower skeletal mass than community controls and substantially more fractures even during childhood *(49)*. (Arguably, this is osteoporosis, although the term is not usually employed for fragility fractures in the pediatric age range.) While low calcium intakes during growth will generally lead to some reduction in bone mass relative to genetic potential, the issue is complex; many populations with low calcium intakes somehow manage to amass a skeleton within the adult range for mineral content *(50)*. This means that they must make better use of their limited calcium intakes – more efficient absorption and renal conservation – than typically occurs in a Caucasian population in Western nations. Some of this must reflect ethnic differences in calcium-handling capacity. For example, African-Americans adolescent girls have been shown, at the same intake as Caucasians, to absorb calcium more efficiently and to conserve it more avidly at the kidney *(51,52)*. The published requirements for calcium intake during growth must, therefore, be understood as representing minimum requirements for bone health in a primarily Caucasian population consuming Western diets. Even Caucasian adolescents, while they gain less bone on low calcium intakes than those supplemented with calcium, are often able to "catch-up," i.e., to extend the period of bone mineral acquisition over a longer period of time; any residual shortfall tends to be seen in those who are tallest, i.e., those with the largest skeletal sizes to fill out *(53)*.

After adult height is achieved, calcium accretion continues during the phase of bone consolidation (which varies from one skeletal site to another, but for most probably ends some time in the late twenties). At the end of consolidation, when the maximum amount of bone has been accumulated, the adult is said to have achieved his or her peak bone mass. However, the timing of peak bone mass varies with skeletal site. The hip achieves peak bone density at approximately age 17–18, whereas the spine can add mass throughout most of the third decade of life in females *(27)*. The skull accumulates bone throughout life, as does the femur shaft *(27,54)*. However, for the most part, the window of opportunity to build bone is largely closed some time before age 30.

Although 60–80% of peak bone mass is genetically predetermined, a number of environmental factors also importantly affect bone mass. The two sources of variability are not mutually exclusive because genetic factors are often expressed in the way the organism responds to its environment (e.g., variation in absorptive efficiency for ingested calcium). Aside from calcium intake, other lifestyle choices that affect peak bone mass include physical activity, intake of other nutrients that alter calcium utilization (see "Nutrient–Nutrient Interactions"), anorexia, and substance abuse.

Adults

The mature female body contains ~25–30 mol (1000–1200 g) calcium and the mature male ~30–40 mol (1200–1600 g). The population coefficient of variation around these means is about 15%. Total body bone mass remains relatively constant over the reproductive years, as decreases in the proximal femur and other sites after age 18 are offset by continued growth at the forearm, femur shaft, total spine, and head. Then, at midlife, menopausal and age-related bone loss sets in. Menopausal loss occurs most rapidly during the 2 years prior to and the 3 years following menopause, and amounts to 5.3% at the upper femur and 10.5% at the lumbar spine *(55)*. The average older adult loses bone at a rate of 0.5–1%/year, rising to as high as 3%/year by age 80 *(56)*. The explanation for bone loss during aging includes a variety of causes, such as declining calcium intakes, declining physical activity, decreased levels of gonadal hormones, decreased circulating levels of $1,25(OH)_2D$, intestinal resistance to $1,25(OH)_2D$, and decreases in calcium absorption and in renal calcium conservation, and perhaps most importantly, intercurrent episodes of illness and hospitalization.

The threshold intake need to maintain adult bone mass during the reproductive years is 20–25 mmol (800–1000 mg)/day. After age 50–60, the threshold intake required to minimize age-related loss rises to 30–40 mmol (1200–1600 mg)/day. Although the matter of the adult calcium requirement would seem largely to have been settled, papers reporting skeletal outcomes for various calcium intakes continue to be published, some finding little effect. Overall, however, more than 90% of the randomized trials in adults show a beneficial effect of higher calcium intake and about 80% of the observational studies are positive as well. Nevertheless individual studies, taken in isolation, can confuse the issue. Publication of results of the calcium and vitamin D arm of the Women's Health Initiative (WHI) is a case in point *(57)*.

WHI found a modest sparing of hip bone loss in the calcium-supplemented group, but no significant reduction in hip fracture risk when analyzed by intention-to-treat. (However, compliance was poor and there was a significant, 29%, reduction in numbers of hip fractures in those complying with the supplement regimen.) This absence of a significant effect by ITT was widely reported as indicating that calcium had little value. However, among other flaws, WHI had no low-calcium control group. Mean intake in the placebo group was already at the recommended intake level. Hence at least half the women were already at or above their respective intake thresholds and had already realized the protective benefit of high calcium intake. They would not have been predicted to respond to further supplementation.[3] Curiously, and despite the largely null effect of the controlled trial, WHI actually provides strong observational evidence in support of existing recommendations. Women entering the trial had calcium intakes nearly twice the national average for their age and sustained a hip fracture rate about half what had been predicted from Medicare statistics. It is not implausible that those two departures from expectation were causally related.

CALCIUM SOURCES

Dietary Considerations

Dietary sources and calcium intakes have changed considerably during human evolution. Early humans derived calcium from roots, tubers, nuts, and greens, as well as the bones of small prey, in quantities believed to exceed 37.5 mmol (1500 g) per day *(59)*, and perhaps up to twice this amount when calculated on the basis of consuming food to meet the caloric demands of a hunter-gatherer of contemporary body size. After domestication of seed-bearing plants, calcium intakes decreased substantially because the staple foods became cereal grains and fruits, the plant parts that contain the least calcium. Consequently, the modern human often consumes insufficient calcium to optimize bone density. The food group that supplies the bulk of the calcium in the Western diet is now the dairy food group, which was not represented at all in the paleolithic diet.

[3] Further treatment of the importance of a low calcium control group can be found in Heaney and Bachmann *(58)*.

Bioavailability

The term "bioavailability" is pharmacologic in origin and has complex connotations. But for mineral ions, and particularly for calcium, these complexities reduce approximately to a simple matter of absorbability. Bioavailability can be measured in several ways, perhaps the most direct and straightforward being the introduction of a suitable isotopic tracer into the calcium source and then the calibrated measurement of the appearance of that tracer in body fluids. These methods permit direct estimation of true unidirectional flux from the intestinal lumen into the body, usually expressed as a decimal fraction of the ingested load. Load size, as discussed earlier, is itself an important determinant of fractional absorption; hence it is not possible to establish a single value for bioavailability for any given calcium source, since its absorption fraction will be dependent on how much was consumed. Clearly, therefore, comparative studies require comparable loads.

A second approach is to measure the small rise in serum total calcium or ECF [Ca^{2+}] following oral ingestion, i.e., a pharmacokinetic approach, using mainly the area under the curve (AUC) of the absorptive rise. As already discussed, the body attempts to damp these absorptive rises; hence they tend to be small and correspondingly require very precise measurement of serum calcium (total or ionized). Pharmacokinetic methods reflect *net* absorption and do not permit direct estimation of absorption fraction, but can be useful in comparing two or more substances, and particularly substances into which it is not possible to introduce a suitable isotopic tracer.

Methods that are even less sensitive measure the increment in urine calcium and/or the decrement in serum PTH, both of which are typically associated with the absorptive rise in serum calcium. These are less sensitive measures both because they are inherently more variable (both within and between subjects), and because the assay methods introduce an additional level of imprecision in their own right.

In general, the isotopic tracer methods have the smallest sample size requirement, the pharmacokinetic methods, an intermediate requirement, and changes in urine calcium or PTH, the largest sample size. Finally, only the isotopic tracer methods produce results that directly translate to true fractional absorption.

Bioavailability is important in this context because not all calcium sources have equally available calcium. As discussed earlier, vegetable greens of the mustard family have an intrinsic bioavailability slightly greater than that of milk, whereas other vegetables, such as beans, sweet potatoes, and at the low end of the spectrum, spinach and rhubarb, exhibit much lower bioavailability for their calcium. Since the range of intrinsic bioavailability values spans something close to a full order of magnitude, it is clear that the available data in food tables do not give a clear picture of the *effective* calcium delivery for each. In the section that follows, I shall show data reflecting both the calcium content of various foods *and their bioavailability.*

Food Sources and Bioavailability

For adults, dairy products supply 72% of the calcium in the US diet, grain products about 11%, and vegetables and fruits about 6% *(60)*. It is difficult for most individuals to ingest enough calcium from foods available in a cereal-based economy without including liberal amounts of dairy products. Ethnic and cultural practices, such as processing corn tortillas with lime, to some extent overcome the inherent limitation of cereal-based foods.

Food manufacturers have recently developed a wider variety of calcium-fortified products that explicitly compensate for their low calcium content. Additionally, many individuals have turned to dietary supplements to meet their calcium needs. However, it is prudent to remember that calcium is not the only nutrient important for health which is supplied by dairy products. Users of milk in the United States compared to nonusers get 35% more vitamin A, 38% more folate, 56% more riboflavin, 22% more magnesium, and 24% more potassium, in addition to 80% more calcium *(61)*.

Aside from gross calcium content, potential calcium sources should be evaluated for bioavailability. Fractional calcium absorption from various dairy products is similar for comparable loads. The calcium from most supplements is absorbed approximately as well as that from milk, since solubility of the salts at neutral pH has little impact on calcium absorption *(62)*. Absorption of one very soluble, complex salt, calcium citrate malate (CCM), is slightly to moderately better than that of most other salts *(63)*.

Several plant constituents form indigestible salts with calcium, thereby decreasing absorption of calcium. The most potent inhibitor of calcium absorption is oxalic acid, found in high concentration in spinach and rhubarb and to a lesser extent in sweet potatoes and beans *(64)*. Calcium absorption fraction from spinach is only 0.04–0.05, compared with 0.27–0.33 from milk ingested at a similar load *(65)*.

Phytic acid, the storage form of phosphorus in seeds, is a modest inhibitor of calcium absorption *(66)*. Fermentation, as occurs during bread making, reduces phytic acid interference because of the phytase present in live yeast *(67)*. Since the early balance studies of McCance and Widdowson *(68)*, who reported negative calcium balance while consuming whole wheat products, it has been assumed that fiber negatively affects calcium balance through either physical entrapment or catonic binding with uronic acid residues *(69)*. However, it is more likely that the phytic acid associated with fiber-rich foods is the component that affected balance, since most purified fibers do not affect calcium absorption appreciably *(70)*. Only concentrated sources of phytate such as wheat bran *(67)* or dried beans *(71)* substantially reduce calcium absorption. For other plants rich in calcium (primarily the *Brassica* genus, which includes broccoli, kale, bok choy, cabbage, mustard, and turnip greens), calcium bioavailability is as good as or better than that from milk *(72)*, despite their high-fiber content (see Fig. 5).

Figure 7 summarizes these concepts graphically, plotting the amount of calcium absorbed from a typical serving of various natural foods. Absorbed calcium in this case is the product of calcium content and measured bioavailability. The figure shows clearly why dairy sources are so important. Foods such as the *Brassica* sp. vegetables exhibit excellent calcium bioavailability (e.g., Fig. 5), but, as Fig. 7 demonstrates, depending on them (and other generally available vegetable sources) to meet one's intake needs would generally not be feasible.

Nutrient–Nutrient Interactions

Several nutrients and food constituents affect aspects of calcium homeostasis by means other than through the straightforward effect on digestibility and absorbability just described. Several dietary components influence urinary calcium excretion. One of the more important, mentioned briefly at the outset, is dietary sodium *(6,7,73)*. Sodium and calcium share some of the same transport systems in the proximal tubule, so that each 100 mmol (2.3 g) increment of sodium excreted by the kidney pulls out approximately 0.5–1.5 mmol

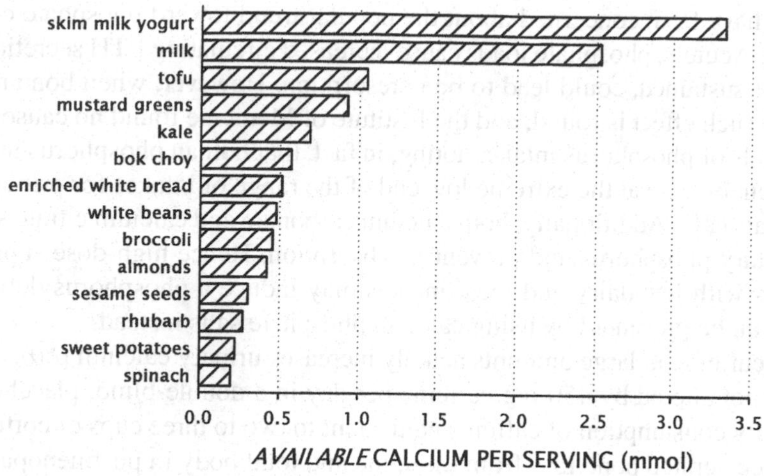

Fig. 7. Available calcium per serving (in mmol) for several natural foods. "Available" for this purpose means the product of calcium content per serving and measured bioavailability (to convert mmol to mg, multiply by 40). (Copyright Robert P. Heaney, 1998. Used with permission.)

(20–60 mg) of accompanying calcium. Because differences in urinary calcium account for about half of the variability in calcium retention, dietary sodium can have a potentially large influence on bone loss. In adult women, each extra gram of sodium per day is projected to produce an additional rate of bone loss of 1% per year if the calcium lost in the urine comes from the skeleton *(74)*. A longitudinal study of postmenopausal women showed a negative correlation between urinary sodium excretion and bone density of the hip *(75)*. The authors concluded, from the range of values available to them, that bone loss could have been prevented either by a daily increase in dietary calcium of 891 mg (~22 mmol) or by halving the daily sodium intake. As experienced clinicians will recognize, the latter option is the less practicable.

Another dietary component that influences urinary calcium retention is protein. Each gram of protein metabolized can increase urinary calcium levels by about 0.025 mmol (1 mg); thus, doubling the amount of purified dietary proteins or amino acids in the diet may increase urinary calcium by about 50% *(4)*. The acid load of the sulfate produced in the metabolism of sulfur-containing amino acids is believed to be partly responsible for this effect. At the other extreme, inadequate protein intakes compromise bone health and may contribute to osteoporosis in the elderly. Because fresh dietary protein is necessary for bone matrix synthesis, protein and calcium actually function synergistically. Thus Hannan et al. *(76)* showed that age-related bone loss was *inversely* associated with protein intake, not directly as might have been predicted from protein's calciuric propensity. Further, Dawson-Hughes and Harris *(77)* showed that bone gain in their trial of calcium supplementation was confined to those with the highest protein intakes. Thus, as discussed earlier (see "Quantitative Operation of the System"), high protein intakes are potentially harmful only in the face of low calcium intakes.

Although widely varying ratios of dietary phosphorus and calcium have not been associated with changes in adult calcium balance *(78)* (presumably because of the offset of increased endogenous secretion of calcium by decreased urinary calcium), some investigators have been concerned about the popular trend toward phosphate consumption in soft drinks. Acutely, phosphate loads cause increased circulating PTH secretion. Elevated PTH levels, if sustained, could lead to bone resorption. However, when bone resorption is measured, no such effect is found, and the Institute of Medicine found no cause for concern in current levels of phosphorus intake, noting, in fact, that human phosphorus intakes, when adjusted for energy, are at the extreme low end of the range of intakes for primates and laboratory animals *(26)*. Additionally, both calcium carbonate and calcium citrate supplements will bind dietary phosphorus and prevent its absorption. Hence high-dose supplement use in individuals with low dairy and meat intakes may induce a phosphorus deficiency state *(79)*, which can be prevented by using calcium phosphate salts instead.

Although caffeine in large amounts acutely increases urinary calcium *(80)*, 24-h urinary calcium was not altered by 450 mg caffeine per day in a double-blind, placebo-controlled trial *(81)*. Daily consumption of caffeine equivalent to two to three cups of coffee was associated with accelerated bone loss from the spine and total body in postmenopausal women who consumed less than 744 mg calcium per day *(82)*, but not in women with higher calcium intakes *(83)*. The relationship between caffeine intake and bone loss in observational studies may be due to a small decrease in calcium absorption *(84)* or to a confounding factor such as a probable inverse association between milk intake and caffeine intake.

Fat intake has a negative impact on calcium balance only during steatorrhea. In this condition, calcium forms insoluble soaps with fatty acids in the gut.

Increased use of calcium supplements and fortified foods has raised concern about high calcium intakes producing relative deficiencies of several minerals. High calcium intakes have produced relative magnesium deficiencies in rats *(85)*; however, calcium intake does not affect magnesium retention in humans *(86)*. Similarly, except for a single report in postmenopausal women *(87)*, decreased zinc retention has not been associated with high calcium intakes *(88)*. The nature of this interaction is complicated and requires further study.

Iron absorption from non-heme sources is decreased by half from radiolabeled test meals in the presence of calcium intakes up to 300 mg (7.5 mmol) Ca/day, above which there is no further reduction. However, up to 12 weeks of calcium supplementation does not change iron status *(89)*, and adolescent girls ingesting high-calcium diets are able to increase total body iron mass quite as well as girls with low calcium intakes *(90)*. This is probably because of compensating upregulation of iron absorption. Single-meal iron absorption studies inevitably exaggerate inhibitory effects that do not appear in the context of the whole diet and of physiological adaptation.

Fortified Foods

The notion of fortifying commonly used foods is an old one. The iodination of table salt is an example and is clearly responsible for virtual elimination of iodine-deficiency goiter in countries that have adopted this practice. As the human population has moved into regions of the world, the soils of which cannot provide the nutrients to which their physiologies have been adapted over the course of hominid evolution, we need to discover what the missing nutrients may be and then find ways to supply them at a population level. Fortification has the advantage that anyone using the fortified foods gets the benefits, without having to make a voluntary decision and without needing to adhere to that decision over the long term. The nutrient concerned simply becomes a part of the food supply, just as it would have been under primitive conditions.

As noted earlier, the portions of plants that are lowest in calcium are the seeds, and, of course, the agricultural revolution has been based on seed crops, principally cereal grains and legumes. More than 60% of the total energy intake of the world's population today comes from these seed food sources, whereas only a tiny fraction of the energy intake of the evolving hominid would have been from such foods. It makes sense, therefore, to enrich the calcium content of the seed foods, and such is beginning to happen in several countries around the world. Others reserve fortification as an instrument of national policy and do not permit voluntary fortification by manufacturers of the foods they produce. Admittedly, voluntary fortification is not always optimal as it often leads to high levels of enrichment of certain foods, rather than a general improvement of most of the food items in the diet. This is a rapidly evolving field, driven less by nutritional science than by market forces, and it is difficult to predict exactly what the aggregate impact of present practices will be.

Calcium is now added as various salts (principally carbonate, phosphate, lactate, and sulfate) to a variety of foods, including ready-to-eat cereals, bread, cereal bars, energy drinks, and fruit juices. Not always has the bioavailability of the calcium in the fortified product been tested. This is not just a theoretical concern. Experience has shown that interactions between the fortificant and other food constituents may affect bioavailability. So, as with natural foods, knowledge of the total calcium content of a fortified food may not be enough. For the next few years, at least, it will become increasingly difficult to assess a person's effective calcium intake, since it will be necessary to ascertain whether or not foods consumed were of a calcium-fortified variety, the level of fortification, and the bioavailability of the aggregate calcium content of the food.

In the best of all possible worlds, the fortification of foods would raise the calcium density of the total diet (i.e., mmol calcium per MJ of energy) to levels approximating that of the primitive diet, i.e., ~4.8 mmol/MJ. At such a time it would no longer be necessary to worry about or assess calcium intake, just as we no longer attempt to assess iodine intake.

Supplements

Calcium supplements will often be necessary in order to achieve desired total calcium intakes, although, with the growing availability of fortified foods, the need for supplements may well decline. Calcium supplements come in a large variety of forms involving different anions and different dosage units. Calcium carbonate and calcium citrate are probably the predominant forms in North America, with the carbonate accounting for the lion's share of the total market. Calcium carbonate has been shown to exhibit good bioavailability (see, for example, Fig. 5). It is economical, it is generally well tolerated, and it exhibits close to the highest calcium density of any of the products available on the market. Most of the calcium supplements on the market today exhibit nearly equivalent bioavailability with some, such as calcium citrate malate or the calcium chelates, exhibiting somewhat better fractional absorption. But generally the differences between the products are so minor as to be negligible or to be easily offset by taking a single extra pill of a less expensive, if less well absorbed, product each week.

However, not all products are equally well formulated, in a pharmaceutical sense. While the pharmaceutics of tablet disintegration and dissolution are well understood, the supplement market, in the United States at least, is not held to those standards, and there was a period of time in the 1980s and the 1990s in which varieties of calcium supplement tablets were widely distributed which simply did not disintegrate in the gastrointestinal tract, and hence enriched no one except their manufacturer. The United States Pharmacopeia (USP) has established disintegration standards for calcium supplements, but adherence to these standards is voluntary, and regulation by the FDA in the United States is minimal. Hence the best course of action in the foreseeable future is to use brand name supplements that adhere to USP standards or have been the subject of suitable bioavailability testing (or both).

Dose Timing

If the calcium is in the food, either naturally or through fortification, then timing is not a relevant issue, since the calcium will come into the body with the other nutrients of the food being consumed. However, if resort is to calcium supplements, then timing can be a factor. Generally the safest course is to take calcium with meals. This replicates the primitive food pattern, and it tends to spread the intake out over the day, so as to optimize absorption (see, for example, Fig. 6). There are obvious problems involved in remembering to take multiple doses of medication, as well as adherence problems with pill-taking generally. (That is one of the reasons why a food fortification policy is likely to produce better population penetration than a strategy based on calcium supplements.)

An argument has been made for taking calcium supplements at bedtime, inasmuch as much of the PTH-mediated bone resorption occurs in the early hours of the morning, and a large calcium dose at bedtime has been shown to suppress PTH secretion. Whether, in the last analysis, this makes any difference to bone mass has not been established. At least one study suggests that this stratagem has little effect *(91)*.

Drug Interference

Calcium is a nutrient and, as such, exhibits little or no interactions with most medications, as is true for most other nutrients as well. Calcium does interfere with iron absorption in single-meal tests, but, as noted above, does not impede the accumulation of total body iron stores in adolescent girls. Similarly, concern about negative interactions between calcium and zinc and magnesium has proved to be unfounded *(86,88)*. This should not be surprising since, once again, calcium is a nutrient that was present in high concentration in the primitive diet. If its presence there had interfered substantially with other nutrients essential for the health of the human organism, we would never have survived as a species.

Calcium does not interfere with the action of calcium channel blockers, except insofar as their effect on the body may be indirectly influenced by the circulating level of PTH [and, correspondingly, *1,25*$(OH)_2D$]. Calcium, on the other hand, may interfere with the absorption of the tetracycline antibiotics, since the tetracyclines strongly adsorb to calcium crystals, which may to some extent be present in the intestinal lumen when the diet is high in calcium. Large doses of calcium have also been reported to interfere with absorption of thyroxine *(92)*, although the effect is small. Nevertheless individuals being treated for hypothyroidism should separate their intakes of thyroxine and calcium by at least 2 h.

Calcium as Co-therapy

Until now the discussion has focused more or less exclusively on calcium as a nutrient. There is a sense, also, in which it can be considered co-therapy particularly in the treatment of disorders such as osteoporosis. Here the knee-jerk reflex has commonly been to think about treatment in terms of *pharmaco*therapy, ignoring the fact that bone is built of mineral, not of drugs or hormones, and that the efficacy of drug or hormone regimens may well depend to a substantial extent on providing adequate raw materials to build or maintain bone in the presence of bone-active pharmacologic agents. All of the modern bone-active agents [bisphosphonates, SERMs, and PTH *(93–98)*] have been tested only in the effective presence of supplemental calcium, and it could be a mistake to conclude that they would remain effective if they were given without additional calcium. The additive effect of calcium is seen most clearly, perhaps, with respect to HRT, where there is extensive experience both with and without supplemental calcium. Figure 8 reproduces the data of a meta-analysis on this topic *(38)* showing the strongly additive effect of the addition of calcium to an HRT regimen.

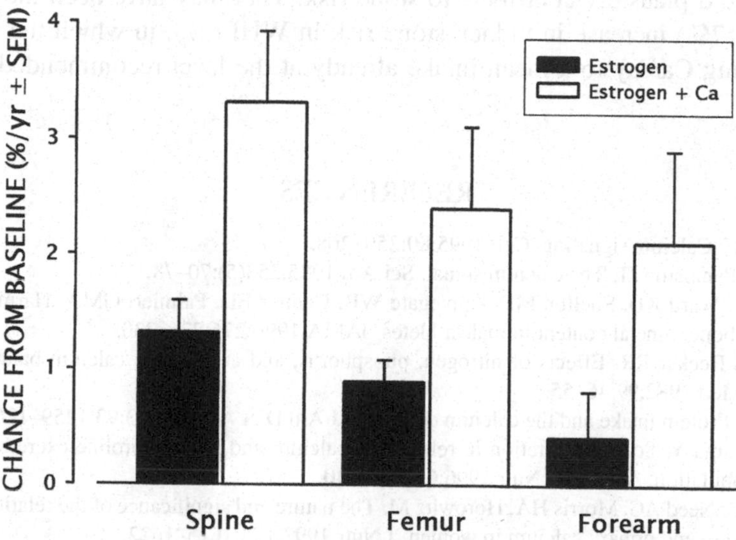

Fig. 8. Change in bone mineral density at three skeletal sites with estrogen replacement in postmenopausal women, both with and without supplementalcalcium. (Redrawn from the data of Nieves et al. (38); Copyright Robert P. Heaney, 2000. Used with permission.)

While 30–40 mmol (1200–1600 mg) calcium per day, the intake recommended for adults over age 50, is probably adequate for skeletal maintenance in an aging population, it may not be sufficient to realize the full effects of the bone-active agents used in treatment of osteoporosis. All antiresorptives are, effectively, PTH antagonists, and hence they lead to increased PTH secretion and correspondingly better peripheral conservation of calcium. But, given prevailing calcium intakes, it is uncertain whether this effect, by itself, is enough to take full advantage of the pharmacotherapy. Hence exact calcium intake requirements for maximal effect are not known. But one anabolic agent, fluoride, has been shown to produce an extraordinary degree of bone hunger, with a consequent requirement for calcium above 60 mmol/day *(99)*.

Toxicity

Too much of any nutrient can produce intoxication and calcium is no exception. However, calcium intoxication, expressed principally as the milk alkali syndrome *(26)*, is extremely rare and has never been reported for food calcium sources. Pastoralist peoples of various ethnic backgrounds regularly consume 150–180 mmol (6000–7200 mg) calcium per day, lifelong, without hint of adverse effects. All reports of calcium toxicity relate to supplement administration, mostly as calcium carbonate.

Additionally, calcium-containing kidney stones can occur in individuals with high supplement intakes *(57)*. Generally, however, the effect is in the opposite direction, with high calcium intakes reducing stone risk by up to 50% *(100,101)*. This is because the complexation of food oxalates by unabsorbed calcium in the gut lumen reduces oxalate absorption and hence lowers the renal oxalate burden *(101,102)*. Mol for mol, oxalate is a much more potent stone risk factor than is calcium. Hence the theoretical increase in stone risk from a high calcium intake is more than offset by the decrease in risk from the reduced oxalate load *(102)*. However, once all the dietary oxalate has been bound, further increases in calcium intake could plausibly contribute to stone risk. That may have been the explanation for the small (17%) increase in kidney stone risk in WHI *(57)*, in which the intervention added ~1000 mg Ca/day to a mean intake already at the level recommended for women over age 50.

REFERENCES

1. Clapham DE. Calcium signaling. Cell 1995;80:259–268.
2. Carafoli E, Penniston JT. The calcium signal. Sci Am 1985;253(5):70–78.
3. Klesges RC, Ward KD, Shelton ML, Applegate WB, Cantler ED, Palmieri GMA, Harmon K, Davis J. Changes in bone mineral content in male athletes. JAMA 1996;276:226–230.
4. Heaney RP, Recker RR. Effects of nitrogen, phosphorus, and caffeine on calcium balance in women. J Lab Clin Med 1982;99:46–55.
5. Heaney RP. Protein intake and the calcium economy. J Am Diet Assoc 1993;93:1259–1260.
6. Itoh R, Suyama Y. Sodium excretion in relation to calcium and hydroxyproline excretion in a healthy Japanese population. Am J Clin Nutr 1996;63:735–740.
7. Nordin BEC, Need AG, Morris HA, Horowitz M. The nature and significance of the relationship between urinary sodium and urinary calcium in women. J Nutr 1993;123:1615–1622.
8. Arnaud CD. Calcium homeostasis: regulatory elements and their integration. Fed Proc 1978;37:2557–2560.
9. Heaney RP, Recker RR. Determinants of endogenous fecal calcium in healthy women. J Bone Miner Res 1994;9:1621–1627.
10. Coluccio LM. Identification of the microvillar 110-kDa calmodulin complex (myosin-1) in kidney. Eur J Cell Biol 1991;56:286–294.
11. Heaney RP, Recker RR, Ryan RA. Urinary calcium in perimenopausal women: normative values. Osteoporos Int 1999;9:13–18.
12. Nemere I, Leathers V, Norman AW. 1,25-dihydroxyvitamin D3-mediated intestinal calcium transport. Biochemical identification of lysosomes containing calcium and calcium-binding protein (calbindin-D28K). J Biol Chem 1986;261:16106–16114.
13. Wasserman RH, Chandler JS, Meyer SA, Smith CA, Brindak ME, Fullmer CS, Penniston JT, Kumar R. Intestinal calcium transport and calcium extrusion processes at the basolateral membrane. J Nutr 1992;122:662–671.
14. Karbach U. Paracellular calcium transport across the small intestine. J Nutr 1992;122:672–677.
15. Hanes DA, Weaver CM, Heaney RP, Wastney M. Absorption of calcium oxalate does not require dissociation in rats. J Nutr 1999;129:170–173.

16. Heaney RP, Recker RR, Stegman MR, Moy AJ. Calcium absorption in women: relationships to calcium intake, estrogen status, and age. J Bone Miner Res 1989;4:469–475.
17. Heaney RP, Saville PD, Recker RR. Calcium absorption as a function of calcium intake. J Lab Clin Med 1975;85:881–890.
18. Heaney RP, Weaver CM, Fitzsimmons ML. The influence of calcium load on absorption fraction. J Bone Miner Res 1990;11:1135–1138.
19. Heaney RP, Berner B, Louie-Helm J. Dosing regimen for calcium supplementation. J Bone Miner Res 2000;15:2291.
20. Wastney ME, Martin BR, Peacock M, Smith D, Jiang X-Y, Jackman LA, Weaver CM. Changes in calcium kinetics in adolescent girls induced by high calcium intake. J Clin Endocrinol Metab 2000;85: 4470–4475.
21. Heaney RP. A unified concept of osteoporosis. Am J Med 1965;39:877–880.
22. Bell NH, Greene A, Epstein S, Oexmann MJ, Shaw S, Shary J. Evidence for alteration of the vitamin D-endocrine system in blacks. J Clin Invest 1985;76:470–473.
23. Aloia JF, Mikhail M, Pagan CD, Arunachalam A, Yeh JK, Flaster E. Biochemical and hormonal variables in black and white women matched for age and weight. J Lab Clin Med 1998;132:383–389.
24. Cosman F, Shen V, Morgan D, Gordon S, Parisien M, Nieves J, Lindsay R. Biochemical responses of bone metabolism to 1,25-dihydroxyvitamin D administration in black and white women. Osteoporos Int 2000;11:271–277.
25. NIH Consensus Conference. Optimal calcium intake. J Am Med Assoc 1994;272:1942–1948.
26. Dietary reference intakes for calcium, magnesium, phosphorus, vitamin D, and fluoride. Washington, D.C.: Food and Nutrition Board, Institute of Medicine, National Academy Press 1997.
27. Matkovic V, Jelic T, Wardlaw GM, Ilich JZ, Goel PK, Wright JK, Andon MB, Smith KT, Heaney RP. Timing of peak bone mass in Caucasian females and its implication for the prevention of osteoporosis. J Clin Invest 1994;93:799–808.
28. Ribot C, Tremollieres F, Pouilles JM, Bonneu M, Germain F, Louvet JP. Obesity and postmenopausal bone loss: the influence of obesity on vertebral density and bone turnover in postmenopausal women. Bone 1988;8:327–331.
29. Alaimo K, McDowell MA, Briefel RR, Bischof AM, Caughman CR, Loria CM, Johnson CL. Dietary intake of vitamins, minerals, and fiber of persons 2 months and over in the United States: Third National Health and Nutrition Examination Survey, Phase 1, 1988–91. Advance data from vital and health statistics; no 258 Hyattsville, Maryland: National Center for Health Statistics 1994.
30. O'Brien KO, Abrams SA, Liang LK, Ellis KJ, Gagel RF. Increased efficiency of calcium absorption during short periods of inadequate calcium intake in girls. Am J Clin Nutr 1996;63:579–583.
31. Nordin BEC, Need AG, Morris HA, Horowitz M. Biochemical variables in pre- and postmenopausal women: reconciling the calcium and estrogen hypotheses. Osteoporos Int 1999;9:351–357.
32. McKenna MJ, Freaney R, Meade A, Muldowney FP. Hypovitaminosis D and elevated serum alkaline phosphatase in elderly Irish people. Am J Clin Nutr 1985;41:101–109.
33. Francis RM, Peacock M, Storer JH, Davies AEJ, Brown WB, Nordin BEC. Calcium malaborption in the elderly: the effect of treatment with oral 25-hydroxyvitamin D_3. Eur J Clin Invest 1983;13:391–396.
34. McKane WR, Khosla S, Egan KS, Robins SP, Burritt MF, Riggs BL. Role of calcium intake in modulating age-related increases in parathyroid function and bone resorption. J Clin Endocrinol Metab 1996;81:1699–1703.
35. Gilsanz V, Gibbens DT, Roe TF, Carlson M, Senac MO, Boechat MI, Huang HK, Schulz FE, Libanati CR, Cann C. Vertebral bone density in children: effect of puberty. Radiology 1988;166:847–850.
36. Genant HK, Cann CF, Ettinger B, Gordan OS, Kolb FO, Reiser U, Arnaud CD. Quantitative computed tomography for spinal mineral assessment. In: Christiansen C, et al. eds., Osteoporosis. Copenhagen, Denmark: Glostrup Hospital, Departnent of Chemistry 1984:65–72.
37. Heaney RP. The bone remodeling transient: implications for the interpretation of clinical studies of bone mass change. J Bone Miner Res 1994;9:1515–1523.
38. Nieves JW, Komar L, Cosman F, Lindsay R. Calcium potentiates the effect of estrogen and calcitonin on bone mass: review and analysis. Am J Clin Nutr 1998;67:18–24.
39. Dawson-Hughes B, Stem DT, Shipp CC, Rasmussen HM. Effect of lowering dietary calcium intake on fractional whole body calcium retention. J Clin Endocrinol Metab 1988;67:62–68.

40. Heaney RP, Barger-Lux MJ, Dowell MS, Chen TC, Holick MF. Calcium absorptive effects of vitamin D and its major metabolites. J Clin Endocrinol Metab 1997;82:4111–4116.
41. Recommended dietary allowances, 10th ed. Washington, D.C.: National Academy Press 1989.
42. Jackman LA, Millane SS, Martin BR, Wood OB, McCabe GP, Peacock M, Weaver CM. Calcium retention in relation to calcium intake and postmenarcheal age in adolescent females. Am J Clin Nutr 1997;66: 327–333.
43. Johnston CC Jr, Miller JZ, Slemenda CW, Reister TK, Hui S, Christian JC, Peacock M. Calcium supplementation and increases in bone mineral density in children. N Engl J Med 1992;327:82–87.
44. Lloyd T, Andon MB, Rollings N, Martel JK, Landis JR, Demers LM, Eggli DF, Kieselhorst K, Kulin HE. Calcium supplementation and bone mineral density in adolscent girls. JAMA 1993;270:841–844.
45. Lee WTK, Leung SSF, Leung DMY, Tsang HSY, Lau J, Cheng JCY. A randomized double-blind controlled calcium supplementation trial, and bone and height acquisition in children. Br J Nutr 1995;74:125–139.
46. Chan GM, Hoffman K, McMurry M. Effects of dairy products on bone and body composition in pubertal girls. J Pediatr 1995;126:551–556.
47. Cadogan J, Eastell R, Jones N, Barker ME. Milk intake and bone mineral acquisition in adolescent girls: randomized, controlled intervention trial. BMJ 1997;315:1255–1260.
48. Lee WTK, Leung SSF, Leung DMY, Cheng JCY. A follow-up study on the effects of calcium-supplement withdrawal and puberty on bone acquisition of children. Am J Clin Nutr 1996;64:71–77.
49. Goulding A, Rockell JEP, Black RE, Grant AM, Jones IE, Williams SM. Children who avoid drinking cow's milk are at increased risk for prepubertal bone fractures. J Am Diet Assoc 2004;104: 250–253.
50. Prentice A, Bates CJ. An appraisal of the adequacy of dietary mineral intakes in developing countries for bone growth and development in children. Nutr Res Rev 1993;6:51–69.
51. Wigertz K, Palacios C, Jackman LA, Martin BR, McCabe LD, McCabe GP, Peacock M, Pratt JH, Weaver CM. Racial differences in calcium retention in response to dietary salt in adolescent girls. Am J Clin Nutr 2005;81:845–850.
52. Abrams SA, O'Brien KO, Liang LK, Stuff JE. Differences in calcium absorption and kinetics between black and white girls aged 5–16 years. J Bone Miner Res 1995;10:829–833.
53. Matkovic V, Goel PK, Badenhop-Stevens NE, Landoll JD, Bin L, Ilich JZ, Skugor M, Nagode LA, Mobley SL, Ha E-J, Hangartner TN, Clairmont A. Calcium supplementation and bone mineral density in females from childhood to young adulthood: a randomized controlled trial. Am J Clin Nutr 2005;81:175–188.
54. Heaney RP, Barger-Lux MJ, Davies KM, Ryan RA, Johnson ML, Gong G. Bone dimensional change with age: interactions of genetic, hormonal, and body size variables. Osteoporos Int 1997;7:426–431.
55. Recker RR, Lappe JM, Davies KM, Heaney RP. Characterization of perimenopausal bone loss: a prospective study. J Bone Miner Res 2000;15:1965–1973.
56. Chapuy MC, Arlot ME, Duboeuf F, Brun J, Crouzet B, Arnaud S, Delmas PD, Meunier PJ. Vitamin D_3 and calcium to prevent hip fractures in elderly women. N Engl J Med 1992;327:1637–1642.
57. Jackson RD, LaCroix AZ, Gass M, Wallace RB, Robbins J, et al. Calcium plus vitamin D supplementation and the risk of fractures. N Engl J Med 2006;354:669–683.
58. Heaney RP, Bachmann GA. Interpreting studies of nutritional prevention. A perspective using calcium as a model. J Women's Health 2005;14:990–997.
59. Eaton SB, Konner M. Paleolithic nutrition. A consideration of its nature and current implications. N Engl J Med 1985;312:283–289.
60. US Department of Agriculture, Nationwide Food Consumption Survey 1987–1988, PB-92-500016. Washington, DC: US Government Printing Office 1989.
61. Fleming KH, Heimbach JT. Consumption of calcium in the US: food sources and intake levels. J Nutr 1994;124:1426S–1430S.
62. Heaney RP, Recker RR, Weaver CM. Absorbability of calcium sources: the limited role of solubility. Calcif Tissue Int 1990;46:300–304.
63. Andon MB, Peacock M, Kanerva RL, DeCastro JAS. Calcium absorption from apple and orange juice fortified with calcium citrate malate (CCM). J Am Coll Nutr 1996;15:313–316.
64. Heaney RP, Weaver CM. Oxalate: Effect on calcium absorption. Am J Clin Nutr 1989;50:830–832.

65. Heaney RP, Weaver CM, Recker RR. Calcium absorbability from spinach. Am J Clin Nutr 1988;47: 707–709.
66. Heaney RP, Weaver CM, Fitzsimmons ML. Soybean phytate content: effect on calcium absorption. Am J Clin Nutr 1991;53:745–747.
67. Weaver CM, Heaney RP, Martin BR, Fitzsimmons ML. Human calcium absorption from whole wheat products. J Nutr 1991;121:1769–1775.
68. McCance RA, Widdowson EM. Mineral metabolism of healthy adults on white and brown bread dietaries. J Physiol 1942;101:44–85.
69. James WPT, Branch WJ, Southgate DAT. Calcium binding by dietary fibre. Lancet 1978;1:638–639.
70. Heaney RP, Weaver CM. Effect of psyllium on absorption of co-ingested calcium. J Am Geriatrics Soc 1995;43:1–3.
71. Weaver CM, Heaney RP, Proulx WR, Hinders SM, Packard PT. Absorbability of calcium from common beans. J Food Sci 1993;58:1401–1403.
72. Heaney RP, Weaver CM, Hinders SM, Martin B, Packard P. Absorbability of calcium from Brassica vegetables. J Food Sci 1993;58:1378–1380.
73. Matkovic V, Ilich JZ, Andon MB, Hsieh LC, Tzagournis MA, Lagger BJ, Goel PK. Urinary calcium, sodium, and bone mass of young females. Am J Clin Nutr 1995;62:417–425.
74. Shortt C, Madden A, Flynn A, Morrissey PA. Influence of dietary sodium intake on urinary calcium excretion in selected Irish individuals. Eur J Clin Nutr 1988;42:595–603.
75. Devine A, Criddle RA, Dick IM, Kerr DA, Prince RL. A longitudinal study of the effect of sodium and calcium intakes on regional bone density in postmenopausal women. Am J Clin Nutr 1995;62: 740–745.
76. Hannan MT, Tucker KL, Dawson-Hughes B, Cupples LA, Felson DT, Kiel DP. Effect of dietary protein on bone loss in elderly men and women: The Framingham Osteoporosis Study. J Bone Miner Res 2000;15:2504–2512.
77. Dawson-Hughes B, Harris SS. Calcium intake influences the association of protein intake with rates of bone loss in elderly men and women. Am J Clin Nutr 2002;75:773–779.
78. Spencer H, Kramer L, Osis D, Norris C. Effect of phosphorus on the absorption of calcium and on the calcium balance in man. J Nutr 1978;108:447–457.
79. Heaney RP. Phosphorus nutrition and the treatment of osteoporosis. Mayo Clin Proc 2004;79:91–97.
80. Hasling C, Søndergaard K, Charles P, Mosekilde L.Calcium metabolism in postmenopausal osteoporotic women is determined by dietary calcium and coffee intake. J Nutr 1992;122:1119–1126.
81. Barger-Lux MJ, Heaney RP, Stegman MR. Effects of moderate caffeine intake on the calcium economy of premenopausal women. Am J Clin Nutr 1990;52:722–725.
82. Harris SS, Dawson-Hughes B. Caffeine and bone loss in healthy postmenopausal women. Am J Clin Nutr 1994;60:573–578.
83. Barrett-Connor E, Chang JC, Edelstein SL. Coffee-associated osteoporosis offset by daily milk consumption. JAMA 1994;271:280–283.
84. Barger-Lux MJ, Heaney RP. Caffeine and the calcium economy revisited. Osteoporos Int 1995;5:97–102.
85. Evans GH, Weaver CM, Harrington DD, Babbs CF Jr. Association of magnesium deficiency with the blood pressure-lowering effects of calcium. J Hypertens 1990;8:327–337.
86. Andon MB, Ilich JZ, Tzagournis MA, Matkovic C. Magnesium balance in adolescent females consuming a low- or high-calcium diet. Am J Clin Nutr 1996;63:950–953.
87. Wood RJ, Zheng JJ. High dietary calcium intakes reduce zinc absorption and balance in humans. Am J Clin Nutr 1997;65:1803–1809.
88. McKenna AA, Ilich JZ, Andon MB, Wang C, Matkovic V. Zinc balance in adolescent females consuming a low- or high-calcium diet. Am J Clin Nutr 1997;65:1460–1464.
89. Minihane AM, Fairweather-Tait SJ, Eagles J. The short and long term effects of calcium supplements on iron nutrition – is there an adaptive response? In: Fischer PWF, L'Abbe MR, Cockell KA, Gibson RS, eds. Trace elements in man and animals – 9: Proceedings of the Ninth International Symposium on Trace Elements in Man and Animals. Ottawa, Canada: NRC Research Press 1997:38–40.
90. Ilich-Ernst JZ, McKenna AA, Badenhop NE, Clairmont AC, Andon MB, Nahhas RW, Goel P, Matkovic V. Iron status, menarche, and calcium supplementation in adolescent girls. Am J Clin Nutr 1998;68: 880–887.

91. Aerssens J, Declerck K, Maeyaert B, Boonen S, Dequeker J. The effect of modifying dietary calcium intake pattern on the circadian rhythm of bone resorption. Calcif Tissue Int 1999;65:34–40.
92. Singh N, Singh PN, Hershman JM. Effect of calcium carbonate on the absorption of levothyroxine. JAMA 2000;283:2822–2825.
93. Liberman UA, Weiss SR, Bröll J, Minne HW, Quan H, Bell NH, Rodriguez-Portales J, Downs RW Jr, Dequeker J, et al. Effect of oral alendronate on bone mineral density and the incidence of fractures in postmenopausal osteoporosis. N Engl J Med 1995;333:1437–1443.
94. Black DM, Cummings SR, Karpf DB, Cauley JA, Thompson DE, Nevitt MC, et al. Randomised trial of effect of alendronate on risk of fracture in women with existing vertebral fractures. Lancet 1996;348:1535–1541.
95. Cummings SR, Black DM, Thompson DE, Applegate WB, Barrett-Connor E, Musliner TA, et al. Effect of alendronate on risk of fracture in women with low bone density but without vertebral fractures. JAMA 1998;280:2077–2082.
96. Harris ST, Watts NB, Genant HK, McKeever CD, Hangartner T, Keller M, Chesnut CH III, Brown J, Eriksen EF, Hoseyni MS, Axelrod DW, Miller PD. Effects of risedronate treatment on vertebral and nonvertebral fractures in women with postmenopausal osteoporosis: a randomized controlled trial. JAMA 1999;282:1344–1352.
97. Ettinger B, Black DM, Mitlak BH, Knickerbocker RK, Nickelsen T, Genant HK, Christiansen C, Delmas PD, Zanchetta JR, et al. Reduction of vertebral fracture risk in postmenopausal women with osteoporosis treated with raloxifene. JAMA 1999;282:637–645.
98. Neer RM, Arnaud CD, Zanchetta JR, Prince R, Gaich GA, Reginster J-Y, Hodsman AB, Eriksen EF, Ish-Shalom S, Genant HK, Wang O, Mitlak BH. Effect of parathyroid hormone (1–34) on fractures and bone mineral density in postmenopausal women with osteoporosis. N Engl J Med 2001;344:1434–1441.
99. Dure-Smith BA, Farley SM, Linkhart SG, Farley JR, Baylink DJ. Calcium deficiency in fluoride-treated osteoporotic patients despite calcium supplementation. J Clin Endocrinol Metab 1996;81:269–275.
100. Curhan GC, Willett WC, Rimm EB, Stampfer MJ. A prospective study of dietary calcium and other nutrients and the risk of symptomatic kidney stones. N Engl J Med 1993;328:833–838.
101. Borghi L, Schianchi T, Meschi T, Guerra A, Allergri F, Maggiore U, Novarini A. Comparison of two diets for the prevention of recurrent stones in idiopathic hypercalciuria. N Engl J Med 2002;346:77–84.
102. Rodgers A. Aspects of calcium oxalate crystallization: theory, in vitro studies, and in vivo implementation. J Am Soc Nephrol 1999;10(Suppl14):S351.

12 Basic Aspects of Vitamin D Nutrition

Reinhold Vieth, PhD, FCACB
and Gloria Sidhom, MD, PhD

CONTENTS

SUMMARY

The serum 25-hydroxyvitamin D [25(OH)D] level measures vitamin D status. Clinical trials show that treatment with vitamin D, 800 IU/day, along with calcium, 1200 mg/day, lowers risk of fractures in older adults, as well as falls. Since the trials showed that a mean serum 25(OH)D of approximately 75 nmol/L (30 ng/mL), from the combination of diet, sunshine, and the vitamin D dosage, was associated with the lower fall and fracture risks, many experts now advise that 25(OH)D in osteoporosis patients should exceed this value. Empirical data show that a daily vitamin D3 dose of 4000 IU (or 28000 once weekly) ensures that the bottom of the bell curve for 25(OH)D in treated adults is at 75 nmol/L. This level of 25(OH)D is associated epidemiologically with health benefits beyond osteoprosis. The natural, physiologic range of serum 25(OH)D in humans due to sun exposure ranges to 225 nmol/L (90 ng/mL) whereas toxicity (hypercalcemia) may become evident beyond 500 nmol/L (200 ng/mL).

Key Words: Nutrition, vitamin D, osteoporosis, vitamin D_2, vitamin D_3, genome, physiology, sunshine, vitamin D-related condition

BASIC ASPECTS OF VITAMIN D-RELATED OSTEOPOROSIS

Introduction

It is well known to anthropologists that as human populations developed technologies making more sedentary lifestyles possible, such changes coincided with a decline in bone quantity, quality, and fracture resistance. These findings have implications for modern populations with their more rapid rates of bone loss and increased risk of osteoporosis and fracture *(1,2)*.

From: *Contemporary Endocrinology: Osteoporosis: Pathophysiology and Clinical Management*
Edited by: R. A. Adler, DOI 10.1007/978-1-59745-459-9_12,

Insufficient supply of the nutrient, vitamin D, is now considered to be one of the most important factors contributing to osteoporosis *(3,4)*. The role played by vitamin D nutrition in the prevention and treatment of osteoporosis is extremely important since it is by far the easiest and cheapest element we can do something about. Thus, it would be of tremendous value and benefit to fully perceive and understand the implications of vitamin D nutrition on bone.

Authentic vitamin D is present in two forms: vitamin D_2 (ergocalciferol) and vitamin D_3 (cholecalciferol). The natural, physiological form of vitamin D in humans and mammals is vitamin D_3 which will be the present focus for discussion. Vitamin D_3 (from here on, vitamin D) is considered the more potent and natural form of vitamin D in primate species including humans *(5,6)*.

During the evolution of our species, requirements for vitamin D were satisfied by the life of the naked ape in the environment for which its genome was optimized through natural selection. The horn of Africa was the original, natural environment for the species, *Homo sapiens*. Our genome, our physiology, and hence our vitamin D requirement are not thought to have changed in the past 100,000 years. However, we have migrated away from tropical climes, and most of us avoid exposing skin to the vitamin D-forming rays of sunshine. Many of us live in regions like Northern Europe or North America, where for most of the year sunshine does not contain the UVB light necessary to produce vitamin D in unprotected skin *(7)*. Thus, one should give serious thought to the question of whether vitamin D-related conditions such as osteoporosis might not at least in part be a harmful side effect of modern human culture.

Primates do not normally need vitamin D in their food because exposure to the sunlight of their normal tropical environment makes it impossible for them to become vitamin D deficient. On the other hand, the "evolution" of vitamin D into an essential nutrient for humans stems from the shift of humans away from the equator, from increased pollution, and from the cultures that avoid exposing the skin surfaces to sunshine.

Vitamin D Activation by the Skin

The skin is a major site of cholesterol synthesis. When 7-dehydrocholesterol, a precursor in the synthetic path to cholesterol, is exposed to ultraviolet B light, the B-ring of the steroid molecule is split open between carbon 9 and carbon 10 to produce a seco-steroid (a fractured steroid) (Fig. 1). It takes about 24 h for this pre-vitamin D to isomerize spontaneously into the mature vitamin D_3 that is useful for the body. If there is sustained exposure to ultraviolet light, an equilibrium is reached in which the pre-vitamin D and vitamin D production are counteracted by deterioration to tachysterol and other compounds. This explains why excess sun exposure does not cause vitamin D intoxication. One to four days are required after sun exposure before rises of vitamin D levels in the circulation are apparent *(8)*.

As age advances, the skin's production of cholesterol decreases, and with this is a partial loss in capacity to produce vitamin D. In humans over 70 years of age, a given amount of sun exposure may generate as little as one fourth of the vitamin D achieved in young subjects. Absorption of vitamin D generated within the skin into the blood is facilitated by vitamin D-binding protein (DBP). Essentially all vitamin D circulates bound to DBP, a protein that can be taken up selectively by the kidney and probably other tissues *(9–11)*.

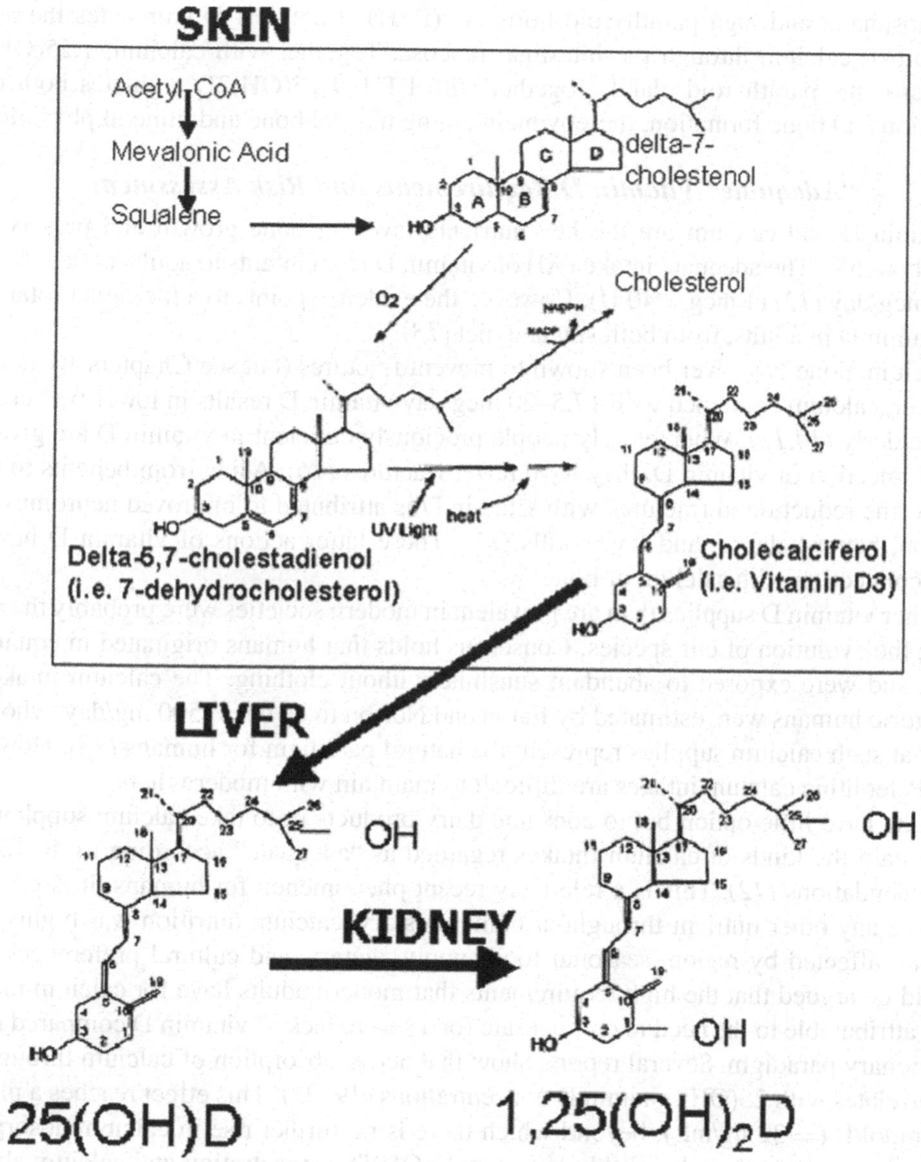

Fig. 1. The molecules in the pathway toward synthesis of the hormone, 1,25-dihydroxyvitamin D [1,25$(OH)_2$D]. The liver metabolizes vitamin D into 25-hydroxyvitamin D [25(OH)D] which is measured to quantify vitamin D nutritional status, which represents long-term exposure of skin to ultraviolet light, or the oral consumption of vitamin D.

Metabolism of Vitamin D

The 25-hydroxylation of vitamin D is the initial step in vitamin D activation (Fig. 1). Enzymes in human liver microsomes and mitochondria convert vitamin D to 25(OH)D. The concentration of this metabolite in blood is the accepted measure of vitamin D nutritional status. The kidney functions as an endocrine gland synthesizing and secreting the hormone, 1,25$(OH)_2$D. Production of 1,25$(OH)_2$D is stimulated by low circulating calcium, low phosphate, and high parathyroid hormone (PTH). 1,25$(OH)_2$D stimulates the active transport of calcium through the intestinal mucosa. Together with calcium, 1,25$(OH)_2$D suppresses the parathyroid gland. Together with PTH, 1,25(OH)2D regulates both bone resorption and bone formation, thereby maintaining normal bone and mineral physiology.

"Adequate" Vitamin D Requirements and Risk Assessment

Vitamin D and calcium are the key nutrients favoring bone growth and preservation throughout life. The adequate intake (AI) of vitamin D from infants to adults under 50 years is 5.0 mcg/day *(12)* (1 mcg = 40 U). However, the evidence points to a far higher total need for vitamin D in adults, from both sun and diet *(13)*.

Calcium alone has never been shown to prevent fractures (but see Chapters 10 and 11). However, calcium combined with 17.5–20 mcg/day vitamin D results in lower fracture risk in the elderly *(14,15)*. When elderly people previously deficient in vitamin D are given an annual injection of vitamin D, they have fewer fractures *(16)*. Aside from benefits to bone density, the reduction in fractures with vitamin D is attributed to improved neuromuscular function, better balance, and fewer falls *(17)*. These latter actions of vitamin D have no direct connection with calcium or bone.

Higher vitamin D supplies than are prevalent in modern societies were probably the norm during the evolution of our species. Consensus holds that humans originated in equatorial Africa and were exposed to abundant sunshine without clothing. The calcium intakes of prehistoric humans were estimated by Eaton and Nelson to be over 1500 mg/day, who contend that such calcium supplies represent the natural paradigm for humans *(18)*. However, these Paleolithic calcium intakes are difficult to maintain with modern diets.

Adults have little option but to consume dairy products or to take calcium supplements to maintain the kinds of calcium intakes regarded as "adequate" according to the dietary recommendations *(12)*. This is a relatively recent phenomenon for humans. It is probable that, like any other nutrient throughout human history, calcium nutrition was highly variable and affected by region, seasonal food supply, dietary, and cultural preferences *(19)*. It could be argued that the high requirements that modern adults have for calcium may be partly attributable to the need to compensate for a severe lack of vitamin D compared to the evolutionary paradigm. Several reports show that active absorption of calcium through the gut correlates with 25(OH) vitamin D concentrations *(19–22)*. This effect reaches a plateau at 80 nmol/L (= 32 ng/mL), beyond which there is no further rise in calcium absorption. The evidence about the relationship between 25(OH)D concentration and calcium absorption suggests that when 25(OH)D concentrations are below 80 nmol/L, the body's ability to absorb calcium is impaired. Recent research suggests that the serum 25(OH)D concentration may be more important than a high calcium intake in maintaining the desired values of serum PTH and calcium metabolism. As long as the 25(OH)D concentration is greater than 45 nmol/L (18 ng/mL) more than 800 mg/day of calcium may be unnecessary for maintaining calcium metabolism *(23)*.

In 1995 the Food and Nutrition Board (FNB) established values for vitamin D intakes that were 15 mcg/day for those over the age of 70 years and lower values for younger adults *(12)*. The 1995 recommendations are being seen as too conservative, and calls are being made to increase recommendations *(24)*, but recommendations for nutrient intake need to be balanced against safety. Risk assessments of vitamin D, using the safe Tolerable upper intake level (UL) method, have been published by the FNB *(12)*, the Scientific

Committee on Food of the European Commission *(25)*, and the Expert Group on Vitamins and Minerals of the United Kingdom *(26)*. The method to establish a UL involves a series formal, standardized steps *(12)*:

(1) Hazard identification—the evaluation of all pertinent information relative to the substance's potential to cause harm in humans. This step identifies the nature of the adverse effect, including its severity and persistence. If the substance causes multiple types of adverse effects, the critical effect is one that meets the severity and persistence criteria at the lowest intake. – For vitamin D the identified hazard is hypercalcemia.
(2) Dose–response assessment—a quantitative evaluation of the relationship between oral intake of the nutrient and the adverse effect. The no observed adverse effect level (NOAEL) and, if possible, the lowest observed adverse effect level (LOAEL) are identified, and a degree of uncertainty is assigned a numerical value, the uncertainty factor (UF).
(3) Calculation of the UL—a simple arithmetic operation: UL = NOAEL ÷ UF (or sometimes UL = LOAEL ÷ UF). The UL is the long-term intake dosage that the public is advised not to exceed.

The evidence from well-conducted human-intervention trials is the appropriate basis for selecting a NOAEL value. The clinical trials have been listed and described by Hathcock et al. *(27)*. The primary criterion for inclusion in their analysis was the use of a vitamin D dose substantially above the current AI (≥ 45 mcg, 1800 IU/day), followed by study design (e.g., randomized, controlled), duration, and sample size. Relevant outcomes included the effects on serum 25(OH)D and the increases in urinary and/or serum calcium.

Serum 25(OH)D level is accepted as the most appropriate indicator of vitamin D status *(12)*. Selection of a NOAEL for vitamin D is aided by consideration of how serum 25(OH)D concentrations relate to toxicity. More specifically, because vitamin D is acquired from multiple sources (cutaneous biosynthesis, foods, supplements), the serum 25(OH)D levels at which hypercalcemia occurs must be examined to define how overall status relates to toxicity (i.e., the critical dose–response relationship). Hathcock et al. found that the serum 25(OH)D levels associated with hypercalcemia from vitamin D are almost exclusively the result of very large intakes of vitamin D. In virtually all instances, serum 25(OH)D levels associated with hypercalcemia exceeded 200 ng/mL = 500 nmol/L *(13)*. To achieve concentrations of 25(OH)D high enough to produce hypercalcemia, adults would need to consume vitamin D_3 in doses much higher than 10,000 IU/day, and this dose has been proposed as the appropriate safe upper limit of vitamin D intake *(27)*.

Regional and Seasonal Variations of Vitamin D

We can use data for modern adults who have abundant exposure of skin to ultraviolet light to infer what the 25(OH)D concentrations would have been in early humans. From this, we can estimate what an oral equivalent may be to early humans' sun-derived daily supply of vitamin D.

For the entire year at the low latitudes, natural for all primates, sunlight penetrates the atmosphere with enough UVB light to disrupt 7-dehydrocholesterol molecules in the skin and produces cholecalciferol (vitamin D) *(28)*. In all studies of healthy non-human primates, circulating 25(OH)D concentrations exceed 80 nmol/L *(29)* (Fig. 2). To estimate the circulating 25(OH)D concentrations prevalent in humans of the late Paleolithic period, focus must be made on people in sun-rich environments who regularly expose most of their

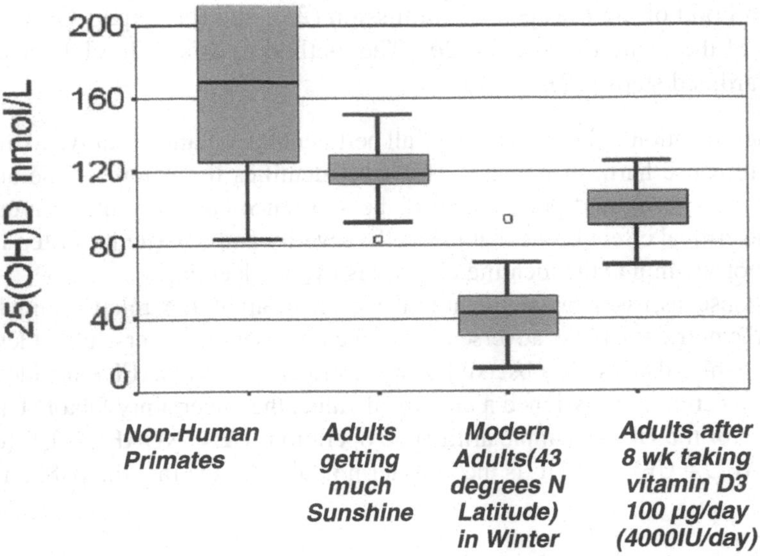

Fig. 2. Evolutionary perspective of circulating vitamin D nutritional status. Boxes show quartile values for 25(OH)D for the groups represented by the figures in the cartoons over the boxes (for example, sitting figure represents modern adult values *(28,47)*). The whiskers indicate the extreme 25(OH)D concentrations and the dots indicate outlier values as determined by SPSS statistical software. For non-human primates, the box extends to beyond the top of the figure.

skin surface to the sun. At least four studies show that UV exposure of the full skin surface of an adult is equivalent to a vitamin D consumption of about 250 mcg/day *(30–33)*. At latitudes beyond 40°, the angle of the sun is so low for much of the year that UVB light penetration to the earth's surface is minimal. For the rest of the year, UV intensity is much lower than at tropical latitudes *(34)*. However, even if modern humans do live in sunny climates, they are not ensured of a serum 25(OH)D concentration that matches the goal now desired, of 75 nmol/L. Culture, clothing, and shelter minimize the natural production of vitamin D by skin. Consequently 25(OH)D concentrations for populations in the Middle East tend to be even lower than they are for people living in America or Europe *(35–39)*.

Since early human evolution occurred under UV-rich conditions, typical 25(OH)D concentrations were surely higher than 100 nmol/L. Levels like this are now seen in lifeguards, farmers, or people who sun tan. This range of 25(OH)D concentration reflects an adult vitamin D input of 200–500 mcg/day *(13)*. Since our genome was selected under these conditions through evolution, it should be evident that our biology was optimized for a vitamin D supply that is far higher than we currently regard as normal.

The question of whether such higher levels of vitamin D nutrition actually make a difference to human health and reduce the risks of osteoporosis needs to be addressed with controlled prospective studies of vitamin D supplementation.

The intensity of ultraviolet light from the sun diminishes during winter months. For example, at the latitude of Rome or Boston (42°N), there is not enough outdoor ultraviolet intensity between November and February to generate any vitamin D in the skin, and this phenomenon is worse at higher latitudes *(34)*. Season of the year affects vitamin D nutritional status. Summer sunshine contains the UVB radiation that disrupts dermal

7-dehydrocholesterol, and this then isomerizes into vitamin D_3 *(40)*. The liver readily hydroxylates vitamin D at carbon 25 producing 25-hydroxyvitamin D (calcidiol). In populations living in temperate latitudes, calcidiol levels rise and fall in annual cycles *(41)*. This affects the rate of change in bone density, which declines more quickly during winter than during summer. Vitamin D supplements (about 20 mcg/day) combined with calcium eliminate the faster fall in bone density during winter *(42,43)*. In a cross-section of young, healthy adults, bone markers are higher in the winter season *(44)*. Likewise, bone turnover markers in both young and old adults are statistically higher in winter *(44,45)*.

Effect of Skin Color on Vitamin D

Deeply pigmented skin is regarded as the original, natural color of the skin of humans *(46,47)*. Dark skin protects against skin cancer and preserves the function of sweat glands needed for thermoregulation. Moreover, dark skin protects circulating micronutrients, especially folic acid, from photodegradation. However, at latitudes farther away from the equator, the process of natural selection favors whiter skin, because this permits dermal generation of sufficient vitamin D when the amount of UVB in sunlight is diminished. Darker skin requires longer exposure. Very black skin requires about 1.5 h, or six times longer than white skin, to reach the equilibrium for vitamin D production *(48)*. Rickets is a well-known consequence of inadequate sunshine, and it was the driving force for the natural selection that has produced the latitudinal gradation of skin color of human populations *(46,49)*. Excessive curvature of long bones is well recognized as a sign of rickets and vitamin D deficiency. However, a misshapen pelvis accompanies both rickets and osteomalacia. Even if a woman did not have rickets during childhood, marginal vitamin D insufficiency caused bouts of osteomalacia that resulted in a progressive reshaping of the pelvis *(29,50,51)*. Thus, the term "sufficient vitamin D" refers only to an amount of vitamin D that is enough to permit and maintain a normally shaped female pelvis that allows natural childbirth.

Vitamin D and Calcium Homeostasis

Plasma calcium concentrations are maintained at a very constant level, and this level is supersaturating with respect to bone mineral. If the plasma becomes less than saturated with respect to calcium and phosphate, then mineralization fails, which results in rickets among children and osteomalacia among adults *(52)*. Of greater immediate importance is the maintenance of the ionic calcium concentration in plasma to sustain normal neuromuscular functions. First, $1,25(OH)_2D$ is the only hormone known to stimulate active intestinal absorption of a nutrient, calcium. Second, $1,25(OH)_2D$ influences the balance of calcium at the intestine in a complex relationship, where at moderate, physiologic concentrations it facilitates bone mineralization, but at larger, pharmacologic concentrations it stimulates resorption *(53)*. Third, the distal renal tubule is responsible for reabsorption of the last 1% of the filtered load of calcium. Parathyroid hormone and $1,25(OH)_2D$ interact to stimulate the reabsorption of the last 1% of the calcium filtered through the glomerulus *(54)*. Because about 7000 mg of calcium are filtered everyday in adults, the last 1% of filtered calcium represents a major contribution to calcium balance. Again, both the parathyroid hormone and the vitamin D hormone are required. Calcium physiologic processes are such that a moderate rise in $1,25(OH)_2D$ can stimulate intestinal mucosa to absorb calcium. If the plasma calcium concentration fails to respond, then the parathyroid glands continue to secrete parathyroid hormone, which increases production of $1,25(OH)_2D$ further to mobilize bone calcium (acting with parathyroid hormone). Under normal circumstances, dietary calcium is used first to maintain ionic calcium; if dietary calcium is inadequate, then internal stores are used through the resorption of bone.

Vitamin D Effects on Bone

Senile osteoporosis has long been thought to be a consequence of prolonged, mild vitamin D deficiency *(3,55,56)*. This view is supported by the modern clinical evidence of fracture prevention with vitamin D in the elderly *(14,15)*. The amounts of vitamin D needed to bring about the kinds of 25(OH)D concentrations associated with abundant sunshine exposure exceed the current official safety limit of 50 mcg/day *(12,57)*. Figure 2 compares circulating 25(OH)D concentrations as they would have been through primate and early human evolution, against levels that are now common for adults, and levels attained with vitamin D intakes far higher than current AIs for the nutrient. In the broader context of this comparison, modern humans are relatively deprived of vitamin D, and even the most recently revised dietary guidelines for this nutrient *(12)* are probably still woefully inadequate for adults.

A major part of the reason why contemporary older adults require calcium intakes at levels attainable only with daily foods or mineral supplements may be because they are relatively vitamin D deprived. Because current nutrient recommendations provide far less vitamin D than what is attainable through sunshine, modern medical thinking effectively maintains adults in a state of relative vitamin D insufficiency, compensated for by high requirements for calcium. In contrast, early humans living in sun-rich environments were relatively vitamin D rich probably at least 100 μg/day. Therefore, early humans may not have required as much calcium to prevent osteoporosis. Of course, early humans had shorter life expectancy.

The one officially recognized indication for use of vitamin D in adults is the treatment and prevention of osteomalacia, bone loss, and fractures. A recent meta-analysis of the use of vitamin D, $1,25(OH)_2D$, and its analogs found no evidence that doses of vitamin D less than 800 IU/day are effective in preventing osteoporotic fractures. That is, prevention of osteoporosis-related fractures required 800 IU/day of vitamin D_3 *(58)*. Furthermore, pharmacological preparations of $1,25(OH)_2D$ and its analogs were no better than conventional, nutritional vitamin D_3. Trivedi et al. added great strength to the vitamin D story with their very simple study, in which 2686 adults (mostly men, age 65–85 years) were randomized to either a placebo or a 100,000 IU vitamin D_3 pill, taken just once every 4 months (826 IU/day, no extra calcium). The vitamin D resulted in a 39% reduction of any first fracture and a 22% reduction in the classic, osteoporosis-type fractures (vertebral, hip, or wrist) *(59)*.

Prevention of fractures is the sin qua non of efficacy in osteoporosis treatment. While it is well accepted that bone loss in women accelerates for a few years after menopause, clinical trials with fracture as an outcome in adults under age 65 are prohibitively difficult because fractures of osteoporosis are too rare at younger ages.

One large cross-sectional study following nurses in the United States showed that early postmenopausal women consuming over 12.5 mcg (500 IU)/day of vitamin D_3 in food or vitamin supplements exhibited 37% fewer hip fractures than women consuming <3.5 mcg (140 IU)/day *(60)*. To support further the effect of vitamin D on bone healthcare data from the large US health survey, NHANES III, showed that in white women under age 50, BMD was steadily higher as 25(OH)D increased to well beyond the normal range *(61)*.

Within the first year of vitamin D treatment for osteoporosis, when bone density cannot have increased by enough to affect its quality, occurrence of fractures is reduced by about one third *(15)*. Vitamin D improves muscle strength and balance. This reduces the occurrence of the falls that cause fractures *(17,22,62,63)*. In the elderly, serum 25(OH)D concentrations correlate positively with muscle strength *(64)*. Vitamin D receptors are present in muscle tissue and they respond to physiologic concentrations of 1,25 dihydroxy vitamin D *(65,66)*. Stimulation of the receptors results in an increase in area of type II fibers *(67)*.

Lastly, it must not be forgotten that bone is accrued in the early years of life. Moreover, its maternal vitamin D status during pregnancy affects the bone density of the child as measured at 9 years of age *(68)*. Several randomized clinical trials now show that for girls especially, vitamin D supplementation increases bone accrual during adolescent years *(69,70)*. The effect of vitamin D treatment confirms the findings in cross-sectional studies that higher 25(OH)D is associated with higher bone density *(71)*. Simple vitamin D nutrition is intimately tied to bone, from the earliest stages of life onward. The doses relevant to children remain virtually unexplored. What we do know is that there is benefit and no harm to adolescents taking 2000 IU/day of vitamin D *(69)*.

Potential Effects of Vitamin D on Other Body Systems

Research in the fields of cell biology and epidemiology over the past two decades is pointing toward vitamin D nutritional status as a means of achieving health benefits well beyond the traditional realm of bone and mineral disease.

Cancer Prevention

Skin is not merely the physiologic source of vitamin D_3 (cholecalciferol), which is produced because of the physiochemical accident that a precursor to cholesterol is unstable in ultraviolet light. The skin is a target organ for this “nutrient” because it possesses the enzymatic machinery to convert vitamin D into 25(OH)D, and this can be metabolized locally in the skin to $1,25(OH)_2D$ *(72,73)*. In 1998, Schwartz et al. *(74)* reported that normal and malignant prostate cancer cells also had the enzymatic machinery to make $1,25(OH)_2D$. This observation helped to crystallize the important role of vitamin D in cancer prevention. Increased exposure to sunlight or vitamin D intake leads to increased production of 25(OH)D by the liver. Higher concentrations of 25(OH)D are used by the prostate cells to make $1,25(OH)_2D$, which helps keep prostate cell proliferation in check and therefore decreases the risk of prostate cells becoming malignant *(40,75)*.

Likewise, breast, colon, lung, brain, and a wide variety of other cells in the body have the enzymatic machinery to make $1,25(OH)_2D$ *(76–81)*. Thus higher concentrations of 25(OH)D provide many tissues in the body with the substrate they need to make $1,25(OH)_2D$ locally, which serves as an autocrine or paracrine regulator to regulate help control cellular growth and maturation and to decrease the risk of malignancy *(82,83)*.

This hypothesis has been further supported by the observation that both prospective and retrospective studies revealed that if the 25(OH)D concentration exceeds 50 nmol/L (20 ng/mL), then there is a ~30–50% decreased risk of developing and dying of colon, prostate, and breast cancers compared to those whose 25(OH)D concentrations are lower than this *(75,83–86)*.

Diabetes Mellitus and Metabolic Syndrome

Vitamin D supplementation during infancy and childhood appears to protect against development of type I diabetes mellitus later in life *(87,88)*. Development of type 1 diabetes was found to be associated with low intake of vitamin D and signs of rickets during the first year of life. The paracrine system supported by vitamin D nutrition is thought to improve the immune function in a way that lowers the risk of developing autoimmune reactions targeted toward the B cells of the pancreas.

In adults 25(OH)D concentrations correlate with insulin resistance and poor glucose tolerance *(89)*. Remarkably, the quality of the correlation between 25(OH)D and insulin response published by Chiu et al. matches the quality of the published correlations between 25(OH)D and parathyroid hormone. The disease relationships with vitamin D suggest that a lack of vitamin D contributes to syndrome X, the combination of hypertension, diabetes, and obesity occurring in the same people *(90)*.

Multiple Sclerosis

Multiple sclerosis is more prevalent in populations that have lower levels of vitamin D nutrition or ultraviolet exposure *(91–94)*. Data from two large, prospective cohort studies suggest that vitamin D may be beneficial as a preventive measure. Dietary information obtained from the Nurses Health Study (NHS) and NHS II was used to evaluate the effect of vitamin D supplementation on the risk of developing MS. Long-term use of a multivitamin (>10 years) resulted in a 41% risk reduction compared with participants who had never used a multivitamin *(95)*. Moreover, in a prospective study, higher 25(OH)D concentrations in serum samples of US military personnel were shown in a case–control study to be preventive of later development of multiple sclerosis, suggesting the desirable goal was to have 25(OH)D exceeding 99 nmol/L (>40 ng/mL) *(96)*.

Australians with a childhood history of high sun exposure (>4 h/day) are one third as likely as those reporting <2 h/day to end up with MS *(97)*. These are associational studies that are highly suggestive, but not conclusive that additional vitamin D will play a role in prevention.

There is little evidence to support the effectiveness of vitamin D in the treatment of MS. One small study suggests that vitamin D supplementation may be helpful *(98–109)*.

Chronic Pain Syndrome

Muscle tenderness and weakness are classic features of vitamin D-deficient infants, and now we know that the same thing occurs in adults. One study showed that low 25(OH)D levels are associated with back and muscle pain that is alleviated through vitamin D supplementation *(99)*.

Immune Function and Influenza

Vitamin D deficiency impairs immune function in laboratory animals *(100)* and in children there is a strong association between pneumonia and rickets *(101)*. The hormone produced from vitamin D, $1,25(OH)_2D$, has profound effects in vitro. It acts as an immune system modulator, preventing excessive expression of inflammatory cytokines and increasing the "oxidative burst" potential of macrophages. It up-regulates the expression of potent anti-microbial proteins, which exist in neutrophils, monocytes, natural killer cells, and in epithelial cells lining the respiratory tract where they play a major role in protecting the lung from infection. Thus, vitamin D reduces the incidence of viral respiratory influenza *(102)*.

Blood Pressure and Cardiovascular Disease

The prevalence of hypertension increases with population distance, north or south, from the equator *(103)*, and in epidemiologic studies, higher 25(OH)D levels correlate with lower diastolic pressure *(104)*. Tanning in vitamin D-forming UVB light lowers blood pressure of patients with mild hypertension *(105)*. One randomized intervention study showed vitamin D at 800 IU/day lowers blood pressure in the elderly *(106)*. The black American population tends to have greater prevalence of hypertension and lower 25(OH)D levels than white Americans *(107)*.

Serum concentrations of a natriuretic peptide associated with severity of cardiovascular disease correlate with serum concentrations of 25(OH)D in patients with congestive heart failure *(108)*. Furthermore, 25(OH)D was lower in patients with congestive heart failure than in control subjects. In addition, patients with cardiovascular heart disease are more likely to develop heart failure if they are vitamin D deficient *(109)*. Patients with peripheral vascular disease and the common complaint of lower leg discomfort (claudication) are often found to be vitamin D deficient. The muscle weakness and pain in these patients has been reported to be not due to the peripheral vascular disease per se, but more related to the vitamin D deficiency *(110)*.

Although the exact mechanism involved in how vitamin D sufficiency protects against cardiovascular heart disease is not fully understood, the relationship could be explained by any or several of a number of mechanisms. Vascular endothelium possesses the 1-hydroxylase and the vitamin D receptor that makes possible autocrine or paracrine relationships *(111,112)*. Renal blood pressure regulation involves $1,25(OH)_2D$ through down-regulating the blood pressure hormone renin in the kidneys *(113)*. Furthermore, there is an inflammatory component to atherosclerosis, and vascular smooth muscle cells have a vitamin D receptor and relax in the presence of $1,25(OH)_2D$ *(114,115)*.

Neurological Disease

Birth in the seasons when 25(OH)D concentrations are lowest is associated with higher risk of schizophrenia, bipolar disorder, autism, Alzheimer's disease, and amyotrophic lateral sclerosis *(116,117)*.These observations are consistent with the view that vitamin D is essential for fetal brain development *(118)*. Life in relatively sun-deprived urban environments is implicated as a risk factor for schizophrenia in later years.

General Well-Being

A subjective sense of well-being is important to patients, but unfortunately has not been a priority area for research funding. There is some evidence beyond anecdotal reports to link vitamin D to a sense of "feeling better." That there are endorphin-like effects of exposure to ultraviolet light has been widely accepted. A recent experiment involving tanning sessions that were provided in a blinded manner, with and without UVA light, gives evidence to demonstrate the phenomenon objectively. Exposure in tanning booths to the same visible light was more desirable if the light spectrum included ultraviolet wavelengths *(119)*. Because changes to serum 25(OH)D happen slowly, the acute desirable sense achieved with ultraviolet light is probably only indirectly related to vitamin D. Humans probably evolved to experience enjoyment from sunshine exposure a means to support behaviors that maintained the vitamin D supply through production in the skin. Seasonal affective disorder is often attributed to a lack of sunlight exposure, and a relationship with vitamin D has been hypothesized *(120–122)*. The best direct comparison between effects of light treatment and vitamin D treatment was reported by Gloth et al. in a trial that randomized subjects to either a month of light treatment or a single large dose of vitamin D (100,000 IU). After the month it was the vitamin D group that exhibited a decline in tests of mental depression *(121)*.

Other clinical trials involving vitamin D supplementation also reported on effects on mood or well-being. In one study, the effect of vitamin D supplementation at either the highest of the officially recommended intake levels, 4200 IU/week (equivalent to 600 IU/day) was compared to supplementation at 28,000 IU/week (equivalent to 4000 IU/day) *(122)*. Male and female treated thyroid clinic outpatients were invited to take part if their serum 25(OH)D concentrations were below 50 nmol/L. The vitamin D-supplementation protocol was started in late November, with questionnaires focusing on depression and well-being evaluated in November and February. By February, participants in the higher vitamin D dose group reported greater improvement in well-being than did those taking the lower dose. In the fracture prevention study of Trivedi et al., healthy men and women were randomized to 5 years of either placebo or vitamin D supplementation. In an analysis of secondary outcomes, the women receiving vitamin D_3 were more likely to report their health as good or excellent by the end of the study *(59)*. Lastly, in the cross-sectional Longitudinal Aging Study of Amsterdam, risk of "depressive symptoms" increased significantly and dramatically as 25(OH)D concentrations declined *(123)*.

BALANCING RISK AND BENEFIT

The highest chronic daily oral intake of vitamin D that will pose no risk of adverse effects for most healthy adults is difficult to define – as for anything with biologic potency. A more realistic approach is to find one dosage that does specify an intake that is indeed safe. It is well accepted that the amount of vitamin D derived from sun exposure – 10,000 IU/day – is safe and probably appropriate. This begs the question of what would happen to people who do obtain this amount of vitamin D from sunshine and then add to that an oral intake. It does appear that a total input of 20,000 IU/day of vitamin D (half of which is orally) will be safe. The results of well-conducted trials of vitamin D lead to the conclusion that the current, safe limitation for vitamin D intake of 2000 IU/day is excessively conservative *(124)*. A daily vitamin D_3 dose of 2000 IU (50 mcg) will raise serum 25(OH)D by about 50 nmol/L, on average, well within the safe range of serum 25(OH)D concentrations that extends to 500 nmol/L. A prolonged physiologic-replacement intake of 10,000 IU/day of vitamin D_3 will raise 25(OH)D by about 200 nmol/L, which approximates the 25(OH)D concentration acquired through sun exposure on the scale seen in lifeguards. The combination of sunshine with 10,000 orally could in theory raise the 25(OH)D concentration to over 400 nmol/L in some individuals. This concentration is still below the 25(OH)D concentrations that characterize adults with hypercalcemia due to excessive vitamin D intake *(124)*. There is no intention here of advising a vitamin D intake of 10,000 IU/day for adults. The purpose is to estimate a dose and the 25(OH)D concentration at which risk is unlikely. That dose is 10,000 IU/day and the 25(OH)D concentration is higher than 500 nmol/L. For essentially all adults, there is no risk associated with the doses of vitamin D supplement proposed for use in the treatment and prevention of osteoporosis.

REFERENCES

1. Robling AG, Stout SD. Histomorphology, geometry, and mechanical loading in past populations. In: Agarwal SC, Stout SD, eds. Bone loss and osteoporosis in past populations: an anthropological perspective. New York: Kluwer Academic Plenum, 2003:189–205.
2. Agarwal SC, Grynpas MD. Bone quantity and quality in past populations. Anat Rec 1996;246(4): 423–432.
3. Heaney RP. Lessons for nutritional science from vitamin D [editorial; comment]. Am J Clin Nutr 1999;69(5):825–826.
4. Parfitt AM. The evolution of vitamin D-related bone disease: The importance of an early stage of increased bone turnover without impaired mineralization. In: Burckhardt P, Dawson-Hughes B, Heaney R, eds. Nutritional Aspects of Osteoporosis. New York: Academic Press, 2001:197–208.
5. Marx SJ, Jones G, Weinstein RS, Chrousos GP, Renquist DM. Differences in mineral metabolism among nonhuman primates receiving diets with only vitamin D_3 or only vitamin D_2. J Clin Endocrinol Metab 1989;69(1282):1282–1289.
6. Trang H, Cole DE, Rubin LA, Pierratos A, Siu S, Vieth R. Evidence that vitamin D3 increases serum 25-hydroxyvitamin D more efficiently than does vitamin D2. American J Clin Nutr 1998;68:854–848.
7. Jablonski NG, Chaplin G. Skin deep. Sci Am 2002;287(4):74–81.
8. Haddad JG, Matsuoka LY, Hollis BW, Hu YZ, Wortsman J. Human plasma transport of vitamin D after its endogenous synthesis. J Clin Invest 1993;91(6):2552–2555.
9. Bikle DD, Halloran BP, Gee E, Ryzen E, Haddad JG. Free 25-hydroxyvitamin D levels are normal in subjects with liver disease and reduced total 25-hydroxyvitamin D levels. J Clin Invest 1986; 78(3):748–752.
10. Vieth R. Simple method for determining specific binding capacity of vitamin D-binding protein and its use to calculate the concentration of "free" 1,25-dihydroxyvitamin D. Clin Chem 1994;40: 435–441.
11. Moestrup SK, Verroust PJ. Megalin- and cubilin-mediated endocytosis of protein-bound vitamins, lipids, and hormones in polarized epithelia. Annu Rev Nutr 2001;21:407–428.
12. Standing Committee on the Scientific Evaluation of Dietary Reference Intakes. Dietary reference intakes: calcium, phosphorus, magnesium, vitamin D, and fluoride. Washington, DC: National Academy Press, 1997.
13. Vieth R. Vitamin D supplementation, 25-hydroxyvitamin D concentrations, and safety. Am J Clin Nutr 1999;69(5):842–856.
14. Chapuy MC, Arlot ME, Duboeuf F, et al. Vitamin D3 and calcium to prevent hip fractures in the elderly women. N Engl J Med 1992;327(23):1637–1642.
15. Dawson-Hughes B, Harris SS, Krall EA, Dallal GE. Effect of calcium and vitamin D supplementation on bone density in men and women 65 years of age or older. N Engl J Med 1997;337(10):670–676.
16. Heikinheimo RJ, Inkovaara JA, Harju EJ, et al. Annual injection of vitamin D and fractures of aged bones. Calcif Tissue Int 1992;51(2):105–110.
17. Pfeifer M, Begerow B, Minne HW, Abrams C, Nachtigall D, Hansen C. Effects of a short-term vitamin D and calcium supplementation on body sway and secondary hyperparathyroidism in elderly women. J Bone Miner Res 2000;15(6):1113–1118.
18. Eaton SB, Nelson DA. Calcium in evolutionary perspective. Am J Clin Nutr 1991;54(1 Suppl): 281S–287S.

19. Heaney RP, Barger-Lux MJ, Dowell MS, Chen TC, Holick MF. Calcium absorptive effects of vitamin D and its major metabolites [In Process Citation]. J Clin Endocrinol Metab 1997;82(12):4111–4116.
20. Devine A, Wilson SG, Dick IM, Prince RL. Effects of vitamin D metabolites on intestinal calcium absorption and bone turnover in elderly women. Am J Clin Nutr 2002;75(2):283–288.
21. Heaney RP, Dowell MS, Hale CA, Bendich A. Calcium absorption varies within the reference range for serum 25-hydroxyvitamin D. J Am Coll Nutr 2003;22(2):142–146.
22. Bischoff HA, Stahelin HB, Dick W, et al. Effects of vitamin D and calcium supplementation on falls: a randomized controlled trial. J Bone Miner Res 2003;18(2):343–351.
23. Steingrimsdottir L, Gunnarsson O, Indridason OS, Franzson L, Sigurdsson G. Relationship between serum parathyroid hormone levels, vitamin D sufficiency, and calcium intake. JAMA 2005;294(18): 2336–2341.
24. Vieth R, Bischoff-Ferrari H, Boucher BJ, et al. The urgent need to recommend an intake of vitamin D that is effective. Am J Clin Nutr 2007;85(3):649–650.
25. Health & Consumer Protection Directorate-General. Opinion of the Scientific Committee on Food on the Tolerable Upper Intake Level of Vitamin D. European Commission, editor. Brussels, Belgium, 1-10-0030, 2002, http://europa.eu.int/comm/food/fs/sc/scf/out157_en.pdf, Accessed on August 11, 2003.
26. Expert Group on Vitamins and Minerals. Safe upper levels for vitamins and minerals. Great Britain: Food Standards Agency, 2003.
27. Hathcock JN, Shao A, Vieth R, Heaney R. Risk assessment for vitamin D. Am J Clin Nutr 2007;85(1): 6–18.
28. Holick MF. The cutaneous photosynthesis of previtamin D3: a unique photoendocrine system. J Invest Dermatol 1981;77(1):51–58.
29. Vieth R. Effects of vitamin D on bone and natural selection of skin color: how much vitamin D nutrition are we talking about? In: Agarwal SC, Stout SD, eds. Bone loss and osteoporosis in past populations: an anthropological perspective. New York: Kluwer Academic Plenum, 2003, in press.
30. Stamp TC. Factors in human vitamin D nutrition and in the production and cure of classical rickets. Proc Nutr Soc 1975;34(2):119–130.
31. Davie MW, Lawson DE, Emberson C, Barnes JL, Roberts GE, Barnes ND. Vitamin D from skin: contribution to vitamin D status compared with oral vitamin D in normal and anticonvulsant-treated subjects. Clin Sci 1982;63(5):461–472.
32. Holick MF. Environmental factors that influence the cutaneous production of vitamin D. Am J Clin Nutr 1995;61(Suppl):638S–645S.
33. Chel VG, Ooms ME, Popp-Snijders C, et al. Ultraviolet irradiation corrects vitamin D deficiency and suppresses secondary hyperparathyroidism in the elderly [In Process Citation]. J Bone Miner Res 1998;13(8):1238–1242.
34. Webb AR, Kline L, Holick MF. Influence of season and latitude on the cutaneous synthesis of vitamin D3: exposure to winter sunlight in Boston and Edmonton will not promote vitamin D3 synthesis in human skin. J Clin Endocrinol Metab 1988;67(2):373–378.
35. Sedrani SH, Elidrissy AW, El Arabi KM. Sunlight and vitamin D status in normal Saudi subjects. Am J Clin Nutr 1983;38(1):129–132.
36. Fonseca V, Tongia R, el Hazmi M, Abu-Aisha H. Exposure to sunlight and vitamin D deficiency in Saudi Arabian women. Postgrad Med J 1984;60(707):589–591.
37. Al Arabi KM, Elidrissy AW, Sedrani SH. Is avoidance of sunlight a cause of fractures of the femoral neck in elderly Saudis? Trop Geogr Med 1984;36(3):273–279.
38. Fuleihan GE, Deeb M. Hypovitaminosis D in a sunny country [letter]. N Engl J Med 1999;340(23): 1840–1841.
39. Alagol F, Shihadeh Y, Boztepe H, et al. Sunlight exposure and vitamin D deficiency in Turkish women [In Process Citation]. J Endocrinol Invest 2000;23(3):173–177.
40. Holick MF. Sunlight and vitamin D for bone health and prevention of autoimmune diseases, cancers, and cardiovascular disease. Am J Clin Nutr 2004;80(6 Suppl):1678S–1688S.
41. Vieth R, Cole DE, Hawker GA, Trang HM, Rubin LA. Wintertime vitamin D insufficiency is common in young Canadian women, and their vitamin D intake does not prevent it. Eur J Clin Nutr 2001;55(12):1091–1097.

42. Dawson-Hughes B, Dallal GE, Krall EA, Harris S, Sokoll LJ, Falconer G. Effect of vitamin D supplementation on wintertime and overall bone loss in healthy postmenopausal women [see comments]. Ann Intern Med 1991;115:505–512.
43. Rosen CJ, Morrison A, Zhou H, et al. Elderly women in northern New England exhibit seasonal changes in bone mineral density and calciotropic hormones. Bone Miner 1994;25(2):83–92.
44. Carnevale V, Modoni S, Pileri M, et al. Longitudinal evaluation of vitamin D status in healthy subjects from southern Italy: seasonal and gender differences. Osteoporos Int 2001;12(12):1026–1030.
45. Rapuri PB, Kinyamu HK, Gallagher JC, Haynatzka V. Seasonal changes in calciotropic hormones, bone markers, and bone mineral density in elderly women. J Clin Endocrinol Metab 2002;87(5): 2024–2032.
46. Jablonski NG, Chaplin G. The evolution of human skin coloration. J Hum Evol 2000;39(1):57–106.
47. Sturm RA, Box NF, Ramsay M. Human pigmentation genetics: the difference is only skin deep. Bioessays 1998;20(9):712–721.
48. Clemens TL, Adams JS, Henderson SL, Holick MF. Increased skin pigment reduces the capacity of skin to synthesis vitamin D3. Lancet 1982;1(8263):74–76.
49. Relethford JH. Hemispheric difference in human skin color [see comments]. Am J Phys Anthropol 1997;104(4):449–457.
50. Harris LJ. Vitamin D and bone. In: Bourne GH, ed. The biochemistry and physiology of bone. New York: Academic Press, 1956:581–622.
51. Vieth R. Would prehistoric human 25-hydroxyvitamin D concentrations be beneficial, and how much vitamin D do we need to ensure desirable nutritional targets? In: Burckhardt P, Heaney R, Dawson-Hughes B, eds. Nutritional aspects of osteoporosis. San Diego: Academic Press, 2001:173–195.
52. Underwood JL, DeLuca HF. Vitamin D is not directly necessary for bone growth and mineralization. Am J Physiol 1984;246(6 Pt 1):E493–E498.
53. Suda T, Ueno Y, Fujii K, Shinki T. Vitamin D and bone. J Cell Biochem 2003;88(2):259–266.
54. Yamamoto M, Kawanobe Y, Takahashi H, Shimazawa E, Kimura S, Ogata E. Vitamin D deficiency and renal calcium transport in the rat. J Clin Invest 1984;74(2):507–513.
55. Bicknell F, Prescott F. Vitamin D. The antirachitic or calcifying vitamin. In: Bicknell F, Prescott F, eds. Vitamins in medicine. London: Whitefriars Press, 1946:630–707.
56. Parfitt AM. Osteomalacia and related disorders. In: Metabolic bone disease and clinically related disorders, 2nd ed. Philadelphia: W. B. Saunders, 1990:329–396.
57. Vieth R, Chan PC, MacFarlane GD. Efficacy and safety of vitamin D(3) intake exceeding the lowest observed adverse effect level. Am J Clin Nutr 2001;73(2):288–294.M
58. Papadimitropoulos E, Wells G, Shea B, et al. Meta-analyses of therapies for postmenopausal osteoporosis. VIII: Meta-analysis of the efficacy of vitamin D treatment in preventing osteoporosis in postmenopausal women. Endocr Rev 2002;23(4):560–569.
59. Trivedi DP, Doll R, Khaw KT. Effect of four monthly oral vitamin D3 (cholecalciferol) supplementation on fractures and mortality in men and women living in the community: randomised double blind controlled trial. BMJ 2003;326:469–475.
60. Feskanich D, Willett WC, Colditz GA. Calcium, vitamin D, milk consumption, and hip fractures: a prospective study among postmenopausal women. Am J Clin Nutr 2003;77(2):504–511.
61. Bischoff-Ferrari HA, Dietrich T, Orav EJ, Dawson-Hughes B. Positive association between 25-hydroxy vitamin d levels and bone mineral density: a population-based study of younger and older adults. Am J Med 2004;116(9):634–639.
62. Bischoff-Ferrari HA, Dietrich T, Orav EJ, et al. Higher 25-hydroxyvitamin D concentrations are associated with better lower-extremity function in both active and inactive persons aged =60 y. Am J Clin Nutr 2004;80(3):752–758.
63. Janssen HC, Samson MM, Verhaar HJ. Vitamin D deficiency, muscle function, and falls in elderly people. Am J Clin Nutr 2002;75(4):611–615.
64. Bischoff HA, Stahelin HB, Tyndall A, Theiler R. Relationship between muscle strength and vitamin D metabolites: are there therapeutic possibilities in the elderly? Z Rheumatol 2000;59(Suppl 1):39–41.
65. Haddad JG, Walgate J, Min C, Hahn TJ. Vitamin D metabolite-binding proteins in human tissue. Biochim Biophys Acta 1976;444(3):921–925.

66. Simpson RU, Thomas GA, Arnold AJ. Identification of 1,25-dihydroxyvitamin D3 receptors and activities in muscle. J Biol Chem 1985;260(15):8882–8891.
67. Bischoff HA, Borchers M, Gudat F, et al. In situ detection of 1,25-dihydroxyvitamin D3 receptor in human skeletal muscle tissue. Histochem J 2001;33(1):19–24.
68. Javaid MK, Crozier SR, Harvey NC, et al. Maternal vitamin D status during pregnancy and childhood bone mass at age 9 years: a longitudinal study. Lancet 2006;367(9504):36–43.
69. El-Hajj Fuleihan G, Nabulsi M, Tamim H, et al. Effect of vitamin D replacement on musculoskeletal parameters in school children: a randomized controlled trial. J Clin Endocrinol Metab 2006;91(2): 405–412.
70. Viljakainen HT, Natri AM, Karkkainen M, et al. A positive dose–response effect of vitamin D supplementation on site-specific bone mineral augmentation in adolescent girls: a double-blinded randomized placebo-controlled 1-year intervention. J Bone Miner Res 2006;21(6):836–844.
71. Lehtonen-Veromaa MK, Mottonen TT, Nuotio IO, Irjala KM, Leino AE, Viikari JS. Vitamin D and attainment of peak bone mass among peripubertal Finnish girls: a 3-y prospective study. Am J Clin Nutr 2002;76(6):1446–1453.
72. Bikle DD, Nemanic MK, Gee E, Elias P. 1,25-Dihydroxyvitamin D3 production by human keratinocytes. Kinetics and regulation. J Clin Invest 1986;78(2):557–566.
73. Abraham S, Lehmann B, Knuschke P, Meurer M. UVB-induced conversion of 7-dehydrocholesterol to 1alpha,25-dihydroxyvitamin D(calcitriol) in cultured keratinocytes is upregulated by tumor necrosis factor-alpha. Exp Dermatol 2005;14(2):154.
74. Schwartz GG, Whitlatch LW, Chen TC, Lokeshwar BL, Holick MF. Human prostate cells synthesize 1,25-dihydroxyvitamin D3 from 25-hydroxyvitamin D3 [In Process Citation]. Cancer Epidemiol Biomarkers Prev 1998;7(5):391–395.
75. Feldman D, Zhao XY, Krishnan AV. Vitamin D and prostate cancer. Endocrinology 2000;141(1):5–9.
76. Holick M. Sunlight and vitamin D. J Gen Intern Med 2002;17(9):733–735.
77. Tangpricha V, Flanagan JN, Whitlatch LW, et al. 25-hydroxyvitamin D-1alpha-hydroxylase in normal and malignant colon tissue. Lancet 2001;357(9269):1673–1674.
78. Cross HS, Bareis P, Hofer H, et al. 25-Hydroxyvitamin D(3)-1alpha-hydroxylase and vitamin D receptor gene expression in human colonic mucosa is elevated during early cancerogenesis. Steroids 2001;66 (3–5):287–292.
79. Mawer EB, Hayes ME, Heys SE, et al. Constitutive synthesis of 1,25-dihydroxyvitamin D3 by a human small cell lung cancer cell line. J Clin Endocrinol Metab 1994;79(2):554–560.
80. Maas RM, Reus K, Diesel B, et al. Amplification and expression of splice variants of the gene encoding the P450 cytochrome 25-hydroxyvitamin D(3) 1,alpha-hydroxylase (CYP 27B1) in human malignant glioma. Clin Cancer Res 2001;7(4):868–875.
81. Tsoukas CD, Provvedini DM, Manolagas SC. 1,25-dihydroxyvitamin D3: a novel immunoregulatory hormone. Science 1984;224(4656):1438–1440.
82. Townsend K, Evans KN, Campbell MJ, Colston KW, Adams JS, Hewison M. Biological actions of extra-renal 25-hydroxyvitamin D-1alpha-hydroxylase and implications for chemoprevention and treatment. J Steroid Biochem Mol Biol 2005.
83. Holick MF. Vitamin D: importance in the prevention of cancers, type 1 diabetes, heart disease, and osteoporosis. Am J Clin Nutr 2004;79(3):362–371.
84. Garland C, Shekelle RB, Barrett-Connor E, Criqui MH, Rossof AH, Paul O. Dietary vitamin D and calcium and risk of colorectal cancer: a 19-year prospective study in men. Lancet 1985;1(8424):307–309.
85. Garland FC, Garland CF, Gorham ED, Young JF. Geographic variation in breast cancer mortality in the United States: a hypothesis involving exposure to solar radiation. Prev Med 1990;19(6):614–622.
86. Ahonen MH, Tenkanen L, Teppo L, Hakama M, Tuohimaa P. Prostate cancer risk and prediagnostic serum 25-hydroxyvitamin D levels (Finland). Cancer Causes Control 2000;11(9):847–852.
87. Hypponen E, Laara E, Reunanen A, Jarvelin MR, Virtanen SM. Intake of vitamin D and risk of type 1 diabetes: a birth-cohort study. Lancet 2001;358(9292):1500–1503.
88. Eva JK. Vitamin D supplement in early childhood and risk for Type I (insulin-dependent) diabetes mellitus. The EURODIAB Substudy 2 Study Group. Diabetologia 1999;42(1):51–54.
89. Chiu KC, Chu A, Go VL, Saad MF. Hypovitaminosis D is associated with insulin resistance and beta cell dysfunction. Am J Clin Nutr 2004;79(5):820–825.

90. Boucher BJ. Inadequate vitamin D status: does it contribute to the disorders comprising syndrome 'X'? Br J Nutr 1998;79(4):315–327.
91. Schwartz GG. Geographic trends in prostate cancer mortality: an application of spatial smoothers and the need for adjustment [letter; comment]. Ann Epidemiol 1997;7(6):430.
92. Hayes CE. Vitamin D: a natural inhibitor of multiple sclerosis. Proc Nutr Soc 2000;59(4):531–535.
93. McGrath J. Does 'imprinting' with low prenatal vitamin D contribute to the risk of various adult disorders? Med Hypotheses 2001;56(3):367–371.
94. Hayes CE, Cantorna MT, DeLuca HF. Vitamin D and multiple sclerosis. Proc Soc Exp Biol Med 1997;216(1):21–27.
95. Munger KL, Zhang SM, O'Reilly E, et al. Vitamin D intake and incidence of multiple sclerosis. Neurology 2004;62(1):60–65.
96. Munger KL, Levin LI, Hollis BW, Howard NS, Ascherio A. Serum 25-hydroxyvitamin D levels and risk of multiple sclerosis. JAMA 2006;296(23):2832–2838.
97. van der Mei IAF, Ponsonby AL, Dwyer T, et al. Past exposure to sun, skin phenotype, and risk of multiple sclerosis: case-control study. BMJ 2003;327(7410):316.
98. Goldberg P, Fleming MC, Picard EH. Multiple sclerosis: decreased relapse rate through dietary supplementation with calcium, magnesium and vitamin D. Med Hypotheses 1986;21(2):193–200.
99. Al Faraj S, Al Mutairi K. Vitamin d deficiency and chronic low back pain in Saudi Arabia. Spine 2003;28(2):177–179.
100. McMurray DN, Bartow RA, Mintzer CL, Hernandez-Frontera E. Micronutrient status and immune function in tuberculosis. Ann N Y Acad Sci 1990;587:59–69.
101. Muhe L, Lulseged S, Mason KE, Simoes EA. Case-control study of the role of nutritional rickets in the risk of developing pneumonia in Ethiopian children. Lancet 1997;349(9068):1801–1804.
102. Cannell JJ, Vieth R, Umhau JC, et al. Epidemic influenza and vitamin D. Epidemiol Infect2006;1–12.
103. Rostand SG. Ultraviolet light may contribute to geographic and racial blood pressure differences. Hypertension 1997;30(2 Pt 1):150–156.
104. Scragg R, Holdaway I, Jackson R, Lim T. Plasma 25-hydroxyvitamin D3 and its relation to physical activity and other heart disease risk factors in the general population. Ann Epidemiol 1992;2(5):697–703.
105. Krause R, Buhring M, Hopfenmuller W, Holick MF, Sharma AM. Ultraviolet B and blood pressure [letter]. Lancet 1998;352(9129):709–710.
106. Pfeifer M, Begerow B, Minne HW, Nachtigall D, Hansen C. Effects of a short-term vitamin D(3) and calcium supplementation on blood pressure and parathyroid hormone levels in elderly women. J Clin Endocrinol Metab 2001;86(4):1633–1637.
107. Harris SS, Dawson-Hughes B. Seasonal changes in plasma 25-hydroxyvitamin D concentrations of young American black and white women [In Process Citation]. Am J Clin Nutr 1998;67(6):1232–1236.
108. Zittermann A, Schleithoff SS, Tenderich G, Berthold HK, Korfer R, Stehle P. Low vitamin D status: a contributing factor in the pathogenesis of congestive heart failure?J Am Coll Cardiol 2003;41(1): 105–112.
109. Zittermann A, Schleithoff SS, Koerfer R. Vitamin D insufficiency in congestive heart failure: Why and what to do about it?Heart Fail Rev 2006;11(1):25–33.
110. Fahrleitner A, Dobnig H, Obernosterer A, et al. Vitamin D deficiency and secondary hyperparathyroidism are common complications in patients with peripheral arterial disease. J Gen Intern Med 2002;17(9): 663–669.
111. Merke J, Milde P, Lewicka S, et al. Identification and regulation of 1,25-dihydroxyvitamin D3 receptor activity and biosynthesis of 1,25-dihydroxyvitamin D3. Studies in cultured bovine aortic endothelial cells and human dermal capillaries. J Clin Invest 1989;83(6):1903–1915.
112. Van Schooten FJ, Hirvonen A, Maas LM, et al. Putative susceptibility markers of coronary artery disease: association between VDR genotype, smoking, and aromatic DNA adduct levels in human right atrial tissue. FASEB J 1998;12(13):1409–1417.
113. Li YC. Vitamin D regulation of the renin-angiotensin system. J Cell Biochem 2003;88(2):327–331.
114. Weishaar RE, Simpson RU. 1,25-dihydroxyvitamin D3 and cardiovascular function in rats. J Clin Invest 1987;76:1706.
115. Weishaar RE, Simpson RU. The involvement of endocrine system in regulating cardiovascular function: emphasis on vitamin D3. Endocr Rev 1989;10(3):351–365.

116. Torrey EF, Miller J, Rawlings R, Yolken RH. Seasonal birth patterns of neurological disorders. Neuroepidemiology 2000;19(4):177–185.
117. Davies G, Welham J, Chant D, Torrey EF, McGrath J. A systematic review and meta-analysis of Northern Hemisphere season of birth studies in schizophrenia. Schizophr Bull 2003;29(3):587–593.
118. McGrath J. Hypothesis: is low prenatal vitamin D a risk-modifying factor for schizophrenia? [In Process Citation]. Schizophr Res 1999;40(3):173–177.
119. Feldman SR, Liguori A, Kucenic M, et al. Ultraviolet exposure is a reinforcing stimulus in frequent indoor tanners implications of a utility model for ultraviolet exposure behavior. J Am Acad Dermatol 2004;51(1):45–51.
120. Lansdowne AT, Provost SC. Vitamin D3 enhances mood in healthy subjects during winter. Psychopharmacology (Berl) 1998;135(4):319–323.
121. Gloth FM III, Alam W, Hollis B. Vitamin D vs broad spectrum phototherapy in the treatment of seasonal affective disorder. J Nutr Health Aging 1999;3(1):5–7.
122. Vieth R, Kimball S, Hu A, Walfish PG. Randomized comparison of the effects of the vitamin D3 adequate intake versus 100 mcg (4000 IU) per day on biochemical responses and the wellbeing of patients. Nutr J 2004;3(1):8.
123. Visser M, Deeg DJ, Puts MT, Seidell JC, Lips P. Low serum concentrations of 25-hydroxyvitamin D in older persons and the risk of nursing home admission. Am J Clin Nutr 2006;84(3):616–622.
124. Hathcock J, Shao A, Vieth R, Heaney R. A risk assessment for vitamin D. American J Clin Nutr 2007;85:6–18.

13 Clinical Aspects of the Use of Vitamin D and Its Metabolites in Osteoporosis

Ian R. Reid, MD

CONTENTS

Key Words: Vitamin D, metabolites, intestinal calcium absorption, osteoblasts, osteoclastogenesis, osteomalacia, hyperparathyroidism, bone loss, parathyroid hormone

INTRODUCTION

The vitamin D compounds regulate intestinal calcium absorption and thus contribute to the maintenance of serum calcium concentrations. They also have direct effects on osteoblasts leading to a stimulation of bone resorption by regulating osteoclastogenesis. In addition, they impact on other aspects of osteoblast activity, the kidney and a variety of other tissues. The clinical syndrome which develops in the presence of severe vitamin D deficiency is osteomalacia, presenting in children as rickets. Osteomalacia is characterized by the presence of unmineralized bone matrix. This occurs in vitamin D deficiency because the low concentrations of both calcium and phosphate in the extracellular fluid are inadequate to sustain the normal formation of hydroxyapatite crystals. Osteomalacia caused by vitamin D deficiency is also characterized by marked hyperparathyroidism, as the body's homeostatic mechanisms struggle to maintain a normal serum calcium concentration in the face of its deficient intestinal absorption. Hyperparathyroidism results in the mobilization of calcium from bone. Clinically apparent osteomalacia in adults is now regarded as a

From: *Contemporary Endocrinology: Osteoporosis: Pathophysiology and Clinical Management*
Edited by: R. A. Adler, DOI 10.1007/978-1-59745-459-9_13,

rarity. However, less marked degrees of vitamin D deficiency are common in those who do not venture outdoors regularly, particularly the frail elderly. These individuals also manifest secondary hyperparathyroidism and the associated acceleration of bone loss, though they often will not have evidence of unmineralized osteoid on bone biopsy. The hyperparathyroidism, however, contributes to the development of osteoporosis, so treatment of vitamin D deficiency becomes an important part of managing osteoporosis in many patients.

Vitamin D is misnamed, since it is not an essential dietary constituent but rather is a hormone precursor synthesized in the skin as a result of sunlight exposure. Body stores are usually assessed from circulating levels of 25-hydroxyvitamin D (25D) and are predominantly determined by sunlight exposure. In addition, 25D concentrations are related to season, physical activity (probably because it reflects time outdoors), gender (lower values in women), age (inversely), fat mass (inversely), skin color (lower values on those with darker skin), and, to some extent, to dietary intake *(1–4)*. There is marked geographic variation in 25D levels, reflecting the effects of these factors as well as differences in customary dress, use of sunscreens, and other lifestyle factors *(5)*. Low values are particularly common in those living in institutions and in those with frailty-related illnesses.

While the importance of vitamin D deficiency in accelerating bone loss is widely accepted, it is uncertain whether other changes in vitamin D metabolism contribute. In advanced old age, there may be a decline in serum concentrations of 1,25-dihydroxyvitamin D as a result of declining renal function, and this is likely to contribute to the rise in parathyroid hormone with age. How important this is to the development of osteoporosis is unclear, and the lack of consistently positive results from trials of treatment using 1α-hydroxylated vitamin D metabolites suggests that this is a relatively small player in most individuals.

The above discussion makes clear the important distinction between supply of the parent compound (i.e., calciferol) and that of its numerous metabolites. There is good evidence for the biological activity of both 25D and 1,25-dihydroxyvitamin D, though the latter is by far the more potent. However, there have been suggestions that other metabolites such as 24,25-dihydroxyvitamin D may also have a role in skeletal metabolism. When calciferol is provided to a vitamin D-deficient individual, all of these metabolites are replaced, and the body's homeostatic mechanisms determine the balance between them. In contrast, when a single active metabolite is administered (e.g., alfacalcidol or calcitriol) levels of other metabolites (such as 25D) may actually be reduced by this intervention, producing an unphysiological balance and a significant risk of hypercalciuria and hypercalcemia. Therefore, when reviewing the evidence from clinical trials, it is very important to draw a distinction between treatment of vitamin D deficiency with calciferol on the one hand and use of its 1α-hydroxylated metabolites on the other.

DEFINITION OF VITAMIN D DEFICIENCY

Recently, there have been attempts to determine the optimal serum 25D concentration, so that an appropriate threshold for intervention can be identified. A number of cross-sectional studies have addressed this by assessing the relationship between serum 25D and parathyroid hormone, using elevation of parathyroid hormone concentrations as a marker of biologically significant vitamin D deficiency *(6)*. Such investigations produce estimates which have wide confidence intervals and some have suggested that the optimal serum 25D concentration may be as high as 100 nmol/L (to convert to μg/L, divide by 2.5) *(7)*. Malabanan et al. *(8)* have addressed this issue by assessing whether the administration of vitamin D resulted in suppression of parathyroid hormone in individuals with a variety of baseline serum 25D concentrations. They found that vitamin D supplementation only caused suppression of parathyroid hormone levels when baseline serum 25D was <50 nmol/L. Lips et al. *(9)* reported a similar threshold following supplementation with 400–600 IU/day of vitamin D, though these subjects also received calcium 500 mg/day. Patel et al. *(10)* have provided data similar to the Malabanan study. Cholecalciferol 800 IU/day increased 25D by 25 nmol/L, while a reciprocal decrease in serum parathyroid hormone (of 6.6 ng/L) was only seen in subjects in the lowest quartile of baseline serum 25D (i.e., 25D < 60 nmol/L).

A further approach to this problem is to assess the relationship between 25D and bone density in a cross-sectional population study. This has been done using the 13,432 participants in NHANES III and showed differences in total hip bone density of about 4% between the lowest and the highest 25D quintiles in whites *(11)*. Most of this difference was between the first and second quintiles which were separated at a 25D concentration of 53 nmol/L. Some prospective epidemiological studies have examined the association between baseline vitamin D status or 25OHD levels and subsequent risk of fracture but have not found a consistent relationship between 25OHD levels and fracture risk *(12–16)*. This question has also been approached by regressing the achieved levels of 25D in clinical studies of vitamin D supplementation against the relative risk of fracture *(17)*. The resulting relationships again have wide confidence intervals but suggest that 25D > 70–80 nmol/L is associated with fewer fractures. However, this analysis did not take into account the fact that some studies co-administered calcium and others did not.

Vitamin D status has also been related to a number of other health states, including dental health, cardiovascular disease, infections, diabetes, and colon cancer *(18)*. Most of these suggestions arise from observational studies, which are confounded by obesity, physical activity, and other health-related behaviors, such as taking vitamin supplements. In general, healthier people are thinner and spend more time outdoors. Like the bone data, these findings are suggestive but not compelling.

It should also be remembered that the circannual variation in 25D means that the threshold for optimal status will vary throughout the year. Our own data show that men need to have a summer peak of >90 nmol/L to ensure that their winter nadir is >50 nmol/L, and for women the summer value must exceed 70 nmol/L *(1,4)*.

In summary, the optimal level of serum 25D for bone health remains an open question with current recommendations spanning a range from 50 to 100 nmol/L *(19)*. The lower end of this range is favored by interventional studies, such as that of Malabanan. If the upper end of this range is accepted, then the majority of older adults would be defined as being deficient. This would lead to a policy of medicating most of the population aged over 50 years, which seems hard to justify in the absence of trial evidence of substantial benefit.

TREATMENT OF VITAMIN D DEFICIENCY

Regimens

The most physiologic way of replacing vitamin D is by exposing individuals to sunlight. We have demonstrated in a randomized controlled trial that spending 30 min/day outdoors results in increases in serum 25D levels from 60 to 78 nmol/L *(20)*. These changes had not plateaued at the end of the 1-month study, suggesting that even greater benefits accrue over time. Supplementation is more commonly undertaken with one of the calciferols, either ergocalciferol (vitamin D_2) or cholecalciferol (vitamin D_3), which are of plant and animal origin, respectively. They have generally been regarded as being equally potent, though several recent studies have suggested that compounds from the vitamin D_3 series have greater biological activity because of longer durations of action following oral administration to humans *(21)*. In a few studies, 25D has been used *(22)*. This would be theoretically attractive in situations where 25-hydroxylation in the liver was likely to be deficient. However, even in advanced liver disease there is usually sufficient capacity to provide adequate hydroxylation of vitamin D, so calciferol is all that is necessary.

Oral or parenteral administration of calciferol is effective. Daily doses between 400 and 1000 international units (IU; 1 μg = 40 IU) per day are typically used. Doses up to several thousand units per day can be administered long term without toxicity *(23)*. A calciferol dose of 1 μg/kg/day increases serum 25D by about 50 nmol/L *(24)*. Other regimens used include 50,000 IU of calciferol once a month by mouth *(25)*, 100,000 IU three-monthly by mouth *(26)*, and 150,000 IU by annual intramuscular injection *(27)*. A single oral dose of up to 500,000 IU of calciferol is effective treatment of established deficiency *(28,29)*. The efficacy of intermittent regimens is attributable to vitamin D being a fat-soluble vitamin which is stored in adipose tissue. The half-life of the decline of 25D after oral loading with calciferol is 90 days *(29)*.

Effects on Bone Density

The effects of vitamin D supplementation on bone density have been studied in a number of contexts. In early postmenopausal women who are not deficient, supplementation has little if any effect on bone density *(30,31)*, and this is also the case even when baseline 25D concentrations are as low as 24–30 nmol/L *(32)*. In older women with sub-optimal serum 25D concentrations, beneficial effects on bone mass of 1–2% are demonstrable *(33,34)*. One study of patients with baseline serum 25D <35 nmol/L demonstrated increases of 4% in spine and hip bone density with calciferol replacement *(28)*.

Effects on Fractures

A number of large studies either with calciferol alone or in combination with calcium have assessed the impact of these interventions on fractures. Heikinheimo et al. *(35)* studied almost 800 elderly men and women, randomized to an annual injection of 150,000 IU vitamin D_2 or to control. Mean baseline levels of 25D were 31 nmol/L in the subjects living independently (two thirds of the cohort) and 14 nmol/L in those in a municipal home. The respective groups increased to 49 and 45 nmol/L with treatment. After a mean follow-up of 3 years, symptomatic fractures were reduced by 25% in the vitamin D-treated subjects ($p = 0.03$). In contrast, Lips et al. showed no difference in fracture incidence in 2578 independently living men and women over the age of 70 years randomized to receive calciferol 400 IU/day or placebo over a period of up to 3.5 years *(36)*. Mean serum 25D concentrations in the third year of the study were 23 nmol/L in the placebo group and 60 nmol/L in the vitamin D group. Trivedi *(37)* randomized 2686 men and women aged 65–85 years living in the general community to 100,000 IU oral vitamin D_3 or placebo every 4 months over 5 years. Relative risks for any fracture were 0.78 ($p = 0.04$) and for hip, wrist/forearm, or vertebral fracture were 0.67 ($p = 0.02$). At year 4, 25D was 74 nmol/L in the intervention group compared with 53 nmol/L in those receiving placebo.

There have also been several large trials of combined treatment with calcium and calciferol in the elderly. In the 3-year study of Chapuy et al. *(38,39)* more than 3000 women aged 69–106 years living in institutions were randomly allocated to take placebo or 1.2 g of elemental calcium plus 800 IU of vitamin D_3 daily. Baseline serum 25D concentrations were 33–40 nmol/L and rose to 100–105 nmol/L in those receiving active therapy. At 18 months, there were 32% fewer non-vertebral fractures in those receiving active treatment ($p = 0.02$) and 43% fewer hip fractures ($p = 0.04$). At the end of 3 years of treatment, the probabilities of non-vertebral fractures and hip fractures were reduced by 24 and 29%, respectively ($p < 0.001$), in those receiving active therapy. Proximal femoral bone mineral density (BMD) increased 2.7% in those receiving active treatment and declined 4.6% in the placebo group ($p < 0.001$). Dawson-Hughes et al. *(40)* have reported similar findings. They randomized 389 men and women aged over 65 years to treatment with either 500 mg of calcium plus 700 IU of calciferol per day or placebo. At the end of 3 years, there had been new non-vertebral fractures in 26 subjects in the placebo group and in 11 in the calcium–vitamin D group ($p = 0.02$). In neither of these studies is it clear whether the calciferol, the calcium, or their combination was the key to success. Larsen et al. *(41)* have reported a community-wide program in which blocks of a municipality were randomized in a factorial design to receive a falls-prevention program or calcium (1 g) and vitamin D (400 IU). They enrolled 9605 individuals (about half of the eligible population) and found a 16% reduction in osteoporotic fractures over 3 years with calcium and vitamin D.

Three large studies have recently been published from Britain. A 2-year, open, randomized study compared a combined intervention of 1 g of calcium plus 800 IU vitamin D_3 daily with dietary and falls-prevention advice in 3314 women aged >70 years with one or more risk factors for hip fracture *(42)*. The study found no significant effect of the calcium/vitamin D intervention on fracture risk (odds ratio for any fracture 1.01, 95% CI 0.71–1.43; odds ratio for hip fracture 0.75, 95% CI 0.31–1.78). However, the findings are limited by the lack of a placebo control, insufficient power to detect a reduction in fracture risk of <30%, and poor adherence (60%) with study medication. The RECORD study recruited 5292 people aged 70 years or older (85% women) with a history of a low-trauma fracture *(43)*. They were randomly assigned to take 800 IU/day vitamin D_3, 1000 mg/day calcium, vitamin D_3 plus calcium, or placebo, and followed for a median period of 45 months. The incidence of new, low-trauma fractures did not differ significantly between participants allocated to calcium and those who were not (hazard ratio 0.94, 95% CI 0.81–1.09). Combined therapy was also ineffective (HR 1.01, 95% CI 0.75–1.36). This study had a low compliance (~50%), there was significant contamination with other therapies for osteoporosis, and it was carried out in a population with prevalent fractures. However, these considerations do not completely explain its negative results. Recently, a further British study has been published, in which 3717 people (76% women, average age 85 years) were randomized to receive ergocalciferol 2.5 mg every 3 months or to act as controls *(44)*. After a median follow-up of 10 months, 3.6% of vitamin D-treated subjects and 2.6% of controls had one or more non-vertebral fractures. Falls and hip fractures were also similar between groups. Baseline 25D was 47 nmol/L and reached 70–80 nmol/L 1–3 months after dosing. However, the study was relatively under-powered, having 50% power to detect a 34% reduction in the incidence of fractures.

Finally, the Women's Health Initiative study recruited 36,282 postmenopausal women, 50–79 years of age, who were randomly assigned to receive 1 g of calcium with 400 IU of vitamin D_3 daily or placebo. Baseline 25D was 47 nmol/L and increased 28% with the intervention. Fractures were ascertained for an average follow-up period of 7.0 years. Intention-to-treat analysis indicated a hazard ratio of 0.88 for hip fracture (95% CI 0.72–1.08), 0.90 for clinical spine fracture (0.74–1.10), and 0.96 for total fractures (0.91–1.02). Censoring data from women when they ceased to adhere to the study medication reduced the hazard ratio for hip fracture to 0.71 (0.52–0.97). There are a number of confounders in this study that need to be considered. The baseline calcium intake was 1150 mg/day, helped to this level by the fact that 30% of subjects were already taking calcium supplements independent of the study. Vitamin D supplements independent of the study were also permitted. Fifty percent of subjects were using hormone replacement therapy and 17% were using a bisphosphonate during the study period. The Women's Health Initiative also had difficulties with compliance, with only 59% taking more than 80% of their study medication at trial end. All these factors militate against the intention-to-treat analysis finding an effect – the high use of supplements and medication effectively made this a study of increasing calcium/vitamin D supplementation in individuals already on a conventional anti-osteoporosis regimen.

The data from these studies indicate that vitamin D deficiency and secondary hyperparathyroidism are common in frail elderly subjects and suggest that these changes contribute to the progressive reduction in bone density which occurs in this age group. These biochemical abnormalities are reversible with physiological doses of vitamin D and calcium, which lead to beneficial effects on bone density, but effects on fracture are equivocal. Bischoff-Ferrari et al. have suggested that anti-fracture efficacy is only attained with a vitamin D dose of at least 700 IU/day and an achieved serum 25D level of 70–80 nmol/L. However, those studies with the greater vitamin D supplement and that achieved the highest 25D levels were also the studies that co-administered calcium, so it is not possible to attribute all the benefit to vitamin D. The present data do suggest, however, that fractures are reduced with high-dose vitamin D and calcium in frail elderly individuals.

Effects on Falls

Severe vitamin D deficiency is associated with myopathy. This has led to the speculation that muscle dysfunction may also occur in less severe states of vitamin depletion. A number of clinical trials have found that vitamin D supplementation reduces falls. Harwood showed a 52% reduction in falls in hip fracture patients given oral or injectable vitamin D *(45)*, and Bischoff-Ferrari et al. *(46)* showed a similar improvement with daily calcium and vitamin D supplements. However, a number of negative studies have also been reported *(47)*. The heterogeneity of patient populations, interventions, and study power may account for these inconsistencies.

VITAMIN D METABOLITES IN POSTMENOPAUSAL OSTEOPOROSIS

Independently of the recognition of the problem of vitamin D deficiency, there has been interest in assessing the active metabolites of vitamin D as pharmaceutical therapies for osteoporosis based on their capacity to increase intestinal calcium absorption and to thereby reduce bone resorption. The agents most studied have been calcitriol and alfacalcidol.

Calcitriol

Two trials in normal women have been reported from Denmark. In early postmenopausal women, those randomized to estrogen/progestin therapy (HRT) had increases in forearm bone mass of ~1% over 1 year, whereas those on placebo or calcitriol lost 2%, the between-groups difference being significant *(48)*. In a similar study in healthy 70-year-old women, bone loss tended to be more marked in the calcitriol-treated group than in those taking placebo, and a loss of vertebral height was only observed in patients taking calcitriol *(49,50)*. More recently, a study from Thailand compared the effects of calcitriol and HRT in early postmenopausal women and showed much more positive changes in bone mass in those receiving estrogen *(51)*. Taken together, these studies suggest that calcitriol has no place in the prevention of normal postmenopausal bone loss and, in European women, may even accelerate it.

A larger number of studies have been carried out in women who already have osteoporosis. Falch et al. *(52)* failed to find any effects of calcitriol on forearm bone mineral content and vertebral fractures over 3 years in 76 women with a history of forearm fracture. A three-center US study resulted in individual reports from each of the centers *(53–55)*. Subjects with at least one vertebral fracture were randomized to calcitriol 0.5 μg/day or placebo, with dose escalation until hypercalciuria or hypercalcemia occurred. The dose titration resulted in the patients of Ott and Chestnut receiving a mean dose of 0.43 μg/day, those of Gallagher 0.62 μg/day, and those of Aloia 0.8 μg/day. The Aloia patients showed between-groups differences in bone density of 2–4% at the various sites (significant using one-tailed tests) but had frequent hypercalciuria and hypercalcemia. The Gallagher group also found beneficial effects (2% between-groups difference in total body BMD at 2 years) and averted major problems with hypercalcemia by restricting dietary calcium intake to 600 mg/day. Ott and Chestnut also had a good safety outcome by restricting calcium intake but bone density changes tended to be more positive in the placebo group than in those receiving calcitriol at the three skeletal sites assessed.

The largest trial of calcitriol in osteoporosis is that of Tilyard *(56)*. Six hundred and twenty-two women with vertebral fractures were randomized to calcitriol 0.5 μg/day or calcium 1 g/day and followed for 3 years. The only end point was vertebral fracture. There were significantly more fractures in the calcium group than in the calcitriol group in both years 2 and 3 – the fracture rate remained stable in the calcitriol group throughout the study but increased threefold in those taking calcium. This apparent deleterious effect of calcium supplementation may be contributed to by the large number of withdrawals in year one. Other issues with this study are that a number of the subjects were vitamin D deficient at entry, the lower fracture rates in calcitriol-treated subjects were only seen in those who had fewer than six fractures at baseline, and the study was not double blind.

More recently, Gallagher *(57)* randomized 489 elderly women to HRT, calcitriol, neither, or both. At 3 years, the increases in BMD were about twice as great in those taking HRT compared with those seen in calcitriol-treated patients, and combination therapy tended to produce the greatest increments in BMD. There was a trend for fracture rates to be lower in the calcitriol groups. Sahota et al. *(58)* have compared calcitriol directly with alendronate and etidronate and shown its effects on markers and bone density to be significantly less than either bisphosphonate. Thus, calcitriol is now little used as a monotherapy for osteoporosis, though occasionally it is sometimes combined with other agents (see below).

The above studies are generally reassuring regarding the safety of calcitriol use, particularly when doses do not exceed 0.5 μg/day. This dose, when used in the absence of calcium supplementation, causes only modest hypercalciuria. None of the more than 200 women treated over a 3-year period by Tilyard developed renal colic, and in the 60 subjects who had renal ultrasonography after 2 years of treatment, no evidence of calcium deposition was seen. In most studies, serum calcium levels have remained stable throughout the trial period, though there have been reports of hypercalcemia in routine clinical use of calcitriol *(59)*. However, the combination of calcitriol with calcium supplementation, or calcitriol doses >0.5 μg/day will result in significant hypercalciuria and hypercalcemia. Such patients require frequent monitoring.

Alfacalcidol

Alfacalcidol (1α-hydroxycholecalciferol) is a synthetic vitamin D compound requiring hydroxylation at position 25 to form calcitriol, its active form. This conversion takes place rapidly in the liver, so it is effectively a pro-drug of calcitriol.

Several studies have failed to demonstrate a beneficial effect of this drug in preventing bone loss in early postmenopausal women *(30,60,61)*. Of the studies in osteoporotic women, many are of short duration, use only forearm bone density measurements, or involve small numbers of patients, possibly accounting for their inconsistent results. Fujita et al. *(62)* compared alfacalcidol with etidronate. Patients were randomized either to alfacalcidol (0.75 μg/day) or to one of two cyclical etidronate regimens (either 200 mg/day or 400 mg/day for the 2-week treatment period). At 1 year, lumbar spine bone density increased 2.4 or 3.4% for the respective etidronate regimens, but showed a non-significant decline (–0.5%) in those receiving alfacalcidol ($p < 0.001$ versus both etidronate groups). Fracture rates (per hundred patients) were the following: low-dose etidronate, 6.9; high-dose etidronate, 5.4; alfacalcidol, 15 ($p = 0.028$ versus high-dose etidronate group). Orimo et al. *(63)* showed that alfacalcidol (1 μg/day) was 1.7% better than placebo at the lumbar spine at 1 year, though there was no treatment effect at the hip. Nuti et al. *(64)* reported similar findings from 148 women studied over 18 months. Shiraki et al. *(65)* and Chen et al. *(66)* reported modest increases in spine BMD of about 2% at 1–2 years with 0.75 μg/day, but these studies are weakened by missing data and being unblinded, respectively. Shiraki et al. *(67)* have also compared alfacalcidol (1 μg/day) and alendronate over 48 weeks. Lumbar spine BMD increased slightly in those receiving the vitamin D metabolite, but substantially more in those on alendronate. No proximal femoral data were reported.

Taken together, these studies suggest a modest beneficial effect of alfacalcidol in postmenopausal osteoporosis. None of the studies established its efficacy definitively, and those using active comparators suggest it is clearly inferior to even a weak bisphosphonate. Most positive data come from studies in Japanese subjects and may not be generalizable to European populations because of genetic and lifestyle (e.g., dietary calcium) differences.

As with calcitriol, the principal safety issues with alfacalcidol are the risks of hypercalciuria and hypercalcemia. In Japanese patients, alfacalcidol 1 μg/day does not elevate serum calcium concentrations unless it is taken in combination with a calcium supplement *(68,69)*. In other groups, there may be hypercalciuria with a dose of only 0.5 μg/day if calcium supplements are also used.

COMBINATION REGIMENS

The combination of vitamin D metabolites with other therapies for osteoporosis has been common, though only recently has evidence to support the practice been forthcoming. Early studies of calcitriol with HRT suggested no benefit from using both together, and similar findings came from the use of calcitriol with a bisphosphonate or calcitonin. Recently, however, studies have shown benefit from the addition of calcitriol to either HRT *(57,70–72)* or a bisphosphonate. Frediani et al. *(73)* randomized women to take calcium, calcitriol 0.5 μg/day, alendronate (10 mg/day), or both. At 2 years, the approximate changes in total body BMD were −2, +2, +4, and +6%, respectively, the combination therapy being significantly better than any of the other interventions. Masud et al. *(74)* compared cyclical etidronate with this regimen plus calcitriol. Again, there was a benefit of more than 2% in the BMD changes at both the spine and the hip. These findings suggest that vitamin D metabolites have small positive effects on bone density when their stimulation of bone resorption is blocked by the co-administration of an anti-resorptive agent.

MALE OSTEOPOROSIS

Orwoll et al. *(75)* studied the effects of calciferol 1000 IU/day plus calcium 1000 mg/day in a placebo-controlled trial in normal men aged 30–87 years. Seventy-seven men were studied over a 3-year period. There was no difference in rates of change of either radial or vertebral BMD between the two groups. However, some of the more recent studies of vitamin D replacement have included men *(35,40)* and they suggest that the beneficial effects are uniform between the sexes. Ebeling *(76)* conducted a randomized, double-blind, placebo-controlled trial of calcitriol 0.5 μg/day versus calcium 1 g/day in osteoporotic men with at least one baseline fracture. The calcium group showed transient positive changes in bone density at the hip and spine, though at 2 years there were no differences between the groups. Over the 2 years of the study, there were 15 vertebral and 6 non-vertebral fractures in the calcitriol group but only a single vertebral fracture in those taking calcium ($p = 0.03$). This suggests that calcitriol should not be used in idiopathic male osteoporosis.

CONCLUSIONS

There is consistent evidence that vitamin D deficiency results in secondary hyperparathyroidism and accelerated bone loss among elderly subjects in many countries. The treatment/prevention of this problem with physiological doses of calciferol (possibly plus calcium) has beneficial effects on bone mass and, possibly, fracture incidence and should be vigorously promoted. The use of vitamin D metabolite (e.g., calcitriol or alfacalcidol) therapy, however, now has little support. There is no evidence to support its use in the prevention of bone loss in normal postmenopausal women. In osteoporotic women, trials have produced variable results, except in Japan where outcomes have been more consistently positive. In those studies in which beneficial effects on BMD have been found, these have generally been less than are seen with HRT or bisphosphonates. Vitamin D metabolites may have effects on BMD which are additive to those of other anti-resorptive agents. There is no conclusive evidence for anti-fracture efficacy of these compounds.

REFERENCES

1. Lucas JA, Bolland MJ, Grey AB, et al. Determinants of vitamin D status in older women living in a subtropical climate. Osteoporos Int 2005;16:1641–1648.
2. Salamone LM, Dallal GE, Zantos D, Makrauer F, Dawson-Hughes B. Contributions of vitamin D intake and seasonal sunlight exposure to plasma 25-hydroxyvitamin D concentration in elderly women. Am J Clin Nutr 1993;58:80–86.
3. Webb AR, Pilbeam C, Hanafin N, Holick MF. An evaluation of the relative contributions of exposure to sunlight and of diet to the circulating concentrations of 25-hydroxyvitamin D in an elderly nursing home population in Boston. Am J Clin Nutr 1990;51:1075–1081.
4. Bolland MJ, Grey AB, Ames RW, et al. Determinants of vitamin D status in older men living in a subtropical climate. Osteoporos Int 2006;17:1742–8.
5. Lips P, Hosking D, Lippuner K, et al. The prevalence of vitamin D inadequacy amongst women with osteoporosis: an international epidemiological investigation. J Intern Med 2006;260:245–254.
6. Steingrimsdottir L, Gunnarsson O, Indridason OS, Franzson L, Sigurdsson G. Relationship between serum parathyroid hormone levels, vitamin D sufficiency, and calcium intake. JAMA 2005;294:2336–41.
7. Dawson-Hughes B, Harris SS, Dallal GE. Plasma calcidiol, season, and serum parathyroid hormone concentrations in healthy elderly men and women. Am J Clin Nutr 1997;65:67–71.
8. Malabanan A, Veronikis IE, Holick MF. Redefining vitamin D insufficiency. Lancet 1998;351:805–806.
9. Lips P, Duong T, Oleksik A, et al. A global study of vitamin D status and parathyroid function in postmenopausal women with osteoporosis: Baseline data from the multiple outcomes of raloxifene evaluation clinical trial. J Clin Endocrinol Metab 2001;86:1212–1221.
10. Patel R, Collins D, Bullock S, Swaminathan R, Blake GM, Fogelman I. The effect of season and vitamin D supplementation on bone mineral density in healthy women: A double-masked crossover study. Osteoporos Int 2001;12:319–325.
11. Bischoff-Ferrari HA, Dietrich T, Orav EJ, Dawson-Hughes B. Positive association between 25-hydroxy vitamin D levels and bone mineral density: a population-based study of younger and older adults. Am J Med 2004;116:634–639.
12. Cummings SR, Browner WS, Bauer D, et al. Endogenous hormones and the risk of hip and vertebral fractures among older women. N Engl J Med 1998;339:733–738.
13. Garnero P, Sornay-Rendu E, Claustrat B, Delmas PD. Biochemical markers of bone turnover, endogenous hormones and the risk of fractures in postmenopausal women: The OFELY study. J Bone Miner Res 2000;15:1526–1536.
14. von Muhlen DG, Greendale GA, Garland CF, Wan L, Barrett-Connor E. Vitamin D, parathyroid hormone levels and bone mineral density in community-dwelling older women: The Rancho Bernardo Study. Osteoporos Int 2005;16:1721–1726.
15. Gerdhem P, Ringsberg K, Obrant K, Akesson K. Association between 25-hydroxy vitamin D levels, physical activity, muscle strength and fractures in the prospective population-based OPRA Study of Elderly Women. Osteoporos Int 2005;16:1425–1431.
16. Jackson RD, LaCroix AZ, Gass M, et al. Calcium plus vitamin D supplementation and the risk of fractures. N Engl J Med 2006;354:669–683.
17. Bischoff-Ferrari HA, Willett WC, Wong JB, Giovannucci E, Dietrich T, Dawson-Hughes B. Fracture prevention with vitamin D supplementation – A meta-analysis of randomized controlled trials. JAMA 2005;293:2257–2264.
18. Bischoff-Ferrari HA, Giovannucci E, Willett WC, Dietrich T, Dawson-Hughes B. Estimation of optimal serum concentrations of 25-hydroxyvitamin D for multiple health outcomes. Am J Clin Nutr 2006;84: 18–28.
19. Dawson-Hughes B, Heaney RP, Holick MF, Lips P, Meunier PJ, Vieth R. Estimates of optimal vitamin D status. Osteoporos Int 2005;16:713–716.
20. Reid IR, Gallagher DJA, Bosworth J. Prophylaxis against vitamin D deficiency in the elderly by regular sunlight exposure. Age Ageing 1986;15:35–40.
21. Armas LAG, Hollis BW, Heaney RP. Vitamin D-2 is much less effective than vitamin D-3 in humans. J Clin Endocrinol Metab 2004;89:5387–5391.

22. Peacock M, Liu GD, Carey M, et al. Effect of calcium or 25OH vitamin D-3 dietary supplementation on bone loss at the hip in men and women over the age of 60. J Clin Endocrinol Metab 2000;85:3011–3019.
23. Vieth R. Vitamin D supplementation, 25-hydroxyvitamin D concentrations, and safety. Am J Clin Nutr 1999;69:842–856.
24. Barger-Lux MJ, Heaney RP, Dowell S, Chen TC, Holick MF. Vitamin D and its major metabolites: Serum levels after graded oral dosing in healthy men. Osteoporos Int 1998;8:222–230.
25. Grey A, Lucas J, Horne A, Gamble G, Davidson JS, Reid IR. Vitamin D repletion in patients with primary hyperparathyroidism and coexistent vitamin D insufficiency. J Clin Endocrinol Metab 2005;90:2122–2126.
26. Zeghoud F, Jardel A, Garabedian M, Salvatore R, Moulias R. Vitamin D supplementation in institutionalized elderly. Effects of vitamin D3 (100,000 IU) orally administered every 3 months on serum levels of 25-hydroxyvitamin D. Rev Rhum Mal Osteoartic 1990;57:809–813.
27. Heikinheimo RJ, Haavisto MV, Harju EJ, et al. Serum vitamin D level after an annual intramuscular injection of ergocalciferol. Calcif Tissue Int 1991;49(Suppl):S87.
28. Adams JS, Kantorovich V, Wu C, Javanbakht M, Hollis BW. Resolution of vitamin D insufficiency in osteopenic patients results in rapid recovery of bone mineral density. J Clin Endocrinol Metab 1999;84:2729–2730.
29. Wu F, Staykova T, Horne A, et al. Efficacy of an oral, 10-day course of high-dose calciferol in correcting vitamin D deficiency. NZ Med J 2003;116:U536.
30. Christiansen C, Christensen MS, McNair P, Hagen C, Stocklund KE, Transbol IB. Prevention of early postmenopausal bone loss: controlled 2-year study in 315 normal females. Eur J Clin Invest 1980;10: 273–279.
31. Hunter D, Major P, Arden N, et al. A randomized controlled trial of vitamin D supplementation on preventing postmenopausal bone loss and modifying bone metabolism using identical twin pairs. J Bone Mineral Res 2000;15:2276–2283.
32. Komulainen MH, Kroger H, Tuppurainen MT, et al. HRT and Vit D in prevention of non-vertebral fractures in postmenopausal women; a 5 year randomized trial. Maturitas 1998;31:45–54.
33. Ooms ME, Roos JC, Bezemer PD, Vandervijgh WJF, Bouter LM, Lips P. Prevention of bone loss by vitamin D supplementation in elderly women: A randomized double-blind trial. J Clin Endocrinol Metab 1995;80:1052–1058.
34. Dawson-Hughes B, Harris SS, Krall EA, Dallal GE, Falconer G, Green CL. Rates of bone loss in postmenopausal women randomly assigned to one of two dosages of vitamin D. Am J Clin Nutr 1995;61:1140–1145.
35. Heikinheimo RJ, Inkovaara JA, Harju EJ, et al. Annual injection of vitamin D and fractures of aged bones. Calcif Tissue Int 1992;51:105–110.
36. Lips P, Graafmans WC, Ooms ME, Bezemer PD, Bouter LM. Vitamin D supplementation and fracture incidence in elderly persons – a randomized, placebo-controlled clinical trial. Ann Intern Med 1996;124:400–406.
37. Trivedi DP, Doll R, Khaw KT. Effect of four monthly oral vitamin D3 (cholecalciferol) supplementation on fractures and mortality in men and women living in the community: randomised double blind controlled trial. [see comment]. BMJ 2003;326:469.
38. Chapuy MC, Arlot ME, Duboeuf F, et al. Vitamin D3 and calcium to prevent hip fractures in the elderly women. N Engl J Med 1992;327:1637–1642.
39. Chapuy MC, Arlot ME, Delmas PD, Meunier PJ. Effect of calcium and cholecalciferol treatment for three years on hip fractures in elderly women. BMJ 1994;308:1081–1082.
40. Dawson-Hughes B, Harris SS, Krall EA, Dallal GE. Effect of calcium and vitamin D supplementation on bone, density in men and women 65 years of age or older. N Engl J Med 1997;337:670–676.
41. Larsen ER, Mosekilde L, Foldspang A. Vitamin D and calcium supplementation prevents osteoporotic fractures in elderly community dwelling residents: A pragmatic population-based 3-year intervention study. J Bone Miner Res 2004;19:370–378.
42. Porthouse J, Cockayne S, King C, et al. Randomised controlled trial of supplementation with calcium and cholecalciferol (vitamin D) for prevention of fractures in primary care. BMJ 2005;330:1003–1006.
43. Grant AM, Anderson FH, Avenell A, et al. Oral vitamin D3 and calcium for secondary prevention of low-trauma fractures in elderly people (Randomised Evaluation of Calcium Or vitamin D, RECORD): a randomised placebo-controlled trial. Lancet 2005;365:1621–1628.

44. Law M, Withers H, Morris J, Anderson F. Vitamin D supplementation and the prevention of fractures and falls: results of a randomised trial in elderly people in residential accommodation. Age Ageing 2006;35:482–486.
45. Harwood RH, Sahota O, Gaynor K, Masud T, Hosking DJ. A randomised, controlled comparison of different calcium and vitamin D supplementation regimens in elderly women after hip fracture : The Nottingham Neck of Femur (NoNOF) Study. Age Ageing 2004;33:45–51.
46. Bischoff-Ferrari HA, Orav EJ, Dawson-Hughes B. Effect of cholecalciferol plus calcium on falling in ambulatory older men and women – a 3-year randomized controlled trial. Arch Int Med 2006;166:424–430.
47. Latham NK, Anderson CS, Reid IR. Effects of vitamin D supplementation on strength, physical performance, and falls in older persons: A systematic review. J Am Geriatr Soc 2003;51:1219–1226.
48. Christiansen C, Christensen MS, Rodbro P, Hagen C, Transbol I. Effect of 1,25-dihydroxy-vitamin D3 in itself or combined with hormone treatment in preventing postmenopausal osteoporosis. Eur J Clin Invest 1981;11:305–309.
49. Jensen GF, Christiansen C, Transbol I. Treatment of postmenopausal osteoporosis. A controlled therapeutic trial comparing oestrogen/gestagen, 1,25-dihydroxy-vitamin D3 and calcium. Clin Endocrinol 1982;16:515–524.
50. Jensen GF, Meinecke B, Boesen J, Transbol I. Does 1,25(OH)2 D3 accelerate spinal bone loss? Clin Orthop 1985;192:215–221.
51. Ongphiphadkanakul B, Piaseu N, Tung SS, Chailurkit L, Rajatanavin R. Prevention of postmenopausal bone loss by low and conventional doses of calcitriol or conjugated equine estrogen. Maturitas 2000;34:179–184.
52. Falch JA, Odegaard OR, Finnanger M, Matheson I. Postmenopausal osteoporosis: no effect of three years treatment with 1,25-dihydroxycholecalciferol. Acta Med Scand 1987;221:199–204.
53. Aloia JF, Vaswani A, Yeh JK, Ellis K, Yasumura S, Cohn SH. Calcitriol in the treatment of postmenopausal osteoporosis. Am J Med 1988;84:401–408.
54. Ott SM, Chesnut CH. Calcitriol treatment is not effective in postmenopausal osteoporosis. Ann Intern Med 1989;110:267–274.
55. Gallagher JC, Goldgar D. Treatment of postmenopausal osteoporosis with high doses of synthetic calcitriol. A randomized controlled study. Ann Intern Med 1990;113:649–655.
56. Tilyard MW, Spears GF, Thomson J, Dovey S. Treatment of postmenopausal osteoporosis with calcitriol or calcium. N Engl J Med 1992;326:357–362.
57. Gallagher JC, Fowler SE, Detter JR, Sherman SS. Combination treatment with estrogen and calcitriol in the prevention of age-related bone loss. J Clin Endocrinol Metab 2001;86:3618–3628.
58. Sahota O, Fowler I, Blackwell PJ, et al. A comparison of continuous alendronate, cyclical alendronate and cyclical etidronate with calcitriol in the treatment of postmenopausal vertebral osteoporosis: A randomized controlled trial. Osteoporos Int 2000;11:959–966.
59. Mathur G, Clifton-Bligh P, Fulcher G, Stiel J, McElduff A. Calcitriol in osteoporosis – is it used safely. Aust N Z J Med 1998;28:348–349.
60. Itoi H, Minakami H, Sato I. Comparison of the long-term effects of oral estriol with the effects of conjugated estrogen, 1-alpha-hydroxyvitamin D-3 and calcium lactate on vertebral bone loss in early menopausal women. Maturitas 1997;28:11–17.
61. Gorai I, Chaki O, Taguchi Y, et al. Early postmenopausal bone loss is prevented by estrogen and partially by 1 alpha-OH-vitamin D-3: Therapeutic effects of estrogen and or 1 alpha-OH-vitamin D-3. Calcif Tissue Int 1999;65:16–22.
62. Fujita T, Orimo H, Inoue T, et al. Double-blind multicenter comparative study of alfacalcidol with etidronate disodium (EHDP) in involutional osteoporosis. Clin Eval 1993;21:261–302.
63. Orimo H, Shiraki M, Hayashi Y, et al. Effects of 1 alpha-hydroxyvitamin D-3 on lumbar bone mineral density and vertebral fractures in patients with postmenopausal osteoporosis. Calcif Tissue Int 1994;54:370–376.
64. Nuti R, Bianchi G, Brandi ML, et al. Superiority of alfacalcidol compared to vitamin D plus calcium in lumbar bone mineral density in postmenopausal osteoporosis. Rheum Int 2006;26:445–453.
65. Shiraki M, Kushida K, Yamazaki K, Nagai T, Inoue T, Orimo H. Effects of 2 years treatment of osteoporosis with 1-alpha-hydroxy vitamin D3 on bone mineral density and incidence of fracture – a placebo-controlled, double-blind prospective study. Endocr J 1996;43:211–220.

66. Chen JT, Shiraki M, Hasumi K, et al. 1-alpha-hydroxyvitamin d-3 treatment decreases bone turnover and modulates calcium-regulating hormones in early postmenopausal women. Bone 1997;20:557–562.
67. Shiraki M, Kushid K, Fukunaga M, et al. A double-masked multicenter comparative study between alendronate and alfacalcidol in Japanese patients with osteoporosis. Osteoporos Int 1999;10:183–192.
68. Orimo H, Shiraki M, Hayashi T, Nakamura T. Reduced occurrence of vertebral crush fractures in senile osteoporosis treated with 1à(OH)-vitamin D3. Bone Miner 1987;3:47–52.
69. Shiraki M, Ito H, Orimo H. The ultra long-term treatment of senile osteoporosis with 1 alpha-hydroxyvitamin D3. Bone Miner 1993;20:223–234.
70. Gutteridge DH, Holzherr M, Will R, et al. Postmenopausal vertebral fractures - advantage of HRT plus calcitriol, over HRT alone, at total body and hip in malabsorbers and normal absorbers of Ca. Bone 1998;23(Suppl):S527.
71. Chen M, Chow SN. Additive effect of alfacalcidol on bone mineral density of the lumbar spine in Taiwanese postmenopausal women treated with hormone replacement therapy and calcium supplementation: a randomized 2-year study. Clin Endocrinol 2001;55:253–258.
72. Mizunuma H, Shiraki M, Shintani M, et al. Randomized trial comparing low-dose hormone replacement therapy and HRT plus 1 alpha-OH-vitamin D-3 (alfacalcidol) for treatment of postmenopausal bone loss. J Bone Miner Metab 2006;24:11–15.
73. Frediani B, Allegri A, Bisogno S, Marcolongo R. Effects of combined treatment with calcitriol plus alendronate on bone mass and bone turnover in postmenopausal osteoporosis two years of continuous treatment. Clin Drug Invest 1998;15:235–244.
74. Masud T, Mulcahy B, Thompson AV, et al. Effects of cyclical etidronate combined with calcitriol versus cyclical etidronate alone on spine and femoral neck bone mineral density in postmenopausal osteoporotic women. Ann Rheum Dis 1998;57:346–349.
75. Orwoll ES, Oviatt SK, McLung MR, Deftos LJ, Sexton G. The rate of bone mineral loss in normal men and the effects of calcium and cholecalciferol supplementation. Ann Intern Med 1990;112:29–34.
76. Ebeling PR, Wark JD, Yeung S, et al. Effects of calcitriol or calcium on bone mineral density, bone turnover, and fractures in men with primary osteoporosis: A two-year randomized, double blind, double placebo study. J Clin Endocrinol Metab 2001;86:4098–4103.

14 The Basic Biology of Estrogen and Bone

Maria Schuller Almeida

CONTENTS

SUMMARY

Estrogens preserve the adult skeleton by suppressing bone turnover and maintaining a focal balance between the rate of bone resorption and formation. Slowing of bone remodeling is due to the attenuating effects of estrogens on the generation of osteoclast and osteoblasts. Maintenance of a focal balance between formation and resorption apparently results from a pro-apoptotic effect on osteoclasts and an anti-apoptotic effect on osteoblasts and osteocytes. Conversely, loss of estrogens leads to a decrease in bone mass due to an increase in bone resorption and formation, with resorption exceeding formation. Bone cells are direct targets of estrogens which bind, predominantly, to the ERα. Estrogens suppress the proliferation of osteoblast progenitors and the apoptosis of osteoblasts and osteocytes and also modulate osteoblast differentiation. The anti-apoptotic actions of estrogens on osteoblasts and osteocytes are mediated by extranuclear kinases and do not require the DNA-binding function of the ER. In cells of the osteoclast lineage, estrogens inhibit the differentiation of osteoclast progenitors and promote the apoptosis of mature osteoclasts. Moreover, estrogens can inhibit osteoclastogenesis indirectly, via the attenuation of the production of osteoclastogenic cytokines by bone marrow mononuclear cells, T lymphocytes, or osteoblast-lineage cells.

From: *Contemporary Endocrinology: Osteoporosis: Pathophysiology and Clinical Management*
Edited by: R. A. Adler, DOI 10.1007/978-1-59745-459-9_14,

Importantly, most of the effects of estrogens on bone cells are mediated via an anti-oxidant mechanism of action.

Key Words: Estrogen, bone, menopause, osteoporosis, estrogen therapy, osteoblasts/ osteocytes, pro-apoptotic effect, osteoclasts, cellular, molecular, 17β-estradiol (E_2), estrone, estriol, postmenopausal

INTRODUCTION

Loss of estrogens at menopause is a major factor for the development of osteoporosis in women. Pioneering work by Fuller Albright *(1)*, validated later by densitometric studies, demonstrated that the accelerated bone loss induced by cessation of ovarian function could be prevented by estrogen therapy *(2,3)*. Estrogens play a key role in the growth and remodeling of the skeleton. In the adult estrogens preserve bone mass by suppressing bone turnover and maintaining a focal balance between the rate of bone formation and resorption. At the cellular level, suppression of bone turnover is a consequence of the attenuating effects of estrogens on the generation of both osteoblast and osteoclast progenitors. Maintenance of a focal balance between formation and resorption by estrogens results from an increase of the life span of osteoblasts/osteocytes and a pro-apoptotic effect on osteoclasts *(4)*.

This chapter will review the recent progress in the understanding of the cellular and molecular mechanisms of action of estrogens on bone cells and the pathogenetic mechanisms responsible for the development of osteoporosis following estrogen deficiency.

GENERAL MECHANISMS OF ESTROGEN ACTION

Endogenous vertebrate estrogens include a large number of molecules, derived from cholesterol, of which the most abundant are 17β-estradiol (E_2), estrone, and estriol. In this review "estrogens" refer to the group of endogenous estrogen molecules. In premenopausal women E_2 produced in the ovaries is the main circulating estrogen. In postmenopausal women estrone, synthesized in several extraovarian sites, including bone, is the most abundant circulating estrogen. E_2, formed by aromatization of testosterone, is the most abundant estrogen in males.

Estrogens act by binding to the estrogen receptor α (ERα) and β (ERβ) that belong to the large family of nuclear receptors *(5)*. ERs are ligand-activated transcription factors that homo- or heterodimerize upon ligand binding and directly bind to specific DNA sequences called estrogen response elements (EREs) in regulatory regions of target genes *(6,7)*. DNA-bound ERs interact with several coregulator proteins to form a multiprotein complex that activates or represses the general transcriptional machinery *(8,9)*. In addition, ERs have the ability to associate indirectly with gene promoters through protein–protein interactions with other transcription factors, as is the case of ER binding to NF-κB. This association inhibits NF-κB activation and the transcription of genes like IL-6 *(10)*. Recently, Cvoro et al. *(11)* reported a novel mechanism of transcriptional repression by estrogen. Specifically, using human osteoblasts and other cells, they showed that TNF-α assembles a transcriptional activation complex at the TNF-α promoter where the unliganded ER interacted with a pre-assembled platform made of c-jun and NF-κB. Importantly, while in the absence of ligand the ER-potentiated TNF-α activation of the TNF-α gene, in the presence of E_2 TNF-α gene expression, is repressed due to the recruitment of glucocorticoid receptor-interacting protein 1 (GRIP1), which behaved as a corepressor. Transcriptional repression of cytokine genes is an important mechanism whereby estrogens affect the skeleton, as will be addressed in more detail later in this chapter.

Within minutes of ligand binding, estrogens are also able to evoke rapid cellular responses that are incompatible with the classical mode of receptor action. These so-called nongenomic or nongenotropic actions of estrogens are due to activation of intracellular signaling cascades, like the mitogen-activated protein kinases (MAPK) or the phosphatidylinositol 3-kinase (PI3K). Such actions are thought to result from ligand binding to ERs localized in the cytoplasm or the plasma membrane *(12)*. Indeed, ERs control an array of genes larger than the one regulated by its direct association with DNA *(13,14)*. In a variety of cell models, including HeLa cells expressing wild-type ERα or the ligand-binding domain of ERα localized to the cell membrane and the OB-6 osteoblastic cell line, among others, treatment with E_2 or estren (a nongenotropic signaling activator) regulated a group of genes distinct from those regulated by classical ER actions *(15)*. Importantly, as will be discussed in more detail below, the effect of sex steroids on the life span of bone cells is mediated by nongenotropic mechanisms of action.

ESTROGENS AND BONE

Estrogens are important regulators of skeletal growth and remodeling. During growth the physiologic actions of these steroids contribute to the sexual dimorphism of the skeleton, the timing of epiphyseal closure, and determination of peak bone mass (see review [*16*]). In the adult, estrogens play a critical role in the maintenance of bone mass. The latter is a consequence of estrogen's ability to attenuate the development of osteoblasts and osteoclasts. On the other hand, acute loss of estrogen increases the rate of remodeling by upregulating osteoblastogenesis and osteoclastogenesis.

Bone remodeling occurs continuously throughout life enabling the localized replacement of old bone with newly formed bone. In the adult skeleton this process is accomplished by temporary anatomic structures, where osteoclasts and osteoblasts assemble called basic multicellular units (BMUs) *(17)*. Each BMU begins at a particular place and advances toward its target which is the region of bone that needs to be repaired. A BMU starts with a team of multinucleated osteoclasts adhering to bone and excavating a tunnel through cortical bone or a trench on the surface of cancellous bone. As the BMU advances, osteoclasts leave the resorption site and osteoblasts are then recruited to fill these cavities with new bone (see detailed review [*18*]). Because the life span of individual cells in a BMU is much shorter than the BMU, new osteoclasts and osteoblasts have to be generated continuously from their progenitors present in the bone marrow as the BMU progresses. As a consequence of this, the balance between the supply of new osteoclasts and osteoblasts and the timing of death of these cells by apoptosis are critical determinants of the initiation of new BMUs and/or extension or shortening of the lifetime of existing ones. The number of each type of cell present in the BMU will, in turn, contribute to the amount of work performed by each cell type and, therefore, is critical for the maintenance of bone homeostasis. Importantly, osteoblast and osteoclast formation is a tightly coupled process due, at least in part, to the dependency of osteoclast precursor development and maturation on support from cells of the stromal/osteoblast lineage through the provision of cytokines and other stimuli. Moreover, the development of osteoblast precursors depends on factors released from the bone matrix by the osteoclast resorption activity *(19)*.

Estrogen deficiency increases the activation frequency ("birth rate") of BMUs, which leads to higher bone turnover. Moreover, loss of estrogen results in a remodeling imbalance by prolonging the resorption phase due to an increase in the life span of osteoclasts *(20)* and shortening the formation phase by promoting osteoblast apoptosis *(4)*. These changes lead to an increase in the volume of bone resorbed beyond the capacity of the osteoblasts to refill it. Furthermore, prolongation of osteoclast life span increases resorption depth and leads to the complete removal of some cancellous elements and loss of trabecular connectivity in cancellous bone *(21,22)*. Concurrently, deeper penetration of osteoclasts in the endocortical surface leads to loss and thinning of cortical bone *(23)*. In women and rodents this acute phase is followed by a long-lasting period of slower bone loss where the dominant microarchitectural change is trabecular thinning. This phase is due to impaired osteoblastic activity which may be secondary to decreased osteoblast formation and increased osteoblast apoptosis.

Estrogens influence skeletal physiology during postnatal life not only in females but also in males. Indeed, decreased BMD has been observed in men and murine models deficient in aromatase and in one man with a truncated, nonfunctional ERα. However, whether this decreased BMD is the result of loss of bone or inability to make bone in the first place is unclear. The reader is directed to excellent reviews on the effects of estrogens on the male skeleton *(24–26)*.

Most, if not all, cell types in the skeleton express ERs. Thus, ERα and ERβ are present in bone marrow stromal cells, osteoblasts, osteocytes, and osteoclasts and their progenitors (see review [27]). Nevertheless, the level of receptor expression in bone cells is low, in both males and females, as compared to reproductive organs *(28,29)*. A review of the literature on the response of the different bone cell types to estrogen indicates that findings are sometimes contradictory. Therefore the results of the different studies will be placed in context of known physiologic functions of estrogen in the skeleton.

Insights from Genetically Modified Mice

During the last decade, several laboratories have generated mice in which the ERs have been deleted or modified in order to elucidate the role of estrogen on its numerous target tissues, including bone. The original ERα knockout mouse model developed by Korach and coworkers *(30,31)* had reduced cortical bone density and cortical bone formation, as well as modestly reduced trabecular bone, in both sexes. Nevertheless, in retrospect these mice were shown to express shortened ERα transcripts that can bind to estrogen *(32,33)*. Complete deletion of ERα ($ER\alpha^{-/-}$) in a different mouse *(34)* resulted in decreased bone remodeling and increased trabecular bone volume in both female and male mice, as well as reduced cortical thickness and density *(35)*. Moreover, the skeletal phenotype was associated with high serum levels of E_2 and T in the females, and higher serum T in the males,

Table 1
Skeletal Phenotype of ER Genetically Modified Mice

Genotype	*Gender*	*Serum sex steroid levels*	*Bone size*	*Bone volume*	*Bone formation*	*Bone resorption*
$ER\alpha^{-/-}$	Female	$E_2 \uparrow$ T $\uparrow$	nc	Tr $\uparrow$ C $\downarrow$	$\downarrow$	$\downarrow$
	Male	E_2 nc T $\uparrow$	$\downarrow$	Tr $\uparrow$ C $\uparrow$	$\uparrow$	$\uparrow$
$ER\beta^{-/-}$	Female	E_2; T nc	nc	Tr $\uparrow$ C nc	nc	$\downarrow$
	Male	E_2; T nc	nc	nc	nc	nc
$ER\alpha\beta^{-/-}$	Female	E_2; T nc	nc	Tr $\downarrow$ C $\downarrow$	$\downarrow$	nc
	Male	E_2 nc T $\uparrow$	nc	Tr $\uparrow$ C $\downarrow$	$\downarrow$	$\downarrow$
$ER\alpha^{-/NERKI}$	Female	$E_2 \uparrow$ T nd	$\downarrow$	Tr nc C $\downarrow$	nd	nd
	Male	E_2; T nc	$\downarrow$	Tr $\downarrow$ C $\downarrow$	$\downarrow$	nc

$\uparrow$ increased or $\downarrow$ decreased as compared to wild-type littermates. nc, no change; nd, not determined; E_2, estradiol; T, testosterone; Tr, trabecular; C, cortical.

when compared to wild-type littermates (Table 1). It was suggested that the increase in trabecular bone results from a compensatory mechanism exerted by the high serum E_2 levels acting through ERβ and high T levels acting through the androgen receptor. In support of this idea, double ER knockout ($ER\alpha\beta^{-/-}$) females show a profound decrease in trabecular bone volume *(35)*.

Deletion of the ERβ gene ($ER\beta^{-/-}$), as opposed to the ERα gene, has dissimilar consequences in male and female mice. While $ER\beta^{-/-}$ males display no bone abnormalities compared with wild-type mice *(35,36)*, $ER\beta^{-/-}$ females have a mild increase in trabecular bone volume associated with a decrease in bone resorption *(35)*. One possible explanation for the observed increase in trabecular bone volume is the removal of the dominant-negative function of ERβ on ERα activity, suggested by in vitro studies *(37,38)*. The skeletal effects of ovariectomy (OVX) followed by E_2 replacement on $ER\alpha^{-/-}$ and $ER\beta^{-/-}$ female mice further demonstrated that ERβ can only partially mediate the E_2 effects on bone, although such effects appear to require much higher doses of E_2 *(39)*.

In agreement with the lack of an effect of ERβ in the male skeleton, male $ER\alpha\beta^{-/-}$ and $ER\alpha^{-/-}$ mice have similar skeletal phenotypes. By contrast, loss of both receptors in the females leads to a striking reduction in trabecular bone volume and an unexpected decrease in bone formation in the presence of unaffected bone resorption. Importantly, sex steroid levels in $ER\alpha\beta^{-/-}$ females are not different from wild type *(35)*.

Jakacka et al. *(40)* have recently generated an ER knock-in (NERKI) mouse model with two substitution mutations in the DNA-binding domain in one of the ERα alleles. The NERKI receptor mutant lacks the ability to bind to DNA and signaling through EREs, but retains the protein–protein interactions and kinase-mediated signaling of estrogen action. Khosla and coworkers have demonstrated that both male and female $ER\alpha^{-/NERKI}$ mice show reduced bone mass and decreased bone size when compared to $ER\alpha^{+/+}$ littermates *(41,42)*. Curiously, the severity of reduction in bone mass was allele dose dependent with respect to classical ERα signaling, with $ER\alpha^{+/NERKI}$ mice exhibiting lower bone mass than $ER\alpha^{+/+}$ but higher than $ER\alpha^{-/NERKI}$ littermates. In both sexes cortical bone was reduced, while trabecular bone was preserved in the females and reduced in male $ER\alpha^{-/NERKI}$ mice. The gender difference observed in the trabecular compartment might be due to a compensatory action of high levels of E_2 acting through the ERβ in the females, while in the males sex steroid levels are normal and ERβ is not relevant for bone, as observed previously in the $ER\alpha^{-/-}$ model. In the male $ER\alpha^{-/NERKI}$ mice the decrease in trabecular bone mass results, most likely, from attenuated bone formation in the presence of unaffected bone resorption (Table 1). Remarkably, $ER\alpha^{-/NERKI}$ female mice showed a severe reduction in osteoblast progenitors as assessed by the number of colony-forming units-osteoblasts (CFU-Ob) in the femur and an impaired ability of mesenchymal stem cells to form mineralized nodules in vitro (Almeida, unpublished observations), suggesting that bone formation might also be compromised in the females.

Overall, the analyses of the skeletal phenotype of ER knockout or mutant mice strongly suggest that ERα is the primary mediator of estrogen action on the skeleton. Moreover, these studies indicate that estrogens acting through classical ERE and/or an intact DNA-binding domain of the ERα are important for bone development and the integrity of the skeleton. Unexpectedly, deletion of ERα leads to a decrease in bone formation and resorption, as opposed to the high remodeling state observed in estrogen-deficient women and mice. Recent work from our laboratory, which will be discussed further below, supports the contention that the decrease in bone formation observed in the absence of the ER might be due to the actions of the unliganded receptor in mediating BMP-induced osteoblastogenesis.

EFFECTS ON CELLS OF THE OSTEOBLASTIC LINEAGE

Loss of estrogens at menopause increases not only osteoclastogenesis and bone resorption but also osteoblastogenesis and bone formation. Conversely, estrogen replacement reduces both osteoclast and osteoblast numbers in cancellous bone *(16)*. Osteoblasts originate from mesenchymal stem cells (MSCs) present in the bone marrow. MSCs can also differentiate to chondrocytes, adipocytes, and stromal and muscle cells, when maintained in the appropriate environment *(43–46)*. The ability of adult MSCs to both self-renew and differentiate is critical for tissue homeostasis and must be maintained under rigorous control. Specifically, the stem cell population would become depleted if cell differentiation overwhelmed self-renewal. Likewise, uncontrolled stem cell self-renewal would expand the stem cell population excessively, with the risk of tumorigenesis (see review [*47*]). Over the last few years, studies in genetically modified mice demonstrated that commitment of MSCs to the osteoblast lineage requires well-orchestrated, sequential, stage-specific input of Indian hedgehog (Ihh), canonical Wnt/β-catenin, and bone morphogenetic protein (BMP) signaling to promote osteogenic, and block chondrogenic, programs of cell fate specification (see review [*48*]). This section emphasizes the role of estrogen on the regulation of osteoblastogenesis at multiple levels, including progenitor cell recruitment, proliferation, differentiation, and apoptosis.

Proliferation

Estrogen affects the supply of osteoblasts to the BMU. Jilka et al. *(49)* in our group have demonstrated that the number of osteoblast progenitors as measured by CFU-OBs is increased after loss of estrogens in mice. The increase in CFU-OB number was still present in mice treated with a bisphosphonate, strongly suggesting that bone resorption (and the release of growth factors from the bone matrix) is not required for the increase in osteoblast precursors. Hence, estrogens must suppress osteoblastogenesis directly. Further studies have elucidated that most CFU-OBs are early transit-amplifying progenitors (i.e., dividing cells with limited self-renewal capacity) and their replication is attenuated by E_2 *(50)*. Thus, suppression of the replication of these progenitor cells may represent a key mechanism of the anti-remodeling effects of estrogen since both osteoblasts and the stromal/osteoblastic cells that are required for osteoclast development originate from a common mesenchymal precursor cell *(51,52)*.

Several other studies using human or rat osteoblastic cell lines have found a consistent inhibitory effect of estrogen on cell proliferation (see review [27]). In contrast, other investigators have reported that estrogen increases osteoblastic cell proliferation in vitro. This discrepancy might be due to different stages of cellular differentiation, cell system heterogeneity, and expression level of the ERs. Nonetheless, a suppressive effect of estrogen on osteoblastic cell proliferation is consistent with the inhibitory action of these steroids on osteoblastogenesis seen in vivo.

Differentiation

In addition to reducing the production of osteoblast progenitors from mesenchymal progenitors, estrogens may affect osteoblast differentiation. In vitro, such effects have been variable, depending on the model system used. In some studies estrogens have been shown to increase some markers of osteoblast differentiation like alkaline phosphatase, osteocalcin, type I collagen, and formation of mineralized nodules. In some other studies, however, estrogens exert suppressive effects on these same markers of osteoblast differentiation (see review [27]). One possible explanation for these discrepancies is that the expression of bone marker genes, osteoblastic matrix formation, and mineralization are dependent not only on the ER isoform expressed by the cells, but also on the stage of osteoblastic differentiation *(53)*. Suppression of osteoblast differentiation as measured by the expression of bone matrix proteins is consistent with a reduction in bone formation promoted by estrogen treatment. Moreover, this evidence suggests that both inhibition of stromal/osteoblastic cell differentiation and osteoblast progenitor self-renewal by estrogen may account for the suppressive effect of this hormone on osteoblastogenesis.

In agreement with a suppressive role of estrogens on osteoblastic cell differentiation, studies from our group and others have recently shown that E_2 attenuated osteoblast progenitor differentiation by decreasing BMP-2-induced activation of Smads and Smad-mediated transcription *(54,55)*. Surprisingly, ICI 182,780, an antagonist of ER which causes its degradation, also attenuated BMP-2-induced differentiation of osteoblast precursor cells *(56)*, suggesting that the unliganded ER might potentiate BMP-induced transcription. In agreement with this hypothesis, overexpression of the ER in an uncommitted osteoblast precursor cell model stimulates BMP-induced transcription (Almeida, unpublished observations). Moreover, at least part of the inhibitory actions of E_2 on osteoblastogenesis may result from a repressive effect of the hormone on the differentiation-promoting actions of the unliganded receptor. Further studies will be required to test this hypothesis.

The antagonistic action of the liganded ER on osteoblastogenesis is dependent on the nature of the ligand, since activation of the ER with estren does not inhibit BMP-induced osteoblastogenesis. In fact, selective activation of kinase-mediated actions of the

ER using estren, or an estradiol–dendrimer conjugate that cannot enter the cell *(57)*, induces osteoblast differentiation in a variety of established cell lines of mesenchymal progenitors or pre-osteoblast, as well as in primary cultures of bone marrow and calvaria cells *(55)*. These effects evidently result from activation of the Src, ERK, PI3K, and JNK kinases and downstream potentiation of both the BMP and Wnt signaling cascades. Consistent with the in vitro findings, estren, but not E_2, stimulated Wnt/β-catenin-mediated transcription in TCF-lacZ transgenic mice. Moreover, E_2 stimulated BMP signaling, in $ER\alpha^{-/NERKI}$ mice, but not in wild-type controls. These data suggest that the ER can either stimulate or repress osteoblast differentiation, depending on whether the activating ligand, and probably the resulting conformation of the receptor, prevent or induce ERE-mediated transcription *(55)*.

Apoptosis

The loss of bone that results from estrogen deficiency is due to an imbalance in the rate of bone resorption and formation, with formation being unable to keep up with resorption. It is now well established that estrogen deficiency increases osteoblast apoptosis, and that this may contribute to the gap between bone formation and resorption noted previously *(4)*. Extensive work by our group has demonstrated that both estrogen and androgen act directly on osteoblasts to induce survival signals, via a kinase-mediated action of the ER *(58)*. The anti-apoptotic effects of sex steroid on osteoblasts are mediated by activation of the Src/Shc/ERK signaling pathway and downregulation of JNK. This activity could be eliminated by nuclear, but not by membrane targeting of the ER. Moreover, estrogen action in osteoblastic cell cultures and murine bone in vivo induces the activation of key transcription factors like Elk-1, CCAAT/enhancer-binding protein-b (C/EBPb), cyclic adenosine monophosphate response element-binding protein (CREB), and suppression of c-jun *(59)*.

EFFECTS ON CELLS OF THE OSTEOCLASTIC LINEAGE

Estrogen deficiency in humans and rodents results in a marked stimulation of bone resorption. This is due to the fact that estrogen affects virtually all aspects of osteoclast development, activity, and life span through the regulation of the production of osteoclastogenic cytokines by bone marrow mononuclear cells and osteoblasts *(60)*. Additionally, estrogens can regulate osteoclastogenesis through direct actions on osteoclasts and their progenitors by controlling their survival, as will be discussed below. Osteoclasts are multinucleated cells derived from hematopoietic progenitors of the myeloid lineage, colony-forming unit-granulocyte/macrophage (CFU-GM) and CFU-M. The development of osteoclasts is controlled by bone marrow stromal and osteoblast-lineage cells, as well as activated T cells, which produce several autocrine and paracrine factors required for osteoclast development, activity, and apoptosis. Among these, receptor activator of NF-κB ligand (RANKL) is indispensable for osteoclast development *(51)*. RANKL binds RANK present on hematopoietic cells, which activates the differentiation of osteoclasts. Osteoblastic lineage cells also secrete osteoprotegerin (OPG) the soluble decoy receptor for RANKL that blocks RANK/RANKL interactions *(61)* and is a potent antagonist of osteoclastogenesis.

Differentiation

Studies of osteoblastic cell lines and rodents have implicated several pro-inflammatory cytokines including interleukin (IL)-1β, IL-6, IL-7, tumor necrosis factor-a (TNF-α), prostaglandins, and macrophage colony-stimulating factor (M-CSF) as mediators of the indirect estrogen actions on osteoclast precursor cells (see reviews [*16,62,63*]). Indeed, estrogen deficiency promotes the upregulation of IL-1, IL-6, IL-7, TNF-α, and M-CSF in humans and animal models. In agreement with these findings, if the production or action of these cytokines is inhibited, the effects of estrogen depletion on osteoclastogenesis are blocked or attenuated. At least in mice, the increase in the above-mentioned cytokines results in an expansion of activated T lymphocytes. Studies by Pacifici and coworkers have implicated T lymphocytes in driving bone loss following estrogen withdrawal. These authors suggest that increased T cell production of TNF is induced by estrogen deficiency via a complex mechanism mediated by antigen-presenting cells and involving the cytokines IFNγ, IL-7, and TGFβ (see review [*63*]). However, in contrast to these findings, Lee et al. *(64)* using three different T lymphocyte deficient mice found that OVX induced the same degree of trabecular bone loss in the absence of T lymphocyte as was found in wild-type mice, whereas cortical bone loss was variable. These results cast doubts on the idea that T lymphocytes are required for the rapid increase in resorptive activity induced by estrogen withdrawal.

At the molecular level, estrogens suppress cytokine production via protein–protein interactions between the ER and other transcription factors. Besides IL-6 expression, as mentioned above, estrogens decrease TNF-α gene expression by blocking JNK activity and the resulting production of c-jun and JunD, and block M-CSF gene expression by regulating phosphorylation of Egr-1 and its interaction with Sp-1 *(65,66)*. Moreover, in a self-amplification fashion TNF-α activates its own expression by a mechanism that requires the unliganded ER, and is antagonized by E_2 treatment *(11)*, as described in a previous section of this review. This mechanism of ER action might further contribute to the increase in TNF levels and osteoclastogenesis that follow estrogen withdrawal.

Riggs and coworkers have suggested that the effect of estrogens on bone can be due to the regulation of RANKL and/or OPG levels. Their suggestion was based on data from clinical studies where they analyzed the expression of RANKL on bone marrow cells from pre- and postmenopausal women and found that estrogens suppress RANKL production by osteoblast-lineage cells and T and B cells *(67)*. However, these studies have not distinguished if estrogens regulate RANKL directly or indirectly through regulation of other cytokines. Although the same group and others demonstrated that estrogen stimulates OPG production in vitro, measurement of levels of circulating OPG in pre- and postmenopausal women was not different in most studies (see review [*62*]). Be that as it may, upregulation of OPG and/or suppression of RANKL by estrogen is a plausible mechanism consistent with the anti-resorptive effect of these steroids on bone.

In addition to their indirect inhibitory effects on bone resorption through cells of the osteoclastic lineage, estrogens might also suppress osteoclastogenesis through direct effects on cells of the osteoclastic lineage *(68)*. Thus, estrogens not only suppress RANKL/M-CSF-induced osteoclast differentiation by blocking AP-1-dependent transcription through a reduction of c-jun expression and decreased phosphorylation *(69,70)* but also induce apoptosis of osteoclast-lineage cells.

Apoptosis

In direct contrast to the anti-apoptotic effects on osteoblasts and osteocytes, estrogen exerts pro-apoptotic effects on mature osteoclasts and their precursors (see review [*71*]).

This effect is associated with reduced expression of IL-1R1 mRNA and increased IL-1 decoy receptor expression *(72)*. In murine bone marrow co-cultures, the pro-apoptotic effect of E_2 seems to be mediated by TGFβ *(20)*. Additionally, downregulation of pro-inflammatory cytokines like M-CSF, IL-1, TNF-α, and RANKL, which in turn promote osteoclast survival *(71)*, also contribute to the pro-apoptotic actions of estrogen on osteoclasts.

Chen et al. *(73)* in our group have recently shown that the pro-apoptotic effect of E_2 on osteoclasts is mediated by ERKs. E_2-induced ERK phosphorylation in osteoclasts was sustained for at least 24 h following exposure to the hormone, in contrast to its transient effect on ERK phosphorylation in osteoblast and osteocytic cells. Interestingly, the pro-apoptotic effect of E_2 on osteoclasts was abrogated by conversion of sustained ERK phosphorylation to transient. On the other hand, prolongation of ERK activation by inducing its retention in the nucleus converted the anti-apoptotic effect of E_2 in osteocytes to a pro-apoptotic one *(73)*.

EFFECTS ON OSTEOCYTES

At the end of their matrix secreting activity some osteoblasts become entrapped within lacunae of the mineralized matrix as osteocytes. Recent evidence suggests that the osteocyte is also a target for estrogen action. Osteocytes are the most abundant cells present in mammalian bone, making up 95% of all bone cells *(74,75)*. Indeed, there are approximately ten times more osteocytes than osteoblasts in an individual bone *(76)*. Osteocytes communicate with one another and with cells at the bone surface via a network of cell dendritic processes that run through canaliculi in the bone matrix *(77)*. Strain-induced flow of interstitial fluid through this network not only promotes the transport of cell signaling molecules, nutrients, and waste products but also seems to mechanically activate the osteocytes *(78)*. It is well recognized that biomechanical strain is a major physiological mechanism responsible for the maintenance of bone mass. On the other hand, reduced physical activity in old age, bed rest, or space flight invariably leads to bone loss *(79)*. Frost's mechanostat theory suggested that mechanical strain, perceived by a hypothetical skeletal mechanostat, leads to changes in bone remodeling in order to adjust bone mass to a level that is appropriate for the current ambient mechanical forces. He also hypothesized that estrogen decreases the minimum effective strain necessary to initiate bone formation *(80)*. Experimental approaches to this question in humans have suggested that estrogens and exercise may exert additive effect on bone mass *(79)*. Moreover, Lanyon and coworkers have shown in mice that the increased bone formation that normally occurs in response to mechanical loading is diminished in estrogen deficiency *(81)*.

One of the consequences of mechanical strain is the maintenance of osteocyte viability. Bellido in our group and other investigators have shown that physiological levels of mechanical strain prevent apoptosis of cultured osteocytic cells *(82,83)*. Conversely, reduced mechanical forces in the murine model of unloading by tail suspension increase the prevalence of osteocyte apoptosis, followed by bone resorption and loss of bone mineral and bone strength *(84)*. The mechanism involved in the promotion of osteocytic cell survival by mechanical strain in vitro is mediated by integrins and downstream activation of the focal adhesion kinase (FAK), Src, and ERKs *(83)*. Interestingly, the ER (α or β) is also required and this function in mechanotransduction is ligand independent, in distinction to the role of ERs as ligand-dependent mediators of the effects of estrogen *(85)*. The involvement of the ER in mediating the anti-apoptotic effect of mechanical strain is consistent with the poor osteogenic response to the loading exhibited by mice lacking the estrogen receptors α or β *(81,86)*. Others have suggested that the ER also mediates the proliferative response of osteoblasts to mechanical loading *(87,88)*.

Importantly, estrogen deficiency increases the prevalence of osteocyte apoptosis in humans *(89)*, rats *(90)*, and mice *(58)*. Death of osteocytes by apoptosis may not only affect bone strength *(91)* but also bone mass, given that osteocytes produce molecules that modulate osteoclast or osteoblast formation *(92,93)*. On the other hand, estrogens inhibit osteocyte apoptosis induced by a variety of stimuli, including etoposide, dexamethasone, or TNF-α in the MLO-Y4 osteocytic cell line *(58)* and by dexamethasone in primary osteocyte cultures *(94)*. Similar to osteoblasts, the anti-apoptotic activity of estrogen in osteocytes requires activation of the Src/Shc/ERK signaling pathway and transcription factors like Elk-1, C/EBPb, and CREB *(58,95)*.

To summarize this section, the effect of estrogens on the skeleton is not only mediated by osteoblasts and osteoclasts but also by osteocytes. Estrogen prolongs the life span of osteocytes and the ER is required to mediate the pro-survival effects of mechanical strain on the same cells. Therefore, increased osteocyte apoptosis and the resulting disruption of the osteocyte network, most likely, contribute to bone fragility that follows estrogen deficiency although this notion has not been tested directly.

ANTI-OXIDANT ACTION OF ESTROGENS IN BONE CELLS

Recently evidence suggests that estrogens exert their beneficial effect on bone by suppressing reactive oxygen species (ROS). ROS are metabolites of molecular oxygen (O_2) that have higher reactivity than O_2 and include unstable oxygen radicals such as superoxide anions, hydroxyl radicals, and nonradical molecules like hydrogen peroxide (H_2O_2). The vast majority of cellular ROS are produced in the mitochondria as by-products of normal aerobic metabolism (see review [96]). Increased oxidative stress causes lipid peroxidation, as well as protein and DNA damage. Therefore, survival is dependent on the ability of cells to adapt to or resist the stress and to repair or replace the damaged molecules. Alternatively, cells may respond to the insult by undergoing apoptosis. Although at high concentrations ROS damage many cell constituents, they also affect many signaling proteins at levels considerably lower than those that cause oxidative injury *(96)*.

One of the mechanisms used by cells to defend against oxidative damage involves the reduction of peroxides to alcohols in a reaction in which glutathione peroxidase oxidizes glutathione (GSH) to the disulfide GSSH, and glutathione reductase (GSR) converts it back into GSH *(97)*. Recent work by Chambers and coworkers *(98,99)* in mice suggested that estrogen suppresses osteoclastogenesis and prevents bone loss following OVX by increasing thiol anti-oxidants in osteoclasts through an increase in glutathione and thioredoxin reductases. Moreover, OVX or orchidectomy (ORX) in mice promotes the upregulation of ROS levels and suppression of GSR activity in the bone marrow and phosphorylation of p53 and $p66^{shc}$ *(100)*. The p53 tumor suppressor and the adapter protein $p66^{shc}$ represent key components of a signal transduction pathway that not only is activated by increased intracellular ROS and converts oxidative signals into apoptosis but also generates ROS in the mitochondria *(101–103)*. Consistent with an involvement of the redox signaling in the bone loss following sex steroid deficiency, E_2, dihydrotestosterone (DHT), or the anti-oxidant *N*-acetyl-cysteine (NAC) prevented the effects of gonadectomy on all markers of oxidative stress *(100)*. Most surprisingly, NAC was as effective as E_2 or DHT in preventing the decrease of BMD, as well as the increase in osteoblast and osteocyte apoptosis caused by either OVX or ORX *(98,100)*. In support of these findings, the beneficial effects of estrogens in several other tissues are shown to result from improved defense against oxidative stress *(104–112)*.

We have recently established a link among E_2, ROS, and the birth and death of bone cells by demonstrating that the pro-apoptotic effect of E_2 on osteoclasts and their ability to suppress osteoclastogenesis, and the anti-apoptotic effect on osteoblasts require GSH. In osteoblasts, the anti-oxidant role of E_2 seems to be mediated by the attenuation of $p66^{shc}$ phosphorylation induced by H_2O_2, via a kinase-mediated mechanism of ER action *(100)*. While oxidative stress promotes osteoblast apoptosis, an increase in ROS, or depletion of GSH increases osteoclast number and resorption in vitro and in vivo by stimulating RANKL and TNF-α expression through ERK and NF-κB activation *(99,113–115)* and leads to osteopenia in mice and, perhaps, in humans *(114,116,117)*. One of the mechanisms that might mediate E_2-induced inhibition of osteoclastogenesis and/or induction of osteoclast apoptosis is the upregulation of GSR and thioredoxin reductase activity and concomitant decrease in ROS in cells of the osteoclastic lineage. The upregulation of GSR activity by E_2 in osteoclasts is mediated by ERKs *(100)*. Moreover, the loss of bone caused by either depletion of GSH or OVX was inhibited by administration of soluble TNF-α receptors and abrogated in mice deleted for TNF-α gene expression *(118)*. These data suggest that the suppressive effect of estrogen on TNF-α levels plays an important role in mediating the anti-oxidant properties of estrogen. In agreement with this, E_2 inhibits the upregulation of TNF-α mRNA, as well as NF-κB activation induced by H_2O_2 in osteoblastic cell cultures (Almeida, unpublished observations). Further, E_2 also blocks the upregulation of TNF-α induced by RANKL in osteoclasts *(98)*. Although further work is needed to clarify the role of oxidative stress in bone cells, in particular in cells of the osteoblastic lineage, the evidence presented here strongly suggest that estrogens increase oxidant defenses in bone, and that the anti-remodeling effect of these steroids may result from anti-oxidant properties.

SUMMARY

Remarkable progress has been achieved in clarifying the mechanisms of the bone-sparing effects of estrogens in vitro and in animal models. Most of the cell types present in bone express ERs and therefore are direct targets of estrogen action. However, the significance of direct estrogen effects on the different bone cells remains to be demonstrated in vivo. The generation of mice with targeted deletion of ER specifically in osteoclasts or osteoblast-lineage cells at different stages of differentiation will aid in elucidating cell autonomous ER function more clearly. The evidence that estrogens exert their beneficial effects on bone by suppressing ROS suggests that postmenopausal osteoporosis should be prevented by therapies that increase oxidant defenses in bone. Finally, the unanticipated role of the unliganded ERs adds up to the functional diversity of these nuclear receptors in different bone cells. A more challenging task will be to demonstrate the relevance of the mechanisms involving the unliganded ERs, described earlier, in animal models.

ACKNOWLEDGMENTS

The author thanks Stavros C. Manolagas and Robert L. Jilka for their comments and suggestions and the NIH (P01 AG13918) for their support.

REFERENCES

1. Reifenstein EC, Albright F. The metabolic effects of steroid hormones in osteoporosis. J Clin Invest 1947;26(1): 24–56.
2. Lindsay R, Hart DM, Aitken JM, MacDonald EB, Anderson JB, Clarke AC. Long-term prevention of postmenopausal osteoporosis by oestrogen. Evidence for an increased bone mass after delayed onset of oestrogen treatment. Lancet 1976;1(7968):1038–1041.
3. Genant HK, Cann CE, Ettinger B, Gordan GS. Quantitative computed tomography of vertebral spongiosa: a sensitive method for detecting early bone loss after oophorectomy. Ann Intern Med 1982;97(5): 699–705.
4. Manolagas SC. Birth and death of bone cells: basic regulatory mechanisms and implications for the pathogenesis and treatment of osteoporosis. Endocr Rev 2000;21(2):115–137.
5. Tsai MJ, O'Malley BW. Molecular mechanisms of action of steroid/thyroid receptor superfamily members. Annu Rev Biochem 1994;63:451–486.
6. Klock G, Strahle U, Schutz G. Oestrogen and glucocorticoid responsive elements are closely related but distinct. Nature 1987;329(6141):734–736.
7. Klein-Hitpass L, Tsai SY, Greene GL, Clark JH, Tsai MJ, O'Malley BW. Specific binding of estrogen receptor to the estrogen response element. Mol Cell Biol 1989;9(1):43–49.
8. McKenna NJ, Lanz RB, O'Malley BW. Nuclear receptor coregulators: cellular and molecular biology. Endocr Rev 1999;20(3):321–344.
9. Chen JD, Li H. Coactivation and corepression in transcriptional regulation by steroid/nuclear hormone receptors. Crit Rev Eukaryot Gene Expr 1998;8(2):169–190.
10. Stein B, Yang MX. Repression of the interleukin-6 promoter by estrogen receptor is mediated by NF-kappa B and C/EBP beta. Mol Cell Biol 1995;15:4971–4979.
11. Cvoro A, Tzagarakis-Foster C, Tatomer D, Paruthiyil S, Fox MS, Leitman DC. Distinct roles of unliganded and liganded estrogen receptors in transcriptional repression. Mol Cell 2006;21(4): 555–564.
12. Manolagas SC, Kousteni S, Chen JR, Schuller M, Plotkin L, Bellido T. Kinase-mediated transcription, activators of nongenotropic estrogen-like signaling (ANGELS), and osteoporosis: a different perspective on the HRT dilemma. Kidney Int 2004;91(Suppl):S41–S49.
13. Rai D, Frolova A, Frasor J, Carpenter AE, Katzenellenbogen BS. Distinctive actions of membrane-targeted versus nuclear localized estrogen receptors in breast cancer cells. Mol Endocrinol 2005;19(6):1606–1617.
14. Pedram A, Razandi M, Aitkenhead M, Hughes CC, Levin ER. Integration of the non-genomic and genomic actions of estrogen. Membrane-initiated signaling by steroid to transcription and cell biology. J Biol Chem 2002;277(52):50768–50775.
15. Almeida M, Han L, O'Brien CA, Kousteni S, Manolagas SC. Classical genotropic versus kinase-initiated regulation of gene transcription by the estrogen receptor alpha. Endocrinology 2006;147(4):1986–1996.
16. Manolagas SC, Kousteni S, Jilka RL. Sex steroids and bone. Recent Prog Horm Res 2002;57:385–409.
17. Frost HM. Bone dynamics in metabolic bone disease. J Bone Joint Surg Am 1966;48(6):1192–1203.
18. Parfitt AM. Targeted and nontargeted bone remodeling: relationship to basic multicellular unit origination and progression. Bone 2002;30(1):5–7.
19. Manolagas SC, Jilka RL, Bellido T, O'Brien CA, Parfitt AM. Interleukin-6-type cytokines and their receptors. In: Bilezikian JP, Raisz LG, Rodan GA, eds. Principles of bone biology. San Diego: Academic Press, 1996:701–713.
20. Hughes DE, Dai A, Tiffee JC, Li HH, Mundy GR, Boyce BF. Estrogen promotes apoptosis of murine osteoclasts mediated by TGF-β. Nat Med 1996;2:1132–1136.
21. Parfitt AM, Mathews CHE, Villanueva AR, Kleerekoper M, Frame B, Rao DS. Relationships between surface, volume and thickness of iliac trabecular bone in aging and in osteoporosis.

Implications for the microanatomic and cellular mechanism of bone loss. J Clin Invest 1983;72: 1396–1409.
22. Eriksen EF, Langdahl B, Vesterby A, Rungby J, Kassem M. Hormone replacement therapy prevents osteoclastic hyperactivity: a histomorphometric study in early postmenopausal women. J Bone Miner Res 1999;14(7):1217–1221.
23. Parfitt AM. Skeletal heterogeneity and the purposes of bone remodeling: Implications for the understanding of osteoporosis. In: Marcus R, Feldman D, Kelsey J, eds. Osteoporosis. San Diego: Academic Press, 1996:315–329.
24. Gennari L, Nuti R, Bilezikian JP. Aromatase activity and bone homeostasis in men. J Clin Endocrinol Metab 2004;89(12):5898–5907.
25. Rochira V, Balestrieri A, Madeo B, Zirilli L, Granata AR, Carani C. Osteoporosis and male age-related hypogonadism: role of sex steroids on bone (patho)physiology. Eur J Endocrinol 2006;154(2): 175–185.
26. Khosla S, Melton LJ III, Riggs BL. Clinical review 144: Estrogen and the male skeleton. J Clin Endocrinol Metab 2002;87(4):1443–1450.
27. Komm B, Bodine PVN. Regulation of bone cell function by estrogens. In: Marcus R, Feldman D, Kelsey J, eds. Osteoporosis. San Diego: Academic Press, 2001:305–337.
28. Benz DJ, Haussler MR, Komm BS. Estrogen binding and estrogenic responses in normal human osteoblast-like cells. J Bone Miner Res 1991;6:531–541.
29. Braidman I, Baris C, Wood L, Selby P, Adams J, Freemont A et al. Preliminary evidence for impaired estrogen receptor-alpha protein expression in osteoblasts and osteocytes from men with idiopathic osteoporosis. Bone 2000;26(5):423–427.
30. Korach K, Taki M, Kimbro KS. The effects of estrogen receptor gene disruption on bone. In: Paoletti R, ed. Women's health and menopause. Amsterdam, The Netherlands: Kluwer Academic and Fondazione Giovanni Lorenzini, 1997:69–73.
31. Vidal O, Lindberg MK, Hollberg K, Baylink DJ, Andersson G, Lubahn DB, et al. Estrogen receptor specificity in the regulation of skeletal growth and maturation in male mice. Proc Natl Acad Sci USA 2000;97(10):5474–5479.
32. Couse JF, Curtis SW, Washburn TF, Lindzey J, Golding TS, Lubahn DB, et al. Analysis of transcription and estrogen insensitivity in the female mouse after targeted disruption of the estrogen receptor gene. Mol Endocrinol 1995;9:1441–1454.
33. Pendaries C, Darblade B, Rochaix P, Krust A, Chambon P, Korach KS, et al. The AF-1 activation-function of ERalpha may be dispensable to mediate the effect of estradiol on endothelial NO production in mice. Proc Natl Acad Sci USA 2002;99(4):2205–2210.
34. Dupont S, Krust A, Gansmuller A, Dierich A, Chambon P, Mark M. Effect of single and compound knockouts of estrogen receptors alpha (ERalpha) and beta (ERbeta) on mouse reproductive phenotypes. Development 2000;127(19):4277–4291.
35. Sims NA, Dupont S, Krust A, Clement-Lacroix P, Minet D, Resche-Rigon M, et al. Deletion of estrogen receptors reveals a regulatory role for estrogen receptors-beta in bone remodeling in females but not in males. Bone 2002;30(1):18–25.
36. Windahl SH, Vidal O, Andersson G, Gustafsson JA, Ohlsson C. Increased cortical bone mineral content but unchanged trabecular bone mineral density in female ERbeta(–/–) mice. J Clin Invest 1999;104(7):895–901.
37. Hall JM, McDonnell DP. The estrogen receptor beta-isoform (ERbeta) of the human estrogen receptor modulates ERalpha transcriptional activity and is a key regulator of the cellular response to estrogens and antiestrogens. Endocrinology 1999;140(12):5566–5578.
38. Pettersson K, Delaunay F, Gustafsson JA. Estrogen receptor beta acts as a dominant regulator of estrogen signaling. Oncogene 2000;19(43):4970–4978.
39. Sims NA, Clement-Lacroix P, Minet D, Fraslon-Vanhulle C, Gaillard-Kelly M, Resche-Rigon M, et al. A functional androgen receptor is not sufficient to allow estradiol to protect bone after gonadectomy in estradiol receptor-deficient mice. J Clin Invest 2003;111(9):1319–1327.
40. Jakacka M, Ito M, Martinson F, Ishikawa T, Lee EJ, Jameson JL. An estrogen receptor (ER)alpha deoxyribonucleic acid-binding domain knock-in mutation provides evidence for nonclassical ER pathway signaling in vivo. Mol Endocrinol 2002;16(10): 2188–2201.

41. Syed F, Modder U, Fraser D, Spelsberg T, Rosen CJ, Krust A, et al. Skeletal effects of estrogen are mediated by opposing actions of classical and non-classical estrogen receptor pathways. J Bone Miner Res 2005;20:1992–2001.
42. Syed FA, Fraser DG, Spelsberg TC, Rosen CJ, Krust A, Chambon P, et al. Effects of loss of classical estrogen response element signaling on bone in male mice. Endocrinology 2007;148(4):1902–1910.
43. Owen M. Marrow stromal stem cells. J Cell Sci Suppl 1988;10:63–76.
44. Aubin JE. Bone stem cells. J Cell Biochem 1998;73–82.
45. Wang X, Hisha H, Taketani S, Adachi Y, Li Q, Cui W, et al. Characterization of mesenchymal stem cells isolated from mouse fetal bone marrow. Stem Cells 2006;24(3):482–493.
46. Muguruma Y, Yahata T, Miyatake H, Sato T, Uno T, Itoh J, et al. Reconstitution of the functional human hematopoietic microenvironment derived from human mesenchymal stem cells in the murine bone marrow compartment. Blood 2006;107(5):1878–1887.
47. Scadden DT. The stem-cell niche as an entity of action. Nature 2006;441(7097):1075–1079.
48. Hartmann C. A Wnt canon orchestrating osteoblastogenesis. Trends Cell Biol 2006;16(3):151–158.
49. Jilka RL, Takahashi K, Munshi M, Williams DC, Roberson PK, Manolagas SC. Loss of estrogen upregulates osteoblastogenesis in the murine bone marrow: evidence for autonomy from factors released during bone resorption. J Clin Invest 1998;101:1942–1950.
50. DiGregorio G, Yamamoto M, Ali A, Abe E, Roberson P, Manolagas SC, et al. Attenuation of the self-renewal of transit amplifying osteoblast progenitors in the murine bone marrow by 17b-estradiol. J Clin Invest 2001;107:803–812.
51. Lacey DL, Timms E, Tan HL, Kelley MJ, Dunstan CR, Burgess T, et al. Osteoprotegerin ligand is a cytokine that regulates osteoclast differentiation and activation. Cell 1998;93(2):165–176.
52. Hsu HL, Lacey DL, Dunstan CR, Solovyev I, Colombero A, Timms E, et al. Tumor necrosis factor receptor family member RANK mediates osteoclast differentiation and activation induced by osteoprotegerin ligand. Proc Natl Acad Sci USA 1999;96(7 Pt 1):3540–3545.
53. Waters KM, Rickard DJ, Riggs BL, Khosla S, Katzenellenbogen JA, Katzenellenbogen BS, et al. Estrogen regulation of human osteoblast function is determined by the stage of differentiation and the estrogen receptor isoform. J Cell Biochem 2001;83(3):448–462.
54. Usui M, Yoshida Y, Tsuji K, Oikawa K, Miyazono K, Ishikawa I, et al. Tob deficiency superenhances osteoblastic activity after ovariectomy to block estrogen deficiency-induced osteoporosis. Proc Natl Acad Sci USA 2004;101(17):6653–6658.
55. Kousteni S, Almeida M, Han L, Bellido T, Jilka RL, Manolagas SC. Induction of osteoblast differentiation by selective activation of kinase-mediated actions of the estrogen receptor. Mol Cell Biol 2007;27(4):1516–1530.
56. Almeida M, Chen X, Han L., Martin-Millan M., Lowe V, Warren A, et al. The liganded versus unliganded estrogen receptor has opposite effects on osteoblast differentiation. J Bone Miner Res 2006;21 (Suppl 1):S95. Ref Type: Abstract.
57. Harrington WR, Kim SH, Funk CC, Madak-Erdogan Z, Schiff R, Katzenellenbogen JA, et al. Estrogen dendrimer conjugates that preferentially activate extranuclear, nongenomic versus genomic pathways of estrogen action. Mol Endocrinol 2006;20(3):491–502.
58. Kousteni S, Bellido T, Plotkin LI, O'Brien CA, Bodenner DL, Han K, et al. Nongenotropic, sex-nonspecific signaling through the estrogen or androgen receptors: dissociation from transcriptional activity. Cell 2001;104:719–730.
59. Kousteni S, Han L, Chen J-R, Almeida M, Plotkin LI, Bellido T, et al. Kinase-mediated regulation of common transcription factors accounts for the bone-protective effects of sex steroids. J Clin Invest 2003;111:1651–1664.
60. Manolagas SC, Jilka RL. Bone marrow, cytokines, and bone remodeling – emerging insights into the pathophysiology of osteoporosis. N Engl J Med 1995;332:305–311.
61. Simonet WS, Lacey DL, Dunstan CR, Kelley M, Chang M-S, Lüthy R, et al. Osteoprotegerin: a novel secreted protein involved in the regulation of bone density. Cell 1997;89:309–319.
62. Clowes JA, Riggs BL, Khosla S. The role of the immune system in the pathophysiology of osteoporosis. Immunol Rev 2005;208:207–227.
63. Weitzmann MN, Pacifici R. Estrogen deficiency and bone loss: an inflammatory tale. J Clin Invest 2006;116(5):1186–1194.

64. Lee SK, Kadono Y, Okada F, Jacquin C, Koczon-Jaremko B, Gronowicz G, et al. T lymphocyte-deficient mice lose trabecular bone mass with ovariectomy. J Bone Miner Res 2006;21(11):1704–1712.
65. Srivastava S, Neale WM, Kimble RB, Rizzo M, Zahner M, Milbrandt J, et al. Estrogen blocks M-CSF gene expression and osteoclast formation by regulating phosphorylation of egr-1 and its interaction with Sp-1. J Clin Invest 1998;102(10):1850–1859.
66. Srivastava S, Weitzmann MN, Cenci S, Ross FP, Adler S, Pacifici R. Estrogen decreases TNF gene expression by blocking JNK activity and the resulting production of c-Jun and JunD. J Clin Invest 1999;104(4): 503–513.
67. Eghbali-Fatourechi G, Khosla S, Sanyal A, Boyle WJ, Lacey DL, Riggs BL. Role of RANK ligand in mediating increased bone resorption in early postmenopausal women. J Clin Invest 2003;111(8): 1221–1230.
68. Oursler MJ. Estrogen regulation of gene expression in osteoblasts and osteoclasts. Crit Rev Eukaryot Gene Expr 1998;8(2):125–140.
69. Shevde NK, Bendixen AC, Dienger KM, Pike JW. Estrogens suppress RANK ligand-induced osteoclast differentiation via a stromal cell independent mechanism involving c-Jun repression. Proc Natl Acad Sci USA 2000;97(14):7829–7834.
70. Srivastava S, Toraldo G, Weitzmann MN, Cenci S, Ross FP, Pacifici R. Estrogen decreases osteoclast formation by down-regulating receptor activator of NF-kappa B ligand (RANKL)-induced JNK activation. J Biol Chem 2001;276(12):8836–8840.
71. Boyce BF, Xing L, Jilka RL, Bellido T, Weinstein RS, Parfit AM, et al. Apoptosis and Bone Cells. In: Bilezikian JP, Raisz LG, Rodan GA, eds. Principles of bone biology. Orlando: Academic Press, 2002:151–168.
72. Sunyer T, Lewis J, Collin-Osdoby P, Osdoby P. Estrogen's bone-protective effects may involve differential IL-1 receptor regulation in human osteoclast-like cells. J Clin Invest 1999;103(10): 1409–1418.
73. Chen JR, Plotkin LI, Aguirre JI, Han L, Jilka RL, Kousteni S, et al. Transient versus sustained phosphorylation and nuclear accumulation of ERKs underlie anti-versus pro-apoptotic effects of estrogens. J Biol Chem 2005;280(6):4632–4638.
74. Marotti G. The structure of bone tissues and the cellular control of their deposition. Ital J Anat Embryol 1996;101(4):25–79.
75. Frost HM. In vivo osteocyte death. J Bone Joint Surg (Am) 1960;42:138–143.
76. Parfitt AM. Bone-forming cells in clinical conditions. In: Hall BK, ed. Bone. Volume 1. The osteoblast and osteocyte. Boca Raton, FL: Telford Press and CRC Press, 1990:351–429.
77. Marotti G, Cane V, Palazzini S, Palumbo C. Structure-function relationships in the osteocyte. Ital J Min Electro Metab 1990;4(2):93–106.
78. Nijweide PJ, Burger EH, Klein-Nulend J. The osteocyte. In: Bilezikian JP, Raisz LG, Rodan GA, eds. Principles of bone biology. San Diego: Academic Press, 2002:93–107.
79. Marcus R. Mechanisms of exercise effects on bone. In: Bilezikian JP, Raisz LG, Rodan GA, eds. Principles of bone biology. San Diego: Academic Press, 2002:1477–1488.
80. Frost HM. The mechanostat: a proposed pathogenic mechanism of osteoporoses and the bone mass effects of mechanical and nonmechanical agents. Bone Miner 1987;2(2):73–85.
81. Lee K, Jessop H, Suswillo R, Zaman G, Lanyon L. Endocrinology: bone adaptation requires oestrogen receptor-alpha. Nature 2003;424(6947):389.
82. Bakker A, Klein-Nulend J, Burger E. Shear stress inhibits while disuse promotes osteocyte apoptosis. Biochem Biophys Res Commun 2004;320(4):1163–1168.
83. Plotkin LI, Mathov I, Aguirre JI, Parfitt AM, Manolagas SC, Bellido T. Mechanical stimulation prevents osteocyte apoptosis: requirement of integrins, Src kinases, and ERKs. Am J Physiol Cell Physiol 2005;289(3):C633–C643.
84. Aguirre JI, Plotkin LI, Stewart SA, Weinstein RS, Parfitt AM, Manolagas SC, et al. Osteocyte apoptosis is induced by weightlessness in mice and precedes osteoclast recruitment and bone loss. J Bone Miner Res 2006;21(4):605–615.
85. Aguirre JI, Plotkin LI, Gortazar AR, Martin MM, O′ Brien CA, Manolagas SC, et al. A novel ligand-independent function of the estrogen receptor is essential for osteocyte and osteoblast mechanotransduction. J Biol Chem 2007;282(35):25501–25508.

86. Lee KC, Jessop H, Suswillo R, Zaman G, Lanyon LE. The adaptive response of bone to mechanical loading in female transgenic mice is deficient in the absence of oestrogen receptor-alpha and -beta. J Endocrinol 2004;182(2):193–201.
87. Lau KH, Kapur S, Kesavan C, Baylink DJ. Up-regulation of the Wnt, estrogen receptor, insulin-like growth factor-I, and bone morphogenetic protein pathways in C57BL/6 J osteoblasts as opposed to C3H/HeJ osteoblasts in part contributes to the differential anabolic response to fluid shear. J Biol Chem 2006;281(14):9576–9588.
88. Damien E, Price JS, Lanyon LE. Mechanical strain stimulates osteoblast proliferation through the estrogen receptor in males as well as females. J Bone Miner Res 2000;15(11):2169–2177.
89. Tomkinson A, Reeve J, Shaw RW, Noble BS. The death of osteocytes via apoptosis accompanies estrogen withdrawal in human bone. J Clin Endocrinol Metab 1997;82(9):3128–3135.
90. Tomkinson A, Gevers EF, Wit JM, Reeve J, Noble BS. The role of estrogen in the control of rat osteocyte apoptosis. J Bone Miner Res 1998;13(8):1243–1250.
91. O'Brien CA, Jia D, Plotkin LI, Bellido T, Powers CC, Stewart SA, et al. Glucocorticoids act directly on osteoblasts and osteocytes to induce their apoptosis and reduce bone formation and strength. Endocrinology 2004;145(4):1835–1841.
92. Winkler DG, Sutherland MK, Geoghegan JC, Yu C, Hayes T, Skonier JE, et al. Osteocyte control of bone formation via sclerostin, a novel BMP antagonist. EMBO J 2003;22(23):6267–6276.
93. Zhao S, Zhang YK, Harris S, Ahuja SS, Bonewald LF. MLO-Y4 osteocyte-like cells support osteoclast formation and activation. J Bone Miner Res 2002;17(11):2068–2079.
94. Gu G, Hentunen TA, Nars M, Harkonen PL, Vaananen HK. Estrogen protects primary osteocytes against glucocorticoid-induced apoptosis. Apoptosis 2005;10(3):583–595.
95. Plotkin LI, Aguirre JI, Kousteni S, Manolagas SC, Bellido T. Bisphosphonates and estrogens inhibit osteocyte apoptosis via distinct molecular mechanisms downstream of extracellular signal-regulated kinase activation. J Biol Chem 2005;280(8):7317–7325.
96. Droge W. Free radicals in the physiological control of cell function. Physiol Rev 2002;82(1):47–95.
97. Dickinson DA, Forman HJ. Glutathione in defense and signaling: lessons from a small thiol. Ann N Y Acad Sci 2002;973:488–504.
98. Lean JM, Davies JT, Fuller K, Jagger CJ, Kirstein B, Partington GA, et al. A crucial role for thiol antioxidants in estrogen-deficiency bone loss. J Clin Invest 2003;112(6):915–923.
99. Lean JM, Jagger CJ, Kirstein B, Fuller K, Chambers TJ. Hydrogen peroxide is essential for estrogen-deficiency bone loss and osteoclast formation. Endocrinology 2005;146(2):728–735.
100. Almeida M, Han L, Martin-Millan M, Plotkin LI, Stewart SA, Roberson PK, et al. Skeletal involution by age-associated oxidative stress and its acceleration by loss of sex steroids. J Biol Chem 2007;282(37):27285–27297.
101. Migliaccio E, Giorgio M, Mele S, Pelicci G, Reboldi P, Pandolfi PP, et al. The p66shc adaptor protein controls oxidative stress response and life span in mammals. Nature 1999;402(6759): 309–313.
102. Trinei M, Giorgio M, Cicalese A, Barozzi S, Ventura A, Migliaccio E, et al. A p53-p66Shc signalling pathway controls intracellular redox status, levels of oxidation-damaged DNA and oxidative stress-induced apoptosis. Oncogene 2002;21(24):3872–3878.
103. Giorgio M, Migliaccio E, Orsini F, Paolucci D, Moroni M, Contursi C, et al. Electron transfer between cytochrome c and p66Shc generates reactive oxygen species that trigger mitochondrial apoptosis. Cell 2005;122(2):221–233.
104. Moor AN, Gottipati S, Mallet RT, Sun J, Giblin FJ, Roque R, et al. A putative mitochondrial mechanism for antioxidative cytoprotection by 17beta-estradiol. Exp Eye Res 2004;78(5):933–944.
105. Chiang K, Parthasarathy S, Santanam N. Estrogen, neutrophils and oxidation. Life Sci 2004;75(20): 2425–2438.
106. Sack MN, Rader DJ, Cannon RO III. Oestrogen and inhibition of oxidation of low-density lipoproteins in postmenopausal women. Lancet 1994;343(8892):269–270.
107. Arnal JF, Clamens S, Pechet C, Negre-Salvayre A, Allera C, Girolami JP, et al. Ethinylestradiol does not enhance the expression of nitric oxide synthase in bovine endothelial cells but increases the release of bioactive nitric oxide by inhibiting superoxide anion production. Proc Natl Acad Sci USA 1996;93(9):4108–4113.

108. Sawada H, Ibi M, Kihara T, Urushitani M, Honda K, Nakanishi M, et al. Mechanisms of antiapoptotic effects of estrogens in nigral dopaminergic neurons. FASEB J 2000;14(9):1202–1214.
109. Chambliss KL, Simon L, Yuhanna IS, Mineo C, Shaul PW. Dissecting the basis of nongenomic activation of endothelial nitric oxide synthase by estradiol: role of ERalpha domains with known nuclear functions. Mol Endocrinol 2005;19(2):277–289.
110. Lu Q, Pallas DC, Surks HK, Baur WE, Mendelsohn ME, Karas RH. Striatin assembles a membrane signaling complex necessary for rapid, nongenomic activation of endothelial NO synthase by estrogen receptor alpha. Proc Natl Acad Sci USA 2004;101(49):17126–17131.
111. Baba T, Shimizu T, Suzuki YI, Ogawara M, Isono KI, Koseki H, et al. Estrogen, insulin, and dietary signals cooperatively regulate longevity signals to enhance resistance to oxidative stress in mice. J Biol Chem 2005;280(16):16417–16426.
112. Lapointe J, Kimmins S, Maclaren LA, Bilodeau JF. Estrogen selectively up-regulates the phospholipid hydroperoxide glutathione peroxidase (PHGPx) in the oviducts. Endocrinology 2005;146(6):2583–2592.
113. Garrett IR, Boyce BF, Oreffo RO, Bonewald L, Poser J, Mundy GR. Oxygen-derived free radicals stimulate osteoclastic bone resorption in rodent bone in vitro and in vivo. J Clin Invest 1990;85(3):632–639.
114. Levasseur R, Barrios R, Elefteriou F, Glass DA, Lieberman MW, Karsenty G. Reversible skeletal abnormalities in gamma-glutamyl transpeptidase-deficient mice. Endocrinology 2003;144(7):2761–2764.
115. Bai XC, Lu D, Liu AL, Zhang ZM, Li XM, Zou ZP, et al. Reactive oxygen species stimulates receptor activator of NF-kappaB ligand expression in osteoblast. J Biol Chem 2005;280(17):17497–17506.
116. Bai XC, Lu D, Bai J, Zheng H, Ke ZY, Li XM, et al. Oxidative stress inhibits osteoblastic differentiation of bone cells by ERK and NF-kappaB. Biochem Biophys Res Commun 2004;314(1):197–207.
117. Basu S, Michaelsson K, Olofsson H, Johansson S, Melhus H. Association between oxidative stress and bone mineral density. Biochem Biophys Res Commun 2001;288(1): 275–279.
118. Jagger CJ, Lean JM, Davies JT, Chambers TJ. Tumor necrosis factor-alpha mediates osteopenia caused by depletion of antioxidants. Endocrinology 2005;146(1):113–118.

15 Estrogens and Estrogen Agonists/Antagonists

Robert Lindsay

CONTENTS

Key Words: Agonists, antagonists, osteoporosis, estrogen deficiency, bone mass, menopause, remodeling, osteoclast recruitment, stress risers, Study of Osteoporotic Fractures, 17beta-estradiol, DXA

INTRODUCTION

The fact that in most cultures osteoporosis occurs more commonly among the female of the species has been known for many years. Bruns *(1)* first demonstrated this for proximal femur fractures in 1882. More than 60 years ago Albright et al. *(2)* noted that vertebral fractures occurred more commonly among women who had had their ovaries removed prior to the average age of menopause. Albright went on to show *(3)* that estrogen intervention could reverse the negative calcium balance that was present among women with osteoporosis. However, it is only comparatively recently that significant data *(4–6)* have been generated that demonstrate beyond all doubt that estrogens by themselves (ET) or in combination with a progestin (HT) can reduce the risk of all fractures among postmenopausal women. However, because of the other effects of ET and HT in those studies, there is still concern about the use of estrogens for osteoporosis prevention and treatment.

PATHOPHYSIOLOGY

In all situations of estrogen deficiency there is an increase in bone remodeling that in many individuals (but likely not all) results in loss of bone mass and disrupts the architecture of the skeleton. This is most obvious after menopause, since all women transition

From: *Contemporary Endocrinology: Osteoporosis: Pathophysiology and Clinical Management*
Edited by: R. A. Adler, DOI 10.1007/978-1-59745-459-9_15,

through menopause around the average age of 51 years. However, in many individuals bone loss begins prior to, and during the menopausal transitions as ovarian function gradually declines. This has been suggested as one reason why Colles' fracture risk increases around the age of 40 years.

In bone biopsy studies Recker et al. *(5)* have shown that increased remodeling across menopause persists into old age. Increased remodeling by itself would lead only to a transient loss of mass if it were caused solely by an increase in the number of remodeling sites within bone tissue. Eventually, over the course of, perhaps, a year or two a new steady state would be reached and bone loss would cease. Thus, for continued bone loss, there must be an imbalance within each remodeling unit, with less new bone formed than removed, or the remodeling process itself sets off a chain of events that exacerbate loss of tissue. Both may be operative. There is some evidence of increased osteoclast recruitment and activity resulting in larger resorption cavities that cannot be completely filled by the osteoblast teams. Excess remodeling can also create so-called stress risers within cancellous bone and may result in micro-cracks that attract osteoclast teams in attempts to repair the damage, but in this circumstance can lead to loss of trabeculae. Because of the increased number of remodeling units, there is stochastically a greater chance of osteoclast teams meeting in the center of a trabecula, another mechanism by which the template for osteoblasts to lay down new bone would be lost. All of these features may contribute to bone loss secondary to estrogen deficiency, but clearly there is considerable heterogeneity in the rate and duration of bone loss among individuals, perhaps related to other risk factors, or remaining endogenous estrogen supply from peripheral conversion of androgens mostly of adrenal origin.

In some studies, there has been evidence for continued biological activity of the low levels of estradiol. For example, in the Study of Osteoporotic Fractures *(6)*, Cummings et al. have shown that individuals with higher levels of circulating 17beta-estradiol have the lower risk of hip fracture, even though these estradiol levels are still low in comparison to premenopausal estradiol levels from the ovary.

It is often stated that there is a phase of more rapid loss of bone most obvious in the spine. In early menopause, the vertebral bodies have a high proportion of surface area to mass, principally because of the high proportion of cancellous bone that is present. As loss occurs and trabeculae are lost, the ratio of surface area to mass must decline and consequently the apparent rate of loss will also decline when measured by DXA. Thus, some of this is an artifact of the measurement, but the remainder is clearly related to the high proportion of surface area since bone remodeling is a phenomenon that occurs on the surfaces of bone. Nonetheless, in many individuals bone loss continues into old age and remains sensitive to estrogen intervention.

The loss of estrogen, as stated, increases bone remodeling (see also Chapter 14). While several mechanisms for this have been proposed, the major final common pathway appears to be a change in the secretory pattern of osteoprotegerin (OPG) and RANK-ligand. Both cytokines are secreted by osteoblasts and other cells of the immune system. RANK-ligand attaches to its receptor (RANK) located on the surface of osteoclasts and preosteoclasts and initiates the change from a mononuclear cell to an active multi-nucleate bone resorbing cell. Estrogens appear to modulate the balance of the secreted products up-regulating the secretion of osteoprotegerin and reducing the secretion of RANK-L. In the absence of estrogen the opposite happens. However, while that explains the increased number of osteoclasts within each bone remodeling unit, it does not adequately explain why there is an increase in the number of remodeling units after menopause or ovariectomy. Since both events contribute to loss of bone mass and more importantly the disruption of architecture that leads to the increased fracture risk among postmenopausal women, there is still some work to be done to fully understand the mechanisms involved in estrogen insufficiency and bone loss, and thus also in understanding the effects of estrogen intervention. Other cytokines have also been implicated in estrogen effects, including Interleukins (1, 6, and 11 in particular), TNF-alpha, lymphotoxin, M-CSF, and GM-CSF. Estrogens may also stimulate secretions of TGF-beta, which inhibits bone resorption and stimulates bone formation. Finally, estrogens also stimulate formation of BMPs, particularly BMP-6 in human osteoblast cell lines.

Clinicians can document the increased remodeling using biochemical markers of bone turnover such as NTX or CTX (see Chapter 6). NTX is usually measured in a second morning fasting urine sample, and CTX is usually estimated in serum from a fasting sample. Both have significant diurnal variability, and there is a food effect for CTX. Thus sampling fasting and between 8 and 10 a.m. (or alternatively at the same time each day for sequential samples) is important. Bone loss may also be detected using BMD testing by DXA. Single time point measurements do not give this information, and serial measurements are required usually at 2-year intervals. The NOF *(7)* recommends BMD testing for all women by age 65, and for younger women if they have risk factors other than age and menopause. The FRAX tool can be used to quantify risk for those whose BMD falls between *T*-scores of –1 and –2.5. A 10-year risk of greater than 20% suggests the need to consider intervention.

Curiously, studies of skeletal sensitivity to hormones conducted in men *(8)* suggest that estrogen is an important regulator of bone physiology here also and may be more important than androgens. Indeed androgens may simply be pro-hormones for the skeleton in both genders.

At any stage in life, estrogen deficiency can result in bone loss. In young women bone loss occurs in any situation with hypothalamic–pituitary–ovarian dysfunction. This is particularly true in settings when loss of estrogen is compounded by other problems. For example, significant osteoporosis can be seen in anorexia nervosa *(9)* where the dietary problems compound the effects of estrogen deficiency. Fortunately, in most settings of estrogen insufficiency in young women, the individual seeks investigation for the amenorrhea that is the presenting symptom. Bone loss, following the use of Depo-Provera as a contraceptive, is simply another example of estrogen insufficiency, and although not proven, may be somewhat ameliorated by the presence of the progestin itself.

EFFECTS OF ESTROGEN INTERVENTION

Clinical Trials with Surrogate Outcomes

Albright's original observational studies set the stage for examination of estrogen as an osteoporosis medication. Albright demonstrated improved calcium balance after the introduction of estrogen in open labeled studies. Henneman and Wallach *(10)*, following up on Albright's patients, observed that patients with osteoporosis treated with estrogen maintained their height, while untreated osteoporosis patients continued to lose height sporadically, presumed to be related to ongoing vertebral collapse.

It was not until the development of techniques that allowed the non-invasive measurement of bone mass that it became possible to undertake controlled clinical trials of estrogen intervention. These early studies measured urine calcium and hydroxyproline as measures of bone turnover, and demonstrated reduced turnover with estrogen use. They also estimated bone mass in peripheral bone (radius, metacarpal bone) using either radiological techniques or single photon absorptiometry and showed that estrogen intervention could prevent the loss of bone that occurred in placebo-treated individuals *(11,12)*. These studies have been repeated multiple times and are conclusive about estrogen effects *(13,14)*. The newer markers of bone turnover, such as NTX, CTX, BAP, and osteocalcin, respond in a similar fashion to estrogen administration as hydroxyproline, confirming the return of bone remodeling to the premenopausal range. The advent of dual energy photon absorptiometry and its offshoot dual energy X-ray absorptiometry allowed studies of the central skeleton which demonstrated both prevention of bone loss in the hip, spine, and total body among women in early menopause and in patients with established osteoporosis.

Perhaps the best known of these studies with surrogate outcomes is a relatively recent one *(15)* – the Postmenopausal Estrogen Progestin Intervention Study (PEPI). This study of early postmenopausal women was an NIH sponsored study that evaluated the effects of conjugated equine estrogens (0.625 mg/day) in combination with medroxyprogesterone acetate or micronized progesterone (HT). This controlled double-blind study demonstrated an increase in bone mass in both spine and hip (by DXA) over the 2 years of the clinical trial. These effects were accompanied by a decline in biochemical markers, as bone remodeling was reduced by CE to premenopausal levels. Additionally the study went on to show that there was loss of bone mass when HT was discontinued confirming the older studies of peripheral bone. It is now clear that any estrogen can exert these effects in estrogen-deprived postmenopausal women. While most clinical trails are of relatively short duration (2–3 years), some studies went on for 5–10 years. All these demonstrate a continuing effect of estrogen in preventing further loss of bone mass.

FRACTURE STUDIES

A large number of observational studies suggested that estrogen intervention would reduce the risk of fractures, especially hip fractures. These studies were unanimous and convincing until the concept of the healthy user effect was raised, curiously, not about fracture prevention but rather more about the effects demonstrated in these observational studies on the prevention of cardiovascular disease. This, in no small way, precipitated the Women's Health Initiative (WHI), which examined the effects of CE with or without a progestin on a variety of disease endpoints including fractures *(16,17)*. Although conducted in a population at relatively low risk of fracture with largely unknown BMD, WHI was robust with over 25,000 women in the two arms of the study and over 5 years of observation overall. Significant reductions were seen in clinical vertebral fractures, hip fractures, and all clinical fractures. This is the only study in this field, in which subjects have been recruited without regard to their risk of fracture, to demonstrate a fracture benefit. In the small percentage of women who did undergo BMD testing at baseline, the vast majority fell into the normal range for young adults. If we assume that that is representative of the entire sample, then this is an extremely robust result in a relatively low-risk population. In pharmacologic studies with fracture endpoints, which are usually phase 3 studies during drug development, the subjects are at much higher risk often with prior fractures and usually with BMD in the osteoporosis range in order to ensure a large number of events during the study and to thereby increase the chance of success.

WHI thus confirmed the observational data and supported the small amount of positive data from other clinical trials, mostly looking at vertebral fractures, although wrist fracture reduction has been noted in one European clinical trial. When evaluated as a function of age, greater reductions were evident in the older individuals or those furthest from menopause, where the risk is greatest and thus where the number of events is greatest. This creates somewhat of a problem, since this is the very population at greatest risk of the negative effects of hormone intervention, DVT, PE, stroke, myocardial infarction, and, in the hormone group only, breast cancer. However, these risks appear much diminished if not absent in the younger (50–60 years) group, and thus HT/ET remains a possible intervention for prevention of bone loss in this population. This is the group with higher prevalence of menopausal symptoms where ET/HT is clearly the treatment of choice, and when used in this setting prevention of bone loss can be expected.

Low Dose ET/HT

Realizing that what had previously been considered "standard" dose ET/HT may have a profile of risk to benefit that would be unacceptable to many individuals, a number of studies of lower doses have been conducted *(18–22)*. Apart from effects on menopausal symptoms and uterine safety, surrogate outcomes, such as BMD and lipids, have been used in such studies. Thus, there are no data that directly test the hypothesis that doses of estrogen lower than 0.625 mg/day can reduce fracture risk. However, the data are extremely suggestive of a positive effect. Doses of conjugated estrogen down to 0.3 mg/day produce positive effects on BMD and bone turnover that are close to those seen with higher doses. For transdermal estrogen, 12.5 mcg/day (roughly one fourth of a standard dose) appears to protect the skeleton *(23)*.

Estrogen Administration by Non-oral Routes

Oral estrogen administration delivers a bolus of estrogen to the liver with induction of hepatic protein synthesis. This is assumed to be responsible for some of the deleterious effects of estrogen by changing lipids and raising clotting factors in circulation. Consequently, there has been interest in delivering estrogens by non-oral routes particularly across the skin, but nasal, vaginal, and rectal routes have been proposed. The most common and the marketed route is transdermal using a patch system with solid-phase technology (estrogen creams also are available, but are labeled as percutaneous and in our experience are not well-tolerated in US patients). Several clinical trials have shown that these systems deliver sufficient estrogen to reduce bone turnover and prevent bone loss. One small study with a 50 mcg patch (i.e., delivering 50 mcg estradiol per day) showed a reduction in radiological vertebral fractures *(24)*. These systems are generally assumed to be safer than the oral route, but much of that argument is based on surrogate outcomes. For those at risk of DVT, CVD, or stroke, however, and who need estrogen, intervention via the transdermal route is a good option.

Clinical Aspects

ET/HT clearly reduces bone loss and prevents fractures. We have shown that the BMD response to ET/HT is improved with an adequate calcium intake (1200 mg/day total intake) and probably also adequate vitamin D 800–100 IU/day (see Chapters 11 and 13). While not tested head to head the results seem little different than those seen with other potent anti-resorptive agents (e.g., bisphosphonates). In individuals with menopausal symptoms unrelieved by simple remedies, HT/ET is clearly the treatment of choice. Clinicians now have the option of tailoring the dose to the patient. Starting at the lowest available dose (0.3 mg/day CEE or equivalent for oral estrogens) and increasing every 4–6 weeks as required seems a logical approach. Patients must be reminded that symptoms will not abate for a few weeks after starting estrogens. For hysterectomized women there seems no logic to adding a progestin, particularly since the HT arm of WHI was associated with increased risk of breast cancer while the ET arm was not.

Asymptomatic women who are in the immediate postmenopausal phase of life can consider ET/HT as an option for prevention of osteoporosis, but they should also consider the benefits and risks of other osteoporosis therapies. Here again initiating treatment at the lowest dose is appropriate and only increasing the dose if bone turnover is not suppressed after perhaps a 6-month time period. It is not known if the side-effect profile is less troublesome with low dose estrogen, although some observational data support that conclusion.

Estrogen Agonist–Antagonists

Estrogen agonist–antagonist is a recently coined term to define the group of molecules previously called selective estrogen receptor modulators (SERMs). This term refers to synthetic compounds that interact with the estrogen receptor to produce a spectrum of effects in estrogen-sensitive tissues. These compounds may variously be estrogen agonists in some tissues, estrogen antagonists in some, and neutral in others. The expression of the effect in each tissue may be dependent on expression of ERalpha and/or beta, as well as a host of co-activator and co-repressor molecules. In a generalization that may not hold in the future, these molecules appear to exhibit anti-estrogenic effects on brain and breast tissue, but estrogenic effects on bone, although perhaps less so than estradiol. Presently only one SERM is marketed for prevention and treatment of osteoporosis – raloxifene. In the pivotal study leading to FDA approval, the MORE study, raloxifene reduced the risk of vertebral fractures over a 4-year period *(25)*. This was extended to 8 years in the CORE study. However, there was no significant reduction overall in the risk of hip or other non-vertebral fractures, in the 8 years of follow-up. Raloxifene also prevents bone loss in women who are close to menopause, and thus is approved for prevention as well as treatment of osteoporosis. The demonstration that raloxifene can reduce the risk of estrogen receptor positive breast cancer in low-risk women and is at least as effective as tamoxifen in women at high risk of breast cancer amplifies the importance of this agent in prevention of osteoporosis, and raloxifene is now approved for this indication. Vertebral fractures occur in women at a younger age than hip fractures. Younger women tend to be more concerned about their own risk of breast cancer, especially since many will have a relative or friend who is a survivor. Raloxifene is therefore a useful agent for prevention of osteoporosis in asymptomatic women in their fifties and early sixties, since these women will obtain two benefits, reduced estrogen receptor positive breast cancer risk and reduced vertebral fracture risk. Agents shown to reduce the risk of hip fracture should be used in older individuals. Side effects of raloxifene include deep vein thrombosis and pulmonary embolism, an increased risk in death from stroke (but not stroke per se), and increase in menopausal symptoms, which for women in early menopause is often the most problematic. Raloxifene does not appear to modulate cardiovascular disease risk.

Other selective estrogen receptor modulators have entered clinical trials and have failed, either because of endometrial stimulation or because of uterine prolapse. Currently, one agent is close the end of development, bazedoxifene, which is being developed as both a single agent and in combination with conjugated estrogens. In this circumstance it is primarily intended to prevent endometrial stimulation by CE and is replacing the progestin in HT. The consequences of this combination on disease endpoints are completely unknown, although it does reduce menopausal symptoms, prevents bone loss, and exerts good control of vaginal bleeding. Arzoxifene is the third SERM in clinical trials, but is yet a few years from clinical use.

REFERENCES

1. Bruns P. Die allgemeine lehre von den knockenbruchen. Deutsche Chirurgie 1882;27:1–400.
2. Albright F, Smith PH, Fraser R. Postmenopausal osteoporosis: its clinical features. JAMA 1941;116:2465.
3. Albright F. The effect of hormones on osteogenesis in Man. Recent Prog Horm Res 1947;1:293–353.
4. Riggs BL, Khosla S, Melton LJ, Sex steroids and the construction and conservation of the adult skeleton. Endocr Rev 2002;23:279–302.
5. Recker RR, Lappe JM, Davies KM, Heaney R. Characterization of postmenopausal bone loss: a prospective study. J Bone Miner Res 2000;15:1965–1973.
6. Cummings SR, Browner WS, Bauer DC, Stone K, Ensrud K, Jamal S, Ettiunger B. Endogenous estrogen and the risk of hip and vertebral fractures among older women. N Engl J Med 339:733–738.
7. National Osteoporosis Foundation. Clinician's guide to prevention and management of osteoporosis,2008.
8. Khosla S, Melton LJ, Atkinson EJ, O'Fallon WM. Relationship of sex steroids to longitudinal changes in bone mineral density and bone resorption in young versus elderly men: effects of estrogen on peak bone mass and on age-related bone loss. J Clin Endocrinol Med 2001;86:3555–3561.
9. Rigotti NA, Nussbaum SR, Herzog DB, et al. Osteoporosis in women with anorexia nervosa. N Engl J Med 1984;311:1601–1606.
10. Henneman PH, Wallch S A. Review of the prolonged use of estrogens and androgens in postmenopausal and senile osteoporosis. Arch Int Med 1957;100:715–723.
11. Lindsay R, Aitken JM, Anderson JB, et al. Long term prevention of postmenopausal osteoporosis by oestrogen. Lancet I 1976;1038–1041.
12. Lindsay R, Hart DM, Purdie D, et al. Comparative effects of oestrogen and a progestin on bone loss in postmenopausal women. Clin Sci Mol Med 1978;54:193–195.
13. Lindsay R, Hart DM, Forrest D, Baird C. Prevention of spinal osteoporosis in oophorectomized women. Lancet II 1980;1151–1154.
14. Christiansen CC, Christiansen MS, McNair P. Prevention of early postmenopausal bone loss. Conducted 2 year study in 315 normal females. Eur J Clin Invest 1980;10:273–279.
15. The Writing Group for PEPI. Effects of hormone therapy on bone mineral density: results from the postmenopausal estrogen/progestin interventions (PEPI) trial A. JAMA 1996;276:1389–1396.
16. Cauley JA, Robbins J, Chen Z, et al. Women's Health Initiative Investigators Effects of estrogen plus progestin on fractures and bone mineral density: the Women's Health Initiative randomized trial. JAMA 2003;290:1729–1738.
17. Women's Health Initiative Steering Committee. Effects of conjugated equine estrogen in post-menopausal women with hysterectomy. The Women's health Initiative randomized controlled trial. JAMA 2004;291:1701–1712.
18. Wells G, Tugwell P, Shea B, et al. Osteoporosis Methodology Group and the Osteoporosis Research Advisory Group. Meat-analyses of therapies for postmenopausal osteoporosis V. meta-analysis of the efficacy of hormone replacement therapy in treating and preventing osteoporosis in postmenopausal women. Endocr Rev 2003;23:529–539.
19. Cosman FC, Dempster D, Lindsay R. Clinical effects of estrogens and anti-estrogens on the skeleton and skeletal metabolism. In: Lindsay R, Demspter D, Jordan C, eds. Estrogen and ant-estrogens. Philadelphia: Lippincott Raven, 1997;151–164.

20. Lindsay R, Gallagher JC, Kleerekoper M, Pickar JH. Effect of lower doses of conjugated equine estrogens with and without medroxyprogesterone acetate on bone in early postmenopausal women. JAMA 2002;287:2668–2676.
21. Rowan JP, Simon JA, Speroff L, Ellman H. Effects of low dose norethindrone acetate plus ethinyl estradiol (0.5 mg/2.5 mcg) in women with postmenopausal symptoms: updated analysis of 3 clinical trials. Clin Ther 2006;28:921–932
22. Rubinacci A, Peruzzi E, Modena AB, et al. Effect of low dose E2/NETA on the reduction of postmenopausal bone loss in women. Menopause 2003;10:241–249.
23. Ettinger B, Ensrud KE, Wallace R, Johnson KC, et al. Effects of ultra-low dose transdermal estradiol on bone mineral density: a randomized clinical trial. Obstet Gynecol 2004;104:443–451.
24. Lufkin EG, Wahner HW, O'Fallon WM. Treatment of postmenopausal osteoporosis with transdermal estrogen. Ann Int Med 1992;117:1–9.
25. Ettinger B, Black DM, Mitlak BH, et al. Reduction in vertebral fracture risk in postmenopausal women with osteoporosis treated with raloxifene. JAMA 1999;282:637–645.

16 Androgen Action in Bone: Basic Cellular and Molecular Aspects

Kristine M. Wiren, PhD

CONTENTS

SUMMARY

The impact of the menopause on skeletal health is obvious, but there remains confusion interpreting the skeletal actions of sex steroids. Thus, the mechanisms by which androgens affect bone homeostasis are becoming the focus of intensified research. As a classic steroid hormone, the biological cellular signaling responses to androgen are mediated through the androgen receptor (AR), a ligand-inducible transcription factor. Androgen effects on bone may also be indirectly modulated and/or mediated by other autocrine and paracrine factors in the bone microenvironment or through steroid metabolic enzymatic activity. ARs have been identified in a variety of cells found in bone, thus clearly identifying bone as a target tissue for androgen action. The direct effects of androgen that influence the complex processes of proliferation, differentiation, mineralization, and gene expression in the osteoblast are being characterized, but much remains controversial. This chapter will review recent progress on characterization of the molecular and cellular mechanisms that underlie androgen action in bone.

Key Words: Androgen, androgen receptor, osteoblast, osteoclast, bone

From: *Contemporary Endocrinology: Osteoporosis: Pathophysiology and Clinical Management*
Edited by: R. A. Adler, DOI 10.1007/978-1-59745-459-9_16,

INTRODUCTION

The obvious impact of the menopause on skeletal health has focused much of the research describing the general action of gonadal steroids on the specific effects of estrogen in bone. However, androgens clearly have important beneficial effects, in both men and women, on skeletal development and on the maintenance of bone mass *(1,2)*. Thus it has been demonstrated that androgens (a) influence growth plate maturation and closure helping to determine longitudinal bone growth during development, (b) mediate regulation of trabecular (cancellous) and cortical bone mass in a fashion distinct from estrogen, leading to a sexually dimorphic skeleton, (c) modulate peak bone mass acquisition, and (d) inhibit bone loss *(2)*. In castrate animals, replacement with nonaromatizable androgens (e.g., 5α-dihydrotestosterone, DHT) yields beneficial effects that are clearly distinct from those observed with estrogen replacement *(3,4)*. In intact females, blockade of the androgen receptor (AR) with the specific AR antagonist hydroxyflutamide results in osteopenia *(5)*. Furthermore, treatment with nonaromatizable androgen alone in females results in improvements in bone mineral density *(6)*. Finally, combination therapy with estrogen and androgen in postmenopausal women is more beneficial than either steroid alone *(7–9)*, indicating non-parallel and distinct pathways of action. Combined, these reports illustrate the distinct actions of androgens and estrogens on the skeleton. Thus, in both men and women it is probable that androgens and estrogens each have important yet distinct functions during bone development, and in the subsequent maintenance of skeletal homeostasis in the adult. With the awakening awareness of the importance of the effects of androgen on skeletal homeostasis, and the potential to make use of this information for the treatment of bone disorders, much remains to be learned.

MOLECULAR MECHANISMS OF ANDROGEN ACTION IN BONE CELLS: THE ANDROGEN RECEPTOR (AR)

Direct characterization of AR expression in a variety of tissues, including bone *(10)*, was made possible by the cloning of the AR cDNA *(11,12)*. The AR is a member of the class I (the so-called classical or steroid) nuclear receptor superfamily, as are the (estrogen receptor) ERα and ERβ isoforms, the progesterone receptor, the mineralocorticoid, and glucocorticoid receptor *(13)*. Steroid receptors are transcription factors with a highly conserved modular design characterized by three functional domains: the transactivation, DNA binding, and ligand binding domains. In the absence of ligand, the AR protein is generally localized in the cytoplasmic compartment of target cells in a large complex of molecular chaperones, consisting of loosely bound heat-shock, cyclophilin, and other accessory proteins *(14)*. Interestingly, in the unliganded form, AR conformation is unique with a relatively unstructured amino-terminal transactivation domain *(15)*. As lipids, androgens can freely diffuse through the plasma membrane to bind the AR to induce a conformational change. Once bound by ligand, the AR dissociates from the multiprotein complex, translocates to the nucleus, and recruits coactivators or corepressors that can display cell-type specific expression *(16)*, allowing the formation of homodimers (or potentially heterodimers) that activate a cascade of events in the nucleus *(17)*. Bound to DNA, the AR influences transcription and/or translation of a specific network of genes, leading to the cellular response to the steroid.

The Androgen Receptor Signaling Pathway

Once bound by ligand, the AR is activated. As shown in Fig. 1, this allows the formation of homodimers (or potentially heterodimers) that bind to DNA at palindromic androgen response elements (AREs) in androgen-responsive gene promoters. Classic ARE sequences are found in the proximal promoter as a motif represented by an inverted repeat separated by 3 bp *(18)* similar to glucocorticoid response elements *(19)*. However, our understanding of hormone binding sites in DNA is becoming better characterized and is more complex than originally described *(20)*. Thus, AR binding sites that influence expression, both positively and negatively, are likely distributed throughout the genome with sequences more complex and diverse than simple ARE repeats. DNA binding of the activated AR organizes a cascade of events in the nucleus leading to transcription and translation of a specific network of genes that is responsible for the cellular response to the steroid *(17)*. In the classic model of steroid action, the latent receptor is converted into a transcriptionally active form by simple ligand binding. Again, this model is now considered an over-simplification, with the understanding that signaling pathways and additional proteins (for example, coactivators or corepressors as described below and shown in Fig. 1) within the cell can influence steroid receptor transduction activity. Furthermore, posttranslational modification of the receptor

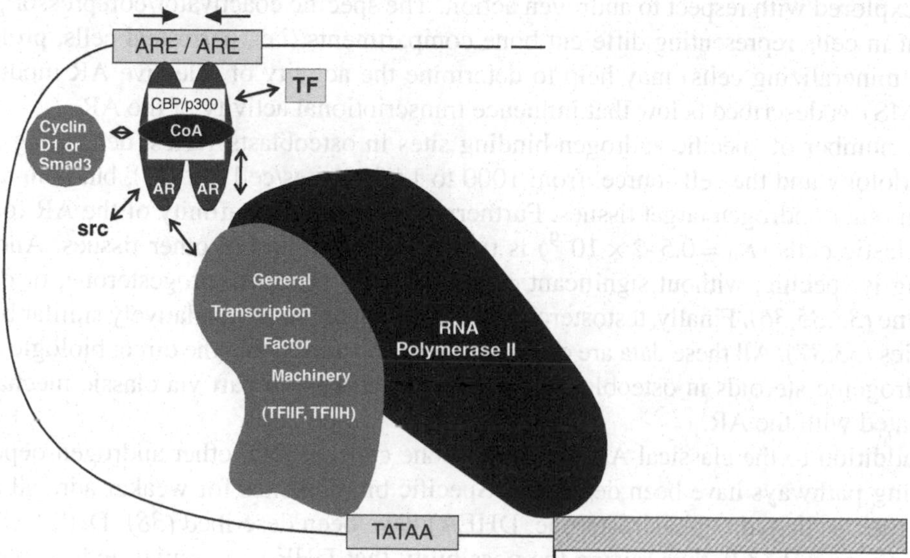

Fig. 1. Model of AR regulation of gene expression. Binding of androgen promotes high-affinity dimerization, followed by DNA binding at the androgen response element (ARE) in an androgen-responsive gene promoter. Coactivators may remodel chromatin through histone acetylase activity to open chromatin structure *(157)* or act as a bridge to attract transcription factors (TFs) that target binding of TATA-binding protein to the TATAA sequence *(13)*. Phosphorylation of receptor may result from activation of SRC by growth factors *(22)*. Smad3 can act as either a coactivator or a corepressor *(158,159)*, while cyclin D1 is a corepressor of AR transactivation *(21)*. AR can also directly contact TFIIH and TFIIF *(160)* in the general transcription machinery. Such interactions between the AR and the general transcription machinery, leading to stable assembly, result in recruitment of RNA polymerase II and subsequent increased gene transcription. Downregulation of gene expression can also be AR mediated.

by acetylation, phosphorylation, and/or ubiquitination can occur *(21)*. For example, steroid receptor phosphorylation can result from signal transduction cascades initiated at the cell membrane, such as from activation of src kinases by growth factors *(22)*. It has been shown that steroid receptor phosphorylation can lead to alterations of the responsiveness of steroid receptors to cognate ligands or, in some cases, even result in ligand-independent activation.

Such potential modification(s) of AR action in bone cells is only poorly characterized; whether the AR in osteoblasts undergoes posttranslational processing that might influence AR activity as described in other tissues *(23,24)*, and the potential functional implications *(25,26)*, are also unknown. Ligand-independent activation of AR has also been described in other tissues *(27)*, but has not been explored in bone. AR activity may also be influenced by receptor modulators, such as the nuclear receptor coactivators or corepressors *(22,28,29)*. These coactivators/corepressors can influence the downstream signaling of nuclear receptors through multiple mechanisms, including histone acetylation/deacetylation, respectively, that result in chromatin remodeling. Such activities may reflect both the cellular context and the particular promoter involved. AR-specific coactivators have been identified *(30)*, many of which interact with the ligand-binding domain of the receptor *(31)*. Expression and regulation of these modulators may thus influence the ability of steroid receptors to regulate gene expression in bone *(18)*, but this remains underexplored with respect to androgen action. The specific coactivator/corepressor profile present in cells representing different bone compartments (i.e., periosteal cells, proliferating or mineralizing cells) may help to determine the activity of selective AR modulators (SARMS) as described below that influence transcriptional activity of the AR.

The number of specific androgen binding sites in osteoblasts varies, depending on the methodology and the cell source, from 1000 to 14,000 sites/cell *(32–35)*, but is in a range seen in other androgen target tissues. Furthermore, the binding affinity of the AR found in osteoblastic cells ($K_d = 0.5–2 \times 10^{-9}$) is typical of that found in other tissues. Androgen binding is specific, without significant competition by estrogen, progesterone, or dexamethasone *(33,35,36)*. Finally, testosterone and DHT appear to have relatively similar binding affinities *(33,37)*. All these data are consistent with the notion that the direct biologic effects of androgenic steroids in osteoblasts are mediated at least in part via classic mechanisms associated with the AR.

In addition to the classical AR present in bone cells, several other androgen-dependent signaling pathways have been described. Specific binding sites for weaker adrenal androgens (such as dehydroepiandrosterone, DHEA) have been described *(38)*; DHEA can also transactivate AR *(39)*, thus raising the possibility that DHEA or similar androgenic compounds may also have direct effects in bone. DHEA and its metabolites may also bind and activate additional receptors, including ER, peroxisome proliferator-activated receptor-α, and pregnane X receptor *(40)*. Bodine et al. *(41)* showed that DHEA caused a rapid inhibition of c-*fos* expression in human osteoblastic cells that was more robust than seen with the classical androgens (DHT, testosterone, androstenedione). In addition, DHEA may inhibit bone resorption by osteoclasts when in the presence of osteoblasts, likely through changes in osteoprotegerin (OPG) and receptor activator of NF-κB ligand (RANKL) concentrations *(42)*. AR may also interact with other transcription factors, such as NF-κB, CREB-binding protein, and different forms of AP-1, to generally repress transcription without DNA binding. Alternatively, androgens may be specifically bound in osteoblastic cells by a novel

63-kDa cytosolic protein *(43)*. In addition, there are reports of distinct AR polymorphisms identified in different races that may have biological impact on androgen responses *(44)*, but to date none have an effect with respect to bone tissue *(45)*. These different isoforms have the potential to interact in distinct fashions with other signaling molecules, such as c-Jun *(46)*. Finally, androgens may regulate osteoblast activity via rapid nongenomic mechanisms *(47,48)* through membrane receptors displayed at the bone cell surface *(49)*. The role and biologic significance of these non-classical signaling pathways in androgen-mediated responses in bone remains controversial, and most data suggest that genomic signaling may be the more significant regulator in bone and other tissues *(50–53)*.

Localization of Androgen Receptor Expression

Clues about the potential sequelae of AR signaling may be derived from a better understanding of the cell types in which receptor expression is documented. In the bone microenvironment, the localization of AR expression in osteoblasts has been described in intact human bone by using immunocytochemical techniques *(10,54)*. In developing bone from young adults, Abu et al. *(10)* showed ARs were predominantly expressed in active osteoblasts at sites of bone formation (Fig. 2). ARs were also observed in osteocytes embedded in the bone matrix. Importantly, both the pattern of AR distribution and the level of expression were similar in males and in females. In addition, expression of the AR has been characterized in cultured osteoblastic cell populations isolated from bone biopsy specimens determined at both the mRNA level and by binding analysis *(35)*. Expression varied according to the skeletal site of origin and age of the donor of the cultured osteoblastic cells: AR expression was higher at cortical and intramembranous bone sites and lower in trabecular bone. This distribution pattern correlates with androgen responsiveness in the bone compartment. AR expression was highest in osteoblastic cultures generated from young adults and somewhat lower in samples from either prepubertal or senescent bone. Again, no differences were found between male and female samples, suggesting that differences in receptor number per se do not underlie development of a sexually dimorphic skeleton. Interestingly, ARs are also expressed in bone marrow stromal *(55)* and mesenchymal precursor cells *(56)*, pluripotent cells that can differentiate into muscle, bone, and fat. Androgen action may modulate precursor differentiation toward the osteoblast and/or myoblast lineage, while inhibiting differentiation toward the adipocyte lineage *(57)*. These effects on stromal differentiation could underlie some of the well-described consequences of androgen administration on body composition including increased muscle mass *(58)*. To date, it has not been established how significant the contribution is, of the increased muscle mass associated with androgen administration, to positively influence bone quality. Bone marrow stomal cells are also responsive to sex steroids during the regulation of osteoclastogenesis.

Because androgens are so important in bone development at the time of puberty, it is not surprising that ARs are also present in epiphyseal chondrocytes *(10,59)*. Noble and coworkers *(54)* described AR expression mainly in the narrow zone of proliferating chondrocytes in the growth plate, with reduced expression in hypertrophied cells. The expression of ARs in such a wide variety of cell types known to be important for bone modeling during development, and remodeling in the adult, provides strong evidence for direct actions of androgens in bone and cartilage tissue. These results also presage the complexity of androgen effects on developing bone tissue.

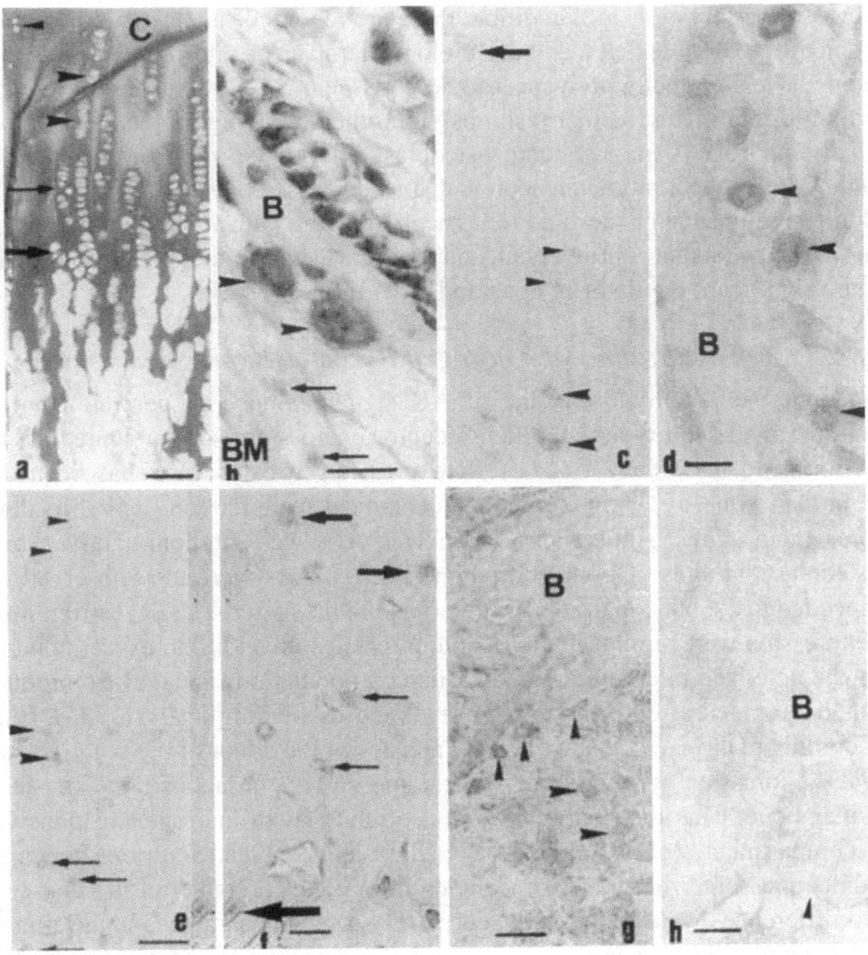

Fig. 2. The localization of AR in normal tibial growth plate and adult osteophytic human bone. (**a**) Morphologically, sections of the growth plate consist of areas of endochondral ossification with undifferentiated (*small arrow head*), proliferating (*large arrow heads*), mature (*small arrow*), and hypertrophic (*large arrow*) chondrocytes. Bar = 80 μm. An inset of an area of the primary spongiosa is shown in (**b**). (**b**) Numerous osteoblasts (*small arrow heads*) and multinucleated osteoclasts (*large arrow heads*) on the bone surface. Mononuclear cells within the bone marrow are also present (*arrows*). Bar = 60 μm. (**c**) In the growth plate, AR is predominantly expressed by hypertrophic chondrocytes (*large arrow heads*). Minimal expression is observed in the mature chondrocytes (*small arrow heads*). The receptors are rarely observed in the proliferating chondrocytes (*arrow*). (**d**) In the primary spongiosa, the AR is predominantly and highly expressed by osteoblasts at modeling sites (*arrow heads*). Bar = 20 μm. (**e**) In the osteophytes, AR is also observed at sites of endochondral ossification in undifferentiated (*small arrow heads*), proliferating (*large arrow heads*), mature (*small arrows*), and hypertrophic-like (*large arrow*) chondrocytes. Bar = 80 μm. (**f**) A higher magnification of (**e**) showing proliferating, mature, and hypertrophic-like chondrocytes (*large arrows*, *small arrows*, and *very large arrows*, respectively). Bar = 40 μm. (**g**) At sites of bone remodeling, the receptors are highly expressed in the osteoblasts (*small arrow heads*) and also in mononuclear cells in the bone marrow (*large arrow heads*). Bar = 40 μm. (**h**) AR is not detected in osteoclasts (*small arrow heads*). Bar = 40 μm. B, Bone; C, cartilage; BM, bone marrow. Adapted from Abu et al. *(10)* and used with permission.

Potential modulation of osteoclast action by androgen is suggested by reports of AR expression in the osteoclast *(60)*. Androgen treatment reduces bone resorption of isolated osteoclasts *(61)*, inhibits osteoclast formation *(62)* including formation stimulated by parathyroid hormone (PTH) *(63)*, and may play a direct role regulating aspects of osteoclast activity based on results in AR null mice *(64)*. Indirect effects of androgen to modulate osteoclasts via osteoblasts are indicated by the increase in osteoprotegerin (OPG) levels following testosterone treatment in osteoblasts *(65)* and increased OPG serum concentrations in skeletally targeted AR-transgenic male mice *(66)*. In addition, DHEA treatment has been shown to increase the OPG/RANKL ratio in osteoblastic cells and to inhibit osteoclast activity in coculture *(67)*. Although androgen may be a less significant determinant of bone resorption in vivo than estrogen *(68,69)*, this remains controversial *(70)*.

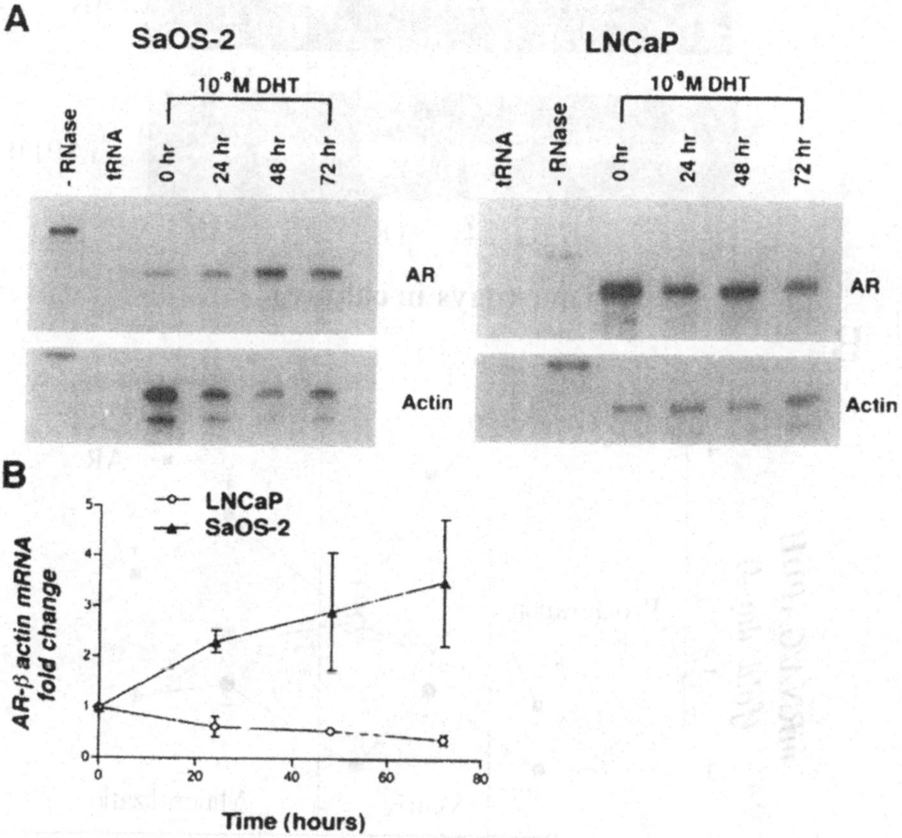

Fig. 3. Dichotomous regulation of AR mRNA levels in osteoblast-like and prostatic carcinoma cell lines after exposure to androgen. (**A**) Time course of changes in AR mRNA abundance after DHT exposure in human SaOS-2 osteoblastic cells and human LNCaP prostatic carcinoma cells. To determine the effect of androgen exposure on hAR mRNA abundance, confluent cultures of either osteoblast-like cells (SaOS-2) or prostatic carcinoma cells (LNCaP) were treated with 10^{-8} M DHT for 0, 24, 48, or 72 h. Total RNA was then isolated and subjected to RNase protection analysis with 50 μg total cellular RNA from SaOS-2 osteoblastic cells and 10 μg total RNA from LNCaP cultures. (**B**) Densitometric analysis of AR mRNA steady state levels. The AR mRNA to β-actin ratio is expressed as the mean ± SE compared to the control value from three to five independent assessments. Adapted from Wiren et al. *(73)* and used with permission.

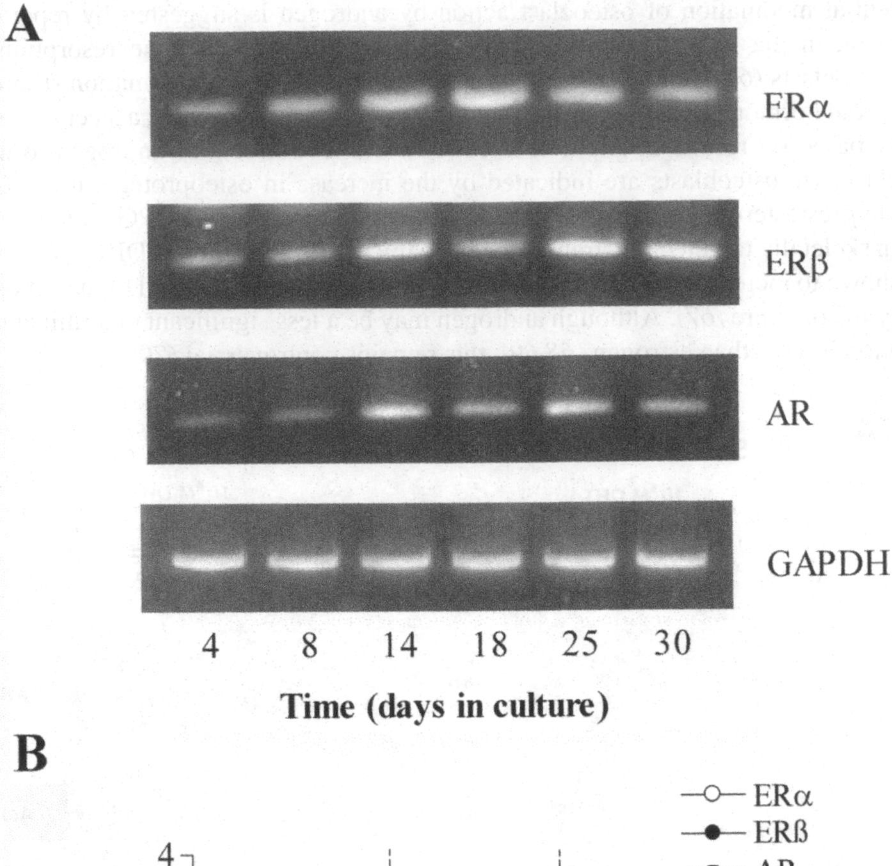

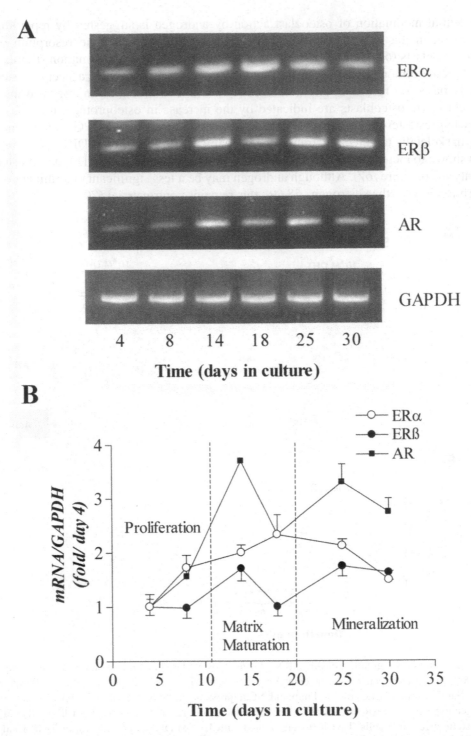

Fig. 4. Expression analyses of ERα, ERβ, and AR during in vitro differentiation in normal rat osteoblastic (rOB) cultures. (**A**) Normal rOB cells were cultured for the indicated number of days during proliferation, matrix maturation, mineralization, and postmineralization stages. Total RNA was isolated and subjected to relative RT-PCR analysis using primers specific for rat ERα, ERβ, and AR or rat GAPDH. Reverse

Regulation of Androgen Receptor Expression

The regulation of AR expression in osteoblasts is incompletely understood. Homologous regulation of AR mRNA by androgen has been described that is tissue specific; up-regulation by androgen exposure is seen in a variety of mesenchymal cells including osteoblasts *(71–74)*, whereas in prostate and smooth muscle tissue, downregulation is observed after androgen exposure *(73,75)* (Fig. 3). The androgen-mediated up-regulation observed in osteoblasts occurs, at least in part, through changes in AR gene transcription *(73,74)*. No effect, or even inhibition, of AR mRNA by androgen exposure in other osteoblastic models has also been described *(35,76)*. Interestingly, a novel property of the AR is that binding of androgen increases AR protein levels that has been shown in osteoblastic cells as well *(74)*. This property distinguishes AR from most other steroid receptor molecules that are downregulated by ligand binding. The elevated AR protein levels may be a consequence of increased stability mediated by androgen binding, resulting from N-terminal and C-terminal interactions *(77)*, but the stability of AR protein in osteoblastic cells has not been determined to date. The mechanism(s) that underlie tissue specificity in autologous AR regulation, and the possible biological significance, is not yet understood. It is possible that AR up-regulation by androgen in bone may result in an enhancement of androgen responsiveness at times when androgen levels are rising or elevated.

Quantitative determination of the level of receptor expression during osteoblast differentiation is difficult to achieve in bone slices. However, analysis of AR, ERα and ERβ mRNA, and protein expression during osteoblast differentiation in vitro demonstrates that each receptor displays distinct differentiation-stage expression patterns in osteoblasts (Fig. 4) *(78)*. The levels of AR expression increase throughout osteoblast differentiation with the highest AR levels seen in mature osteoblast/osteocytic cultures. These results suggest that an important compartment for androgen action may be mature, mineralizing osteoblasts, and indicate that osteoblast differentiation and steroid receptor regulation are intimately associated. Given that the osteocyte is the most abundant cell type in bone, and a likely mediator of focal bone deposition and response to mechanical strain *(79)*, it is not surprising that androgens may also augment the osteo-anabolic effects of mechanical strain in osteoblasts *(80)*.

Fig. 4. (continued) transcription was conducted with PCR carried out for 40 cycles for the steroid receptors, with parallel reactions performed using GAPDH primers for 25 cycles (all in the linear range). Bands for rat ERα at the predicted 240 bp, rat ERβ at 262 bp, rat AR at 276 bp, and GAPDH at 609 bp are shown. (**B**) Analyses of ERα, ERβ, and AR mRNA relative abundance. Semi-quantitative analysis of mRNA steady-state expression by relative RT-PCR was performed after scanning the negative image of the photographed gels. Data are expressed in arbitrary units as the ratio of receptor abundance to GAPDH expression, then normalized to expression values at day 4 in pre-confluent cultures. Data represent mean ± SEM. Adapted from Wiren et al. *(78)* and used with permission.

EFFECTS OF ANDROGENS ON OSTEOBLASTIC CELLS

Evidence suggests that androgens act directly on the osteoblast and there are reports, some in clonal osteoblastic cell lines, of modulatory effects of gonadal androgen treatment on proliferation, differentiation, matrix production, and mineral accumulation *(81)*. Not surprisingly, androgen has been shown to influence bone cells in a complex fashion.

Androgens and Osteoblast Proliferation

As an example, the effect of androgen on osteoblast proliferation has been shown to be biphasic in nature, with enhancement following short or transient treatment but significant inhibition following longer treatment. As a case in point, Kasperk et al. *(82,83)* demonstrated in osteoblast-like cells in primary culture (murine, passaged human) that a variety of androgens in serum-free medium increase DNA synthesis ([^{3}H]thymidine incorporation) and cell counts. Testosterone and nonaromatizable androgens (DHT and fluoxymesterone) were nearly equally effective regulators. Yet the same group *(84)* reported that prolonged DHT treatment inhibited normal human osteoblastic cell proliferation (cell counts) in cultures pretreated with DHT. Hofbauer et al. *(85)* examined the effect of DHT exposure on proliferation in hFOB/AR-6, an immortalized human osteoblastic cell line stably transfected with an AR expression construct (with ~4000 receptors/cell). In this line, DHT treatment inhibited cell proliferation by 20–35%. Consistent with stimulation, Somjen et al. *(86)* have demonstrated increased creatine kinase-specific activity in male osteoblastic cells after exposure to DHT for 24 h. Although these various studies employed different model systems and culture conditions, it appears that exposure time is an important variable. Clear time dependence for the response to androgen has been shown by Wiren et al. *(87)*, where osteoblast proliferation was stimulated at early treatment times, but with more prolonged DHT treatment osteoblast viability decreased (Fig. 5). This result was AR dependent (inhibitable by coincubation with flutamide) and was observed in both normal rat calvarial osteoblasts and in AR stably transfected MC-3T3 cells. In mechanistic terms, reduced viability was associated with overall reduction in mitogen-activated (MAP) kinase signaling and with inhibition of *elk-1* gene expression, protein abundance, and extent of phosphorylation. The inhibition of MAP kinase activity after chronic androgen treatment again contrasts with stimulation of MAP kinase signaling and AP-1 transactivation observed with brief androgen exposure *(87)* that may be mediated through non-genomic mechanisms *(47,88,89)*.

Androgens and Osteoblast Apoptosis

As a component of control of osteoblast survival, it is also important to consider the process of programmed cell death or apoptosis *(90)*. In particular, as the osteoblast population differentiates in vitro, the mature bone cell phenotype undergoes apoptosis *(91)*. With respect to the effects of androgen exposure, chronic DHT treatment has been shown to result in enhanced osteoblast apoptosis in both proliferating osteoblastic (at day 5) and mature osteocytic cultures (day 29) *(92)*. In this report, inhibition observed with DHT treatment was opposite to inhibitory effects on apoptosis seen with E_2 treatment (Fig. 6). An androgen-mediated increase in the Bax/Bcl-2 ratio was also observed, predominantly through inhibition of Bcl-2, and was dependent on functional AR. Overexpression of *bcl-2* or RNAi knockdown of *bax* abrogated the effects of DHT, indicating that increased

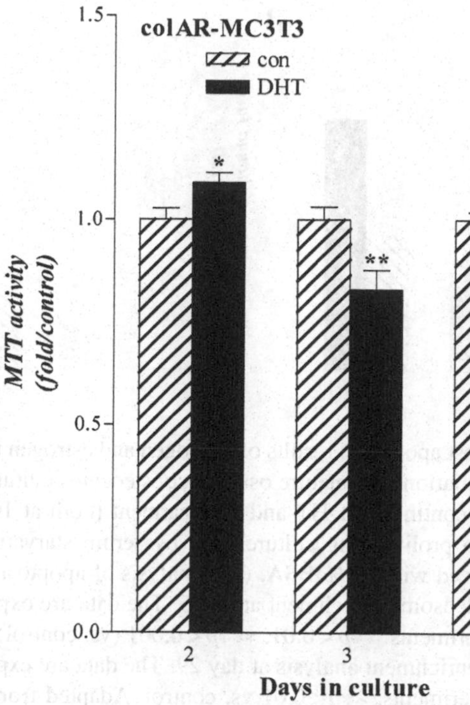

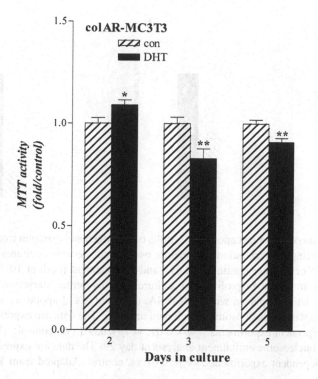

Fig. 5. Complex effect of androgen on DNA accumulation in osteoblastic cultures. Kinetics of DHT response in proliferating colAR-MC3T3 cultures measured with colorimetric [3-(4,5-dimethylthiazol-2-yl)-2,5-diphenyltetrazolium bromide] (MTT) assay. Cultures of stably transfected colAR-MC3T3 continuously with 10^{-8} M DHT for 2 days led to increased MTT accumulation, but longer treatment for 3 or 5 days resulted in inhibition. Data are mean ± SEM of six to eight dishes with six wells/dish. $*p < 0.05$; $**p < 0.01$ (vs. control). Adapted from Wiren et al. *(87)* and used with permission.

Bax/Bcl-2 was necessary and sufficient for androgen-enhanced apoptosis. The increase in the Bax/Bcl-2 ratio was at least in part a consequence of reductions in Bcl-2 phosphorylation and protein stability, consistent with inhibition of MAP kinase pathway activation after DHT treatment as noted above. In vivo analysis of calvaria in AR-transgenic male mice demonstrated enhanced TUNEL staining in both osteoblasts and osteocytes and was observed even in areas of new bone growth *(92)*. This may not be surprising, given an association between new bone growth and apoptosis *(93)*, as has been observed in other remodeling tissues and/or associated with development and tissue homeostasis *(94)*. Apoptotic cell death could thus be important in making room for new bone formation and matrix deposition, which may have clinical significance by influencing bone homeostasis and bone mineral density *(95)*. Thus, mounting evidence suggests that chronic androgen treatment does not increase osteoblast number or viability in the mature bone compartment. It is interesting to speculate that the inhibitory action of androgens in osteoblasts at the endosteal surface is important for the relative maintenance of cortical width (which is similar between males and females), given the strong stimulation at the periosteal surface, such that the skeleton does not become excessively large and/or heavy during development.

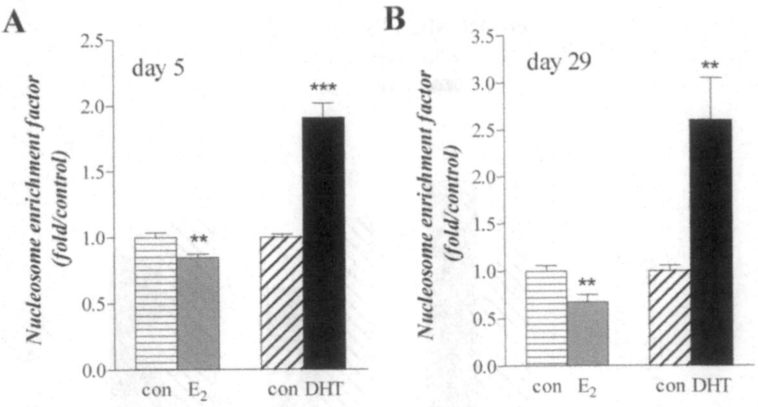

Fig. 6. Characterization of osteoblast apoptosis: results of androgen and estrogen treatment during proliferation (day 5) and during differentiation into mature osteoblast/osteocytes cultures (day 29). Apoptosis was assessed at day 5 or 29 after continuous DHT and E_2 treatment (both at 10^{-8} M). Apoptosis was induced by etoposide treatment in proliferating cultures and by serum starvation for 48 h in confluent cultures before isolation, replaced with 0.1% BSA. (**A**) Analysis of apoptosis after evaluating DNA fragmentation by cytoplasmic nucleosome enrichment at day 5. The data are expressed as mean ± SEM ($n = 6$) from two independent experiments. $**p < 0.01$, $***p < 0.001$ (vs. control). (**B**) Analysis of apoptosis by cytoplasmic nucleosome enrichment analysis at day 29. The data are expressed as mean ± SEM ($n = 6$) from two independent experiments. $**p < 0.01$ vs. control. Adapted from Wiren et al. *(92)* and used with permission.

Effects of Androgens on the Differentiation of Osteoblastic Cells

Osteoblast differentiation is often characterized by changes in alkaline phosphatase activity and/or alterations in the expression of important extracellular matrix proteins, such as type I collagen, osteocalcin, and osteonectin. Enhanced osteoblast differentiation, as measured by increased matrix production, has been shown to result from androgen exposure. Androgen treatment in both normal osteoblasts and transformed clonal human osteoblastic cells (TE-89) appears to increase the proportion of cells expressing alkaline phosphatase activity, thus representing a shift toward a more differentiated phenotype *(82)*. Kasperk et al. subsequently reported dose-dependent increases in alkaline phosphatase activity in both high and low-alkaline phosphatase subclones of SaOS2 cells *(96)* and human osteoblastic cells *(84)*. However, there are also reports in a variety of model systems of androgens either inhibiting *(85)* or having no effect on alkaline phosphatase activity *(71,97)*, which may reflect both the complexity and the dynamics of osteoblastic differentiation. There are also reports of androgen-mediated increases in type I α-1 collagen protein and mRNA levels *(37,96–98)* in certain circumstances and increased osteocalcin mRNA or protein secretion *(84,98)*. Consistent with increased collagen production, androgen treatment has also been shown to stimulate mineral accumulation in a time and dose-dependent manner *(71,84,99)*. However, transgenic mice with targeted overexpression of AR in the osteoblast lineage showed decreased levels of most bone markers in vivo in total RNA extracts derived from long bone samples, including decreased collagen, osterix, and osteocalcin gene expression *(66)*. These results suggest that, under certain conditions, androgens may enhance osteoblast differentiation and could thus play an important role in the regulation of bone matrix production and/or organization. On the other hand, many positive anabolic effects of androgen may be limited to distinct osteoblastic populations, for example, in the periosteal compartment *(2,66)*.

Interaction with Other Factors to Modulate Bone Formation and Resorption

The effects of androgens on osteoblast activity must certainly also be considered in the context of the very complex endocrine, paracrine, and autocrine milieu in the bone microenvironment. Systemic and/or local factors can act in concert, or can antagonize, to influence bone cell function. This has been well described with regard to modulation of the effects of estrogen on bone (see, for example, *(100–102)*). Androgens have also been shown to regulate well-known modulators of osteoblast proliferation or function. The most extensively characterized growth factor influenced by androgen exposure is transforming growth factor-β (TGF-β). TGF-β is stored in bone (the largest reservoir for TGF-β) in a latent form and has been shown to be a mitogen for osteoblasts. Androgen treatment can increase TGF-β activity in osteoblastic cultures: the expression of some TGF-β mRNA transcripts (apparently TGF-β2) was increased but no effect on TGF-β1 mRNA abundance was observed *(41,83)*, but also see *(103)*. At the protein level, specific immunoprecipitation analysis reveals DHT-mediated increases in TGF-β activity to be predominantly TGF-β2 *(41,84)*. DHT has also been shown to inhibit both TGF-β gene expression and TGF-β-induced early gene expression that correlates with growth inhibition in this cell line *(85)*. The TGF-β-induced early gene has been shown to be a transcription factor that may mediate some TGF-β effects *(104)*. These results are consistent with the notion that TGF-β may mediate androgen effects on osteoblast proliferation. On the other hand, TGF-β1 mRNA levels are increased by androgen treatment in human clonal osteoblastic cells (TE-89), under conditions where osteoblast proliferation is slowed *(37)*. Thus, the specific TGF-β isoform may determine osteoblast responses. It is interesting to note that in vivo, orchiectomy (ORX) drastically reduces bone content of TGF-β levels, and testosterone replacement prevents this reduction *(105)*. These data support the findings that androgens influence cellular expression of TGF-β and suggest that the bone loss associated with castration is related to a reduction in growth factor abundance induced by androgen deficiency.

Other growth factor systems may also be influenced by androgens. Conditioned media from DHT-treated normal osteoblast cultures are mitogenic, and DHT pretreatment increases the mitogenic response to fibroblast growth factor and to insulin-like growth factor II (IGF-II) *(83)*. In part, this may be due to slight increases in IGF-II binding in DHT-treated cells *(83)*, as IGF-I and IGF-II levels in osteoblast-conditioned media are not affected by androgen *(83,106)*. Although most studies have not found regulation of IGF-I or IGF-II abundance by androgen exposure *(33,83,106)*, there is a report that IGF-I mRNA levels are significantly up-regulated by DHT *(107)*. Androgens may also modulate expression of components of the AP-1 transcription factor *(41)* or AP-1 transcriptional activation *(87)*. Thus, androgens may modulate osteoblast differentiation via a mechanism whereby growth factors or other mediators of differentiation are regulated by androgen exposure.

Androgens may modulate responses to other important osteotropic hormones/regulators. Testosterone and DHT specifically inhibit the cAMP response elicited by PTH or parathyroid hormone-related protein (PTHrP) in the human clonal osteoblast-like cell line SaOS-2, while the inactive or weakly active androgen 17α-epitestosterone had no effect, via an effect on effector G_s-adenylyl cyclase *(108–110)*. The production of prostaglandin E_2 (PGE_2), another important regulator of bone metabolism, is also affected by androgens. Pilbeam and Raisz showed that androgens (both DHT and testosterone) were potent inhibitors of both parathyroid hormone and interleukin-1-stimulated PGE_2 production in cultured neonatal mouse calvaria *(111)*. The effects of androgens on parathyroid hormone action and PGE_2 production suggest that androgens could act to modulate (reduce) bone turnover in response to these agents.

Finally, both androgen *(112)* and estrogen *(101,113)* can inhibit production of interleukin-6 by osteoblastic cells (but see *(114)*). In stromal cells of the bone marrow, androgens have been shown to have potent inhibitory effects on the production of interleukin-6 and the subsequent stimulation of osteoclastogenesis by marrow osteoclast precursors *(115)*. Interestingly, adrenal androgens (androstenediol, androstenedione, DHEA) have similar inhibitory activities on interleukin-6 gene expression and protein production by stromal cells *(115)*. Moreover, androgens inhibit the expression of the genes encoding the two subunits of the IL-6 receptor (gp80 and gp130) in the murine bone marrow, another mechanism which may blunt the effects of this osteoclastogenic cytokine in intact animals *(116)*. In these aspects, the effects of androgens seem to be very similar to those of estrogen, which may also inhibit osteoclastogenesis via mechanisms that involve interleukin-6 inhibition and/or OPG/RANKL ratio changes.

METABOLISM OF ANDROGENS IN BONE

Sex steroids, ultimately derived from cholesterol, are synthesized predominantly in gonadal tissue, the adrenal gland, and placenta as a consequence of enzymatic conversions. After peripheral metabolism, androgenic activity is represented in a variety of steroid molecules that include testosterone (Fig. 7). There is evidence in a range of tissues that the eventual cellular effects of testosterone may not be the result (or not only the result) of direct action of testosterone, but may also reflect the effects of sex steroid metabolites formed as a consequence of local enzyme activities.

The most important testosterone metabolites in bone are 5α-DHT (the result of 5α reduction of testosterone) and estradiol (formed by the aromatization of testosterone). Testosterone and DHT are the major and most potent androgens, with androstenedione (the major circulating androgen in women) and DHEA as immediate androgen precursors that exhibit weak androgen activity *(39)*. In men, the most abundant circulating androgen metabolite is testosterone while concentrations of other weaker androgens-like androstenedione and DHEA-sulfate are similar between males and females. Downstream metabolites of DHT and androstenedione are inactive at the AR and include 5α-androstane-3α or 3β,17β-diol (3αβ-androstanediol), and 5α-androstanedione. Data suggest that aromatase cytochrome P450 (the product of the CYP19 gene), 17β-hydroxysteroid dehydrogenase (17β-HSD), and 5α-reductase activities are all present in bone tissue, at least to some measurable extent in some compartments, but the biologic relevance of each remains somewhat controversial.

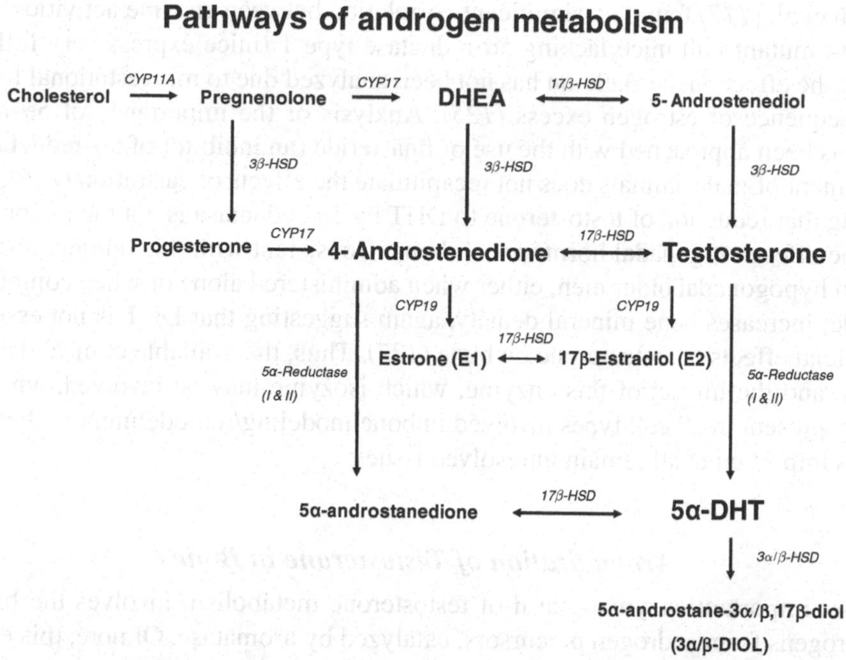

Fig. 7. Principle conversions and major enzyme activities involved in androgen synthesis and metabolism. Steroid hormone synthesis involves metabolism of cholesterol, with dehydrogenation of pregnenolone producing progesterone that can serve as a precursor for the other gonadal steroid hormones. DHEA, dehydroepiandrosterone; CYP11A, cytochrome P450 cholesterol side chain cleavage enzyme; CYP17, cytochrome P450 17α hydroxylase/17,20 lyase; 17β-HSD, 17β-hydroxysteroid dehydrogenase; CYP19, aromatase cytochrome P450.

5α-Reductase Activity in Osteoblasts

5α-reductase is an important activity with regard to androgen metabolism in general, since testosterone is converted to the more potent androgen metabolite DHT via 5α-reductase action *(117)*. 5α-Reductase activity was first described in crushed rat mandibular bone *(118)* with similar findings reported in crushed human spongiosa *(119)*. Two different 5α-reductase genes encode type 1 and type 2 isozymes in many mammalian species *(120)*; human osteoblastic cells express the type 1 isozyme *(121)*. Essentially the same metabolic activities were reported in experiments with human epiphyseal cartilage and chondrocytes *(122)*. In general, the K_m values for bone 5α-reductase activity are similar to those in other androgen responsive tissues *(33,119)*. However, the cellular populations in many of these studies were mixed and hence the specific cell type responsible for the activity is unknown. Interestingly, Turner et al. *(123)* found that periosteal cells do not have detectable 5α-reductase activity, raising the possibilities that the enzyme may be functional in only selected skeletal compartments and that testosterone may be the active androgen metabolite at this clinically important site.

From a clinical perspective, the general importance of this enzymatic pathway is uncertain, as patients with 5α-reductase type 2 deficiency have normal bone mineral density *(124)* and Bruch et al. *(117)* found no significant correlation between enzyme activities and bone volume. In mutant null mice lacking 5α-reductase type 1 (mice express very little type 2 isozyme), the effect on the skeleton has not been analyzed due to midgestational fetal death as a consequence of estrogen excess *(125)*. Analysis of the importance of 5α-reductase activity has been approached with the use of finasteride (an inhibitor of 5α-reductase activity); treatment of male animals does not recapitulate the effects of castration *(126)*, strongly suggesting that reduction of testosterone to DHT by 5α-reductase is not the major determinant in the effects of gonadal hormones on bone. Consistent with this finding, testosterone therapy in hypogonadal older men, either when administered alone or when combined with finasteride, increases bone mineral density, again suggesting that DHT is not essential for the beneficial effects of testosterone on bone *(127)*. Thus, the available clinical data remain uncertain, and the impact of this enzyme, which isozyme may be involved, whether it is uniformly present in all cell types involved in bone modeling/remodeling, or whether local activity is important at all remain unresolved issues.

Aromatization of Testosterone in Bone

Another important enzymatic arm of testosterone metabolism involves the biosynthesis of estrogens from androgen precursors, catalyzed by aromatase. Of note, this enzyme is well known to be both expressed and regulated in a very pronounced tissue-specific manner *(128)* and also demonstrates species differences, given the low levels in mice. Modest levels of aromatase activity have been reported in bone from mixed cell populations derived from both sexes *(129–131)* and from osteoblastic cell lines *(33,132,133)*. Aromatase expression in intact bone has also been documented by in situ hybridization and immunohistochemical analysis *(131)*. Aromatase mRNA is expressed predominantly in lining cells, chondrocytes, and some adipocytes; however, there is no detectable expression in osteoclasts, or in cortical bone in mice *(66)*. At least in vertebral bone, the mesenchymal distal promoter I.4 is predominantly utilized *(134)*. The enzyme kinetics in bone cells seem to be similar to those in other tissues, although the V_{max} may be increased by glucocorticoids *(133)*. Whether the level of aromatase activity in bone is high enough to produce physiologically relevant concentrations of steroids remains an open question; nevertheless in males only 15% of circulating estrogen is produced in the testes, with the remaining 85% produced by peripheral metabolism that could include bone as one site of conversion *(135)*.

Aromatase catalyzes the metabolism of adrenal and testicular C19 androgens (androstenedione and testosterone) to C18 estrogens (estrone and estradiol), thus producing the potent estrogen estradiol (E2) from testosterone, and the weaker estrogen estrone (E1) from its adrenal precursors androstenedione and DHEA *(129)*. Typically in the circulation, E2 will make up to 40% of total estrogen, E1 will make up an additional 40%, with estriol (E3) comprising the remaining 20% of total estrogen *(136)*. In addition to aromatase itself, osteoblasts contain enzymes that are able to inter-convert estradiol and estrone (17β-HSD) and to hydrolyze estrone sulfate, the most abundant estrogen in the circulation, to estrone (steroid sulfatase) *(132,137)*. Nawata et al. *(129)* have reported that dexamethasone and 1α,25$(OH)_2D_3$ synergistically enhance aromatase activity and aromatase mRNA expression in human osteoblast-like cells. In addition, both leptin and 1α,25$(OH)_2D_3$ treatment increased aromatase activity in human mesenchymal stem cells during osteogenesis, but not during adipogenesis *(138)*. Additional studies are needed to better define expression, given the potential importance of the enzyme, and its regulation by a variety of mechanisms (including androgens and estrogens) in other tissues *(128,139)*.

The clinical impact of aromatase activity and an indication of the importance of conversion of circulating androgen into estrogen are shown in reports of women and men with aromatase deficiencies, who present with a skeletal phenotype *(140)*. Interestingly, natural mutation is remarkably rare with only seven males and six females reported to date. The presentation of men with aromatase deficiency is very similar to that of a man with estrogen receptor-α (ERα) deficiency *(141)*, namely an obvious delay in bone age, lack of epiphyseal closure, and tall stature with high bone turnover and osteopenia *(135)*, suggesting that aromatase (and likely estrogen action) has a substantial role to play during skeletal development in the male. In addition, estrogen therapy of males with aromatase deficiency has been associated with an increase in bone mass *(135)*, particularly in the growing skeleton *(142)*. Inhibition of aromatization pharmacologically with nonsteroidal inhibitors (such as vorozole or letrozole) results in modest decreases in bone mineral density and changes in skeletal modeling in young growing orchidectomized males *(143)*, and less dramatically so in boys with constitutional delay of puberty treated for 1 year *(144)*, suggesting short-term treatment during growth has limited negative consequences in males. Inhibition of aromatization in older orchidectomized males resembles castration with similar increases in bone resorption and bone loss, suggesting that aromatase activity likely plays a role in skeletal maintenance in males *(145)*. These studies herald the importance of aromatase activity (and estrogen) in the mediation of some androgen action in bone in both males and females. The finding of these enzymes in bone clearly raises the difficult issue of the origin of androgenic effects in the skeleton; do they arise solely from direct androgen effects (as is suggested by the actions of nonaromatizable androgens such as DHT) or also from the local or other site production of estrogenic intermediates? The results described above would seem to indicate that both steroids appear to be important to both male and female skeletal health.

17β-Hydroxysteroid Dehydrogenase Activity in Osteoblasts

The 17β-HSDs (most of which are dehydrogenase-reductases, except type 5 that is an aldo–keto reductase) have been shown to catalyze either the last step of sex steroid synthesis or the first step of their degradation (to produce weak or potent sex steroids via oxidation or reduction, respectively) and can thus also play a critical role in peripheral steroid metabolism. The oxidative pathway forms 17-ketosteroids, while the reductive pathway forms 17β-hydroxysteroids. The enzyme reversibly catalyzes the formation of androstenediol (an estrogen) from DHEA, in addition to the biosynthesis of estradiol from estrone, the synthesis of testosterone from androstenedione, and the production of DHT from 5α-androstanedione all via the reductive activity of 17β-HSD. Of the 13 enzyme isotypes of 17β-HSD activity *(136)*, types 1–4 have been demonstrated in human osteoblastic cells *(146)*.

The administration of testosterone can stimulate bone formation and inhibit bone resorption, likely through multiple mechanisms that involve both androgen and estrogen receptor-mediated processes. However, there is substantial evidence that some, if in fact not most, of the biologic actions of androgens in the skeleton are mediated by AR. Both in vivo and in vitro systems reveal the effects of the nonaromatizable androgen DHT to be essentially the same as those of testosterone (vida infra). In addition, blockade of the AR with the receptor antagonist flutamide results in osteopenia as a result of reduced bone formation *(5)*. In addition, complete androgen insensitivity results in a significant decrease in bone mineral density in spine and hip sites *(124)* even in the setting of strong compliance with estrogen treatment *(147)*. These reports clearly indicate that androgens, independent of estrogenic metabolites, have primary effects on osteoblast function. However, the clinical reports of subjects with aromatase deficiency also highlight the relevance of metabolism of androgen to bio-potent estrogens at least in the circulation, to influence bone development and/or maintenance. It thus seems likely that further elucidation of the regulation of steroid metabolism, and the potential mechanisms by which androgenic and estrogenic effects are coordinated, will have physiological, pathophysiological, and therapeutic implications.

Drugs with Androgenic Activity

In addition to the endogenous steroid metabolites highlighted in Fig. 7, there are also a variety of drugs with androgenic activity. These include anabolic steroids, such as nonaromatizable oxandrolone, that bind and activate AR (albeit with lower affinity than testosterone *(148)*), and a class of drugs under extensive development referred to as SARMs that demonstrate tissue-specific agonist or antagonist activities with respect to AR transactivation *(149)*. These orally active nonsteroidal nonaromatizable SARMS are being developed to target androgen action in bone, muscle, fat and to influence libido but to not exacerbate prostate growth, hirsutism, and acne. Several have recently been identified with beneficial effects on bone mass *(150–152)*, and provide a new alternative to androgen replacement therapy.

GENDER SPECIFICITY IN THE ACTIONS OF SEX STEROIDS

Although controversial, there may be gender-specific responses in osteoblastic cells to sex steroids. In most mammals, there is a marked gender difference in morphology that results in a sexually dimorphic skeleton. The mechanisms responsible for these differences are necessarily complex, and presumably involve both androgenic and estrogenic actions on the skeleton. It is becoming increasingly clear that estrogens are particularly important for the regulation of epiphyseal function and act to reduce the rate of longitudinal growth via influences on chondrocyte proliferation and function, as well as on the timing of epiphyseal closure *(153)*. Androgens, on the other hand, appear to have many opposite effects to estrogen on the skeleton. For example, androgens tend to promote long bone growth, chondrocyte maturation, and metaphyseal ossification, opposite to effects of estrogen. Another notable example is the effect of AR activation in cortical bone in males, which can stimulate bone formation at the periosteal surface but inhibit formation at the endosteum *(66)*. Thus, the most dramatic effect of androgens is on bone size, in particular cortical thickness *(154)*. This difference of course has important biomechanical implications, with thicker bones being stronger bones *(155)*. Furthermore, the response of the adult skeleton (to the same intervention) results in distinct responses in males and females. For example, in a model of disuse osteopenia, antiorthostatic suspension results in significant reduction in bone formation rate at the endosteal perimeter in males. In females, however, a decrease in bone formation rate occurred along the periosteal perimeter *(156)*. Gender-specific responses in vivo and in vitro (for example, see *(86)*), and the mechanism(s) that underlie such responses in bone cells, may thus have significant implications in treatment options for metabolic bone disease.

CONCLUSION

Thus, the effects of androgens on bone health are both complex and pervasive. Androgens influence skeletal modeling and remolding by multiple mechanisms through effects on osteoblasts, osteoclasts, and even perhaps an influence on the differentiation of pluripotent stem cells toward distinct lineages. The specific effects of androgen on bone cells are mediated directly through an AR-signaling pathway, but there are also indirect contributions to overall skeletal health through aromatization and ER signaling. The effects of androgens are particularly dramatic during growth in boys, particularly at the periosteum, but almost certainly play an important role during this period in girls as well. Throughout the rest of life, androgens affect skeletal function and maintenance in both sexes. Nevertheless, given this importance, relatively little has been done to unravel the mechanisms by which androgens influence the physiology and pathophysiology of bone, and there is still much to be learned about the roles of androgens at all levels. The interaction of androgens and estrogens and how their respective actions can be utilized for specific diagnostic and therapeutic benefit are important but unanswered issues. With an increase in the understanding of the nature of androgen effects will come greater opportunities to use their positive actions in the prevention and treatment of a wide variety of bone disorders.

REFERENCES

1. Vanderschueren D, Vandenput L, Boonen S, Lindberg M, Bouillon R, Ohlsson C. Androgens and bone. Endocr Rev 2004;25:389–425.
2. Wiren K. Androgens and bone growth: it's location, location, location. Curr Opin Pharmacol 2005;5: 626–632.
3. Turner R, Hannon K, Demers L, Buchanan J, Bell N. Differential effects of gonadal function on bone histomorphometry in male and female rats. J Bone Miner Res 1989;4(4):557–563.
4. Turner R, Wakley G, Hannon K. Differential effects of androgens on cortical bone histomorphometry in gonadectomized male and female rats. J Orthopaedic Res 1990;8:612–617.
5. Goulding A, Gold E. Flutamide-mediated androgen blockade evokes osteopenia in the female rat. J Bone Miner Res 1993;8(6):763–769.
6. Coxam V, Bowman B, Mecham M, Roth C, Miller M, Miller S. Effects of dihydrotestosterone alone and combined with estrogen on bone mineral density, bone growth, and formation rates in ovariectomized rats. Bone 1996;19:107–114.
7. Miller B, De Souza M, Slade K, Luciano A. Sublingual administration of micronized estradiol and progesterone, with and without micronized testosterone: effect on biochemical markers of bone metabolism and bone mineral density. Menopause 2000;7:318–326.
8. Castelo-Branco C, Vicente J, Figueras F, et al. Comparative effects of estrogens plus androgens and tibolone on bone, lipid pattern and sexuality in postmenopausal women. Maturitas 2000;34:161–168.
9. Raisz L, Wiita B, Artis A, et al. Comparison of the effects of estrogen alone and estrogen plus androgen on biochemical markers of bone formation and resorption in postmenopausal women. J Clin Endocrinol Metab 1996;81:37–43.
10. Abu E, Horner A, Kusec V, Triffitt J, Compston J. The localization of androgen receptors in human bone. J Clin Endocrinol Metab 1997;82:3493–3497.
11. Chang C, Kokontis J, Liao S. Structural analysis of complementary DNA and amino acid sequences of human and rat androgen receptors. Proc Natl Acad Sci USA 1988;85:7211–7215.
12. Lubahn D, Joseph D, Sullivan P, Willard H, French F, Wilson E. Cloning of human androgen receptor complementary DNA and localization to the X chromosome. Science 1988;240:324–326.
13. Mangelsdorf D, Thummel C, Beato M, et al. The nuclear receptor superfamily: the second decade. Cell 1995;83:835–839.
14. Picard D. Chaperoning steroid hormone action. Trends Endocrinol Metab 2006;17:229–235.

15. Shen H, Coetzee G. The androgen receptor: unlocking the secrets of its unique transactivation domain. Vitam Horm 2005;71:301–319.
16. Kumar S, Saradhi M, Chaturvedi N, Tyagi R. Intracellular localization and nucleocytoplasmic trafficking of steroid receptors: an overview. Mol Cell Endocrinol 2006;246:147–156.
17. Chang C, Saltzman N, Yeh S, et al. Androgen receptor: an overview. Crit Rev Eukaryot Gene Expr 1995;5:97–125.
18. Haussler M, Haussler C, Jurutka P, et al. The vitamin D hormone and its nuclear receptor: molecular actions and disease states. J Endocrinol 1997;154(Suppl):S57–S73.
19. Denison S, Sands A, Tindall D. A tyrosine aminotransferase glucocorticoid response element also mediates androgen enhancement of gene expression. Endocrinology 1989;124:1091–1093.
20. Carroll J, Meyer C, Song J, et al. Genome-wide analysis of estrogen receptor binding sites. Nat Genet 2006;38:1289–1297.
21. Leader J, Wang C, Fu M, Pestell R. Epigenetic regulation of nuclear steroid receptors. Biochem Pharmacol 2006;72:1589–1596.
22. Kraus S, Gioeli D, Vomastek T, Gordon V, Weber M. Receptor for activated C kinase 1 (RACK1) and Src regulate the tyrosine phosphorylation and function of the androgen receptor. Cancer Res 2006;66: 11047–11054.
23. Kemppainen J, Lane M, Sar M, Wilson E. Androgen receptor phosphorylation, turnover, nuclear transport, and transcriptional activities. J Biol Chem 1992;267:968–974.
24. Ikonen T, Palvimo J, Kallio P, Reinikainen P, Janne O. Stimulation of androgen-regulated transactivation by modulators of protein phosphorylation. Endocrinology 1994;135:1359–1366.
25. Blok L, de Ruiter P, Brinkmann A. Androgen receptor phosphorylation. Endocrin Res 1996;22(3): 197–219.
26. Wang L, Liu X, Kreis W, Budman D. Phosphorylation/dephosphorylation of androgen receptor as a determinant of androgen agonistic or antagonistic activity. Biochem Biophys Res Commun 1999;259: 21–28.
27. Dehm S, Tindall D. Ligand-independent androgen receptor activity is activation function-2 independent and resistant to antiandrogens in androgen refractory prostate cancer cells. J Biol Chem 2006; 281: 27882–27893.
28. He B, Gampe Jr R, Hnat A, et al. Probing the functional link between androgen receptor coactivator and ligand-binding sites in prostate cancer and androgen insensitivity. J Biol Chem 2006;281: 6648–6663.
29. Yoon H, Wong J. The corepressors silencing mediator of retinoid and thyroid hormone receptor and nuclear receptor corepressor are involved in agonist- and antagonist-regulated transcription by androgen receptor. Mol Endocrinol 2006;20:1048–1060.
30. MacLean H, Warne G, Zajac J. Localization of functional domains in the androgen receptor. J Steroid Biochem Mol Biol 1997;62(4):233–242.
31. Yeh S, Chang C. Cloning and characterization of a specific coactivator, ARA_{70}, for the androgen receptor in human prostate cells. Proc Natl Acad Sci USA 1996;93:5517–5521.
32. Masuyama A, Ouchi Y, Sato F, Hosoi T, Nakamura T, Orimo H. Characteristics of steroid hormone receptors in cultured MC3T3-E1 osteoblastic cells and effect of steroid hormones on cell proliferation. Calcif Tissue Int 1992;51:376–381.
33. Nakano Y, Morimoto I, Ishida O, et al. The receptor, metabolism and effects of androgen in osteoblastic MC3T3-E1 cells. Bone Miner 1994;26:245–259.
34. Liesegang P, Romalo G, Sudmann M, Wolf L, Schweikert H. Human osteoblast-like cells contain specific, saturable, high-affinity glucocorticoid, androgen, estrogen, and 1a,25-dihydroxycholecalciferol receptors. J Androl 1994;15:194–199.
35. Kasperk C, Helmboldt A, Borcsok I, et al. Skeletal site-dependent expression of the androgen receptor in human osteoblastic cell populations. Calcif Tissue Int 1997;61:464–473.
36. Colvard D, Eriksen E, Keeting P, et al. Identification of androgen receptors in normal human osteoblast-like cells. Proc Natl Acad Sci USA 1989;86:854–857.
37. Benz D, Haussler M, Thomas M, Speelman B, Komm B. High-affinity androgen binding and androgenic regulation of a1(I)-procollagen and transforming growth factor-β steady state messenger ribonucleic acid levels in human osteoblast-like osteosarcoma cells. Endocrinology 1991;128:2723–2730.

38. Meikle A, Dorchuck R, Araneo B, et al. The presence of a dehydroepiandrosterone-specific receptor binding complex in murine T cells. J Steroid Biochem Mol Biol 1992;42:293–304.
39. Mo Q, Lu S, Simon N. Dehydroepiandrosterone and its metabolites: differential effects on androgen receptor trafficking and transcriptional activity. J Steroid Biochem Mol Biol 2006;99:50–58.
40. Webb S, Geoghegan T, Prough R, Michael Miller K. The biological actions of dehydroepiandrosterone involves multiple receptors. Drug Metab Rev 2006;38:89–116.
41. Bodine P, Riggs B, Spelsberg T. Regulation of c-fos expression and TGF-β production by gonadal and adrenal androgens in normal human osteoblastic cells. J Steroid Biochem Mol Biol 1995;52(2): 149–158.
42. Wang Y, Wang L, Li da J, Wang W. Dehydroepiandrosterone inhibited the bone resorption through the upregulation of OPG/RANKL. Cell Mol Immunol 2006;3:41–45.
43. Wrogemann K, Podolsky G, Gu J, Rosenmann E. A 63-kDa protein with androgen-binding activity is not from the androgen receptor. Biochem Cell Biol 1991;69:695–701.
44. Pettaway C. Racial differences in the androgen/androgen receptor pathway in prostate cancer. J Natl Med Assoc 1999;91:653–660.
45. Van Pottelbergh I, Lumbroso S, Goemaere S, Sultan C, Kaufman J. Lack of influence of the androgen receptor gene CAG-repeat polymorphism on sex steroid status and bone metabolism in elderly men. Clin Endocrinol (Oxf) 2001;55:659–666.
46. Grierson A, Mootoosamy R, Miller C. Polyglutamine repeat length influences human androgen receptor/c-Jun mediated transcription. Neurosci Lett 1999;277:9–12.
47. Kang H, Cho C, Huang K, et al. Nongenomic androgen activation of phosphatidylinositol 3-kinase/Akt signaling pathway in MC3T3-E1 osteoblasts. J Bone Miner Res 2004;19:1181–1190.
48. Kousteni S, Chen J, Bellido T, et al. Reversal of bone loss in mice by nongenotropic signaling of sex steroids. Science 2002;298:843–846.
49. Lieberherr M, Grosse B. Androgens increase intracellular calcium concentration and inositol 1,4,5-triphosphate and diacylglycerol formation via a pertussis toxin-sensitive G-protein. J Biol Chem 1994;269:7217–7223.
50. Centrella M, McCarthy T, Chang W, Labaree D, Hochberg R. Estren (4-estren-3alpha,17beta-diol) is a prohormone that regulates both androgenic and estrogenic transcriptional effects through the androgen receptor. Mol Endocrinol 2004;18:1120–1130.
51. van der Eerden B, Emons J, Ahmed S, et al. Evidence for genomic and nongenomic actions of estrogen in growth plate regulation in female and male rats at the onset of sexual maturation. J Endocrinol 2002;175:277–288.
52. Sims N, Clement-Lacroix P, Minet D, et al. A functional androgen receptor is not sufficient to allow estradiol to protect bone after gonadectomy in estradiol receptor-deficient mice. J Clin Invest 2003;111:1319–1327.
53. Hewitt S, Collins J, Grissom S, Hamilton K, Korach K. Estren behaves as a weak estrogen rather than a nongenomic selective activator in the mouse uterus. Endocrinology 2006;147:2203–2214.
54. Tomkinson A, Gevers E, Wit J, Reeve J, Noble B. The role of estrogen in the control of rat osteocyte apoptosis. J Bone Miner Res 1998;18:1243–1250.
55. Gruber R, Czerwenka K, Wolf F, Ho G, Willheim M, Peterlik M. Expression of the vitamin D receptor, of estrogen and thyroid hormone receptor alpha- and beta-isoforms, and of the androgen receptor in cultures of native mouse bone marrow and of stromal/osteoblastic cells. Bone 1999;24:465–473.
56. Sinha-Hikim I, Taylor W, Gonzalez-Cadavid N, Zheng W, Bhasin S. Androgen receptor in human skeletal muscle and cultured muscle satellite cells: up-regulation by androgen treatment. J Clin Endocrinol Metab 2004;89:5245–5255.
57. Singh R, Artaza J, Taylor W, Gonzalez-Cadavid N, Bhasin S. Androgens stimulate myogenic differentiation and inhibit adipogenesis in C3H 10T1/2 pluripotent cells through an androgen receptor-mediated pathway. Endocrinology 2003;144:5081–5088.
58. Herbst K, Bhasin S. Testosterone action on skeletal muscle. Curr Opin Clin Nutr Metab Care 2004;7: 271–277.
59. Carrascosa A, Audi L, Ferrandez M, Ballabriga A. Biological effects of androgens and identification of specific dihydrotestosterone-binding sites in cultured human fetal epiphyseal chondrocytes. J Clin Endocrinol Metab 1990;70:134–140.

60. van der Eerden B, van Til N, Brinkmann A, Lowik C, Wit J, Karperien M. Gender differences in expression of androgen receptor in tibial growth plate and metaphyseal bone of the rat. Bone 2002;30:891–896.
61. Pederson L, Kremer M, Judd J, et al. Androgens regulate bone resorption activity of isolated osteoclasts in vitro. Proc Natl Acad Sci USA 1999;96:505–510.
62. Huber D, Bendixen A, Pathrose P, et al. Androgens suppress osteoclast formation induced by RANKL and macrophage-colony stimulating factor. Endocrinology 2001;142:3800–3808.
63. Chen Q, Kaji H, Sugimoto T, Chihara K. Testosterone inhibits osteoclast formation stimulated by parathyroid hormone through androgen receptor. FEBS Lett 2001;491:91–93.
64. Kawano H, Sato T, Yamada T, et al. Suppressive function of androgen receptor in bone resorption. Proc Natl Acad Sci USA 2003;100:9416–9421.
65. Chen Q, Kaji H, Kanatani M, Sugimoto T, Chihara K. Testosterone increases osteoprotegerin mRNA expression in mouse osteoblast cells. Horm Metab Res 2004;36:674–678.
66. Wiren K, Zhang X-W, Toombs A, et al. Targeted overexpression of androgen receptor in osteoblasts: unexpected complex bone phenotype in growing animals. Endocrinology 2004;145:3507–3522.
67. Wang Y, Wang L, Li D, Wang W. Dehydroepiandrosterone inhibited the bone resorption through the upregulation of OPG/RANKL. Cell Mol Immunol 2006;3:41–45.
68. Falahati-Nini A, Riggs B, Atkinson E, O' Fallon W, Eastell R, Khosla S. Relative contributions of testosterone and estrogen in regulating bone resorption and formation in normal elderly men. J Clin Invest 2000;106:1553–1560.
69. Oh K, Rhee E, Lee W, et al. Circulating osteoprotegerin and receptor activator of NF-kappaB ligand system are associated with bone metabolism in middle-aged males. Clin Endocrinol (Oxf) 2005;62: 92–98.
70. Leder B, LeBlanc K, Schoenfeld D, Eastell R, Finkelstein J. Differential effects of androgens and estrogens on bone turnover in normal men. J Clin Endocrinol Metab 2003;88:204–210.
71. Takeuchi M, Kakushi H, Tohkin M. Androgens directly stimulate mineralization and increase androgen receptors in human osteoblast-like osteosarcoma cells. Biochem Biophys Res Commun 1994;204(2):905–911.
72. Zhuang Y, Blauer M, Pekki A, Tuohimaa P. Subcellular location of androgen receptor in rat prostate, seminal vesicle and human osteosarcoma MG-63 cells. J Steroid Biochem Mol Biol 1992;41:693–696.
73. Wiren K, Zhang X-W, Chang C, Keenan E, Orwoll E. Transcriptional up-regulation of the human androgen receptor by androgen in bone cells. Endocrinology 1997;138:2291–2300.
74. Wiren K, Keenan E, Zhang X, Ramsey B, Orwoll E. Homologous androgen receptor up-regulation in osteoblastic cells may be associated with enhanced functional androgen responsiveness. Endocrinology 1999;140:3114–3124.
75. Lin M, Rajfer J, Swerdloff R, Gonzalez-Cadavid N. Testosterone down-regulates the levels of androgen receptor mRNA in smooth muscle cells from the rat corpora cavernosa via aromatization to estrogens. J Steroid Biochem Mol Biol 1993;45:333–343.
76. Hofbauer L, Hicok K, Schroeder M, Harris S, Robinson J, Khosla S. Development and characterization of a conditionally immortalized human osteoblastic cell line stably transfected with the human androgen receptor gene. J Cell Biochem 1997;66:542–551.
77. Langley E, Kemppainen J, Wilson E. Intermolecular NH2-/carboxyl-terminal interactions in androgen receptor dimerization revealed by mutations that cause androgen insensitivity. J Biol Chem 1998;273: 92–101.
78. Wiren K, Chapman Evans A, Zhang X. Osteoblast differentiation influences androgen and estrogen receptor-alpha and -beta expression. J Endocrinol 2002;175:683–694.
79. Seeman E. Osteocytes–martyrs for integrity of bone strength. Osteoporos Int 2006;17:1443–1448.
80. Liegibel U, Sommer U, Tomakidi P, et al. Concerted action of androgens and mechanical strain shifts bone metabolism from high turnover into an osteoanabolic mode. J Exp Med 2002;196:1387–1392.
81. Notelovitz M. Androgen effects on bone and muscle. Fertil Steril 2002;77 Suppl 4:S34–S41.
82. Kasperk C, Wergedal J, Farley J, Linkart T, Turner R, Baylink D. Androgens directly stimulate proliferation of bone cells in vitro. Endocrinology 1989;124:1576–1578.
83. Kasperk C, Fitzsimmons R, Strong D, et al. Studies of the mechanism by which androgens enhance mitogenesis and differentiation in bone cells. J Clinic Endocrinol Metab 1990;71:1322–1329.

84. Kasperk C, Wakley G, Hierl T, Ziegler R. Gonadal and adrenal androgens are potent regulators of human bone cell metabolism in vitro. J Bone Miner Res 1997;12:464–471.
85. Hofbauer L, Hicok K, Khosla S. Effects of gonadal and adrenal androgens in a novel androgen-responsive human osteoblastic cell line. J Cell Biochem 1998;71(1):96–108.
86. Somjen D, Katzburg S, Kohen F, et al. Responsiveness to estradiol-17beta and to phytoestrogens in primary human osteoblasts is modulated differentially by high glucose concentration. J Steroid Biochem Mol Biol 2006;99:139–146.
87. Wiren K, Toombs A, Zhang X-W. Androgen inhibition of MAP kinase pathway and Elk-1 activation in proliferating osteoblasts. J Mol Endocrinol 2004;32:209–226.
88. Kousteni S, Han L, Chen J, et al. Kinase-mediated regulation of common transcription factors accounts for the bone-protective effects of sex steroids. J Clin Invest 2003;111:1651–1664.
89. Zagar Y, Chaumaz G, Lieberherr M. Signaling cross-talk from Gbeta4 subunit to Elk-1 in the rapid action of androgens. J Biol Chem 2004;279:2403–2413.
90. Wyllie A, Kerr J, Currie A. Cell death: the significance of apoptosis. Int Rev Cytol 1980;68:251–307.
91. Lynch M, Capparelli C, Stein J, Stein G, Lian J. Apoptosis during bone-like tissue development in vitro. J Cell Biochem 1998;68:31–49.
92. Wiren KM, Toombs AR, Semirale AA, Zhang X. Osteoblast and osteocyte apoptosis associated with androgen action in bone: requirement of increased Bax/Bcl-2 ratio. Bone 2006;38:637–651.
93. Palumbo C, Ferretti M, De Pol A. Apoptosis during intramembranous ossification. J Anat 2003;203: 589–598.
94. Lanz R, Chua S, Barron N, Soder B, DeMayo F, O'Malley B. Steroid receptor RNA activator stimulates proliferation as well as apoptosis in vivo. Mol Cell Biol 2003;23:7163–7176.
95. Miura M, Chen X, Allen M, et al. A crucial role of caspase-3 in osteogenic differentiation of bone marrow stromal stem cells. J Clin Invest 2004;114:704–713.
96. Kasperk C, Faehling K, Borcsok I, Ziegler R. Effects of androgens on subpopulations of the human osteosarcoma cell line SaOS2. Calcif Tissue Int 1996;58(5):376–382.
97. Gray C, Colston K, Mackay A, Taylor M, Arnett T. Interaction of androgen and 1,25-dihydroxyvitamin D3: effects on normal rat bone cells. J Bone Miner Res 1992;7(1):41–46.
98. Davey R, Hahn C, May B, Morris H. Osteoblast gene expression in rat long bones: effects of ovariectomy and dihydrotestosterone on mRNA levels. Calcif Tissue Int 2000;67:75–79.
99. Kapur S, Reddi A. Influence of testosterone and dihydrotestosterone on bone-matrix induced endochondral bone formation. Calcif Tissue Int 1989;44:108–113.
100. Horowitz M. Cytokines and estrogen in bone: anti-osteoporotic effects. Science 1993;260:626–627.
101. Kassem M, Harris S, Spelsberg T, Riggs B. Estrogen inhibits interleukin-6 production and gene expression in a human osteoblastic cell line with high levels of estrogen receptors. J Bone Miner Res 1996;11(2):193–199.
102. Kawaguchi H, Pilbeam C, Vargas S, Morse E, Lorenzo J, Raisz L. Ovariectomy enhances and estrogen replacement inhibits the activity of bone marrow factors that stimulate prostaglandin production in cultured mouse calvariae. J Clin Invest 1995;96:539–548.
103. Wang X, Schwartz Z, Yaffe P, Ornoy A. The expression of transforming growth factor-beta and interleukin-1beta mRNA and the response to 1,25(OH)2D3' 17 beta-estradiol, and testosterone is age dependent in primary cultures of mouse-derived osteoblasts in vitro. Endocrine 1999;11:13–22.
104. Subramaniam M, Harris S, Oursler M, Rasmussen K, Riggs B, Spelsberg T. Identification of a novel TGF-beta-regulated gene encoding a putative zinc finger protein in human osteoblasts. Nucleic Acids Res 1995;23:4907–4912.
105. Gill R, Turner R, Wronski T, Bell N. Orchiectomy markedly reduces the concentration of the three isoforms of transforming growth factor beta in rat bone, and reduction is prevented by testosterone. Endocrinology 1998;139(2):546–550.
106. Canalis E, Centrella M, McCarthy T. Regulation of insulin-like growth factor-II production in bone cultures. Endocrinology 1991;129:2457–2462.
107. Gori F, Hofbauer L, Conover C, Khosla S. Effects of androgens on the insulin-like growth factor system in an androgen-responsive human osteoblastic cell line. Endocrinology 1999;140(12):5579–5586.
108. Fukayama S, Tashjian H. Direct modulation by androgens of the response of human bone cells (SaOS-2) to human parathyroid hormone (PTH) and PTH-related protein. Endocrinology 1989;125:1789–1794.

109. Gray A, Feldman H, McKinlay J, Longcope C. Age, disease, and changing sex hormone levels in middle-aged men: results of the Massachusetts male aging study. J Clin Endocrinol Metab 1991;73:1016–1025.
110. Vermeulen A. Clinical review 24: Androgens in the aging male. J Clin Endocrinol Metab 1991;73: 221–224.
111. Pilbeam C, Raisz L. Effects of androgens on parathyroid hormone and interleukin-1-stimulated prostaglandin production in cultured neonatal mouse calvariae. J Bone Miner Res 1990;5(11):1183–1188.
112. Hofbauer L, Khosla S. Androgen effects on bone metabolism: recent progress and controversies. Eur J Endocrinol 1999;140(4):271–286.
113. Passeri G, Girasole G, Jilka R, Manolagas S. Increased interleukin-6 production by murine bone marrow and bone cells after estrogen withdrawal. Endocrinology 1993;133(2):822–828.
114. Rifas L, Kenney J, Marcelli M, et al. Production of interleukin-6 in human osteoblasts and human bone marrow stromal cells: evidence that induction by interleukin-1 and tumor necrosis factor-alpha is not regulated by ovarian steroids. Endocrinology 1995;136(9):4056–4067.
115. Bellido T, Jilka R, Boyce B, et al. Regulation of interleukin-6, osteoclastogenesis, and bone mass by androgens. J Clin Invest 1995;95:2886–2895.
116. Lin S, Yamate T, Taguchi Y, et al. Regulation of the gp80 and gp130 subunits of the IL-6 receptor by sex steroids in the murine bone marrow. J Clin Invest 1997;100(8):1980–1990.
117. Bruch H, Wolf L, Budde R, Romalo G, Scheikert H. Androstenedione metabolism in cultured human osteoblast-like cells. J Clin Endocrinol Metab 1992;75(1):101–105.
118. Vittek J, Altman K, Gordon G, Southren A. The metabolism of 7alpha-3H-testosterone by rat mandibular bone. Endocrinology 1974;94(2):325–329.
119. Schweikert H, Rulf W, Niederle N, Schafer H, Keck E, Kruck F. Testosterone metabolism in human bone. Acta Endocrinol 1980;95:258–264.
120. Russell D, Wilson J. Steroid 5a-reductase: two genes/two enzymes. Annu Rev Biochem 1994;63:25–61.
121. Issa S, Schnabel D, Feix M, et al. Human osteoblast-like cells express predominantly steroid 5alpha-reductase type 1. J Clin Endocrinol Metab 2002;87:5401–5407.
122. Audi L, Carrascosa A, Ballabriga A. Androgen metabolism by human fetal epiphyseal cartilage and its chondrocytes in primary culture. J Clin Endocrinol Metab 1984;58:819–825.
123. Turner R, Bleiberg B, Colvard D, Keeting P, Evans G, Spelsberg T. Failure of isolated rat tibial periosteal cells to 5a reduce testosterone to 5a-dihydroxytestosterone. 5 1990;7:775–779.
124. Sobel V, Schwartz B, Zhu Y, Cordero J, Imperato-McGinley J. Bone Mineral Density in the Complete Androgen Insensitivity and 5{alpha}-Reductase-2 Deficiency Syndromes. J Clin Endocrinol Metab 2006;91:3017–3023.
125. Mahendroo M, Cala K, Landrum C, Russell D. Fetal death in mice lacking 5a-reductase type 1 caused by estrogen excess. Mol Endocrinol 1997;11:917–927.
126. Rosen H, Tollin S, Balena R, et al. Bone density is normal in male rats treated with finasteride. Endocrinology 1995;136:1381–1387.
127. Amory J, Watts N, Easley K, et al. Exogenous testosterone or testosterone with finasteride increases bone mineral density in older men with low serum testosterone. J Clin Endocrinol Metab 2004;89:503–510.
128. Simpson E, Mahendroo M, Means G, et al. Aromatase cytochrome P450, the enzyme responsible for estrogen biosynthesis. Endocr Rev 1994;15:342–355.
129. Nawata H, Tanaka S, Tanaka S, et al. Aromatase in bone cell: Association with osteoporosis in postmenopausal women. J Steroid Biochem Mol Biol 1995;53:165–174.
130. Schweikert H, Wolf L, Romalo G. Oestrogen formation from androstenedione in human bone. Clin Endocr 1995;43:37–42.
131. Sasano H, Uzuki M, Sawai T, et al. Aromatase in human bone tissue. J Bone Miner Res 1997;12: 1416–1423.
132. Purohit A, Flanagan A, Reed M. Estrogen synthesis by osteoblast cell lines. Endocrinology 1992;131(4):2027–2029.
133. Tanaka S, Haji Y, Yanase T, Takayanagi R, Nawata H. Aromatase activity in human osteoblast-like osteosarcoma cell. Calcif Tissue Int 1993;52:107–109.
134. Shozu M, Simpson E. Aromatase expression of human osteoblast-like cells. Mol Cell Endocrinol 1998;139:117–129.
135. Gennari L, Nuti R, Bilezikian J. Aromatase activity and bone homeostasis in men. J Clin Endocrinol Metab 2004;89:5898–5907.

136. Lin S, Shi R, Qiu W, et al. Structural basis of the multispecificity demonstrated by 17beta-hydroxysteroid dehydrogenase types 1 and 5. Mol Cell Endocrinol 2006;248:38–46.
137. Muir M, Romalo G, Wolf L, Elger W, Schweikert H. Estrone sulfate is a major source of local estrogen formation in human bone. J Clin Endocrinol Metab 2004;89:4685–4692.
138. Pino A, Rodriguez J, Rios S, et al. Aromatase activity of human mesenchymal stem cells is stimulated by early differentiation, vitamin D and leptin. J Endocrinol 2006;191:715–725.
139. Abdelgadir S, Resko J, Ojeda S, Lephart E, McPhaul M, Roselli C. Androgens regulate aromatase cytochrome P450 messenger ribonucleic acid in rat brain. Endocrinology 1994;135:395–401.
140. Jones M, Boon W, Proietto J, Simpson E. Of mice and men: the evolving phenotype of aromatase deficiency. Trends Endocrinol Metab 2006;17:55–64.
141. Smith E, Boyd J, Frank G, et al. Estrogen resistance caused by a mutation in the estrogen-receptor gene in a man. N Engl J Med 1994;331(16):1056–1061.
142. Bouillon R, Bex M, Vanderschueren D, Boonen S. Estrogens are essential for male pubertal periosteal bone expansion. J Clin Endocrinol Metab 2004;89:6025–6029.
143. Vanderschueren D, Van Herck E, Nijs J, Ederveen A. Aromatase inhibition impairs skeletal modeling and decreases bone mineral density in growing male rats. Endocrinology 1997;138:2301–2307.
144. Wickman S, Kajantie E, Dunkel L. Effects of suppression of estrogen action by the p450 aromatase inhibitor letrozole on bone mineral density and bone turnover in pubertal boys. J Clin Endocrinol Metab 2003;88:3785–3789.
145. Vanderschueren D, Van Herck E, De Coster R, Bouillon R. Aromatization of androgens is important for skeletal maintenance of aged male rats. Calcif Tissue Int 1996;59:179–183.
146. Feix M, Wolf L, Schweikert H. Distribution of 17beta-hydroxysteroid dehydrogenases in human osteoblast-like cells. Mol Cell Endocrinol 2001;171:163–164.
147. Marcus R, Leary D, Schneider D, Shane E, Favus M, Quigley C. The contribution of testosterone to skeletal development and maintenance: lessons from the androgen insensitivity syndrome. J Clin Endocrinol Metab 2000;85:1032–1037.
148. Kemppainen J, Langley E, Wong C, Bobseine K, Kelce W, Wilson E. Distinguishing androgen receptor agonists and antagonists: distinct mechanisms of activation by medroxyprogesterone acetate and dihydrotestosterone. Mol Endocrinol 1999;13:440–454.
149. Omwancha J, Brown T. Selective androgen receptor modulators: in pursuit of tissue-selective androgens. Curr Opin Investig Drugs 2006;7:873–881.
150. Miner J, Chang W, Chapman M, et al. An orally active selective androgen receptor modulator is efficacious on bone, muscle, and sex function with reduced impact on prostate. Endocrinology 2007;148:363–373.
151. Allan G, Lai M, Sbriscia T, et al. A selective androgen receptor modulator that reduces prostate tumor size and prevents orchidectomy-induced bone loss in rats. J Steroid Biochem Mol Biol 2007;103:76–83.
152. Kearbey J, Gao W, Narayanan R, et al. Selective androgen receptor modulator (SARM) treatment prevents bone loss and reduces body fat in ovariectomized rats. Pharm Res 2007;24:328–335.
153. Turner R, Riggs B, Spelsberg T. Skeletal effects of estrogen. Endocrine Rev 1994;15:275–300.
154. Kasra M, Grynpas M. The effects of androgens on the mechanical properties of primate bone. Bone 1995;17:265–270.
155. Seeman E. Periosteal bone formation–a neglected determinant of bone strength. N Engl J Med 2003;349:320–323.
156. Bateman T, Broz J, Fleet M, Simske S. Differing effects of two-week suspension on male and female mouse bone metabolism. Biomed Sci Instrum 1997;34:374–379.
157. Spencer T, Jenster G, Burcin M, et al. Steroid receptor coactivator-1 is a histone acetyltransferase. Nature 1997;389:194–198.
158. Kang H, Huang K, Chang S, Ma W, Lin W, Chang C. Differential modulation of androgen receptor-mediated transactivation by Smad3 and tumor suppressor Smad4. J Biol Chem 2002;277:43749–43756.
159. Hayes S, Zarnegar M, Sharma M, et al. SMAD3 represses androgen receptor-mediated transcription. Cancer Res 2001;61:2112–2118.
160. Lee D, Chang C. Molecular communication between androgen receptor and general transcription machinery. J Steroid Biochem Mol Biol 2003;84:41–49.

17 Androgen Actions on Bone: Clinical Aspects

Androgen and Bone

Stefan Goemaere, MD, *Guy T'Sjoen,* MD, PHD, *and Jean-Marc Kaufman,* MD, PHD

CONTENTS

SUMMARY

Androgen actions in target tissues depend on plasma concentration of bio-available androgen, on local androgen metabolism and on the presence and activity of sex steroids receptors (AR and partially ER) in association with regulatory co-factors, as well as on non-genomic pathways. As evidenced by androgen receptor insensitivity syndromes, androgens appear to play an important role in the development of the male skeletal phenotype, especially bone size. It is also probable that androgens participate in the later maintenance of adult bone remodelling/mass/structure. The old concept that androgens are responsible for skeletal abnormalities in hypogonadism is only partially erroneous. The declining sex steroid levels in the elderly may adversely affect the preservation of skeletal integrity and indicates that aromatisation of testosterone to estradiol is an important mediator of bone metabolism in the elderly. Androgens and estrogens have actions in bone development and maintenance and the complex interplay between both has only partially elucidated.

Clinical studies on the skeletal effects of hypogonadism and testosterone and non-aromatizable androgen therapy confirm the indisputable evidence of androgen action in bone.

From: *Contemporary Endocrinology: Osteoporosis: Pathophysiology and Clinical Management*
Edited by: R. A. Adler, DOI 10.1007/978-1-59745-459-9_17,

The interventional studies indicate only favorable effects in those men with pre-treatment serum testosterone levels clearly below the range of young men. Substitutive or pharmacologic treatment with androgens for the prevention or reversion of bone loss or increased fracture risk in aging men can only be considered if there is convincing evidence for androgen deficiency, although there is no precise definition of the "physiological" androgen requirements in elderly men. Avoiding side-effects and improving the dosing regimens of the presently available androgen treatments provide options for further developments. Selective androgen receptor modulators may present novel opportunities in the prevention or treatment of metabolic bone disorders.

Key Words: Androgens, male, female, bone acquisition, bone maintenance; bone mass, bone size, bone structure, transsexuals, androgen treatment, selective androgen receptor modulators

INTRODUCTION

Evidence for the importance of androgen actions on bone can be drawn from studies of gonadal dysfunction or testosterone replacement. Bone loss and increased bone turnover have been observed following orchidectomy in animals and men. As described in Chapter 16, the skeletal effects of androgens are mediated through direct activation of the androgen receptor (AR) or alternatively the oestrogen receptor α (ERα) following aromatization of testicular and/or adrenal androgens to oestrogens, with non-genomic pathways sometimes playing a minor role. In light of the presence of AR, ER and operational metabolic pathways in a variety of cells and tissues, androgens act on many cells and tissues and their effects on bone may be even more complex (and indirect) due to the interdependence and functional relationships between tissues and organs. For instance, bone–neuro–muscular relationships are operative in a functional system adaptive to locomotive function. In this biological system, the androgen actions on the skeleton should be interpreted as a modulation of the controlling feedback systems, keeping a balance to adapt men and women to growth, maintaining function and aging. In the first part of this chapter, androgen metabolism in humans is described in depth. The second part reviews the effect on growth and attaining peak bone mass, bone size and structure. In the third part, maintenance and change/loss of the bone are described relative to blood and tissue androgen levels. Finally, clinical effects of androgens on bone are discussed.

ANDROGEN METABOLISM IN HUMANS

Androgens in the Systemic Circulation in Men

Testosterone T, dihydrotestosterone (DHT), androstenedione, dehydroepiandrosterone (DHEA) and its sulphate (DHEAS) are the major androgens in the systemic circulation. T is secreted almost exclusively by the testes, while only about 20% of circulating DHT originates from direct testicular secretion, the rest derived from 5α-reduction of T in peripheral tissues *(1)*. Peripheral conversion of DHEA and T provides 15% of androstenedione, the remainder from direct secretion by the testes and the adrenals in approximately equal parts *(2,3)*. DHEA and DHEAS originate almost exclusively from the adrenals. Biologically, the most important plasma androgen is T. It is largely bound to plasma proteins. Only

1–2% is free, 40–50% is loosely bound to albumin and 50–60% is specifically and strongly bound to sex hormone-binding globulin (SHBG) *(4,5)*. The serum-free T (FT) and the albumin-bound T represent the fractions readily available for biological action. The non-SHBG-bound T, i.e. the combined free and albumin-bound T, is often referred to as the "bioavailable T" (bioT). As described in Chapter 16, androgenic actions of T are mediated via binding to the nuclear androgen receptor (AR), either directly or after 5α-reduction to DHT, whereas part of the physiologic actions of T results from its aromatization to oestradiol, which binds to oestrogen receptors (ER). The AR does not bind androstenedione, DHEA or DHEAS; it is assumed that the androgenic effects of these steroids are attributable to their transformation to T in the tissues. T can also exert rapid, non-genomic effects, in part via binding to a G protein-coupled membrane receptor for the SHBG–T complex that initiates a cyclic AMP-mediated, transcription-independent signalling pathway affecting calcium channels *(6–8)*.

In the early 1970s, several authors reported an age-associated decline of serum T levels from the fourth or fifth decade of life. Although controversial, a decline of one-third from age 25 to 75 years has now been confirmed by a large series of cross-sectional studies *(9)* and by several longitudinal studies *(10–14)*.

There is an age-associated increase in SHBG levels by about 1.2% per year *(13)* so that the decrease in FT and bioT serum levels is larger than that in total serum T *(13–21)*. Cross-sectional studies do not show substantial changes in serum levels of DHT in aging men, although due to the increase in SHBG, there may be a modest decrease in the free fraction *(16,21)*. Plasma androstenedione levels significantly decline with age *(22)*. The androgenic activity of androstenedione is dependent on biotransformation to T *(3)*. Plasma DHEA and DHEAS are secreted almost exclusively by the adrenals. Only about 10% of DHEA is derived from the gonads, while about 50–70% derives from desulphatation of DHEAS in peripheral tissues *(23)*. The blood conversion rate to T is about 0.6%; hence, its contribution to plasma T levels is negligible in adult men. However, as this conversion occurs in peripheral tissues where T may act locally, contribution of DHEA to tissular androgenic activity is not predicted by serum levels. DHEAS is by far the most abundant androgen in plasma. Its hormonal and metabolic effects are essentially attributable to its transformation to T and oestrogens in tissues *(24)*. However, the contribution to the global androgenic effect is probably modest.

Tissue Levels of Androgens and Androgenic Action in Men

Although T itself exerts androgenic and anabolic actions through binding to the nuclear androgen receptor (AR) in target cells, it is essentially a prohormone, being reduced to the more active androgen DHT in tissues expressing 5α-reductase, whereas a fraction of T can be aromatized to oestradiol in tissues expressing the cytochrome P450 aromatase enzyme. Hence, the action of T is a complex result of tissue availability and locally achieved T concentrations, of local intracellular T metabolism, of expression of AR and/or oestrogen receptors (ER), as well as the expression of a number of co-activators and repressors of these receptors.

Sex Steroid (Androgen and Oestrogen) Receptors in Bone

Both the AR and the ER (ERα and/or ERβ) are expressed in a wide range of tissues, including bone *(25)*. The distribution of the androgen receptor in the skeleton is wide both at cellular and organ levels. Little gender difference is observed in androgen receptor levels, suggesting a widespread androgen action. The presence of specific high-affinity androgen receptors was first reported for osteoblast-like cells *(26–31)* and also shown in other bone cells *(25,28,32,33)*. Site specificity of AR expression has been reported *(31)*.

T and DHT bind to the same receptor, but the affinity of DHT for the AR is greater than that of T and in many tissues, DHT mediates most androgenic effects of T. In muscle, however, T itself is the active androgen *(34)*. Aging leads to a decrease in AR concentration in different tissues *(35–37)*. Androgen sensitivity may be modulated by functional AR receptor polymorphisms, such as the variation in functionally important polyglutamine and polyglycine tracts, encoded by a polymorphic trinucleotide CAG repeat and GGC repeat, respectively *(38–41)*. In conclusion, androgen action in target tissues depends on plasma concentration of bio-available androgen, on local androgen metabolism and on the presence and activity of sex steroid receptors and (AR and partially ER) in association with regulatory co-factors.

ANDROGEN EFFECTS ON BONE ACQUISITION

The risk of developing osteoporosis in later life is related to bone deposition during childhood, puberty and early adulthood *(42)*. It is estimated that 60% of the fracture risk in older adults is explained by the peak bone mass attained at skeletal maturity *(43)*. By the end of the adolescent period 90% of the adult BMC *(44,45)* is acquired, and 25% of the total BMC at maturity is acquired in just 2 years of adolescence *(45)*.

Androgen as a Determinant of Peak Bone Mass, Bone Size and Bone Structure

Sex Steroid Effects on Bone in Boys and Men: General Aspects

The combined androgenic and oestrogenic actions result in the genesis and maintenance of gender differences. Effects of androgens and oestrogens on bone metabolism (bone acquisition and maintenance) are clearly demonstrated; however, their relative contributions are not yet completely elucidated. See Chapters 14 and 15 for a review of oestrogens in bone. Compared to oestrogens, the skeletal role of androgens remains less clear, e.g. serum oestrogen levels in older men correlate better with bone mineral density than do the androgen levels in most *(46–53)* but not all *(54,55)* cross-sectional studies. Also, in some longitudinal studies, oestrogens were shown to play a more dominant role in the attainment of peak bone mass in young men, as well as in bone loss in older men *(56,57)*. However, studies in osteoporotic men do not consistently confirm these correlations and do not suggest lower oestrogen levels as a pathophysiological mechanism. Another finding in the cross-sectional studies of men with idiopathic and secondary osteoporosis is higher levels of sex hormone-binding globulin (SHBG) *(58,59)*. Higher SHBG levels may be predictive of fracture *(58,60–62)*.

Skeletal size, shape and internal structure are determined by embryonic development and growth before and during sexual maturation. These phases are characterized by endosteal resorption and periosteal expansion in cortical bone and remodelling of the trabecular network throughout life, during which complex intercellular communication among bone takes place. Androgens influence proliferation and function of osteoblasts, osteoclasts and chondrocytes *(63)*, endochondral bone formation and fracture healing *(64,65)* and bone maturation *(66)*. Numerous experimental approaches and strong clinical evidence illustrate that androgens have independent skeletal actions by stimulating osteoblast proliferation, differentiation and lifespan *(67)*. In addition, androgens suppress osteoclast function, activity and lifespan *(68)* through complex endocrine, paracrine and autocrine action *(69)*. More recently, the apoptotic effects of sex hormones on osteoclasts and anti-apoptotic effects on osteoblasts and osteocytes have been shown to be mediated through non-genotropic actions *(68,69)*.

In human studies on the differential effects of androgens and oestrogens, where T deficiency occurs with maintenance of normal oestradiol levels, there is a limited increase in bone resorption *(70)* in the short term. Congenital male hypogonadism, e.g. idiopathic hypogonadotropic hypogonadism *(71,72)* or Klinefelter's syndrome *(73)*, is associated with osteoporosis. Osteopenia and osteoporosis in males are a consequence of various forms of acquired male hypogonadism, e.g. castration *(74)*, hyperprolactemia *(75)*, anorexia nervosa *(76)* or treatment with gonadotropin-releasing hormone analogues *(77–79)*. Gonadal insufficiency during adolescence is associated with skeletal deficits *(80,81)*. At least partial restitution of bone mass and bone mineral density is reported by testosterone replacement, in particular in hypogonadal men with still open growth plates *(71,82–84)*. The major gender differences in bone size have been proposed to be a consequence of increased periosteal bone formation stimulated by the androgens. In animal studies *(85–87)* using non-aromatizable androgens and in various clinical androgen deficiency states, cortical bone and puberty are the preferred place and time for androgen action. The differential periosteal effects leading to larger bone size in men at peak bone mass appear to decrease later fracture risk in men compared to women *(88)*.

Androgen Effects on the Acquisition of Bone Mass and Bone Density

Androgens play an essential role in the male pubertal growth and radial bone expansion *(89,90)*. Direct stimulatory action of T on periosteal bone via the (AR) leads to greater bone diameter and cortical thickness in men compared to women *(91,92)*, thus contributing to the observed sexual dimorphism of bone architecture. Free T is a positive predictor, whereas free oestradiol is a negative predictor of the cortical bone size in young healthy men *(93)*. Androgen insensitivity abolishes the typical male skeletal morphology. The resulting female bone phenotype of the (partially) inactive AR or the androgen insensitivity syndrome (AIS) is apparent from both animal *(94–96)* and human *(96–101)* studies. The lumbar spine areal bone density is decreased by 1 SD in complete human AIS, the deficit being even greater in case of poor oestrogen replacement therapy compliance *(97)*. Controlling for the increased stature in AIS by calculating the apparent volumetric bone mineral density (BMAD) revealed an even more decreased BMAD at the lumbar spine (*Z* score -1.30 ± 0.43) and the proximal femur (*Z* score -1.38 ± 0.28) *(97,101)*. In contrast to complete blockade of oestrogen action, bone length is not affected in AIS. This suggests that only oestrogen, possibly acting via the growth hormone (GH)–IGF-I axis, is required for longitudinal bone growth *(90,102)*.

The genetic component of peak bone mineral mass (PBM) is evident from family resemblance in aBMD; daughters of women with osteoporotic fracture have relatively lower BMD *(103)*. PBM accounts for about half of the BMD variation in old age and may influence the osteoporosis risk *(104,105)*. The majority of bone mass accumulation is achieved in late adolescence followed by a period of consolidation *(106,107)*, referring to increased bone mass after the cessation of linear growth at the end of puberty. The PBM is dependent on genetic and environmental factors. There is a wide age range (third to fourth decade) during which the peak bone mass/density is attained depending on localization *(108,109)*. Measurement of areal BMD (aBMD) by DXA is a planar measurement dependent on bone size, incorporating information about bone width and height but not depth. Therefore, bigger bones with similar density within the periosteal envelope (volumetric BMD, vBMD) will be reported as having a higher aBMD; volumetric BMD (vBMD) is a better measure of mineral status since bone size is taken into account. Studies on peak vBMD, measured by QCT *(112–114)* or mathematically estimated *(114–116)*, illustrate that in late puberty during the rapid accrual of bone mineral within the periosteal envelope, there is a gradual but slight increase in vBMD (approximately 10–30%) *(117,118)*, compared to the more manifest changes in bone size and mass during the pubertal transition up to the age of 16 years.

Androgen Effects on the Acquisition of Bone Size

The increase in the vertebral bone size is steeper in boys than in girls *(118)*, resulting in a greater vertebral size in men compared to women *(112,113,119,120)*. The greater bone size is determined by a greater vertebral width with an identical vertebral height *(112,120,121)*. Reduced vertebral size (width and volume) has been linked with increased vertebral fracture risk later in the life of men and women *(122–125)*. The vBMD at the femoral neck is almost constant during growth because the increase in bone mass and bone volume is proportional *(110,111,113–115,118,126,127)*. Bone width at the appendicular skeleton, at the femoral neck *(128,129)* and the metacarpals *(130,131)* is observed to be greater in boys than girls due to the greater periosteal apposition at puberty *(131)*. Similarly, at the distal radius, the vBMD in boys does not change during growth due to the proportional increases of bone mass and bone size *(118,130)*. In contrast to boys, bone size at the distal radius does not change during growth in girls *(118)*. The small increase in vBMD in girls is due to a bone mass accrual within the periosteal envelope mainly due to endosteal apposition as estimated by pQCT *(132)*. This lesser periosteal apposition in bone translates into a lower bone strength, since indices of bone strength (section modulus and strength strain index) are size dependent and therefore greater in boys than girls *(133)*. Hence, at the distal radius, the gender differences in bone size and vBMD during growth illustrate the sexual dimorphism of the growing skeleton. Viewing the continuous increase in bone size during puberty (except for the radius in girls) with the little increase in vBMD, it is speculated that the observed increases in bone mass during and after the consolidation phase *(118)* after the closure of epiphyseal growth plates and cessation of longitudinal growth are due to increases in bone size from an increased periosteal apposition *(124,128,134–138)*.

As the timing of peak bone mass development depends mainly on bone size development, it would be more accurate to examine the timing of peak vBMD. At the lumbar spine, peak vBMD was achieved at age 22 and 29 in men and women, respectively *(106,118)*. At the metacarpals, cortical thickness increases more rapidly in boys to peak at 25 years *(139)*. In women, the increase is more gradual and peaks later at 45 years. At the femoral neck, peak vBMD is already achieved at 12 year in both sexes, which is much earlier than at the distal radius, which peaks at 19 in women *(118)*. All these observations illustrate that bone development is region specific *(115,140–143)*. Indeed, trabecular and cortical bone respond differently to metabolic and mechanical stimuli *(140,144)*. Growth of the legs is more rapid than that of the spine before puberty, while the converse is true at puberty *(117,145)*.

Androgen Effects on Bone Structure

Although BMD by DXA is non-invasive and the results correlate with existing vertebral deformities *(146)* and the development of clinical fractures *(147)*, the correlation is imperfect. Subjects with similar bone mineral density measurements may have different degrees of perturbation of the bone architecture as determined by histomorphometry *(148–150)*. To circumvent the limitations of DXA and to assess the importance of the microarchitecture of bone in determining its strength and resistance to fracture, techniques based on quantitative computed tomography (QCT) and magnetic resonance imaging (MRI) have been developed.

The trabecular architecture of men with severe testosterone deficiency differs from eugonadal men. A deterioration of the plate-like structures into a rod-shaped, thin and disconnected network, characteristic of osteoporosis, is illustrated by a 36% decreased surface/curve ratio at the distal tibia *(151)*. Similarly, the erosion index was significantly increased by 36% in hypogonadal compared to eugonadal men, in contrast to no significant difference in spine and hip BMD *(151)*. Trabecular bone effects may be site independent *(152)*. The architectural abnormalities in hypogonadal men may result in less mechanically competent bone with increased susceptibility to fracture. The 40–60% variation of the mechanical bone strength explained by its mass or density may be supplemented by an additional 25–40% via the bone architecture indices as determined by high-resolution CT or MRI *(153–156)*.

Androgen Effects on Bone in Women

Androgen receptors in bone have been demonstrated in women *(28)*, but bone effects of hypoandrogenism in women are not well established. In male and female patients with adrenal insufficiency (Addison's disease), variable effects on aBMD have been described *(157–160)*. The reduced BMD, reported mainly in postmenopausal women, has been attributed to the subtle over-replacement with corticosteroids and/or the reduction in adrenal androgen production *(160,161)*. Androgen levels in young *(162)* and late menopausal women *(163)* have been correlated with trabecular bone density. Women with osteoporosis have been reported to have decreased DHEAS values *(164)*. Recent data suggest that androgen deficiency contributes to osteopenia in women with hypopituitarism *(165)*. Conversely, increased BMD has been reported to be associated with hyperandrogenism in women *(166,167)*. In lean women with polycystic ovary syndrome (PCOS), significantly higher BMD compared to control women has been described in the upper skeleton *(168)*. In healthy adult women, circulating androgen concentrations are reported to be independent predictors of BMD *(169,170)*, and androgen administration improves BMD in older osteoporotic women *(171–173)*.

As in men, female patients with isolated hypogonadotropic hypogonadism of prepubertal origin, gonadal dysgenesis or delayed puberty have a decrease in the cortical and trabecular bone envelope and peak bone mass development *(174–176)*. During normal puberty, the increasing levels of sex steroids result in closely associated bone growth and rapid accumulation of true BMD *(177,178)*. Girls with early menarche (before 12 years) showed higher BMD at the end of the adolescent period than did subjects with late menarche (after 14 years) *(179)*.

Interactions of Androgens with Factors Determining Peak Bone Mass

GROWTH DURING NORMAL, PRECOCIOUS AND DELAYED PUBERTY

No sexual dimorphism is observed before sexual maturity: skeletal size and volumetric BMD are similar in pre-pubertal girls and boys. Before puberty, growth is more rapid in the legs than in the trunk *(180)*. By that time, vBMD is constant due to the proportional increase of bone size and bone mass *(115)*. Puberty plays a dual role in growth: height velocity is markedly accelerated, while the rate of skeletal maturation is also increased with resultant fusion of epiphyseal cartilages. Puberty can be considered as a growth-promoting event as well as the final height-limiting process. This concept is illustrated by the early exposure to sex steroids, such as in central precocious puberty or congenital adrenal hyperplasia, resulting in accelerated growth and subsequent short adult height *(181–184)*. Since growth of the bone regions precedes the increase in bone mass, this results in a continuously more advanced size than BMC in all regions of the skeleton *(180)*. This temporal imbalance has been one of the explanatory factors for the peak of fracture risk around 14 years in boys and 11 years of age in girls *(185)*, being the ages of the peak size and mass accrual velocities. It is hypothesized that differences in growth pattern between skeletal regions may predispose to site-specific deficits in bone size, bone mass and vBMD in adult life as a consequence of adverse health factors or diseases which intervene during one of the growth phases *(180)*. The appendicular skeleton is more at risk before puberty, while the axial skeleton is more at risk during the late pubertal phase *(186,187)*. The contribution of growth-related factors is suggested by observations that the offspring of men with osteoporosis and/or fractures have reduced aBMD and vBMD at the site of fracture of their fathers *(188,189)*. Between the start and the end of puberty, growth produces bigger bones, with a 200% increase in bone volume and a 300% increase in BMC, but with only a slightly denser skeleton as indicated by a 30–40% increase in the calculated vBMD from the DXA measurements *(180)*. Both cortical and trabecular bone mineral mass and areal bone density increase rapidly *(190–192)*. The mean age for the onset of puberty in boys is 11.5 years, although 9.5–13.5 years is considered to be normal *(193)*. In approximately 3% of boys, puberty begins after the age of 13.5 either as a consequence of a pathologic condition or more frequently due to constitutionally delayed puberty. Because of the later onset and longer duration of the growth spurt in boys, they acquire 10% greater body weight and 25% greater peak bone mass compared to girls *(179)*. The greater bone mass in males is due to a greater bone size. Testosterone promotes long bone growth, chondrocyte maturation, metaphyseal ossification, periosteal new bone formation and an increase in calcium incorporation into bone *(194)*. Oestrogen appears to increase endosteal bone apposition, while androgens have little activity in this regard. This explains the larger cortical bone and thicker cortex seen in young adult male as compared to women.

Young men with idiopathic hypogonadotropic hypogonadism have reduced cortical and trabecular bone density. Although their bone mineral density increases with androgen therapy, neither cortical nor trabecular bone mineral density reaches normal values *(193,195)*. These and other DXA studies *(196–198)* suggest that the timing of puberty is critical for the optimal development of peak bone mineral mass/density in boys, as demonstrated by a reduced aBMD in men presenting with constitutionally delayed puberty. A cross-sectional large-scale pQCT study revealed that the age at peak height velocity (PHV), as a marker of pubertal timing, is associated with cortical and trabecular vBMD and previous fractures in young adult men *(199)*. Similarly, girls with delayed menarche are reported to have increased fractures *(200)* and weak negative correlations exist between age at menarche and the cortical aBMD *(179,201)*.

INTERACTIONS OF SEX STEROIDS WITH GROWTH HORMONE AND IGF-I

Several hormones may interact to determine the pubertal growth spurt. Besides the sex steroids (androgens and oestrogens) of gonadal and adrenal origin, there are specific effects of growth hormone (GH) and insulin-like growth factor-I (IGF-I), permissive actions of thyroid hormones and interactions with insulin. In animal studies, GH has been shown to regulate bone size and shape *(202)*. Pre-pubertal growth is predominantly controlled by GH, and adult stature is less influenced by pubertal growth than by the height at onset of puberty *(203)*. In the absence of GH and IGF-I secretion, gonadal steroids have limited growth-promoting effects *(204,205)*. Both sex steroids *(206–211)* effectively stimulate GH secretion. During spontaneous puberty, the priming effect of sex steroids on integrated GH concentrations is due to increased amplitude of GH secretory episodes while the frequency is unaffected *(212,213)*.

During normal puberty the characteristic rise in plasma concentrations of IGF-I levels correlated with oestradiol in both sexes *(214)*. A rise in IGF-I can be induced by androgen *(214,215)* as well as oestrogen *(216,217)* treatment in hypogonadal patients. The experimental and clinical evidence that increased sex steroid secretion is associated with GH and IGF-I and accelerated growth and bone maturation has been reviewed previously *(218)*.

Androgens need to interact with the growth hormone (GH)/insulin-like growth hormone-I (IGF-I) axis for the full expression of the skeletal sexual dimorphism *(219)*.

ANDROGEN INTERACTIONS WITH MUSCULAR FUNCTION AND EXERCISE

In addition to the hormonal control of pubertal skeletal growth, other regulatory mechanisms may operate on skeletal development through general body growth, body weight and muscle mass *(220)*. The increase in muscle size and strength, through increased mechanically induced bone deformation or strain, leads to increased bone modelling (e.g. mass increases) and (micro)architectural adaptations (e.g. size, geometry changes) of the bone tissue *(221)*. Bone strength and mass normally adapt to the largest voluntary loads on bone. The major loads come from muscles, not body weight. Both androgens and GH are essential for the increase in muscle mass during growth and its maintenance into adulthood. The interactions between those factors and bone mass, size, geometry and subsequent bone strength are often referred to as the "muscle–bone mechanostat" *(220,222)*. Applied strains increase fluid flow in bone *(223)*, and strain magnitude is the principal transducing mechanism to which bone apposition is assigned in the "mechanostat model" *(224,225)*. The peak strains and loading rates are increased with jogging and running *(226)*, which explain the increase in bone mass with exercise in young people *(227)*. High-frequency shock waves are generated in the limb when the foot contacts the ground at the end of the swing phase *(228,229)*. Exercise during growth has been shown to lead to larger increases in bone mass *(230–233)* and biomechanical strength indices of bones *(232–235)*. Intervention studies have also shown to affect bone size in young subjects before and during puberty *(236,237)*.

Supporting cross-sectional reports, longitudinal studies in adolescents engaged in normal levels of physical activity demonstrate significant positive relationships between physical activity scores with bone mineral accrual *(238)*, peak bone mass *(43,239,240)* and indices of bone strength *(241)*. Impact loading and more importantly muscle force dominate the postnatal structural development *(242,243)*, adapting the bone to the usage. The modelling includes the interplay of bone size and shape development *(232,244,245)* by bone accruing at the periosteum to maximize bone strength for a given amount of bone mass, as bending strength increases with the bone radius to the power of 4 *(246)*. In general, exercise during growth is widely recommended as a key strategy in the primary prevention of osteoporosis. However, it still needs to be proven that in contrast to the larger effects of intensive training in young athletes, a moderate exercise program in normally active children *(247)* results in benefits large enough to reduce the risk of fracture.

In adult male athletes, total and free T concentrations are influenced by the intensity, the duration and the type of physical activity *(248)*. Acutely and transiently increased serum T levels have been observed in short-term resistance or endurance exercise *(249,250)*. However, studies in endurance athletes have reported either normal *(251,252)* or reduced *(253–255)* levels of circulating total and free T, nevertheless remaining within the normal ranges *(256)*. In contrast to the reported low bone mass in female runners and ballet dancers with hypoestrogenism due to strenuous physical activity and calorie restriction *(257–258)*, the incidence of low T levels in male athletes has rarely been associated with low BMD *(252,255,259)*.

ANDROGENS AND THE GENETIC PEAK BONE MASS POTENTIAL

Although reproductive, nutritional and life-style factors influence bone mineral density (BMD), family and twin studies suggest that BMD is largely heritable and under multigenetic control *(260,261)*. Heritability estimates for BMD average about 60–70% in humans.

Genetic Syndromes with Decreased Androgen Levels Klinefelter's syndrome is usually due to the XXY karyotype. Clinically, the major symptoms are small and firm testes, increased plasma gonadotropins, infertility and a variable degree of hypotestosteronaemia. Klinefelter subjects with normal T levels have normal bone structure, while in hypotestosteronaemic Klinefelter subjects, variable degrees of osteoporosis have been observed *(73)*. As in other forms of hypogonadism, a consistent correlation between the serum T levels and the decreased bone mineral content has been observed, independent of the type of hypogonadism *(262)*. Other genetic syndromes with low testosterone levels are various forms of hypogonadotropic hypogonadism such as Kallmann syndrome *(263)*.

Genetic Syndrome with Increased Androgen Levels: Androgen Insensitivity Syndrome A unique opportunity to evaluate the consequences of decreased androgen action is provided by androgen receptor mutations, producing impaired to complete lack of response to endogenous and exogenous androgens *(264)*. In these androgen insensitivity syndromes (AIS), individuals possess a normal male 46,XY genotype and functioning testes *(265,266)*. Subjects with complete AIS are phenotypic females with normal breast development during puberty, absent androgen-dependent body hair and primary amenorrhoea. Beginning at puberty, high serum levels of both T and oestradiol *(267,268)* are observed until gonadectomy is performed to prevent malignancy. Individuals with partial forms of AIS show variable degrees of virilization and sexual ambiguity. Anthropometric features, such as height and the dimensions of bone and teeth, are intermediate between typical male and female patterns *(266)*. In isolated case reports and small series *(98–100)*, a high prevalence of low BMD is described at the lumbar spine and the proximal femur. The extent of BMD reduction reaches 1–2 SD *(97)*. Also subnormal spinal BMD is observed in women with complete AIS receiving oestrogens after gonadectomy, raising questions about the timing and dosage of this supplementation. Women with partial AIS have superior BMD *(97)*. These observations are compatible with the hypothesis of independent participation of androgens in skeletal acquisition and maintenance *(97)*.

Androgen-Sensitive Gene Regulation: Variants of the Androgen Receptor (AR) A polymorphic CAG repeat, located on exon 1 of the androgen receptor (AR) on the X chromosome, which encodes a polyglutamine (CAG) repeat in the AR protein affects AR transactivation capacity. Initially, high number of CAG repeats has been reported to be associated with quantitative ultrasound measurements at the phalanges in men *(269)* and with lumbar spine BMD in women *(270)*. However, this effect has not been confirmed in middle-aged Finnish men *(271)* and in elderly men *(272)*. An effect of CAG-repeat length AR polymorphism on sex steroid levels has not been illustrated in middle-aged men *(271)*, and only reported in the elderly men study *(273)*. Following the description of aromatase gene defects, the consequence of gene polymorphisms on the expression of this particular gene, being present in the bone tissue *(274)*, has been the subject of some additional studies. A tetranucleotide repeat polymorphism $(TTTA)_n$ in intron 4 of the human aromatase cytochrome P-450 (*CYP19*) gene has been described *(275)*. In women a higher number of TTTA repeats (>11) has been reported to be associated with higher oestradiol levels and breast cancer risk *(276)*, higher lumbar BMD and lower incidences of spine fractures *(277)*. In men, however, no association with prevalent femoral, forearm or lumbar BMD or with biochemical markers of bone turnover has been documented in adult *(271)* or elderly men *(278)*. In the latter study, a relationship of the CYP19 genotype and clinical fracture history and their first-degree relatives have been reported *(278)*. Studies on the effect of the TTTA repeat polymorphism on bone loss in aging showed independent contribution of a short-repeat CYP19 genotype to an increased bone loss at the forearm *(278)* or the lumbar spine *(279)*.

EFFECTS OF ANDROGEN ON BONE MAINTENANCE AND BONE LOSS

Introduction

Once perceived as a female disease, osteoporosis is a significant cause of morbidity and mortality in elderly men. Men exhibit slow bone loss with aging, resulting in overall losses of about 25–30% in both cortical and trabecular bone between the age of 25 and

75 years. Because men do not have the equivalent of menopause, they lack the early, accelerated bone loss phase that is induced by the precipitous fall of serum oestrogens in women after menopause. With aging, there is a slow decline in the serum levels of the biologically active fractions of T and oestradiol. There is convincing evidence that aromatization from androgens to oestrogens is an important pathway mediating the actions of testosterone on bone physiology. Oestrogen is probably the dominant sex steroid regulating bone resorption in men, but both androgens and oestrogens are important in maintaining bone formation.

Bone Loss in Hypogonadal Adult Men

In circumstances of acute hypogonadism, castrated men have a pattern of rapid bone loss similar to that of women after menopause *(74,280,281)*. Similarly, drug-induced androgen deprivation such as in patients with prostate cancer treated with gonadotropin-releasing hormone (GnRH) analogues and/or anti-androgens results in a severe hypogonadism *(282,283)*, increased bone turnover *(284,285)*, bone loss within a few months of treatment *(285,286)* and increased fracture risk *(287,288)*. Bone loss in male hypogonadism has been reported to be more intense in the trabecular compared to the cortical bone compartment *(289,290)*. Several studies describe a correlation between the bone mineral density and the serum T *(73,291)*. Hypogonadism is not an uncommon finding in men with low bone mass and a wide variety of causes of gonadal failure are associated with osteoporosis *(292,293)*. Increased fracture risk has been reported to be associated with abnormal gonadal function in adult men *(294)*.

Bone Loss and Age-Associated Decreases in Androgen Levels in Men

Bone Changes from Adult Life to Old Age

By old age because of endosteal resorption, there is extensive loss of cortical bone compared to peak bone mass. The endosteal resorption associated with aging is partially offset by periosteal apposition, which is three times greater in men than in women *(295,296)*. The rate of periosteal expansion has been shown to be stable in men, while progressively reduced in women *(297,298)*. This effect contributes further to the already existing greater bone size in adult men and to the lower loss of bone strength during aging in men compared to women. Bone formed on the periosteal surface is mechanically advantageous because it increases the cross-sectional movement of inertia and the bending strength of the long bone *(299)*.

Changing Serum Androgen Levels and Aging Symptoms

In women the menopause signals the irreversible end of reproductive life as well as the end of cyclic ovarian activity and consequent low sex hormone levels in *all* postmenopausal women. In men, fertility persists until very old age and the age-associated decrease in T levels is slowly progressive. In the majority of men T levels are still within the normal range for young men until the 8th decade *(300)*. Subnormal T levels are thus not a generalized feature of aging and androgen deficiency in the elderly is only partial. Therefore, the terms partial androgen deficiency of the aging male (PADAM) or late-onset hypogonadism have been proposed as more appropriate than the terms andropause or male climacteric. The clinical relevancy of the age-related decrease in androgen levels has not been well established. There are some similarities between the symptomatology of aging and that of androgen deficiency in young hypogonadal men, as well as an association between the severity of symptoms and androgen levels. However, aging is accompanied by a decline of almost all physiologic functions such as cardiac output, pulmonary ventilatory capacity, renal clearance and growth hormone secretion. Such changes plus alterations in lifestyle such as retirement or relative sedentarism may contribute to the symptomatology of aging. The age-related decreases in growth hormone and IGF-1 levels are associated with changes in lean body mass, bone density and abdominal adiposity, similar to the changes observed in hypogonadal states.

Hormonal Aging and Bone Integrity: Senile Osteoporosis

In the view of the multifactorial origin of aging symptoms, strong correlations with free (FT) or bioavailable (BioT) T levels can hardly be expected and meaningful multivariate regression analysis becomes difficult. Furthermore, cross-sectional association studies cannot establish causality, whereas long-term prospective observational studies are rare. Aging in men is associated with continuous loss of bone and an exponential increase in the incidence of fractures of the hip *(301,302)* and the spine *(303,304)*. Moreover, the morbidity and the mortality from fractures are more severe in older men than in older women *(305,306)*. Acquired profound hypogonadism in men induces high bone turnover and accelerated bone loss *(74)*, such as in elderly men treated with androgen deprivation therapy for prostate cancer *(307,308)*. However, the importance of an age-related partial androgen deficiency in age-related osteoporosis in men is not definitely established. Although the complex role of T in the regulation of bone metabolism is not fully elucidated, there is good evidence that besides direct androgen actions, aromatization to oestrogen plays an important role in the preservation of adult skeletal integrity *(309,310)*. Indeed, cross-sectional studies, in which age and BMI (or body weight) are major confounders, have yielded inconsistent results as to the association of serum T levels with BMD in elderly men. Some studies do not show an independent association *(311–313)*, while others show weak but significant positive correlations, in particular with FT or bioT *(314–319)*. On the other hand, in a series of recent cross-sectional studies, multivariate analysis consistently indicated that (F or bio)oestradiol is a better predictor of prevalent aBMD in elderly men than is (F or bio)T *(314,318–326)*. Biochemical indices of bone turnover increase moderately with aging in men and are inversely related to prevalent aBMD in the elderly *(327,328)*, with markers of bone resorption more clearly (negatively) associated with serum levels of oestradiol than with those of T *(319,324,326,327,329)*.

Cohort studies have shown that bioavailable oestradiol is negatively associated with prospectively assessed bone loss, without independent association of serum (bioavailable) T *(319,325,329)*. Moreover, prospectively assessed bone changes in elderly men are also found to be associated with a polymorphism of the *CYP19* gene that encodes the aromatase enzyme, independently of serum oestradiol levels, suggesting indirectly that local aromatization of T in bone might play a role *(325,331)*. Whereas there has been a report of association of a CAG-repeat polymorphism of the AR with bone mineral density assessed by ultrasound in men aged 20–50 years *(332)*, in community-dwelling men over age 70 years, no association was found between this polymorphism and either BMD or biochemical indices of bone turnover *(333)*. The important role of aromatization of T to oestrogen in the regulation of bone metabolism in elderly men has been elegantly demonstrated in a short-term intervention study with selective manipulation of T and oestradiol levels *(334)*. There is evidence indicating that there may be a threshold level for the association of bioavailable oestradiol with bone loss and indices of bone metabolism *(322,330,335–337)*, although other studies did not demonstrate such a threshold *(325)*.

As to the association of sex steroid levels with fracture risk in elderly men, little data are available. In case–control studies, there was a higher prevalence of low serum T in men recruited following a hip fracture *(338–340)*, but T levels assessed following a serious event should be interpreted with caution. In the Rancho Bernardo study, lower oestradiol levels, but not serum T concentrations, were associated with a higher prevalence of vertebral fracture in older men *(349)*. In a case–control study of men aged 67.7±6.8 years as part of the Rotterdam Study, there was no significant association between vertebral fracture and either (bio)oestradiol or (bio)T *(342)*. In the Swedish part of the MrOs study, FT was the modest and independent predictor of previous osteoporosis-related fractures in elderly men *(343)*. In community-dwelling men over age 70 years, an aromatase gene polymorphism, associated with longitudinal changes in BMD, was also significantly associated with self-reported clinical fractures at the spine, the hip and/or the wrist and with the occurrence of these fractures in their first-degree relatives. There was no association of fracture history with circulating bioavailable oestradiol *(325)*. In summary, the evidence suggests that declining sex steroid levels in the elderly may adversely affect the preservation of skeletal integrity. Aromatization of T to oestradiol is a likely regulator of bone metabolism in elderly men. The skeletal effects of relative T deficiency in the elderly may be modulated by aromatase activity, which in turn is affected by factors such as adiposity and heredity.

Interrelations with Body Composition Changes During Aging

Aging is associated with important changes in body composition *(344–346)*. Similar to age-associated changes, a decrease in lean body mass and an increase in fat mass are observed in hypogonadal men as compared to age and BMI-matched controls *(347)*. A reduction of muscle mass by about 30% between age 30 and 80 years *(348)* is accompanied by a proportional decrease in muscle strength *(350)*. This decreased muscle strength contributes to frailty and is a risk factor for falls, hip fractures and loss of independence. The similarity of low muscle mass in hypogonadal young men raises the hypothesis that the age-associated decrease in androgen levels may possibly be responsible for the sarcopenia of elderly men. Few data concerning the correlation between endogenous androgen levels and muscle mass in elderly men are available. However, in an already mentioned study *(346)* involving middle-aged and elderly community-dwelling men, no correlation was found between T or FT levels and lean mass. Similar negative findings were reported by van den Beld et al. *(314)* and by Roy et al. *(351)* in men aged 20–90 years old who observed nevertheless a positive association of (F)T levels with muscle strength. Szulc et al. *(326)*, in a cross-sectional analysis in men aged 51–85 years, found that low FT is associated with lower muscle mass, functional impairment in the legs and occurrence of falls in the past year. In a subgroup analysis on fall incidence in the community-based study of elderly men aged 65–99 years (the MrOs study), lower bioT levels in men were associated with lower physical performance and increased fall risk *(352)*. In institutionalized healthy elderly men, Abassi et al. *(353)* observed a correlation between T levels and severity of sarcopenia. Also Baumgartner et al. *(354)* observed a positive association of FT with muscle mass, but not with muscle strength. Confounding effects such as age-associated decrease in physical inactivity and decreased GH may obscure the potential causal relationship between the age-related decline of androgen levels and body composition changes.

BONE AND TREATMENTS WITH ANDROGENS AND RELATED DRUGS

Steroidal androgens are used in both men and women for a large variety of diseases including osteoporosis, frailty, hypogonadism and sexual dysfunction *(358)*. A number of side effects limit broad-scaled use of presently available androgens *(356)*. Classical androgen therapy can be provided by parenteral administration of testosterone or testosterone esters (implants, injectable or transdermal) or by the stimulation of endogenous testosterone production [human chorionic gonadotropin (hCG), aromatase inhibitor]. Preparations for buccal administration have also been made available.

Androgen Treatment in Childhood

Long-acting T ester injections, dosed at 100–250 mg/month, have been used to induce and control pubertal growth in hypopituitary boys *(357–362)*. The dosage directly affects the rate of bone maturation and can reduce the total pubertal height gain. The impact on the adult stature or the final adult height is not clear *(309)*. Other factors such as age at onset of GH therapy and height at onset of puberty may modulate the effects of treatment. In excessively tall boys, administration of long-acting esters of T at high dosage of 500 mg twice monthly has resulted in a reduction in the predicted final height *(363)*. T is also used for puberty induction in boys with delayed puberty. For this indication the possible benefit of association with an aromatase inhibitor is being investigated *(364)*.

Androgen Treatment in Adults

TESTOSTERONE AND CLASSIC ANDROGEN TREATMENTS

Androgen therapy may have two potential bone effects. First, the treatment can be intended to achieve specific anabolic effects in men who are not hypogonadal, e.g. to prevent or mitigate sarcopenia or senile osteoporosis. Second, the substitution in men who are hypogonadal may improve their quality of life by alleviating symptoms, believed to be at least in part the consequence of androgen deficiency. The distinction between these two goals can sometimes be blurred because in the elderly there is no generally accepted definition of hypogonadism *(300)*. The actual operational definitions are based on the descriptive symptoms in addition to the serum T levels. However, the relationship between symptoms and T levels has never been firmly established in long-term longitudinal studies. No single controlled study is of sufficient size and duration to allow an evaluation of relevant clinical endpoints, such as fracture, long-term functionality, quality of life, long-term safety or survival *(300)*. For extensive literature on this topic, one can refer to a number of reviews *(300–372)* and systematic reviews *(373–375)* that have been published in recent years.

Androgen Replacement in Hypogonadal Adult Men T therapy increases bone mineral density in hypogonadal men and the response in trabecular bone (e.g. spine) appears to be more prominent than that in cortical bone (e.g. radius) *(71)*. Treatment with T for 18 months increased spine BMD by about 6% in a group of adult men with hypogonadism, but the increase in radial BMD was insignificant *(376)*. The adequacy of androgen replacement (dose and application) influenced the BMD response to T at the lumbar spine, the proximal femur *(377)* and the distal radius *(378)*. Also trabecular bone architecture parameters, as assessed by magnetic resonance microimaging (μMRI), improved by 7.5–11% following 24 months of T treatment *(379)*. The increased bone remodelling rate associated with hypogonadism declines with T replacement, as assessed by biochemical markers of bone resorption. There are little published data in the area of secondary hypogonadism, such as glucocorticoid excess, renal insufficiency, post-transplantation or alcoholism. In small studies, T therapy for 1 year improved spine BMD by 4–5%, but not hip or total body BMD in men receiving long-term glucocorticoid treatment *(380,381)*. This effect was not confined to non-aromatizable androgens, such as nandrolone *(380)*. In a study including cases with secondary hypogonadism of pituitary origin *(378)*, an inferior trabecular vBMD response at the distal radius was observed, probably due to confounding factors, e.g. growth hormone deficiency. No significant BMD or body composition changes were observed in young men following androgen replacement for mild Leydig cell insufficiency after cytotoxic chemotherapy *(382)*.

Apart from the increase in bone mass, other additional positive effects of androgen replacement therapy include increase in muscle strength and lean body mass *(383,384)*, which may help to promote bone health and reduce fracture risk. These effects, similar to the BMD effects, seem to be independent of the 5α-reduction of T to DHT *(385,386)*. This suggests that adding finasteride or dutasteride to T therapy in order to avoid the prostate hyperplasia *(386)* would not compromise the therapeutic benefits. Specific data on the anti-fracture efficacy or fall reduction capacity are not available. The optimal route and the dose of androgen administration for prevention or treatment of bone loss are uncertain. Transdermal applications appear to be as effective as intramuscular administration in improving bone mass *(376,387)*. An adequate dosage should be accompanied by a reduction in the biochemical markers of bone turnover.

Androgen Therapy in Eugonadal Men and Elderly Men Anabolic effects can be obtained in eugonadal young and older men by administrating "supraphysiological" doses of androgens *(387–390)*. At present, it is not possible to make a clear distinction between "replacement therapy" and "pharmacological treatment" because serum T levels vary by age *(300)*. Mid or upper physiological range levels in young may be clearly supraphysiological in some of the elderly men. In contrast to beneficial effects on muscle strength *(391)* and body composition *(392)*, studies on the effects on bone mass and biochemical remodelling indices are inconclusive *(392–394)*. In a study of men over 65 years of age *(395)*, reduced bone resorption markers were found only in a subgroup with subnormal pre-treatment T levels. Data on bone formation markers, e.g. osteocalcin and alkaline phosphatase, have been widely inconsistent *(380,381,383,386,393,395–397)*. In contrast to dihydrotestosterone (DHT), chorionic gonadotropin (rhCG) increased serum N-terminal propeptide of type I procollagen (S-PINP) *(398)*. T treatment increased BMD at the spine, but this increase was not significantly different from placebo at 3 years *(395)* in elderly men with low normal to moderately low serum testosterone levels. The spinal BMD effects were inversely related to the baseline serum testosterone level, being significant only in men with the lowest T levels (between 100 and 300 ng/dl). This study *(395)* also showed no effect on femoral BMD. In contrast, other T studies showed a positive increase of 1.9% compared with a placebo group *(386,397)*. Meta-analyses found only borderline relative BMD effects over placebo of 3 and 2% for lumbar spine and femur neck, respectively *(392)*. Sensitivity analysis revealed heterogeneity among the studies, which disappeared after taking the contribution of the T preparation into account. The highest effects were found with T esters. Overall the reported BMD and bone marker effects are difficult to interpret. Other potential beneficial effects on fatigue, depression, reduced muscle mass, haematopoiesis and sexual dysfunction are not fully established *(399)*. In conclusion, these interventional data indicate favourable effects only in those men with pre-treatment serum T levels clearly below the range of young men. Thus replacement or pharmacologic treatment with androgens for the prevention or the reversion of bone loss in aging men can be considered only if there is convincing evidence for androgen deficiency *(300)*. However, for now there is no precise definition of the "physiological" androgen requirements in elderly men. Moreover, alternative treatments, i.e. bisphosphonates and teriparatide, should also be considered when evaluating the treatment options (see Chapter 24).

Androgens (and Anti-androgens) in Transsexual Individuals In the interpretation of BMD results in transsexuals, one should take into account that previous endogenous effects of androgens and/or oestrogens on the skeleton, such as greater height, size and shape of hands, feet, jaws and pelvis in biological men or lower height and broader hips in biological women, will not change after hormonal treatment.

In male-to-female transsexual persons, oestrogens will be most effective in a milieu devoid of androgen. Thus anti-androgen therapy may be added. Both components are usually prescribed 2 years before and oestrogens are continued after sex-changing surgery. BMD loss induced by T deprivation was prevented in male-to-female transsexual persons by cross-sex hormones *(400)*. Histomorphometric studies of trans-iliac bone biopsies *(401)* indicate that anti-androgen and oestrogen treatment in male-to-female transsexuals is not associated with bone loss and may suppress bone turnover. In female-to-male transsexual persons, the principal hormone treatment is a T preparation. In one study, T was unable to prevent lumbar bone mineral loss associated with a decline in oestrogen levels *(402)*, but in other studies, a significant increase in mean femoral neck BMD *(403)* and an increase in mean spine BMD *(403,404)* were reported. A bone histomorphometric study showed intact trabecular bone structure and increased cortical thickness with low bone turnover indices *(405)*. An inverse relationship between serum LH and FSH levels and BMD has been described in both male-to-female and female-to-male transsexuals *(400)*. Beneficial bone effects of the cross-genotype sex hormone treatment confirm the findings in case reports of abnormal sexual differentiation,: e.g. XX male with androgen insensitivity syndrome and XY female with congenital adrenal hyperplasia *(406)*.

OTHER ANDROGENS AS TREATMENT OPTION

Dehydroepiandrostenedione (DHEA) and its water-soluble sulphate (DHEAS) are adrenal androgenic steroid hormones and serve as precursors in the biosynthesis of steroid hormones (T and oestradiol) and as weak androgens. Great variability of the serum levels exists within the population and an age-related decrease to 20% of its peak values is described in men and women *(407)*. Low serum concentration has been associated with cardiovascular risk in men *(408)* and breast cancer in women *(409)*. In aging women, however, epidemiological studies have demonstrated that endogenous DHEA concentrations are correlated with vigour, feelings of well-being and functional independence *(410)*. In men, the presence of the more potent androgen T (even at low levels) renders the use of extra DHEA in men unlikely to be affective. Physiological DHEA replacement raises the serum T and DHEA levels to reproductive age levels *(411)* and is assumed to yield clinical benefits without side effects associated with androgen therapy *(412–414)*. However, pilot studies *(412,415,416)* in men and women have not provided sufficient proof for any relevant effect on psychosexual function, body composition, muscle mass/strength, physical activity or quality of life.

Androgen Treatment in Women

During the menopausal transition, apart from the decline in ovarian oestrogen production, there is also a decline in ovarian and adrenal androgen production. Associated with these hormonal decreases are age-related loss of bone mass, muscle mass and muscle strength with subsequent physical impairment and functional dependence. Without knowing the different pathogenic contribution of these hormonal deficiencies, but based on Albright's hypothesis of the need for bone-forming effects of T *(417)*, androgens and anabolic steroids have been used to treat severe postmenopausal osteoporosis. Albright and Reifenstein *(418)* used testosterone propionate and methyltestosterone, and later other investigators used anabolic steroids such as methandrostenolone and stanozolol *(419–421)*. However, the reported beneficial bone effects were outweighed by the virilizing side effects, leading to the development of synthetic anabolic steroid with fewer virilizing effects *(422)*. The anabolic steroid nandrolone decanoate improves BMC at the distal radius *(423–427)* and BMD of the spine *(171)* in older osteoporotic women. Addition of androgenic steroids to hormonal regimens for hormonal substitution in postmenopausal women has been reported to increase BMD beyond the effect with oestrogen alone *(172)*.

Selective Androgen Receptor Modulators (SARMs)

Several shortcomings of classical androgen treatment need to be eliminated, e.g. the abnormally high T levels immediately after injection, skin irritation of transdermal forms, uncertain long-term prostate safety, cross-reactivity with other steroid hormone receptors, and also the absence of an acceptable oral preparation. The bone-related effect of classical androgens is obscured by conversion to oestrogens by aromatization. Notwithstanding the important role of ER in the male skeleton *(428)*, pure androgen action on bone could be an additional treatment option as suggested by the effects of non-aromatizable androgens in trabecular bone *(429)* and the severe osteopenia in male androgen receptor knockout mice *(96,430)*. Therefore, a number of non-steroidal, oral selective androgen receptor modulators (SARMs) with significant effect on muscle, bone and sexual function, but with reduced severity of side effects (e.g. on the prostate), are under development *(431)*. In animal models *(432–434)*, drugs of this class have exhibited anti-resorptive effects on trabecular bone formation effects on cortical bone, leading to improved bone strength. In addition muscle maintenance and growth and sexual function were improved, without or with only minimal stimulation of prostate tissue. This tissue selectivity may provide an interesting therapeutic option if clinical studies find SARMs to be safe and effective.

CONCLUSION

Clinical studies on the skeletal effects of hypogonadism and T therapy support the indisputable evidence of androgen action in bone. Even more specific evidence is provided by the effects of non-aromatizable androgens on bone mass, bone remodelling and bone cell biology. The clinical significance of the androgen actions, via steroid receptor as well as non-genomic pathways, has been partially elucidated and some have to be differentiated from oestrogens. As evidenced by androgen receptor insensitivity syndromes, androgens appear to play an important role in the development of the male skeletal phenotype, especially bone size. It is also probable that androgens participate in the later maintenance of adult bone remodelling/mass. The old concept that androgens are responsible for skeletal abnormalities in hypogonadism is only partially erroneous. Both androgens and oestrogens have actions in bone, and development and maintenance require an interplay between the two. The potential therapeutic usefulness of androgens requires further study. The development of selective androgen receptor modulators may present novel opportunities in the prevention or the treatment of metabolic bone disorders.

REFERENCES

1. Hammond GL, Ruokonen A, Kontturi M, Koskela E, Vihko R. Simultaneous radioimmunoassay of 7 steroids in human spermatic and peripheral venous-blood. J Clin Endocrinol Metab 1977;45:16–24.
2. Horton R, Tait J. Androstenedione production, and conversion rates in peripheral blood and studies on the possible site of its interconversion to testosterone. J Clin Invest 1966;45:301–307.
3. Horton R, Tait J. The in vivo conversion of dehydroisoandrosterone to plasma androstenedione and testosterone. J Clin Endocrinol Metab 1967;27:79–82.
4. Vermeulen A, Verdonck L. Studies on the binding of testosterone to human plasma. Steroids 1968;11:609–635.
5. Dunn JF, Nisula BC, Rodbard D. Transport of Steroid-Hormones – Binding of 21 endogenous steroids to both testosterone-binding globulin and corticosteroid-binding globulin in human-plasma. J Clin Endocrinol Metab 1981;53:58–68.
6. Rosner W, Hryb DJ, Khan MS, Nakhla AM, Romas NA. Sex hormone-binding globulin – binding to cell-membranes and generation of a 2nd messenger. J Androl 1992;13:101–106.
7. Porto CS, Abreu LC, Gunsalus GL, Bardin CW. Binding of sex-hormone-binding globulin (SHBG) to testicular membranes and solubilized receptors. Mol Cell Endocrinol 1992;89:33–38.
8. Benten WPM, Lieberherr M, Giese G, Wrehlke C, Stamm O, Sekeris CE, Mossmann H, Wunderlich F. Functional testosterone receptors in plasma membranes of T cells. FASEB J 1999;13:123–133.
9. Vermeulen A. Androgens in the aging male. J Clin Endocrinol Metab 1991;713:221–224.
10. Morley JE, Kaiser FE, Perry HM, Patrick P, Morley PMK, Stauber PM, Vellas B, Baumgartner RN, Garry PJ. Longitudinal changes in testosterone, luteinizing hormone, and follicle-stimulating hormone in healthy older men. Metab Clin Exp 1997;46:410–413.
11. Harman SM, Metter EJ, Tobin JD, Pearson J, Blackman MR. Longitudinal effects of aging on serum total and free testosterone levels in healthy men. J Clin Endocrinol Metab 2001;86:724–731.
12. Zmuda JM, Cauley JA, Kriska A, Glynn NW, Gutai JP, Kuller LH. Longitudinal relation between endogenous testosterone and cardiovascular disease risk factors in middle-aged men – a 13-year follow-up of former multiple risk factor intervention trial participants. Am J Epidemiol 1997;146:609–617.
13. Feldman HA, Longcope C, Derby CA, Johannes CB, Araujo AB, Coviello AD, Bremner WJ, Mckinlay JB. Age trends in the level of serum testosterone and other hormones in middle-aged men: longitudinal results from the Massachusetts Male Aging Study. J Clin Endocrinol Metab 2002;87:589–598.

14. Lapauw B, Goemaere S, Crabbe P, Kaufman JM, Ruige JB. Is the effect of testosterone on body composition modulated by the androgen receptor gene CAG repeat polymorphism in elderly men? Eur J Endocrinol 2007;159:459–468.
15. Deslypere JP, Vermeulen A. Leydig-cell function in normal men – effect of age, life-style, residence, diet, and activity. J Clin Endocrinol Metab 1984;59:955–962.
16. Vermeulen A, Kaufman JM, Giagulli VA. Influence of some biological indexes on sex hormone-binding globulin and androgen levels in aging or obese males. J Clin Endocrinol Metab 1996;81:1821–1826.
17. Ferrini RL, Barrett-Connor E. Sex hormones and age: A cross-sectional study of testosterone and estradiol and their bioavailable fractions in community-dwelling men. Am J Epidemiol 1998;147: 750–754.
18. Simon D, Preziosi P, Barrett-Connor E, Roger M, Saintpaul M, Nahoul K, Papoz L. The influence of aging on plasma sex-hormones in men – the Telecom-Study. Am J Epidemiol 1992;135:783–791.
19. Kaufman JM, Vermeulen A. Declining gonadal function in elderly men. Bailliere Clin Endocrinol Metab 1997;11:289–309.
20. Vermeulen A, Verdonck L, Kaufman JM. A critical evaluation of simple methods for the estimation of free testosterone in serum. J Clin Endocrinol Metab 1999;84:3666–3672.
21. Gray A, Feldman HA, Mckinlay JB, Longcope C. Age, disease, and changing sex-hormone levels in middle-aged men – results of the Massachusetts Male Aging Study. J Clin Endocrinol Metab 1991;73:1016–1025.
22. Vermeulen A. Dehydroepiandrosteronesulfate and aging. Ann NY Acad Sci 1995;774:121–127.
23. Longcope C. Adrenal and gonadal androgen secretion in normal females. Clin Endocrinol Metab 1986;15:213–228.
24. Labrie F, Belanger A, Cusan L, Candas B. Physiological changes in dehydroepiandrosterone are not reflected by serum levels of active androgens and estrogens but of their metabolites: intracrinology. J Clin Endocrinol Metab 2003;82:2403–2409.
25. Riggs BL, Khosla S, Melton LJ. Sex steroids and the construction and conservation of the adult skeleton. Endocr Rev 2002;23:279–302.
26. Colvard D, Eriksen E, Keeting P, Wilsone EM, Lubahn DB, French FS, Riggs BL, Spelsberg TC. Evidence of steroid receptors in human osteoblast-like cells. Proc Natl Acad Sci USA 1989;86:854–857.
27. Benz DJ, Haussler MR, Thomas MA, Speelman B, Komm BS. High-affinity androgen binding, and androgenic regulation for $\alpha 1(1)$ procollagen and transforming growth factor-β steady state messenger ribonucleic acid levels in human osteoblast-like osteosarcoma cells. Endocrinology 1991;128: 2723–2730.
28. Abu EO, Horner A, Kusec V, Triffitt JT, Compston JE. The localization of androgen receptors in human bone. J Clin Endocrinol Metab 1997;82:3493–3497.
29. Orwoll ES, Stribrska L, Ramsay EE, Keenan EJ. Androgen receptors in osteoblast-like cells lines. Calcif Tissue Int 1991;49:182–187.
30. Benz DJ, Haussler MR, Thomas MA, Speelman B, Komm BS. High-affinity androgen binding and androgenic regulation of α_1(I)-procollagen and transforming growth factor-β steady state messenger ribonucleic acid levels in human osteoblast-like osteosarcoma cells. Endocrinology 1991; 128:2723–2730.
31. Kasperk C, Helmboldt A. Borcsok I, Heuthe S, Cloos O, Niethard F, Ziegler R. Skeletal site dependent expression of the androgen receptor in human osteoblastic populations. Calcif Tissue Int 1997;61: 464–473.
32. Carrascosa A, Audi L, Ferrandez AM, Ballabriga A. Biological effects of androgens and identification of specific dihydrotestosterone-binding sites in cultured human fetal epiphyseal chondrocytes. J Clin Endocrinol Metab 1990;70:134–140.
33. Bellido T, Jilka RJ, Boyce BF, Girasole G, Broxmeyer H, Dalrymple SA, Murray R, Manolagas SC. Regulation of interleukin-6, osteoclastogenesis and bone mass by androgens: the role of the androgen receptor. J Clin Invest 1995;95:2886–2895.
34. Deslypere JP, Vermeulen A. Influence of age on steroid concentrations in skin and striated muscle in women and in cardiac muscle and lung tissue in men. J Clin Endocrinol Metab 1985;61:648–653.
35. Rajfer J, Namkung PC, Petra PH. Identification, partial characterization and age-related changes of a cytoplasmic androgen receptor in the rat penis. J Steroid Biochem 1980;13:1489–1492.

36. Roehrborn CG, Lange JL, George FW, Wilson JD. Changes in amount and intracellular distribution of androgen receptor in human foreskin as a function of age. J Clin Invest 1987;79:44–47.
37. Roth GS, Hess GD. Changes in the mechanisms of hormone and neurotransmitter action during aging: current status of the role of receptor and post-receptor alterations. A review. Mech Ageing Dev 1982;20:175–194.
38. Irvine RA, Ma H, Yu MC, Ross RK, Stallcup MR, Coetzee GA. Inhibition of p160-mediated coactivation with increasing androgen receptor polyglutamine length. Hum Mol Genet 2000;9:267–274.
39. Kazemiesfarjani P, Trifiro MA, Pinsky L. Evidence for a repressive function of the long polyglutamine tract in the human androgen receptor – possible pathogenetic relevance for the (CAG)(n)-expanded neuronopathies. Hum Mol Genet 1995;4:523–527.
40. Giovannucci E, Stampfer MJ, Krithivas K, Brown M, Dahl D, Brufsky A, Talcott J, Hennekens CH, Kantoff PW. The CAG repeat within the androgen receptor gene and its relationship to prostate cancer. Proc Natl Acad Sci USA 1997;94:8272.
41. Nelson WG, De Marzo AM, Isaacs WB. Prostate cancer. N Engl J Med 2003;349:366–381.
42. Eisman J, Kelly P, Morrison N, Pocock N, Yeoman R, Birmingham J, Sambrook P. Peak bone mass and osteoporosis prevention. Osteoporos Int 1993;3:56–60.
43. Heaney RP, Abrams S, Dawson-Hughes B, Looker A, Marcus R, Matkovic V, Weaver C. Peak bone mass. Osteoporos Int 2000;11:985–1009.
44. Martin A, Bailey D, McKay H, Whiting S. Bone Mineral and calcium accretion during puberty. Am J Clin Nutr 1997;66:611–615.
45. Bailey D, Martin A, McKay H, Whiting S, Mirwald R. Calcium accretion in girls and boys during puberty: a longitudinal analysis. J Bone Miner Res 2000;15:2245–2250.
46. Slemenda CW, Longcope C, Zhou L, Hui SL, Peacock M, Johnston CC. Sex steroids and bone mass in older men: positive associations with androgens. J Clin Invest 1997;100:755–759.
47. Greendale GA, Edelstein S, Barret-Connor E. Endogenous sex steroids and bone mineral density in older women and men: the Rancho Bernardo study. J Bone Miner Res 1997;12:1833–1843.
48. Khosla S, Melton LJ III, Atkinson EJ, O'Fallon WM, Klee GG, Riggs BL. Relationship of serum sex steroid levels and bone turnover markers with bone mineral density in men and women: a key role for bioavailable estrogens. J Clin Endocrinol Metab 1998;83:2266–2274.
49. Ongphiphadhanakul B, Rajatanavin R, Chaprasertyothin S, Piaseu N, Chailurkit L. Serum oestradiol and oestrogen-receptor gene polymorphism are associated with bone mineral density independently of serum testosterone in normal males. Clin Endocrinol (Oxford) 1998;19:803–809.
50. Gilberg P, Johansson AG, Ljunghall S. Decreased estradiol levels and free androgen index and elevated sex hormone-binding globulin in male idiopathic osteoporosis. Calcif Tissue Int 1999;64:209–213.
51. Center JR, Nguyen TV, Sambrook PN, Eisman JA. Hormonal and biochemical parameters in the determination of osteoporosis in elderly men. J Clin Endocrinol Metab 1999;84: 3626–3635.
52. Amin S, Zhang Y, Sawin CT, Evens SR, Hannan MT, Kiel DP, Wilson PWF, Felson DT. Association of hypogonadism and estradiol levels with bone mineral density in elderly men from the Framingham study. Ann Intern Med 2000;133:951–963.
53. Szulc P, Munoz F, Claustrat B, Garnero P, Marchand F, Duboeuf F, Delmas PD. Bioavailable estradiol may be an important determinant of osteoporosis in men. the MINOS study. J Clin Endocrinol Metab 2001;86:192–199.
54. Scopacasa F, Horowitz M, Wishart JM, Morris HA, Chatterton BE, Need AG. The relation between bone density, free androgen index, and estradiol in men 60 to 70 years old. Bone 2000;27:145–149.
55. Martinez Diaz Guerra G, Hawkins F, Rapado A, Ruiz diaz MA, Diaz. Hormonal and anthropometric predictors of bone mass in healthy elderly men: major effect of sex hormone binding globulin, parathyroid hormone and body weight. Osteoporosis Int 2001;12:178–184.
56. Khosla S, Melton LJ III, Riggs BL. Estrogens and bone health in men. Calcif Tissue Int 2001;69:189–192.
57. Goemaere S, Zmierczak H, Van Pottelbergh I, Toye K, Daems M, Kaufman JM. Free or bioavailable estradiol is a determinant of bone loss in community-dwelling elderly men: a longitudinal study. J Bone Miner Res 2001;10:Abstract S355.
58. Legrand E, Hedde C, Gallois Y, Degasne I, Boux De Casson F, Mathieu E, Basle MF, Chappard D, Audran M. Osteoporosis in men: a potential role for the sex hormone binding globulin. Bone 2001;29:90–95.

59. Van Den Beld AW, De Jong FH, Grobbee DE, Pols HAP, Lamberts SWJ. Measures of bioavailable serum testosterone and estradiol and their relationships with muscle strength, bone density, and body composition in elderly men. J Clin Endocrinol Metab 2000;85:3275–3282.
60. Lormeau C, Soudan B, D'Herbomez M, Pigny P, Duquesnoy B, Cortet B. Sex hormone-binding globulin, estradiol, and bone turnover markers in male osteoporosis. Bone 2004;34:933–939.
61. Center JR, Nguyen TV, Sambrook PN, Eisman JA. Hormonal and biochemical parameters and osteoporotic fractures in elderly men. J Bone Miner Res 2000;15:1405–1411.
62. Evans SF, Davie MW. Low body size and elevated sex hormone binding globulin distinguish men with idiopathic vertebral fracture. Calcif Tissue Int 2002;70:9–15.
63. Rubenstein HS, Salomon ML, The growth depressing effect of large doses of testosterone propionate in the castrate albino rat. Endocrinology 1941;28:112–114.
64. Clein LJ, Kowalewski K. Some effects of cortisone and an anabolic steroid on healing of experimental fractures. Can J Surg 1962;5:108–117.
65. Wiancko KB, Kowalewski K. Strength of callus in fractured humerus rat treated with anti-anabolic and anabolic compounds. Acta Endocrinol (Copenh) 1961;36:310–318.
66. Chesnut CH, Ivey, Gruber HE, Matthews M, Nelp WB, Sisom K, Baylink DJ. Stanozolol in postmenopausal osteoporosis: therapeutic efficacy and possible mechanism of action. Metabolism 1983;32:571–580.
67. Manolagas SC. Birth and death of bone cells: basic regulatory mechanisms and implications for the pathogenesis and treatment of osteoporosis. Endocr Rev 2000;21:115–137.
68. Kousteni S, Bellido T, Plotkin LI, O'Brien Ca, Bodenner DL, Han K, DiGregorio GB, Katzenellenbogen JA, Katzenellenbogen BS, Roberson PK, Weinstein RS, Jilka RL, Manolagas SC. Nongenotropic, sex-nonspecific signaling through the estrogen and androgen receptors: dissociation of transcriptional activity. Cell 2001;104:719–730.
69. Kousteni S, Chen JR, Bellido T, Han L, Ali AA, O'Brien CA, Plotkin L, Fu Q, Mancino AT, Wen Y, Vertino AM, Powers CC, Stewart SA, Ebert R, Parfitt AM, Weinstein RS, Jilka RL, Manolagas SC. Reversal of bone loss in mice by nongenotropic signaling of sex steroids. Science 2002;298: 843–846.
70. Falahati-Nini A, Riggs BL, Atkinson EJ, O'Fallon WM, Eastell E, Khosla S. Relative contributions of testosterone and estrogen in regulating bone resorption and formation in normal elderly men. J Clin Invest 2000;106:1533–1560.
71. Finkelstein JA, Klibanski A, Neer RM, Doppelt SH, Rosenthal DI, Serge GV, Crowley WF Jr. Increases in bone density during treatment of mean with idiopathic hypogonadism hypogonadism. J Clin Endocrinol Metab 1989;69:776–783.
72. Guo CY, Jones TH, Eastell R. Treatment of isolated hypogonadotropic hypogonadism effect on bone mineral density and bone turnover. J Clin Endocrinol Metab 1997;82:658–665.
73. Foresta C, Ruzza G, Mioni R, Meneghello A, Baccichetti C. Testosterone and bone loss in Klinefelter. Horm Metabol Rex 1983;15:56–57.
74. Stepan JJ, Lachman M, Zverina J, Pacovsky V, Baylink DJ. Castrated men exhibit bone loss: effect of calcitonin treatment of biochemical indices of bone remodelling. J Clin Endocrinol Metab 1989;69: 523–527.
75. Greenspan SL, Oppenheim DS, Klibanski A. Importance of gonadal steroids to bone mass in men with hyperprolactemic hypogonadism. Ann Intern Med 1989;110:526–531.
76. Rigotti NA, Neer RM, Jameson L. Osteopenia and bone fractures in a man with anorexia nervosa and hypogonadism. JAMA 1986;256:385–388.
77. Goldray D, Weisman Y, Jaccard N, Merdler C, Chen J, Matzkin H. Decreased bone density in elderly men treated with gonadotropin-releasing hormone agonist decapeptyl (D-Trp^6-GnRH). J Clin Endocrinol Metab 1993;76:288–290.
78. Stoch SA, Parker RA, Chen L, Bubley G, Ko YJ, Vincelette A, Greenspan SL. Bone loss in men with prostate cancer treated with gonadotropin-releasing hormone agonists. J Clin Endocrinol Metab 2001;2787–2791.
79. Diamond TH, Higano CS, Smith MR, Guise TA, Singer FR. Osteoporosis in men with prostate carcinoma receiving androgen-deprivation therapy: recommendations for diagnosis and therapies. Cancer 2004;100:892–899.

80. Finkelstein JS, Klibanski A, Neer RM, Greenspan SL, Rosenthal DI, Crowley WF Jr. Osteoporosis in men with idiopathic hypogonadotropic hypogonadism. Ann Int Med 1987;106:354–361.
81. Finkelstein JS, Neer RM, Biller BMK, Crawford JD, Klibanski A. Osteopenia in men with a history of delayed puberty. N Engl J Med 1992;326:600–604.
82. Katznelson L, Finkelstein JA, Schoenfeld DA, Rosenthal DI, Anderson EJ, Klibanski A. Increase in bone density and lean body mass during testosterone administration in men with acquired hypogonadism. J Clin Endocrinol Metab 1996;81:4358–4365.
83. Behre HM, Kliesch S, Leifke E, Link TM, Neischlag E. Long-term effect of testosterone therapy on bone mineral density in hypogonadal men. J Clin Endocrinol Metab 1997;82:2386–2390.
84. Snyder PJ, Peachey H, Berlin JA, Hannoush P, Haddad G, Dlewati A, Santanna J, Loh L, Lenrow DA, Holmes JH, Kapoor SC, Atkinson LE, Strom BL. Effects of testosterone replacement in hypogonadal men. J Clin Endocrinol Metab 2000;85:2670–2677.
85. Venken K, De Gendt K, Boonen S, Ophoff J, Bouillon R, Swinnen JV, Verhoeven G, Vanderschueren D. Relative impact of androgen and estrogen receptor in the effects of androgens on trabecular and cortical bone in growing mice: a study in the androgen receptor knock-out mouse model. J Bone Miner Res 2006;21:576–585.
86. Turner RT, Hannon KS, Demers LM, Buchaman J, Bell NH. Differential effects of gonadal function in bone histomorphometry in male and female rats. J Bone Miner Res 1989;4: 557–563.
87. Vanderschueren D, Van Herck E, Nijs J, Ederveen AG, De Coster R, Bouillon R. Aromatase inhibition impairs skeletal modelling and decreases bone mineral density in growing male rats. Endocrinology 1997;6:2301–2307.
88. Martin RB. Aging and changes in cortical mass and structure. In: Orwoll ES, ed. Osteoporosis in men: the effects of gender on skeletal health. San Diego: Academic Press, 1999:111–128.
89. Rogol AD. Androgens and puberty. Mol Cell Endocrinol 2002;198:25–29.
90. Vanderschueren D, Vandeput L, Boonen S, Lindberg MK, Bouillon R, Ohlsson C. Androgen and bone. Endocr Rev 2004;25:389–425.
91. Turner RT, Wakley GK, Hannon KS. Differential effects of androgens on cortical bone histomorphometry in gonadectomized male and female rats. J Orthop Res 1990;8:612–617.
92. Zhang XZ, Kaly DN, Erbas B, Hopper JL, Seeman E. The effects of gonadectomy on bone size, mass and volumetric density in growing rats are gender-, site- and growth hormone-specific. J Bone Miner Res 1999;14:802–809.
93. Lorentson M, Swanson C, Andersson N, Mellströ m D, Ohlsson C. Free testosterone is a positive, whereas free estradiol is a negative predictor of corticol bone size in young Swedish men: The GOOD study. J Bone Miner Res 2005;20:1334–1341.
94. Vanderschueren D, Van Herck E, Suiker AM, Visser WJ, Schot LP, Chung K, Lucas RS, Einhorn RA, Bouillon R. Bone and mineral metabolism in the androgen-resistant (testicular feminized) male rat. J Bone Miner Res 1993;8:801–809.
95. Vandeput L. Swinnen JV, Boonen S. Van Herck E, Erben RG, Bouillon R, Vanderschueren D. Role of the androgen receptor in skeletal homeostasis: the androgen-resistant testicular feminized male mouse model. J Bone Miner Res 2004;19:1462–1470.
96. Kawano H, Sato T, Yamada T, Matsumoto T, Sekine K, Watanabe T, Nakamura T, Fukuda T, Yoshimura K, Yoshizawa T, Aihara K, Yamamoto Y, Nakamichi Y, Metzger D, Chambon P, Nakamura K, Kawaguchi H, Kato S. Suppressive function of androgen receptor in bone resorption. Proc Natl Acad Sci USA 2003;100:9416–9421.
97. Marcus R, Leary D, Schneider DL, Shane E, Favus M, Quigley CA. The contribution of testosterone to skeletal development and maintenance: lessons from the androgen insensitivity syndrome. J Clin Endocrinol Metab 2000;85:1032–1037.
98. Munoz-Torres M, Jodar E, Quesada M, Escobar-Jemenez F. Bone mass in androgen-insensitivity syndrome: response to hormonal replacement therapy. Calcif Tissue Int 1995;57:94–96.
99. Soule SG, Conway G, Prelevic GM, Prentice M, Ginsburg J, Jacobs HS. Osteopenia as a feature of the androgen insensitivity syndrome. Clin Endocrinol (Oxf) 1995;43:671–675.
100. Bertelloni S, Baroncelli GI, Federico G, Cappa M, Lala R, Saggese G. Altered bone mineral density in patients with complete androgen insensitivity syndrome. Horm Res 1998;50:309–314.

101. Schwartz BD, Zhy Y-S, Cordero J, Imperato-McGinley J. 5α-reductase deficiency and complete androgen insensitivity: natural models to suggest a direct role for androgens on bone density in men (Abstract OR23-1). Proc of the 81th annual Meeting of the Endocrine Society (1999).
102. Riggs BL, Khosla S, Melton LJ III. Sex steroids and the construction and conservation of the adult skeleton. Endocr Rev 2002;23:279–302.
103. Tabensky A, Duan Y, Edmonds J, Seeman E. The contribution of reduced peak accrual of bone and age-related bone loss to osteoporosis at the spine and hip: insights from the daughters of women with vertebral and hip fractures. J Bone Miner Res 2001;16:1101–1107.
104. Hui SL, Slemenda C, Johnston CC Jr. The contribution of bone loss to postmenopausal osteoporosis. Osteoporos Int 1990;1:30–34.
105. Kelly PJ, Morrison NA, Sambrook PN, Nguyen TV, Eisman JA. Genetic influences on bone turnover, bone density and fracture. Eur J Endocrinol 1995;133:265–271.
106. Matkovic V, Jelic T, Wardlaw GM, Ilich JZ, Goel PK, Wright JK, Andon MB, Smith KT, Heaney RP. Timing of peak bone mass in Caucasian females and its implication for the prevention of osteoporosis: inference from a cross-sectional model. J Clin Invest 1999;93:788–808.
107. Parsons TJ, Prentice A, Smith EA, Cole TJ, Compston JE. Bone mineral mass consolidation in young British adults. J Bone Miner Res 1992;11:264–274.
108. Recker R, Davies M, Hinders SM, Heaney RP, Stegman MR, Kimmel DB. Bone gain in young adult women. JAMA 1992;268:2403–2408.
109. Slosman DO, Rizzoli R, Pichard C, Donath A, Bonjour JP. Longitudinal measurement of regional and whole body bone mass in young healthy adults. Osteoporos Int 1994;4:185–190.
110. Kroger H, Kotaniemi A, Vainio P, Alhava E. Bone densitometry of the spine and femur in children by dual-energy X-ray absorptiometry. Bone Miner 1992, 17:75–85.
111. Gilsanz V, Skaggs DL, Kovanlikaya A, Sayre J, Loro ML, Kaufman F, Korenman SG. Differential effect of race on the axial and appendicular skeleton of children. J Clin Endocrinol Metab 1994;83: 1420–1427.
112. Gilsanz V, Boechat MI, Roe RF, Loro ML, Sayre JW, Goodman WG. Gender differences in vertebral body size in children and adolescents. Radiology 1999;190:673–677.
113. Mora S, Pitukcheewanont P, Kaufman FR, Nelson JC, Gilsanz V. Biochemical markers of bone turnover and the volume and the density of bone in children at different stages of sexual development. J Bone Miner Res 1997;14:1664–1671.
114. Katzman DK, Bachrach LK, Carter DR, Marcus R. Clinical and anthropometric correlates of bone mineral acquisition in healthy adolescent girls. J Clin Endocrinol Metab 1996;73:1332–1339.
115. Lu PW, Cowell CT, Lloyd-Jones SA, Briody JN, Howmen-Giles R. Volumetric bone mineral density in normal subjects, aged 5–27 years. J Clin Endocrinol Metab 2000;81:1586–1590.
116. Boot AM, de Ridder MAJ, Pols HAP, Krenning EP, de Muinck Keizer-Schrama SMPF. Bone mineral density in children and adolescents: relation to puberty, calcium intake and physical activity. J Clin Endocrinol Metab 1997;82:57–62.
117. Bass S, Delmas PD, Pearce G, Hendrich E, Tabensky A, Seeman E. The differing tempo of growth in bone size, mass and density in girls is region-specific. J Clin Invest 1988;104:795–804.
118. Henry YM, Fatayerji D, Eastell R. Attainment of peak bone mass at the lumbar spine, femoral neck and radius in men and women: relative contributions of bone size and volumetric bone mineral density. Osteoporos Int 2004;15:263–273.
119. Gilsanz V, Kovanlikaya A, Costin G, Roe TF, Sayre J, Kaufman F. Differential effect of gender on the sizes of the bones in the axial and appendicular skeleton. J Clin Endocrinol Metab 1984;82:1603–1607.
120. Taylor J, Twomey LT. Sexual dimorphism in human vertebral body shape? J Anat 1986;138:281–286.
121. Veldhuizen AG, Baas P, Webb PJ. Observations on the growth of the adolescent spine. J Bone Joint 1999;68B:724–728.
122. Vega E, Ghiringhelli G, Mautalen C, Valzacchie GR, et al. Bone mineral density and bone size in men with primary osteoporosis and vertebral fractures. Calcif Tissue Int 1995;62:465–469.
123. Gilsanz V, Luiza Loro M, Roe TF, Sayre J, Gilsanz R, Schulz EE. Vertebral size in elderly women with osteoporosis. J Clin Invest 1996;95:2332–2337.
124. Seeman E, Duan Y, Fong C, Edmonds J. Fracture site-specific deficits in bone size and volumetric density in men with spine and hip fractures. J Bone Miner Res 2001;16:120–127.

125. Duan Y, Parfitt AM, Seeman E. Vertebral bone mass, size and volumetric density in women with spinal fractures. J Bone Mineral Res 1999;14:1796–1802.
126. Hangartner T, Gilsanz V. Evaluation of cortical bone by computed tomography. J Bone Miner Res 1996;11:1518–1525.
127. Faulkner RA, Bailey DA, Drinkwater DT, McKay HA, Arnold C, Wilkinson AA. Bone densitometry in Canadian children 8–17 years of age. Calcif Tissue Int 1991;59:344–351.
128. Beck TJ, Ruff CB, Scott WW Jr, Plato CC, Tobin JD, Quan CA. Sex differences in geometry of the femoral neck with aging: a structural analysis of bone mineral data. Calcif Tissue Int 1998;50:24–29.
129. Peacock M, Carey GLM, Ambrosius W, Turner Ch, Hui S, Johnston CC Jr. Bone mass and structure at the hip in men and women over the age of 60 years. Osteoporos Int 1996;8:231–239.
130. Zamberlan N, Radetti G, Paganini C, Rossini M, Braga V, Adami S. Evaluation of the cortical thickness and bone density by roentgen microdensitometry in growing males and females. Eur J Pediatr 1996;155:377–382.
131. Garn SM. Changes at the subperiosteal surface. In: The earlier gain and later loss of cortical bone. Springfield: CC Thomas, 1992.
132. Rauch F, Neu C, Manz F, Schoenau E. The development of metaphyseal cortex – implications for distal radius fractures during growth. J Bone Miner Res 2001;16:1547–1555.
133. Schoenau E, Neu CM, Rauch F, Manz F. The development of bone strength at the proximal radius during childhood and adolescence. J Clin Endocrinol Metab 2001;86:613–618.
134. Israel H. Progressive enlargement of the vertebral body as part of the process of human skeletal aging. Age Aging 1990;2:71–79.
135. Mosekilde L, Mosekilde L. Sex difference in age related changes in vertebral body size, density and biomechanical competence in normal individuals. Bone 1992;11:67–73.
136. Garn SM, Sullivan TV, Decker SA, Larkin FA, Hawthorne VM. Continuing bone expansion and increasing bone loss over a two-decade period in men and women from a total community sample. Am J Hum Biol 1988;4:57–67.
137. Ruff CD, Hayes WC. Sex differences in age-related remodeling of the femur and tibia. J Orthoped Res 1999;6:886–896.
138. Libanati C, Baylink DJ, Lois-Wenzel E, Srinivasan N, Mohan S. Studies on the potential mediators of skeletal changes occurring during puberty in girls. J Clin Endocrinol Metab 1995;84:2807–2814.
139. Garn SM, Rhomann CG, Nolan P Jr. The developmental nature of bone changes during aging. In: Birren JE, ed. Relations of development and aging. N.H.: Ayer North Stratford, 1980:41–61.
140. Haapasalo H, Kannus P, Sievanen H, Pasanen M, UusiRasi K, Heinonen A, Oja P, Vuori I. Development of mass, density, and estimated mechanical characteristics of bones in Caucasian females. J Bone Miner Res 1996;11:1751–1760.
141. Bonjour JP, Thientz G, Buchs B, Slosman D, Rizzoli R. Critical years and stages of puberty for spinal and femoral bone mass accumulation during adolescence. J Clin Endocrinol Metab 1992;73: 555–556.
142. Geusens P, Cantatore F, Nijs J, Proesmans W, Emma F, Dequeker J. Heterogeneity of growth of bone in children at the spine, radius and total skeleton. Growth Dev Aging 1999;55:249–256.
143. Hui SL, Zhou L, Evans R, Slemenda CW, Peacock M, Weaver CM, McClintock C, Johnston CC. Rates of growth and loss of bone mineral in the spine and femoral neck in white females. Osteoporos Int 1992;9:200–205.
144. Parfitt AM. The physiology and clinical significance of bone histomorphometric data. In: Recker RR, ed. Bone histomorphometry: techniques and interpretation, Boca Raton: CRC Press, 143–223.
145. Bradney M, Karlson MK, Duan Y, Stuckey S, Bass S, Seeman E. Heterogeneity in the growth of the axial and appendicular skeleton in boys: implications for the pathogenesis of bone fragility in men. J Bone Miner Res 1996;15:1871–1878.
146. Mann T, Oviatt SK, Wilson D, Nelson D, Orwoll ES. Vertebral deformity in men. J Bone Miner Res 1992;7:1259–1265.
147. Marshall D, Johnell O, Wedel H. Meta-analysis of how well measures of bone mineral density predict occurrence of osteoporotic fractures. Br Med J 1996;312:1254–1259.
148. Kleerekoper M,Villanueva AR,Stanciu J, Rao DS, Parfitt AM. The role of three-dimensional trabecular microstructure in the pathogenesis of vertebral compression fractures. Calcif Tissue Int 1985;37:594–597.

149. Recker RR. Architecture and vertebral fracture. Calcif Tissue Int 1993;53:S139–S142.
150. Legrand E, Chappard D, Basle MF, Audran M. Evaluation of trabecular microarchitecture. Prospects for predicting the risk of osteoporosis and fracture. Rev Rhum Engl Ed 1999;66:543–547.
151. Benito M, Gomberg B, Wehrli FW, Weening RH, Zemel B, Wright AC, Song HK, Cucchiara A, Snyder PJ. Deterioration of trabecular architecture in hypogonadal men. J Clin Endocrinol Metab 2003;88: 1497–1502.
152. Ito M, Nakamura T, Tsurusaki K, Uetani M, Hayashi K. Effects of menopause on age-dependent bone loss in the axial and appendicular skeletons in healthy Japanese women. Osteoporos Int 1999;10:377–383.
153. Majumdar S, Kothari M, Augat P, Newitt DC, Link TM, Lin JC, Lang T, Lu Y, Genant HK. High-resolution magnetic resonance imaging: three-dimensional trabecular bone architecture and biomechanical properties. Bone 1998;22:445–454.
154. Gordon CL, Webber CE, Nicholson PS. Relation between image-based assessment of distal radius trabecular structure and compressive strength. Can Assoc Radiol J 1998;49:390–397.
155. Oden ZM, Selvitelli DM, Hayes WC, Myers ER. The effect of trabecular structure on DXA-based predictions of bone failure. Calcif Tissue Int 1998;63:67–73.
156. Ulrich D, van Rietbergen B, Laib A, Ruegsegger P. The ability of three-dimensional structural indices to reflect mechanical aspects of trabecular bone. Bone 1999;25:55–60.
157. Devogelaer JP, Crabbé J, Deuxchaisnes CN de. Bone mineral density in Addison's disease: evidence of an effect on adrenal androgens on bone mass. Br Med J 1987;294:798–800.
158. Florkowski CM, Holmes SJ, Elliot JR, Donald RA, Espiner EA. Bone mineral density is reduced in female but not male subjects with Addison's disease. NZ Med J 1994;107:52–53.
159. Zelissen PMJ, Croughs RJM, Van Rijk JK, Raymakers JA. Effects of glucocorticoids replacement therapy on bone mineral density in patients with Addison's disease. Ann Intern Med 1994;120:207–210.
160. Valero Ma, Leon M, Ruiz Valdepenas MPR, Larrodera L, Lopez MB, Papapietro K, Jara A, Hawkins F. Bone density and turnover in Addison's disease: effect of glucocorticoid treatment. Bone Miner 1994;26:9–17.
161. Braatvedt GD, Joyce M, Evans M, Clearwater J, Reid IR. Bone mineral density in patients with Addison's disease. Osteoporos Int 1999;10:435–440.
162. Buchanan JR, Myers C, Lloyd T, Leuenberger P, Demers LM. Determinants of peak trabecular bone density in women: the role of androgens, estrogen, and exercise. J Bone Miner Res 1988;3:673–680.
163. Deutsch S, Benjamin F, Seltzer V, Tafreshi M, Kocheril G, Frank A. The correlation of serum estrogen and androgens with bone density in the late menopause. Int J Gynaecol Obstet 1987;25:217–222.
164. Haden ST, Glowacki J, Hurwitz S, Rosen C, LeBoff MS. Effects of age and serum dehydroepiandrosterone sulphate, IGF-I and IL-6 levels in women. Calcif Tissue 2000;66:414–418.
165. Miller KK, Biller BMK, Hier J, Arena E, Klibansky A. Androgens and bone density in women with hypopituitarism. J Clin Endocrinol Metab 2002;87:2770–2776.
166. Dixon JE, Rodin A, Murby B, Chapman MG, Fogelman I. Bone mass in hirsute women with androgen excess. Clin Endocrinol 1989;30:271–277.
167. Dagogo-Jack S, Al-Ali N, Qurttom M. Augmentation of bone mineral density in hirsute women. J Clin Endocrinol Metab 1997;82:2821–2825.
168. Good C, Tulchinsky M, Mauger D, Derners LM, Legro RS. Bone mineral density and body composition in lean women with polycystic ovary syndrome. Fertil Steril 1990;72:21–25.
169. Slemenda C, Longcope C, Peacock M, Hui S, Johnston C. Sex steroids, bone mass, and bone loss. A prospective study of pre-, peri- and postmenopausal women. J Clin Invest 1996;97:14–21.
170. Greendale G, Edelstein S, Barrett-Connor E. Endogenous sex steroids and bone mineral density in older women: the Rancho Bernardo Study. J Bone Miner Res 1997;12:1833–1843.
171. Need GA, Horowitz M, Bridges A, Diprad A, Morris HA, Nordin CN. Effects of nandrolone decanoate and anti-resorptive therapy on vertebral density in osteoporotic women. Arch Intern Med 1989;149: 57–60.
172. Christiansen C, Riis BJ. 17β-estradiol and continuous norethisterone: a unique treatment for established osteoporosis in elderly women. J Clin Endocrinol Metab 1990;71:836–841.
173. Raisz LG, Wiita B, Artis A, Bowen A, Schwartz S, Trahiotis M, Shoukri K, Smith J. Comparison of the effects of estrogen alone and estrogen plus androgen on biochemical markers of bone formation and resorption in postmenopausal women. J Clin Endocrinol Metab 1996;81:37–43.

174. Cann CE, Martin MC, Genant HK, Jaffe RB. Decreased spinal mineral content in amenorrheic women. JAMA 1994;251:626–629.
175. Guleki B, Davies MC, Jacobs HS. Effects of treatment on established osteoporosis in young women with amenorrhea. Clin Endocrinol 1994;41:275–281.
176. Davies MC, Guleki B, Jacobs HS. Osteoporosis in Turner's syndrome and other forms of primary amenorrhea. Clin Endocrinol 1995;43:741–746.
177. Bonjour JP, Theintz G, Buchs B, Slosmans D, Rizzoli. Critical years and stages of puberty for spinal and femoral bone mass accumulation during adolescence. J Clin Endocrinol Metab 1991;73: 555–563.
178. Theintz G, Buchs B, Rizzoli R, Slosman D, Clavien H, Sizonenko PC, Bonjour JP. Longitudinal monitoring of bone mass accumulation in healthy adolescents; evidence for a marked reduction after 16 year of age at the levels of lumbar spine and femoral neck in female subjects. J Clin Endocrinol Metab 1992 75:1060–1065.
179. Takahaski Y, Minamitani K, Kobayashi Y, Minagawa M, Yasuda T, Niimi H. Spinal and femoral bone mass accumulation during normal adolescence: comparison with female patients with sexual precocity and with hypogonadism. J Clin Endocrinol Metab 1996;81:1248–1253.
180. Bradney M, Karlsson MK, Duan Y, Stuckey S, Bass S, Seeman E. Heterogeneity in the growth of the axial and appendicular skeleton in boys: Implications for the pathogenesis of bone fragility in men. J Bone Miner Res 2000;15:1871–1878.
181. Sigurjonsdottir TJ, Hayles AB. Precocious puberty: a report of 96 cases. Am J Dis Child 1968, 115:309.
182. Jones-Klingensmith G, Carcia SC, Jones HW, Migeon CJ, Blizzard RM. Glucocorticoid treatment of girls with congenital adrenal hyperplasia: effect on height, sexual maturation and fertility. J Pediatr 1977,90:996.
183. Urban MD, Lee PA, Migeon CJ. Adult height and fertility in men with congenital virilizing adrenal hyperplasia. N Engl J Med 1978;299:1392.
184. Di Martino-Nardi J, Stoner E, O'Connell A, New MI The effect of treatment on final height in classical congenital adrenal hyperplasia. Acta Endocrinol (Copenh) (Suppl) 1986;279:305.
185. Cooper C, Dennison EM, Leufkens HG, Bishop NJ, van Staa TP. Epidemiology of childhood fractures in Britain. A study using the general practice research database. J Bone Miner Res 2004;19: 1976–1981.
186. Seeman E, Karlsson M, Duan Y. On exposure to anorexia nervosa, the temporal variation in axial and appendicular skeleton development predisposes to site-specific deficits in bone size and density: a cross-sectional study. J Bone Miner Res 2000;15:2259–2265.
187. Bass S, Bradney M, Pearce G, Hendrich E, Stuckey S, Seeman E. Short stature and delayed puberty: influence of selection bias on leg length and reduced energy intake on trunk length in gymnasts. J Pediatr 2000;136:149–155.
188. Ristevski S, Yeung S, Poon C, Wark J, Ebeling P. Osteopenia is common in young first-degree male relatives of men with osteoporosis. ANZBMS, Australia: Annual Scientific Meeting, 7:65.
189. Van Pottelbergh I, Goemaere S, Zmierczak H, De Bacquer D, Kaufman JM. Deficient acquisition of bone during maturation underlies idiopathic osteoporosis in men: evidence from a three-generation family study. J Bone Miner Res 2003;18:303–311.
190. Gilsanz V, Gibbens DT, Roe TF, Carloson M, Senac MO, Boechat MI, Huang HK, Schulz EE, Libanati CR, Cann CC. Vertebral bone density in children: effect of puberty. Radiology 1988;166:847–850.
191. Krabbe S. Christiansen C, RØ dbro P, TransbØ l I. Effect of puberty on rates of bone growth and mineralization: with observations in male delayed puberty. Arch Dis Child 1979;54:950–953.
192. Krabbe S, Christiansen C. Longitudinal study of calcium metabolism in male puberty. I. Bone mineral content and serum levels of alkaline phosphatase, phosphate and calcium. Acta Pediatr Scan 1984;73:745–749.
193. Rosenfield RL. Diagnosis and management of delayed puberty. J Clin Endocrinol Metab 1990;70: 559–562.
194. Seeman E. From density to structure: growing up and growing old on the surfaces of bone. J Bone Miner Res 1997;12:509–521.
195. Tanner JM, Davies PSW. Clinical longitudinal standards for height and height velocity for North American children. J Pediatr 1985;107:317–329.

196. Bertolloni S, Baroncelli GI, Ferdeghini M, Perri G, Saggese G. Normal volumetric bone mineral density an bone turnover in young men with histories of constitutional delay of puberty. J Clin Endocrinol Metab 1998;83:4280–4283.
197. Finkelstein JS, Klibanski A, Neer RM. A longitudinal evaluation of bone mineral density in adults with histories of delayed puberty. J Clin Endocrinol Metab 1996;81:1152–1155.
198. Yap F, Hogler W, Briody J, Moore B, Howman-Giles R, Cowell CT. The skeletal phenotype of men with previous constitutional delay of puberty. J Clin Endocrinol Metab 2004;89:4306–4311.
199. Kindblom JM, Lorentzon M, Norjavaara E, Hellqvist A, Nilsson S, Mellströ m D, Ohlsson C. Pubertal timing predicts previous fractures and BMD in young adult men: the GOOD study. J Bone Miner Res 2006;21:790–795.
200. Warren MP, Brooks-Gunn J, Hamilton LH, Warren LF, Hamilton WG. Scoliosis and fractures in young ballet dancers: relation with delayed menarche and secondary amenorrhea. N Engl J Med 1986;314: 1348–1353.
201. Dhuper S, Warren MP, Brooks-Gunn J, Fox R. Effects of hormonal status on bone density in adolescent girls. J Clin Endocrinol Metab 1990;71:1083–1088.
202. Sims AN, Clement-Lacroix P, De Ponte F, Bouali Y, Binart N, Moriggl R, Goffin V, Coschigano K, Gaillard-Kelly M, Kopchick J, Baron R, Kelly PA. Bone homeostasis in growth hormone receptor-null mice in restored by IGF-I but independent from stat5. J Clin Invest 2000;106:1095–1103.
203. Tanner JM, Whitehouse RH, Marubini E, Resele LF. The adolescent growth spurt of boys and girls of the Harpenden growth study. Ann Hum Biol 1976;3:109–126.
204. Blizzard RM, Thompson RG, Baghdassarian A, Kowarski A, Migeon CJ, Rodriguez A. The interrelationship of steroids, growth hormone and other hormones on pubertal growth. In: Grumbach MM, Grave GD, Mayer FE, eds. The control of the onset of puberty. New York: John Wiley & Sons, 1974:342.
205. Laron Z, Pertzelan A, Mannheimer S. Genetic pituitary dwarfism with high serum concentration of GH. A new inborn error of metabolism. Israel J Med Sci 1966;2:15.
206. Martin LG, Clark JW, Connor TB. Growth hormone secretion enhanced by androgens. J Clin Endocrinol Metab 1968;28:425
207. Martin LG, Grossman MS, Connor TB, Levitsky LL, Clark JW, Camitta FD. Effect of androgen on growth hormone secretion and growth in boys with short stature. Acta Endocrinol (Copenh) 1979;91: 201–212.
208. Illig R, Prader A. Effect of testosterone on growth hormone secretion in patients with anorchia and delayed puberty. J Clin Endocrinol Metab 1970;20:615.
209. Wiedeman E, Schwartz F, Frantz AG. Acute and chronic estrogen effects upon serum somatomedin activity, growth hormone and prolactin in man. J Clin Endocrinol Metab 1976;42:942–952.
210. Moll G, Rosenfield RL, Fang VS. Administration of low-dose estrogen rapidly and directly stimulates growth hormone production. Am J Dis Child 1986;140:124–127.
211. Meyer WJ, Furlanetto RW, Walker PA. The effect of sex steroids on radioimmunoassayable plasma somatomedin-C concentrations. J Clin Endocrinol Metab 1982;55:1184–1187.
212. Ho YK, Evans WS, Blizzard RM, Veldhuis JD, Merriam GR, Samojlik E, Furlanetto R, Rogol AD, Kaiser DL, Thorner MO. Effects of sex and age on the twenty-four-hour profile of growth hormone secretion in man: importance of endogenous estradiol concentrations. J Clin Endocrinol Metab 1987;64: 51–58.
213. Mauras N, Blizzard RM, Link K, Johnson ML, Rogol AD, Veldhuis JD. Augmentation of growth hormone secretion during puberty: evidence for a pulse amplitude-modulated phenomenon. J Clin Endocrinol Metab 1987;64:596–601.
214. Rosenfield RL, Furlanetto R, Bock D. Relationship of somatomedin-C concentrations to pubertal changes. J Pediatr 1983;103:723–728.
215. Parker MW, Johanson AJ, Rogol AD, Kaiser DL, Blizzard RM. Effects of testosterone on somatomedin-C concentrations in prepubertal boys. J Clin Endocrinol Metab 1984;58:87–90.
216. Ross JL, Cassorla FG, Skerda MC, Valk IM, Loriaux DL, Cutler GB. A preliminary study of the effect of estrogen dose on growth in Turner's syndrome. N Engl J Med 1983;39:1104–1106.
217. Cuttler L, Van Vliet G, Conte FA, Kaplan SL, Grumbach M. Somatomedin-C levels in children and adolescents with gonadal dysgenesis: differences from age-matched normal females and effect of chronic replacement therapy. J Clin Endocrinol Metab 1985;60:1087–1092.

218. Bourguignon JP. Linear growth as a function of age at onset of puberty and sex steroid dosage: therapeutic implications. Endocr Rev 1988;9:467–488.
219. Styne DM. The regulation of pubertal growth. Horm Res 2003;60(suppl 1):22–26.
220. Frost HM. Bone "mass" and the "mechanostat": a proposal. Anat Rec 1987;219:1–9.
221. Frost HM. A determinant of bone architecture. The minimum effective strain. Clin Orthop Relat Res 1983;175:286–292.
222. Ferretti JL, Capozza RF, Cointry GR, Garcia SL, Plotkin H, Alvarez Filgueira ML, Zanchetta JR. Gender-related differences in the relationship between densitometric values of whole-body bone mineral density and lean body mass in humans between 2 and 87 years of age. Bone 1998;22:683–690.
223. Knothe-Tate M, Steck R, Forwood M, Niederer P. In vivo demonstration of load-induced fluid flow in the rat tibia and its potential implications for processes associated with functional adaptation. J Exp Biol 2000;203:2737–2745.
224. Frost HM. The mechanostat: a proposed pathogenic mechanism of osteoporoses and the bone mass effects of mechanical and nonmechanical agents. Bone Miner 1987;2:73–85.
225. Burr DB. Orthopedic principle of skeletal growth, modelling, and remodelling. In: Carlson D, Goldstein S, eds. Bone biodynamics in orthodontic and orthopedic treatment. Ann Arbor, MI, USA: University of Michigan, 15–51.
226. Biewener AA, Taylor CR. Bone strain: a determinant of gait and speed? J Exp Biol 1986;123:383–400.
227. Turner CH. Three rules for bone adaptation to mechanical stimuli. Bone 1998;23:399–407.
228. Dickinson JA, Cook SD, Leinhardt TM. The measurements of shock waves following heel strike in running. J Biochem 1985;18:415–422.
229. Smeathers JE. Transient vibrations caused by heel strike. Proc Inst Mech Engin 1989;203:181–186.
230. Vuori I. Peak bone mass and physical activity: a short review. Nutr Rev 1996;54:S11–S14.
231. Fuchs RK, Bauer JJ, Snow CM. Jumping improves hip and lumbar spine bone mass in prepubescent children: a randomized controlled trial. J Bone Miner Res 2001;16:148–156.
232. Bradney M, Pearce G, Naughton G, Sullivan C, Bass S. Beck T, Carlson J, Seeman E. Moderate exercise during growth in prepubertal boys: changes in bone mass, volumetric density and bone strength. A controlled prospective study. J Bone Miner Res 1998;13:1814–1821.
233. MacKelvie KJ, Petit MA, Khan KM, Beck TJ, McKay HA. Bone mass and structure are enhanced following a 2-year randomized controlled trial of exercise in prepubertal boys. Bone 2004;34: 755–764.
234. Petit MA, McKay HA, MacKelvie KJ, Heinonen A, Khan KM, Beck TJ. A randomized school-based jumping intervention confers site and maturity-specific benefits on bone structural properties in girls: A hip structural analysis study. J Bone Miner Res 2002;17:363–372.
235. Bass SL, Saxon L, Daly RM, Turner CH, Robling AG, Seeman E, Stuckey S. The effect of mechanical loading on the size and shape of bone in pre-, peri- and postpubertal girls: a study in tennis players. J Bone Miner Res 2002;12:2274–2280.
236. Fuchs RK, Bauer JJ, Snow CM. Jumping improves hip and lumbar spine bone mass in prepubescent children: a randomized controlled trial. J Bone Miner Res 2001;16:148–156.
237. Nordstrom P, Pettersson U, Lorentzon R. Type of physical activity, muscle strength and pubertal stage as determinants of bone mineral density and bone area in adolescent boys. J Bone Miner Res 1998;13: 1141–1148.
238. Bailey DA, McKay HA, Mirwald RL, Crocker PR, Faulkner RA. A six-year longitudinal study of the relationship of physical activity to bone mineral accrual in growing children: the university of Saskatchewan bone mineral accrual study. J bone Mineral Res 1999;14:1672–1679.
239. Chesnut CH III. Is osteoporosis a pediatric disease? Peak bone mass attainment in the adolescent female. Public Health Rep 1989;104:50–54.
240. Gustavsson A, Thorsen K, Nordstrom P. A 3 year longitudinal study on the effect of physical activity on the accrual of bone mineral density in healthy adolescent males. Calcif Tissue Int 2003;73:108–114.
241. Forwood MR, Baxter-Jones AD, Beck TJ, Mirwald RL, Howard A, Bailey DA. Physical activity and strength of the femoral neck during the adolescent growth spurt. A longitudinal analysis. Bone 2006:38:576–583.
242. Frost HM. On our age-related bone loss: insights from a new paradigm. J Bone Miner Res. 1997;12: 1539–1546.

243. Lu RW, Taylor SK, O'Connor JJ, Walker PS. Influence of muscle activity on the forces in the femur: an in vivo study. J Biochem 1997;30:1101–1106.
244. Rauch F, Bailey D, Baxter-Jones A, Mirwald R, Faulkner R. The "muscle-bone unit" during the pubertal growth spurt. Bone 2004;34:771–775.
245. Ward KA, Roberts SA, Adams JE, Mughal MZ. Bone geometry and density in the skeleton of pre-pubertal gymnasts and school children. Bone 2005;36:1012–1018.
246. Turner CH, Burr DB. Basic biomechanical measurement of bone: a tutorial. Bone 1993:14:595–608.
247. Hind K, Burrows M. Weight-bearing exercise and bone mineral accrual in children and adolescents. A review of controlled trials. Bone 2007;40:14–27.
248. Galbo H, Hummer L, Petersen IB, Christiensen NJ, Bie N. Thyroid and testicular responses to graded and prolonged exercise in men. Eur J Appl Physiol 1977;36:101–106.
249. Hakkinen K, Pakarinen A. Acute hormonal responses to two different fatiguing heavy-resistance protocols in male athletes. J Appl Physiol 1993:74:882–887.
250. Fahrner CL, Hackney AC. Effects of endurance exercise of free testosterone concentration and the binding affinity of sex hormone binding globulin (SHBG). Int J Sports Med 1998;19:12–15.
251. MacConnie SE, Barkan A, Lampman RM, Schork MA, Beitins IZ. Decreased hypothalamic gonadotrophin-releasing hormone secretion in male marathon runners. N Engl J Med 1986;315:411–417.
252. MacDougall JD, Webber CE, Martin J, Ormerod S, Chesley A, Younglai EV, Gordon L, Blimkie CJR. Relationship among running mileage, bone density, and serum testosterone in male runners. J Appl Physiol 1992;73:1165–1170.
253. Wheeler GD, Singh M, Pierce WD, Epling WF, Cumming DC. Endurance training decreases serum testosterone levels in men without change in luteinizing hormone pulsatile release. J Clin Endocrinol Metab 1991;72:422–425.
254. De Souza MJ, Arce JC, Pescatello LS, Sherzer HS, Luciano A. Gonadal hormones and semen quality in male runners. Int J Sports Med 1994;15:383–391.
255. Smith R, Rutherford OM. Spine and total bone mineral density and serum testosterone levels in male athletes. Eur J Appl Physiol Occup Physiol 1993;67:330–334.
256. Hoogeveen AR, Zonderblad ML. Relationship between testosterone, cortisol and performance in professional cyclists. Int J Sports Med 1996;17:423–428.
257. Cann CE, Martin MC, Genant HK, Jaffe RB. Decreased spinal mineral content in amenorrheic women. JAMA 1984;251;626–629.
258. Robinson TL, Snow-Harter C, Taffe G, Gillis D, Shaw J, Marcus R. Gymnast exhibit higher bone mass than runners despite similar prevalence of amenorrhea and oligomenorrhea. J Bone Miner Res 1995;10:26–35.
259. Maïmoun L, Lumbroso S, Manetta J, Paris F, Leroux JL, Sultan C. Testosterone is significantly reduced in endurances athletes without impact on bone mineral density. Horm Res 2003;59:285–292.
260. Guéguen R, Jouanny P, Guilleming F, Kuntz C, Pourel J, Siest G. Segregation analysis and variance components analysis of bone mineral density in healthy families. J Bone Miner Res 1995;10: 2017–2022.
261. Pocock NA, Eisman JA, Hopper JL, Yates MG, Sambrook PN, Eberl S. Genetic determinants of bone mass in adults: a twin study. J Clin Invest 1987;80:706–710.
262. Benoit FL, Theil GB, Watten RH. Titel Metabolism 1963;12:1072–1082.
263. Taylor HS, Block K, Bick DP, Shering RJ. Layman LC. Mutation analysis of the EMX2 gen in Kallmann's syndrome. Fertility and Sterility 1999;72:910–914.
264. Brown TR, Lubahn DB, Wilson EM, Joseph DR, French FS, Migeon CJ. Deletion of the steroid-binding domain of the human androgen receptor gene in one family with complete androgen insensitivity: evidence for further genetic heterogeneity in this syndrome. Proc Natl Acad Sci USA 1988;85:8152–8155.
265. Morris JM. The syndrome of testicular feminization in male pseudohermaphrodites. Am J Obstet Gynecol 1953;65:1192–1211.
266. Quigley CA, De Bellis A, Marschke KB, El-Awady MK, Wilson EM, French FS. Androgen receptor defects: historical, clinical and molecular perspectives. Endocr Rev 1995;16:271–316.
267. French FS, Baggett B, Van Wyk JJ, Talbert LS, Hubbard WR, Johnston FR, Weaver RP. Testicular feminization: clinical, morphological and biochemical studies. J Clin Endocrinol Metab 1965;25: 661–677.

268. MacDonald PC, Madden JD, Brenner PF, Wilson JD, Siiteri PK. Origin of estrogen in normal men and in women with testicular feminization. J Clin Endocrinol Metab 1979;49:905–916.
269. Zitzmann M, Brune M, Kornmann B, Gromoll J, Junker R, Nieschlag E. The CAG repeat polymorphism in the androgen receptor gene affects bone density and bone metabolism in healthy males. Clin Endocrinol 2001;55:649–657.
270. Sowers M, Willing M, Burns T, Deschenes S, Hollis B, Curtchfield M, Jannausch M. Genetic markers, bone mineral density and serum osteocalcin levels. J Bone Miner Res 1999;14:1411–1419.
271. Remes T, Väisänen SB, Mahonen A, Huuskonen J, Kröger H, Jurvelin JS, Penttilä IM, Rauramaa R. Aerobic exercise and bone mineral density in middle-aged Finnish men: a controlled randomized trial with reference to androgen receptor, aromatase, and estrogen receptor α gene polymorphisms Bone 2003;32:412–420.
272. Van Pottelbergh I, Lumbroso S, Goemaere S, Sultan C, Kaufman JM. Lack of influence of the androgen receptor gene CAG-repeat polymorphism on sex steroid status and bone metabolism in elderly men. Clin Endocrinol 2001;55:659–666.
273. Crabbe P, Bogaert V, De Bacquer D, Goemaere S, Zmierczak H, Kaufman JM. Part of the interindividual variation in serum testosterone levels in healthy men reflects differences in androgen sensitivity and feedback set point: contribution of the androgen receptor polyglutamine tract polymorphism. J Clin Endocrinol Metab 2007;92:3604–3610.
274. Simpson ER, Zhao Yn, Agarwal VR, Michael MD, Bulun SE, Hinshelwood MM, Graham-Lorence S, Sun T, Fisher CR, Qin K, Mendelson CR. Aromatase expression in health and disease. Recent Prog Horm Rex 1997;52:185–213.
275. Polymeropoulos MH, Xiao H, Rath DS, Merril CR. Tetranucleotide repeat polymorphism at the human cytochrome P-450 gene (CYP19). Nucl Acids Res 1991;19:4792–4792.
276. Haiman CA, Hankinson SE, Spiegelman D, De Vivo I, Colditz GA, Willett WC, Speizer FE, Hunter DJ. A tetranucleotide repeat polymorphism in CUP19 and breast cancer risk. Int J Cancer 2000;87: 204–210.
277. Masi L, Becherini L, Gennari L, Amedei A, Colli E, Falchetti A, Farci M, Silvestri S, Gonnelli S, Brandi ML. Polymorphism of the aromatase gene in postmenopausal Italian women: distribution and correlation with bone mass and fracture risk. J Clin Endocrinol Metab 2001;86:2263–2269.
278. Van Pottelbergh I, Goemaere S, Kaufman JM. Bioavailable estradiol and an aromatase gene polymorphism are determinants of bone mineral density changes in men over 70 years of age. J Clin Endocrinol Metab 2003;88:3075–3081.
279. Gennari L, Becherini L, Merlotti D, Masi L, Lucani B, Gonnelli S, Falchetti A, Dal Conto N, Nuti R, Gennari C, Brandi ML. Body mass index and circulating testosterone modulate the effect of aromatase gene polymorphism on bone in elderly men. J Bone Miner Res 2002 15(suppl 1): M121 (abstract).
280. Eriksson S, Eriksson A, Stege R, Carlström K. Bone mineral density in patients with prostatic cancer treated with orchidectomy and with estrogens. Calcif Tissue Int 1995;57:97–99.
281. Daniell HW. Osteoporosis after orchiectomy for prostate cancer. J Urol 1997;157:439–444.
282. Moul JW. Contemporary hormonal management of advanced prostate cancer. Oncology 1998;12: 499–505.
283. Robson M, Dawson N. How is androgen-dependent metastatic prostate cancer best treated? Hematol Oncol Clin North Am 1996;10:727–747.
284. Hoff AO, Gagel RF. Osteoporosis in breast and prostate cancer survivors. Oncology 2005;19: 651–658.
285. Maillefert JF, Sibilia J, Michel F, Saussine C, Javier RM, Tavernier C. Bone mineral density in men treated with synthetic gonadotropin-releasing hormone agonists for prostatic carcinoma. J Urol 1999;161: 1219–1222.
286. Higano CS. Understanding treatments for bone loss and bone metastases in patients with prostate cancer: a practical review and guide for the clinician. Urol Clin North Am 2004;31:331–352.
287. Townsend MF, Sanders WH, Northway RO, Graham SD Jr. Bone fractures associated with luteinizing hormone-releasing hormone agonists used in the treatment of prostate carcinoma. Cancer 1997;79: 545–550.
288. Shahinian VB, Kuo YF, Freeman JL, Goodwin JS. (2005) Risk of fracture after androgen deprivation for prostate cancer. N Engl J Med 2005;352:154–164.

289. Jackson JA, Kleerkper M, Parfitt AM, Rao DS, Villanueva AR, Frame B. Bone histomorphometry in hypogonadal and eugonadal men with spinal osteoporosis. J Clin Endocrinol Metab 1987;65:53–58.
290. Francis RM, Peacock M, Aaron JE, Selby PL, Taylor GA, Thompson J, Marshall DH, Horsman A. Osteoporosis in hypogonadal men: role of decreased plasma 1,25 dihydroxyvitamin D, Calcium malabsorption, and low bone formation. Bone 1986;7:261–268.
291. Horowitz M, Wishart JM, O'Loughlin PD, Morris HA, Need AG, Nordin BE. Osteoporosis and Klinefelter's syndrome. Clin Endocrinol 1992;36:113–118.
292. Orwoll ES, Klein RF. Osteoporosis in men. Endocr Rev 1995;16:87–116.
293. Kelepouris N, Harper KD, Gannon F, Kaplan JG. Severe osteoporosis in men. Ann Intern Med 1995;123:452–460.
294. Stanley HL, Schmitt BP, Poses RM, Deiss WP. Does hypogonadism contribute to the occurrence of a minimal trauma hip fracture in elderly men? J Am Geriatr Soc 1991;39:766–771.
295. Bass S, Delmas PD, Pearce G, Hendrich E, Tabensky A, Seeman E. The differing tempo of growth in bone size, mass and density in girls is region-specific. J Clin Invest 1999;104:795–804.
296. Garn SM. The course of bone gain and the phases of bone loss. Orthop Clin North Am. 1972;3:503–520.
297. Szulc P, Seeman E, Duboeuf F, Sornay-Rendu E. Delmas PD. Bone fragility: failure of periosteal apposition to compensate for increased endocortical resorption in postmenopausal women. J Bone Mineral Res 2006;21:1856–1863.
298. Szulc P. Delmas PD, Bone loss in elderly men: increased endosteal bone loss and stable periosteal apposition. The prospective MINOS study. Osteoporos Int 2007;18:495–503.
299. Schönau E, Neu CM, Rauch F, Manz F. The development of bone strength at the proximal radius during childhood and adolescence. J Clin Endocrinol Metab 2001;86:613–618.
300. Kaufman JM, Vermeulen A. The decline of androgen levels in elderly men and its clinical and therapeutic implications. Endocr Rev 2005;26:833–876.
301. Oden A, Dawson A, Dere W, Johnell O, Jonsson B, Kanis JA. Lifetime risk of hip fractures is underestimated. Osteoporosis Int 1998;8:599–603.
302. Cooper C, Campion G, Melton LJ. Hip-fractures in the elderly – A worldwide projection. Osteoporosis Int 1992;2:285–289.
303. Felsenberg D, Silman AJ, Lunt M, Armbrecht G, Ismail AA, Finn JD, Cockerill WC, Banzer D, Benevolenskaya LI, Bhalla A, Bruges AJ, Cannata JB, Cooper C, Dequeker J, Eastell R, Felsch B, Gowin W, Havelka S, Hoszowski K, Jajic I, Janott J, Johnell O, Kanis JA, Kragl G, Lopes VA, Lorenc R, Lyritis G, Masaryk P, Matthis C, Miazgowski T, Parisi G, Poor G, Raspe HH, Reid DM, Reisinger W, Scheidt-Nave C, Stepan JJ, Todd CJ, Weber K, Woolf AD, Yershova OB, Reeve J, O'Neill TW. Incidence of vertebral fracture in Europe: results from the European Prospective Osteoporosis Study (EPOS). J Bone Miner Res 2002;17:716–724.
304. Van der Klift M, De Laet CEDH, McCloskey EV, Hofman A, Pols HAP. The incidence of vertebral fractures in men and women: The Rotterdam Study. J Bone Miner Res 2002;17:1051–1056.
305. Center JR, Nguyen TV, Schneider D, Sambrook PN, Eisman JA. Mortality after all major types of osteoporotic fracture in men and women: an observational study. Lancet 1999;353:878–882.
306. Poor G, Atkinson EJ, Lewallen DG, OFallon WM, Melton LJ. Age-related hip fractures in men: Clinical spectrum and short-term outcomes. Osteoporosis Int 1995;5:419–426.
307. Stoch SA, Parker RA, Chen LP, Bubley G, Ko YJ, Vincelette A, Greenspan SL. Bone loss in men with prostate cancer treated with gonadotropin-releasing hormone agonists. J Clin Endocrinol Metab 2001;86:2787–2791.
308. Mittan D, Lee S, Miller E, Perez RC, Basler JW, Bruder JM. Bone loss following hypogonadism in men with prostate cancer treated with GnRH analogs. J Clin Endocrinol Metab 2002;87:3656–3661.
309. Riggs BL, Khosla S, Melton LJ. Sex steroids and the construction and conservation of the adult skeleton. Endocr Rev 2002;23:279–302.
310. Khosla S, Melton LJ III, Riggs BL. Clinical review 144: Estrogen and the male skeleton. J Clin Endocrinol Metab 2002;87:1443–1450.
311. Meier DE, Orwoll ES, Keenan EJ, Fagerstrom RM. Marked decline in trabecular bone mineral content in healthy men with age: lack of association with sex steroid levels. J Am Geriatr Soc 1987;35:189–197.
312. Drinka PJ, Olson J, Bauwens S, Voeks SK, Carlson I, Wilson M. Lack of association between free testosterone and bone density separate from age in elderly males. Calcif Tissue Int 1993;52:67–69.

313. Clarke BL, Ebeling PR, Jones JD, Wahner HW, O'Fallon WM, Riggs BL, Fitzpatrick LA. Changes in quantitative bone histomorphometry in aging healthy men. J Clin Endocrinol Metab 1996;81: 2264–2270.
314. van den Beld AW, de Jong FH, Grobbee DE, Pols HA, Lamberts SW. Measures of bioavailable serum testosterone and estradiol and their relationships with muscle strength, bone density, and body composition in elderly men. J Clin Endocrinol Metab 2000;85:3276–3282.
315. Rudman D, Drinka PJ, Wilson CR, Mattson DE, Scherman F, Cuisinier MC, Schultz S. Relations of endogenous anabolic hormones and physical activity to bone mineral density and lean body mass in elderly men. Clin Endocrinol 1994;40:653–661.
316. Murphy S, Khaw KT, Cassidy A, Compston JE. Sex hormones and bone mineral density in elderly men. Bone Miner 1993;20:133–140.
317. Kenny AM, Gallagher JC, Prestwood KM, Gruman CA, Raisz LG. Bone density, bone turnover, and hormone levels in men over age 75. J Gerontol A Biol Sci Med Sci 1998;53:M419–M425.
318. Greendale GA, Edelstein S, Barrett-Connor E. Endogenous sex steroids and bone mineral density in older women and men: the Rancho Bernardo Study. J Bone Miner Res 1997;12:1833–1843.
319. Khosla S, Melton LJ III, Atkinson EJ, O'Fallon WM, Klee GG, Riggs BL. Relationship of serum sex steroid levels and bone turnover markers with bone mineral density in men and women: a key role for bioavailable estrogen. J Clin Endocrinol Metab 1998;83:2266–2274.
320. Slemenda CW, Longcope C, Zhou LF, Hui SL, Peacock M, Johnston CC. Sex steroids and bone mass in older men – Positive associations with serum estrogens and negative associations with androgens. J Clin Invest 1997;100:1755–1759.
321. Center JR, Nguyen TV, White CP, Eisman JA. Male osteoporosis predictors: Sex hormones and calcitropic hormones. J Bone Miner Res 1997;12(supplement):F569.
322. Ongphiphadhanakul B, Rajatanavin R, Chanprasertyothin S, Piaseu N, Chailurkit L. Serum oestradiol and oestrogen-receptor gene polymorphism are associated with bone mineral density independently of serum testosterone in normal males. Clin Endocrinol 1998;49:803–809.
323. Amin S, Zhang YQ, Sawin DT, Evans SR, Hannan MT, Kiel DP, Wilson PWF, Felson DT. Association of hypogonadism and estradiol levels with bone mineral density in elderly men from the Framingham study. Ann Int Med 2000;133:951–963.
324. Szulc P, Munoz F, Claustrat B, Garnero P, Marchand F, Duboeuf F, Delmas PD. Bioavailable estradiol may be an important determinant of osteoporosis in men: The MINOS study. J Clin Endocrinol Metab 2001;86:192–199.
325. Van Pottelbergh I, Goemaere S, Kaufman JM. Bioavailable estradiol and an aromatase gene polymorphism are determinants of bone mineral density changes in men over 70 years of age. J Clin Endocrinol Metab 2003;88:3075–3081.
326. Szulc P, Claustrat B, Marchand F, Delmas PD. Increased risk of falls and increased bone resorption in elderly men with partial androgen deficiency: The MINOS study. J Clin Endocrinol Metab 2003;88: 5240–5247.
327. Goemaere S, Van P, I, Zmierczak H, Toye K, Daems M, Demuynck R, Myny H, De Bacquer D, Kaufman JM. Inverse association between bone turnover rate and bone mineral density in community-dwelling men >70 years of age: no major role of sex steroid status. Bone 2001;29:286–291.
328. Szulc P, Kaufman JM, Delmas PD. Biochemical assessment of bone turnover and bone fragility in men. Osteoporos Int 2007;18:1451–1461.
329. Khosla S, Melton LJ III, Riggs BL. Clinical review 144: estrogen and the male skeleton. J Clin Endocrinol Metab 2002;87:1443–1450.
330. Khosla S, Melton LJ, Atkinson EJ, O'Fallon WM. Relationship of serum sex steroid levels to longitudinal changes in bone density in young versus elderly men. J Clin Endocrinol Metab 2001;86:3555–3561.
331. Gennari L, Masi L, Merlotti D, Picariello L, Falchetti A, Tanini A, Mavilia C, Del Monte F, Gonnelli S, Lucani B, Gennari C, Brandi ML. A polymorphic CYP19 TTTTA repeat influences aromatase activity and estrogen levels in elderly men: effects on bone metabolism. J Clin Endocrinol Metab 2004;89: 2803–2810.
332. Zitzmann M, Brune M, Kornmann B, Gromoll J, Junker R, Nieschlag E. The CAG repeat polymorphism in the androgen receptor gene affects bone density and bone metabolism in healthy males. Clin Endocrinol 2001;55:649–657.

333. Van Pottelbergh I, Lumbroso S, Goemaere S, Sultan C, Kaufman JM. Lack of influence of the androgen receptor gene CAG-repeat polymorphism on sex steroid status and bone metabolism in elderly men. Clin Endocrinol 2001;55:659–666.
334. Falahati-Nini A, Riggs BL, Atkinson EJ, O'Fallon WM, Eastell R, Khosla S. Relative contributions of testosterone and estrogen in regulating bone resorption and formation in normal elderly men. J Clin Invest 2000;106:1553–1560.
335. Doran PM, Riggs BL, Atkinson EJ, Khosla S. Effects of raloxifene, a selective estrogen receptor modulator, on bone turnover markers and serum sex steroid and lipid levels in elderly men. J Bone Miner Res 2001;16:2118–2125.
336. Center JR, Nguyen TV, Sambrook PN, Eisman JA. Hormonal and biochemical parameters in the determination of osteoporosis in elderly men. J Clin Endocrinol Metab 1999;84:3626–3635.
337. Gennari L, Merlotti D, Martini G, Gonnelli S, Franci B, Campagna S, Lucani B, Dal Canto N, Valenti R, Gennari C, Nuti R. Longitudinal association between sex hormone levels, bone loss, and bone turnover in elderly men. J Clin Endocrinol Metab 2003;88:5327–5333.
338. Stanley HL, Schmitt BP, Poses RM, Deiss WP. Does hypogonadism contribute to the occurrence of a minimal trauma hip fracture in elderly men? J Am Geriatr Soc 1991;39:766–771.
339. Boonen S, Vanderschueren D, Cheng XG, Verbeke G, Dequeker J, Geusens P, Broos P, Bouillon R. Age-related (type II) femoral neck osteoporosis in men: Biochemical evidence for both hypovitaminosis D- and androgen deficiency-induced bone resorption. J Bone Miner Res 1997;12:2119–2126.
340. Jackson JA, Riggs MW, Spiekerman AM. Testosterone deficiency as a risk factor for hip fractures in men: a case–control study. Am J Med Sci 1992;304:4–8.
341. Barrett-Connor E, Mueller JE, von Muhlen DG, Laughlin GA, Schneider DL, Sartoris DJ. Low levels of estradiol are associated with vertebral fractures in older men, but not women: the Rancho Bernardo Study. J Clin Endocrinol Metab 2000;85:219–223.
342. Goderie-Plomp HW, Van der Klift M, de Ronde W, Hofman A, de Jong FH, Pols HAP. Endogenous sex hormones, sex hormone-binding globulin, and the risk of incident vertebral fractures in elderly men and women: The Rotterdam Study. J Clin Endocrinol Metab 2004;89:3261–3269.
343. Mellstrom Dn Johnell, Ljunggren O, Eriksson AL, Lorentzon M, Mallmin H, Holmberg A, Redlund-Johnell I, Orwoll E, Ohlsson C. Free testosterone is an independent predictor of BMD and prevalent fractures in elderly men: MrOS Sweden. J Bone Miner Res 2006;21:529–535.
344. Tenover JS. Androgen administration to aging men. Endocrin Metab Clin North Am 1994;23:877–892.
345. Swerdloff RS, Wang C. Androgens and aging in men. Exp Gerontol 1993;28:435–446.
346. Vermeulen A, Goemaere S, Kaufman JM. Sex hormones, body composition and aging. Aging Male 2003;2:8–16.
347. Katznelson L, Rosenthal DI, Rosol MS, Anderson EJ, Hayden DL, Schoenfeld DA, Klibanski A. Using quantitative CT to assess adipose distribution in adult men with acquired hypogonadism. Am J Roentgenol 1998;170:423–427.
348. Tzankoff SP, Norris AH. Effect of muscle mass decrease on age-related BMR changes. J Appl Physiol 1977;43:1001–1006.
349. Forbes GB, Reine JC. Adult lean body mass declines with age: some longitudinal observations. Metabolism 1970;19:653–667.
350. Larsson L, Grimby G, Karlsson J. Muscle strength and speed of movement in relation to age and muscle morphology. J Appl Physiol 1979;46:451–456.
351. Roy TA, Blackman MR, Harman SM, Tobin JD, Schrager M, Metter EJ. Interrelationships of serum testosterone and free testosterone index with FFM and strength in aging men. Am J Physiol Endocrinol Metab 2002;283:E284–E294.
352. Orwoll E, Lambert LC, Marshall LM, Blank J, Barrett-Connor E, Cauly J, Ensrud K, Cummings SR. Endogenous testosterone levels, physical performance and fall risk in older men. Arch Intern Med 2006;166:2124–2131.
353. Abbasi AA, Drinka PJ, Mattson DE, Rudman D. Low circulating levels of insulin-like growth factors and testosterone in chronically institutionalized elderly men. J Am Geriatr Soc 1993;41:975–982.
354. Baumgartner RN, Waters DL, Gallagher D, Morley JE, Garry PJ. Predictors of skeletal muscle mass in elderly men and women. Mech Ageing Dev 1999;107:123–136.
355. Orwoll ES. Androgens: basic biology and clinical implication. Calcif Tissue Int 2001;69:185–188.

356. Bahsin S, Bremmer WJ. Clinical review 85: emerging issues in androgen replacement therapy. J Clin Endocrinol Metab 1997;82:3–8.
357. Aynsley-Green A, Zachmann, M, Prader. Interrelation of the therapeutic effects of growth hormone and testosterone on growth in hypopituitarism. J Pediatr 1976;89:992–999.
358. Burns EC, Tanner JM, Preece MA, Cameron N. Final height and pubertal development in 55 children with idiopathic growth hormone deficiency, treated for between 2 and 15 years with human growth hormone. Eur J Pediatr 1981;137:155–164.
359. Bourguignon PJ, Vandeweghe M, Vanderschueren-Lodeweyckx, Malvaux P, Wolter R, Du Caju M, Ernould C. Pubertal growth and final height in hypopituitary boys: a minor role of bone age at onset of puberty. J Clin Endocrinol Metab 1986;63:376–382.
360. Ranke MB, Butenandt O. Idiopathic growth hormone deficiency: final height to treatment with growth hormone and effects of puberty and sex steroids. In: Firsch H, Laron Z, eds. Induction of puberty in hypopituitarism. Serono Symposia review 16, Aris-Serono Symposia, Rome, p 85.
361. Lenko HL, Leisti S, Perheentupa J. The efficacy of growth hormone in different types of growth failure. An analysis of 101 cases. Eur J Pediatr 1982;138:241–249.
362. Joss E, Zuppinger K, Scharz HP, Roten H. Final height of patients with pituitary growth failure and changes in growth variables after long-term hormonal therapy. Pediatr Res 1983;17:676–679.
363. Zachmann M, Ferrandez A, Mürset G, Prader A. Testosterone treatment of excessively tall boys. J Pediatr 1976;88:116–123.
364. Wickman S, Sipila I, Ankarberg-Lindgren C, Norjavaara E, Dunkel L. A specific aromatase inhibitor and potential increase in adult height in boys with delayed puberty: a randomised controlled trial. Lancet 2001;357:1743–1748.
365. Jain P, Rademaker AW, McVary KT. Testosterone supplementation for erectile dysfunction: results of meta-analysis. J Urol 2000;164:371–375.
366. Bhasin S, Singh AB, Mac RP, Carter B, Lee MI, Cunningham GR. Managing the risks of prostate disease during testosterone replacement therapy in older men: recommendations for a standardized monitoring plan. J Androl 2003;24:299–311.
367. Rhoden EL, Morgentaler A. Medical progress: risk of testosterone-replacement therapy and recommendations for monitoring. N Engl J Med 2004;350:482–492.
368. Bhasin S. Testosterone supplementation for aging-associated sarcopenia. J Gerontol A Biol Sci 2004;58:1002–1008.
369. Basaria S, Dob AS. Hypogonadism and androgen replacement therapy in elderly men. Am J Med 2001;110:563–572.
370. Snyder PJ. Effects of age on testiscular function and consequences of testosterone treatment. J Clin Endocrinol Metab 2001;86:2369–2372.
371. Tan RS, Culberson JW. An integrative review on current evidence of testosterone replacement for the andropause. Maturitas 2003;45:15–27.
372. Vastag B. Many questions, few answers for testosterone replacement therapy. JAMA 2003;289: 971–972.
373. Liu PY, Swerdloff RS, Veldhuis JD. The rationale, efficacy and safety of androgen therapy in older men: future research and current practice recommendations. J Clin Endocrinol Metab 2004;89: 4789–4796.
374. Gruenewald DA, Matsumoto AM. Testosterone supplementation therapy for older men: potential benefits and risks. J Am Geriatr Soc 2003;51:101–115.
375. Liberman C, Blazer D. Testosterone and aging: clinical research directions. Washington DC: The National Academic Press.
376. Behre HM, Kliesch S, Leifke E, Link TM, Nieschlag E. Long-term effect of testosterone therapy on bone mineral density in hypogonadal men. J Clin Endocrinol Metab 1997;82:2386–2390.
377. Aminorroaya A, Kelleher S, Conway AJ, Ly LP, Handelsman DJ. Adequacy of androgen replacement influences bone density response to testosterone in androgen-deficient men. Eur J Endocrinol 2005;152:881–886.
378. Schubert M, Bullmann C, Minneman T, Reiners C, Krone W, Jockenhövel F. Osteoporosis in male hypogonadism: responses to androgen substitution differ among men with primary and secondary hypogonadism. Horm Res 2003;60:21–28.

379. Benito M, Vasilic B, Wehrli FW, Bunker B, Wald M, Bomberg B, Wright AC, Zemel B, Cucchiara, Snyder PJ. Effect of testosterone replacement of trabecular architecture in hypogonadal men. J Bone Mineral Res 2005;20:1785–1791.
380. Crawford BAL, Liu PY, Kean MT, Bleasel JF, Handelsman DJ. Randomized placebo-controlled trial of androgen effects on muscle and bone in men requiring long-term systemic glucocorticoid treatment. J Clin Endocrinol Metab 2003;88:3167–3176.
381. Reid IR, Wattie DJ, Evans MC, Stapleton JP. Testosterone therapy in glucocorticoid-treated men. Arch Intern Med 1996;156:1173–1177.
382. Howell SJ, Radford JA, Adams JE, Smets EMA, Warburton R, Shalet SM. Randomized placebo-controlled trial of testosterone replacement in men with mild Leydig cell insufficiency following cytotoxic chemotherapy. Clin Endocrinol 2001; 315–324.
383. Sih R, Morley JE, Kaiser FE, Perry HM, Patrick P, Ross C. Testosterone replacement in older hypogonadal men: a 12 month randomized controlled study. J Clin Endocrinol Metab 1997;82:1661–1667.
384. Wang C, Alexander G, Berman N, Salehian B, Davidson T, McDonald V, Steiner B, Hull L, Callegari C, Swerdloff RS. Testosterone replacement therapy improves mood in hypogonadal men – a clinical research center study. J Clin Endocrinol Metab 1996;81:3578–3583.
385. Page ST, Amory JK, DuBois Bowman F, Anawalt BD, Matsumoto AM, Bremmer WJ, Tenover JL. Exogenous testosterone (T) alone or with finasteride increases physical performance, grip strength and lean body mass in older men with low serum T. J Clin Endocrinol Metab 2005;90:1502–1510.
386. Amory JK, Watts NB, Easley KA, Sutton PR, Anawalt BD, Matsumoto AM, Bremmer WJ, Tenover JL. Exogenous testosterone or testosterone with finasteride increase bone mineral density in older men with low serum testosterone. J Clin Endocrinol Metab 2004;89:503–510.
387. Wang C, Swerdloff RS, Iranmanesh A, Dobs A, Snyder PJ, Cunningham G, Matsumoto AM, Weber T, Berman N and the Testosterone Gel Study Group. Effects of transdermal testosterone gel on bone turnover markers and bone mineral density in hypogonadal men. Clin Endocrinol 2001;54:739–750.
388. Bhasin S, Storer TW, Berman N, Callegari C, Clevenger B, Phillips J, Bunnell TJ, Tricker R, Shirazi A, Casaburi R. The effects of supraphysiologic doses of testosterone on muscle size and strength in normal men. N Engl J Med 1996;335:1–7.
389. Bhasin S, Woodhouse L, Casaburi R, Singh AB, Bhasin D, Berman N, Chen XH, Yarasheski KE, Magliano L, Dzekov C, Dezkov J, Bross R, Phillips J, Sinha-Hikim I, Shen RQ, Storer TW. Testosterone dose–response relationships in healthy young men. Am J Physiol Endocrinol Metab 2001;281: E1172–E1181.
390. Bhasin S, Woodhouse L, Casaburi R, Singh AB, Mac RP, Lee MI, Yarasheski KE, Sinha-Hikim I, Dzekov C, Dzekov J, Magliano L, Storer TW. Older men are as responsive as young men to the anabolic effects of graded doses of testosterone on the skeletal muscle. J Clin Endocrinol Metab 2005;90:678–688.
391. Ottenbacher KJ, Ottenbacher ME, Ottenbacher AJ, Acha AA, Ostir GV. Androgen treatment and muscle strength in elderly men: a meta-analysis. J Am Geriatr Soc 2006;54:1666–1673.
392. Isidori AM, Giannetta E, Greco EA, Gianfrilli D, Bonifacio V, Isidori A, Lenzi A, Fabbri A. Effects of testosterone on body composition, bone metabolism and serum lipid profile in middle-aged men: a meta-analysis. Clin Endocrinol 2005;63:280–293.
393. Tenover JS. Effects of testosterone supplementation in aging male. J Clin Endocrinol Metab 1992;75:1092–1098.
394. Morley JE, Perry HM, Kaiser FE, Kraenzle D, Jensen J, Houston K, Mattammal M, Perry HM. Effects of testosterone replacement therapy in old hypogonadal males: a preliminary study. J Am Geriatr Soc 1993;41:149–152.
395. Snyder PJ, Peachey H, Hannoush P, Berlin JA, Loh L, Holmes JH, Dlewati A, Staley J, Santanna J, Kapoor SC, Attie MF, Haddad JG, Strom BL. Effect of testosterone treatment on bone mineral density in men over 65 years of age. J Clin Endocrinol Metab 1999;84:1966–1972.
396. Christmas, O'Connor KG, Harman SM, Tobin JD, Munzer T, Bellantoni MF, Clair CS, Pabst KM, Sorkin JD, Blackman MR. Growth hormone and sex steroid effects on bone metabolism and bone mineral density in healthy aged women and men. J Gerontol A Biol Sci Med Sci 2002;57:M12–M18.
397. Kenney AM, Prestwood KM, Gruman CA, Marcello KM, Raisz LG. Effects of transdermal testosterone on bone and muscle in older men with low bioavailable testosterone levels. J Gerontol A Biol Sci Med Sci 2001;56:266–272.

398. Meier C, Miu PY, Ly LP, de Winter-Modezelewski J, Jimenez M, Handelsman DJ, Seibel MJ. Recombinant human chorionic gonadotropin but not dehydrotestosterone alone stimulates osteoblastic collagen synthesis in older men with partial age-related androgen deficiency. J Clin Endocrinol Metab 2004;89:3033–3041.
399. Seidman SN, Klein DF. AA2500 testosterone gel normalizes androgen levels in aging males with improvements in body composition and sexual function. J Clin Endocrinol Metab 2004;89:6358–6359.
400. van Kesteren, P, Lips, P, Gooren, LJ, Asscheman H, Megens J. Long term follow-up of bone mineral density in transsexuals treated with cross-sex hormones. Clin Endocrinol 1998;48:347–354.
401. Lips P, Asscheman H, Uitewaal P, Netelenbos JC, Gooren L. The effect of cross-gender hormonal treatment on bone metabolism in male-to-female transsexuals. J Bone Miner Res 1989;4:657–662.
402. van Kesteren P, Lips P, Deville W, Popp-Snijders C, Asscheman H, Megens J, Gooren L. The effect of one-year cross-sex hormonal treatment on bone metabolism and serum insulin-like growth factor-1 in transsexuals. J Clin Endocrinol Metab 1996;81:2227–2232.
403. Turner A, Chen TC, Barber TW, Malabanan AO, Holick MF, Tangpricha V. Testosterone increases bone mineral density in female-to-male transsexuals: a case series of 15 subjects. Clin Endocrinol (Oxf) 2004;61:560–566.
404. Goh HHV, Ratman SS. Effects of hormone deficiency, androgen therapy and calcium supplementation on bone mineral density in female transsexuals. Maturitas 1997;26:45–52.
405. Lips P, van Kesteren PJ, Asscheman H, Gooren LJ. The effect of androgen treatment on bone metabolism in female-to-male transsexuals. J Bone Miner Res 1996;11:1769–1773.
406. Vered I, Kaiserman I, Sela BA, Sack J. Cross genotype sex hormone treatment in two cases of hypogonadal osteoporosis. J Clin Endocrinol Metab 1997;82:576–578.
407 Orenteich N, Brind JL, Rizer Vogelman JH. Age changes and sex differences in serum dehydroepiandrosterone sulfate concentrations through adulthood. J Clin Endo Metab 1984;59:551–555.
408. Barrett-Connor E, Khaw K, Yen SSC. A prospective study of DS, mortality and cardiovascular risk. N Engl J Met 1986;315:1519–1924.
409. Helzsouer KJ, Gordon GB, Alberg A, Bush TL, Comstock GW. Relationship of prediagnostic serum levels of DHEA and DS to the risk of developing premenopausal breast cancer. Cancer Res 1992;52:1–4.
410. Carwoord EH, Bancroft J. Steroid hormones, the menopause, sexuality and well-being of women. Psychol Med 1996;26:925.
411. Morales A, Nolan J, Nelson J, Yen S. Effects of replacement dose of dehydroepiandrostenedione in men and women of advancing age. J Clin Endocrinol Metab 1994;78:1360–1367.
412. Morales AJ, Haubrich RH, Hwang JY, Asakura H, Yen SS. The effect of six months treatment with a 100 mg daily dose of dehydroepiandrostenedione (DHEA) on circulating sex steroids, body composition, muscle strength in age-advanced men and women. Clin Endocrinol 1998;49:421–432.
413. Yen SSC, Morales AJ, Khorram O. Replacement of DHEA in aging men and women. Ann NY Acad Sci 1995;774:128–142.
414. Mortola JF, Yen SSC. The effects of oral dehydroepiandrostenedione on endocrine-metabolic parameters in postmenopausal women. J Clin Endocrinol Metab 1990;71:696–704.
415. Pecheron G, Hogrel JY, Denot-ledunois S, Fayet G, Forette F, Baulieu EE, Fardeau M, Marini JF. Effect of 1-year oral administration of dehydroepiandrosterone to 60- to 80-year old individuals on muscle function and cross-sectional area: a double-blind placebo-controlled trial. Arch Intern Med 2003;163; 720–727.
416. Dayal M, Sammel MD, Zhao J, Hummel AC, Vandenbourne K, Barnhart KT. Supplementation of DHEA: effect on muscle size, strength, quality of life and lipids. J Women's Health 2005;14:391–400.
417. Albright F, Smith PH, Richardson AM. Postmenopausal osteoporosis: its clinical features. J Am Med Assoc 1941;116:2465–2474.
418. Riggs BL, Jowsey J, Goldsmith RS, Kelly PJ, Hoffman DL, Arnaud CD. Short and long-term effects of estrogen and synthetic anabolic hormone in postmenopausal osteoporosis. J Clin Invest 1972;51: 1659–1663.
419. Chesnut CH, Nelp WB, Baylink DJ, Demay JD. Effect of methandrostenolone on postmenopausal bone wasting as assessed by changes in total mineral mass. Metabolism 1977;26:276–277.
420. Aloia JF, Kappoor A, Vaswani A, Cohn SH. Changes in body composition following therapy of osteoporosis with methandrostenolone. Metabolism 1983;30:1076–1079.

421. Chesnut C, Ivey JL, Gruber HE, Matthews M, Nelp WB, Sisom K, Baylink DJ. Stanozolol in postmenopausal osteoporosis: therapeutic efficacy and possible mechanisms of action. Metabolism 1983;32:571–580.
422. Kopera H. The history of anabolic steroids and a review of clinical experience with anabolic steroids. Acta Endocrinol 1985;Suppl 271:11–18.
423. Dequeker J, Geusens P. Anabolic Steroids and osteoporosis. Acta Endocrinologica 1985;Suppl 271: 45–52.
424. Geusens P, Dequeker J. Long-term effect of nandrolone decanoate, 1α-hydroxyvitamin D_3, or intermittent calcium infusion therapy on bone mineral content, bone remodeling and fracture rate in symptomatic osteoporosis: a double-blind controlled study. Bone Mineral 1986;1:347–357.
425. Need AG, Chatterton BE, Walker CJ, Steuer TA, Horowitz M, Nordin BEC. Comparison of calcium, calcitriol ovarian hormones and nandrolone in the treatment of osteoporosis. Maturitas 1986;8:275–280.
426. Need AG, Morris HA, Hartley TF, Horowitz M, Nordin BEC. Effects of nandrolone decanoate on forearm mineral density and calcium metabolism in osteoporotic postmenopausal women. Calcif Tissue Int 1987;41:7–10.
427. Johansen JS, Hassager C, Podenphant J, Riis BJ, Hartwell D, Thomsen K, Christiansen C. Treatment of postmenopausal osteoporosis: is the anabolic steroid nandrolone decanoate a candidate ? Bone Miner 1989:6:77–86.
428. Grumbach MM. Estrogen, bone, growth and sex: a sea change in conventional wisdom. J Pediatr Endocrinol Metab 2000;13(suppl 6):1439–1455.
429. Wackley GK, Schutte HD Jr, Hannon KS, Turner RT. Androgen treatment prevents loss of cancellous bone in the orchidectomized rat. J Bone Miner Res 1991;6:325–330.
430. Sato T, Matsumoto T, Kawano H, Watanabe T, Uematsu Y, Sekine K, Fukuda T, Aihara K, Krust A, Yamada T, Nakamichi Y, Yamamoto Y, Nakamura T, Yoshimura K, Yoshizawa T, Metzger D, Chambon P, Kato S. Brain masculinization requires androgen receptor function. Proc Natl Acad Sci USA 2004;101:1673–1678.
431. Negro-Vilar A. Selective androgen receptor modulators (SARMs): a novel approach to androgen therapy for the new millennium. J Clin Endocrinol Metab 1999;84:3459–3462.
432. Allan G, Lai MT, Sbriscia T, Linton O, Haynes-Johnson D, Bhattacharjee S, Dodds R, Fiordeliso J, Lanter J, Sui J, Lundeen S. A selective androgen receptor modulator that reduces prostate tumor size and prevents orchidectomy-induced bone loss in rats. J Steroid Bioch Molec Biol 2007;103:76–83.
433. Kearbey JD, Gao W, Narayanan R, Fisher SJ, Wu Di, Miller DD, Dalton JT. Selective androgen receptor modulator (SARM) treatment presents bone loss and reduces body fat in ovariectomized rats. Pharmaceutical Res 2007;24:328–335.
434. Miner JN, Chang W, Chapman MS, Finn PD, Hong MH, Lopez FJ, Marschke KB, Rosen J, Schrader W, Turner R, van Oeveren A, Viveros H, Zhi L, Negro-Vilar A. An orally active selective androgen receptor modulator in efficacious on bone, muscle and sex function with reduced impact on prostate. Endocrinology 2007;148:363–373.

18 Salmon Calcitonin: An Update on Its Clinical Utility in Osteoporosis

Charles H. Chesnut III, MD
and Moise Azria, PhD

Contents

Key Words: Salmon Calcitonin, Osteoporosis, metabolic bone disease, antiresorptive osteoporosis therapies, antifracture efficacy, SCT, nasal spray, oral formulation

From: *Contemporary Endocrinology: Osteoporosis: Pathophysiology and Clinical Management*
Edited by: R. A. Adler, DOI 10.1007/978-1-59745-459-9_18,

INTRODUCTION

Salmon calcitonin (SCT) has been available as a therapeutic agent for metabolic bone disease for more than 30 years, approved in more than 70 countries worldwide for the treatment of postmenopausal osteoporosis.

As one of the first available antiresorptive osteoporosis therapies, the efficacy and the favorable safety profile of SCT have been established over decades. As well, the past 5 years have provided new insights into the effects of SCT in preserving bone quality (trabecular microarchitecture) as a possible mechanism for its antifracture efficacy.

SCT is commercially available as an injectable form and as a nasal spray. A new oral formulation has been recently developed and data from the first clinical trials indicate a potential utility in osteoporosis.

This review will summarize important aspects of pharmacological and clinical trial data for SCT, with focus on the widely used nasal spray formulation. The evidence for salmon calcitonin nasal spray (SCT-NS) will be discussed in the light of new data, and the future perspectives for the oral formulation of SCT will be evaluated.

PHYSIOLOGY AND PHARMACOLOGY

Calcitonin (CT) is a 32-amino-acid peptide secreted by the C cells of the thyroid in mammals and by the ultimobranchial glands in submammals. The hormone was discovered by Copp and Cameron *(1)* in 1961 as a substance lowering blood calcium. Synthetic or recombinant calcitonins from different species, including human calcitonin, porcine calcitonin, eel calcitonin derivative and salmon calcitonin, have been used for medical purposes. SCT is by far the most widely used preparation in the clinical practice, due to its 40–50 times higher intrinsic potency when compared to human calcitonin and its improved analgesic properties *(2)*. However, even 45 years after its discovery, the physiologic role of calcitonin is not fully understood. Calcitonin acts in collaboration with parathyroid hormone and 1,25-dihydroxycholecalciferol to mediate and "fine-tune" the short-term calcium homeostasis, particularly at times of "calcium stress" such as pregnancy and the postprandial state *(3)*. Initial findings of osteopenia in calcitonin knockout mice (CT/CGRP$^{-/-}$) *(4)*, were not corroborated *(5)* and no bone pathologies have been associated with hypo- or hypersecretion of calcitonin in humans *(6)*. In healthy subjects with normal calcium levels only subtle, transient calcium-lowering effects are observed following the administration of SCT *(7,8)*. In hypercalcemic states, however, calcitonin, when used at high doses by parenteral route, leads to marked, though mostly transient, reductions of elevated calcium levels. In these conditions, the calcium-lowering effect of SCT is characterized by a rapid onset of action, i.e., usually within 2 h *(9)*. The calcium-lowering effect is primarily due to the reduction of bone resorption by inhibition of osteoclast activity and possibly osteoclast number and secretory activity *(10)*. An increase in renal calcium excretion has also been described and may contribute to the fast onset of the calcium-lowering effect of SCT in hypercalcemic stages *(11,12)*.

The inhibition of bone resorption by calcitonin is mediated in part by binding to osteoclast membrane receptors. It has been estimated that one osteoclast holds approximately one million calcitonin receptors *(13)*. Flattening of the osteoclast-ruffled borders and withdrawal of osteoclasts from sites of active bone resorption occur upon exposure to calcitonin in vitro *(14–18)*. The inhibitory effects of calcitonin on osteoclasts are reversible. Cell apoptosis, as reported with bisphosphonates, has not been observed with calcitonin for either osteoclasts, osteoblasts, or osteocytes *(19,20)*. Whether calcitonin exerts a stimulatory effect on osteoblast-mediated bone formation is as yet uncertain. The existence of calcitonin receptors on osteoblasts has been suggested *(21–24)* and findings in some clinical trials have indicated a possible stimulatory effect on bone formation. Regulation of both bone resorption and formation has also been suggested based on results in genetically modified mouse models *(25)*. Physiologic downregulation of calcitonin receptor sites has been reported *(26)*; however, neither downregulation nor the development of calcitonin antibodies appears to be of clinical relevance *(27,28)*.

GENETIC ASPECTS

One of the candidate genes for osteoporotic fracture is the calcitonin gene. The calcitonin gene complex (an α and β gene, including the calcitonin receptor gene) is located on chromosome 11 *(29)*. An association has been described between specific calcitonin gene receptor genotypes and phenotypes of modestly increased bone mineral density (BMD) in Japanese populations *(30)* and in patients with juvenile idiopathic arthritis *(31)*. An association has also been described between specific calcitonin gene receptor genotypes and increased femoral neck BMD and reduced osteoporotic fracture risk in postmenopausal women *(32)*. Currently unexplored, however, is whether certain genetic profiles might be associated with a higher fracture risk or if there is any relevant pharmacogenetic predetermination of the responsiveness to SCT treatment.

PHARMACEUTICAL SCT FORMULATIONS

SCT is commercially available as an injectable formulation for intravenous, intramuscular, or subcutaneous use, and as nasal spray. An oral SCT preparation is currently under clinical development. In this new oral formulation of SCT, the 5-CNAC-disodium salt functions as a carrier which provides bioavailability for the salmon calcitonin peptide. The oral calcitonin formulations have been developed and enabled using Emisphere's Eligen® technology *(33)*.

EFFICACY OF SCT IN POSTMENOPAUSAL OSTEOPOROSIS

Injectable SCT was first introduced to the market in 1974 and was approved by the FDA in 1984. Effects on lumbar spine BMD have been reported in a number of smaller controlled clinical trials *(34–36)*. Efficacy in vertebral fracture risk reduction was shown in one randomized controlled clinical trial *(34)* and risk reduction in hip fracture was reported in the retrospective Mediterranean Osteoporosis Study *(37)*.

SCT-NS is currently the most widely used formulation due to its evidence-based efficacy for vertebral fracture prevention and its superior tolerability profile and convenience for the daily, long-term administration. The efficacy profile of SCT-NS is established through results from randomized controlled clinical studies, which have demonstrated a reduction in markers of bone turnover, a moderate effect on bone mineral density, the preservation of bone microarchitecture, and, most importantly, a reduction in vertebral fracture risk. SCT-NS was approved for treatment of postmenopausal osteoporosis by the FDA in the United States in 1995.

EFFECT OF SCT-NS ON BONE RESORPTION MARKERS

In a recent single-dose study, the bone turnover marker serum CTX-1 showed a marked maximum suppression of 55% within 1 h after SCT-NS administration *(38)*, which was reversible over 24 h. Continued, long-term use of SCT-NS leads to a gradual decrease in overnight fasting serum CTX-1 levels over time (Fig. 1) as demonstrated in a recent study *(39)* with marker response as the primary endpoint. In this study by Srivastava et al., SCT-NS (200 IU/day) showed a statistically significant reduction of 34% in serum CTX-1 vs. baseline and vs. placebo at 6 months in elderly, postmenopausal women with high bone turnover. Serum CTX-1 reductions vs. placebo were 25.5% at 2 years in the Qualitative Effects of Salmon Calcitonin Study (QUEST) *(40)* ($p = 0.02$; last observation carried forward analysis) and 12.3% at 5 years in the Prevent Recurrence of Osteoporotic Fracture Study (PROOF) ($p < 0.01$) for the 200 IU/day dose groups *(28)*.

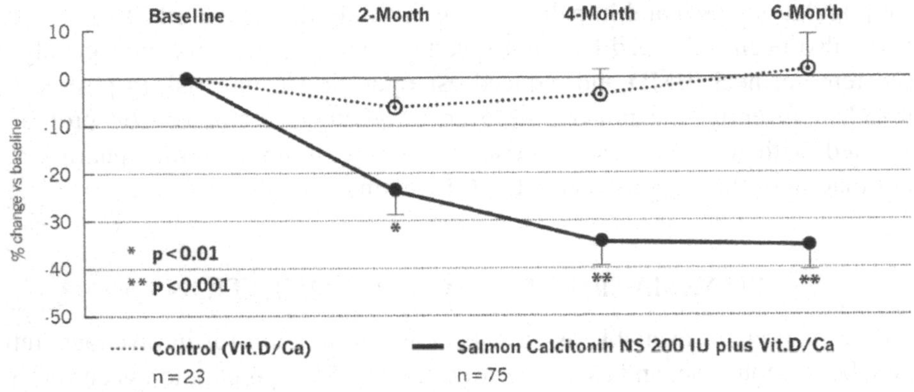

Fig. 1. Sustained gradual suppression of serum CTX-1 fasting levels during SCT-NS sustained, long-term treatment [adapted from Srivastava et al. *(39)*].

Bone turnover markers return to baseline levels within 3 months of SCT treatment discontinuation *(41)*. This underlines the potentially beneficial reversibility of osteoclast inhibition exerted by SCT as compared to bisphosphonate therapy where prolonged bone turnover suppression after treatment discontinuation is observed.

It is debatable whether the therapeutic response to SCT is dependent on the degree of bone turnover: Civitelli et al. *(42)* reported that a higher level of baseline bone resorption did result in greater increases in spine bone mineral content for injectable calcitonin. Such a relationship between baseline bone turnover and trabecular microarchitecture was however not seen with SCT-NS in the more recent QUEST study *(43)*. Lastly, as might be expected with normal coupling mechanisms, decreases in markers of bone formation including bone-specific alkaline phosphatase have been noted in most studies. Effects on bone formation were however of distinctly lower magnitude than effects on markers of bone resorption. Such suppression of bone resorption without a significant decrease in bone formation may favorably contribute to the therapeutic effect of SCT-NS.

EFFECTS OF SCT-NS ON BONE MINERAL DENSITY

Effects on BMD are less pronounced with SCT-NS than with other antiresorptive treatments, especially bisphosphonates and strontium ranelate. Early studies in postmenopausal women, which included BMD as primary endpoint, have demonstrated improvements in a range of 3% vs. baseline in lumbar spine BMD *(44)*. Similar results were obtained in a study of 208 postmenopausal women with established osteoporosis, which showed a dose-dependent increase in lumbar spine BMD and an overall statistically significant relative fracture risk reduction vs. placebo (RR 0.23, 95% CI 0.07–0.77) *(45)*. Studies in early menopausal women have typically shown a stabilization of BMD at the lumbar spine *(46,47)*. No data with fracture endpoints are available for this patient population and SCT-NS is not currently FDA approved for the prevention of osteoporosis. In the two recent, randomized, placebo-controlled clinical trials in women with established postmenopausal osteoporosis, QUEST and PROOF, BMD was assessed as a secondary endpoint. In QUEST, a nonsignificant difference in lumbar spine BMD of 0.8% was noted between SCT-NS and placebo at 2 years, despite significant favorable effects on bone microarchitecture. In PROOF, BMD increased during the 5 years by only approximately 1.5% vs. baseline ($p < 0.01$) and by approximately 1% vs. placebo ($p < 0.05$; 200 IU/day dose group), despite a marked and statistically significant reduction in the occurrence of new vertebral fractures for SCT-NS vs. placebo.

ANTIFRACTURE EFFICACY OF SCT-NS: THE PROOF STUDY

The aforementioned Overgaard study *(45)* noted a significant ($p = 0.046$) reduction in the rate of overall fractures in postmenopausal osteoporotic women receiving 50, 100, and 200 IU SCT-NS (pooled dosages) as compared to placebo. However, the number of fractures in this study was small, and the main evidence for the antifracture efficacy of SCT-NS is derived from the PROOF study *(28)*, which was a confirmative large-scale multicenter trial initiated in 1991.

The Prevent Recurrence of Osteoporotic Fracture Study (PROOF) was a 5-year multicenter double-blind, placebo-controlled trial in 1255 postmenopausal osteoporotic women, the majority of whom had 1–5 prevalent vertebral fractures and a lumbar spine BMD *T* score <–2.0. Subjects were randomized to placebo nasal spray or 100, 200, or 400 IU/day SCT-NS (Miacalcic®/Miacalcin®). All patients received 1000 mg calcium and 400 IU vit. D_2. The intent to treat analysis demonstrated an absolute risk reduction (ARR) of 8.2% and a relative risk reduction (RRR) of 33% for new vertebral fractures over 5 years (RR 0.67, 95% CI 0.47–0.97; $p < 0.05$) for the 200 IU/day dose group. In women with 1–5 prevalent vertebral fractures at baseline, the RRR for new vertebral fractures was 38, 40, and 36% (all $p < 0.05$) at 3, 4, and 5 years, respectively (Fig. 2).

There was an apparent dose response for the 200 IU/day dose group (RRR 35%, $p = 0.03$) over the 100 IU/day dose group (RR 15%, $p = 0.37$), but not for the 400 IU/day dose group (RRR 16%, $p = 0.32$). The reasons for the lack of an effect for the 400 IU dosage are unclear, particularly as significant effects of the 400 IU dosage were seen on bone turnover (as noted below) and BMD. A preplanned per-protocol analysis in patients defined as "3-year valid completers" (stayed on treatment for at least 3 years or had an

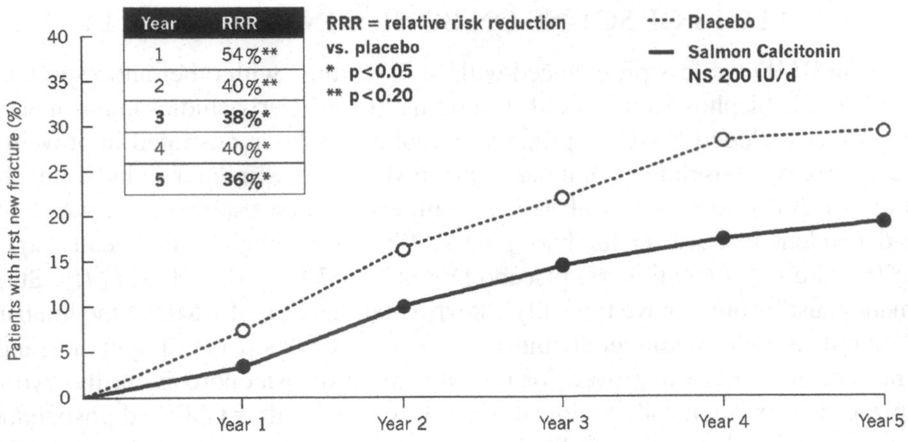

Fig. 2. PROOF study: vertebral fracture relative risk reduction over 5 years in patients with 1–5 prevalent vertebral fractures at baseline.

incident fracture prior to 3 years, had 1–5 prevalent fractures, did not take forbidden medications, and were at least 75% compliant with study medication) suggested that a plateau for the antifracture efficacy is reached at a daily dose of 200 IU. For these "3-year valid completers" the RRR was lower for the 100 IU/day dose group (i.e., RRR 9%, $p=0.64$), whereas similar levels of RRR were achieved for new vertebral fractures in the 200 and the 400 IU/day dose groups (RRR 34%, $p=0.04$ for 200 IU/day and RRR 29%, $p=0.09$ for 400 IU/day at 5 years). At 4 years there was a statistical significant RRR of 37% in the 200 IU/day dose group and 36% in the 400 IU/day dose group ($p<0.05$ in both groups). The results for bone resorption markers again raised the question of why there was not an effect on fractures for the 400 IU dosage, as serum CTX-1 decreased to a similar extent vs. placebo in both the 200 IU/day dose group (–12%, $p<0.01$) and in the 400 IU/day dose group (–14%, $p<0.01$), whereas no significant effect was found in the 100 IU/day dose group.

PREFERENTIAL EFFECTS OF SCT-NS IN ELDERLY PATIENTS AT THE LUMBAR SPINE

The mean age in the PROOF study cohort was 68.2 years in the placebo group and 69.0 years in the SCT-NS 200 IU/day dose group. When fracture risk data from the PROOF study were analyzed in a post hoc analysis over different age groups (i.e., ≤ or >age 70) and for the thoracic spine vs. the lumbar spine, a particular therapeutic benefit was apparent in elderly women and at the lumbar spine.

At 5 years the absolute risk reduction (ARR) for the total study cohort was 8.2% ($p=0.02$) compared to 14.3% ($p=0.01$) in the subgroup of women above age 70. The corresponding RRR was 33% ($p=0.02$) for the total study cohort compared to 44% ($p=0.03$) in women above age 70. As shown in Fig. 3, an increase in RRR with age was observed primarily for the lumbar spine. A significant fracture risk reduction was demonstrated for the thoracic spine alone in the total study cohort (ARR 6.4%, $p=0.04$; RRR 33%, $p=0.06$), but not for lumbar spine alone. In patients above age 70 however, both ARR and RRR were

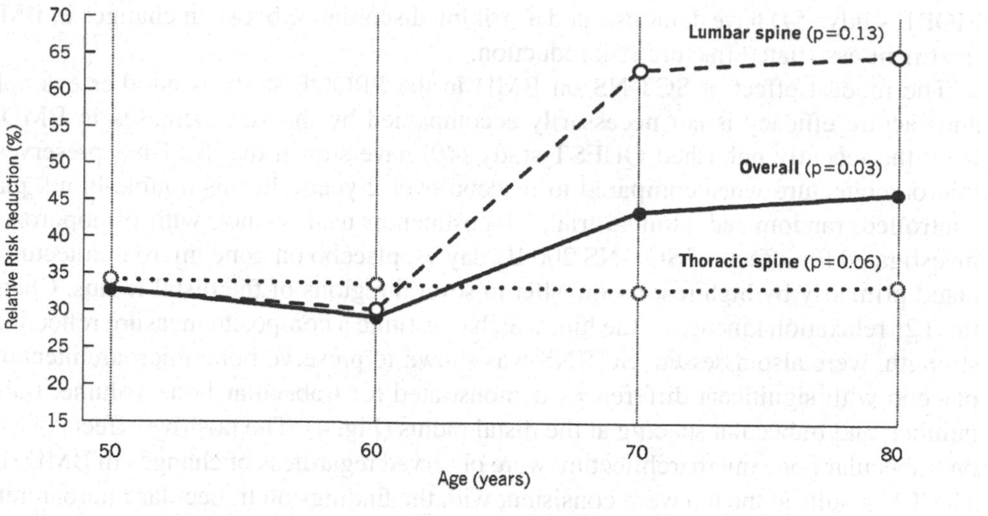

Fig. 3. Relative risk reduction at 5 years for vertebral fractures by region and age (post hoc analysis of data from the PROOF study).

significant at the lumbar spine (ARR 10.4%, $p = 0.01$; RRR 64%, $p = 0.017$). The clinical relevance of a preferential effect on lumbar spine fractures in the elderly population relates to a greater impairment of quality of life status reported for lumbar spine fractures. As well, such impairment may be greater in elderly (age >70) individuals *(48)*.

NONVERTEBRAL FRACTURE RISK REDUCTION WITH SCT-NS

The number of hip fractures or the number of upper extremity fractures within the individual dose groups of the PROOF study was small and did not allow drawing meaningful conclusions on fracture risk reduction. However, a number of observations are warranted.

For hip fractures, a nonsignificant 48% RRR was found for the 200 IU/day dose at 5 years. Post hoc analyses indicated a statistically significant RRR of 68% ($p < 0.05$) for the pooled 100 and 200 IU/day dose groups *(49)* and an RRR of 54% ($p = 0.08$) when all dose groups were pooled. For combined hip plus upper extremity fractures, an RRR of 37% ($p = 0.14$) was observed at 5 years for the 200 IU/day dose group and an RRR of 43% ($p = 0.02$) for the pooled dose groups. Similar subgroup analyses on the potential for nonvertebral fracture risk reduction have been used and validated as an appropriate analysis in other trials of osteoporosis on antiresorptive agents *(50,51)*.

POSSIBLE MECHANISMS FOR SCT-NS-MEDIATED ANTIFRACTURE EFFICACY: THE QUEST STUDY

In recent years, BMD has been questioned as being the predominant predictor of fracture risk and a more integrative concept has been favored, which includes material properties, bone turnover, bone geometry, and bone microarchitecture as the determinants of bone strength *(52)*. Doubts have emerged on BMD being a good predictor and mediator of fracture risk reduction in patients on antiresorptive therapy *(53)*. Post hoc analyses from the

MORE study *(54)* have demonstrated a striking discordance between changes in BMD and treatment-associated fracture risk reduction.

The modest effect of SCT-NS on BMD in the PROOF study is another example that antifracture efficacy is not necessarily accompanied by marked increases in BMD. Data from the recently published QUEST study *(40)* have shown that SCT-NS preserves bone microarchitecture when compared to placebo over 2 years. In this double-blind, placebo-controlled, randomized, clinical trial, 91 postmenopausal women with osteoporosis were investigated for effects of SCT-NS 200 IU/day vs. placebo on bone microarchitecture, evaluated primarily by high-resolution MRI in several regions of the distal radius. Changes in the $T2^*$ relaxation kinetics of the hip, which constitute a composite measure reflecting bone strength, were also assessed. SCT-NS was shown to preserve bone microarchitecture over placebo with significant differences demonstrated for trabecular bone volume, trabecular number, and trabecular spacing at the distal radius (Fig. 4). The positive effects of SCT-NS on trabecular bone microarchitecture were observed regardless of changes in BMD (Fig. 5). The $T2^*$ results at the hip were consistent with the findings on trabecular microarchitecture at the distal radius.

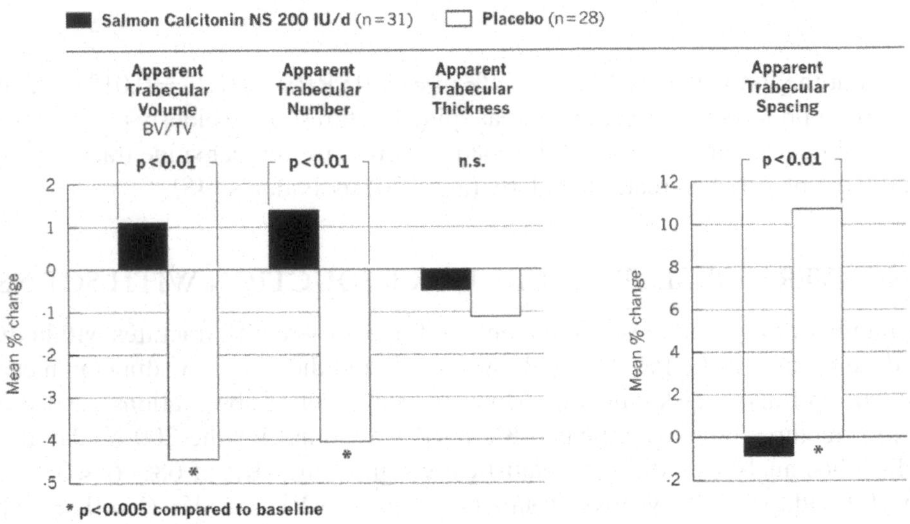

Fig. 4. Radius MRI: change in parameters for trabecular microarchitecture from baseline to 24 months.

Iliac crest bone biopsies, with two-dimensional histomorphometry and three-dimensional micro-CT, were also obtained in the QUEST study (Fig. 6).

In addition to providing information on SCT-NS's effect on trabecular microarchitecture, the QUEST trial confirmed the utility of the MRI technology as a research and possibly clinical tool for the osteoporosis field, demonstrated a heterogeneous therapeutic response to SCT-NS across differing skeletal sites, and confirmed that therapeutic benefit could be achieved with an antiresorptive therapy such as SCT-NS even in the absence of a substantial effect on BMD. As well, a post hoc analysis of the QUEST study has further confirmed the importance of SCT-NS's effect on trabecular microarchitecture; placebo subjects with a low trabecular number at baseline subsequently demonstrated a significant decrease in trabecular number over 2 years, as compared to a nonsignificant loss in those placebo patients with

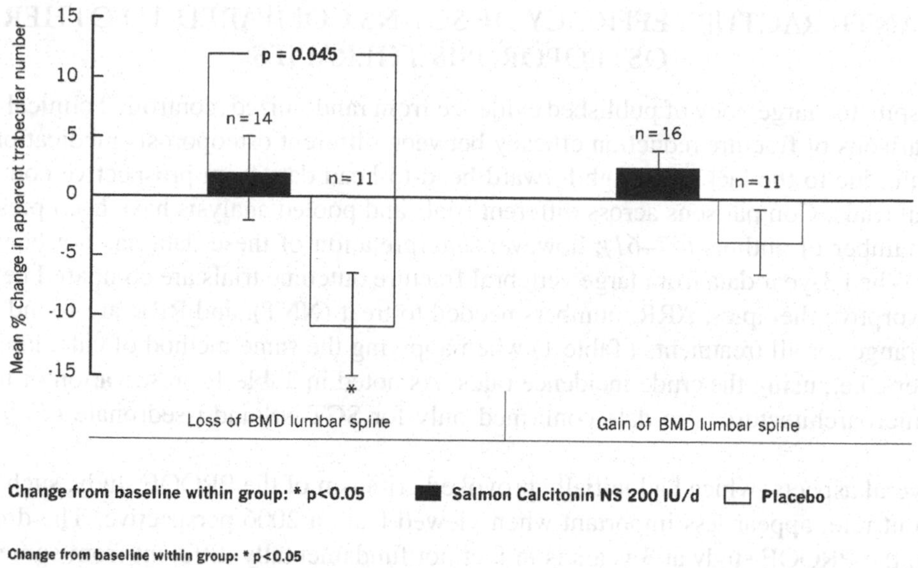

Fig. 5. Radius MRI: trabecular number as a function of lumbar spine BMD from baseline to 24 months.

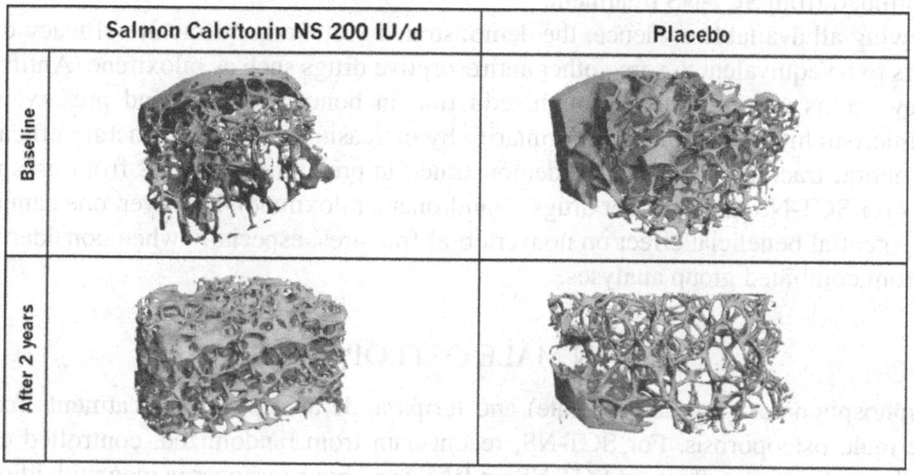

Fig. 6. Clinical examples (QUEST study; micro-CT of iliac crest biopsies). Changes in bone microarchitecture. Patient on SCT-NS (left panel), patient on placebo (right panel).

a high trabecular number at baseline. SCT-NS patients however preserved their trabecular number regardless of their baseline value *(55)*.

Lastly, the QUEST study was not designed or powered to assess the effects of SCT-NS on fracture (as mediated by its preservative effect on trabecular microarchitecture); however, previous studies have confirmed a relationship between trabecular microarchitecture, biomechanical integrity, and osteoporotic fracture risk. In addition, MRI analysis in a recent study has confirmed a significant positive effect of SCT on compressive stress and on trabecular microarchitecture in an animal model *(56)*.

ANTIFRACTURE EFFICACY OF SCT-NS COMPARED TO OTHER OSTEOPOROSIS THERAPIES

Despite the large body of published evidence from randomized, controlled clinical trials, comparisons of fracture reduction efficacy between different osteoporosis medications are difficult, due to the lack of straightforward head-to-head data from prospective controlled clinical trials. Comparisons across different trials and pooled analysis have been presented by a number of authors *(57–61)*; however, interpretation of these data has not been uniform. When 3-year data from large vertebral fracture outcome trials are compared between antiresorptive therapies, ARR, numbers needed to treat (NNT), and RRR are found in the same range for all treatments (Table 1) when applying the same method of calculating the numbers, i.e., using the crude incidence rates. As noted in Table 1, preservation of trabecular microarchitecture is to date confirmed only for SCT-NS and risedronate *(40,62)*.

Several aspects, which had initially provoked criticism of the PROOF study, such as the drop-out rate, appear less important when viewed from a 2006 perspective. The drop-out rate in the PROOF study at 3 years is in fact not fundamentally different from some other studies. It is furthermore unlikely that discontinuations would have confounded the study results in favor of SCT-NS, as placebo participants, who prematurely discontinued from the PROOF study, showed a greater decrease in lumbar spine BMD than did patients that discontinued from SCT-NS treatment.

Viewing all available evidence, the demonstrated vertebral antifracture efficacy of SCT appears to be equivalent to some other antiresorptive drugs such as raloxifene. Antifracture efficacy seems to be exerted through reduction in bone resorption and preservation of bone microarchitecture rather than primarily by increasing BMD. Antifracture efficacy for nonvertebral fractures has not been demonstrated in predefined analyses from prospective studies for SCT-NS and for other drugs (ibandronate, raloxifene). However, one cannot rule out a potential beneficial effect on nonvertebral fractures, especially when considering the data from combined group analyses.

SCT IN MALE OSTEOPOROSIS

Bisphosphonates (e.g., alendronate) and teriparatide are approved treatments for idiopathic male osteoporosis. For SCT-NS, recent data from randomized, controlled clinical trials showed positive effects of SCT-NS on BMD and bone turnover in men with idiopathic osteoporosis. In two placebo-controlled trials over 12 or 18 months ($n = 28$ and 40) *(63,64)*, SCT-NS led to statistically significant increases in lumbar spine BMD when compared to placebo. Effects on femoral neck BMD were not consistent and meaningful fracture data are not currently available. Male patients were also included within studies on the analgesic efficacy of SCT in vertebral fracture-associated pain syndromes *(65,66)*.

SCT IN CORTICOSTEROID-INDUCED OSTEOPOROSIS

Results from few, smaller studies indicate that injectable calcitonin may reduce the rate of bone loss at lumbar spine and radius in patients both initiating and receiving corticosteroid therapy. Data on bone loss prevention are conflicting with SCT-NS. There are no data with fracture as an endpoint *(67)*.

Table 1
Three-Year Vertebral Fracture Results in Postmenopausal Women with Osteoporosis and Prevalent Baseline Vertebral Fractures from Large Randomized, Controlled, Double-Blind Clinical Trials with Antiresorptive Drugs

Drug (dose/day)	*Study*	*Pts. (n) treated active treatment placebo*	*Percentage of randomized pts. completing 3 years*	*Pts (%) with VFx at baseline*	*Rate of new VFx at 3 years:[a] active treatment placebo crude rate/ (published)*	*Crude rate (published)*			*Lumbar spine BMD increase vs. placebo*	*Preservation of bone quality*
						ARR[b]	*NNT[c]*	*RRR[d]*		
Alendronate (10 mg)[e]	FIT (94)	1022, 1005	87[f]	100	8.0%, 15.0%	7.1%	14	47%**	6.2%	No published clinical data
Ibandronate (2.5 mg)	BONE (51)	982, 982	66	94	3.8%/(4.7%)[g], 7.5%/(9.6%)	3.7%	27 (20)[g]	49% (52%***)	5.2%	No published clinical data
Raloxifene (60 mg)	MORE (95)	769, 770	78[h]	90	14.7%, 21.2 %	6.5%	15 (16)[i]	31%* (30%)	2.6%	No published clinical data
Risedronate (5 mg)	VERT-NA (96)	813, 815	60	80	8.8%/(11.3%)[j], 13.7%/(16.3%)	5.0%	20	36% (41%**)	4.3%	Borah et al. (Bone 2004)
VERT-MN (97)	407, 407	62	100	15.4%/ (18.1%)[j], 25.7%/ (29.0%)	10.3%	10	40% (49%***)	5.9%		

(*Continued*)

Table 1
(conitnued)

S-Calcitonin (200 IU)	PROOF (28)	316, 311	65	79	13.6%, 21.2%	7.6.%	13 (11)[i]	36%* (38%*)[i]	0.6%	Chesnut et al. (JBMR, 2005)
Strontium ranelate (2 g)[k]	SOTI (98,99)	719, 723	76	88	20.9%, 32.8%	11.9	8 (9)	36% (41%)***	8.1%[l]	No published clinical data

[a]New vertebral fractures as defined by X-ray morphometry.

[b]Crude ARR (%) = (rate of new vertebral fractures on placebo) – (crude rate of new vertebral fractures on active treatment).

[c]Crude NNT = 100/ARR; published NNT provided in parentheses, if different from calculated crude rates.

[d]Crude RRR (%) = 100 × (rate of new fractures on placebo – rate of new fractures on active treatment)/rate of new fracture on placebo; published RRR provided in parentheses, if different from calculated crude rates.

[e]Daily dose was 5 mg/day for the years 0–2 and 10 mg/day for the third year.

[f]Eighty-nine percentage of surviving study patients (98%) were reported to be taking study medication at the closeout visit (combined alendronate and placebo).

[g]Percentage of patients with incident VFx in the *BONE* journal publication refer to a life-table analysis (VFx rate at 3 years for placebo 9.6% and for ibandronate 2.5 mg/day 4.7%). RRR of new vertebral fractures was provided as adjusted analysis (adjustment for baseline BMD) at 62% RRR and as unadjusted analysis at 52% RRR.

[h]Proportion refers to all raloxifene dose groups (i.e., 3977/5129 pts.).

[i]Refers to subgroup of patients with 1–5 vertebral fractures at baseline.

[j]Percentage of patients with incident VFx in the *VERT-MN* journal publication refer to Kaplan–Meier estimate.

[k]Number (n) of patients with fractures was not provided in publications; calculations are on percentages as published by Meunier et al.

[l]Value numerically adjusted for strontium content (unadjusted 14.4% vs. placebo).

* $p<0.05$; ** $p<0.01$: *** $p<0.001$.

Analgesic Effects of SCT

The analgesic potency of calcitonin in bone-related pain has been described early on in a number of case series. Numerous calcitonin-binding sites have been detected in the CNS, especially in the hypothalamus *(68–70)*, and it is therefore assumed that the analgesic effects of salmon calcitonin are at least to some extent mediated centrally, with serotonergic pathways involved *(71–73)*.

In controlled clinical trials, the analgesic efficacy of SCT was demonstrated for various pain-related endpoints, including the reduction in pain scores on visual analogue scale (VAS), the reduction in concomitant analgesic medication, and the improvement of early patient mobilization following acute vertebral fractures. Injectable salmon calcitonin has been shown superior to placebo in acute vertebral fractures *(74)* and in metastatic bone disease *(75,76)*. In addition a number of non-controlled studies have indicated that injectable calcitonin provides analgesic effects in Paget's disease *(77,78)*.

For SCT-NS, a number of well-designed, placebo-controlled clinical trials have demonstrated substantial analgesic effects, especially in pain associated with acute vertebral fractures. Analgesic effects of SCT-NS have also been investigated in the postoperative setting following femoral/hip arthroplasty *(79,80)*. Overall, the pain relieving effects of nasal spray and injectable SCT appear comparable *(81,82)*.

Blau et al. *(83)* found that in 13 out of 14 placebo-controlled trials, statistically significant improvement in vertebral fracture pain or function-related endpoints was reported for the calcitonin-treated patients (with various SCT formulations). In another recent systematic review on pain related to acute vertebral compression fractures, Knopp et al. presented a combined analysis of five double-blind, placebo-controlled clinical trials. A marked and statistically significant early onset pain reduction was shown for SCT with a mean weighted VAS difference vs. placebo of 3.08 (95% CI 2.64, 3.52) on a 10-point VAS scale at 1 week and with a sustained effect over 4 weeks treatment (MWD 4.03; 95% CI 3.70–4.35) *(65,84–87)*.

Safety of SCT-NS

Salmon calcitonin has a well-established, excellent safety profile, based on numerous clinical trials and a long-standing postmarketing experience. The safety experience for SCT-NS pertains to more than 20 years of broad utilization in clinical practice with an estimated exposure of several million patient years. The only contraindication is related to known hypersensitivity to ingredients of SCT-NS. When hypersensitivity is suspected, skin testing is recommended prior to the first administration of SCT-NS. Systemic side effects such as flush or nausea, which are not uncommon with the injectable forms, are rarely seen with the nasal spray formulation *(88)*. In clinical trials, adverse event rates were generally comparable between SCT-NS and placebo. For SCT-NS, the most frequent adverse events involve local, transient (nasal) reactions, such as stinging or tingling of the nasal passage, sneezing, rhinitis, nasal mucosal erythema, and, occasionally, minor bleeding. In earlier studies, these local reactions were reported in fewer than 10% of patients receiving SCT-NS *(89,90)*. In the PROOF study, the rate of rhinitis events was 22% in the combined SCT-NS dose groups, compared to 15% in the placebo group ($p < 0.01$). However, 97% of those reactions were reported as mild or moderate.

Because salmon calcitonin is a peptide, the possibility of allergic reactions exist; however, the evidence on severe allergic reactions is anecdotal. Overall, SCT-NS is widely regarded as very safe and compares favorably vs. other antiresorptive or anabolic osteoporosis drugs in terms of side effects, contraindications, precautions, and interactions with other treatments. Due to the transient inhibition of osteoclasts and based on the long-standing clinical experience, there appears to be no potential for detrimental effects on bone structure during long-term treatment.

CURRENT THERAPEUTIC RECOMMENDATIONS FOR DOSING IN OSTEOPOROSIS

SCT-NS is recommended at a dose of 200 IU/day for treatment of established postmenopausal osteoporosis to prevent further progression of the disease. Given the comparatively modest effect of SCT-NS on BMD, the clinical monitoring of therapeutic response to SCT-NS is primarily confirmed by preservation of bone mineral density at spine and hip (i.e., no significant loss of BMD), a significant decrease in markers of bone resorption, and the absence of further clinical skeletal fractures.

For injectable forms of SCT, dosing recommendations for subcutaneous administration range from 50 IU every second day to 100 IU/day, depending on the indication and the severity of disease.

THE ORAL SCT FORMULATION

In recent years, an oral SCT preparation has been developed, which is expected to provide superior bioavailability and higher systemic SCT levels. To protect SCT from intestinal degradation, the active peptide hormone is combined with a caprylic acid derivative. An initial study in healthy subjects has demonstrated a rapid and reproducible dose-dependent increase in serum SCT levels after oral intake, with a corresponding biological response in markers of bone resorption *(91)*. A more recent 3-month dose ranging study in 277 postmenopausal women confirmed the effective absorption from the gastrointestinal tract, resulting in dose-dependent, sustained responses in bone resorption markers *(92)*. In addition to the effects on bone turnover, recent data indicated a benefit of oral SCT in reducing cartilage degradation in osteoarthritis *(93)*.

CONCLUSIONS AND SUMMARY

More than 30 years after its market introduction, SCT is a well-established, effective, and safe treatment for postmenopausal osteoporosis.

The favorable benefit to risk profile of SCT has recently been confirmed by the major health authorities and is also reflected by the approved use of SCT over decades in more than 70 countries worldwide. The vertebral antifracture efficacy is evidence based for SCT-NS. Fracture prevention appears to be mediated through preservation of bone microarchitecture and decreased bone resorption, with only moderate effects on BMD. Future indications, especially for the new oral formulation of SCT, may include both osteoporosis and osteoarthritis.

REFERENCES

1. Copp DH, Cameron EC. Demonstration of a hypocalcemic factor (calcitonin) in commercial parathyroid extract. Science 1961;134:2038.
2. Azria M, Copp D, Zanelli J. 25 years of salmon calcitonin: from synthesis to therapeutic use. Calcif Tissue Int 1995;57(6):405–408.
3. Woodrow JP, Noseworthy CS, Fudge NJ, Hoff AO, Gagel RF, Kovacs CS. Calcitonin/calcitonin gene-related peptide protect the maternal skeleton from excessive resorption during lactation (abstract). J Bone Miner Res 2003, 18(Suppl 2):S37.
4. Hoff A, Thomas M, Cote G. Generation of a calcitonin knockout mouse model (abstract). Bone 1998;23:1062.
5. Hoff AO, Catala-Lehnen P, Thomas PM, Priemel M, Rueger JM, Nasonkin I, Bradley A, Hughes MR, Ordonez N, Cote GJ, Amling M, Gagel RF. Increased bone mass is an unexpected phenotype associated with deletion of the calcitonin gene. J Clin Invest 2002;110(12):1849–1857.
6. Hirsch PF, Baruch H. Is calcitonin an important physiological substance ? Endocrine 2003;21(3):201–208.
7. Thamsborg G. Effect of nasal salmon calcitonin on calcium and bone metabolism. Dan Med Bull 1999;46(2):118–126.
8. Buclin T, Randin J, Jacquet A, Azria M, Attinger M, Gomez F, Burckhardt P. The effect of rectal and nasal administration of salmon calcitonin in normal subjects. Calcif Tissue Int 1987;41(5):252–258.
9. Wisneski L. Salmon calcitonin in the acute management of hypercalcemia. Calcif Tissue Int 1990;46(Suppl): S26–S30.
10. Zaidi M, Inzerillo A, Troen B, et al. Molecular and clinical pharmacology of calcitonin. In: Bilezikian J, Raisz L, Rodan G, eds. Principles of bone biology. San Diego: Academic press, 2002:1423–1440.
11. Ralston SH, Coleman R, Fraser WD, Gallagher SJ, Hosking DJ, Iqbal JS, McCloskey E, Sampson D. Medical management of hypercalcemia. Calcif Tissue Int 2004;74(1):1–11.
12. Hoskin D. Gilson D. Comparison of the renal and skeletal actions of calcitonin in the treatment of severe hypercalcemia of malignancy. Quart J Med 1984;211:359–368.
13. Nicholson G, Moseley J, Sexton P, Mendelsohn F, Martin T. Abundant calcitonin receptors in isolate rat osteoclasts, biochemical, and autoradiographic characterization. J Clin Invest 1986;78:355–360.
14. Holtrop N, Raisz L, Simmons H. The effects of parathyroid hormone, colchicines and calcitonin on the ultrastructure and the activity of osteoclasts in organ culture. J Cell Biol 1974;346–355.
15. Yumita S, Nicholson G, Rowe D, Kent G, Martin T. Biphasic effect of calcitonin on tartrate-resistant acid phosphatase activity in isolated rat osteoclasts. J Bone Miner Res 1991;6:591–597.
16. Zaidi M, Inzerillo A, Moonga B, Bevis P, Huang C. Forty years of calcitoninwhere are we now? A tribute to the work of Iain Macinttyre, FRS. Bone 2002;30(5):655–663.
17. Chambers T, Moore A. The sensitivity of isolated osteoclasts to morphological transformation by calcitonin. J Clin Endocrinol Metab 1983;57:819–824.
18. Chambers T, Magnus C. Calcitonin alters behaviour of isolated osteoclasts. J Pathol 1982;136(1):27–39.
19. Vaananen K. Mechanism of osteoclast mediated bone resorption-rationale for the design of new therapeutics. Adv Drug Deliv Rev 2005;57(7):959–971.
20. Selander KS, Harkonen PL, Valve E, Monkkonen J, Hannuniemi R, Vaananen HK. Calcitonin promotes osteoclast survival in vitro. Mol Cell Endocrinol 1996;122(2):119–129.
21. Plotkin L, Weinstein R, Parfitt A, Robertson P, Manolagas S, Bellido T. Prevention of osteocyte and osteoblast apoptosis by bisphosphonates and calcitonin. J Clin Invest 1999;104:1363–1374.
22. Farley JR, Tarbaux NM, Hall SL, Linkhart TA, Baylink DJ. The anti-bone-resorptive agent calcitonin also acts in vitro to directly increase bone formation and bone cell proliferation. Endocrinology 1988;123(1):159–167.
23. Wallach S, Farley JR, Baylink DJ, Brenner-Gati L. Effects of calcitonin on bone quality and osteoblastic function. Calcif Tissue Int 1993;52(5):335–339.
24. Furuichi H, Fukuyama R, Izumo N, Fujita T, Kohno T, Nakamuta H, Koida M. Bone-anabolic effect of salmon calcitonin on glucocorticoid-induced osteopenia in rats. Biol Pharm Bull 2000;23(8):946–951.
25. Voss A, Liese S, Priemel M, Catala-Lehnen P, Schilling AF, Mueldner C, Haberland M, Rueger JM, Emeson RB, Gagel RF, Schinke T, Amling M. Uncovering the physiologic function of calcitonin using genetically modified mouse models (abstract). J Bone Miner Res 2005;(Suppl.):1162.

26. Takahashi S, Goldring S, Katz M, Hilsenbeck S, Williams R, Roodman GD. Downregulation of calcitonin receptor mRNA expression by calcitonin during human osteoclast-like cell differentiation. J Clin Invest 1995;95(1):167–171.
27. Singer FR, Aldred JP, Neer RM, Krane SM, Potts JT Jr, Bloch KJ. An evaluation of antibodies and clinical resistance to salmon calcitonin. J Clin Invest 1972;51(9):2331–2338.
28. Chesnut CH III, Silverman S, Andriano K, Genant H, Gimona A, Harris S, Kiel D, LeBoff M, Maricic M, Miller P, Moniz C, Peacock M, Richardson P, Watts N, Baylink D. A randomized trial of nasal spray salmon calcitonin in postmenopausal women with established osteoporosis: the prevent recurrence of osteoporotic fractures study. PROOF Study Group. Am J Med 2000;109(4):267–276.
29. Kittur S, Hoppener J, Anatonarakis S, Daniels J, Meyers D, Maestry N, Jaansen M, Korneluk R, Nelkin B, Kazaziam H. Linkage map of the short arm of human chromosome 11: location of the genes for catalase, calcitonin, and insulin-like growth factor II. Proc Natl Acad Sci 1985;83:5064–5067.
30. Nakamura M, Morimoto S, Zhang Z, Utusnomiya H, Inagami T, Ogihara T, Kakudo K. Calcitonin receptor gene polymorphism in Japanese women; Correlation with body mass and bone density, Calcif Tissue Int 2001;68:211–215.
31. Masi L, Cimaz R, Simonini G, Bindi G, Stagi S, Gozzini A, Malentacchi C, Brandi ML, Falcini F. Association of low bone mass with vitamin d receptor gene and calcitonin receptor gene polymorphisms in juvenile idiopathic arthritis. J Rheumatol 2002;29(10):2225–2231.
32. Taboulet J, Frenkian M, Frendo JL, Feingold N, Jullienne A, de Vernejoul MC. Calcitonin receptor polymorphism is associated with a decreased fracture risk in post-menopausal women. Hum Mol Genet 1998;7(13):2129–2133.
33. Emisphere Technologies, Inc. is located in Tarrytown, NY and can be found at www.emisphere.com.
34. Rico H, Hernandez ER, Revilla M, Gomez-Castresana F. Salmon calcitonin reduces vertebral fracture rate in postmenopausal crush fracture syndrome. Bone Miner 1992;16(2):131–138.
35. Mazzuoli GF, Passeri M, Gennari C, Minisola S, Antonelli R, Valtorta C, Palummeri E, Cervellin GF, Gonnelli S, Francini G. Effects of salmon calcitonin in postmenopausal osteoporosis: a controlled double-blind clinical study. Calcif Tissue Int. 1986;38(1):3–8.
36. Meschia M, Brincat M, Barbacini P, Maini MC, Marri R, Crosignani PG. Effect of hormone replacement therapy and calcitonin on bone mass in postmenopausal women. Eur J Obstet Gynecol Reprod Biol 1992;47(1):53–57.
37. Kanis JA, Johnell O, Gullberg B, Allander E, Dilsen G, Gennari C, Lopes Vaz AA, Lyritis GP, Mazzuoli G, Miravet L, et al. Evidence for efficacy of drugs affecting bone metabolism in preventing hip fracture. BMJ 1992;305(6862):1124–1128.
38. Zikan V, Stepan J. Plasma type 1 collagen cross-linked C-telopeptide: a sensitive marker of acute effects of salmon calcitonin on bone resorption. Clin Chim Acta 2002;316(1–2):63–69.
39. Srivastava AK, Libanati C, Hohmann O, Kriegman A, Baylink DJ. Acute effects of calcitonin nasal spray on serum C-telopeptide of type 1 collagen (CTx) levels in elderly osteopenic women with increased bone turnover. Calcif Tissue Int 2004;75(6):477–481.
40. Chesnut CH III, Majumdar S, Newitt DC, Shields A, Van Pelt J, Laschansky E, Azria M, Kriegman A, Olson M, Eriksen EF, Mindeholm L. Effects of salmon calcitonin on trabecular microarchitecture as determined by magnetic resonance imaging: results from the QUEST study. J Bone Miner Res 2005;20(9):1548–1561.
41. Overgaard K, Hansen MA, Nielson VA, et al. Discontinuous calcitonin treatment of established osteoporosis – effects of withdrawal of treatment. Am J Med 1990;89:1–6.
42. Civitelli R, Gonnelli S, Zacchei F, Bigazzi S, Vattimo A, Avioli LV, Gennari C. Bone turnover in postmenopausal osteoporosis. Effect of calcitonin treatment. J Clin Invest 1988;82(4): 1268–1274.
43. Chesnut CH III, personal communication, 2005.
44. Overgaard K, Riis BJ, Christiansen C, Podenphant J, Johansen JS. Nasal calcitonin for treatment of established osteoporosis. Clin Endocrinol (Oxf) 1989;30(4):435–442.
45. Overgaard K, Hansen MA, Jensen SB, Christiansen C. Effect of salcatonin given intranasally on bone mass and fracture rates in established osteoporosis: a dose–response study. BMJ 1992;305(6853):556–561.
46. Overgaard K, Riis BJ, Christiansen C, Hansen MA. Effect of salcatonin given intranasally on early postmenopausal bone loss. BMJ 1989;299(6697):477–479.

47. Reginster JY, Denis D, Deroisy R, Lecart MP, De Longueville M, Zegels B, Sarlet N, Noirfalisse P, Franchimont P. Long-term (3 years) prevention of trabecular postmenopausal bone loss with low-dose intermittent nasal salmon calcitonin. J Bone Miner Res 1994;9(1):69–73.
48. Silverman SL. Quality-of-life issues in osteoporosis. Curr Rheumatol Rep 2005;7(1):39–45.
49. Chesnut CH, Richardson P, Mindeholm L. Salmon calcitonin nasal spray (SCNS): effect on hip fractures in postmenopausal women (abstract). Osteoporos Int 2002;13(Suppl. 1):P128SA.
50. Delmas PD, Genant HK, Crans GG, Stock JL, Wong M, Siris E, Adachi JD. Severity of prevalent vertebral fractures and the risk of subsequent vertebral and nonvertebral fractures: results from the MORE trial. Bone 2003;33(4):522–532.
51. Chesnut C III, Skag A, Christiansen C, Recker R, Stakkestad J, Hoiseth A, Felsenberg D, Huss H, Gilbride J, Schimmer R, Delmas P. Oral ibandronate osteoporosis vertebral fracture trial in North America and Europe (BONE). J Bone Miner Res 2004;19(8):1241–1249.
52. Rubin CD. Emerging concepts in osteoporosis and bone strength. Curr Med Res Opin 2005;21(7): 1049–1056.
53. Cefalu C. Is bone mineral density predictive of fracture risk reduction ? Curr Med Res Opin 2004; 20 (3):341–349
54. Sarkar S, Mitlak BH, Wong M, Stock JL, Black DM, Harper KD. Relationships between bone mineral density and incident vertebral fracture risk with raloxifene therapy. J Bone Miner Res 2002;17(1): 1–10.
55. Olson M, Mindeholm L, Eriksen EF, Majumdar S, Azria M, Chesnut C. Trabecular number as risk factor in osteoporosis and the role of nasal spray calcitonin (NS-CT) in its modification(abstract). Osteoporos Int 2006:17(Suppl. 1):S12–S13.
56. Jiang Y, Zhao J, Geusens P, Liao EY, Adriaensens P, Gelan J, Azria M, Boonen S, Caulin F, Lynch JA, Ouyang X, Genant HK. Femoral neck trabecular microstructure in ovariectomized ewes treated with calcitonin: MRI microscopic evaluation. J Bone Miner Res 2005;20(1):125–130.
57. Lufkin E, Sarkar S, Kulkarni M, Ciaccia A, Siddhanti S, Stock J, Plouffe L. Antiresorptive treatment of postmenopausal osteoporosis: review of randomized clinical studies and rationale for the Evista alendronate comparison (EVA) trial. Curr Med Res Opin 2004;20(3):351–357.
58. Marcus R, Wong M, Heath H, Stock J. Antiresorptive treatment of postmenopausal osteoporosis: comparison of study designs and outcomes in clinical trials with fracture as endpoint. Endocr Rev 2002;23:16–37.
59. Boonen S, Body J, Boutsen Y, Devogelaer J, Goemaere S, Kaufman J, Rozenberg S, Reginster J. Evidence-based guidelines for the treatment of postmenopausal osteoporosis: a consensus document of the Belgian Bone Club. Osteoporos Int 2005;16:239–254.
60. Altkorn D, Vokes T. Treatment of postmenopausal osteoporosis. JAMA 2001;285:1415–1418.
61. Hamdy R, Chesnut CH III, Holick M, Leib E, Lewiecki M, Maricic M, Watts N. Review of treatment modalities for postmenopausal osteoporosis. South Med J 2005;98(10):1000–1014.
62. Borah B, Dufresne TE, Chmielewski PA, Johnson TD, Chines A, Manhart MD. Risedronate preserves bone architecture in postmenopausal women with osteoporosis as measured by three-dimensional microcomputed tomography. Bone 2004;34(4):736–746
63. Trovas GP, Lyritis GP, Galanos A, Raptou P, Constantelou E. A randomized trial of nasal spray salmon calcitonin in men with idiopathic osteoporosis: effects on bone mineral density and bone markers. J Bone Miner Res 2002;17(3):521–527.
64. Toth E, Csupor E, Meszaros S, Ferencz V, Nemeth L, McCloskey EV, Horvath C. The effect of intranasal salmon calcitonin therapy on bone mineral density in idiopathic male osteoporosis without vertebral fracturesan open label study. Bone 2005;36(1):47–51.
65. Pun KK, Chan LW. Analgesic effect of intranasal salmon calcitonin in the treatment of osteoporotic vertebral fractures. Clin Ther 1989;11(2):205–209.
66. Lyritis GP, Paspati I, Karachalios T, Ioakimidis D, Skarantavos G, Lyritis PG. Pain relief from nasal salmon calcitonin in osteoporotic vertebral crush fractures. A double blind, placebo-controlled clinical study. Acta Orthop Scand 1997;275(Suppl.):112–114.
67. Cranney A, Welch V, Adachi JD, Homik J, Shea B, Suarez-Almazor ME, Tugwell P, Wells G. Calcitonin for the treatment and prevention of corticosteroid-induced osteoporosis. Cochrane Database Syst Rev 2000;2:CD001983.

68. Sexton PM. Central nervous system binding sites for calcitonin and calcitonin gene-related peptide. Mol Neurobiol 1992;5:251–273.
69. Fischer JA, Tobler PH, Kaufmann M, Born W, Henke H, Cooper PE, Sagar SM, Martin JB. Calcitonin: regional distribution of the hormone and its binding sites in the human brain and pituitary. Proc Natl Acad Sci. USA 1981;78:7801–7895.
70. Laurian L, Oberman Z, Graff E, Gilard S, Moerer E, et al. Calcitonin-induced increase in ACTH, β-endorphin and cortisol secretion. Hormone Metab Res 1986;18:268–271.
71. Colado M, Ormazabal M, Goicoechea C, Lopez F, Alfaro M, Martin M. Involvement of central serotonergic pathways in analgesia elicited by salmon calcitonin in the mouse. Eur J Pharmacol 1994;252:291–297.
72. Clementi G, Prato A, Conforto G, Scapagnini U. Role of serotonin in the analgesic activity of calcitonin. Eur J Pharmacol 1984;98:449–451.
73. Silverman SL, Azria M. The analgesic role of calcitonin following osteoporotic fracture. Osteoporos Int 2002;13(11):858–867.
74. Lyritis GP, Tsakalakos N, Magiasis B, Karachalios T, Yiatzides, Tsekoura M. Analgesic effect of salmon calcitonin in osteoporotic vertebral fractures: A double-blind placebo-controlled clinical study. Calcif Tissue Int 1991;49:369–372.
75. Gennari C, Nami R, Francini G, et al. Calcitonin and metastatic bone disease: effects on bone pain and osteolysis. Proceedings of International Symposium "Calcitonin: the many-sided hormone". Athens 1982:74
76. Lussier D, Huskey AG, Portenoy RK. Adjuvant analgesics in cancer pain management. Oncologist 2004;9(5):571
77. Grunstein HS, Clifton, Bligh P, Posen S. Paget's disease of bone: experiences with 100 patients treated with salmon calcitonin. Med J Aust 1981;2:278–280.
78. Kuhlencordt F, Ringe JD, Kruse HP. Behandlung der osteodystrophia deformans paget mit lachs-calcitonin. Dtsch Med Wochenschr 1981;106:1620–1623.
79. Peichl P, Marteau R, Griesmacher A, Kumpan W, Schedl R, Prosquil E, Fasol P, Broll H. Salmon calcitonin nasal spray treatment for postmenopausal women after hip fracture with total hip arthroplasty. J Bone Miner Metab 2005;23(3):243–252.
80. Huusko TM, Karppi P, Kautiainen H, Suominen H, Avikainen V, Sulkava R. Randomized, double-blind, clinically controlled trial of intranasal calcitonin treatment in patients with hip fracture. Calcif Tissue Int 2002;71(6):478–484.
81. Combe B, Cohen C, Aubin F. Equivalence of nasal spray and subcutaneous formulations of salmon calcitonin. Calcif Tissue Int 1997;61(1):10–15
82. Maksymowych WP. Managing acute osteoporotic vertebral fractures with calcitonin. Can Fam Physician 1998;44:2160–2166.
83. Blau LA, Hoehns JD. Analgesic efficacy of calcitonin for vertebral fracture pain. Ann Pharmacother 2003;37(4):564–570.
84. Knopp JA, Diner BM, Blitz M, Lyritis GP, Rowe BH. Calcitonin for treating acute pain of osteoporotic vertebral compression fractures: a systematic review of randomized, controlled trials. Osteoporosis Int 2005;16(10):1281–1290.
85. Lyritis GP, Paspati I, Karachalios T, Ioakimidis D, Skarantavos G, Lyritis PG. Pain relief from nasal salmon calcitonin in osteoporotic vertebral crush fractures. A double blind, placebo-controlled clinical study. Acta Orthop Scand Suppl 1997;275:112–114.
86. Arinoviche R, Arriagada M, Jacobelli S, Massardo L, Rivero S, Aris H, Valenzuela M, Rojas C, Carvallo A, Gatica H, et al. (Calcitonin in acute pain due to vertebral fracture in osteoporosis. Cooperative study) Rev Med Chil 1987;115(11):1039–1043.
87. Lyritis GP, Ioannidis GV, Karachalios T, Roidis N, Kataxaki E, Papaioannou N, Kaloudis J, Galanos A. Analgesic effect of salmon calcitonin suppositories in patients with acute pain due to recent osteoporotic vertebral crush fractures: a prospective double-blind, randomized, placebo-controlled clinical study. Clin J Pain 1999;15(4):284–289.
88. Plosker GL, McTavish D. Intranasal salcatonin (salmon calcitonin): a review of its pharmacological properties and role in the management of postmenopausal osteoporosis. Drugs Aging 1991;8:378–400.
89. Clissold S, Fitton A, Chrisp P. Intranasal salmon calcitonin. A review of its pharmacological properties and potential utility in metabolic bone disorders associated with aging. Drugs Aging 1991;1:405–423.

90. Foti R, Martorana U, Broggini M. Long-term tolerability of nasal spray formulation of salmon calcitonin. Curr Ther Res 1995;56:429–435.
91. Buclin T, Cosma Rochat M, Burckhardt P, Azria M, Attinger M. Bioavailability and biological efficacy of a new oral formulation of salmon calcitonin in healthy volunteers. J Bone Miner Res 2002;17(8):1478–1485.
92. Tanko LB, Bagger YZ, Alesandersen P, Devogelaer JP, Reginster JY, Chick R, Olson M, Benmammar H, Mindeholm L, Azria M, Christiansen C. Safety and efficacy of a novel salmon calcitonin (sCT) technology-based oral formulation in healthy postmenopausal women: acute and 3-month effects on biomarkers of bone turnover. J Bone Miner Res 2004;19(9):1531–1538.
93. Bagger YZ, Tanko LB, Alexandersen P, Karsdal MA, Olson M, Mindeholm L, Azria M, Christiansen C. Oral salmon calcitonin induced suppression of urinary collagen type II degradation in postmenopausal women: a new potential treatment of osteoarthritis. Bone 2005;37(3):425–430.

19 Bisphosphonate Mechanisms of Action

Alfred A. Reszka

CONTENTS

SUMMARY

The nitrogen-containing bisphosphonates are potent and highly effective non-hormonal anti-osteoporotic agents for clinical use in the treatment of post menopausal or glucocorticoid-induced osteoporosis, Paget's disease, metastatic bone disease and hypercalcemia of malignancy, among others. The Potency of the nitrogen-containing bisphosphonates can partially be attributed to their specific targeting to bone-associated osteoclasts with intermittent dosing at monthly or yearly intervals, the nitrogen-containing bisphosphonates may also label the osteoblast surface, where they remain insert, awaiting the next resorption cycles that will eventually initials at these sites. Through current or future resorption cycles these bisphosphonates can be liberated from the bone surface and taken into the osteoclast interior, where they exert their pharmacological effects as inhibitors of the isoprenoid biosynthetic enzyme, farnesyl diphosphate synthase. This chapter will discuss the utility of this class of drug as effective antifracture agents with a focus on their intriguing mechanism of action.

Key Words: Bisphosphonates, mechanism of action, osteoclast, mevalonate, bone resorption, apoptosis

INTRODUCTION

Osteoporosis and Fracture Risk

Osteoporosis is a reduction in bone mass and bone microarchitecture leading to increased bone fragility and fracture risk. The most common cause of osteoporosis is increased bone turnover with excessive bone resorption (destruction) that exceeds bone formation. Among women, this is often caused by estrogen deficiency following menopause. A second large

From: *Contemporary Endocrinology: Osteoporosis: Pathophysiology and Clinical Management*
Edited by: R. A. Adler, DOI 10.1007/978-1-59745-459-9_19,

and independent contributor is glucocorticoid use. Later in life, a combination of vitamin D insufficiency, reduced 1,25$(OH)_2$-vitamin D_3 production, and inadequate calcium nutrition contribute to bone loss in both men and women. Both menopause and glucocorticoid use cause an imbalance between the processes of bone resorption (removal) and formation, leading to bone loss. A woman can experience a loss of up to 5% of her bone mass per year during the first 5 years postmenopause. There exists a correlation between the reduction in bone mineral density *(1–4)* and the increased bone turnover *(5–7)* with increased fracture risk.

Incidence of fracture increases with age and associated increased risk of trauma with falls, which is an independent contributor. The most common fractures occur in the spine, and their frequency increases progressively in women and men beginning in the sixth and seventh respective decades of life. The most serious fractures are of the hip. The incidence of these increases steadily, reaching a rate of about 5% per year in the ninth decade of life. Approximately 70–75% of all hip fractures occur in women, likely due to their earlier and more dramatic bone loss, gender-based differences in bone mass, and greater longevity. The increase in men occurs about a decade later than in women.

With the continued increase in life expectancy due to medical and other advancements and increase in the population worldwide, it is projected that the incidence of osteoporotic fractures will reach epidemic proportions within the next couple of decades if effective means to combat them are not implemented.

Bisphosphonates as Therapy for Osteoporosis and Other Bone-Destructive Conditions

The bisphosphonates (BPs), in particular alendronate (ALN), risedronate (RIS), and zoledronate (ZOL; noted in its salt form) are the only non-hormonal agents shown to suppress both spinal and non-vertebral osteoporotic fractures. Ibandronate (IBA) reduces the risk of vertebral fractures but has not demonstrated the effect on non-vertebral fracture risk. Because they do not work via endocrine receptors, BPs can be and are widely used for the treatment and prevention of both postmenopausal and glucocorticoid-induced osteoporosis and Paget's disease without risk of off-target effects in other organs or changes in endocrine function. Indeed, they can be and are used for the treatment of bone metastases, where intravenous pamidronate (PAM) and ZOL are standard therapy. BPs suppress bone turnover by reducing the number of bone remodeling sites where excessive osteoclastic bone resorption takes place. Two major molecular mechanisms have been identified that explain how BPs suppress osteoclastic bone resorption. For the older, less potent BPs (BPs that require substantially higher dosing), specifically etidronate and clodronate, the molecule is taken up by the osteoclast and converted into a toxic ATP analog. For the more potent and most frequently used BPs, the molecule is also taken up by the osteoclast but it is not metabolized. Instead these bisphosphonates target and inhibit an enzyme called farnesyl diphosphate synthase (FPPS), a component of the mevalonate to cholesterol biosynthetic pathway. This property of the N-BPs and other physicochemical aspects of BPs in general are the subject of this chapter.

BISPHOSPHONATE PHYSICAL PROPERTIES

BP Structure

BPs are analogs of pyrophosphate (P–O–P) in which the central oxygen has been substituted by carbon (P–C–P) (Fig. 1). P–C–P bonds are not enzymatically cleaved, and this minimizes the possibility for hepatic or cellular metabolism, and none has been detected for ALN in pharmacokinetic studies *(8,9)*. All clinically used BPs are derivatives of the basic structure, shown in Fig. 1, and they can be broadly broken down according to their intracellular mechanisms (Fig. 2), as discussed below. A main common feature relates to the P–C–P backbone that, by adhering to the hydroxyapatite component of bone, localizes these compounds in the target tissue. The human skeleton has a large surface area and virtually an unsaturable capacity for the binding of the BPs. Thus, for the highly potent N-BPs, the number of potential binding sites is immense, and the total skeletal burden is very low (measured in the low parts per million).

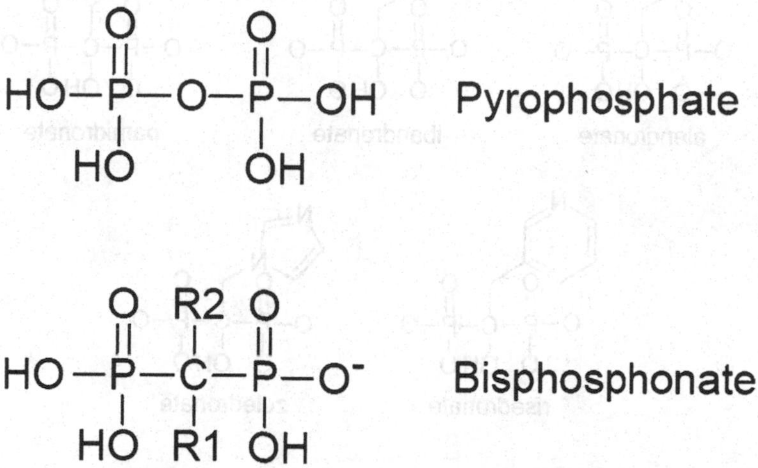

Fig. 1. Structures of (top) pyrophosphate and (bottom) a basic bisphosphonate. Note that in the basic structure, substitutions at R^1 are generally considered to affect binding to bone, while substitutions at R^2 affect potency.

Effect of BP Structure on Physicochemical Interactions with Bone

BINDING TO NATURAL BONE

The affinity of BPs for natural bone and for hydroxyapatite is shown in Table 1. The direct binding affinity of ALN for human bone has recently been measured by Scatchard analysis (K_d of 110 μM), and comparable affinity was calculated from on (69/M/min) and off (0.033/min) rates *(10)*. The measurement of an off rate is an interesting feature, as it demonstrates that this BP, as a representative of the entire class, does not irreversibly bind to the bone surface. Instead, it binds, releases, and rebinds. The key to measuring the off rate relates to the initial application of a radioactively tagged BP onto the bone surface and then to saturate the bone with excess non-tagged BP. When the radiolabeled BP is released, the excess untagged BP binds to the bone in its place, and the radiolabel becomes effectively

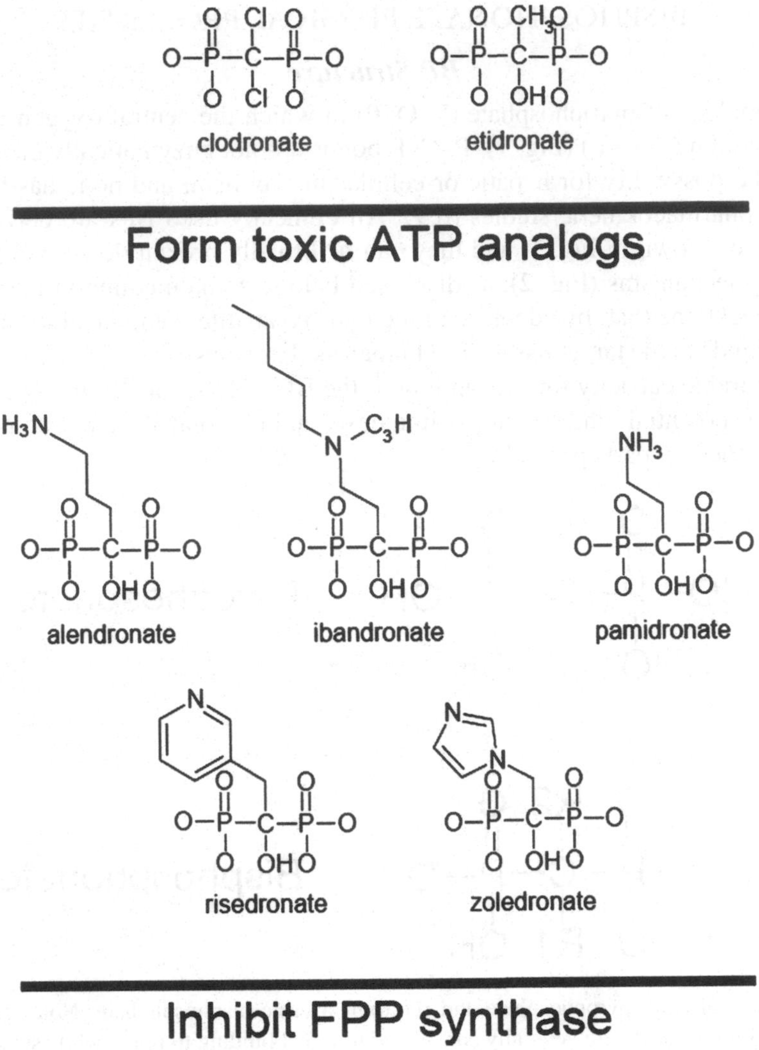

Fig. 2. Structures of BPs-lacking nitrogen (top), which inhibit bone resorption by inducing osteoclast apoptosis and N-BPs (bottom), which can inhibit function or induce osteoclast apoptosis, depending on dose.

trapped in solution, away from the bone. This can be achieved in the laboratory setting, and it enables the released BP to be quantified by scintillation counting. The rate at which the radiolabel accumulates in solution indicates the "off rate." In the human body, there is no excess BP sitting in solution ready to bind onto the bone surface in place of the released BP. Thus, the BP that releases from the bone can follow any of three major paths: (1) it can reattach in the same or an adjacent site, (2) it can redistribute to other sites on bone, or (3) it can be excreted in the urine. Which of these activities occurs is in part affected by the affinity of the BP for the bone surface.

The affinity of ALN for bone is slightly different from that of other BPs, as each has its own unique structure. Therefore competition binding assays were used to measure the binding of a series of clinically tested and used BPs to human bone. In these studies, the

Table 1
Binding Affinities of BPs for Natural Bone and Hydroxyapatite

Bisphosphonate	*Relative affinity for natural bone (μM)[a]*	*Estimated affinity for hydroxyapatite (μM)[b]*
Clodronate	806	1.39
Etidronate	90.7	0.84
Risedronate	84.6	0.46
Ibandronate	116	0.42
Alendronate	60.9	0.34
Zoledronate	80.8	0.29
Pamidronate	82.7	nd
Tiludronate	173	nd

[a]Based on Leu et al. *(10)*
[b]Calculated from Nancollas et al. *(14)*

competing BPs had no radioactive tag, and they were mixed with radioactive ALN prior to applying to the human bone. Their ability to compete with ALN for binding sites is a measure of their affinity for bone and is represented by a loss of (ALN) radioactivity that can effectively bind in their presence. By these analyses, it was shown that most BPs bearing a hydroxyl (OH) at R^1 (Fig. 2) bind in a relatively narrow (70–170 μM) range *(10)*. In this regard, etidronate, a BP-lacking nitrogen, fell in line with the other hydroxyl-bearing N-BPs (ALN, IBA, PAM, RIS, and ZOL). In agreement with the relative binding affinities measured toward human bone, others have measured similar affinities toward mouse long bones *(11–13)*. Two BPs that stand out as significantly different in terms of binding affinity are tiludronate (228 μM) and especially clodronate (1182 μM), both of which lack an R^1 hydroxyl group, and both of which display significantly weaker affinity for human bone vs. the hydroxyl-bearing BPs.

With respect to clodronate, the substantially weaker binding affinity for bone has negative consequences on the potency of the drug. Clodronate can approach the antiresorptive potency of ALN and RIS in in vitro analyses whereby concentrations are kept at a constant (i.e., with excess solution-based drug available for binding to bone in areas where release has occurred). However, clodronate loses roughly 10-fold potency when retention on the bone surface is required for continued anti-osteoclastic activity *(10)*. The latter state is achieved through simply coating the bone with the BP and then washing it prior to subsequent application of osteoclasts. Here the BP must rebind to the bone surface in order to have an antiresorptive effect. This state more closely resembles that seen in vivo. In contrast to clodronate, ALN and RIS maintain equal relative potency regardless of whether concentration is kept constant or requires binding/rebinding to bone. This feature is most likely attributable to the fact that both ALN and RIS, like the other hydroxyl-bearing BPs, adhere to bone through what is called "tridentate" binding *(11)*. An amine at R^1, as an alternative to a hydroxyl at this site, is also effective in increasing BP affinity to rodent bone. It is important to note here that the widely used N-BPs only have a hydroxyl at R^1. For these BPs, the nitrogen is a component of the side chain attached at R^2, where it does not contribute significantly to binding affinity. The lack of an effect of the R^2 substituents to meaningfully alter binding affinity toward bone is interesting, given that they do seem to have some minor impact on binding to pure hydroxyapatite in vitro, as discussed below.

Binding to Pure Hydroxyapatite

Hydroxyapatite in pure form is related to hydroxyapatite in bone, although it lacks both surface and embedded protein components, such as type I collagen. This may be important, since BP affinity toward hydroxyapatite is ~100- to ~600-fold higher than it is for natural bone (Table 1). Binding affinities of BPs for the pure chemical components of hydroxyapatite have not been measured directly, although constant composition kinetic studies of crystal growth, coupled with a pseudo Langmuir adsorption isotherms, have been performed to estimate binding affinity *(14)*. These studies suggest a narrow range for binding affinities (0.3–1.4 μM, as shown in Table 1). The differences in reported affinity for pure hydroxyapatite vs. human bone are likely attributable to differences in methodology (direct binding vs. crystal growth) and the composition of the binding surface (natural bone vs. hydroxyapatite crystal). In the constant composition kinetic analyses of pure hydroxyapatite, clodronate remained at the weak end of the affinity spectrum (1.4 μM). This BP and etidronate showed small, but significant affinity differences vs. the reference BP, RIS, which bound with two- to three-fold higher affinity. Meanwhile, ALN and ZOL showed small (1.35- and 1.58-fold, respectively), but significantly higher binding affinities vs. RIS. The statistically significant differences likely arise from the highly controlled conditions in these experiments and the lack of protein that is normally found in bone. In general, the rank ordering for affinity of the various BPs for hydroxyapatite differs vs. that for bone, although in both model systems, clodronate falls at the weak end of the spectrum.

BP Effects on Zeta Potential

Zeta potential is measured by assessing the electrophoretic mobilities of particles in suspension under constant ionic conditions. General applications for zeta potential include estimation of the stability of colloidal suspensions, although several groups have also applied them to the study of bone. The zeta potential of natural bone is most heavily influenced by the organic (e.g., protein) component. This conclusion comes from observations that removal of the mineral component from bone has little effect of zeta potential, while removal of the organic matrix results in a much smaller zeta potential *(15)*. Thus, collagen (and likely other bone matrix proteins), rather than hydroxyapatite mineral, is implicated as the constituent of whole bone dominating the zeta potential.

Recently, the zeta potential of pure hydroxyapatite was assessed in the absence or presence of various BPs *(14)*. Depending on the pH, the hydroxyl-bearing BPs were found to alter the zeta potential of pure hydroxyapatite crystals in the range of ~ –9 to +6 mV under mildly acidic conditions and ~ –5 to +>10 mV at neutral pH (after adjusting for pH effects on the crystals in the absence of BP treatment). At neutral pH, clodronate, etidronate, and RIS tended to reduce zeta potential, while ALN and IBA tended to increase it. Etidronate is especially interesting in this context, as it has also been tested for in vivo effects on the zeta potential of natural bone in gonad-intact and oophorectomized rats. For context, etidronate's effect on pure hydroxyapatite in vitro is to reduce zeta potential by ~ –9 mV at neutral pH. However, in the bone of gonad-intact rats, etidronate only modestly reduced zeta potential by –0.59 mV after 6 weeks of treatment at high dose (5 mg/kg, s.c. twice weekly), and this effect diminished and lost significance after continued dosing to 16 weeks *(16)*. In the context of ovariectomy, etidronate showed a positive effect to maintain bone mass in these studies, but it had only a minor (–0.11 mV), non-significant effect on zeta potential, despite the high dosing. There have been no similar in vivo reports for the highly potent N-BPs, which are dosed at levels far below those for etidronate. In the absence of these data, it is difficult to assign significance to the in vitro effects of the BPs on zeta potential of hydroxyapatite. Nonetheless, the preliminary findings are interesting, and they warrant follow-up in more relevant systems.

Summary of Physicochemical Properties of BPs

Overall, substituents at the R^1 position of the BP, in particular the presence of a hydroxyl group, have the potential to positively affect BP binding to natural human bone or to pure hydroxyapatite. Meanwhile, substituents at R^2 appear to have only a minor impact on binding affinity. These substituents may alter BP effects on zeta potential of hydroxyapatite in vitro. However, such effects on natural bone may be greatly reduced by the effects of the proteinaceous components. Perhaps a more relevant role for the substituents attached at R^2 relate to the positioning of a nitrogen atom 3–4 positions away from the central carbon of the P–C–P backbone. This plays a critical role in determining intracellular potency, with consequent effects on dosing and efficacy, as discussed in sections below.

Impact of BP Structure on Pharmacokinetics

Absorption and Bioavailability

The P–C–P backbone endows the entire BP class with several common properties, especially regarding pharmacokinetics. The highly charged phosphonate moieties limit absorption in the gut to around 0.6–2%, depending on the BP and the dose. ALN and RIS show linear oral bioavailability. However, IBA exhibits an interesting, non-linear bioavailability that changes across the range used to treat osteoporosis. This is reflected in the area under the curve (AUC) for IBA, as measured at 50, 100, and 150 mg oral doses, whereby the systemic exposure ratios were 130 and 191% (relative to the 50-mg dose) for the 100- and 150-mg doses, respectively *(17)*. This suggests that, although the 150 mg monthly tablet contains 60-fold more IBA vs. daily (2.5 mg), systemic exposure of the monthly dose should be at least ~115-fold higher or more. Thus the 150 mg monthly tablet results in four-fold greater cumulative BP exposure vs. the 2.5 mg daily tablet. This would differ from the systemic exposures for weekly ALN and RIS, which are linear in the dosing range surrounding daily and weekly doses *(18,19)*, resulting in the same cumulative exposure.

ALN entry into the blood stream from the gut was found to be by paracellular transport, and renal excretion is the only route for elimination from the body, in part by glomerular filtration and by a secretory process that remains to be elucidated *(20)*. The hydrophilic phosphonate moieties limit the penetration of BPs through cellular lipid bilayer membranes to undetectable levels, thus distribution is limited to an extracellular compartment and, 1 day after a dose, is essentially limited to the surface of bone. The bioavailable BP is thus rapidly cleared from the circulation with an end result of about 50% binding to the bone mineral, as reported for ALN *(21)*. The remainder is excreted in the urine, which is the sample material used for most pharmacokinetic analyses. A head-to-head comparison of ALN and RIS showed that the initial uptake over the first 24 h was not different between the two BPs, as suggested by urinary excretion *(22)*. It is likely that initial bone uptake of all BPs in clinical use is similar. This suggests a similar initial pharmacokinetic profile for these, and perhaps other, BPs. During this first 24 h period, the circulating BP half-life is approximately 1–2 h, and the bulk of the BP not retained on the bone surface is excreted during what is called the first elimination phase.

HALF-LIVES

Understanding the initial pharmacokinetic profile of the BPs should take into account the physicochemical parameters (described above) and the distribution of the BPs over the bone surface. BPs bind to the mineral surface of bone, perhaps with the affinity being influenced by the presence of protein in and on the bone. Because the resting surfaces of bone are covered with cells (osteoblasts and lining cells), the most exposed sites are those undergoing active bone resorption. It was shown that these are the preferential sites for ALN uptake in bone at pharmacologically relevant doses in animals *(23–25)*. At suprapharmacological doses (far above those used to treat humans), ALN is more or less evenly distributed over the bone surface. Due to its much lower antiresorptive potency, pharmacologically relevant doses of etidronate are high, and these result in a uniform distribution over the bone surface when dosed appropriately.

Before bone formation is initiated at a given BP-coated site, the drug can be released from the surface through both simple and facilitated release. With respect to simple release, ALN has an observed off rate of 0.033/min at neutral pH in vitro *(10)*. Any BP that is released through this process has the possibility of rebinding to nearby sites, or it can escape back into the circulation where it is either distributed to another site on the bone surface or excreted into the urine. BP on the surface of bone may also be incorporated into newly formed bone, from which it is released only through osteoclast-mediated bone resorption. Both simple and facilitated release relate to the intermediate and terminal elimination phases, as discussed below.

Intermediate half-lives The intermediate elimination phases exclusively represent BP that has bound and then later been released from the bone surface. The effect of time post-dose on estimated half-life can be illustrated by two pharmacokinetic studies of ALN and RIS, whereby sampling and intermediate half-life calculations were conducted over a period of time as short as 7 days or out to 180 days *(18,21)*. The earliest intermediate elimination phase calculated for ALN (30 mg, IV) was estimated after 4–7 days post-dose, whereby the half-life was calculated at 0.8 days. Measurements of ALN release into the urine between days 9 and 16 post-dose yielded a half-life of 6.6 days. Meanwhile the last intermediate elimination phase was measured between days 30 and 180, whereby a half-life of 35.6 days was measured. Consistent with the findings for ALN, a 7 day study of RIS at the 2.5 mg dose (p.o.) yielded a half-life of 5.6 days *(18)*. Longer sampling could not be achieved for this dose, as the RIS in the urine fell below the limit of detection. The 5 mg dose of RIS was detected in urine for 28 days, and the data yielded a half-life of 9 days. A comparison of the half-lives estimated for these BPs shows a clear trend whereby measurements immediately following initial administration yield half-lives that are considerably shorter than those that are calculated weeks to months post-dose. This in some way reflects the dynamic nature of bone remodeling and the location of administered BP over time.

Changes in estimated half-life, as measured over time, are in part controlled by the osteoclast and its interactions with both the BP and the mineral surface. The fundamental means by which the osteoclast demineralizes the bone surface is through secretion of acid into the resorption lacuna. This is important, as the process also provides a means to release the BP from the mineral surface as well *(23)*. Thus, an initial step in the process is the release of BP into the resorption lacuna as a part of the process of bone resorption by the osteoclast. Roughly two decades ago it was documented by microradiography that following radioactive ALN administration in vivo, the BP can be detected inside the osteoclast after 4 h *(23,25)*. This step involves transcytosis, a process for the removal of liberated mineral and proteinaceous components of bone through the osteoclast's interior in vesicular enclosures *(26,27)*. The vesicles, considered to be part of the extracellular space, collect contents from the resorption lacuna, traverse the cytoplasm, and then fuse at the ventral membrane to release into the local environment. These vesicles, although located in the cell's interior, provide a barrier that helps to keep the N-BP from its intended target(s) within the cytoplasm. Nonetheless, it was shown in vitro that osteoclasts that have lost the ability to take up material from their surroundings, due to a mutation that blocks transcytosis (e.g., osteoclasts from the oc/oc mouse), do not respond to tiludronate *(28)*. A response could be produced, however, by microinjecting this BP into the cells. The current model thus holds that during the transcytosis process, some BP can penetrate the vesicular membrane to enter into the cytoplasm. A recent study suggests that this is a result of acidification of the vesicle, coupled with the process of pinocytosis *(29)*. Once within the cytoplasm, there still remains a lag period before the BPs can have their effect. Overall, the time from first administration to first signs of inhibition is 16–24 h *(30,31)*. By this time, the osteoclast's capacity to facilitate BP release begins to be diminished, and this slows the process of releasing the BP from the bone surface. The osteoclastogenesis that results from the small rise in circulating parathyroid hormone levels means that each resorption site can have several osteoclasts, each displaying a different degree of inhibition related to the time the osteoclast has been exposed to BP. This makes the inhibition process somewhat asynchronous, and thus the decline in markers of bone resorption is more gradual. Moreover, recently formed osteoclasts will be fully active until they have taken up sufficient BP to inhibit resorption. This mechanism differs from that for RANK ligand inhibitors, such as denosumab, which has been demonstrated to achieve a more immediate suppression of C-telopeptides vs. ALN through its effects on both existing, active osteoclasts and their precursors *(32)*.

The degree to which a BP reduces bone turnover therefore relates to how much of the administered dose is retained on the surface of the skeleton, with better control of turnover associated with better skeletal retention. This has been documented in clinical studies of PAM in both cancer patients and those with rheumatoid arthritis, whereby lower bone turnover rates, assessed by release of C-telopeptides and N-telopeptides of type I collagen, were associated with high retention of the initially bound PAM, while high bone turnover was associated with reduced retention *(33,34)*. This is in part (a) a reflection of the activity of the osteoclasts that liberate the BP from the bone surface, (b) the efficacy of the BP to inhibit the osteoclast, and (c) the completion of the bone resorption cycle at the site of

BP attachment. Termination of the resorption cycle is called "reversal," which is followed by bone formation, which seals the BP into an inactive compartment. The association of higher skeletal retention with greater efficacy can be explained through two equally compelling models. In the first, the efficacy of the BP slows the osteoclasts and hampers their ability to liberate the BP from the bone. In the second, the greater skeletal retention leads to better BP access to inhibit the osteoclasts, which reduces bone turnover more effectively. The models are not mutually exclusive, and elements of both are likely to come into play.

A parallel comparison of the events at the bone remodeling unit to the pharmacokinetics of the BPs during the first days to weeks suggests that the shortest half-lives correspond to periods when the osteoclasts are least affected by the BPs. Half-lives extend as osteoclast activities decline through the binding of the BPs to their intracellular targets. Half-lives extend even further as bone formation initiates over the site of the adherent BP, thus effectively sealing it into the bone along the cement line. The period of time necessary for these sites to be revisited by new resorption cycles is the ultimate controlling element that determines terminal half-life, which is discussed below.

Terminal half-life The terminal half-life of the BP is a measure of the rate at which BP buried in bone is released back into circulation and excreted. In the final elimination phase for ALN, which was measured between 10 and 18 months post-dose, the release of BP into the urine over time reached true linearity. Having reached final linearity, one can estimate the terminal half-life, which is calculated at 10.9 years for ALN in humans *(21)*. No other BP has been studied for an equivalent time, although the terminal half-life for PAM, derived using data from a 6-month study, was modeled based on the 18-month data for ALN *(35)*.

Mechanistically, the terminal half–life of a BP is a reflection of the general state of bone turnover, which itself is influenced by the BP. Rates of turnover from both cortical and cancellous bone surfaces therefore determine not only the relative uptake and distribution of BPs when initially administered but also the subsequent release of BPs into the bloodstream. The cancellous bone takes up a relatively larger proportion of the absorbed BP than the cortical bone, since cancellous bone is subject to substantially higher turnover. Thus, the mechanistic insights showing how BPs distribute to the bone surface, and the subsequent events that govern their release can explain why accurate assessments of terminal half-life in pharmacokinetic analysis require a substantial follow-up. Indeed, the half-life estimated from modeling of bone turnover at the various compartments is comparable to that obtained in the 18-month pharmacokinetic analysis of ALN. From the modeling, an estimation of the total body burden of ALN after 10 years of treatment with an averaged daily dose of 10 mg orally has been calculated to be 75 mg *(36)*. Similar calculations could also be applied to other BPs, taking into account relative dosing, antiresorptive efficacy and duration of treatment.

MECHANISM OF ACTION

N-BP Action at the Molecular Level

Although tested clinically for over a decade, the molecular target for the N-BPs, was not described until the late 1990s. Prior to this, BPs were shown to affect several biochemical pathways. For example, numerous BPs were found to inhibit the activity of several protein tyrosine phosphatases *(37–41)*. These actions occurred usually at the upper range of pharmacologically relevant concentrations and failed to correlate with the pharmacological potency of these agents. Although these phosphatase inhibitory activities could be involved in the mechanism of action of some BPs, more compelling proof was obtained for a different molecular target responsible for BP inhibition of osteoclastic bone resorption, as described below.

N-BP Inhibition of the Cholesterol Biosynthetic Pathway

Over 15 years ago it was shown that certain BP derivatives (isoprenoid [phosphinylmethyl] phosphonates) weakly inhibit the cholesterol biosynthetic enzyme, squalene synthase *(42)*. The search for more potent inhibitors that might block cholesterol production revealed that the N-BPs incadronate (YM175) and IBA potently inhibit squalene synthase *(43)*. Subsequent studies examined the structure–activity relationship for inhibition of squalene synthase *(44–46)*. In vivo testing showed that certain compounds suppressed serum cholesterol in rodents *(44)*. Other cholesterol lowering bisphosphonates were shown to trigger degradation of hydroxymethylglutaryl coenzyme A *(47–49)*. In the same context, utility of squalene synthase inhibition by bisphosphonate was also used for the development of an assay to measure ZOL levels in animals and clinical serum samples *(50)*. Other N-BPs, such as ALN and PAM, do inhibit cholesterol synthesis, although this effect is mediated through targeting of an enzyme upstream of squalene synthase in the cholesterol biosynthetic pathway. Due to the pharmacokinetics and distribution to bone, these effects are limited to osteoclasts.

Although cholesterol itself is important for osteoclast signaling and survival, the osteoclast relies on low-density lipoprotein (LDL) as an external source rather than through internal synthetic pathways *(51,52)*. Indeed, restoration of cholesterol in the ALN-treated osteoclast does nothing to interfere with its inhibitory action on bone resorption *(53)*. This then lead to a search for other possible enzymes that could account for N-BP antiresorptive effects.

Farnesyl Diphosphate Synthase as the Molecular Target of the N-BPs

The ability of ALN and PAM to inhibit sterol biosynthesis upstream of squalene synthase *(43)* suggested that the relevant molecular target for inhibition would lie upstream of squalene synthase in the mevalonate pathway *(54)* (Fig. 3). After it was firmly established that replacement of downstream metabolites from this pathway could block N-BP action in osteoclasts (see below), the exact targeted enzyme was pursued. In these studies, the key enzyme inhibited by N-BPs was found to be farnesyl diphosphate synthase (FPPS) *(51,55,56)*. FPPS catalyzes the formation of FPP through the sequential condensation of two isopentenyl diphosphates (IPPs) and one dimethylallyl diphosphate (DMAPP) (Fig. 3). FPP itself is a substrate for squalene synthase, and thus inhibition of FPPS prevents accumulation of metabolites that are required for cholesterol synthesis.

Affinities of the various N-BPs for FPPS fall into the low-to-mid nanomolar range. The general rank ordering for potency against this enzyme in vitro correlates with the rank ordering for potency in vivo *(55)*. This and the fact that a key metabolite below FPPS in this metabolic pathway is critical for osteoclast function and survival (discussed below) strongly suggested that this enzyme was the key target for N-BP action.

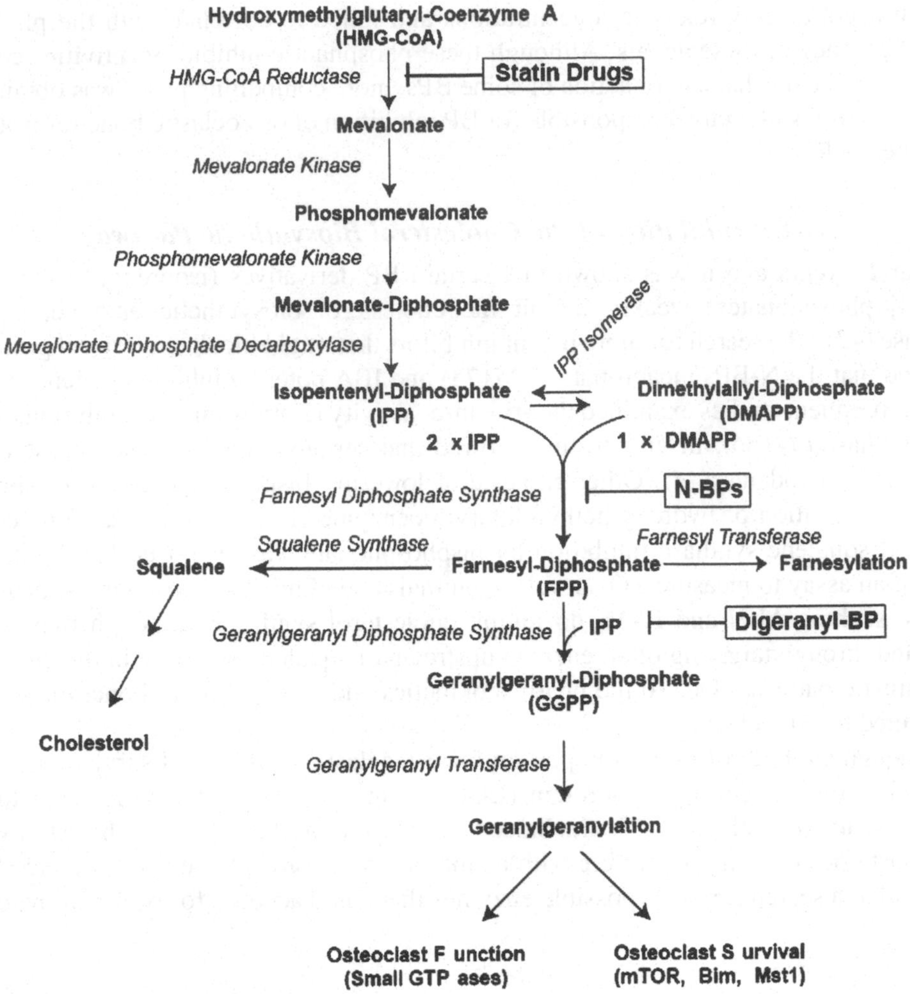

Fig. 3. Schematic of the mevalonate pathway. All enzymes are listed in *italics*, while metabolites are in **bold**. The target of inhibition (farnesyl diphosphate synthase) for the N-BPs is enclosed within a box, as is the target for the statins, which is shown for reference. A new BP (digeranyl-BP), which targets geranylgeranyl diphosphate synthase, is also shown.

Modeling of FPPS inhibition using RIS showed that modifications (e.g., addition of a methyl group) to the structure of the R^2 side chain can give rise to analogs with markedly less potent inhibition of the enzyme, making them less effective inhibitors of bone resorption in vivo *(55)*. The variable that confers potency against FPPS appears to relate to the position of the nitrogen group relative to the phosphonate groups. Interestingly, a modification in one of the phosphonate groups of RIS, while drastically reducing FPPS inhibition, gave rise to a new compound with new activity against type II geranylgeranyl transferase *(57)*. This derivative has substantially less antiresorptive activity than RIS in vivo, likely due to reduced binding to bone *(13)*. Other modifications of RIS can confer specificity for isopentenyl diphosphate isomerase in addition to FPPS *(58)*. Interestingly, a new BP-lacking nitrogen (digeranyl BP) has been shown to specifically target geranylgeranyl diphosphate (GGPP) synthase (Fig. 3), an enzyme immediately downstream of FPPS in the isoprenoid biosynthetic branch pathway that controls protein geranylgeranylation *(59)*. The in vivo effects of this BP-lacking nitrogen on bone turnover remain to be determined.

Early modeling of the interaction between N-BPs and FPPS suggested binding to the DMAPP/geranyl diphosphate (GPP) site *(60)*, where it would act as a transition-state analog. Enzymological studies suggest that inhibition of FPPS is complex *(61)*. Both competitive and non-competitive inhibitions have been reported, depending on the substrate used in the assay, IPP or GPP, respectively. Recent crystallographic studies have revealed exactly how the N-BP docks into FPPS. Binding is in the "allylic" site, which is normally occupied by DMAPP and in the second reaction, GPP. Structures derived using bacterial FPPS show that RIS binding into this site is enhanced in the presence of IPP *(62)*, which binds in the adjacent site. The binding of RIS mimics a "carbocation intermediate" to inhibit the enzyme, which is consistent with the original model. The microbial enzyme is smaller than that found in higher eukaryotes, and thus it was important to see the results refined. A more recent study with ALN, IBA, PAM, and ZOL bound to human FPPS confirmed that IPP binds to and stabilizes the N-BP-FPPS complex *(63)*. Importantly, this study revealed that the potent N-BPs promote the formation of a closed conformation of the enzyme in the presence of IPP. This effect can be attributed to the relative positioning of the nitrogen group of the N-BP, which contributes to interactions within the catalytic pocket of FPPS, including the formation of salt bridges and hydrogen bonds. As the most potent binder ZOL was found to create the best transition-state mimetic, while the weaker binding PAM did not make strong interactions or adopted more than one conformation within the enzyme active site. Interestingly, this study also revealed that the OH group at the R^1 position, known for its ability to enhance binding to bone *(10,12)*, also contributes to the binding of N-BPs to FPPS through the formation of a hydrogen bond and a polar contact with the enzyme. Thus, although the nitrogen at R^2 appears to have its greatest effect on binding to FPPS, the hydroxyl at R^1 appears to play a role in binding to bone and another role in stabilizing the N-BP interaction with FPPS. It may be for this reason that all current clinically used N-BPs have both the nitrogen in the chain attached at R^2 and the hydroxyl group attached at R^1.

Inhibition of FPPS Blocks Protein Isoprenylation and Sterol Synthesis

FPPS is responsible for the production of isoprenoid lipids FPP (15 carbon) and FPP is an immediate precursor for geranylgeranyl diphosphate (GGPP) (20 carbon). While FPP, formed by the condensation of two IPPs and one DMAPP, is primarily used to synthesize cholesterol, it also can be used for (15 carbon) protein isoprenylation (Fig. 3). FPP can also be condensed with a fourth IPP to form geranylgeranyl diphosphate (GGPP) by GGPP synthase, a distinct enzyme separate from FPPS. While the clinically tested N-BPs do not inhibit this enzyme directly, digeranyl BP (as noted above) directly inhibits the enzyme, which, in comparison to ZOL, shows a high specificity for blocking GGPP synthesis *(59)*. This is interesting, as a loss of GGPP synthesis in the osteoclast is critical for N-BP effects on suppressing osteoclastic bone resorption *(53)* and inducing osteoclast apoptosis *(64)*. GGPP, like FPP, is a substrate for protein isoprenylation, and both isoprenoids exhibit specificity in regard to the proteins to which they can be coupled. Isoprenylation involves the transfer of a farnesyl or geranylgeranyl lipid group onto a cysteine amino acid residue in characteristic carboxy-terminal (e.g., CAAX) motifs *(65,66)*. Most of the isoprenylated proteins identified to date are small GTPases that are geranylgeranylated, and specific CAAX motifs are responsible for directing which lipids are attached to each respective protein *(65)*. Geranylgeranylated signaling proteins are important for the regulation of a variety of cell processes required for osteoclast function, including cytoskeletal regulation, formation of the ruffled border, and regulation of apoptosis *(67–70)*. Interestingly, and counter to expectations, loss of geranylgeranylation of several of these proteins, specifically Rac, Cdc42, and Rho GTPases, leads to unregulated activation *(71)* (and not inactivation) of the proteins. Regardless of whether the GTPases are constitutively activated or inactivated, the result is the same: osteoclast inhibition.

The ability of the N-BPs to inhibit the cholesterol biosynthetic pathway and protein isoprenylation was actually first demonstrated in J774 macrophages *(43,54)*. The relevance of this model relates to the fact that J774 cells come from the same lineage as osteoclasts and that these cells, like osteoclasts, undergo apoptosis in response to N-BP treatment. In these early studies, it was recognized that N-BP inhibition of the cholesterol biosynthetic pathway and isoprenylation was important *(54)*. Using a more relevant system, it was later discovered that ALN inhibits incorporation of [^{14}C]mevalonate into either isoprenylated proteins or sterols in purified murine or rabbit osteoclasts *(51,72)*. The relevance of this effect was proven through the ability of a GGPP precursor, geranylgeraniol (GGOH), to block ALN effects on the osteoclast *(30,53,64)*, as discussed in detail below.

Evidence for Molecular Mechanisms In Vivo

The molecular actions of the N-BPs, described above, have been confirmed in vivo using surrogate markers *(73,74)*. In one study, the well-documented feedback regulation of HMG-CoA reductase expression by cholesterol biosynthetic intermediates was examined *(73)*. The N-BPs ALN, IBA, PAM, and RIS suppressed expression of HMG-CoA reductase in osteoclasts from the proximal tibia. Neither etidronate not clodronate could elicit any similar response. The effect of the N-BPs on HMG-CoA reductase was attributable to the accumulation of metabolites upstream of FPPS, as the effect could be blocked by co-treatment with a statin, which blocks their synthesis. In the second study, osteoclasts were examined for the in vivo actions of ALN on geranylgeranylation of the small GTPase, Rap1A *(74)*. In osteoclasts purified after ALN, but not clodronate, treatment, geranylgeranylation of the Rap1A was suppressed. One consistent observation in both studies was that N-BP effects were only seen in the osteoclast. This is congruent with the fact that ALN, and likely all other potent N-BPs, targets to the osteoclast on bone *(23,25)*. It is also consistent with the model whereby the bone surface must be acidified in order to facilitate release of the BP and transcytosis for their uptake, since only the osteoclasts can achieve these effects.

We still await the ultimate proof of a cause–effect relationship between N-BP inhibition of FPPS and inhibition of the osteoclast in vivo. Such evidence could come from transgenic animals overexpressing wild-type or mutated forms of FPPS. Although obtained in a model quite unrelated to bone, a recent study in *Leishmania major* has demonstrated that overexpression of FPPS can confer resistance to the antiprotozoal activity of RIS *(75)*. This establishes the concept that simple enzyme overexpression can alter the pharmacological response. The prediction in vertebrate animals would be that overexpression of wild-type or mutated FPPS could exhibit N-BP resistance in a setting such as ovariectomy or other challenges that lead to rapid bone loss. Although such an experiment would provide overwhelming individual proof for the known mechanism, the collective evidence from in vitro and in vivo studies provides a sound basis for accepting the current theories.

Mechanism of Action at the Cellular Level

The relationship between molecular action and antiresorptive effects has been documented for BPs lacking and containing nitrogen. For the non-N-BPs, which are intracellularly metabolized to form toxic analogs of ATP, the mechanism is accepted based on the ability of the toxic analogs to reproduce the effects of the parent BPs when administered to the osteoclast *(76)*. Perhaps the best documentation for a cause–effect relationship has been established for the N-BPs, where inhibition of FPPS and consequential effects on the osteoclast (loss of resorption, induction of apoptosis) can be overcome simply by reintroducing the critical lost metabolite. Among the downstream metabolites that could specifically restore the three major processes leading to cholesterol synthesis, farnesylation, or geranylgeranylation, only GGOH, a lipid alcohol that can replenish GGPP, prevents the N-BP effect *(53)*. Other metabolites downstream of FPPS that feed into farnesylation or sterol synthesis are without effect. The observation that farnesol, which is readily metabolized to form FPP, cannot restore osteoclast survival or function was unexpected *(31,53)*. FPP, like GGPP, is sufficient to block N-BP-induced macrophage apoptosis *(54)*. The reasons for farnesol not being metabolized to GGPP during N-BP treatment remain to be elucidated. Interestingly, the upstream metabolite, mevalonate, can also partially rescue inhibition of resorption, although this effect disappears with increasing concentration of ALN *(53,54)*.This is consistent with competitive inhibition of FPPS by N-BPs *(61)*. By this token, lower concentrations of N-BP may show a disproportionate loss of activity, since upstream metabolite accumulation could result in more effective competition for the allylic binding site within FPPS. In the context of the in vivo finding that N-BPs can also suppress HMG-CoA reductase expression *(73)*, this feedback mechanism might serve as a secondary method to increase efficacy by preventing excessive accumulation of such metabolites.

N-BP Effects on Downstream Intracellular Signaling

In addressing the downstream cellular mechanisms related to suppression of bone resorption, substantial evidence has accumulated to link loss of geranylgeranylation to induction of osteoclast apoptosis, disruption of the actin cytoskeleton and altered membrane trafficking *(30,31,72,77,78)*. The original observation that osteoclasts undergo apoptosis in response to N-BP treatment *(79)*, remained for several years the primary model for BP action in vitro and in vivo. The apoptotic action of both N-BPs and BPs-lacking nitrogen results from intracellular action within the osteoclast, as opposed to other indirect actions that could be mediated via osteoblasts, which in turn could control osteoclast survival *(31)*. That N-BPs cause apoptosis by interfering with geranylgeranylated proteins in osteoclasts was demonstrated by blocking the effect simply by restoring GGPP levels in the osteoclast through the addition of GGOH. Induction of osteoclast apoptosis by ALN and RIS, but not BPs lacking nitrogen, can be blocked by addition of GGOH, but not farnesol. For reasons unknown, farnesol feeds only into the farnesylation pathway and cannot restore geranylgeranylation *(31)*. This effect of farnesol was unexpected, since it feeds into the metabolic pathways downstream of the site of inhibition and upstream of the step required for synthesis of GGPP. In contrast to the osteoclast, both FPP and GGPP can prevent N-BP-induced apoptosis in other cell types, perhaps suggesting easier conversion of FPP to GGPP in these cells *(54,80–82)*.

The signaling pathways involving geranylgeranylated small GTPases that are affected by bisphosphonates and that lead to osteoclast apoptosis remain to be determined. Perhaps most proximal to the GTPases is the mammalian target of rapamycin (mTOR)/ribosomal protein S6 kinase (S6K) signaling pathway *(83)*. Signaling through this path is suppressed when geranylgeranylation is blocked in the osteoclast (Fig. 3). Furthermore, specific inhibition of mTOR by rapamycin causes induction of osteoclast apoptosis over a similar time course to that of the N-BPs. Signaling through mTOR represents a relatively novel pathway downstream of RANK, TNFα, and IL-1 signaling in the osteoclast *(84,85)*. Downstream of phosphoinositol-3 kinase, signaling through the Akt kinase to mTOR was originally implicated in maintaining osteoclast survival, putatively through the regulation of protein translation, which itself was shown to be critical for osteoclast differentiation and survival. More recent evidence suggests that Akt is actually dispensable for survival, whereas mTOR, and its signaling to the Bcl-2 family member Bim, form the critical pathway required for the survival of the osteoclast *(85)*. Bim is a pro-apoptotic mammalian regulator of cell death. Akt, in turn, is critical for differentiation, which N-BPs can inhibit in vitro. Not only can N-BPs suppress signaling from survival cytokines, such as TNFα and RANK ligand, to mTOR *(84)* but also specific inhibition of protein geranylgeranylation with a geranylgeranylation inhibitor and/or the withdrawal of cholesterol from the osteoclast *(52)* can lead to both suppression of mTOR signaling and the induction of osteoclast apoptosis. This illustrates both the importance of this signaling pathway as well as its reliance on both protein isoprenylation and cellular cholesterol content for proper functioning. The caveat here is that FPP is critical for osteoclast isoprenylation alone, whereas LDL is critical for maintaining cholesterol levels in the osteoclast.

Downstream consequences of N-BP inhibition of mTOR signaling include induction of (pro-apoptotic) Bim expression and suppression of protein translation. The latter effect in the osteoclast triggers the rapid induction of caspases, leading to osteoclast apoptosis *(83)*. With regard to Bim, knock-down of its expression extends osteoclast survival after cytokine withdrawal *(85)*. Meanwhile, increased Bim expression can cause caspase activation. Caspase 3 is the major effector caspase activated in osteoclasts undergoing apoptosis following treatment with a range of bisphosphonates in vitro *(82)*. A downstream effector of the caspases is a kinase named MST1, which acts as both a substrate for caspases 3, 7, and 9 and an activator of these caspases *(83,86,87)*. MST1 acts as a pro-apoptotic signaling intermediate downstream of the bisphosphonates that is activated during osteoclast apoptosis by several N-BPs, and clodronate *(31)*. Caspase cleavage of MST1 results in the formation of an unregulated, highly active kinase species shown to cause nuclear condensation *(88)*. High Mst1 activity also leads to caspase 3 and 9 activation, thus creating a sort of pro-apoptotic cycle *(83)*. What lies downstream of MST1 in the osteoclast, other than its feedback activation of the caspases, remains to be determined.

Dose-dependent Effects of N-BPs on Osteoclast Apoptosis

A general theory for BP action (including N-BPs and non-N-BPs) could hold that these agents act through the induction of osteoclast apoptosis. This was reasonably based on a key study demonstrating suprapharmacological N-BP doses lead to induction of osteoclast apoptosis in vivo *(79)*. In this model, a decreased osteoclast number would reduce the number of sites of resorption, and thus generally reduce turnover. The application of this model to low dose (daily and weekly administered N-BPs) is compelling at first glance, as a reduction in osteoclast numbers is clearly seen over time. However, previous studies reported that pharmacologically relevant ALN treatment initially increased osteoclast number *(89,90)*. Further, in vitro studies have demonstrated that inhibition of apoptosis can block the antiresorptive effects on BPs lacking nitrogen, such as clodronate and etidronate, although it has no effect on the N-BPs, ALN, and RIS *(30)*. Moreover, osteoclasts inhibited by ALN in vitro can be re-activated 24–48 h after N-BP treatment by the addition of the downstream metabolite, GGOH. This shows clearly that these osteoclasts are inactive but viable. The finding that suppression of resorption is seen prior to osteoclast apoptosis suggests direct inhibition of osteoclast function by the N-BP, rather than osteoclast apoptosis, is responsible.

One critical question tied to this model for the cellular action of N-BPs relates to whether or not one consistent mechanism is applied with all administered doses. There is strong evidence of ALN-induced osteoclast apoptosis in vivo when the dose was extremely high *(79)*. There is other compelling evidence that low-dose ALN increases osteoclast numbers, at least initially. A recent study addressing this issue compared the daily, weekly, monthly, and yearly equivalent doses of ALN, IBA, and ZOL in rats in vivo *(91)*. Interestingly, low-dose administration of the N-BPs, ALN, and IBA, at daily or weekly equivalents showed no induction of osteoclast apoptosis. Instead, the affected osteoclasts adopted a sort of flattened morphology, which might be tied to their inactivated state. Total osteoclast numbers increased, as previously reported, which might be attributable to the documented increase in parathyroid hormone that is commonly seen after antiresorptive treatment. Recent clinical evidence has shown that postmenopausal women treated with ALN for three years have increased osteoclast numbers and a slowed apoptotic process, which is consistent with the in vivo data *(92)*. In stark contrast to the effects of daily and weekly N-BP, the higher doses associated with monthly and yearly administration of IBA and ZOL, respectively, caused a striking and significant rise in the induction of osteoclast apoptosis. This suggests the distinct possibility that different cellular mechanisms can come into play, depending on the administered dose of the BP.

In summary, the data are thus consistent with all previous observations on N-BP effects on osteoclast apoptosis and number in vivo. They suggest a model whereby low-dose, more frequently administered N-BPs (ALN, RIS, and IBA daily, along with ALN and RIS weekly) act to reduce bone turnover by reducing osteoclast activity. With time, the reduced bone turnover reduces the number of bone remodeling units, and thus reduces overall osteoclast numbers. In contrast, high-dose, less frequently administered N-BPs (IBA monthly and ZOL yearly) appear to act by the rapid induction of osteoclast apoptosis. In this regard, they share the effect with the non-N-BPs, etidronate and clodronate, which only act via this mechanism. It is quite possible that the apoptotic effect diminishes over time and switches to a more inhibitory mechanism until the next dose of N-BP is administered. In this regard, it is not an inherent qualitative difference in the properties of each N-BP that controls the osteoclast response, but rather it is the dose of the N-BPs that dictates the outcome.

Non-apoptotic Mechanisms for Low-dose N-BP Inhibition of Osteoclast Function

Decades ago it was reported that BP administration causes the osteoclasts to change morphology and appear inactive *(93)*. The changes in the osteoclast are numerous *(94)* and include disruption of the cytoskeleton, including actin and vinculin, as well as disruption of the ruffled border *(23,28,93,95)*. The actin cytoskeleton is required for adhesion of the osteoclast to the bone surface, cell migration, and formation of the ruffled border. The ruffled border is a highly convoluted membrane structure situated above the resorption lacuna that is responsible for excretion of acid and proteases onto the bone surface. The ruffled border is also the point of invagination, whereby membrane vesicles form to engulf the released bone mineral, peptides and other partially digested bone constituents as a first step in the transcytosis process. As mentioned above, all BPs are rapidly taken up by the skeleton and localize preferentially on exposed mineral at bone resorption surfaces. Osteoclasts, the bone resorbing cells, attach to the exposed mineral and start the bone resorption process. The result of the intracellular action of N-BPs, shown for PAM and ALN *(23,96)*, is disappearance of the ruffled border. At high doses of N-BP, osteoclast morphology can also shift toward the generation of large and plump cells *(73)*. These plump cells contain a higher than usual number of nuclei, and they may be in transition toward the induction of apoptosis *(91)*. At low dose, there is more of a trend toward a flattening of the osteoclast along the bone surface. Clinical data from postmenopausal women treated for three years with ALN show both more normal osteoclasts and more giant multinucleated osteoclasts *(92)*. In this regard, the giant osteoclasts, in the context of an overall increase in osteoclast number, represent a slowing of the apoptotic process. The disappearance of the ruffled border in otherwise normal-appearing osteoclasts may therefore reflect the morphology of the inhibited, non-apoptotic osteoclast. As noted above, the ruffled border is a convoluted membrane, which faces the bone surface and is a hallmark of active osteoclasts. Ruffled border formation is a process that is highly dependent on cytoskeletal function, strongly regulated by geranylgeranylated GTP binding proteins, such as Rac, Rho, which appear to be abnormally activated after N-BP treatment *(71)*. The vesicles normally located above the ruffled border (that disappear after N-BP treatment) are needed for the formation of the ruffled border itself, and the trafficking of these vesicles is largely under the control of the Rabs, which are also geranylgeranylated proteins. It remains to be determined whether the Rabs are constitutively activated or inactivated by the lack of geranylgeranylation. In either case, the effect would likely lead to loss of function, and thus loss of the ruffled border. Disappearance of the ruffled border in the absence of signs of apoptosis, therefore, provides morphological evidence for mechanism-based osteoclast inactivation and could explain the lack of acid extrusion caused by ALN in isolated osteoclasts *(97)*. N-BP suppression acid extrusion may limit intracellular exposure to the N-BP. This then might reduce the likelihood that the osteoclast undergoes apoptosis.

Mode of Action at the Tissue Level

Osteoporosis and other types of bone loss are associated with increased bone turnover and elevated levels of bone resorption. Osteoclastic bone resorption is a 2-week process that begins the bone remodeling process. Resorption itself can be effectively slowed or controlled by inhibiting osteoclast generation, reducing osteoclast activity or both. ALN is one of the most effective inhibitors of bone resorption. ALN improvement of mechanical strength, reflected in a reduction in fracture risk, is caused by an increase in bone mass and mineralization (discussed above) as well as by an improvement in microarchitecture, attributable to a reduction in bone turnover. A higher number of bone remodeling sites, where excessive osteoclastic destruction of bone takes place, leads to loss of bone tissue, formation of areas of stress concentration, decreased strength, and increased fracture risk. By reducing turnover, bisphosphonates reverse this condition. Effects on bone turnover can be estimated by measuring either cross-linked C-terminal or N-terminal telopeptides of type I collagen degradation products or deoxypyridinoline (formed in type I bone collagen) in the urine or in the blood. These degradation products come as a result of proteolytic activity within the resorption lacuna, followed by their release during transcytosis and subsequent extra-skeletal metabolism. ALN-induced suppression of these markers can be detected within days, and maximal effects are reached within a few weeks whereupon levels stabilize and remain reduced at a stable level for the duration of treatment, followed up to 10 years for ALN so far *(98)*. Bone formation is also reduced, albeit about 3 months later than resorption, as part of the reduction in bone turnover, reaching a nadir at 3–6 months. This is a reflection of the so-called "coupling" between resorption and formation whereby, through mechanisms that have not been fully elucidated, changes in resorption engender changes in formation in the same direction. Another mechanism for increased bone strength is the increase in average mineralization associated with lower bone turnover *(99–101)*. This has been described in ALN-treated baboons *(99)* and, more importantly, in osteoporotic women treated with ALN and RIS *(100–103)*. Lower turnover lengthens the life span of the bone remodeling BMU (basic multicellular unit), thus permitting it to mineralize more completely and increase mineral content. This is a process that can take years to fully complete. The effect is to reduce the proportion of incompletely mineralized, recently formed bone. The mineralization of mature bone is not increased. BMD or BMC measures the combined BP effects on bone volume and mineralization. The initial rise in bone mass measured by dual beam X-ray absorptiometry is caused by the continued rebuilding of preexisting BMUs that were initiated prior to N-BP treatment. BPs subsequently reduce the number of new BMUs, and at individual BMUs, they act by decreasing the depth of resorption and possibly increasing wall width during the formation phase *(104)*. A continuous increase in spinal BMD was observed during 10 years treatment of postmenopausal women with ALN *(98)* and 5 years treatment with RIS *(105)*. Increases in BMD and mineralization are associated with improvements in bone strength. Increased bone strength following BP treatment has been documented in experimental animals by ex vivo biomechanical testing *(106–110)* and is reflected in the reduction in fracture risk observed in clinical trials.

Very high doses of ALN and RIS (six times above clinical dosing), when administered for a period of 1 year, were reported to suppress bone turnover in dogs by up to 95% and cause accumulation of microcracks in both cortical and cancellous bone *(111)*. In this study, microcracks are defined by the presence of microscopic streaks in bone sections that stain with basic fuchsin. Interestingly, the amount of microcracks in dog bones was not associated with any extrinsic biomechanical property, although it was associated with an increase in compressive strength. The clinical relevance of these findings with suprapharmacological doses of N-BPs is uncertain. The best comparator for this type of modeling comes from the 5 and 10-year data for RIS and ALN, which show no increase in non-vertebral fracture risk *(98,105)*. This is consistent with the finding that the microcracks in dog bones do not progress during multi-year treatment with high doses of BPs. This suggests either absence of microcrack accumulation at the usual osteoporosis treatment dose of these N-BPs or a lack of relevance of microcracks to fracture risk. Consistent with the latter, untreated elderly women with and without femoral neck fractures were found to have the same degree of microcrack accumulation *(112)*, suggesting that microcracks themselves are not predictors of fracture risk.

SUMMARY

In conclusion, the potent N-BPs show a high degree of specificity in binding to bone and in targeting the osteoclast. Effects on osteoclast-mediated bone resorption are a function of their concentration on the surface of bone undergoing resorption and their intrinsic potency. Recent data have identified the mevalonate pathway enzyme, FPPS, as the primary molecular target of N-BPs in the osteoclast. These agents bind into the allylic pocket of this enzyme to form a carbocation transition state analog that blocks function. Inhibition of this enzyme has indirect effects leading to reduction of protein isoprenylation in osteoclasts. The deregulated small GTPases become constitutively activated, leading to osteoclast disregulation, thus reducing bone resorption. The specific loss of protein geranylgeranylation, and not farnesylation, is responsible for osteoclast inactivation. Because of the low bioavailability of N-BPs, the osteoclasts are the only non-gastrointestinal cells exposed to high enough concentrations to allow N-BP inhibition of FPPS. The response to such treatments is primarily osteoclast inhibition, which can eventually lead to a reduction in osteoclast numbers as the number of remodeling units is reduced. However, clinical data suggest that osteoclast numbers remain elevated to 3 years, suggesting that N-BP itself or its effects can slow osteoclast apoptosis. High-dose N-BPs, either administered orally or intravenously, may still show the same specificity for the osteoclast. However, the resulting higher intracellular concentrations of drug appear to cause a greater shift toward an apoptotic response. It remains to be determined if these effects are seen in the clinic. It is quite possible that the lower levels of N-BP found on non-resorbed surfaces are sufficient to achieve a more inhibitory (vs. apoptotic) effect. Thus, these high-dose regimens may act through two or more cellular mechanisms, and the mechanisms may even change over time between doses. This may explain why the high doses are able to achieve a lasting effect on resorption. Regardless of whether the osteoclasts are inhibited or experience cell death, resorption levels decline. Importantly, it is possible that one intracellular mechanism, inhibition of FPPS, is capable of controlling all osteoclast responses to N-BP treatment. Gaps in our understanding of the intracellular downstream mechanisms still exist, and this makes these very interesting and powerful antiresorptive drugs worthy of further scientific exploration in years to come.

REFERENCES

1. Jensen GF, Christiansen C Boesen J Hegedus V Transbol I. Epidemiology of postmenopausal spinal and long bone fractures. A unifying approach to postmenopausal osteoporosis. Clin Orthop 1982;166:75–81.
2. Melton LJ III. Epidemiology of fractures. In:Riggs BL, Melton LJ III, eds. Osteoporosis: etiology, diagnosis, and management. New York: Raven Press, 1988:133–154.
3. Hochberg MC, Ross PD, Black D, Cummings SR, Genant HK, Nevitt MC, Barrett Connor E, Musliner T, Thompson D. Larger increases in bone mineral density during alendronate therapy are associated with a lower risk of new vertebral fractures in women with postmenopausal osteoporosis. Fracture Intervention Trial Research Group. Arthritis Rheum 1999;42(6):1246–1254.

4. Nevitt MC, Ross PD, Palermo L, Musliner T, Genant HK, Thompson DE. Association of prevalent vertebral fractures, bone density, and alendronate treatment with incident vertebral fractures: effect of number and spinal location of fractures. The Fracture Intervention Trial Research Group. Bone 1999;25(5):613–619.
5. Adachi JD. The correlation of bone mineral density and biochemical markers to fracture risk. Calcif Tissue Int 1996;59(Suppl 1):16–19.
6. Ravn P, Rix M, Andreassen H, Clemmesen B, Bidstrup M, Gunnes M. High bone turnover is associated with low bone mass and spinal fracture in postmenopausal women. Calcif Tissue Int 1997;60(3): 255–260.
7. Hochberg MC, Greenspan S, Wasnich RD, Miller P, Thompson DE, Ross PD. Changes in bone density and turnover explain the reductions in incidence of nonvertebral fractures that occur during treatment with antiresorptive agents. J Clin Endocrinol Metab 2002;87(4):1586–1592.
8. Cocquyt V, Kline WF, Gertz BJ, Van Belle SJ, Holland SD, DeSmet M, Quan H, Vyas KP, Zhang KE, De Greve J, Porras AG. Pharmacokinetics of intravenous alendronate. J Clin Pharmacol 1999;39(4):385–393.
9. Porras AG, Holland SD, Gertz BJ. Pharmacokinetics of alendronate. Clin Pharmacokinet 1999;36(5):315–328.
10. Leu CT, Luegmayr E, Freedman LP, Rodan GA, Reszka AA. Relative binding affinities of bisphosphonates for human bone and relationship to antiresorptive efficacy. Bone 2006;38(5):628–636.
11. van Beek E, Hoekstra M, van de Ruit M, Lowik C, Papapoulos S. Structural requirements for bisphosphonate actions in vitro. J Bone Miner Res 1994;9(12):1875–1882.
12. van Beek E, Lowik C, Que I, Papapoulos S. Dissociation of binding and antiresorptive properties of hydroxybisphosphonates by substitution of the hydroxyl with an amino group. J Bone Miner Res 1996;11(10):1492–1497.
13. van Beek ER, Lowik CW, Ebetino FH, Papapoulos SE. Binding and antiresorptive properties of heterocycle-containing bisphosphonate analogs: structure-activity relationships. Bone 1998;23(5): 437–442.
14. Nancollas GH, Tang R, Phipps RJ, Henneman Z, Gulde S, Wu W, Mangood A, Russell RG, Ebetino FH. Novel insights into actions of bisphosphonates on bone: differences in interactions with hydroxyapatite. Bone 2006;38(5):617–627.
15. Otter M, Goheen S, Williams WS. Streaming potentials in chemically modified bone. J Orthop Res 1988;6(3):346–359.
16. Kowalchuk RM, Corcoran TA, Pollack SR, Steinberg ME. Effects of etidronate and oophorectomy on the zeta potential of rat bone. Clin Orthop Relat Res 1996;328:241–249.
17. Reginster JY, Wilson KM, Dumont E, Bonvoisin B, Barrett J. Monthly oral ibandronate is well tolerated and efficacious in postmenopausal women: results from the monthly oral pilot study. J Clin Endocrinol Metab 2005;90(9):5018–5024.
18. Mitchell DY, Eusebio RA, Sacco-Gibson NA, Pallone KA, Kelly SC, Nesbitt JD, Brezovic CP, Thompson GA, Powell JH. Dose-proportional pharmacokinetics of risedronate on single-dose oral administration to healthy volunteers. J Clin Pharmacol 2000;40(3):258–265.
19. Schnitzer T, Bone HG, Crepaldi G, Adami S, McClung M, Kiel D, Felsenberg D, Recker RR, Tonino RP, Roux C, Pinchera A, Foldes AJ, Greenspan SL, Levine MA, Emkey R, Santora AC II, Kaur A, Thompson DE, Yates J, Orloff JJ. Therapeutic equivalence of alendronate 70 mg once-weekly and alendronate 10 mg daily in the treatment of osteoporosis. Alendronate Once-Weekly Study Group. Aging (Milano) 2000;12(1):1–12.
20. Lin JH. Bisphosphonates: a review of their pharmacokinetic properties. Bone 1996;18(2):75–85.
21. Khan SA, Kanis JA, Vasikaran S, Kline WF, Matuszewski BK, McCloskey EV, Beneton MN, Gertz BJ, Sciberras DG, Holland SD, Orgee J, Coombes GM, Rogers SR, Porras AG. Elimination and biochemical responses to intravenous alendronate in postmenopausal osteoporosis. J Bone Miner Res 1997;12(10):1700–1707.
22. Phipps R, Lindsay R, Burgio D, Sun A, Russell D, Kuzmak B, Keck B, Christiansen C. Head-to-head comparison of risedronate and alendronate pharmacokinetics at clinical doses. Bone 2004;34:S81–S82.
23. Sato M, Grasser W, Endo N, Akins R, Simmons H, Thompson DD, Golub E, Rodan GA. Bisphosphonate action. Alendronate localization in rat bone and effects on osteoclast ultrastructure. J Clin Invest 1991;88(6):2095–2105.

24. Azuma Y, Sato H, Oue Y, Okabe K, Ohta T, Tsuchimoto M, Kiyoki M. Alendronate distributed on bone surfaces inhibits osteoclastic bone resorption in vitro and in experimental hypercalcemia models. Bone 1995;16(2):235–245.
25. Masarachia P, Weinreb M, Balena R, Rodan GA. Comparison of the distribution of 3H-alendronate and 3H-etidronate in rat and mouse bones. Bone 1996;19(3):281–290.
26. Salo J, Lehenkari P, Mulari M, Metsikko K, Vaananen HK. Removal of osteoclast bone resorption products by transcytosis. Science 1997;276(5310):270–273.
27. Palokangas H, Mulari M, Vaananen HK. Endocytic pathway from the basal plasma membrane to the ruffled border membrane in bone-resorbing osteoclasts. J Cell Sci 1997;110(Pt 15):1767–1780.
28. Murakami H, Takahashi N, Sasaki T, Udagawa N, Tanaka S, Nakamura I, Zhang D, Barbier A, Suda T. A possible mechanism of the specific action of bisphosphonates on osteoclasts: tiludronate preferentially affects polarized osteoclasts having ruffled borders. Bone 1995;17(2):137–144.
29. Thompson K, Rogers MJ, Coxon FP, Crockett JC. Cytosolic entry of bisphosphonate drugs requires acidification of vesicles after fluid-phase endocytosis. Mol Pharmacol 2006;69(5):1624–1632.
30. Halasy-Nagy JM, Rodan GA, Reszka AA. Inhibition of bone resorption by alendronate and risedronate does not require osteoclast apoptosis. Bone 2001;29(6):553–559.
31. Reszka AA, Halasy Nagy JM, Masarachia PJ, Rodan GA, Bisphosphonates act directly on the osteoclast to induce caspase cleavage of mst1 kinase during apoptosis. A link between inhibition of the mevalonate pathway and regulation of an apoptosis-promoting kinase. J Biol Chem 1999;274(49): 34967–34973.
32. McClung MR, Lewiecki EM, Cohen SB, Bolognese MA, Woodson GC, Moffett AH, Peacock M, Miller PD, Lederman SN, Chesnut CH, Lain D, Kivitz AJ, Holloway DL, Zhang C, Peterson MC, Bekker PJ. Denosumab in postmenopausal women with low bone mineral density. N Engl J Med 2006;354(8): 821–831.
33. Cremers SC, Lodder MC, Den Hartigh J, Vermeij P, Van Pelt P, Lems WF, Papapoulos SE, Dijkmans BA. Short term whole body retention in relation to rate of bone resorption and cartilage degradation after intravenous bisphosphonate (pamidronate) in rheumatoid arthritis. J Rheumatol 2004;31(9): 1732–1737.
34. Cremers SC, Papapoulos SE, Gelderblom H, Seynaeve C, den Hartigh J, Vermeij P, van der Rijt CC, van Zuylen L. Skeletal retention of bisphosphonate (pamidronate) and its relation to the rate of bone resorption in patients with breast cancer and bone metastases. J Bone Miner Res 2005;20(9): 1543–1547.
35. Cremers S, Sparidans R, Den HJ, Hamdy N, Vermeij P, Papapoulos S. A pharmacokinetic and pharmacodynamic model for intravenous bisphosphonate (pamidronate) in osteoporosis. Eur J Clin Pharmacol 2002;57(12):883–890.
36. Rodan G, Reszka A, Golub E, Rizzoli R. Bone safety of long-term bisphosphonate treatment. Curr Med Res Opin 2004;20(8):1291–1300.
37. Schmidt A, Rutledge SJ, Endo N, Opas EE, Tanaka H, Wesolowski G, Leu CT, Huang Z, Ramachandaran C, Rodan SB, Rodan GA. Protein-tyrosine phosphatase activity regulates osteoclast formation and function: inhibition by alendronate. Proc Natl Acad Sci USA 1996;93(7):3068–3073.
38. Endo N, Rutledge SJ, Opas EE, Vogel R, Rodan GA, Schmidt A. Human protein tyrosine phosphatase-sigma: alternative splicing and inhibition by bisphosphonates. J Bone Miner Res 1996;11(4):535–543.
39. Opas EE, Rutledge SJ, Golub E, Stern A, Zimolo Z, Rodan GA, Schmidt A. Alendronate inhibition of protein-tyrosine-phosphatase-meg1. Biochem Pharmacol 1997;54(6):721–727.
40. Murakami H, Takahashi N, Tanaka S, Nakamura I, Udagawa N, Nakajo S, Nakaya K, Abe M, Yuda Y, Konno F, Barbier A, Suda T. Tiludronate inhibits protein tyrosine phosphatase activity in osteoclasts. Bone 1997;20(5):399–404.
41. Skorey K, Ly HD, Kelly J, Hammond M, Ramachandran C, Huang Z, Gresser MJ, Wang Q. How does alendronate inhibit protein-tyrosine phosphatases? J Biol Chem 1997;272(36):22472–22480.
42. Biller SA, Forster C, Gordon EM, Harrity T, Scott WA, Ciosek CP Jr. Isoprenoid (phosphinylmethyl)phosphonates as inhibitors of squalene synthetase. J Med Chem 1988;31(10):1869–1871.
43. Amin D, Cornell SA, Gustafson SK, Needle SJ, Ullrich JW, Bilder GE, Perrone MH. Bisphosphonates used for the treatment of bone disorders inhibit squalene synthase and cholesterol biosynthesis. J Lipid Res 1992;33(11):1657–1663.

44. Ciosek CP Jr, Magnin DR, Harrity TW, Logan JV, Dickson JK Jr, Gordon EM, Hamilton KA, Jolibois KG, Kunselman LK, Lawrence RM. Lipophilic 1,1-bisphosphonates are potent squalene synthase inhibitors and orally active cholesterol lowering agents in vivo. J Biol Chem 1993;268(33): 24832–24837.
45. Magnin DR, Biller SA, Dickson JK Jr, Logan JV, Lawrence RM, Chen Y, Sulsky RB, Ciosek CP Jr, Harrity TW, Jolibois KG, Kunselman LK, Rich LC, Slusarchyk DA. 1,1-Bisphosphonate squalene synthase inhibitors: interplay between the isoprenoid subunit and the diphosphate surrogate. J Med Chem 1995;38(14):2596–2605.
46. Amin D, Cornell SA, Perrone MH, Bilder GE. 1-Hydroxy-3-(methylpentylamino)-propylidene-1,1-bisphosphonic acid as a potent inhibitor of squalene synthase. Arzneimittelforschung 1996;46(8): 759–762.
47. Berkhout TA, Simon HM, Patel DD, Bentzen C, Niesor E, Jackson B, Suckling KE. The novel cholesterol-lowering drug SR-12813 inhibits cholesterol synthesis via an increased degradation of 3-hydroxy-3-methylglutaryl-coenzyme A reductase. J Biol Chem 1996;271(24):14376–14382.
48. Berkhout TA, Simon HM, Jackson B, Yates J, Pearce N, Groot PH, Bentzen C, Niesor E, Kerns WD, Suckling KE. SR-12813 lowers plasma cholesterol in beagle dogs by decreasing cholesterol biosynthesis. Atherosclerosis 1997;133(2):203–212.
49. Jackson B, Gee AN, Guyon-Gellin Y, Niesor E, Bentzen CL, Kerns WD, Suckling KE. Hypocholesterolaemic and antiatherosclerotic effects of tetra-iso-propyl 2-(3,5-di-tert-butyl-4-hydroxyphenyl)ethyl-1,1-diphosphonate (SR-9223i). Arzneimittelforschung 2000;50(4):380–386.
50. Risser F, Pfister CU, Degen PH. An enzyme inhibition assay for the quantitative determination of the new bisphosphonate zoledronate in plasma. J Pharm Biomed Anal 1997;15(12):1877–1880.
51. Bergstrom JD, Bostedor RG, Masarachia PJ, Reszka AA, Rodan G. Alendronate is a specific, nanomolar inhibitor of farnesyl diphosphate synthase. Arch Biochem Biophys 2000;373(1):231–241.
52. Luegmayr E, Glantschnig H, Wesolowski GA, Gentile MA, Fisher JE, Rodan GA, Reszka AA. Osteoclast formation, survival and morphology are highly dependent on exogenous cholesterol/lipoproteins. Cell Death Differ 2004;11(Suppl 1):S108–S118.
53. Fisher JE, Rogers MJ, Halasy JM, Luckman SP, Hughes DE, Masarachia PJ, Wesolowski G, Russell RG, Rodan GA, Reszka AA. Alendronate mechanism of action: geranylgeraniol, an intermediate in the mevalonate pathway, prevents inhibition of osteoclast formation, bone resorption, and kinase activation in vitro. Proc Natl Acad Sci USA 1999;96(1):133–138.
54. Luckman SP, Hughes DE, Coxon FP, Graham R, Russell G, Rogers MJ. Nitrogen-containing bisphosphonates inhibit the mevalonate pathway and prevent post-translational prenylation of GTP-binding proteins, including Ras. J Bone Miner Res 1998;13(4):581–589.
55. Dunford JE, Thompson K, Coxon FP, Luckman SP, Hahn FM, Poulter CD, Ebetino FH, Rogers MJ. Structure-activity relationships for inhibition of farnesyl diphosphate synthase in vitro and inhibition of bone resorption in vivo by nitrogen-containing bisphosphonates. J Pharmacol Exp Ther 2001;296(2): 235–242.
56. van Beek E, Pieterman E, Cohen L, Lowik C, Papapoulos S. Nitrogen-containing bisphosphonates inhibit isopentenyl pyrophosphate isomerase/farnesyl pyrophosphate synthase activity with relative potencies corresponding to their antiresorptive potencies in vitro and in vivo. Biochem Biophys Res Commun 1999;255(2):491–494.
57. Coxon FP, Helfrich MH, Larijani B, Muzylak M, Dunford JE, Marshall D, McKinnon AD, Nesbitt SA, Horton MA, Seabra MC, Ebetino FH, Rogers MJ. Identification of a novel phosphonocarboxylate inhibitor of Rab geranylgeranyl transferase that specifically prevents Rab prenylation in osteoclasts and macrophages. J Biol Chem 2001;276(51):48213–48222.
58. Thompson K, Dunford JE, Ebetino FH, Rogers MJ. Identification of a bisphosphonate that inhibits isopentenyl diphosphate isomerase and farnesyl diphosphate synthase. Biochem Biophys Res Commun 2002;290(2):869–873.
59. Wiemer AJ, Tong H, Swanson KM, Hohl RJ. Digeranyl bisphosphonate inhibits geranylgeranyl pyrophosphate synthase. Biochem Biophys Res Commun 2007;353(4):921–925.
60. Martin MB, Arnold W, Heath HT III; Urbina JA, Oldfield E. Nitrogen-containing bisphosphonates as carbocation transition state analogs for isoprenoid biosynthesis. Biochem Biophys Res Commun 1999;263(3):754–758.

61. Dunford JE, Ebetino FH, Rogers MJ. The mechanism of inhibition of farnesyl diphosphate synthase by nitrogen-containing bisphosphonates. Bone 2002;30(3):40S.
62. Hosfield DJ, Zhang Y, Dougan DR, Broun A, Tari LW, Swanson RV, Finn J. Structural basis for bisphosphonate-mediated inhibition of isoprenoid biosynthesis. J Biol Chem 2004;279(10):8526–8529.
63. Rondeau JM, Bitsch F, Bourgier E, Geiser M, Hemmig R, Kroemer M, Lehmann S, Ramage P, Rieffel S, Strauss A, Green JR, Jahnke W. Structural basis for the exceptional in vivo efficacy of bisphosphonate drugs. ChemMedChem 2006;1(2):267–273.
64. Reszka AA, Halasy-Nagy JM, Masarachia PJ, Rodan GA. Bisphosphonates act directly on the osteoclast to induce caspase cleavage of mst1 kinase during apoptosis. A link between inhibition of the mevalonate pathway and regulation of an apoptosis-promoting kinase. J Biol Chem 1999;274(49):34967–34973.
65. Zhang FL, Casey PJ. Protein prenylation: molecular mechanisms and functional consequences. Annu Rev Biochem 1996;65:241–269.
66. Sinensky M. Recent advances in the study of prenylated proteins. Biochim Biophys Acta 2000;1484(2–3):93–106.
67. Ridley AJ, Paterson HF, Johnston CL, Diekmann D, Hall A. The small GTP-binding protein rac regulates growth factor-induced membrane ruffling. Cell 1992;70(3):401–410.
68. Ridley AJ, Hall A. The small GTP-binding protein rho regulates the assembly of focal adhesions and actin stress fibers in response to growth factors. Cell 1992;70(3):389–399.
69. Zhang D, Udagawa N, Nakamura I, Murakami H, Saito S, Yamasaki K, Shibasaki Y, Morii N, Narumiya S, Takahashi N, Suda T. The small GTP-binding protein, rho p21, is involved in bone resorption by regulating cytoskeletal organization in osteoclasts. J Cell Sci 1995;108(Pt 6):2285–2292.
70. Clark EA, King WG, Brugge JS, Symons M, Hynes RO. Integrin-mediated signals regulated by members of the rho family of GTPases. J Cell Biol 1998;142(2):573–586.
71. Dunford JE, Rogers MJ, Ebetino FH, Phipps RJ, Coxon FP. Inhibition of protein prenylation by bisphosphonates causes sustained activation of Rac, Cdc42, and Rho GTPases. J Bone Miner Res 2006;21(5):684–694.
72. Coxon FP, Helfrich MH, Van't Hof R, Sebti S, Ralston SH, Hamilton A, Rogers MJ. Protein geranylgeranylation is required for osteoclast formation, function, and survival: inhibition by bisphosphonates and GGTI-298. J Bone Miner Res 2000;15(8):1467–1476.
73. Fisher JE, Rodan GA, Reszka AA. In vivo effects of bisphosphonates on the osteoclast mevalonate pathway. Endocrinology 2000;141(12):4793–4796.
74. Frith JC, Monkkonen J, Auriola S, Monkkonen H, Rogers MJ. The molecular mechanism of action of the antiresorptive and antiinflammatory drug clodronate: evidence for the formation in vivo of a metabolite that inhibits bone resorption and causes osteoclast and macrophage apoptosis. Arthritis Rheum 2001;44(9):2201–2210.
75. Ortiz-Gomez A, Jimenez C, Estevez AM, Carrero-Lerida J, Ruiz-Perez LM, Gonzalez-Pacanowska D. Farnesyl diphosphate synthase is a cytosolic enzyme in Leishmania major promastigotes and its overexpression confers resistance to risedronate. Eukaryot Cell 2006;5(7):1057–1064.
76. Frith JC, Monkkonen J, Blackburn GM, Russell RG, Rogers MJ. Clodronate and liposome-encapsulated clodronate are metabolized to a toxic ATP analog, adenosine 5'-(beta, gamma-dichloromethylene) triphosphate, by mammalian cells in vitro. J Bone Miner Res 1997;12(9):1358–1367.
77. Rogers HL, Marshall D, Rogers MJ. Effects of bisphosphonates on osteoclasts in vitro, studies by scanning electron microscopy. Bone 2002;30(3):43S.
78. Alakangas A, Selander K, Mulari M, Halleen J, Lehenkari P, Monkkonen J, Salo J, Vaananen K. Alendronate disturbs vesicular trafficking in osteoclasts. Calcif Tissue Int 2002;70(1):40–47.
79. Hughes DE, Wright KR, Uy HL, Sasaki A, Yoneda T, Roodman GD, Mundy GR, Boyce BF. Bisphosphonates promote apoptosis in murine osteoclasts in vitro and in vivo. J Bone Miner Res 1995;10(10):1478–1487.
80. Luckman SP, Coxon FP, Ebetino FH, Russell RG, Rogers MJ. Heterocycle-containing bisphosphonates cause apoptosis and inhibit bone resorption by preventing protein prenylation: evidence from structure-activity relationships in J774 macrophages. J Bone Miner Res 1998;13(11):1668–1678.
81. Shipman CM, Croucher PI, Russell RG, Helfrich MH, Rogers MJ. The bisphosphonate incadronate (YM175) causes apoptosis of human myeloma cells in vitro by inhibiting the mevalonate pathway. Cancer Res 1998;58(23):5294–5297.

82. Benford HL, Frith JC, Auriola S, Monkkonen J, Rogers MJ. Farnesol and geranylgeraniol prevent activation of caspases by aminobisphosphonates: biochemical evidence for two distinct pharmacological classes of bisphosphonate drugs. Mol Pharmacol 1999;56(1):131–140.
83. Glantschnig H, Rodan GA, Reszka AA. Alendronate mechanism of action: the role of geranylgeranylation in p70S6 kinase-dependent osteoclast survival. Bone 2002;30(3):41S.
84. Glantschnig H, Fisher JE, Wesolowski G, Rodan GA, Reszka AA. M-CSF, TNFalpha and RANK ligand promote osteoclast survival by signaling through mTOR/S6 kinase. Cell Death Differ 2003;10(10): 1165–1177.
85. Sugatani T, Hruska KA. Akt1/Akt2 and mammalian target of rapamycin/Bim play critical roles in osteoclast differentiation and survival, respectively, whereas Akt is dispensable for cell survival in isolated osteoclast precursors. J Biol Chem 2005;280(5):3583–3589.
86. Graves JD, Gotoh Y, Draves KE, Ambrose D, Han DK, Wright M, Chernoff J, Clark EA, Krebs EG. Caspase-mediated activation and induction of apoptosis by the mammalian Ste20-like kinase Mst1. EMBO J 1998;17(8):2224–2234.
87. Graves JD, Draves KE, Gotoh Y, Krebs EG, Clark EA. Both phosphorylation and caspase-mediated cleavage contribute to regulation of the Ste20-like protein kinase Mst1 during CD95/Fas-induced apoptosis. J Biol Chem 2001;276(18):14909–14915.
88. Lee KK, Ohyama T, Yajima N, Tsubuki S, Yonehara S. MST, a physiological caspase substrate, highly sensitizes apoptosis both upstream and downstream of caspase activation. J Biol Chem 2001;276(22):19276–19285.
89. Seedor JG, Quartuccio HA, Thompson DD. The bisphosphonate alendronate (MK-217) inhibits bone loss due to ovariectomy in rats. J Bone Miner Res 1991;6(4):339–346.
90. Bikle DD, Morey Holton ER, Doty SB, Currier PA, Tanner SJ, Halloran BP. Alendronate increases skeletal mass of growing rats during unloading by inhibiting resorption of calcified cartilage. J Bone Miner Res 1994;9(11):1777–1787.
91. Fisher JE, Reszka A. Evidence that High-Dose, Intermittent Ibandronate and Zoledronate Inhibit Osteoclastic Bone Resorption through a Mechanism Independent of the Mevalonate Pathway. J Bone Miner Res 2006;21(Suppl. 1):S414.
92. Weinstein RS, Roberson PK, Manolagas SC. Giant osteoclast formation and long-term oral bisphosphonate therapy. N Engl J Med 2009;(1):53–62.
93. Schenk R, Merz WA, Muhlbauer R, Russell RG, Fleisch H. Effect of ethane-1-hydroxy-1,1-diphosphonate (EHDP) and dichloromethylene diphosphonate (Cl 2 MDP) on the calcification and resorption of cartilage and bone in the tibial epiphysis and metaphysis of rats. Calcif Tissue Res 1973;11(3):196–214.
94. Sato M, Grasser W. Effects of bisphosphonates on isolated rat osteoclasts as examined by reflected light microscopy. J Bone Miner Res 1990;5(1):31–40.
95. Selander K, Lehenkari P, Vaananen HK. The effects of bisphosphonates on the resorption cycle of isolated osteoclasts. Calcif Tissue Int 1994;55(5):368–375.
96. Kim TW, Yoshida Y, Yokoya K, Sasaki T. An ultrastructural study of the effects of bisphosphonate administration on osteoclastic bone resorption during relapse of experimentally moved rat molars. Am J Orthod Dentofacial Orthop 1999;115(6):645–653.
97. Zimolo Z, Wesolowski G, Rodan GA. Acid extrusion is induced by osteoclast attachment to bone. Inhibition by alendronate and calcitonin. J Clin Invest 1995;96(5):2277–2283.
98. Bone HG, Hosking D, Devogelaer JP, Tucci JR, Emkey RD, Tonino RP, Rodriguez-Portales JA, Downs RW, Gupta J, Santora AC, Liberman UA. Ten years' experience with alendronate for osteoporosis in postmenopausal women. N Engl J Med 2004;350(12):1189–1199.
99. Meunier PJ, Boivin G. Bone mineral density reflects bone mass but also the degree of mineralization of bone: therapeutic implications. Bone 1997;21(5):373–377.
100. Boivin GY, Chavassieux PM, Santora AC, Yates J, Meunier PJ. Alendronate increases bone strength by increasing the mean degree of mineralization of bone tissue in osteoporotic women. Bone 2000;27(5):687–694.
101. Roschger P, Rinnerthaler S, Yates J, Rodan GA, Fratzl P, Klaushofer K. Alendronate increases degree and uniformity of mineralization in cancellous bone and decreases the porosity in cortical bone of osteoporotic women. Bone 2001;29(2):185–191.

102. Durchschlag E, Paschalis EP, Zoehrer R, Roschger P, Fratzl P, Recker R, Phipps R, Klaushofer K. Bone material properties in trabecular bone from human iliac crest biopsies after 3- and 5-year treatment with risedronate. J Bone Miner Res 2006;21(10):1581–1590.
103. Zoehrer R, Roschger P, Paschalis EP, Hofstaetter JG, Durchschlag E, Fratzl P, Phipps R, Klaushofer K. Effects of 3- and 5-year treatment with risedronate on bone mineralization density distribution in triple biopsies of the iliac crest in postmenopausal women. J Bone Miner Res 2006;21(7):1106–1112.
104. Boyce RW, Wronski TJ, Ebert DC, Stevens ML, Paddock CL, Youngs TA, Gundersen HJ. Direct stereological estimation of three-dimensional connectivity in rat vertebrae: effect of estrogen, etidronate and risedronate following ovariectomy. Bone 1995;16(2):209–213.
105. Ste-Marie LG, Sod E, Johnson T, Chines A. Five years of treatment with risedronate and its effects on bone safety in women with postmenopausal osteoporosis. Calcif Tissue Int 2004;75(6):469–476.
106. Balena R, Toolan BC, Shea M, Markatos A, Myers ER, Lee SC, Opas EE, Seedor JG, Klein H, Frankenfield D, Quartuccio H, Fioravanti C, Brown JCE, Hayes WC, Rodan GA. The effects of 2-year treatment with the aminobisphosphonate alendronate on bone metabolism, bone histomorphometry, and bone strength in ovariectomized nonhuman primates. J Clin Invest 1993;92(6):2577–2586.
107. Guy JA, Shea M, Peter CP, Morrissey R, Hayes WC. Continuous alendronate treatment throughout growth, maturation, and aging in the rat results in increases in bone mass and mechanical properties. Calcif Tissue Int 1993;53(4):283–288.
108. Lafage MH, Balena R, Battle MA, Shea M, Seedor JG, Klein H, Hayes WC, Rodan GA. Comparison of alendronate and sodium fluoride effects on cancellous and cortical bone in minipigs. A one-year study. J Clin Invest 1995;95(5):2127–2133.
109. Mosekilde L, Thomsen JS, Mackey MS, Phipps RJ. Treatment with risedronate or alendronate prevents hind-limb immobilization-induced loss of bone density and strength in adult female rats. Bone 2000;27(5):639–645.
110. Toolan BC, Shea M, Myers ER, Borchers RE, Seedor JG, Quartuccio H, Rodan G, Hayes WC. Effects of 4-amino-1-hydroxybutylidene bisphosphonate on bone biomechanics in rats. J Bone Miner Res 1992;7(12):1399–1406.
111. Mashiba T, Turner CH, Hirano T, Forwood MR, Johnston CC, Burr DB. Effects of suppressed bone turnover by bisphosphonates on microdamage accumulation and biomechanical properties in clinically relevant skeletal sites in beagles. Bone 2001;28(5):524–531.
112. Mori S, Harruff R, Ambrosius W, Burr DB. Trabecular bone volume and microdamage accumulation in the femoral heads of women with and without femoral neck fractures. Bone 1997;21(6):521–526.

20 Bisphosphonates – Treatment of Osteoporosis

Ann Cranney

Contents

Key Words: Bisphosphonates, non-nitrogen-containing bisphosphonates, etidronate, tiludronate, clodronate, nitrogen-containing bisphosphonates, alendronate, risedronate, zolendronate, pamidronate, ibandronate, osteoclastic bone resorption, bone mass, Paget's disease of bone, fibrous dysplasia, osteogenesis imperfect, corticosteroid-induced osteoporosis, metastatic cancer, multiple myeloma

INTRODUCTION

Bisphosphonates are inorganic pyrophosphate (P–O–P) analogues, in which the bridging oxygen atom is replaced by carbon. The P–C–P moiety is responsible for the binding of bisphosphonates to hydroxyapatite bone mineral surfaces *(1)*. Bisphosphonates can be grouped

From: *Contemporary Endocrinology: Osteoporosis: Pathophysiology and Clinical Management*
Edited by: R. A. Adler, DOI 10.1007/978-1-59745-459-9_20,

into two main groups, depending whether or not they contain a nitrogen side chain. Non-nitrogen-containing bisphosphonates include etidronate, tiludronate, and clodronate *(2)*. Nitrogen-containing bisphosphonates such as alendronate, risedronate, zolendronate, pamidronate, and ibandronate are more potent than non-nitrogen bisphosphonates.

Bisphosphonates inhibit osteoclastic bone resorption, increase bone mass, and decrease the risk of fractures. These agents are poorly absorbed (approximately 1%) and are either excreted in the urine or avidly taken up by bone on actively resorbing sites *(2)*. Bisphosphonates can accumulate in bone, hence the potential concerns relating to their long-term safety *(3)*.

In addition to being used for the treatment of osteoporosis, bisphosphonates have been used to treat other conditions associated with abnormal bone remodeling, such as Paget's disease of bone *(4–6)*, fibrous dysplasia *(7,8)*, osteogenesis imperfecta, corticosteroid-induced osteoporosis *(9–11)*, and to treat skeletal consequences of metastatic cancer and multiple myeloma *(12,13)*. Orthopedic applications include the protection of loosening of joint prostheses and preservation of bone architecture after osteonecrosis *(14,15)*.

This chapter summarizes the results of randomized controlled trials (RCTs) and meta-analyses that have evaluated the BMD and fracture efficacy of different bisphosphonates. The results of observational studies that provided long-term safety data are also reviewed.

ETIDRONATE

Etidronate is a first-generation bisphosphonate that is approved for the treatment of post-menopausal osteoporosis in Canada and Europe, but has not been approved by the Food and Drug Administration (FDA). With etidronate there is a 10- to 100-fold difference in doses that inhibit mineralization when compared to doses that inhibit bone resorption *(3)*. Due to concerns about impaired mineralization, a cyclical regimen has been used (400 mg of oral etidronate daily for 2 weeks every 3 months). Randomized controlled trials demonstrated that intermittent cyclical etidronate increased in lumbar spine (4–5%) and femoral neck bone mineral density (BMD) (2%). A meta-analysis of nine trials found that cyclical etidronate decreased the risk of incident vertebral fractures after 2–3 years of treatment [RR 0.63 (95% CI 0.44, 0.92)]. Combining data from seven trials that evaluated non-vertebral fractures showed no effect on non-vertebral fractures [RR 0.99 (95% CI 0.69, 1.42)] or hip fractures. The etidronate trials were not powered to assess non-vertebral and hip fractures *(16–18)*.

CLODRONATE

Clodronate is a non-nitrogen-containing bisphosphonate of intermediate potency between etidronate and the nitrogen-containing bisphosphonates, which is not approved by the FDA for treatment of osteoporosis *(19)*. Clodronate can be given either orally or intravenously and has been used to treat hypercalcemia of malignancy or multiple myeloma and to prevent the skeletal complications of metastatic bone disease *(12,13)*. Various cyclical or continuous regimens of clodronate have been used for the treatment of postmenopausal osteoporosis *(20,21)*. A 3-year RCT of oral clodronate 800 mg/day in 5596 women 75 years of age found that clodronate decreased the incidence of osteoporosis-related non-hip fractures by 29% [HR 0.71 *(95%* CI *0.57–0.87)*], although there was no effect on hip fractures. Interestingly, the reduction in fracture risk was reported to be similar in women with normal or osteopenic BMD and women with osteoporosis *(22)*.

PAMIDRONATE

Pamidronate, a nitrogen-containing bisphosphonate, has not been approved for the treatment of postmenopausal osteoporosis, but is approved for the treatment of Paget's disease and hypercalcemia of malignancy *(23,24)*. Intravenous pamidronate is used off-label to treat osteoporosis in patients who have difficulty in tolerating oral bisphosphonates. Although there is evidence that pamidronate increases BMD in patients with postmenopausal and corticosteroid-induced osteoporosis, there are no fracture data with pamidronate *(23, 25–28)*. The usual dose of pamidronate is 90 mg given intravenously (IV) for the first dose, followed by 30 mg IV every 3 months, which can be infused in over an hour.

ALENDRONATE

Alendronate is a nitrogen-containing bisphosphonate that is 100–1000 times more potent than etidronate *(29)*. Alendronate is approved for the treatment of postmenopausal osteoporosis and corticosteroid-induced osteoporosis and the prevention of bone loss in postmenopausal osteoporosis *(30)*. The approved treatment dose is 10 mg daily or 70 mg weekly. In the RCTs, after 3 years of alendronate the BMD of the lumbar spine increased by 8 and 6% for the femoral neck relative to control *(31)*.

The fracture intervention trial (FIT) was conducted to assess the effect of alendronate on fractures in 6459 postmenopausal women with low hip BMD (*T*-score $\leq$2.0) *(32,33)*. The FIT consisted of a 3-year vertebral fracture arm which included women with prevalent fractures and low femoral neck BMD ($n = 2027$), and a 4-year clinical fracture arm which included women with low BMD, some of who did not meet BMD criteria for osteoporosis ($n = 4432$). Women were randomized to either placebo or alendronate 5 mg daily which was increased to 10 mg after the second year. The results of the vertebral fracture arm trial demonstrated a 47% reduction in radiographic vertebral fractures [RR 0.53 (95% CI 0.41, 0.68)], a 48% reduction in wrist fractures, and a 51% reduction in hip fractures *(32)*. In the clinical fracture trial, there was a significant 44% reduction in morphometric vertebral fractures [RR 0.56 (95% CI 0.39, 0.80)] with alendronate. The overall reduction in clinical fractures was non-significant [RR 0.86 (95% CI 0.73, 1.01)]. However, there was a significant interaction between BMD and non-vertebral fractures in the clinical fracture trial, as women with a baseline femoral neck *T*-score < -2.5 had a 36% reduction in non-vertebral fractures, [RR 0.64 (95% CI 0.50, 0.82)] (33). Meta-analyses of randomized trials have confirmed that alendronate consistently reduced the risk of vertebral, non-vertebral, and hip fractures, with smaller effects on non-vertebral than vertebral fractures *(34,35)*.

A secondary analysis of pre-treatment levels of bone turnover and anti-fracture efficacy revealed that the non-vertebral fracture efficacy of alendronate was greater in women with higher pre-treatment levels of bone turnover (N-terminal propeptide of type 1 collagen) *(36)*. Although fracture trials were not conducted using weekly alendronate, trials of weekly alendronate have demonstrated comparable increases in mean lumbar spine BMD and reductions in bone turnover markers, compared to daily alendronate *(37)*.

Long-term therapy was evaluated in a 10-year follow-up trial of 247 women (initial sample 994) who participated in the all three extension studies. After 10 years of alendronate, lumbar spine BMD increased by 13.7%, trochanteric BMD by 10.3%, and total hip by 6.7%. Women who continued alendronate had small increases in the lumbar spine BMD and maintained gains in total hip BMD, although most of the BMD increase occurred within the initial 5 years. In this trial, after discontinuation of alendronate therapy, bone turnover markers increased after a year, but remained below baseline levels *(38)*. However, clinical fracture rates could not be assessed and a limitation of this trial was the small number of women followed beyond 5 years.

The extension study of the fracture intervention trial long-term extension (FLEX) re-randomized postmenopausal women enrolled in FIT, who had taken alendronate for mean of 5 years to either 5 or 10 mg of alendronate or placebo for an additional 5 years *(39)*. Of 2852 women who were contacted, 1195 were eligible and of these, 1099 were enrolled in the trial. The mean age of women was 73 years, 34% had prevalent vertebral fractures and 60% a history of clinical fractures since menopause. The average total hip BMD was 0.73 gm/cm^2 (*T*-score –1.9). The primary outcome of this trial was BMD and fractures were an exploratory outcome. In FLEX, the mean difference in lumbar spine BMD in women randomized to alendronate (5 and 10 mg arms combined) compared to placebo was 3.74% (95% CI 3.03–4.45), $p < 0.001$, and mean difference in BMD at the total hip was 2.36% (95% CI 1.8–2.9), $p < 0.001$ with a decline of 3.38% in total hip BMD in the placebo group. Similar statistically significant differences were noted at the femoral neck, trochanter, forearm, and total body. The differences in BMD seen between 5 and 10 mg alendronate groups were small. Overall BMD gains at each site were significantly greater in the group treated for 10 years compared to women who took alendronate for 5 years followed by placebo (e.g., lumbar spine BMD increase of 14.8% versus 10.99%, difference of 3.81% and difference of 2.57% at the total hip, $p < 0.001$). Clinical vertebral fracture risk was decreased [RR 0.45 (95% CI 0.24, 0.85)] in women who continued alendronate for 10 years compared to those who discontinued alendronate, but the risk of new morphometric vertebral fractures was not different [RR 0.86 (95% CI 0.6–1.22)]. In addition, the risk of non-vertebral fractures was similar in the women who discontinued alendronate compared to those women who were treated for 10 years [RR 1.00 (95% CI 0.76–1.32)] (40).

Bone turnover markers (serum C-telopeptide, bone-specific alkaline phosphatase, and serum N-propeptide of Type 1 collagen) increased gradually over the 5-year period in women who stopped alendronate after 5 years, but still remained below FIT pre-treatment levels by the end of the FLEX trial. The changes in bone markers and BMD results suggested a residual effect of alendronate and are in contrast to changes in BMD after discontinuation of estrogen or intermittent parathyroid hormone *(41)*. Only 18 iliac crest biopsy specimens were suitable, and in this sample, there were no significant differences in trabecular parameters between alendronate and placebo groups, and dual-labels of tetracycline were present in all specimens.

RISEDRONATE

Risedronate is a nitrogen-containing pyridinyl bisphosphonate that is approved for the treatment and prevention of postmenopausal osteoporosis. Fracture trials have demonstrated that risedronate 5 mg is effective in reducing the risk of incident vertebral and non-vertebral fractures in women with prevalent vertebral fractures *(42,43)*. In the vertebral fracture efficacy with risedronate therapy (VERT) trials, lumbar spine BMD increased by 5–6% and total hip BMD by 1.6–3.1% after 3 years. There was a significant 40–50% reduction in morphometric vertebral fractures in both trials and a 39% significant reduction in non-vertebral fractures in the North American study. A reduction in hip fractures was seen in the Hip Intervention Program (HIP) trial of 9331 older women. This 3-year study consisted of two subgroups of women: (i) 5445 women aged 70–79 years with low hip BMD and (ii) 3886 women aged 80–89 years with at least one risk factor for hip fracture, but who did not have low BMD. The overall risk of hip fractures was significantly reduced in the risedronate arm by 30% (2.8% versus 3.9%; RR 0.7, 95% CI 0.6, 0.9). However, the risk of hip fracture was significantly reduced only in the group of women with low BMD and prevalent fractures, but not in the older group of women with clinical risk factors, but normal BMD *(44)*.

Meta-analyses using either summary or individual-patient data from the risedronate RCTs have shown that risedronate reduces the risk of vertebral and non-vertebral fractures with relative risk reductions ranging from 36 to 55% for vertebral and 27–41% for non-vertebral fractures *(45–47)*. The results of the pooled individual-patient data analysis with the 5 mg dose for non-vertebral fractures resulted in a relative risk of [RR 0.59 (95% CI 0.27, 0.77)] *(45)* and a relative risk of [RR 0.45 (95% CI 0.31, 0.57)] for vertebral fractures after 3 years *(46)*. In a 2-year blinded extension trial of the risedronate multinational vertebral fracture trial ($n = 265$ women of original 1226), BMD was either maintained or increased, with an increase in lumbar spine BMD of 9.3% over 5 years. The risk of new vertebral fractures was reduced in years 4 and 5 by 59%, although the reduction in non-vertebral fractures in years 4 and 5 was non-significant *(48)*.

A second 2-year extension open label study of 136 women who all received risedronate 5 mg found that lumbar spine BMD increased in years 6 and 7, and femoral neck BMD was stable. There was also no change in the rate of vertebral or non-vertebral fractures between years 4 and 5 and years 6 and 7. The risk of non-vertebral fractures was similar in both risedronate and placebo/risedronate treatment arms *(49)*. Women who changed from placebo to risedronate during years 6 and 7 had a significant reduction in vertebral fractures, compared to years 1–5. Bone biopsy data were limited, and qualitative bone parameters including mineralization were normal in risedronate-treated subjects *(50,51)*.

Watts et al. completed a 1-year open label follow-up study of the North American vertebral fracture study, in 759 women out of the initial 2458 women randomized (818 completed the 3-year trial). In the year off risedronate, the BMD of the lumbar spine and femoral neck declined, and bone turnover markers returned to levels seen in control patients *(52)*.

Similar to alendronate, a trial of once weekly risedronate 35 mg resulted in similar increases in BMD to once daily 5 mg of risedronate *(53)*.

A 2-year non-inferiority randomized trial compared the efficacy of monthly risedronate 150–5 mg daily with intermediate outcomes. The increases in lumbar spine BMD after 1 year and changes in bone turnover markers were similar in both groups *(54)*.

IBANDRONATE

Ibandronate is a nitrogen-containing bisphosphonate and has been approved by the FDA for the treatment of postmenopausal osteoporosis at an oral dose of 2.5 mg daily, 150 mg monthly, or 3 mg intravenously every 3 months. The higher potency of ibandronate translates into the need for less frequent dosing intervals and a variety of dosing regimens have been evaluated in clinical trials *(55)*. In a 1-year prevention trial in 627 postmenopausal women, Stakestaad found a dose–response increase in lumbar spine BMD with doses of 0.5, 1 or 2 mg of IV ibandronate every 3 months, compared to control ($p < 0.0001$) *(56)*. McClung et al., in a 2-year trial randomized 653 postmenopausal women to one of four arms: calcium or oral ibandronate 0.5 mg, 1.0 mg, or 2.5 mg daily. BMD of the spine and total hip increased by 1.9% and total hip by 1.8%, respectively, with 2.5 mg daily of ibandronate versus control ($p < 0.001$). Bone turnover markers were suppressed to pre-menopausal levels *(57)*.

Eight randomized trials of ibandronate were conducted in postmenopausal women with osteoporosis *(58–65)*. In a 1-year randomized trial of 520 older postmenopausal women with BMD *T*-scores < –2.5, Adami et al. *(63)* compared 1 and 2 mg doses of ibandronate given IV every 3 months versus control. There was a dose–response effect on BMD of the lumbar spine with ibandronate 2 mg (5.0%), 1 mg (2.8%) versus – 0.04 % in the control arm. Two large randomized placebo-controlled trials evaluated the effect of different dosages of oral or intravenous ibandronate on fractures *(58,59)*. In a 3-year double-blind fracture trial in postmenopausal women with prevalent vertebral fractures ($n = 2946$) Chestnut et al. evaluated the efficacy of daily 2.5 mg of ibandronate and intermittent ibandronate (20 mg every 2 days for 12 doses every 3 months) versus placebo on incident vertebral fractures (ibandronate osteoporosis vertebral fracture trial) *(58)*. The mean lumbar spine *T*-score was –2.8 and femoral neck *T*-score was –2.0 with a primary outcome of morphometric vertebral fractures. Ibandronate given daily or intermittently resulted in LS BMD increases of 6.5 and 5.7%, respectively, versus 1.3% in placebo ($p < 0.0001$) *(58)*. There was a significant reduction in both morphometric (50–62%) and clinical vertebral fractures (48%), but no effect on non-vertebral fractures, except in a post-hoc analysis of women with femoral neck BMD *T*-score < –3.0 and/or lumbar spine BMD *T*-score < –2.5 and a history of clinical fractures.

In another 3-year trial of 2962 postmenopausal women, Recker et al. evaluated the fracture efficacy of two IV doses of ibandronate given intermittently (0.5 mg and 1.0 mg every 3 months) versus control. In this trial, 1 mg ibandronate IV significantly increased LS BMD by 4.0% (95% CI 3.5, 4.5) and total hip by 3.6% (95% CI 3.2, 4.0) compared to placebo ($p < 0.001$). However, there were no differences in vertebral fractures in the ibandronate arms versus controls and no effect on non-vertebral fractures. The lack of an effect on fractures suggested that 1 mg every 3 months is an ineffective dose *(59)*.

In a non-inferiority trial (DIVA, Dosing IntraVenous Administration) 2 mg IV every 2 months or 3 mg IV every 3 months of ibandronate was compared to an active control of 2.5 mg ibandronate daily. The mean lumbar spine BMD increase was 5.1% in the 2 mg IV arm, 4.8% in the 3 mg IV arm versus 3.8% in the 2.5 mg daily arm. Increases in total hip and femoral neck were also greater in IV arms *(61)*.

In another 2-year non-inferiority trial (MOBILE, Monthly Oral iBandronate In Ladies), 1609 postmenopausal women with osteoporosis were randomized to different oral monthly doses, 50/50, 100, 150 mg compared with 2.5 mg daily. All monthly regimens proved non-inferior to 2.5 mg daily and the 150 mg dose was superior to 2.5 mg daily dose based on the increase in LS BMD and suppression of bone turnover *(66)*.

ZOLEDRONATE

Zoledronate is a potent third-generation bisphosphonate that has been used primarily in oncology patients. Extended dosing intervals have been evaluated in clinical trials of zoledronate as a result of its higher potency *(67)*. A 1-year RCT of 351 postmenopausal women (mean age 64 years) compared the efficacy of different regimens of intermittent IV zoledronate, 0.25, 0.5, or 1 mg every 3 months, 2 mg every 6 months, or one 4 mg dose versus placebo on BMD. The increases in BMD with zoledronate ranged from 4.3 to 5.1% at the lumbar spine and 3.1–3.5% at the femoral neck compared to placebo ($p<0.001$). Bone turnover markers were suppressed by 3 months and remained suppressed by 12 months *(67)*.

Fracture efficacy of 5 mg of intravenous zoledronic acid given yearly was evaluated in a 3-year double-blind placebo-controlled randomized fracture trial (HORIZON PFT: Health Outcomes and Reduced Incidence with Zoledronic Acid Once Yearly, Pivotal Fracture Trial). A total of 7765 postmenopausal women were randomized to either zoledronic acid or placebo. All patients received daily calcium 1000–1500 mg/day and vitamin D 400–1200 IU/day. This trial included women aged 65–89 with either low femoral neck BMD *T*-score $\leq$2.5 with or without a vertebral fracture, or *T*-score of $\leq$1.5 with at least two mild vertebral fractures or one moderate vertebral fracture. Sixty-four percent of women had prevalent vertebral fractures at baseline and the mean age was 73 years. There were two strata in this trial: (1) women on no current osteoporosis therapy ($n=3045$) and (2) women on SERMS, calcitonin, HT, or tibolone ($n=3039$). The mean increase in lumbar spine BMD was 6.71% (95% CI, 5.69–7.74) and 6.02% (95%, CI 5.77–6.28) at the total hip when compared to placebo, $p<0.001$ after 3 years. In the combined results from Stratum 1 and 2, there was a 41% reduction in hip fractures (2.5% versus 1.4%), (95% CI 17–58), NNT 98, a 70% reduction in morphometric vertebral fractures (10.9% versus 3.3%), (95% CI 62–75), NNT 14. For the secondary endpoints, there was a 25% reduction in non-vertebral fractures [RR 0.75 (95 % CI 0.64, 0.87)], a 33% reduction in clinical fractures, and a 67% reduction in clinical vertebral fractures, $p<0.001$ *(68)*.

The HORIZON recurrent fracture trial randomized 2127 older men and women with a prevalent hip fracture to either yearly IV zoledronic acid 5 mg or calcium and vitamin D with a primary outcome of recurrent fracture. In contrast to pivotal fracture trial, this trial was event-based driven and the mean follow-up period was 1.9 years. The median age of participants was 76 years and 76% of participants were female. With zoledronic acid, there was a 35% risk reduction (8.6 versus 13.9%), absolute risk reduction of 5.3% in new clinical fractures [HR 0.65, 95% CI, 16–50), $p=0.0012$ and a significant reduction in clinical vertebral (46%), non-vertebral (27%), and non-significant reduction in hip fractures (30%, HR 0.70; 95% CI 0.41–1.19). This was also the first trial of an anti-resorptive to demonstrate a significant 28% reduction in mortality rate (HR 0.72; 95% CI 0.56–0.93, $p=0.0117$) *(69)*.

COMPARATIVE EFFICACY

A 3-year randomized double-blind head-to-head trial followed by a 1-year extension study of alendronate 70 mg versus risedronate 35 mg weekly was conducted in 1053 postmenopausal women with low bone mineral density *(70,71)*. The mean lumbar spine

T-score of participants was –2.24. The primary endpoint of this trial was a comparison of the change in BMD of the trochanter, between alendronate and risedronate. Secondary endpoints included differences in BMD change at total hip, femoral neck and lumbar spine, and bone turnover markers. After 12 months, there were larger BMD increases with alendronate when compared to risedronate at the trochanter (3.4% versus 2.1%) and at the lumbar spine (3.7% versus 2.6%), $p < 0.001$. Significantly more women had a BMD increase of 3% at the hip trochanter site, total hip and lumbar spine with alendronate compared to risedronate. Alendronate produced significantly greater reductions in bone turnover markers at 3 months. Tolerability was similar for both bisphosphonates. However, the correlation of differences in BMD response with differences in fracture risk reduction between the two bisphosphonates is unclear *(70)*.

Head-to-head fracture trials of bisphosphonates have not been feasible due to the large number of participants needed to demonstrate differences in fracture reduction *(72)*. As a result, data from observational studies have been used to compare effectiveness of different bisphosphonates. An example is an observational cohort (risedronate and alendronate cohort -REAL) of women aged 65 and older created from commercially available data sets was used to compare the effectiveness of risedronate to alendronate in reducing non-vertebral fractures, after 1 year of treatment. The authors reported that risedronate was more effective in reducing non-vertebral and hip fractures *(73)*. Limitations of this type of analysis include that it was not possible to adjust for all potential confounding variables, since it was not an analysis of a prospective cohort study. Although observational studies can be very useful in generating hypotheses and providing preliminary data on relative effectiveness, randomized head-to-head trials remain the gold standard when evaluating drug efficacy *(74)*.

RELATIONSHIP BETWEEN BMD, BONE TURNOVER, AND FRACTURE REDUCTION

A number of studies have explored the relationship between the changes in BMD and fracture reduction seen after treatment with bisphosphonates. The proportion of fracture risk reduction that is explained by BMD varies with most studies suggesting that the effect of treatment on BMD only accounts for a small fraction of the observed reduction in vertebral and non-vertebral fractures *(75–81)*. Discrepancies between studies can be explained by the inclusion of different trials or differences in methodology *(82)*. The small reductions in vertebral fracture risk that occur without an associated increase in BMD suggest that suppression of bone turnover has an independent effect on fracture risk. In addition, the vertebral fractures are reduced within the first year of treatment with bisphosphonates, prior to significant increases in BMD, suggesting that effects on bone turnover and microarchitecture are important contributors to fracture reduction *(42,43,83–85)*. Eastell et al. analyzed the risedronate trials and reported a significant relationship between changes in bone turnover markers at 3–6 months with vertebral fracture incidence at 3 years. There appeared to be a threshold, below which further decreases in bone resorption (55–60% in C-telopeptide) were not associated with a further decrease in vertebral fracture risk. This threshold was not evident for non-vertebral fractures *(86)*. Other studies have not identified a specific plateau and the exact relationship between BMD, bone markers, and fracture reduction with bisphosphonates is not fully understood *(83)*.

BISPHOSPHONATES IN COMBINATION WITH OTHER ANTI-RESORPTIVE AGENTS OR ANABOLIC AGENTS

Randomized trials of combination therapy of bisphosphonates with other anti-resorptive agents (hormone therapy, raloxifene) have been conducted in postmenopausal women using surrogate endpoints of BMD and bone turnover markers *(87–90)*. Trials of combined therapies have noted additive effects on BMD, when compared to either agent alone. For example, Greenspan in a 3-year factorial trial randomized 373 older women to either hormone therapy (HT), alendronate 10 mg daily, both HT and alendronate combined, versus no treatment. Combination therapy resulted in significantly greater increases in the lateral lumbar (11.8%), posterior–anterior lumbar spine (10.4%), and total hip BMD (5.9%) compared to either alendronate or HT alone ($p < 0.001$) *(87)*.

Anabolic agents such as intermittent PTH *(1–34)* and *(1–84)* target the osteoblast and enhance bone formation, so it was hypothesized that a combination of intermittent PTH and bisphosphonates may have a synergistic action on bone density. In an RCT trial of 238 postmenopausal women with osteoporosis, alendronate 10 mg combined with 100 μg of PTH *(1–84)* was compared to 100 μg of PTH alone versus alendronate alone. BMD results showed that the combination therapy was not significantly better than monotherapy with PTH *(1–84)*, suggesting that alendronate in combination with PTH seemed to blunt the increase in LS BMD, when compared to PTH *(1–84)* alone *(91)*. In contrast, sequential therapy of PTH *(1–84)* followed by a bisphosphonate has been shown to maintain BMD changes *(92)*. The same blunting effect may not be applicable to other anti-resorptive agents when used in combination with PTH *(93)*.

ADVERSE EVENTS

Side-effects with IV bisphosphonates include acute phase reactions manifested by fever, myalgias, headache, and lymphopenia. These reactions are usually transient and decrease in severity with repeated dosing *(61,67,94)*. Hypocalcemia has been reported with IV administration of bisphosphonates *(95–97)*. Laboratory abnormalities described with bisphosphonates include elevated serum PTH, phosphate levels. Increases in serum creatinine have been noted in clinical trials, but have not been associated with differences in long-term renal function *(69)*.

Skin rashes and ocular reactions, such as episcleritis or uveitis, have also been reported to occur after administration of bisphosphonates *(98–100)*.

In the HORIZON trials, adverse events were higher in the zoledronate-treated group and were primarily due to post-dose symptoms of pyrexia, myalgia, flu-like symptoms, headache, and bone pain or musculoskeletal pain which occurred with 3 days (31.6 versus 6.2% of placebo group). Changes in renal function that occurred in the zoledronic acid group were transient and there were no differences in serum creatinine between groups at 3 years. Arrhythmias occurred more frequently in the zoledronic acid group (6.9% versus 5.3% of participants, $p = 0.03$). Serious atrial fibrillation (defined as resulting in hospitalization, disability, or life-threatening) was more common in the zolendronic acid group (1.3% versus 0.5%), $p < 0.001$, which translates into an NNH of 129. In most cases, the cases of atrial fibrillation occurred more than 39 days post-infusion *(68)*. The incidence of stroke did not differ between groups and overall cases of atrial fibrillation did not differ between groups. The mechanism for atrial fibrillation is uncertain and it is also not clear if this is an adverse event associated with other bisphosphonates since serious atrial fibrillation events were an inconsistent finding across trials. There was a trend to an increase in serious atrial fibrillation (1.5% versus 1.0%) on re-analysis of serious adverse events in the fracture intervention trial; however, there was no evidence on re-analysis of the risedronate trials or the zoledronic acid recurrent fracture trial *(69,101)*.

Although less frequent than with the intravenous bisphosphonates, use of oral bisphosphonates can be associated with flu-like illness and these are more frequently reported with monthly regimens of ibandronate and risedronate.*(54,60)*

The most common side-effects associated with oral nitrogen-containing bisphosphonates are gastrointestinal and include esophageal erosions and ulcerative esophagitis which can occur especially, if these agents are not taken properly. Although not reported in clinical trials, serious esophageal events were noted with daily alendronate when initially marketed *(32,102)*. Esophageal side-effects can be minimized by taking the bisphosphonates on an empty stomach, with a full glass of water when sitting upright. The risk of esophagitis appears to be lower with the once weekly versus daily preparations *(103–107)*.

It is believed that bone remodeling targets microdamage in bone to help maintain integrity of the skeleton. A potential concern given the long half-life of potent bisphosphonates in bone matrix is that over suppression of bone turnover could result in impaired bone strength, and increased risk of fractures, as a consequence of microdamage accumulation *(108,109)*. Case reports of adynamic bone disease or atypical fractures associated with bisphosphonates have been published, but it is not clear if other metabolic bone diseases were ruled out *(110,111)*. Histomorphometric studies of bone biopsies taken before and after treatment with bisphosphonates have not shown any evidence of adynamic bone or microcracks, and RCTs have not demonstrated an increased risk of fractures with long-term bisphosphonate use *(112,113)*.

OSTEONECROSIS OF THE JAW

A potential complication related to the use of bisphosphonates, osteonecrosis of the jaws (ONJ) became apparent in 2003 after a series of case reports and chart reviews *(114–117)*. ONJ is characterized by an area of exposed bone in the maxillofacial area that does not heal over a 2-month period after being identified by a health-care provider, in a patient who has been exposed to bisphosphonates and who has not received radiation to the area *(118)*. The exact mechanism underlying the development of ONJ is uncertain and there is no clear evidence relating ONJ to suppression of bone turnover. Potential mechanisms that have been postulated relate to the antiangiogenic properties of nitrogen-containing bisphosphonates, the preferential accumulation of bisphosphonates in the jaw, which is an active remodeling site or perhaps direct toxicity of bisphosphonates on the oral epithelium *(118–120)*. Most cases of ONJ have been described in cancer patients treated exposed to higher cumulative doses of IV pamidronate or zoledronate for metastatic bone cancer or multiple myeloma (estimated incidence of 1–10 per 100 patients). Other risk factors for ONJ include comorbid conditions, a history of dental extraction, glucocorticoids, pre-existing dental or periodontal disease, poor fitting dental applications, and oral bone manipulating surgery. Woo summarized 368 cases of bisphosphonate-associated ONJ and reported that 60% of the cases occurred after dentoalveolar surgery and 4% ($n = 15$) of cases occurred in patients who

Table 1
Bisphosphonates and Fracture Efficacy: Relative Risk Reduction

Bisphosphonate	*Doses in trials*	*Vertebral fractures*	*Non-vertebral fractures*	*Hip fractures*
Etidronate	400 mg for 2 weeks every 3 months	37%	No overall reduction	No overall reduction
Pamidronate	30 mg IV every 3 months	No data	No data	No data
Alendronate	5 or 10 mg/day	40–48%	20–49%	25–50%
Risedronate	5 mg/day	40–50%	20–40%	20–36%
Ibandronate	2.5 mg/day or 20 mg every 2 days × 12 doses every 3 months	50–60%	No overall reduction in two trials	Not assessed
Zoledronate	5 mg IV annually	70%	25%	41%
Clodronate	800 mg/day	No data	20–29% reduction in clinical fractures	No reduction

were receiving treatment for osteoporosis. Over 80% of patients had myeloma or metastatic cancers and other risk factors for osteonecrosis including chemotherapy, corticosteroids, and/or radiation *(121)*. A literature review of bisphosphonate-associated ONJ determined that there were 57 cases associated with treatment for osteoporosis (most with oral alendronate, 2 with risedronate, 1 received both alendronate and risedronate, and 2 received either IV pamidronate or zoledronic acid), and 7 cases who were receiving treatment for Paget's disease *(118)*.

Osteonecrosis of the jaw was not reported as an adverse event in the bisphosphonate trials, but ONJ has only recently been adjudicated in clinical trials of bisphosphonates *(68)*. The incidence of ONJ in bisphosphonate treatment for osteoporosis is unknown, with estimates ranging from 1 in 10,000 to 1 in 100,000 patient treatment years *(122)*. It is difficult to determine incidence given the lack of prospective cohort studies and the uncertainty surrounding case ascertainment *(118,123)*.

CONCLUSIONS

Bisphosphonates are effective in the prevention and treatment of postmenopausal osteoporosis and are generally well tolerated. Nitrogen-containing bisphosphonates (alendronate, risedronate, ibandronate, and zoledronic acid) increase BMD of the lumbar spine and proximal femur, suppress bone turnover markers, and reduce the risk of clinical and morphometric vertebral fractures in postmenopausal women with osteoporosis or low bone mass. Non-vertebral fracture and hip fracture efficacy in postmenopausal women with osteoporosis or prevalent vertebral fractures have been also confirmed in clinical trials of alendronate, risedronate, and zoledronic acid.

Based on long-term data, it appears safe to continue bisphosphonates for up to 10 years, without an increased risk of fracture. Long-term therapy is indicated in those women at high risk of fracture, i.e., those with severe osteoporosis or prevalent vertebral fractures. Bone turnover remains suppressed up to 5 years after discontinuing alendronate, although this does not be the case with other bisphosphonates *(52)*. The maintenance of BMD and continued suppression of bone turnover has been felt to be a surrogate marker suggesting continued fracture efficacy.

Given that the rate of non-vertebral and morphometric vertebral fractures are similar for 5 versus 10 years of treatment with alendronate, it would seem reasonable to consider a drug holiday after 5 years, in individuals who are not at high risk for fractures, and who have had a good response to alendronate. BMD and bone turnover markers can be used to re-evaluate if therapy should be resumed after a drug holiday *(36)*.

Additional epidemiologic studies and surveillance, including improved case ascertainment will help clarify the risks of osteonecrosis of the jaw and other potential harms.

REFERENCES

1. Rodan GA, Reszka AA. Osteoporosis and bisphosphonates. J Bone Joint Surg Am 2003;85-A(Suppl 3):8–12.
2. Reszka AA, Rodan GA. Nitrogen-containing bisphosphonate mechanism of action. Mini-Rev Med Chem 2004;4(7):711–719.
3. Russell RG. Bisphosphonates: from bench to bedside. Ann N Y Acad Sci 2006;1068:367–401.
4. Brown JP, Chines AA, Myers WR, Eusebio RA, Ritter-Hrncirik C, Hayes CW. Improvement of pagetic bone lesions with risedronate treatment: a radiologic study. Bone 2000;26(3):263–267.
5. Hosking D, Lyles K, Brown JP, Fraser WD, Miller P, Diaz CM, et al. Long-term control of bone turnover in Paget's disease with zoledronic acid and risedronate. J Bone Miner Res 2007;22(1):142–148.
6. Reid IR, Miller P, Lyles K, Fraser W, Brown JP, Saidi Y, et al. Comparison of a single infusion of zoledronic acid with risedronate for Paget's disease. N Engl J Med 2005;353(9):898–908.
7. Chapurlat RD, Hugueny P, Delmas PD, Meunier PJ. Treatment of fibrous dysplasia of bone with intravenous pamidronate: long-term effectiveness and evaluation of predictors of response to treatment. Bone 2004;35(1):235–242.
8. Chapurlat RD. Medical therapy in adults with fibrous dysplasia of bone. J Bone Miner Res 2006;21(Suppl 2):114–119.
9. Adachi JD, Roux C, Pitt PI, Cooper C, Moniz C, Dequeker J, et al. A pooled data analysis on the use of intermittent cyclical etidronate therapy for the prevention and treatment of corticosteroid induced bone loss. J Rheumatol 2000;27(10):2424–2431.
10. Adachi JD, Bensen WG, Brown J, Hanley D, Hodsman A, Josse R, et al. Intermittent etidronate therapy to prevent corticosteroid-induced osteoporosis. N Engl J Med 1997;337(6):382–387.
11. Saag KG. Glucocorticoid-induced osteoporosis. Endocrinol Metab Clin North Am 2003;32(1):135–157.
12. McCloskey EV, Dunn JA, Kanis JA, MacLennan IC, Drayson MT. Long-term follow-up of a prospective, double-blind, placebo-controlled randomized trial of clodronate in multiple myeloma. Br J Haematol 2001;113(4):1035–1043.
13. Kanis JA, Powles T, Paterson AH, McCloskey EV, Ashley S. Clodronate decreases the frequency of skeletal metastases in women with breast cancer. Bone 1996;19(6):663–667.
14. Lai KA, Shen WJ, Yang CY, Shao CJ, Hsu JT, Lin RM. The use of alendronate to prevent early collapse of the femoral head in patients with nontraumatic osteonecrosis. A randomized clinical study. J Bone Joint Surg Am 2005;87(10):2155–2159.
15. Wilkinson JM, Eagleton AC, Stockley I, Peel NF, Hamer AJ, Eastell R. Effect of pamidronate on bone turnover and implant migration after total hip arthroplasty: a randomized trial. J Orthop Res 2005;23(1):1–8.

16. Watts NB, Harris ST, Genant HK, Wasnich RD, Miller PD, Jackson RD, et al. Intermittent cyclical etidronate treatment of postmenopausal osteoporosis. N Engl J Med 1990;323(2):73–79.
17. Storm T, Thamsborg G, Steiniche T, Genant HK, Sorensen OH. Effect of intermittent cyclical etidronate therapy on bone mass and fracture rate in women with postmenopausal osteoporosis. N Engl J Med 1990;322(18):1265–1271.
18. Cranney A, Guyatt G, Krolicki N, Welch V, Griffith L, Adachi JD, et al. A meta-analysis of etidronate for the treatment of postmenopausal osteoporosis. Osteoporos Int 2001;12(2):140–151.
19. Kanis JA, McCloskey EV. Clodronate. Cancer 1997;80(8 Suppl):1691–1695.
20. Filipponi P, Cristallini S, Policani G, Schifini MF, Casciari C, Garinei P. Intermittent versus continuous clodronate administration in postmenopausal women with low bone mass. Bone 2000;26(3):269–274.
21. Filipponi P, Cristallini S, Rizzello E, Policani G, Fedeli L, Gregorio F, et al. Cyclical intravenous clodronate in postmenopausal osteoporosis: results of a long-term clinical trial. Bone 1996;18(2):179–184.
22. McCloskey EV, Beneton M, Charlesworth D, Kayan K, Detakats D, Dey A, et al. Clodronate reduces the incidence of fractures in community-dwelling elderly women unselected for osteoporosis: results of a double-blind, placebo-controlled randomized study. J Bone Miner Res 2007;22(1):135–141.
23. Cauza E, Etemad M, Winkler F, Hanusch-Enserer H, Partsch G, Noske H, et al. Pamidronate increases bone mineral density in women with postmenopausal or steroid-induced osteoporosis. J Clin Pharm Ther 2004;29(5):431–436.
24. Coukell AJ, Markham A. Pamidronate. A review of its use in the management of osteolytic bone metastases, tumour-induced hypercalcaemia and Paget's disease of bone. Drugs Aging 1998;12(2): 149–168.
25. Brumsen C, Papapoulos SE, Lips P, Geelhoed-Duijvestijn PH, Hamdy NA, Landman JO, et al. Daily oral pamidronate in women and men with osteoporosis: a 3-year randomized placebo-controlled clinical trial with a 2-year open extension. J Bone Miner Res 2002;17(6):1057–1064.
26. Peretz A, Body JJ, Dumon JC, Rozenberg S, Hotimski A, Praet JP, et al. Cyclical pamidronate infusions in postmenopausal osteoporosis. Maturitas 1996;25(1):69–75.
27. Lees B, Garland SW, Walton C, Ross D, Whitehead MI, Stevenson JC. Role of oral pamidronate in preventing bone loss in postmenopausal women. Osteoporos Int 1996;6(6):480–485.
28. Boutsen Y, Jamart J, Esselinckx W, Devogelaer JP. Primary prevention of glucocorticoid-induced osteoporosis with intravenous pamidronate and calcium: a prospective controlled 1-year study comparing a single infusion, an infusion given once every 3 months, and calcium alone. J Bone Miner Res 2001;16(1):104–112.
29. Lourwood DL. The pharmacology and therapeutic utility of bisphosphonates. Pharmacotherapy 1998;18(4):779–789.
30. Porras AG, Holland SD, Gertz BJ. Pharmacokinetics of alendronate. Clin Pharmacokinet 1999;36(5):315–328.
31. Liberman UA, Weiss SR, Broll J, Minne HW, Quan H, Bell NH, et al. Effect of oral alendronate on bone mineral density and the incidence of fractures in postmenopausal osteoporosis. The Alendronate Phase III Osteoporosis Treatment Study Group. N Engl J Med 1995;333(22):1437–1443.
32. Black DM, Cummings SR, Karpf DB, Cauley JA, Thompson DE, Nevitt MC, et al. Randomised trial of effect of alendronate on risk of fracture in women with existing vertebral fractures. Fracture Intervention Trial Research Group. Lancet 1996;348(9041):1535–1541.
33. Cummings SR, Black DM, Thompson DE, Applegate WB, Barrett-Connor E, Musliner TA, et al. Effect of alendronate on risk of fracture in women with low bone density but without vertebral fractures: results from the Fracture Intervention Trial. JAMA 1998;280(24):2077–2082.
34. Papapoulos SE, Quandt SA, Liberman UA, Hochberg MC, Thompson DE. Meta-analysis of the efficacy of alendronate for the prevention of hip fractures in postmenopausal women. Osteoporos Int 2005;16(5):468–474.
35. Liberman UA, Hochberg MC, Geusens P, Shah A, Lin J, Chattopadhyay A, et al. Hip and non-spine fracture risk reductions differ among antiresorptive agents: Evidence from randomised controlled trials. Int J Clin Pract 2006;60(11):1394–1400.
36. Bauer DC, Garnero P, Hochberg MC, Santora A, Delmas P, Ewing SK, et al. Pretreatment levels of bone turnover and the antifracture efficacy of alendronate: the fracture intervention trial. J Bone Miner Res 2006;21(2):292–299.

37. Rizzoli R, Greenspan SL, Bone G III, Schnitzer TJ, Watts NB, Adami S, et al. Two-year results of once-weekly administration of alendronate 70 mg for the treatment of postmenopausal osteoporosis. J Bone Miner Res 2002;17(11):1988–1996.
38. Bone HG, Hosking D, Devogelaer JP, Tucci JR, Emkey RD, Tonino RP, et al. Ten years' experience with alendronate for osteoporosis in postmenopausal women. N Engl J Med 2004;350(12): 1189–1199.
39. Ensrud KE, Barrett-Connor EL, Schwartz A, Santora AC, Bauer DC, Suryawanshi S, et al. Randomized trial of effect of alendronate continuation versus discontinuation in women with low BMD: results from the Fracture Intervention Trial long-term extension. J Bone Miner Res 2004;(8):1259–1269.
40. Black DM, Schwartz AV, Ensrud KE, Cauley JA, Levis S, Quandt SA, et al. Effects of continuing or stopping alendronate after 5 years of treatment: the Fracture Intervention Trial Long-term Extension (FLEX): a randomized trial. JAMA 2006;296(24):2927–2938.
41. Greenspan SL, Emkey RD, Bone HG, Weiss SR, Bell NH, Downs RW, et al. Significant differential effects of alendronate, estrogen, or combination therapy on the rate of bone loss after discontinuation of treatment of postmenopausal osteoporosis. A randomized, double-blind, placebo-controlled trial. [summary for patients in Ann Intern Med. 2002;137(11):I31; PMID: 12459003]. Ann Intern Med 2002;137(11):875–883.
42. Harris ST, Watts NB, Genant HK, McKeever CD, Hangartner T, Keller M, et al. Effects of risedronate treatment on vertebral and nonvertebral fractures in women with postmenopausal osteoporosis: a randomized controlled trial. Vertebral Efficacy With Risedronate Therapy (VERT) Study Group. JAMA 1999;282(14):1344–1352.
43. Reginster JY. Risedronate increases bone mineral density and reduces the vertebral fracture incidence in postmenopausal women. Clin Exp Rheumatol 2001;19(2):121–122.
44. McClung MR, Geusens P, Miller PD, Zippel H, Bensen WG, Roux C, et al. Effect of risedronate on the risk of hip fracture in elderly women. Hip Intervention Program Study Group. N Engl J Med 2001;344(5):333–340.
45. Harrington JT, Ste-Marie LG, Brandi ML, Civitelli R, Fardellone P, Grauer A, et al. Risedronate rapidly reduces the risk for nonvertebral fractures in women with postmenopausal osteoporosis. Calcif Tissue Int 2004;74(2):129–135.
46. Adachi JD, Rizzoli R, Boonen S, Li Z, Meredith MP, Chesnut CH III. Vertebral fracture risk reduction with risedronate in post-menopausal women with osteoporosis: a meta-analysis of individual patient data. Aging Clin Exp Res 2005;17(2):150–156.
47. Cranney A, Tugwell P, Adachi J, Weaver B, Zytaruk N, Papaioannou A, et al. Meta-analyses of therapies for postmenopausal osteoporosis. III. Meta-analysis of risedronate for the treatment of postmenopausal osteoporosis. [Review] [21 refs]. Endocr Rev 2002;23(4):517–523.
48. Sorensen OH, Crawford GM, Mulder H, Hosking DJ, Gennari C, Mellstrom D, et al. Long-term efficacy of risedronate: a 5-year placebo-controlled clinical experience. Bone 2003;32(2):120–126.
49. Mellstrom DD, Sorensen OH, Goemaere S, Roux C, Johnson TD, Chines AA. Seven years of treatment with risedronate in women with postmenopausal osteoporosis. Calcif Tissue Int 2004;75(6): 462–468.
50. Ste-Marie LG, Sod E, Johnson T, Chines A. Five years of treatment with risedronate and its effects on bone safety in women with postmenopausal osteoporosis. Calcif Tissue Int 2004;75(6):469–476.
51. Miller PD, Roux C, Boonen S, Barton IP, Dunlap LE, Burgio DE. Safety and efficacy of risedronate in patients with age-related reduced renal function as estimated by the Cockcroft and Gault method: a pooled analysis of nine clinical trials. J Bone Miner Res 2005;20(12):2105–2115.
52. Watts NB, Chines A, Olszynski WP, McKeever CD, McClung MR, Zhou X, et al. Fracture risk remains reduced one year after discontinuation of risedronate. Osteoporos Int 2008;19(3): 365–372.
53. Brown JP, Kendler DL, McClung MR, Emkey RD, Adachi JD, Bolognese MA, et al. The efficacy and tolerability of risedronate once a week for the treatment of postmenopausal osteoporosis. Calcif Tissue Int 2002;71(2):103–111.
54. Delmas PD, McClung MR, Zanchetta JR, Racewicz A, Roux C, Benhamou CL, et al. Efficacy and safety of risedronate 150 mg once a month in the treatment of postmenopausal osteoporosis. Bone 2008;42(1):36–42.

55. Pyon EY. Once-monthly ibandronate for postmenopausal osteoporosis: review of a new dosing regimen. Clin Ther 2006;28(4):475–490.
56. Stakkestad JA, Benevolenskaya LI, Stepan JJ, Skag A, Nordby A, Oefjord E, et al. Intravenous ibandronate injections given every three months: a new treatment option to prevent bone loss in postmenopausal women [see comment]. Ann Rheum Dis 2003;62(10):969–975.
57. McClung MR, Wasnich RD, Recker R, Cauley JA, Chesnut CH III, Ensrud KE, et al. Oral daily ibandronate prevents bone loss in early postmenopausal women without osteoporosis. J Bone Miner Res 2004;1:11–18.
58. Chesnut CH III, Skag A, Christiansen C, Recker R, Stakkestad JA, Hoiseth A, et al. Effects of oral ibandronate administered daily or intermittently on fracture risk in postmenopausal osteoporosis. J Bone Miner Res 2004;8:1241–1249.
59. Recker R, Stakkestad JA, Chesnut CH III, Christiansen C, Skag A, Hoiseth A, et al. Insufficiently dosed intravenous ibandronate injections are associated with suboptimal antifracture efficacy in postmenopausal osteoporosis. Bone 2004;34(5):890–899.
60. Miller PD, McClung MR, Macovei L, Stakkestad JA, Luckey M, Bonvoisin B, et al. Monthly oral ibandronate therapy in postmenopausal osteoporosis: 1-year results from the MOBILE study. J Bone Miner Res 2005;20(8):1315–1322.
61. Delmas PD, Adami S, Strugala C, Stakkestad JA, Reginster JY, Felsenberg D, et al. Intravenous ibandronate injections in postmenopausal women with osteoporosis: one-year results from the dosing intravenous administration study. Arthritis Rheum 2006;54(6):1838–1846.
62. Ravn P, Neugebauer G, Christiansen C. Association between pharmacokinetics of oral ibandronate and clinical response in bone mass and bone turnover in women with postmenopausal osteoporosis. Bone 2002;30(1):320–324.
63. Adami S, Felsenberg D, Christiansen C, Robinson J, Lorenc RS, Mahoney P, et al. Efficacy and safety of ibandronate given by intravenous injection once every 3 months. Bone 2004;34(5):881–889.
64. Riis BJ, Ise J, von Stein T, Bagger Y, Christiansen C. Ibandronate: a comparison of oral daily dosing versus intermittent dosing in postmenopausal osteoporosis. J Bone Miner Res 2001;16(10):1871–1878.
65. Thiebaud D, Burckhardt P, Kriegbaum H, Huss H, Mulder H, Juttmann JR, et al. Three monthly intravenous injections of ibandronate in the treatment of postmenopausal osteoporosis. Am J Med 1997;103(4):298–307.
66. Reginster JY, Adami S, Lakatos P, Greenwald M, Stepan JJ, Silverman SL, et al. Efficacy and tolerability of once-monthly oral ibandronate in postmenopausal osteoporosis: 2-year results from the MOBILE study. Ann Rheum Dis 2006;65(5):654–661.
67. Reid IR, Brown JP, Burckhardt P, Horowitz Z, Richardson P, Trechsel U, et al. Intravenous zoledronic acid in postmenopausal women with low bone mineral density. N Engl J Med 2002;346(9):653–661.
68. Black DM, Delmas PD, Eastell R, Reid IR, Boonen S, Cauley JA, et al. Once-yearly zoledronic acid 5 mg for treatment of postmenopausal osteoporosis. N Engl J Med 2007;356(18):1809–1822.
69. Lyles KW, Colon-Emeric CS, Magaziner JS, Adachi JD, Pieper CF, Mautalen C, et al. Zoledronic Acid and Clinical Fractures and Mortality after Hip Fracture. N Engl J Med 2007;357:1799–1809.
70. Rosen CJ, Hochberg MC, Bonnick SL, McClung M, Miller P, Broy S, et al. Treatment with once-weekly alendronate 70 mg compared with once-weekly risedronate 35 mg in women with postmenopausal osteoporosis: a randomized double-blind study. J Bone Miner Res 2005;20(1):141–151.
71. Bonnick S, Saag KG, Kiel DP, McClung M, Hochberg M, Burnett SA, et al. Comparison of weekly treatment of postmenopausal osteoporosis with alendronate versus risedronate over two years. J Clin Endocrinol Metab 2006;91(7):2631–2637.
72. Wehren LE, Hosking D, Hochberg MC. Putting evidence-based medicine into clinical practice: comparing anti-resorptive agents for the treatment of osteoporosis. Curr Med Res Opin 2004;20(4):525–531.
73. Silverman SL, Watts NB, Delmas PD, Lange JL, Lindsay R. Effectiveness of bisphosphonates on nonvertebral and hip fractures in the first year of therapy: The risedronate and alendronate (REAL) cohort study. Osteoporos Int 2007;18(1):25–34.
74. Black DM, Rosen CJ. Is risedronate or alendronate more effective at preventing nonvertebral fractures in women with osteoporosis? Nat Clin Pract Rheumatol 2007;3(7):378–379.
75. Wasnich RD, Miller PD. Antifracture efficacy of antiresorptive agents are related to changes in bone density. J Clin Endocrinol Metab 2000;85(1):231–236.

76. Hochberg MC, Ross PD, Black D, Cummings SR, Genant HK, Nevitt MC, et al. Larger increases in bone mineral density during alendronate therapy are associated with a lower risk of new vertebral fractures in women with postmenopausal osteoporosis. Fracture Intervention Trial Research Group. Arthritis Rheum 1999;42(6):1246–1254.
77. Watts NB, Cooper C, Lindsay R, Eastell R, Manhart MD, Barton IP, et al. Relationship between changes in bone mineral density and vertebral fracture risk associated with risedronate: greater increases in bone mineral density do not relate to greater decreases in fracture risk. J Clin Densitom 2004;7(3):255–261.
78. Cummings SR, Karpf DB, Harris F, Genant HK, Ensrud K, LaCroix AZ, et al. Improvement in spine bone density and reduction in risk of vertebral fractures during treatment with antiresorptive drugs. Am J Med 2002;112(4):281–289.
79. Hochberg MC, Greenspan S, Wasnich RD, Miller P, Thompson DE, Ross PD. Changes in bone density and turnover explain the reductions in incidence of nonvertebral fractures that occur during treatment with antiresorptive agents. J Clin Endocrinol Metab 2002;87(4):1586–1592.
80. Watts NB, Geusens P, Barton IP, Felsenberg D. Relationship between changes in BMD and nonvertebral fracture incidence associated with risedronate: reduction in risk of nonvertebral fracture is not related to change in BMD. J Bone Miner Res 2005;20(12):2097–2104.
81. Delmas PD, Seeman E. Changes in bone mineral density explain little of the reduction in vertebral or nonvertebral fracture risk with anti-resorptive therapy. Bone 2004;34(4):599–604.
82. Delmas PD, Li Z, Cooper C. Relationship between changes in bone mineral density and fracture risk reduction with antiresorptive drugs: some issues with meta-analyses. J Bone Miner Res 2004;19(2): 330–337.
83. Bauer DC, Black DM, Garnero P, Hochberg M, Ott S, Orloff J, et al. Change in bone turnover and hip, non-spine, and vertebral fracture in alendronate-treated women: the fracture intervention trial. J Bone Miner Res 2004;8:1250–1258.
84. Borah B, Dufresne TE, Chmielewski PA, Johnson TD, Chines A, Manhart MD. Risedronate preserves bone architecture in postmenopausal women with osteoporosis as measured by three-dimensional microcomputed tomography. Bone 2004;34(4):736–746.
85. Recker R, Masarachia P, Santora A, Howard T, Chavassieux P, Arlot M, et al. Trabecular bone microarchitecture after alendronate treatment of osteoporotic women. Curr Med Res Opin 2005;21(2):185–194.
86. Eastell R, Barton I, Hannon RA, Chines A, Garnero P, Delmas PD. Relationship of early changes in bone resorption to the reduction in fracture risk with risedronate. J Bone Miner Res 2003;18(6):1051–1056.
87. Greenspan SL, Resnick NM, Parker RA. Combination therapy with hormone replacement and alendronate for prevention of bone loss in elderly women: a randomized controlled trial. JAMA 2003;289(19):2525–2533.
88. Harris ST, Eriksen EF, Davidson M, Ettinger MP, Moffett JA Jr, Baylink DJ, et al. Effect of combined risedronate and hormone replacement therapies on bone mineral density in postmenopausal women. J Clin Endocrinol Metab 2001;86(5):1890–1897.
89. Johnell O, Scheele WH, Lu Y, Reginster JY, Need AG, Seeman E. Additive effects of raloxifene and alendronate on bone density and biochemical markers of bone remodeling in postmenopausal women with osteoporosis [see comment]. J Clin Endocrinol Metab 2002;87(3):985–992.
90. Wimalawansa SJ. A four-year randomized controlled trial of hormone replacement and bisphosphonate, alone or in combination, in women with postmenopausal osteoporosis. Am J Med 1998;104(3):219–226.
91. Black DM, Greenspan SL, Ensrud KE, Palermo L, McGowan JA, Lang TF, et al. The effects of parathyroid hormone and alendronate alone or in combination in postmenopausal osteoporosis. N Engl J Med 2003;349(13):1207–1215.
92. Cosman F, Nieves J, Zion M, Woelfert L, Luckey M, Lindsay R. Daily and cyclic parathyroid hormone in women receiving alendronate. N Engl J Med 2005;353(6):566–575.
93. Canalis E, Giustina A, Bilezikian JP. Mechanisms of anabolic therapies for osteoporosis. N Engl J Med 2007;357(9):905–916.
94. Tyrrell CJ, Collinson M, Madsen EL, Ford JM, Coleman T. Intravenous pamidronate: infusion rate and safety. Ann Oncol 1994;5(Suppl 7):S27–S29.
95. Rosen CJ, Brown S. Severe hypocalcemia after intravenous bisphosphonate therapy in occult vitamin D deficiency. N Engl J Med 2003;348(15):1503–1504.

96. Champallou C, Basuyau JP, Veyret C, Chinet P, Debled M, Chevrier A, et al. Hypocalcemia following pamidronate administration for bone metastases of solid tumor: three clinical case reports. J Pain Symptom Manage 2003;25(2):185–190.
97. Reid IR, Brown JP, Burckhardt P, Horowitz Z, Richardson P, Trechsel U, et al. Intravenous zoledronic acid in postmenopausal women with low bone mineral density. N Engl J Med 2002;346(9):653–661.
98. Rey J, Daumen-Legre V, Pham T, Bernard P, Dahan L, Acquaviva PC, et al. Uveitis, an under-recognized adverse effect of pamidronate. Case report and literature review. Joint Bone Spine 2000;67(4):337–340.
99. Stewart GO, Stuckey BG, Ward LC, Prince RL, Gutteridge DH, Constable IJ. Iritis following intravenous pamidronate. Aust N Z J Med 1996;26(3):414–415.
100. Fraunfelder FW, Fraunfelder FT, Jensvold B. Scleritis and other ocular side effects associated with pamidronate disodium. Am J Ophthalmol 2003;135(2):219–222.
101. Cummings SR, Schwartz AV, Black DM. Alendronate and atrial fibrillation. N Engl J Med 2007;356(18):1895–1896.
102. Eisman JA, Rizzoli R, Roman-Ivorra J, Lipschitz S, Verbruggen N, Gaines KA, et al. Upper gastrointestinal and overall tolerability of alendronate once weekly in patients with osteoporosis: results of a randomized, double-blind, placebo-controlled study. Curr Med Res Opin 1920;5:699–705.
103. Lanza F, Schwartz H, Sahba B, Malaty HM, Musliner T, Reyes R, et al. An endoscopic comparison of the effects of alendronate and risedronate on upper gastrointestinal mucosae. Am J Gastroenterol 2000;95(11):3112–3117.
104. Lanza FL. Gastrointestinal adverse effects of bisphosphonates: Etiology, incidence and prevention. Treat Endocrinol 2002;1(1):37–43.
105. Taggart H, Bolognese MA, Lindsay R, Ettinger MP, Mulder H, Josse RG, et al. Upper gastrointestinal tract safety of risedronate: A pooled analysis of 9 clinical trials. Mayo Clin Proc 2002;77(3): 262–270.
106. Cryer B, Bauer DC. Oral bisphosphonates and upper gastrointestinal tract problems: What is the evidence? Mayo Clin Proc 2002;77(10):1031–1043.
107. Bauer DC, Black D, Ensrud K, Thompson D, Hochberg M, Nevitt M, et al. Upper gastrointestinal tract safety profile of alendronate: the fracture intervention trial. Arch Intern Med 2000;160(4):517–525.
108. Li J, Mashiba T, Burr DB. Bisphosphonate treatment suppresses not only stochastic remodeling but also the targeted repair of microdamage. Calcif Tissue Int 2001;69(5):281–286.
109. Mashiba T, Hui S, Turner CH, Mori S, Johnston CC, Burr DB. Bone remodeling at the iliac crest can predict the changes in remodeling dynamics, microdamage accumulation, and mechanical properties in the lumbar vertebrae of dogs. Calcif Tissue Int 2005;77(3):180–185.
110. Ott SM. Long-term safety of bisphosphonates. J Clin Endocrinol Metab 2005;90(3):1897–1899.
111. Odvina CV, Zerwekh JE, Rao DS, Maalouf N, Gottschalk FA, Pak CY. Severely suppressed bone turnover: a potential complication of alendronate therapy. J Clin Endocrinol Metab 2005;90(3): 1294–1301.
112. Recker R, Ensrud K, Diem S, Cheng E, Bare S, Masarachia P, et al. Normal bone histomorphometry and 3D microarchitecture after 10 years alendronate treatment of postmenopausal women. J Bone Miner Res 2004;19:S1–S45. Ref Type: Abstract
113. Chapurlat RD, Arlot M, Burt-Pichat B, Chavassieux P, Roux JP, Portero-Muzy N, et al. Microcrack frequency and bone remodeling in postmenopausal osteoporotic women on long-term bisphosphonates: a bone biopsy study. J Bone Miner Res 2007;22(10):1502–1509.
114. Ruggiero SL, Mehrotra B, Rosenberg TJ, Engroff SL. Ten years of alendronate treatment for osteoporosis in postmenopausal women. N Engl J Med 2004;351(2):190–192; author reply.
115. Marx RE, Sawatari Y, Fortin M, Broumand V. Bisphosphonate-induced exposed bone (osteonecrosis/osteopetrosis) of the jaws: risk factors, recognition, prevention, and treatment. J Oral Maxillofac Surg 2005;63(11):1567–1575.
116. Woo SB, Hellstein JW, Kalmar JR. Narrative [corrected] review: bisphosphonates and osteonecrosis of the jaws. Ann Intern Med 2006;144(10):753–761.
117. Carter G, Goss AN, Doecke C. Bisphosphonates and avascular necrosis of the jaw: a possible association. Med J Aust 2005;182(8):413–415.
118. Khosla S, Burr D, Cauley J, Dempster DW, Ebeling PR, Felsenberg D, et al. Bisphosphonate-associated osteonecrosis of the jaw: report of a Task Force of the American Society for Bone and Mineral Research. J Bone Miner Res 2007;22(10):1479–1491.

119. Bilezikian JP. Osteonecrosis of the jaw – do bisphosphonates pose a risk? N Engl J Med 2006;355(22): 2278–2281.
120. Reid IR, Bolland MJ, Grey AB. Is bisphosphonate-associated osteonecrosis of the jaw caused by soft tissue toxicity? Bone 2007;41(3):318–320.
121. Lenz JH, Steiner-Krammer B, Schmidt W, Fietkau R, Mueller PC, Gundlach KK. Does avascular necrosis of the jaws in cancer patients only occur following treatment with bisphosphonates? J Craniomaxillofac Surg 2005;33(6):395–403.
122. Sambrook P, Olver I, Goss A. Bisphosphonates and osteonecrosis of the jaw. Aust Fam Physician 2006;35(10):801–803.
123. Shane E, Goldring S, Christakos S, Drezner M, Eisman J, Silverman S, et al. Osteonecrosis of the jaw: more research needed. J Bone Miner Res 2006;21(10):1503–1505.

21 Basic Aspects of PTH in Skeletal Health

J. M. Hock, BDS PHD

CONTENTS

SUMMARY

We review in vivo studies of parathyroid hormone (PTH) anabolic actions at the cellular and molecular level, include updated information obtained from genetically modified mice, and new information on human skeletal responses to PTH that now better guides the use of animal models. Molecular mechanisms that underlie the anabolic effects of PTH are still not fully understood. Trabecular bone increases as bone formation processes dominate. This response has been intensively studied in mice and rats. Lifetime treatment of rats at higher doses increased the frequency of osteosarcoma, but the relevance of this finding to humans remains unknown. Cortical bone mass may increase or remain unchanged, as both bone resorption and bone formation are stimulated in remodeling of osteonal bone. The net effect is to increase bone strength. This response has been best demonstrated in rabbits and monkey models. In PTH-responsive osteoporotic humans, the complex of responses translate into reduction in fracture rate.

Key Words: Teriparatide, anabolic, bone remodeling, bone strength, animal models

INTRODUCTION

Small clinical trials using once daily administration of the synthetic fragment human parathyroid hormone (hPTH) 1–34 in the early 1970s suggested PTH could be used as an anabolic therapy for osteoporosis *(1,2)*. Since these initial clinical trials, numerous studies in animal models and humans have demonstrated that PTH anabolic effect is dependent on its intermittent administration. Continuous infusion of PTH results in decreased bone mass due to a change in bone balance to favor bone resorption *(1–6)*. PTH uniformly stimulates

From: *Contemporary Endocrinology: Osteoporosis: Pathophysiology and Clinical Management*
Edited by: R. A. Adler, DOI 10.1007/978-1-59745-459-9_21,

bone turnover. Whether this results in bone mass gain, loss, or equilibrium is determined by pharmacologic regimen or the presence of disease. For example, prolonged exposure to PTH as a consequence of hyperparathyroidism shifts bone distribution from cortical bone to trabecular bone, resulting in thinned cortical bone *(1–9)*. Work with transgenic mice expressing a constitutively activated PTH1 G-protein-coupled receptor (PTH1R) implicated both upregulation and distribution of PTHR1 as a key step in determining outcomes at specific bone sites *(10)*. In mice, PTH appears to regulate bone marrow organogenesis *(11)*, specifically the hematopoietic stem cell niche, a previously unrecognized function of this hormone; see review *(12)*. Despite a wealth of in vitro research on the cell and molecular actions of PTH, we still do not understand the mechanisms that result in these multiple effects in vivo.

The aims of this chapter are to review in vivo studies of PTH anabolic actions at the molecular and cellular level and to include updated information obtained by the increasing use of mouse strains and genetically modified mice, as well as new information on the skeletal response to PTH in humans that has better guided the use of animal models.

CELL AND MOLECULAR ACTIONS

PTH Regulation of Osteoblasts

Although in vitro work assumes osteoblasts are the primary target of PTH, in vivo data suggest pluripotential proliferating stromal and hematopoietic cells that give rise to osteoblasts and osteoclasts, respectively, are more likely candidates targeted by PTH to control the size of the cell pool and their lineage commitment in the skeleton *(13–19)*. The size of the cell pools which will determine differentiated cell numbers appears to be PTH dose dependent. PTH-induced changes in the timing and sequence of activation of terminally differentiated osteoblasts and osteoclasts will regulate bone turnover and the accumulation or loss of bone.

If the targets are pluripotential proliferating cells, then outcomes may either regulate continued cell cycle or exit from the cell cycle, or entry into specific cell lineages in bone marrow. Studies in young and old rats provide no evidence to support intermittent PTH as a stimulator of osteoblast proliferation *(20–23)*. When 5-bromo-2-deoxyuridine (BrdUrd) was given to label cells in S-phase in 2-h intervals ranging from 2 h prior to PTH to 6 h after PTH injection, an increased percent of labeled osteoblasts was observed 3 days later *(14)*. The 2-h labeling period is too short to label entry into S-phase, so it likely labels cells already in S-phase *(24,25)*, supporting the hypothesis that PTH recruits proliferating cells into the osteoblast lineage, rather than stimulating entry into the cell cycle. In young rats, there are large pools of pluripotential proliferating cells underlying the growth plates, the metaphyseal cortical endosteal surface and the diaphyseal periosteal surfaces *(26,27)*, which may be regulated by PTH *(14–16,28)*. The large numbers of pluripotential proliferating cells in young rats and mice suggest PTH recruits these cells into the osteoblast differentiation pathway to increase the number of osteoblasts *(14–16)*. Because continuous exposure to PTH will increase proliferation of these same pluripotential cells into a putative fibroblast lineage *(21,29,30)*, one critical PTH mechanism controls the transition between cell cycle exit and entry into osteoblast lineage.

The mechanism determining the balance between continued cycling of bone marrow mesenchymal stromal/stem progenitors (MSC) versus exit and entry into the osteoblast lineage appears to depend on duration of exposure to PTH. Continuous PTH infusion into rats combined with ^{3}H-thymidine labeling of cycling cells in S-phase showed an increase in percent ^{3}H-thymidine-labeled fibroblasts and marrow fibrosis adjacent to unlabeled bone surface cells *(21,29,30)*. A similar observation was made in genetically modified mice with constitutive activation of PTHR1 *(10,31)*. The increase in S-phase cycling marrow fibroblasts was abrogated by Trapidil, an inhibitor of platelet-derived growth factor-A, PDGF-A *(30)*, a growth factor secreted by osteoblasts *(32)*. When PTH infusion was discontinued, ^{3}H-thymidine-labeled fibroblasts entered the osteoblast lineage to increase bone-forming surfaces *(30)*.The sequence of upregulation of PTHR1 followed by rapid downregulation of the receptor, such as is seen with intermittent PTH treatment *(20)*, may signal entry of cycling stromal cells into the osteoblast lineage.

In older animals with closed growth plates and few proliferating progenitors *(33)*, PTH and its analogs may increase osteoblast number by activating quiescent bone surface osteocytes *(21)*. This hypothesis is supported by a number of studies, including electron microscopy *(34)*; thymidine autoradiography *(21,35,36)*; and histomorphometry in both humans and animals. The early increase in bone-forming surfaces (Fig. 1), after initiating once daily PTH injections in humans to increase bone mass, is more consistent with recruitment of pluripotential stromal cells into the osteoblast lineage, than stimulation of cell cycle entry *(1,37,38)*.

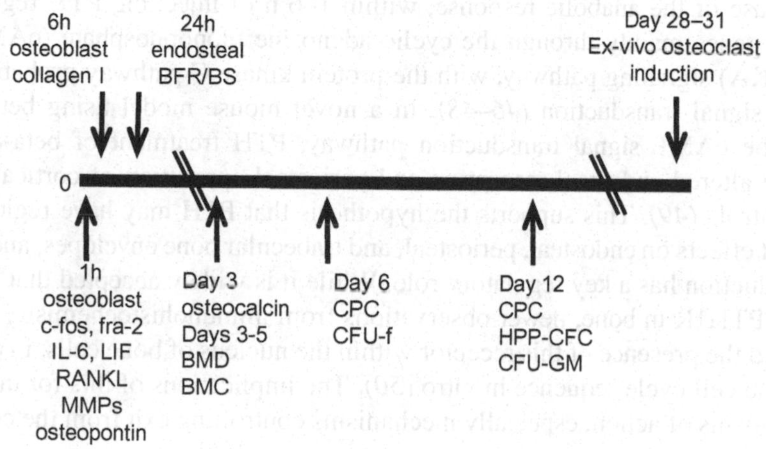

Fig. 1. Selected time-dependent changes in bone and hematopoietic cells after once daily PTH treatment in young rats for up to 31 days. BFR/BS bone formation rate on endosteal trabecular surfaces; MMPs metalloproteases; BMD bone mineral density; BMC bone mineral content; CPC hematopoietic committed progenitor cells; CFU-f alkaline phosphatase-positive fibroblastic colony forming units derived from stromal cells, and used as surrogate marker for osteoprogenitor cells; HPP-CFC (hematopoietic) highly proliferating potential-colony-forming cells; CFU-GM (hematopoietic) myeloid precursor colony-forming units, which are considered to contain the precursors of osteoclasts. Note the immediate activation of osteoblast function, and gene expression for cytokines associated with signal transduction to osteoclasts. Induction of both osteoblast and osteoclast precursors appears to be a late event in the young growing rat model. Cartoon based on data in following work *(14,20,78,89,92,100,174)*.

An alternate hypothesis to explain how PTH increases osteoblast number is inhibition of osteoblast apoptosis, based on PTH-inhibition of etoposide-induced apoptosis and reduced percent of trabecular cells positive for terminal deoxynucleotidyl transferase biotin-dUTP nick end labeling (TUNEL) by bone histomorphometry of mice treated with once daily PTH *(39–41)*. The inhibitory effect on osteoblast apoptosis occurring in metaphyseal secondary spongiosa may be a direct effect of PTH or an indirect effect associated with PTH-induced changes in bone turnover. Time–response studies show an initial stimulation of apoptosis followed by inhibition of apoptosis after once daily PTH in rats and mice *(42,43)* and link this biphasic response to the stage of differentiation of the osteoprogenitors at the time of PTH administration *(42,43)*. Because rat and mouse osteoblasts have a half-life of 7–14 days, entry into terminal osteoblast differentiation inevitably predicts apoptotic processes of the 80% of osteoblasts that do not adopt an osteocyte phenotype. Upregulation of caspase 3 expression, a key irreversible step in apoptosis, has been linked to cell cycle arrest and terminal osteoblast differentiation *(44,45)*. A finding of decreased osteoblast apoptosis may be due to a change in relative ratio of an increase in newly PTH-recruited osteoprogenitors to decreased or unchanged numbers of terminal osteoblasts. Apart from an early study on the cortical surface of very young, growing rabbits *(25)*, there have been no studies of PTH-regulated osteoprogenitor proliferation and apoptosis in animal models with osteonal bone, in which the response to PTH is independent of the growth and development skeletal processes always present in rats and mice.

Time-dependent changes activated following PTH treatment (Fig. 1), and the implications for the mechanisms operating during induction of the response, compared to those operating later after several remodeling cycles have not been widely appreciated. During the early phase of the anabolic response, within 1–6 h of injection, PTH regulates many osteoblastic genes mainly through the cyclic adenosine monophosphate (cAMP)–protein kinase A (PKA) signaling pathway, with the protein kinase C pathway probably also contributing to signal transduction *(46–48)*. In a novel mouse model using beta-arrestin, a protein in the cAMP signal transduction pathway, PTH treatment of beta-arrestin null female mice altered endosteal resorption and periosteal apposition of cortical bone compared to controls *(49)*. This supports the hypothesis that PTH may have regional-specific and different effects on endosteal, periosteal, and trabecular bone envelopes, and that cAMP signal transduction has a key regulatory role. While it is widely accepted that PTH signals through the PTH1R in bone, newer observations from immunohistochemistry of rat bones have reported the presence of this receptor within the nucleus of bone cells, in close association with the cell cycle sequence in vitro *(50)*. The implications of this for understanding PTH mechanisms of action, especially mechanisms controlling exit from the cell cycle, are unknown.

Downstream of exit from the cell cycle, PTH regulates multiple genes associated with osteoblast differentiation and function. PTH-stimulated proteins include transcription factors, matrix proteins required for new bone formation, proteins associated with matrix degradation and turnover, and osteoclast differentiation proteins. Studies in young mice *(42)* and rats *(51)* indicate that PTH upregulates cell differentiation in trabecular bone in a dose-dependent manner by transient and selective stimulation of the AP-1 complex of transcription factors c-*fos*, c-*jun*, and c-*myc*. Of these early response genes, c-*fos* shows the greatest magnitude of change in response to PTH *(42)* (Fig. 2) and is linked to downstream upregulation of both Runx2 and osterix expression. In vitro, exposure to PTH *(1–34)* and

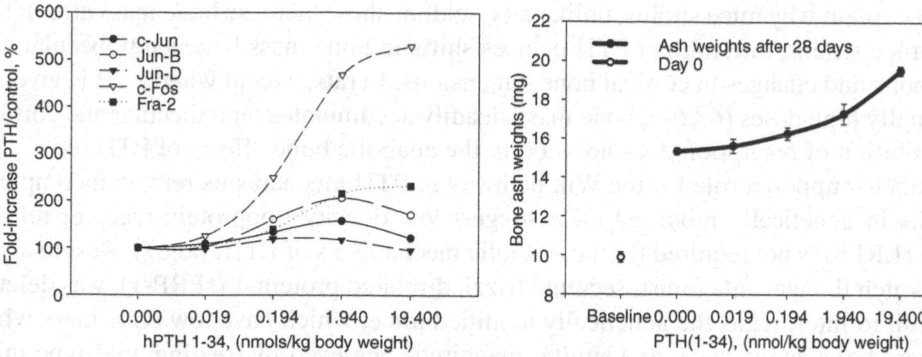

Fig. 2. Left graph: Dose-dependent effects of rhPTH 1–34 on expression of AP-I gene family members in femur metaphysis of young male Balb/C mice treated with once daily injections for 3 days. Expression of c-fos, assessed using RNAse protection assays, was markedly higher than the other genes; fra-2 expression peaks about 30 mins after c-fos has peaked (data not shown). No difference in magnitude was detected when genes were examined after 7days, compared to 1 or 3 days *(42)*. Right graph: dose-dependent effects of rhPTH 1–34 on bone mass, expressed as ash weight of femurs of young male Balb/C mice treated once daily with rhPTH 1–34 for 28 days. Day 0 value shows ash weight in baseline group, to account for growth of young rapidly growing mice. Data adapted from those reported in Ref. *(175)*.

PTH-related peptide (PTHrP) *(1–34)* rapidly induces c-fos gene expression in bone cell lines *(52,53)*. The magnitude of c-fos increase has been interpreted as osteoblastic in origin, and predictive of the magnitude of the anabolic response. New data suggest multiple pathways activated by PTH contribute to the magnitude of c-fos expression.

Mouse strains vary in their responsiveness to anabolic actions of PTH. Although some strains exhibit localized changes in bone mass in response to PTH *(42)*, none exhibit an overall increment in skeletal bone mass *(54)*, suggesting that there is a redistribution of bone within the skeleton necessitating activation of both formation and resorption *(55)*. Studies of c-fos deficient mice suggested that c-fos was essential for PTH anabolic effect on bone mass; bone mass decreased in PTH-treated c-fos–/– mice, compared to vehicle-treated controls or treatment of c-fos intact mice *(56)*. While absence of c-fos abrogated the PTH effect, a reduced magnitude in PTH-induced c-fos gene expression did not. In neurofibromin 1 haplo-insufficient (*Nf1* +/–) mice, which exhibit deregulation of ras signal transduction *(57)*, PTH decreased c-fos expression by 50% but increased bone mass equivalently to that of PTH-treated wild-type mice *(58)*. It is possible that osteoclasts and other cells, in addition to osteoprogenitors, contribute to PTH-stimulated changes in c-fos. Osteoclasts obtained from Nf1+/– mice and NF1 humans exhibit hyper-responsiveness to RANKL and enhanced stimulation of M-CSF-induced p21ras-GTP and phosphorylation of PI3 kinase *(57)*. When host c-fos +/+ mice with allogeneic grafts of vertebral bodies ("vossicles") resected from c-fos null or +/+ mice were treated with PTH, c-fos–/– vossicles exhibited an anabolic response. While osteoprogenitors are thought to be derived only from the vossicle, osteoclast progenitors circulate and are more likely host derived, suggesting a role for osteoclasts in mouse PTH responsiveness. When osteoclast induction in the vossicle model was blocked by osteoprotegerin (OPG), the anabolic response was blunted *(59)*. Osteoclast activation in mouse PTH mechanisms suggests induction of bone turnover, similar to that exhibited by animals with osteonal bone and humans *(37,60–62)*.

This may explain why mice strains, unlike rats, seldom show increase bone mass after PTH. In most mice strains, intermittent PTH induces shifts in bone mass between trabecular and cortical bone and changes in cortical bone dimensions. In rats, except when PTH is given at exceptionally high doses *(63,64)*, bone mass steadily accumulates on trabecular and cortical bone; inhibition of resorption does not modify the anabolic bone effects of PTH *(65)*.

The data to support a role for the Wnt pathway in PTH mechanisms remain incomplete, but results in genetically modified mice suggest low density lipoprotein receptor-related protein 5 (LRP5) is not required for the anabolic mechanisms of PTH *(66,67)*. Results from mice in which the wnt antagonist, secreted frizzled-related protein-1 (sFRP-1), was deleted are difficult to interpret as the genetically modified mice, which have low bone mass when young, gain bone as they age, to a similar magnitude achieved by treating wild-type mice with PTH. As sFRP-1 age and gain bone, the anabolic effect of PTH becomes attenuated. The reason for this is not known, but may reflect changes in microarchitecture, availability of stem and progenitor cell pools, availability of bone surfaces for osteoblastic stimulation and osteoclast regulation in the genetically modified mice.

Interestingly, effects on mRNA expression of osteocalcin, growth factors, such as IGF-I, TGFβ, FGF-2, and their receptors, are not detectable until a few days after initiation of treatment *(14,68,69)*. Deletion of IGF-I, IRS-1 (insulin receptor substrate-1) which is activated after IGF-I binds to its receptor or FGF2 in genetically modified mice greatly reduced the anabolic effect of PTH *(70–73)*. Expression of mRNA for the Nr4A family, representing genes for nerve-growth inducible factors occurs within 0.5–1 h *(74)*. Expression of the bone matrix proteins, osteopontin and osteonectin, is upregulated within an hour of PTH injection in vivo, while sclerostin expression is downregulated at 4 h *(75)*. Which gene profiles are required for the later stimulatory effects of PTH on collagen I gene expression require at 6 h are still not known. Translation of the collagen gene upregulation into increased bone-forming surface requires about 24 h, based on histomorphometry and in situ histohybridization *(14,76)*.

Data from proteomics technologies demonstrate additional mechanisms either integral to the anabolic effects of PTH or in addition to those effects. When mice were given PTH or vehicle once daily for 3 or 11 days, the most abundant and stable PTH-upregulated serum protein peaks were identified as hemoglobin-alpha and hemoglobin-beta *(77)*. These proteins, which are associated with calcium homeostasis and calcium influx into erythroid cells, were previously identified at high levels in hyperparathyroidism. Proteomics data suggest the hypothesis that protein profiles observed in hyperparathyroidism may be *qualitatively* equivalent to the characteristic profile of regulated proteins at therapeutic doses of PTH.

Much less is known of the PTH-regulated genes associated with continuous infusion or with animal models of hyperparathyroidism. Experimentally, it is interesting that ADAMTS-1 mRNA expression increased by 35-fold within 1 h of a single injection, but by only sevenfold in cells continuously exposed to PTH *(78)*. The different regimens of PTH may govern not only the duration of exposure, but also the intensity of the gene expression response profile.

In vitro, PTH acts on differentiated osteoblasts to inhibit expression and synthesis of matrix proteins, including collagen 1, osteocalcin, and alkaline phosphatase *(79–81)*. Following continuous infusion of PTH in adult rats, peritrabecular fibrosis and focal resorption were observed, together with hypercalcemia and increased calcitonin *(5,6,29)*.

Over-activation due to a missense mutation in the alpha-subunit of Gs, a protein in a key pathway activated by the PTH1 receptor, was associated with malfunction of mature osteoblasts, manifest as abnormal matrix composition and collagen organization *(31,82)*. The histopathology of fibrosis of hyperparathyroidism and fibrous dysplasia appear to have common features *(31)*. The fibrosis subsequent to PTH regulation of collagen synthesis may be mediated by a changing ratio between IGF-I and IGF-binding proteins, such that IGF-I is suppressed and the IGF-binding proteins dominate in osteoblasts. IGF-I observed in osteoblasts of rats treated with once daily PTH was not detected in bone lining cells during PTH infusion *(83,84)*. Continuous infusion increased the intensity of staining for IGF-binding proteins, IGF-BP3, BP4, and BP5 *(85)*. These shifts in distribution and magnitude of IGF-1 and IGF-binding proteins associated with different PTH regimens suggest that these may play a role in cell fate determination of the multi-potential progenitors in close proximity to active osteoblasts.

Prolonged exposure to PTH in cultured bone cells alters several nuclear matrix (NM) proteins that mediate nuclear architecture, including NuMA and topoisomerase IIα and IIβ, which are structural components of the mitotic chromosome scaffold *(86,87)*. The PTH-induced upregulation of NMP4/NP, an architectural transcription factor which binds directly to the collagen and collagenase promoters, may be a critical mechanism regulating expression of type I collagen *(88)*. These PTH-induced changes in osteoblast microarchitecture via regulation of the NM may modify the profile of transcribed genes that determine a catabolic response *(86)*. Importantly, HMG1 box protein and its receptor, RAGE, which have a role in innate immunity, are upregulated 16 h after exposure to PTH in UMR107 osteoblastic osteosarcoma cells, but downregulated in primary osteoblasts and MC3T3.E1 osteoblast cell line. These data support the existence of a novel mechanism to link skeletal and immune cells, in addition to the time-dependent effects of the RANKL/OPG/RANK pathways regulated by PTH *(89)*. Because innate immunity plays a role in cancer biology, further investigation of the differentially PTH-regulated links between normal or cancerous skeletal and immune cells may illuminate a mechanism to explain promotion of osteosarcoma in rats after long-term PTH therapy.

A consistent finding has been the upregulated expression of both matrix degrading proteins, such as matrix metalloproteinases (MMPs), their inhibitor, TIMP, and ADAMTS-1 (*a* *d*isintegrin *a*nd *m*etalloprotease with *t*hrombo*s*pondin motifs) in addition to cytokines associated with regulating matrix degradation and turnover, such as interleukin-6 (IL-6) and IL-11 *(20,86,90–92)*. Over-expression of TIMP in transgenic mice enhanced the osteoblastic response to PTH, and greatly increased bone mass while blocking the osteoclastic effects *(93)*. This suggests matrix metalloproteinases are important in regulating the magnitude of bone response to PTH. Actions of matrix degrading enzymes to recondition the bone surface may lead to cell detachment resulting in osteoblast apoptosis. Cell detachment in vivo is suggested by the finding of a transient increase in apoptosis in proliferating cells and osteocytes of young rat metaphysis during the initial response to PTH *(42)*. Together, these observations of upregulated MMPs and transient increases in apoptosis are consistent with mechanisms activating bone turnover. Another consequence of activation of matrix degrading enzymes may be that reconditioned bone surface can serve as an attractant for newly differentiating osteoblasts to increase bone-forming surfaces (anabolic action) or as an attractant for differentiating osteoclasts to continue resorption of old surfaces (catabolic action) *(94)*.

Regulation of Osteoclasts

As discussed earlier in this chapter, mouse models and human data on biomarker changes over time clearly show a role for osteoclasts in the PTH stimulation of bone turnover relevant to cortical bone and shifts in bone between its cortical and trabecular compartments. Current dogma holds that stromal cells and osteoblast lineage cells regulate osteoclast differentiation through cell–cell contact by controlling synthesis of OPG and RANKL, the ligand for the osteoclast progenitor receptor, RANK *(95,96)*. These two secreted proteins compete for binding to RANK, a TNF receptor family member *(96)*. If RANKL binding to RANK predominates, as seen following PTH treatment of cultured osteoblast-like osteosarcoma cells transfected with the PTH1 receptor *(97)*, osteoclast progenitors differentiate into osteoclasts *(96)*. In a variety of bone cells lines, PTH downregulates OPG, a potent inhibitor of osteoclast formation and function, via a cAMP/PKA pathway *(95)*. In young rats, mRNA expression for RANKL increases while that for OPG decreases within 1 h of injection *(89)*. The significance of this time dependence is not known, but is likely part of the mechanisms by which PTH activates bone turnover. In vitro data *(95,96)* suggest that increased resorption plays a key role in the mechanisms activated by PTH. Additional evidence that osteoclasts are integral to PTH mechanisms was obtained from microarrays showing genes typically associated with osteoclast induction are upregulated in a time-dependent manner by PTH treatment in mice and rats. In young rats, upregulated genes within 1 h of PTH injection, include immediate early genes, IL-6 and LIF and RANKL, RGS2, ADAMS-T, and matrix metalloproteinases, such as collagenase 9 (gelatinase B), while expression of the PTH receptor, histone H4, and OPG are decreased *(20,51,86,89–91,98)*.

One limitation of these studies is our lack of knowledge of how changes in activation frequency may favor formation (anabolic effect of intermittent PTH) or resorption (catabolic effect of continuous PTH). A mathematical model that assumes a longer delay in osteoclast activation (due to a requirement for signals from the osteoblast to osteoclast progenitors) than the delay required for osteoblast differentiation argues that osteoblast function will predominate with intermittent PTH, while resorption will be greater with continuous PTH *(99)*. This speculation is supported by preliminary unpublished data that show that the ex vivo induction of osteoclasts was delayed in mice given once daily injections of PTH until 28–31 days, whereas under conditions of continuous infusion, increased ex vivo induction of osteoclasts was detected within 14 days *(100)*.

Mediators of PTH Actions

Candidate agents, implicated as mediators in regulation of the osteoblast axis by PTH, include growth hormone (GH), growth factors, prostaglandins, and 1,25-dihydroxyvitamin D. GH has been evaluated either as a direct regulator of bone cell biology or as a stimulator of insulin-like growth factor-I (IGF-I), which stimulates osteoblast proliferation and differentiation in vitro *(13)*. Studies in young and old rats suggest that GH or GH-dependent IGF-I is required for the anabolic effect of PTH during the "adolescence" phase of skeletal growth but is not necessary after skeletal maturation in this species *(101,102)*. Although in vitro studies suggest that IGF-I is a mediator of PTH effects on skeletal growth and maturation processes via its stimulatory effects on osteoblasts *(32)*, and knockout of IGF-I abrogates the effect of PTH on bones of young mice, its role in animals which have completed growth or in humans remains uncertain *(103)*. Because

IGF-I inhibits collagenase *(104)*, IGF-I may mediate a different aspect of the anabolic mechanism, namely regulating the process by which osteoblasts condition the bone surface as a prerequisite to attract osteoclast progenitors to bone. Since skeletal cells secrete the six known IGF-binding proteins (IGFBPs) and two of the four known IGFBP-related proteins, there are likely additional levels of regulation if IGF-I mediates actions of PTH in vivo *(105,106)*.

The hypothesis that local IGF-I may mediate bone turnover is supported by work on genetically modified mice. PTH treatment of IGF-I–/– CD1 mice led to changes in trabecular and cortical bone compartments, such that only endocortical bone showed responsiveness. In vitro assays of colony formation by bone marrow stromal cells showed equivalence although PTH increased IGF-I and IGF-1R receptor expression *(107)*. This suggests that the mechanism is not direct regulation of osteoblast progenitors or osteoblast lineage recruitment. Mice with global knockout of IGF-I failed to respond to PTH *(70,108)*, although there were increases in bone PTHR1, IGF-1R, and osteoblast markers expression. In serum, IGF-1 circulates as a 150 kDa protein complex which includes IGF-1, IGF-BP3, and the acid-labile subunit protein (ALS). PTH treatment of mice with targeted knockout of either the liver IGF-I gene (LID) or the acid-labile subunit (ALSKO) decreased cross-sectional cortical area and increased trabecular bone volume, consistent with a shift in bone between the two compartments, typical of activation of bone turnover *(109)*. The double knockout, LID + ALSKO, did not respond to PTH suggesting circulating IGF-I may be needed. The anabolic effect of PTH declines as mice age, suggesting any systemic IGF-I effects may be GH mediated, and explaining why serum IGF-I increases have not been detected in serum of humans treated with PTH in clinical trials (C Rosen, personal communication, 2007).

In vitro studies and studies of genetically modified mice have demonstrated PTH-induced regulation of gene expression of other growth factors [e.g., fibroblast growth factor-2 (FGF-2) and transforming growth factor-β (TGF-β)] *(72,110)*. The effects of FGF2 in intact rats are dose-dependent and occur at higher doses than those needed to induce an increase in bone mass *(69)*. The anabolic effect of PTH was greatly reduced in FGF2-null mice *(71,72,111)*. Because PTH upregulates a gene expression profile associated with anabolism but this does not translate into increased BMD in IGF-1 or FGF2 null mice, these growth factors may regulate protein complexes, or modifications, needed to fully execute the anabolic bone response to PTH. In vitro, there is strong evidence to support an intermediary role for prostaglandins in the actions of PTH in bone *(81)*. In contrast, treatment of young rats with indomethacin failed to block the anabolic effect of PTH *(112)*, suggesting that prostaglandins are not mediators of the anabolic effects of PTH in vivo. It remains possible, however, that prostaglandins may mediate effects on remodeling and bone turnover in animals with osteonal skeletons.

The vitamin D metabolite, 1,25-dihydroxyvitamin D [$1,25(OH)_2D3$], and PTH operate in mutual feedback loops. Because PTH raises serum $1,25(OH)_2D3$ in vivo and interacts with $1,25(OH)_2D$ in several molecular pathways in cultured bone cells, $1,25(OH)_2D3$ may mediate or contribute to PTH mechanisms of action in vivo. However, experiments in young and aged rats failed to show that $1,25(OH)_2D3$ contributed to the anabolic effects of PTH *(113,114)*. In the PATH study of PTH treatment of osteoporotic humans supplemented with vitamin D at 400 IU, change in serum $1,25(OH)_2D$ was the best predictor of trabecular bone density by CT because it accounted for 25% of the variance in BMD (Sellmeyer et al. 2007.

Osteoporosis International. In press). This suggests that there may be PTH–1,25$(OH)_2$D interactions in humans that are not detectable in rat models.

PRECLINICAL STUDIES

Animal Models

Numerous studies in rats over the past two decades have demonstrated that PTH augments bone mass by stimulating bone formation and increases the resistance of bones to fracture at all sites tested [see reviews by *(2,115)*]. In mature ovariectomized (OVX) rats, treatment with PTH or one of its analogs increased bone mineral density (BMD) by more than two- to fourfold in the spine and long bones after 6 months *(116,117)*. The use of rat models for studies of PTH anabolism is limited by the weak contribution of PTH regulation of osteoclasts, which are better studied in mice, animals with osteonal bone, or humans. In humans, 45–55% of the skeleton is osteonal Haversian cortical bone. In osteonal skeletons, PTH-induced bone mass gain, based on dual X-ray absorptiometry (DXA) measures, was in the range of 8–15% in OVX monkeys after 18 months *(118)* (Fig. 3) and in osteoporotic women after 2–3 years *(1,119–121)*.

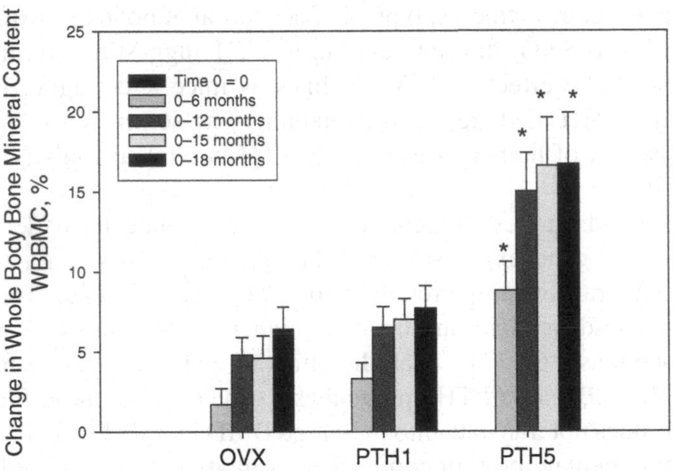

Fig. 3. Change in whole body mineral content of adult, ovariectomized monkeys treated once daily with vehicle (OVX) or rhPTH 1–34 at 1 (PTH1) or 5 (PTH5) µg/kg/day for up to 18 months. Data are shown as the percent change from baseline for each time point measured and were re-graphed from data in *(118,136)*. Values for PTH5 are significantly different ($*p < 0.05$) from those of OVX or PTH1, which were not significantly different from each other at any time point. Note the time course and rapid increase in whole body bone mineral content in PTH5 monkeys.

Anabolic Versus Catabolic Effects of PTH

Dosing regimens, duration of treatment, and the dose magnitude of in vivo studies determine if the outcome is anabolic, in which there is a gain in bone mass due to pronounced stimulation of bone formation, or catabolic, in which stimulation of resorption, combined with a reduction in bone surfaces available for stimulation of formation, results in a net loss of bone mass over time *(1,2,122)*. Catabolic actions of PTH in bone may be induced by continuous infusion, irrespective of animal model *(1,3,4,29,123–128)*. Between these two extremes, PTH may stimulate activation frequency to accelerate bone turnover, but because there is coordinated upregulation of both formation and resorption, bone mass itself remains unchanged. Even though bone mass is unchanged, bone is redistributed and matrix renewed, as bone architecture may show dramatic changes under conditions of increased turnover.

The anabolic effect of PTH has been demonstrated in a wide variety of animals *(4,61,118,129,130)* as well as humans *(1,121)* when administered intermittently. In contrast to rats, in which extensive anabolic PTH dose responses may be conducted without stimulating prolonged hypercalcemia, humans and animals with osteonal skeletons exhibit a narrow dose response within the normocalcemic range *(1,2,121,125–128)*. Interestingly, mechanisms underlying the length of time between PTH injections that would still increase bone mass and enhance biomechanical properties have not been studied extensively. In young rats, the anabolic effect on bone-forming surfaces was lost by about 48 h *(131)*. This must only be one aspect of the anabolism as studies in rats and osteoporotic humans given PTH once weekly showed increased bone mass, and a transient initial activation of bone markers *(64,132)*. This beneficial effect may be due to the increasing replacement of old bone matrix with more resilient new matrix due to PTH stimulation of bone remodeling, especially in cortical bone *(133,134)*.

Comparative Effects of PTH on Modeling and Remodeling

In rats and mice, PTH stimulates bone formation at sites of new metaphyseal bone to modify trabecular three-dimensional geometry. These effects reflect normal growth processes as well as stimulation of bone modeling in which bone formation occurs on quiescent surfaces without prior resorption *(122)*. When PTH is given to rats for prolonged periods of time, skeletal abnormalities due to changes in bone morphology occur *(135)*. Such nonphysiologic responses have not been reported in animals with osteonal bone or in humans to date. One hypothesis based on work in transgenic mice with constitutively active PTHR1 speculates that PTH depletes the bone marrow stromal stem cells, delays the natural transition from bone to marrow with age, and deregulates differentiation of stromal progenitors in marrow adipocytes *(11)*. If prolonged treatment with PTH depletes the marrow stromal stem cell compartment in mice and rats, so that only transit-amplifying progenitors are available to respond to PTH, bone formation will continue but will be deregulated because physiological processes required to maintain or increase bone marrow and bone marrow cell phenotypes, including adipocytes and osteoclasts, are disrupted by the loss of key stem cells as these rodent species age.

In humans and animals with osteonal bone structure, remodeling dominates over modeling, so that PTH stimulates significant restructuring of bone via intratrabecular tunneling and intracortical remodeling, in addition to stimulating apposition of new matrix on endosteal surfaces *(122)*. The overall effect is a positive bone balance in the skeleton *(118,129,130,136,137)*. These changes observed in osteonal models mimic the processes that have been associated with development and maturation of the skeleton in young humans. Bone turnover due to remodeling, which is an integrated sequence of bone formation and resorption, may blunt the increment of bone gain possible with modeling *(125–128)*. This may explain why the gains in bone mass in human and animals with osteonal skeletons are never as dramatic as the extraordinary increments reported in rats.

Comparative Effects of PTH on Trabecular and Cortical Bone

The anabolic effects of PTH to increase trabecular bone have been amply demonstrated in many animal models and in humans. It is only recently that our understanding of PTH effects on cortical bone has improved. The findings of decreased cortical bone mass in early clinical trials *(138–140)* and increased cortical porosity in canine models with Haversian remodeling *(123,141)* have raised concern that PTH treatment might lead to reduced cortical bone mass and strength. Rat studies have uniformly shown that PTH, PTHrP, and their analogs increase cortical thickness and area via endocortical appositional bone growth, to increase resistance of bones to fracture *(117,142–145)*. Recent studies in animals with Haversian remodeling have provided valuable data on the response to PTH at both cortical and trabecular sites, which have important clinical implications. Treatment of adult OVX monkeys with hPTH 1–34 at 5 μg/kg once daily for 12 or 18 months increased whole body bone mineral content (WBBMC) compared to controls within the first 6 months of treatment *(118)* (Fig. 3). Observed increases in spinal bone mass and femur neck bone volume were associated with significantly improved biomechanical properties at both sites *(129,146)* (Fig. 4). Histomorphometry confirmed that the gain in bone mass was due to increased bone surface apposition which occurred early in treatment *(60,130,136)*. PTH-treated monkeys exhibited significant remodeling of their trabeculae, such that trabecular number and connectivity increased as the bone formation rate increased *(61)*.

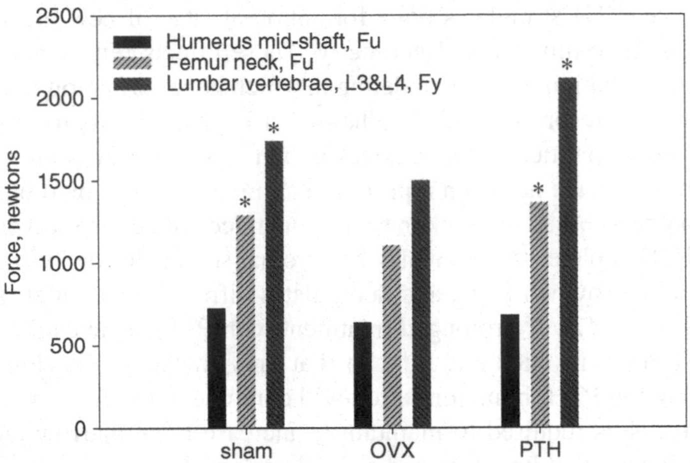

Fig. 4. Biomechanical properties of strength, shown as ultimate force (Fu) for midshaft humerus and femur neck, and as yield force for lumbar vertebrae, L3 and L4 resected from adult, sham-operated (sham), and ovariectomized monkeys, treated once daily with vehicle (OVX) or rhPTH 1–34 at 5 μg/kg/day (PTH) for up to 18 months. PTH values are significantly different ($*p < 0.05$) from either OVX or sham in the femur neck and spine. Data adapted from report *(146,166)*.

Studies of intact rabbits and the OVX monkey model show complex responses in cortical osteonal bone following PTH treatment *(129,130)*. There is significant stimulation of endocortical bone formation while periosteal formation remains equivalent or slightly higher than controls. Unique to osteonal bone, there is an increase in forming osteons and an increase in porosity of intracortical bone as a reflection of the increase in remodeling transients *(129,130)*. Analyses of the localization of the porosities showed that they occurred predominantly in the endocortical zone, which also exhibits increased appositional bone growth. As this zone is closest to the neutral axis, the cross-sectional moment of inertia, stiffness, and ultimate force characteristics of strength remained stable in the mid-cortex of the long bones *(129,130)*.

One clinical concern was that if the increase in porosity occurs prior to deposition of PTH-induced new bone formation, an osteoporotic patient with thinned cortical bone may be susceptible to fracture early in treatment. In rats, increases in bone matrix proteins and bone-forming surfaces have been demonstrated within 24 h of the first injection of hPTH 1–34 while resorption measures remained unchanged *(13)* (Fig. 1). More recently, the time sequence of events has been studied in cortical bone of intact rabbits treated with hPTH 1–34 for 1 remodeling cycle *(147)*. The percent fluorochrome-labeled (new) osteons and endocortical bone formation increased within the first cycle. The increase in porosity was not significant until the end of the first cycle, at 70 days, while the increase in cortical area due to appositional bone formation occurred prior to 35 days. Collectively, these data suggest that PTH "braces" the bone by immediately stimulating formation at both modeling and remodeling sites, so that an initial period of increased susceptibility to fracture would not be predicted.

Occurrence of Osteosarcoma in Rats Treated With PTH

An unexpected observation of longer term preclinical studies was the increased frequency of osteosarcoma in rats given PTH 1–34 for 2 years, starting at 6 weeks *(135,148,149)*. The increase in incidence of rat osteosarcoma was time and PTH dose dependent, because it could be abrogated by starting treatment when rats were older or by reducing PTH dose *(148)*. Osteosarcoma is a metastatic bone cancer occurs spontaneously in rats, dogs, and humans at frequencies of 1:1000; 1:10,000; and 1:250,000 *(150–153)*; and rapidly metastasizes to the lungs. In humans, osteosarcoma is a rare cancer most commonly occurring in adolescents and young adults (Fig. 5).

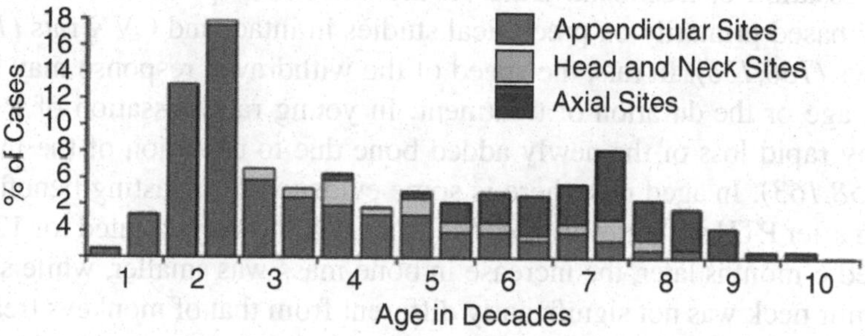

Fig. 5. US SEER data showing incidence of osteosarcoma throughout life span of humans. Note that approximately 65% of humans with osteosarcoma present before 30 years of age, and over 30% present in the second decade of life.

Osteosarcoma is associated with an early and dramatic breakdown in genomic integrity, due to multiple chromosomal recombinations, translocations, and gain and loss of DNA on individual chromosomes. Research to ascertain why PTH promoted the frequency of metastatic osteosarcoma in rats needs to consider loss of regulation of mechanisms that maintain genomic integrity in the bone organ, especially in inbred species. Because of the normal underlying risk of spontaneous osteosarcoma in rats, mice, dogs, and humans, it is most unlikely that PTH induces osteosarcomagenesis. There are multiple rat and human osteosarcoma osteoblast-like cell lines, such as ROS 17/2.8, UMR106, SaOS, U2OS, MG63, that exhibit PTHR1 and respond with increased proliferation to PTH *(154,155)*. Xenografts of these cell lines remain localized and do not result in metastatic osteosarcoma. Many of the osteoblast-like cell lines derived from rat, mouse, and human osteosarcoma, recapitulate multiple aspects of osteoblast differentiation when stimulated with PTH in vitro; such responses are not associated with cell dedifferentiation typical of osteosarcoma. Thus, there is no easy explanation for the increase in osteosarcoma frequency in rats treated with hPTH 1–34 for most of their life.

Pharmacokinetic studies of PTH given intravenously or via the hepatic vein show bioavailability of PTH is very different in different species *(156)*. This species differences in PTH bioavailability means that extrapolation of responses to dose and duration of treatment from animals to humans should be made cautiously. To date, a single case of osteosarcoma has been reported in older women with a complex medical history, who had been treated with hPTH 1–34 (teriparatide) for more than a year *(157)*. Because the human osteosarcoma incidence is 1:250,000, and more than 300,000 patients have been treated with hPTH1–34, a single case falls within the calculated probability of spontaneous osteosarcoma and cannot be attributed to PTH treatment at this time *(157)*. Thus, the relevance of the increased incidence of osteosarcoma observed in rats treated with PTH for most of their lifetime to the promotion of osteosarcoma in humans remains unknown.

Consequences of Stopping PTH Treatment

One important issue involving PTH therapy is the possible loss of previously gained BMD after cessation of treatment. Data on the skeletal response to withdrawal of PTH were initially based primarily on preclinical studies in intact and OVX rats *(158–162)* and OVX monkeys *(130,136)*. In rats, the speed of the withdrawal response may be dependent on either the age or the duration of treatment. In young rats, cessation of PTH treatment is followed by rapid loss of the newly added bone due to cessation of the increased bone formation *(158,163)*. In aged rats, there is some evidence for a lasting beneficial effect on bone strength after PTH withdrawal *(164,165)*. In OVX monkeys treated for 12 months, and then examined 6 months later, the increase in bone mass was smaller, while strength at the spine and femur neck was not significantly different from that of monkeys treated at equivalent doses for 18 months *(146,164–166)*. An unexpected finding was the favorable shift in mineral distribution and size in quantitative computed tomography (QCT) images that correlated with the retention of improved biomechanical properties of bone after withdrawal of treatment *(164–166)*.

Comparisons of the response to withdrawal in ovariectomized rats and monkeys suggest that the incremental gain due to bone modeling during PTH treatment decreases after two or more remodeling cycles *(146,159,162,165–168)*. In osteonal skeletons, there is a residual benefit associated with the remodeling processes because PTH alters bone geometry and "rejuvenates" the matrix by turnover and mineralization of new matrix *(133,134)*. Following withdrawal, active bone-forming surfaces revert to quiescent status *(61,130)*, so that it is likely that, as the bone turnover rate returns to its pretreatment levels, the next fraction of bone to be targeted for turnover will be the older fraction of bone *(125–128,169)*. In humans, withdrawal of PTH results in loss of BMD in the subsequent 12 months *(170)*.

CONCLUSIONS AND FUTURE DIRECTIONS

The extensive research using in vitro approaches and animal models, briefly reviewed here, has provided new insights into the effects of PTH at each organizational level of osteonal bone (Table 1). Clinical trials have demonstrated that PTH strengthens bones and increases bone mass at trabecular bone-rich sites with little or no effect on bone mass of cortical bone-rich sites *(1,121,171–173)*. A large Phase 3 clinical trial reported a 65–69% reduction in vertebral fractures and a 54% reduction in non-vertebral fractures *(121)*. Nonetheless, there are still unanswered questions that will drive future research. While our knowledge of genetic regulation and signal transduction in bone cells has expanded, there is still limited understanding of the gene patterns and signal transduction pathways that differentially induce and regulate modeling, growth processes, and remodeling in vivo to change bone shape or regulate the spatial distribution of bone within a bone organ. Additionally, the cellular and mineralization events associated with intermittent intervals of PTH delivery and PTH withdrawal have yet to be determined. Information is lacking on the differences in cell and molecular responses to intermittent PTH required to promote osteoblast differentiation and function and those associated with continuous infusion of PTH that activate osteoclast differentiation and function. Importantly, with the discovery of PTH as a regulator of hematopoietic stem cells, and PTH regulation of protein pathways linking skeletal cells and innate immunity, we need to think beyond the conventional interpretations that only consider PTH effects regulating skeletal physiology and calcium homeostasis. New

Table 1
The Effects of PTH at Each Organizational Level of Osteonal Bone

	Cells →	**Tissue** →	**Organ** →	**Skeleton**
	1000s up-and down regulated genes ↑↑ Osteoblasts differentiate to increase number Regulation of bone cell apoptosis Delay in ↑ osteoclast activation	↑ Bone formation rate ↑ Trabecular & endocortical bone ↑ New osteons ↑ Cortical & trabecular remodeling	↑ BMC, ↑ BMD ↑ Cross-sectional moment of inertia	↑ Whole body BMC ± calcium absorption
	↓ **Outcomes**	↓ **Outcomes**	↓ **Outcomes**	↓ **Outcomes**
	↑ Bone forming surfaces Quiescent surfaces decrease	Bone structuring and replacement improves geometry & connectivity ↑ Cortical width	↑ Resistance to fracture ↑ Bone quality	↑ Bone balance and strength

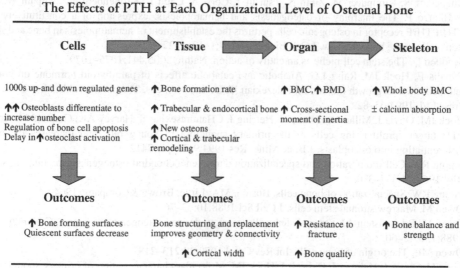

Black up arrows indicate upregulation in measures, with double arrows indicating a marked increase. Horizontal grey arrows show progression from cell level up to whole skeletal level. Down grey arrows indicate the outcomes or sequelae to the responses at each level.

animal models, microarray technology, proteomics, the advances in bioinformatics and in functional pathway mapping should help elucidate much of the mystery still surrounding this bone and calcium-regulating hormone.

REFERENCES

1. Cosman F, Lindsay R. Is parathyroid hormone a therapeutic option for osteoporosis? A review of the clinical evidence. Calcif Tissue Int 1998;62:475–480.
2. Dempster DW, Cosman F, Parisien M, Shen V, Lindsay R. Anabolic actions of parathyroid hormone on bone. Endocr Rev 1993;14:690–709.
3. Podbesek R, Eduoard C, Meunier PJ, Parsons JA, Reeve J, Stevenson RW, Zanelli JM. Effects of two treatment regimes with synthetic human parathyroid hormone fragment on bone formation and the tissue balance of trabecular bone in greyhounds. Endocrinology 1983;112:1000–1006.
4. Hock JM, Gera I. Effects of continuous and intermittent administration and inhibition of resorption on the anabolic response of bone to parathyroid hormone. J Bone Miner Res 1992;7:65–72.
5. Ibrahim M, Forte L, Thomas M. Maintainance of normocalcemia by continuous infusion of the synthetic bovine parathyroid hormone (1–34) in parathyroidectomized rats 1982;34(6):553–557.
6. Kitazawa R, Imai Y, Fukase M, Fujita T. Effects of continuous infusion of parathyroid hormone and parathyroid hormone-related peptide on rat bone in vivo: comparative study by histomorphometry. Bone Miner 1991;12:157–166.
7. Parisien M, Silverberg S, Shane E, Cruz Ldl, Lindsay R, Bilezekian J, Dempster D. The histomorphometry of bone in primary hyperparathyroidism: preservation of cancellous bone structure. J Clin Endocrinol Metab 1990;70:930–938.
8. Heath H. Primary hyperparathyroidism, hyperparathyroid bone disease, and osteoporosis. Chapter 45. In: Marcus R, ed. Osteoporosis. NY: Academic Press Inc., 1996:885–897.
9. Christiansen P, Steiniche T, Brixen K, Hessov I, Melsen F, Heickerndorff L, Mosekilde L. Primary hyperparathyroidism: effect of parathyroidectomy on regional bone mineral density in Danish patients: a three-year follow-up study. Bone 1999;5:589–595.
10. Calvi L, Sims N, Hunzelman J, Knight M, Giovannetti A, Saxton J, Kronenberg H, Baron R, Schipani E. Activated parathyroid hormone/parathyroid hormone related protein receptor in osteoblastic cells differentially affects cortical and trabecular bone. J Clin Invest 2001;107:277–286.
11. Kuznetsov S, Riminucci M, Ziran N, Tsutsui T, Corsi A, Calvi L, Kronenberg H, Schipani W, Robey P, Bianco P. The interplay of osteogenesis and hematopoiesis: expression of a constitutively active PTH/PTHrP receptor in osteogenic cells perturbs the establishment of hematopoiesis in bone and skeletal stem cells in the bone marrow. J Cell Biol 2004;167:1113–1122.
12. Scadden D. The stem cell niche as an entity of action. Nature 2006;441:1075–1079.
13. Canalis E, Hock JM, Raisz LG. Anabolic and catabolic effects of parathyroid hormone on bone and interactions with growth factors. In: Bilezekian JP, Levine MA, eds. The parathyroids. New York: Raven Press Ltd, 1994:65–82.
14. Hock JM, Onyia J, Miller B, Hulman J, Herring J, CHandrasekhar S, Harvey AK, Gunness M. Anabolic PTH targets proliferating cells of the primary spongiosa in young rats, and increases the number differentiating into osteoblasts. J Bone Miner Res 1994;9(Suppl):S412.
15. Young RW. Cell proliferation and specialization during endochondral osteogenesis in young rats. J Cell Biol 1962;14:357–370.
16. Young RW. Specialization of bone cells. Boston, MA: Little, Brown &Company, 1964.
17. Owen M. Marrow stromal stem cells. J Cell Sci 1988;10:63–76.
18. Owen M, Friedenstein AJ. Stromal stem cells: marrow-derived osteogenic precursors. Ciba Fdn Sympos 1988;136:42–60.
19. Owen ME. The origin of bone cells. Int Rev Cytol 1970;28:213–218.
20. Long H, Onyia J, Hulman J, Bidwell J, Hock JM. Molecular characterization of primary spongiosa cells from the distal femurs of young rats. J Bone Miner Res 1995;10:S312.
21. Dobnig H, Turner R. Evidence that intermittent treatment with parathyroid hormone increases bone formation in adult rats by activation of bone lining cells. Endocrinology 1995;136:3632–3638.

22. Feister H, Swartz D, Odgren P, Holden J, Hock J, Onyia J, Bidwell J. Topoisomerase II expression in osseous tissue. J Cell Biochem 1997;67:451–465.
23. Feister H, Yang X, Onyia J, Miles R, Hock J, Bidwell J. Parathyroid hormone regulates the expression of NuMA and topoisomerase II-alpha in bone. Bone 1998;23(Suppl):S207 (TO215).
24. Owen ME, Cave J, Joyner CJ. Clonal analysis in vitro of osteogenic differentiation of marrow CFU-f. J Cell Sci 1987;87:731–738.
25. Bingham P, Brazell I, Owen M. The effect of parathyroid extract on cellular activity and plasma calcium levels in vivo. J Endocrinol 1969;45:387–400.
26. Kember NF. Cell division in endochondral ossification. A study of cell proliferation in rat bones by the method of triated thymidine autoradiography. J Bone Joint Surg 1960;42:824–839.
27. Kimmel DB, Jee WSS. Bone cell kinetics during longitudinal bone growth in the rat. Calcif Tissue Int 1980;32:123–133.
28. Yamaguchi T, Bradley A, McMahon A, Jones S. A wnt5 pathway underlies outgrowth of multiple structures in the vertebrate embryo. Development 1999;126:1211–1223.
29. Dobnig H, Turner R. The effects of programmed administration of human parathyroid hormone fragment (1–34) on bone histomorphometry and serum chemistry in rats. Endocrinology 1997;138: 4607–4612.
30. Turner R, Evans G, Cavolina J, Halloran B, Morey-Holton E. Programmed administration of parathyroid hormone increases bone formation and reduces bone loss in hindlimb-unloaded ovariectomized rats. Endocrinology 1998;139:4086–4091.
31. Bianco P, Riminucci M, Kuznetsov S, Robey P. Multipotential cells in the bone marrow stroma: regulation in the context of organ physiology. Crit Rev Eukaryot Gene Expr 1999;9:159–173.
32. Canalis E, Centrella M, Burch W, McCarthy T. Insulin-like growth factor I mediates selective anabolic effects of parathyroid hormone in bone cultures. J Clin Invest 1989;83:60–65.
33. Fedarko NS, Vetter UK, Weinstein S, Robey PG. Age-related changes in hyaluronan, proteoglycan, collagen and osteonectin synthesis in human bone cells. J Cell Physiol 1992;151:215–227.
34. Leaffer D, Sweeney M, Kellerman L, Avnur Z, Krstenansky J, Vickery B, Caufield J. Modulation of osteogenic cell ultrastructure by RS-23581, an analog of human parathyroid hormone (PTH)-related peptide-(1–34) and bovine PTH-(1–34). Endocrinology 1995;136:3624–3631.
35. Lotinun S, Sibonga J, Turner R. Evidence that the cells responsible for marrow fibrosis in a rat model for hyperparathyroidism are preosteoblasts. Endocrinology 2005;146:4074–4081.
36. Lotinun S, Sibonga J, Turner R. Triazolopyrimidine (Trapidil) a platelet-derived growth factor antagonist, inhibits parathyroid hormone disease in an animal model for chronic hyperparathyroidism. Endocrinology 2003;144:2000–2007.
37. Hodsman A, Fraher L, Osbye T, Adachi J, Steer B. An evaluation of several biochemical markers for bone formation and resorption in a protocol utilizing cyclical parathyroid hormone and calcitonin therapy for osteoporosis. J Clin Invest 1993;91:1138–1148.
38. Meng X, Liang X, Birchman R, Wu D, Dempster D, Lindsay R, Shen V. Temporal expression of the anabolic action of PTH in cancellous bone of ovariectomized rats. J Bone Miner Res 1996;11: 421–429.
39. Jilka R, Weinstein R, Bellido T, Roberson P, Parfitt A, Manolagos S. Increased bone formation by prevention of osteoblast apoptosis with parathyroid hormone. J Clin Invest 1999;104:439–446.
40. Manolagas S. Editorial: cell number versus cell vigor – what really matters to a regenerating skeleton? Endocrinology 1999;140:4377–4381.
41. Manolagas S. Birth and death of bone cells: basic regulatory mechanisms and implications for the pathogenesis and treatment of osteoporosis. Endocr Rev 2000;21:115–137.
42. Stanislaus D, Devanarayan V, Hock J. In vivo comparison of AP-1 gene activation in response to hPTH 1–34 and hPTH 1–84 in the distal femur metaphyses of young mice. Bone 2000;27:819–826.
43. Chen H, Demiralp B, Schneider A, Koh A, Silve C, Wang C, McCauley L. Parathyroid hormone and parathyroid hormone-related hormone exert both pro- and anti-apoptotic effects in mesenchymal cells. J Biol Chem 2002;277:19374–19381.
44. Miura M, Chen X, Allen M, Bi Y, Gronthos S, Seo B, Lakhani S, Flavell R, Feng X, Robey P, Young M, Shi S. A crucial role for caspase-3 in osteogenic differentiation of bone marrow stromal stem cells. J Clin Invest 2004;114:1704–1713.

45. Mogi M, Togari A. Activation of caspases is required for osteoblastic differentiation. J Biol Chem 2003;278:47477–47482.
46. Morley P, Whitfield J, Willick G. Anabolic effects of PTH on bone. Trends Endocrinol Metab 1997;8:225–231.
47. Kronenberg H. PTH: mechanisms of action. 3rd ed. Philadelphia, PA: American Society of Bone and Mineral Research, 1996.
48. Whitfield J, Morley P. Anabolic treatments for osteoporosis. Boca Raton, FL: CRC Press LLC, 1998.
49. Bouxsein M, Pierroz D, Glatt V, Goddard D, Cavat F, Rizzoli R, Ferrari S. Beta-Arrestin 2 regulates the differential response of cortical and trabecular bone to intermittent PTH in female mice. J Bone Miner Res 2005;20:635–643.
50. Watson P, Fraher L, Hendy G, Chung U, Kisiel M, Natale B, Hodsman A. Nuclear localization of the type 1 PTH/PTHrP receptor in rat tissues. J Bone Miner Res 2000;15:1033–1044.
51. Liang J, Hock J, Sandusky G, Santerre R, Onyia J. Immunohistochemical localization of selected early response genes expressed in trabecular bone of young rats given hPTH 1–34. Calcif Tissue Int 1999;65:369–373.
52. McCauley L, Koh A, Beecher C, Rosol T. Proto-oncogene c-fos is transcriptionally regulated by parathyroid hormone (PTH) and PTH-related protein in a cyclic adenosine monophosphate-dependent manner in osteoblastic cells. Endocrinology 1997;138:5427–5433.
53. Tyson D, Swarthout J, Partridge N. Increased osteoblastic c-fos expression by parathyroid hormone requires protein kinase A phosphorylation of the cyclic adenosine 3′,5′-monophosphate response element-binding protein at serine 133. Endocrinology 1999;140:1255–1261.
54. Zeng Z, Cole H, SMith S, Bryant H, Sato M. Bone effects in mice of ovariectomy and recombinant human PTH (1–34) are highly strain dependent. Bone 1998;23(Suppl 5):S448.
55. Hock J. Discrimination around osteoblasts? PTH analog may reveal site specific differences in mice. Bone 2000;27:467–469.
56. Demiralp B, Chen H, Koh A, Keller E, McCauley L. Anabolic actions of parathyroid hormone during bone growth are dependent on c-fos. Endocrinology 2002;143:4038–4047.
57. Yang F, Chen S, Robling A, Yu X, Nebesio T, Yan J, Morgan T, Li X, Yuan J, Hock J, Ingram D, Clapp D. Hyperactivation of p21ras and PI3K cooperate to alter murine and human neurofibromatosis type 1–haploinsufficient osteoclast functions. J Clin Invest 2006;116:2880–2891.
58. Yu X, Milas J, Watanabe N, Rao N, Murthy S, Potter O, Wenning M, Clapp W, Hock J. Neurofibromatosis type 1 gene haploinsufficiency reduces AP-1 gene expression without abrogating the anabolic effect of parathyroid hormone. Calcif Tissue Int 2006;78:162–170.
59. Koh A, Demiralp B, Neiva K, Hooten J, Nohutcu R, Shim H, Datta N, Taichman R, McCauley L. Cells of the osteoclast lineage as mediators of the anabolic actions of parathyroid hormone in bone. Endocrinology 2005;146:4584–4596.
60. Jerome C, Johnson C, Lees C. Parathyroid hormone (PTH) increases axial and appendicular bone mass without cortical bone loss in ovariectomized cynomolgus monkeys. J Bone Miner Res 1995;10(Suppl 1):S416.
61. Jerome C, Burr D, Bibber TV, Hock J, Brommage R. Treatment with human parathyroid hormone (1–34) for 18 months increases cancellous bone volume and improves trabecular architecture in ovariectomized cynomolgus monkeys (Macaca fascicularis). Bone 2000;28:150–159.
62. Finkelstein J, Leder B, Burnett S, Wyland J, Lee H, Paz Adl, Gibson K, Neer R. Effects of teriparatide, alendronate or both on bone turnover in men. J Clin Endocrinol Metab 2006;91:2882–2887.
63. Jerome CP. Anabolic effect of high doses of human parathyroid hormone (1–38) in mature intact female rats. J Bone Miner Res 1994;9:933–942.
64. Okimoto N, Tsurukami H, Osazaki Y, Nishida S, Sakai A, Ohnishi H, Hori M, Yasukawa K, Nakamura T. Effects of a weekly injection of human parathyroid hormone (1–34) and withdrawal on bone mass, strength, and turnover in mature ovariectomized rats. Bone 1998;22:523–531.
65. Hock JM, Hummert JR, Boyce R, Fonseca J, Raisz LG. Resorption is not essential for the stimulation of bone growth by human parathyroid hormone 1–34 in rats in vivo. J Bone Miner Res 1989;4:449–458.
66. Iwaniec U, Wronski T, Liu J, Rivera M, Arzaga R, Hansen G, Brommage R. Parathyroid hormone stimulates bone formation in mice deficient in Lrp5. J Bone Miner Res 2007;22:394–402.

67. Sawakami K, Robling A, Ai M, Pitner N, Liu D, Warden S, Li J, Maye P, Rowe D, Duncan R, Warman M, Turner C. The Wnt co-receptor LRP5 is essential for skeletal mechanotransduction but not for the anabolic bone response to parathyroid hormone treatment. J Biol Chem 2006;281: 23698–23711.
68. Falla N, Marder P, Cain R, Mann L, Hock J. Anabolic intermittent treatment with hPTH 1–34 selectively upregulates multiple growth factor receptors in cells of the metaphyseal but not diaphyseal marrow of young rats. J Bone Miner Res 1966;11(S1):S417(T470).
69. Pfeilshifter J, Laukhuf F, Muller-Beckmann B, Blum W, Pfister T, Ziegler R. Parathyroid hormone increases the concentration of insulin-like growth factor-1 and transforming growth factor beta-1 in rat bone. J Clin Invest 1995;96:767–774.
70. Bikle D, Sakata T, Leary C, Elalieh H, Ginzinger D, Rosen C, Beamer W, Majumdar S, Halloran B. Insulin-like growth factor I is required for the anabolic actions of parathyroid hormone on mouse bone. J Bone Miner Res 2002;17:1570–1578.
71. Hurley M, Okada Y, Xiao L, Tanaka Y, Ito M, Okimoto N, Nakamura T, Rosen C, Doetschman T, Coffin J. Impaired bone anabolic response to parathyroid hormone in Fgf2–/– and Fgf2+/– mice. Biochem Biophys Res Commun 2006;341:989–994.
72. Hurley M, Tetradis S, Huang Y, Hock J, Kream B, Raisz L, Sabbieti M. Parathyroid hormone regulates the expression of fibroblast growth factor-2 mRNA and fibroblast growth factor receptor mRNA in osteoblastic cells. J Bone Miner Res 1999;14:776–783.
73. Yamaguchi M, Ogata N, Shinoda Y, Akune T, Kamekura S, Terauchi Y, Kadowaki T, Takahashi H, Hoshi K, Chung U, Nakamura K, Kawaguchi H. Insulin receptor substrate-1 is required for bone anabolic function of parathyroid hormone in mice. Endocrinology 2005;146:2620–2628.
74. Pirih F, Aghaloo T, Bezouglaia O, Nervina J, Tetradis S. Parathyroid hormone induces the NR4A family of nuclear orphan receptors in vivo. Biochem Biophys Res Commun 2005;332:494–503.
75. Keller H, Kneissel M. SOST is a target gene for PTH in bone. Bone 2005;37:148–158.
76. Onyia J, Bidwell J, Herring J, Hulman J, Hock J. In vivo, human parathyroid hormone fragment (hPTH 1–34) transiently stimulates immediate early response gene expression, but not proliferation, in trabecular bone cells of young rats. Bone 1995;17:479–484.
77. Prahalad A, Hickey R, Huang J, Hoelz D, Dobroleck L, Murthy S, Winata T, Hock J. Serum proteome profiles identifies parathyroid hormone physiologic response. Proteomics 2006;6:3482–3493.
78. Miles R, Sluka J, Halladay D, Snaterre R, Hale L, Bloem L, Thirunavukkarasu K, Galvin R, Hock J, Onyia J. ADAMTS-1: a cellular disintegrin and metalloprotease with thrombospondin motifs is a target for parathryroid hormone in bone. Endocrinology 2000;141:4533–4542.
79. Bogdanovic Z, Huang Y, Dodig M, Clark S, Lichtler A, Kream B. Parathyroid hormone inhibits collagen synthesis and the activity of rat col1a1 transgenes mainly by a cAMP-mediated pathway in mouse calvariae. J Cell Biochem 2000;77:149–158.
80. Dietrich J, Canalis E, Maina D, Raisz L. Hormonal control of bone collagen synthesis in vitro: effects of parathyroid hormone and calcitonin. Endocrinology 1976;98:943–949.
81. Tetradis S, Nervina J, Nemoto K, Kream B. Parathryoid hormone induces expression of the inducible cAMP early repressor in osteoblastic MC3T3-E1 cells and mouse calvariae. J Biol Chem 1998; 269:9392–9396.
82. Riminucci M, Fisher L, Shenker A, Spiegel A, Bianco P, Robey P. Fibrous dysplasia in bone in the McCune-Albright syndrome: abnormalities in bone formation. Am J Pathol 1997;151:1587–1600.
83. Watson P, Fraher L, Kisiel M, DeSousa D, Hendy G, Hodsman A. Enhanced osteoblast development after continuous infusion of hPTH (1–84) in the rat. Bone 1999;24:89–94.
84. Watson P, Lazowski D, Han V, Fraher L, Steer B, Hodsman A. Parathyroid hormone restores bone mass and enhances osteoblast insulin-like growth factor I gene expression in ovariectomized rats. Bone 1995;16:357–365.
85. Hodsman A, Watson P, Drost D, Fraher L, Holdsworth D, Thornton M, Hock J, Bryant H. The addition of a raloxifene analog (LY117018) allows for reduced PTH (1–34) dosing during reversal of osteopenia in ovariectomized rats. J Bone Miner Res 1999;14:675–679.
86. Feister H, Onyia J, Miles R, Yang X, Galvin R, Hock J, Bidwell J. The expression of the nuclear matrix proteins NuMA, topoisomerase II-alpha and -beta in bone and osseous cell culture: regulation by parathyroid hormone. Bone 2000;26:227–234.

87. Bidwell J, ALvarez M, Feister H, Onyia J, Hock J. Nuclear matrix proteins and osteoblast gene expression. J Bone Miner Res 1998;13:155–167.
88. Alvarez M, Thunyakitpisal P, Morrison P, Onyia J, Hock J, Bidwell J. PTH-responsive osteoblast nuclear matrix architectural transcription factor binds to the rat type I collagen promoter. J Cell Biochem 1998;69:336–352.
89. Onyia J, Miles R, Halladay D, Chandrasekhar S, Martin T. In vivo demonstration that parathyroid hormone (hPTH 1–38) inhibits the expression of osteoprotegerin (OPG) in bone with the kinetics of an immediate early gene. J Bone Miner Res 2000;14(S1):S166.
90. Greenfield E, Horowitz M, Lavish S. Stimulation by parathyroid hormone of interleukin 6 and leukemia inhibitory factor expression in osteoblasts is an immediate-early gene response induced by cAMP signal transduction. J Biol Chem 1996;271:10984–10989.
91. Greenfield EM, Gornik SA, Horowitz MC, Donahue HJ, Shaw SM. Regulation of cytokine expression in osteoblasts by parathyroid hormone: rapid stimulation of interleukin-6 and leukemia inhibitory factor mRNA. J Bone Miner Res 1993;8:1163–1171.
92. Miles R, Sluka J, Santerre R, Hale L, Bloem L, Boguslawski G, Thirunavukkarasu K, Hock J. Dynamic regulation of RGS2 in bone: potential new insights into PTH signaling mechanisms. Endocrinology 2000;141:28–36.
93. Merciris D, Schiltz C, Legoupil N, Marty-Morieux C, Vernejoul Md, Geoffroy V. Over-expression of TIMP-1 in osteoblasts increases the anabolic response to PTH. Bone 2007;40:75–83.
94. Jiminez M, Balbin M, Lopez J, Alvarez J, Komori T, Lopez-Otin C. Collagenase 3 is a target of Cbfa1, a transcription factor of the runt gene family involved in bone formation. Mol Cell Biol 1999;19: 4431–4442.
95. Kanzawa M, Sugimoto T, Kanatani M, Chihara K. Involvement of osteoprotegerin/osteoclastogenesis inhibitory factor in the stimulation of osteoclast formation by parathryoid hormone in mouse bone cells. Eur J Endocrinol 2000;142:661–664.
96. Suda T, Takahashi N, Udagawa N, Jimi E, Gillespie M, Martin T. Modulation of osteoclast differentiation and function by new members of the tumor necrosis factor receptor and ligand families. Endocr Rev 1999;20:345–357.
97. Itoh K, Udagawa N, Matsuzaki K, Takami M, Amano H, Shinki T, Ueno Y, Takahashi N, Suda T. Importance of membrane or matrix-associated forms of M-CSF and RANKL/ODF in osteoclastogenesis supported by SaOS-4/3 cells expressing recombinant PTH/PTHrP receptors. J Bone Miner Res 2000;15:1766–1775.
98. Miles R, Sluka J, Santerre R, Hale L, Bloem L, Thirunavukkarasu K, Hock J, Onyia J. ADAMTS-1: a cellular disintegrin and metalloprotease with thrombospondin motifs is a target for PTH in bone. Endocrinology 2000;14:4533–4542.
99. Kroll M. Parathyroid hormone temporal effects on bone formation and resorption. Bull Math Biol 2000;62:163–188.
100. Galvin R, Babbey L, Bryan P, Cain R, Hulman J, Hock J. Human PTH (1–34) administered by once daily dosing is anabolic in mice and increases ex vivo osteoclast differentiation. J Bone Miner Res 1999;14(Suppl 1):S414.
101. Gunness M, Hock J. Anabolic effect of parathyroid hormone is not modified by supplementation with insulinlike growth factor I (IGF-I) or growth hormone in aged female rats fed an energy-restricted or ad libitum diet. Bone 1995;16:199–207.
102. Hock JM, Canalis E, Centrella M. Transforming growth factor-beta stimulates bone matrix apposition and bone cell replication in cultured fetal rat calvariae. Endocrinology 1990;126:421–426.
103. Rosen C. The cellular and clinical parameters of anabolic therapy for osteoporosis. Crit Rev Eukaryot Gene Expr 2003;13:25–38.
104. Canalis E, Rydziel S, Delaney A, Varghese S, Jeffrey J. Insulin-like growth factors inhibit interstitial collagenase synthesis in bone cell cultures. Endocrinology 1995;136:1348–1354.
105. Moriwake T, Tanaka H, Kanzaki S, Higuchi J, Seino Y. 1,25-Dihydroxyvitamin D3 stimulates the secretion of insulin-like growth factor binding protein 3 (IGFBP-3) by cultured human osteosarcoma cells. Endocrinology 1992;130:1071–1073.
106. LaTour D, Mohan S, Linkhart T, Baylink D, Strong D. Inhibitory insulin-like growth factor-binding protein: cloning, complete sequence, and physiological regulation. Mol Endocrinol 1990;4: 1806–1814.

107. Wang L, Quarles L, Spurney R. Unmasking the osteoinductive effects of a G-protein-coupled receptor (GPCR) kinase (GRK) inhibitor by treatment with PTH(1–34). J Bone Miner Res 2004;19: 1661–1670.
108. Miyakoshi N, Kasukawa Y, Linkhart T, Baylink D, Mohan S. Evidence that anabolic effects of PTH on bone require IGF-I in growing micc. Endocrinology 2001;142:4349–4356.
109. Yakar S, Bouxsein M, Canalis E, Sun H, Glatt V, Gundberg C, Cohen P, Hwang D, Boisclair Y, Leroith D, Rosen C. The ternary IGF-I complex influences postnatal bone acquisition and the skeletal response to intermittent parathyroid hormone. J Endocrinol 2006;189:289–299.
110. Wu Y, Kumar R. Parathyroid hormone regulates transforming growth factor beta1 and beta2 synthesis in osteoblasts via divergent signaling pathways. J Bone Miner Res 2000;15:879–884.
111. Okada Y, Montero A, Zhang X, Sobue T, Lorenzo J, Doetschman T, Coffin J, Hurley M. Impaired osteoclast formation in bone marrow cultures of FGF2 null mice in response to parathyroid hormone. J Biol Chem 2003;278:21258–21266.
112. Gera I, Hock JM, Gunness-Hey M, Fonseca J, Raisz LG. Indomethacin does not inhibit the anabolic effect of parathyroid hormone on the long bones of rats. Calcif Tissue Int 1987;40:206–211.
113. Riond J, Fischer IG-v, Kuffer B, Toromanoff A, Forrer R. Influence of the dosing frequency of parathyroid hormone (1–38) on its anabolic effect in bone and on the balance of calcium, phosphorus and magnesium. Z Ernahrungswiss 1998;37:183–189.
114. Gunness-Hey M, Gera I, Fonseca J, Raisz LG, Hock JM. 1,25-dihydroxyvitamin D3 alone or in combination with parathyroid hormone does not increase bone mass in young rats. Calcif Tissue Int 1988;43:284–288.
115. Wronski TJ, Cintron M Dann LM Horner SL. Temporal relationship between bone loss and increased bon turnover in ovariectomized rats. Calcif Tiss Int 1988;179–184.
116. Sato M, Zeng G, Turner C. Biosynthetic human parathyroid hormone (1–34) effects on bone quality in aged ovariectomized rats. Endocrinology 1997;138:4330–4337.
117. Stewart A, Cain R, Burr D, Jacob D, Turner C, Hock J. Six month daily administration of PTH and PTHrP peptides to adult ovariectomized rats markedly enhances bone mass and biomechanical properties: A comparison of human PTH (1–34), PTHrP (1–36) and SDZ-PTH-893. J Bone Miner Res 2000;15: 1517–1525.
118. Brommage R, Hotchkiss CE, Lees CJ, Stancill MW, Hock JM, JeromeCP . Daily treatment with human recombinant parathyroid hormone-(1–34), LY333334, for 1 year increases bone mass in ovariectomized monkeys. J Clin Endocrinol Metab 1999;84:3757–3763.
119. Hodsman AB, L. J. Fraher, P. H. Watson, T. Ostbye, L. W. Stitt, J. D. Adachi, D. H. Taves, D. Drost. A randomized controlled trial to compare the efficacy of cyclical parathyroid hormone versus cyclical parathyroid hormone and sequential calcitonin to improve bone mass in postmenopausal women with osteoporosis. J Clin Endocrinol Metab 1997;82:620–628.
120. Lindsay R, Nieves J, Formica C, Henneman E, Woelfert L, Shen V, Dempster D, Cosman F. Randomised controlled study of effect of parathyroid hormonc on vertebral-bone mass and fracture incidence among post-menopausal women on oestrogen with osteoporosis. Lancet 1997;350:550–555.
121. Rosen C, Bilezekian J. Anabolic therapy for osteoporosis. J Clin Endocrinol Metab 2001;86:957–964.
122. Hock J. Stemming bone loss by suppressing apoptosis: invited commentary. J Clin Invest 1999;104: 371–373.
123. Malluche H, Sherman D, Meyer W, Ritz E, Norman A, Massry S. Effects of long-term infusion of physiologic doses of 1–34 PTH on bone. Am J Physiol 1982;242:F197–F201.
124. Cosman F, Shen V, Herrington B, Lindsay R. Response of the parathyroid gland to infusion of parathyroid hormone (1–34): Demonstration of suppression of endogenous secretion using immunoradiometric intact PTH (1–84) assay. J Clin Endocrinol Metab 1991;73:1345–1351.
125. Parfitt A. The actions of parathyroid hormone on bone: relation to remodeling and turnover, calcium homeostasis and metabolic bone disease. Part 1: mechanisms of calcium transfer between blood and bone and their cellular basis: morphologic and kinetic approaches to bone turnover. Metabolism 1976;25: 809–844.
126. Parfitt A. The actions of parathyroid hormone on bone in relation to bone remodeling and turnover, calcium homeostasis, and metabolic bone disease. II. PTH and bone cells: bone turnover and plasma calcium regulation. Metabolism 1976;25:909–955.

127. Parfitt A. The actions of parathyroid hormone on bone: relation to bone remodeling and turnover, calcium homeostasis and metabolic bone disease. Part III: PTH and osteoblasts, the relationship between bone turnover and bone loss and the state of the bones in primary hyperparathyroidism. Metabolism 1976;25:1033–1068.
128. Parfitt A. The actions of parathyroid hormone on bone: relation to bone remodeling and turrnover, calcium homeostasis and metabolic bone disease. Part IV: the state of the bones in uremic hyperparathyroidism – the mechanisms of skeletal resistance to PTH in renal failure and pseudohyperparathyroidism and the role of PTH in osteoporosis, osteopetrosis and osteofluorosis. Metabolism 1976;25:1157–1187.
129. Hirano T, Burr D, Cain R, Hock J. Changes in geometry and cortical porosity in adult ovary intact rabbits after 5 months treatment with LY333334 (hPTH 1–34). Calcif Tissue Int 2000;66:456–460.
130. Burr D, Hirano T, Turner C, Cain R, Hock J. Intermittently administered hPTH (1–34) treatment increases intracortical bone turnover and porosity without reducing bone strength in the humerus of ovariectomized cynomolgus monkeys. Calcif Tissue Int 2000;66:157–165.
131. Gunness-Hey M, Hock JM. Loss of anabolic effect of parathyroid hormone on bone after discontinuation of hormone in rats. Bone 1990;10:447–452.
132. Fujita T, Onoue T, Morii H, Morita R, Norimatsu H, Orimo H, Takahashi H, Yamamoto K, Fukunaga M. Effect of intermittent weekly dose of human parathyroid (1–34) on osteoporosis: a randomized double-masked prospective study using three dose levels. Osteoporosis Int 1999;9:296–306.
133. Paschalis E, Burr D, Mendelsohn R, Hock J, Boskey A. Bone mineral and collagen quality in humeri of ovariectomized cynomolgus monkeys given rhPTH(1–34) for 18 months. J Bone Miner Res 2003;18:769–775.
134. Paschalis E, Glass E, Donley D, Eriksen E. Bone mineral and collagen quality in iliac crest biopsies of patients given teriparatide: new results from the fracture prevention trial. J Clin Endocrinol Metab 2005;90:4644–4649.
135. Sato M, Vahle J, Schmidt A, Westmore M, Smith S, Rowley E, Ma L. Abnormal bone architecture and biomechanical properties with near-lifetime treatment of rats with PTH. Endocrinology 2002;143: 3230–3242.
136. Brommage R, Hotchkiss C, Lees C, Stancill M, Hock J, Jerome C. Effects of continuation or withdrawal of treatment with parathyroid hormone (1–34) on biochemical parameters and bone mineral density in ovariectomized monkeys. J Bone Min Res 1999;14(Suppl 1):S275.
137. Brommage R, Hotchkiss C, Lees C, Hock J, Jerome C. Effects of continuation or withdrawal of PTH (1–34) treatment on spine and proximal tibia BMD in ovariectomized monkeys. J Bone Miner Res 1999;14(Suppl 1):S275.
138. Hesp R, Hulme P, Williams D, Reeve J. The relationship between changes in femoral bone density and calcium balance in patients with involutional osteoporosis treated with human parathyroid hormone fragment (hPTH 1–34). Metab Bone Dis Relat Res 1981;2:331–334.
139. Hodsman A, Steer B, Fraher L, Drost D. Bone densitometric and histomorphometric responses to sequential human parathyroid hormone (1–38) and salmon calcitonin in osteoporotic patients. Bone Miner 1991;14:67–83.
140. Reeve J, Davies U, Hesp R, McNally E, Katz D. Treatment of osteoporosis with human parathyroid peptide and observation on effect of sodium fluoride. Br Med J 1990;301:314–317.
141. Boyce R, Paddock C, Franks A, Jankowsky M, Eriksen E. Effects of intermittent hPTH (1–34) alone and in combination with 1,25(OH)2D3 or risedronate on endosteal bone remodeling in canine cancellous and cortical bone. J Bone Miner Res 1996;11:600–613.
142. Mosekilde L, Sogaard CH, McOsker JE, Wronski TJ. PTH has a more pronounced effect on vertebral bone mass and biomechanical competence than antiresorptive agents (estrogen and bisphosphonate)-assessed in sexually mature ovariectomized rats. Bone 1994;15:401–408.
143. Mosekilde L, Danielsen C, Soogaard C, McOsker J, Wronski T. The anabolic effects of parathyroid hormone on cortical bone mass, dimensions and strength – assessed in a sexually mature, ovariectomized rat model. Bone 1995;16:223–230.
144. Mosekilde L, Danielsen CC, Gasser J. The effect of vertebral bone mass and strength of long-term treatment with antiresorptive agents (estrogen and calcitonin), human parathyroid hormone (1–38), and combination therapy, assessed in aged ovariectomized rats. Endocrinology 1994;134:2126–2134.
145. Agerbaek MO, Eriksen EF, Kragstrup J, Mosekilde L, Melsen F. A reconstruction of the remodelling cycle in normal human cortical iliac bone. Bone Mineral 1991;12:101–112.

146. Turner C, Wang T, Hock J, Hotchkiss C, Jerome C, Brommage R. In monkeys, treatment with PTH 1–34, LY333334, increases bone strength at trabecular bone sites without compromising the strength of cortical bone. London, UK: Freund Publishing House Inc., 1999.
147. Mashiba T, Burr D, Turner C, Sato M, Cain R, Hock J. Effects of human parathyroid hormone (1–34) LY333334, on bone mass, remodeling and mechanical properties of cortical bone during the first remodeling cycle in rabbits. Bone 2000;28:538–547.
148. Vahle J, Long G, Sandusky G, Westmore M, Ma Y, Sato M. Bone neoplasms in F344 rats given teriparatide (rhPTH 1–34) are dependent on duration of treatment and dose. Toxicol Pathol 2004;32: 426–438.
149. Vahle J, Sato M, Long G, Young J, Francis P, Engelhardt J, Westmore M, Y Lina, Nold J. Skeletal changes in rats given daily subcutaneous injections of recombinant human parathyroid hormone (1–34) for 2 years and relevance to human safety. Toxicol Pathol 2002;30:312–321.
150. Franks L, Rowlatt C, Chesterman F. Naturally occurring bone tumors in C57BL-Lcrf mice. J Natl Cancer Inst 1973;50:431–438.
151. Litvinov N, Soloviev J. Pathology of tumors in laboratory animals. Tumours of the rat. Tumours of bone. ARS Sci Publ 1990;99:659–676.
152. Withrow S, Powers B, Straw R, Wilkins R. Comparative aspects of osteosarcoma. Dog versus Man. Clin Orthop 1991;270:159–168.
153. Surveillance Research Program National Cancer Institute SEER∗Stat software (www.seer.cancer.gov/seerstat) version 6.1.4.
154. Chaudhary L, Avioli L. Identification and activation of mitogen-activated protein (MAP) kinase in normal human osteoblastic and bone marrow stromal cells: attenuation of MAP kinase activation by cAMP, parathyroid hormone and foskolin. Mol Cell Biochem 1998;178:59–68.
155. Onishi T, Hruska K. Expression of p27Kip1 in osteoblast-like cells during differentiation with parathyroid hormone. Endocrinology 1997;138:1995–2004.
156. Jones K, Owusu-Ababio G, Vick A, Khan M. Pharmacokinetics and hepatic extraction of recombinant human parathyroid hormone, hPTH (1–34) in rat, dog and monkey. J Pharm Sci 2006;95:2499–2506.
157. Harper K, Krege J, Marcus R, Mitlak B. Comments on initial experience with teriparatide in the United States. Curr Med Res Opin 2006;22:1927.
158. Gunness-Hey M, Hock JM. Loss of anabolic effect of parathyroid hormone on bone after discontinuation of hormone in rats. Bone 1989;10:447–452.
159. Shen V, Birchman R, Liang X, Wu D, Dempster D, Lindsay R. Accretion of bone mass and strength with parathyroid hormone prior to the onset of estrogen deficiency can provide temporary beneficial effects in skeletally mature rats. J Bone Miner Res 1998;13:883–890.
160. Lindsay R, Cosman F, Shen V, Nieves J, Dempster D. Bone mass increments induced by PTH treatment can be maintained by estrogen. J Bone Miner Res 1995;10(Suppl 1):S200.
161. Lindsay R, Cosman F, Nieves J, Dempster D, Shen V. A controlled clinical trial of the effects of 1–34 hPTH in estrogen-treated osteoporotic women. J Bone Miner Res 1993;8(Suppl 1):S130.
162. Shen V, Dempster DW, Mellish RWE, Birchman R, Horbert W, Lindsay R. Effects of combined and separate intermittent administration of low-dose human parathyroid hormone fragment (1–34) and 17-beta estradiol on bone histomorphometry in ovariectomized rats with established osteopenia. Calcif Tissue Int 1992;50:214–220.
163. Yamamoto N, Takahashi H, Tanizawa T, Endo N, Nishida S, Kinto N. Discrepancy of response of hPTH administration and its withdrawal between trabecular and cortical bone sites in OVX rats. Bone 1995;17(Suppl 4):279S–283S.
164. Okimoto N. Effects of a weekly injection of human parathyroid hormone (1–34) and withdrawal on bone mass, strength and turnover in mature ovariectomized rats. Bone 1998;22:523–531.
165. Mosekilde L, Thomsen J, McOsker J. No loss of biomechanical effects after withdrawal of short-term PTH treatment in an aged, osteopenic, ovariectomized rat model. Bone 1997;20:429–437.
166. Sato M, Westmore M, Clendenon J, Smith S, Hannum B, Zeng GQ, Brommage R, Turner CH. Three-dimensional modeling of the effects of parathyroid hormone on bone distribution in lumbar vertebrae of ovariectomized monkeys. Osteoporosis Int. 2000;11:871–880.
167. Shen V, Birchman R, Xu R, Otter M, Wu D, Lindsay R, Dempster D. Effects of reciprocal treatment with estrogen and estrogen plus parathyroid hormone on bone structure and strength in ovariectomized rats. J Clin Invest 1995;96:2331–2338.

168. Shen V, Dempster DW, Birchman R, Xu R, Lindsay R. Loss of cancellous bone mass and connectivity in ovariectomized rats can be restored by combined treatment with parathyroid hormone and estradiol. J Clin Invest 1993;91:2479–2487.
169. Eriksen E, Mosekilde L, Melsen F. Trabecular bone remodeling and balance in primary hyperparathyroidism. Bone 1986;7:213–221.
170. Black D, Bilzekian J, Ensrud K, Greenspan S, Palermo L, Hue T, Lang T, McGowan J, Rosen C. One year of alendronate after one year of parathyroid hormone (1–84) for osteoporosis. N Engl J Med 2005;353:555–565.
171. Neer R, Arnaud C, Zanchetta J, Prince R, Gaich G, Reginster J, Hodsman A, Eriksen E, Ish-Shalom S, Genant H, Wang O, Mitlak B. Effect of parathyroid hormone (1–34) on fractures and bone mineral density in post menopausal women with osteoporosis. N Engl J Med 2001;344:19.
172. Black D, Greenspan S, Ensrud K, Palermo L, McGowan J, Lang T, Garnero P, Bouxsein M, Bilezekian J, Rosen C. The effects of parathyroid hormone and alendronate alone and in combination in postmenopausal osteoporosis. N Engl J Med 2003;349:1207–1215.
173. Slovik DM, Neer RM, Potts JT. Short-term effects of synthetic human parathyroid hormone (1–34) administration on bone mineral metabolism in osteoporotic patients. J Clin Invest 1981;68:1261–1271.
174. Hock JM, Miller B, Cottrell S, Onyia J, McAndrews-Hill M, Williams D. Regulation of marrow stromal fibroblasts and hematopoietic cells by intermittent PTH. Bone 2000;27:209–218.
175. Stanislaus D, Yang X, Liang J, Wolfe J, Cain R, Onyia J, Falla N, Marder P, Bidwell J, Hock J. In vivo regulation of apoptosis in metaphyseal trabecular bone of young rats by synthetic human parathyroid hormone fragment, hPTH 1–34. Bone 2000; Submitted for review.

22 Clinical Use of Parathyroid Hormone in Osteoporosis

John P. Bilezikian, MD

Contents

Summary

The availability of parathyroid hormone (PTH) as an anabolic agent for the treatment of osteoporosis has expanded our therapeutic options. By stimulating processes directly associated with bone formation, PTH reduces fracture incidence. It does so by improving bone qualities in addition to increasing bone mass. Approved forms of PTH include the full-length molecule PTH(1-84) available in a number of countries outside the United States and the human recombinant fragment PTH(1-34) available throughout the world, including the United States. The 1-34 fragment of PTH, known generically as teriparatide, has emerged as a major approach to selected patients with osteoporosis. The means by which teriparatide reduces fracture risk is by increasing bone density and bone turnover, improving microarchitecture, and increasing bone size. The incidence of vertebral and non-vertebral fractures is reduced. A current concept in the mechanism of teriparatide action is related to its effect to stimulate processes associated with bone formation before it stimulates processes associated with bone resorption. This chronology has led to the concept of the anabolic window,

From: *Contemporary Endocrinology: Osteoporosis: Pathophysiology and Clinical Management*
Edited by: R. A. Adler, DOI 10.1007/978-1-59745-459-9_22,

the period of time when teriparatide is maximally anabolic. Newer approaches to the use of teriparatide alone and in combination with antiresorptive agents have led to ways in which the anabolic window can be expanded. Since teriparatide or PTH(1-84) is used for a limited period of time, it should be followed by an antiresorptive agent to maintain the densitometric gains achieved during its use.

Key Words: Osteoporosis, antiresorptive agents, parathyroid hormone, teriparatide, bone quality, bone density, anabolic window

INTRODUCTION

Until 2002, antiresorptive agents defined our pharmacological approach to osteoporosis. With the introduction of teriparatide, PTH(1-34), and more recently PTH(1-84) as treatments for osteoporosis, we now have available a class of drugs that reduce fracture risk by completely different mechanisms. By stimulating bone formation to a greater extent and earlier than bone resorption, teriparatide and PTH(1-84) improve not only bone mineral density (BMD) but also other properties of bone. These other properties include skeletal microarchitecture and bone size. These features confer upon PTH, the potential to reconstruct the skeleton *(1)*. Since PTH and antiresorptives operate by completely different mechanisms, the rationale for combination therapy is attractive. Further work has provided new insights into how antiresorptive agents and PTH can be used in sequence or in combination for maximal therapeutic benefits.

Parathyroid Hormone as an Anabolic Agent

In primary hyperparathyroidism, a disorder of chronic, continuous secretion of excess PTH, catabolic effects are seen commonly at cortical sites such as the distal one-third radius. Nevertheless, even in primary hyperparathyroidism, a clue to the anabolic actions of PTH can be appreciated by its salutary effects at the cancellous skeleton such as the lumbar spine *(2)*. The typical pattern of bone density in primary hyperparathyroidism is relative well-conserved lumbar spine density with preferential reduction of bone density at the distal one-third radius. This is particularly noteworthy in postmenopausal women with primary hyperparathyroidism who are not receiving estrogens. In these individuals one would expect early and preferential reduction of lumbar spine bone density since sex steroid deficiency is classically associated with rapid cancellous bone loss.

Greater insight into the anabolic potential of PTH came with the recognition that this property could be distinguished from its catabolic proclivities when PTH is used in low doses and intermittently *(3)*. Subsequent animal and then human studies confirmed the point that PTH is a potent anabolic agent when it is used intermittently and in low doses.

PTH is currently available in many countries as the recombinant human PTH(1-34) fragment known as teriparatide. The full-length molecule, human recombinant PTH(1-84), is also available in Europe. Teriparatide leads to a rapid increase in bone formation markers followed sometime thereafter by increases in bone resorption markers. The discordant chronology of PTH actions on these two turnover phases, that are generally tightly linked, suggest that PTH may initially stimulate processes associated with bone formation and only later promote those associated with generally increased bone turnover. This sequence

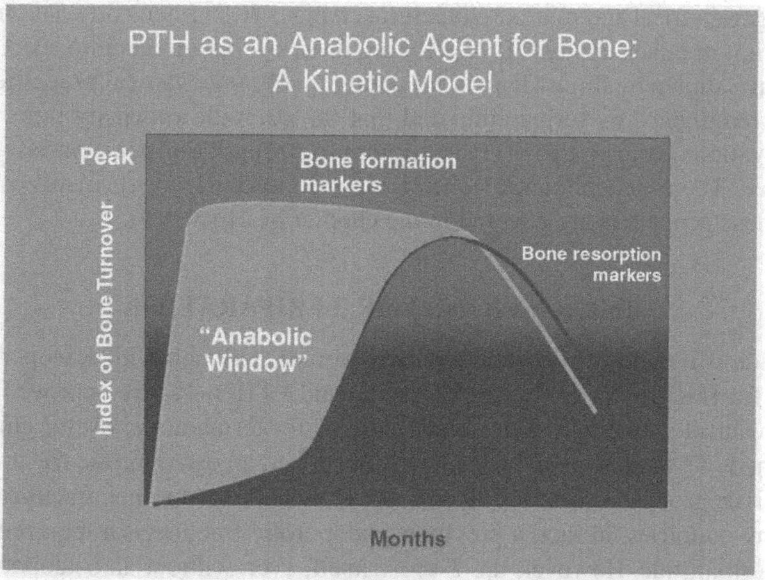

Fig. 1. The anabolic window. Based on the difference in kinetics of changes between bone formation and bone resorption markers, an "anabolic window" is formed during which the actions of parathyroid hormone are believed to be maximally anabolic.

of events with bone formation preceding bone resorption has led to the concept of the "anabolic window," a period of time when the actions of PTH are maximally anabolic *(4)* (Fig. 1). Although the concept of the anabolic window is supported by many observations, in many different clinical trials, the mechanistic basis is not clear. Hodsman et al. *(5)* and more recently Lindsay et al. *(6)* have analyzed biopsies 1 month after therapy with PTH using the quadruple labeling tetracycline technique. While remodeling-based processes seem to be stimulated most prominently by PTH, other histomorphometric features argue for an element of modeling-based bone formation to help account for its actions. Evidence for substantially increased bone formation on previously quiescent surfaces helps to make the point that, at least in part, PTH stimulates bone modeling directly. The extent to which bone remodeling or generally increased bone turnover facilitates modeling-based processes stimulated by PTH is not clear.

The beneficial effects of teriparatide on properties of the skeleton, such as bone density, microarchitecture, collagen maturity, bone geometry, and overall bone strength are demonstrated by a variety of techniques *(7–13)*. At a cortical skeletal site, such as the distal one-third radius, PTH typically does not increase bone density. In fact, there may be a small decline in BMD in association with an increase in cortical porosity. However, this does not translate into decreased bone strength because the increased porosity occurs only in the inner one-third of bone, where the mechanical effect is minimal. Even more importantly, other positive effects of teriparatide at cortical bone, such as changes in bone geometry and microarchitecture, adequately compensate for any increase in cortical porosity. PTH stimulates periosteal apposition which leads to increases in cortical area, cortical thickness, and an overall increase in cross-sectional area *(8–11)*. Moreover, microarchitectural changes due to teriparatide are evident at cortical sites such as the distal one-third radius as well. These geometrical and microarchitectural changes strengthen cortical bone despite the small reduction in bone density *(10,11)*. Taking these overall effects into account, Keaveny et al. *(13)* have shown by finite element modeling that biomechanical properties of the vertebrae are strengthened by teriparatide and that the strength to density ratio is improved. These observations indicate that PTH is improving strength through a variety of effects of bone qualities. The exact cellular, biochemical, and molecular mechanisms by which PTH influences these properties are covered in the chapter by Hock *(14)*.

INDICATIONS FOR TERIPARATIDE

Teriparatide is indicated in postmenopausal women and men with osteoporosis who are at high risk for fracture. In Europe, teriparatide and PTH(1-84) are approved for use only in postmenopausal women. To help select patients for teriparatide, useful guidelines have been published *(1)*. Patients who have already sustained an osteoporotic fracture are among the highest risk group because the likelihood of sustaining another fracture is very high *(15)*. In many countries, in fact, a previous osteoporotic fracture is a requirement for coverage with teriparatide. However, the *T*-score itself, even without an osteoporotic fracture, can confer high risk, especially if the *T*-score is very low (i.e., <–3.0). Age of the patient is also important because it confers greater risk for any given *T*-score. A 75-year-old woman with a *T*-score of –2.5 is at greater risk for a fracture than a 55-year-old woman with the same *T*-score. While these indications are straightforward, it is not always clear when teriparatide or PTH(1-84) should be used since the major clinical trials with the two major bisphosphonates, alendronate and risedronate, also were shown to be effective in patients whose osteoporosis was just as severe as those for whom teriparatide is indicated. This discussion has to take into account the fact that favor a bisphosphonate (cost, oral route of administration) versus those that would favor teriparatide (actual incremental gains in bone tissue per se).

Other potential candidates for PTH therapy are patients in whom one might consider a bisphosphonate but who cannot tolerate the drug. In addition, patients who fracture while on antiresorptive therapy could be considered to be at even higher risk and thus be candidates for teriparatide. In the United States, teriparatide is approved for 2 years of therapy; in Europe, approval is limited to 18 months.

TERIPARATIDE AS MONOTHERAPY IN POSTMENOPAUSAL OSTEOPOROSIS

In the randomized, double-blind, pivotal clinical trial of Neer et al. *(16)*, women with severe osteoporosis were treated with subcutaneous injections of placebo, 20 or 40 μg of teriparatide. High risk was defined in this population by the fact that the average number of fragility fractures per patient was over 2. Over a follow-up period of 21 months, BMD increased by an average of 10–14%. Total hip BMD also improved, but more slowly and to a smaller extent (approximately 3%) in comparison to the lumbar spine. At 20 μg of teriparatide, BMD did not change at the distal radius. The most important findings of the teriparatide trial by Neer et al. were significant reductions in new vertebral and nonvertebral fractures (Fig. 2). This drug also is associated with dramatic improvements in microarchitectural features of bone (Fig. 4) and other properties as shown above. By post

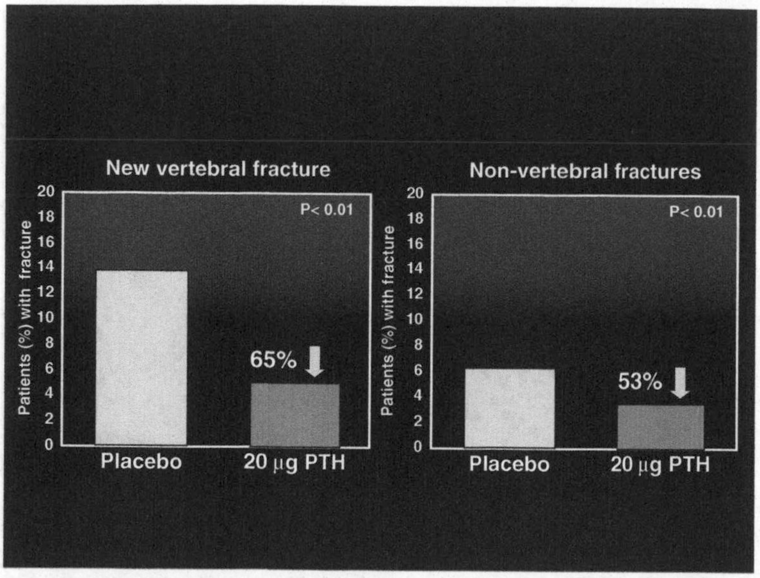

Fig. 2. Fracture incidence reduced with teriparatide. Fracture incidence after treatment with teriparatide. As shown for the registered 20 µg dose teriparatide reduces the incidence of vertebral and non-vertebral fractures significantly. Adapted from Ref. *(16)*.

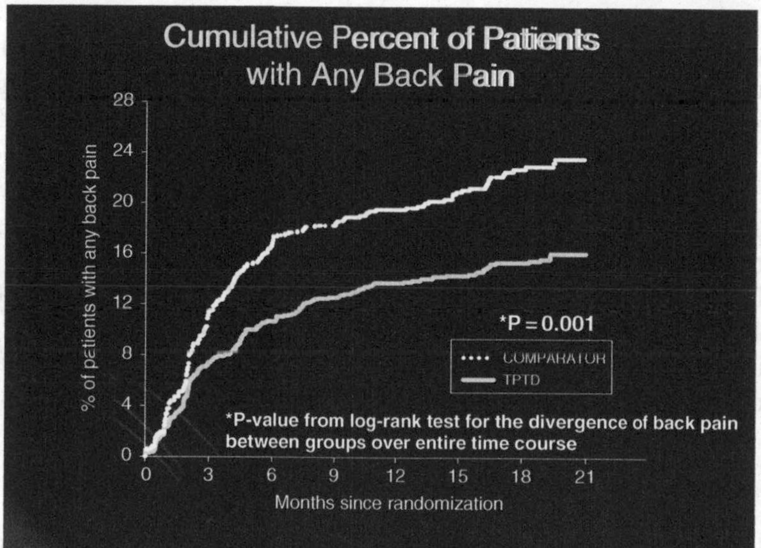

Fig. 3. Reduced back pain with teriparatide. The effect of teriparatide on bone pain in comparison to alendronate. Adapted from Ref. *(19)*.

hoc analysis, the reduction in fracture incidence due to teriparatide was not related to the number, severity, or site of previous fractures *(17)*. Further post hoc analysis of this cohort demonstrated that the fracture risk reduction was largely independent of age and initial

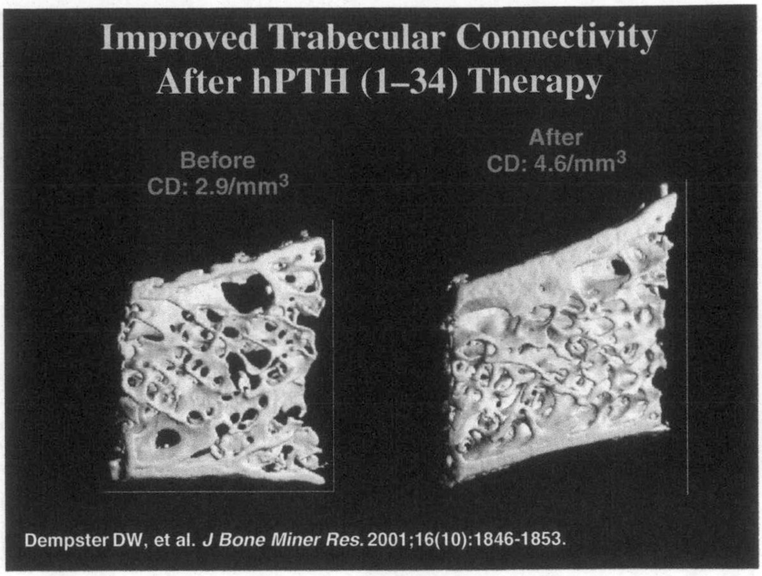

Fig. 4. Microarchitectural changes with teriparatide. After therapy with teriparatide there are marked changes in trabecular and cortical architecture as shown in this study by Dempster et al. J Bone Min Res 2001;16:1846–1853 (adapted).

BMD *(18)*. Moreover, in a comparator trial with alendronate, Miller et al. *(19)* have shown that teriparatide is associated with a significant reduction in back pain (Fig. 3). Miller et al. *(20)* also recently showed that teriparatide is effective across a range of renal function down to estimated GFRs as low as 30 ml/min *(20)*. In an observational cohort from this trial, fracture reduction was sustained for up to 30 months after teriparatide discontinuation, although many individuals in the original and treatment groups received bisphosphonate therapy during this follow-up period *(21)*.

Chen et al. *(22)* have recently related the change in BMD with teriparatide to the reduction in fracture risk. Similar to analyses relating change in bone mineral density to reduction in fracture risk for antiresorptive agents *(23–25)*, teriparatide-mediated increases in spine BMD accounted for only 30–40% of the reduction in vertebral fracture risk.

PTH(1-84) IN POSTMENOPAUSAL OSTEOPOROSIS

PTH(1-84) has been studied less intensively than teriparatide and is not currently available in the United States. It is available in Europe. In a dose-finding clinical trial, subjects were administered placebo or one of three doses of PTH(1-84): 50, 75, or 100 μg for 12 months *(26)*. There were time- and dose-related increases in lumbar spine BMD. Similar to the teriparatide studies, bone turnover markers rose quickly. Histomorphometric analysis of bone biopsy specimens confirms an anabolic response to PTH(1-84) with an increase in bone formation and improvements in cancellous architecture *(27)*. In contrast to the study by Neer et al. in which the average number of fragility fractures per study subject was >2, the prevalence of baseline fragility fractures in the phase III PTH(1-84) study was only 19%. Nevertheless, a reduction in new vertebral fracture incidence was seen with PTH(1-84) in women both with and without prior vertebral fractures *(27)*. A reduction in non-vertebral fractures was not demonstrated. The results of the pivotal trial with PTH (1-84) were recently published confirming these preliminary observations *(28)*. There was no reduction in non-vertebral fracture risk.

TERIPARATIDE IN MEN WITH OSTEOPOROSIS

In the first randomized, double-blinded controlled trial of teriparatide in men, Kurland et al. studied 23 men with 400 U/day of teriparatide (equivalent to 25 μg/day) or placebo for 18 months *(29)*. The men who received teriparatide demonstrated an impressive 13.5% increase in lumbar spine bone density. Hip BMD increased significantly but more slowly and to a smaller extent in comparison to the lumbar spine. Cortical bone density at the distal radius did not change as compared to placebo. Bone turnover markers rose quickly and substantially in the men treated with teriparatide, with bone formation markers rising and peaking earlier than bone resorption markers. In a larger trial of 437 men that was the counterpart of the pivotal trial of Neer et al. in postmenopausal women, Orwoll et al. *(30)* followed a protocol that was essentially identical to the study of Neer et al. BMD increased significantly in the 20 μg treatment group by 5.9% at the lumbar spine and by 1.5% at the femoral neck. These increases were independent of gonadal status. Although fractures could not be assessed during the short 11-month trial, they were assessed in a follow-up observational period of 30 months. Two hundred and seventy-nine men from the original cohort had lateral thoracic and lumbar spine X-rays, 18 months after treatment was stopped. In the combined teriparatide treatment groups (20 and 40 μg), the risk of vertebral fracture was reduced by 51% ($p = 0.07$). Significant reductions were seen in the combined group as compared to placebo when only moderate or severe fractures were considered [6.8% versus 1.1%; $p<0.02$] *(31)*. As was the case in the observational follow-up period in postmenopausal women, a substantial number of male study subjects in all groups (25–30%) reported use of antiresorptive therapy during the follow-up period. Men treated with placebo utilized antiresorptive therapy to a greater extent than those who were treated with either dose of teriparatide (36% versus 25%).

SEQUENTIAL AND COMBINATION THERAPY WITH TERIPARATIDE AND AN ANTIRESORPTIVE AGENT

Previous Use of an Antiresorptive

As many as 50% of patients who are considered candidates for teriparatide have previously been treated with bisphosphonates or other antiresorptives. Cosman et al. *(32)* treated postmenopausal women, previously given estrogen for at least 1 year, with teriparatide. Increases in vertebral BMD began with no delay and increased in a linear fashion during the entire 3-year study. Ettinger et al. *(33)* studied the influence of raloxifene or alendronate, prior to treatment with teriparatide. Fifty-nine postmenopausal women with *T*-scores ≤–2.0 had been treated for an average of 28 months either with raloxifene or alendronate. In most respects, subjects were well matched in terms of age, BMI, and *T*-scores. Similar to the study of Lindsay et al. for estrogen, raloxifene did not impede the effects of teriparatide to increase BMD rapidly and linearly. In contrast, alendronate was associated with a 6-month delay before BMD in the lumbar spine began to increase. After 18 months, lumbar spine BMD increased by 10.2% in the prior raloxifene-treated group compared to only 4.1% in the prior alendronate-treated subjects ($p<0.05$). The alendronate-treated group showed an initial decline in hip BMD at 6 months, but at 18 months, mean total hip BMD was not different from baseline. During teriparatide treatment, bone markers in prior alendronate patients increased later and peaked at about one-third lower levels as compared to prior raloxifene-treated patients.

These results imply that the potency of the antiresorptive to control bone turnover can determine the early response to teriparatide. Cosman et al. *(34)* have helped to refine this point in a study of teriparatide in postmenopausal women who also had previously received alendronate for the same period of time. In contrast to the study of Ettinger et al., their subjects responded to teriparatide with rapid increases in BMD. To account for these differences, it is noteworthy that the baseline bone turnover markers prior to the initiation of teriparatide therapy were markedly different in the two studies. In the study by Ettinger et al., bone turnover markers were almost completely suppressed. In comparison, in the study of Cosman et al., bone turnover markers were less suppressed and more in the range that one tends to find in subjects after alendronate therapy. Therefore, it is distinctly possible that it is not so much the specific antiresorptive used prior to teriparatide that dictates the subsequent densitometric response to teriparatide, but rather the extent to which bone turnover is reduced. To support this idea, the response to teriparatide has been shown to be a function of the level of baseline bone turnover in subjects not previously treated with any therapy for osteoporosis: the higher the level of turnover, the more robust the densitometric response to teriparatide *(29)*. A study that has recently been complete is testing both alendronate and risedronate in a head-to-head study of how these two bisphosphonates may affect subject patient behavior when then given teriparatide. The results are expected soon.

Concurrent Use of Anabolic and Antiresorptive Therapy

It is attractive to consider combination therapy with an antiresorptive and PTH as potentially more beneficial than monotherapy given that their mechanisms of action are quite different from each other. If bone resorption is being inhibited (antiresorptive) while bone formation is being stimulated (anabolic), combination therapy might give better results than with either agent alone. Despite the intuitive appeal of this reasoning, important data to the contrary have been provided by Black et al. *(35)* and by Finkelstein et al. *(36)*. These two groups independently completed trials using a form of PTH alone, alendronate alone, or the combination of a PTH form and alendronate. Black et al. studied postmenopausal women with 100 μg of PTH(1-84). The study of Finkelstein et al. involved men treated with 40 μg of teriparatide. Both studies utilized DXA and QCT to measure areal or volumetric BMD, respectively. With either measurement, monotherapy with PTH exceeded densitometric gains with combination therapy or alendronate alone at the lumbar spine. Measurement of trabecular bone by QCT, in fact, showed that combination therapy was associated with substantially smaller increases in BMD than monotherapy with PTH (Fig. 5). Bone turnover markers followed the expected course for anabolic (increases) or antiresorptive (decreases)

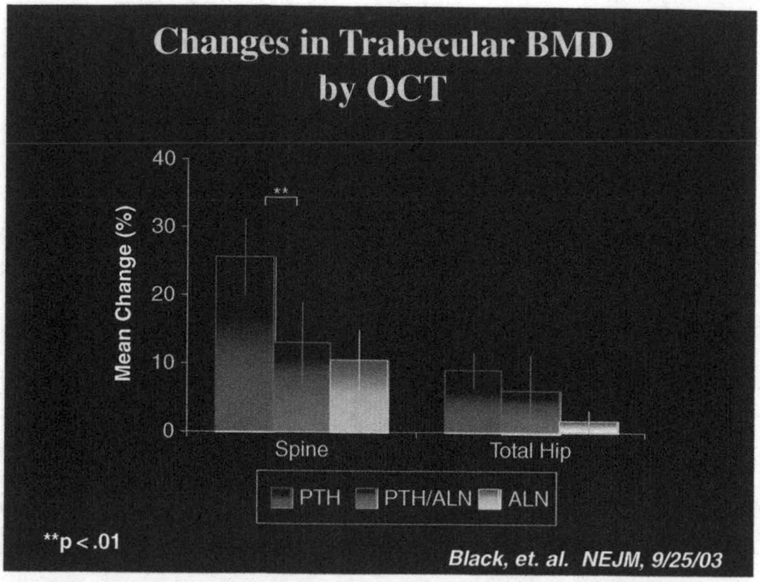

Fig. 5. The effect of combination therapy with PTH(1-84) and alendronate on bone density of the lumbar spine. The use of monotherapy with PTH(1-84) is clearly superior in increasing lumbar spine BMD by QCT than combination therapy or monotherapy with alendronate. Adapted from Ref. *(35)*.

therapy alone. However for combination therapy, bone markers followed the course of alendronate, not PTH therapy, with reductions in bone formation and bone resorption markers. This suggests that the impaired response to combination therapy, in comparison to PTH alone, might be due to the dominating effects of the antiresorptive agent to suppress bone dynamics when both drugs are used together. Since we do not have data referent to other aspects of bone quality, such as actual bone strength, it may be premature to reach the conclusion that combination therapy is necessarily not as good as or even inferior to monotherapy. For example, if an antiresorptive were not as powerfully suppressive as is alendronate on bone turnover, would the delay still be appreciated? Recent data by Deal et al. argue, to this point, that under certain circumstances, combination therapy can appear to be beneficial to monotherapy *(37)*. In a 6-month clinical trial, Deal et al. *(37)* showed that combination therapy with teriparatide and raloxifene may have more beneficial effects on hip bone density than monotherapy with teriparatide in postmenopausal osteoporosis. Bone formation markers increased similarly in both groups. Bone resorption markers, however, were reduced in the combination group. BMD increased to a similar extent in the lumbar spine and femoral neck in both groups, but the increase in total hip BMD was significantly greater in subjects treated with both teriparatide and raloxifene (Fig. 6). The effect of raloxifene, a less potent antiresorptive than alendronate, appears to allow teriparatide to stimulate bone formation, unimpeded, but does impair the ability of teriparatide to stimulate bone resorption. These actions may, thus, expand the anabolic window over that which is seen with teriparatide alone.

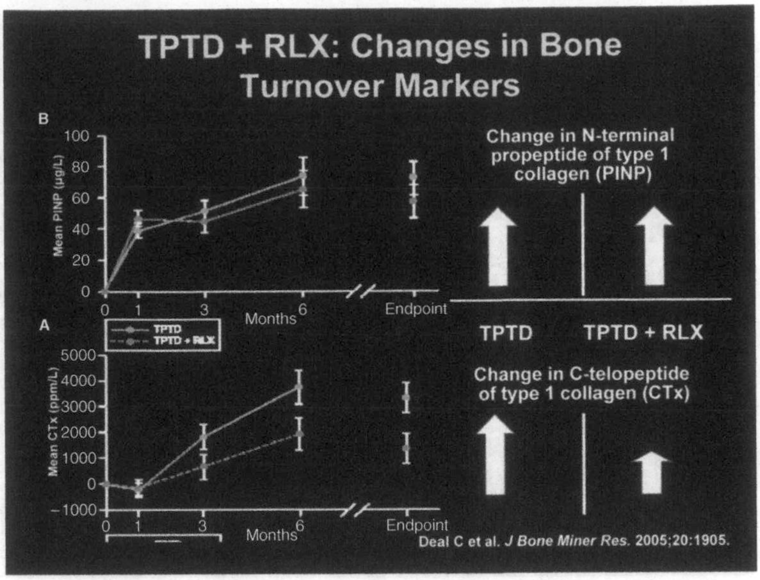

Fig. 6. The effect of combination therapy with teriparatide and raloxifene on indices of bone formation and bone resorption. Adapted from Deal et al. *(37)*.

CONSEQUENCES OF DISCONTINUING ANABOLIC THERAPY WITH PTH

Since teriparatide is approved for a very limited period of time, there are obvious concerns regarding the consequences of discontinuing therapy after this relatively short period of time. Some a priori concerns relate to the fact that new bone matrix is not fully mineralized following PTH therapy *(38)*. Therefore, this new bone matrix could be at risk for resorption if a period of consolidation with an antiresorptive is not used.

Published data addressing this concern were initially based on observational trials *(35)*. These studies, using either bisphosphonate *(21,39,40)* or estrogen *(41,42)* therapy following PTH, suggested that antiresorptive treatment may be necessary to maintain densitometric gains achieved during PTH administration. With a stronger experimental design, the PaTH study has provided prospective data in a rigorously controlled, blinded fashion to address this issue *(43)*. Postmenopausal women who had received PTH(1-84) for 12 months were randomly assigned to an additional 12 months of therapy with 10 mg of alendronate daily or placebo. In subjects who received alendronate, there was a further 4.9% gain in lumbar spine BMD while those who received placebo experienced a substantial decline. By QCT analysis, the net increase over 24 months in lumbar spine BMD among those treated with alendronate after PTH(1-84) was 30%. In those who received placebo after PTH(1-84), the net change in bone density was only 13% (Fig. 7). There were similar dramatic differences in hip BMD when those who followed PTH with alendronate were compared to those who were treated with placebo (13% versus 5%). The results of this study establish the importance of following PTH or teriparatide therapy with an antiresorptive.

Continued fracture efficacy over a longer period of time, well after the pivotal clinical trial was completed, was reported in the 30-month observational cohort following the trial

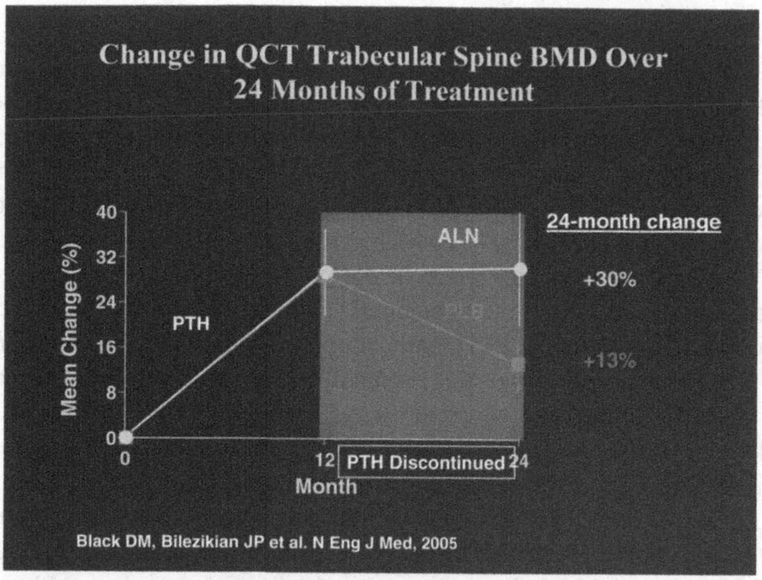

Fig. 7. Discontinuation of PTH(1-84) therapy after 1 year. As shown, the group of women who received alendronate were able to maintain their gains in trabecular spine BMD while those who were not treated had substantial declines. Adapted from Ref. *(43)*.

of Prince et al. *(21)*. Subjects were given the option of switching to a bisphosphonate or not taking any further medications following teriparatide. A majority (60%) were treated with antiresorptive therapy after PTH discontinuation. Gains in bone density were maintained in those who chose to begin antiresorptive therapy immediately after teriparatide. Reductions in BMD were progressive throughout the 30-month observational period in subjects who elected not to follow teriparatide with any therapy. In a group who did not begin antiresorptive therapy until 6 months after teriparatide discontinuation, major reductions in BMD were seen during these first 6 months but no further reductions were observed after antiresorptive initiation *(39)*. Despite these densitometric data, the effect of previous therapy with teriparatide and/or subsequent therapy with a bisphosphonate on fracture prevention persisted for as long as 31 months after teriparatide discontinuation. Non-vertebral fragility fractures were reported by proportionately fewer women previously treated with PTH (with or without a bisphosphonate) as compared with those treated with placebo (with or without a bisphosphonate; $p<0.03$). In a logistic regression model, bisphosphonate use for 12 months or longer was said to add little to overall risk reduction of new vertebral fractures in this post-treatment period. However, it is hard to be sure of this conclusion as the data were not separately analyzed into those who did or did not follow teriparatide treatment with an antiresorptive. Also, the above findings were in an observational study in which participants self-selected for the use of antiresorptive therapy after PTH treatment, making the results even more difficult to interpret. One might anticipate a residual but transient protection against fracture after PTH treatment without follow-up antiresorptive therapy which could wane over time. Additional studies are needed to address fracture outcomes specifically. However, based particularly on the PaTH trial, the importance of following PTH or teriparatide therapy with an antiresorptive to maintain increases in bone mass is clear.

SAFETY OF PTH

Overall, PTH is well tolerated. In the teriparatide trials, hypercalcemia occurred but in a very small percentage of subjects. The recent postmarketing experience would suggest that the incidence of verified hypercalcemia is even lower than initially reported *(44)*. With PTH(1-84), hypercalcemia occurred to a substantially greater extent *(29)*. An explanation for the greater incidence of hypercalcemia may relate, at least in part, to the inclusion criteria in which subjects in the PTH(1-84) could be enrolled even if their serum calcium was as much as 0.5 mg/dL above the upper limits of normal *(29)*. Hypercalcemia is generally corrected by reducing the amount of supplemental calcium and vitamin D. Hypercalcemia in the teriparatide trial did not occur to a significant degree while it did occur more commonly in the PTH(1-84) trial. Again, a partial explanation for these different observations may relate to the inclusion criteria in which subjects in the PTH(1-84) trial could be enrolled even if an element of hypercalciuria was present. Osteosarcoma has been seen in rats that have been given very high doses of either teriparatide or PTH(1-84) for prolonged periods of time *(45)*. It is considered unlikely that this animal toxicity is related to human skeletal physiology *(46,47)*, but in the United States, a warning is included in the labeling instructions. Over 300,000 individuals have been treated with teriparatide worldwide. Based on the epidemiology of osteosarcoma in the general population, one might expect that a case would have appeared by now. In fact, a case has recently been reported in whom a malignant process was diagnosed and variably read as osteosarcoma *(48)*. The case could not be completely studied and the diagnosis of osteosarcoma is still not clear. Even if this is a case of osteosarcoma, the expected incidence of osteosarcoma in the adult population, independent of the use of teriparatide, could well account for this observation.

FUTURE PERSPECTIVES

In the future, PTH may be modified for easier and more targeted delivery. Parathyroid hormone-related protein (PTHrP) has also been studied as an anabolic skeletal agent. In a small sample of postmenopausal women, subcutaneous administration of PTHrP resulted in a 4.7% increase in lumbar spine density after only 3 months of treatment *(49)*. Less frequent administration of PTH, such as once weekly, might also be an effective treatment option *(50)*. Cosman et al. *(34)* have reported on the use of cyclical 3-month courses of teriparatide against a backdrop of continued alendronate use. In comparison to regular, uninterrupted teriparatide use, the cyclic administration of teriparatide was associated with similar densitometric gains. Of further interest was the observation that with sequential 3-month cycles of teriparatide, bone formation markers that fell quickly when teriparatide was stopped, were stimulated to the same degree with each cycle. On the other hand, bone resorption markers showed smaller increases with successive cycles. This observation gives credence to the idea that the anabolic window is actually expanded when teriparatide is used in this context *(51)*. Cosman et al. *(52)* have shown that during long-term alendronate therapy, a rechallenge with PTH after 12 months off PTH increases bone formation, bone resorption, and BMD to a similar extent as during the first course of PTH administration. These data suggest that a future paradigm might be a second course of PTH given 12 months after a first course of therapy in patients who remain at high fracture risk. Apart from forms and ways to administer exogenous PTH, Gowen et al. *(53)* described an oral calcilytic molecule that antagonizes the parathyroid cell calcium receptor, thus stimulating the endogenous release of PTH. This approach could represent a novel endogenous delivery system for intermittent PTH administration.

CONCLUSIONS

Although antiresorptives remain the mainstay of osteoporosis treatment, the advent of anabolic skeletal agents is changing our approach to therapy. Parathyroid hormones as both the full-length molecule [PTH(1-84) and its truncated variant [PTH(1-34) have emerged as promising treatment options. For the first time, a drug is available that significantly improves microarchitectural, geometric, and other properties of bone. These changes in bone quality induced by anabolic therapy are attractive considering the goal of therapy for osteoporosis, namely to improve the basic underlying abnormalities that give rise to skeletal fragility.

REFERENCES

1. Hodsman AB, Bauer DC, Dempster D, Dian L, Hanley DA, Harris ST, Kendler D, McClung MR, Miller PD, Olszynski WP, Orwoll E, Yuen CK. Parathyroid hormone and teriparatide for the treatment of osteoporosis: a review of the evidence and suggested guidelines for its use. Endocr Rev, 2005; 26(5):688–703.
2. Dempster DW, Parisien M, Silverberg SJ, Liang XG, Schnitzer M, Shen V, Shane E, Kimmel DB, Recker R, Lindsay R, Bilezikian JP. On the mechanism of cancellous bone preservation in postmenopausal women with mild primary hyperparathyroidism. J Clin Endocrinol Metab, 1999;84(5):1562–1566.
3. Sato M, Zeng GQ, Turner CH. Biosynthetic human parathyroid hormone(1-34) effects on bone quality in aged ovariectomized rats. Endocrinology 1997;138:4330–4337.
4. Rubin M, Bilezikian J. The anabolic effects of parathyroid hormone therapy. Clin Geriatric Med 2002;19:415–432.
5. Hodsman AB, Fraher LJ, Ostbye T, Adachi JD, Steer BM. An evaluation of several biochemical markers for bone formation and resorptoin in a protocol utilizing cylical parathyroid hormone and calcitonin therapy for osteoporosis. J Clin Invest 1993;91:1138–1148.
6. Lindsay R, Zhou H, Cosman F, Nieves J, Dempster DW, Hodsman AB. Effects of one-month treatment with PTH(1-34) on bone formation on cancellous, endocortical, and periosteal surfaces of the human ilium. J Bone Miner Res 2007;22:495–502.
7. Jiang Y, Zhao JJ, Mitlak BH, Wang O, Genant HK, Eriksen EF. Recombinant human parathyroid hormone (1-34) [teriparatide] improves both cortical and cancellous bone structure. J Bone Miner Res 2003;18(11):1932–1941.
8. Burr DB, Hirano T, Turner CH, Hotchkiss C, Brommage R, Hock JM. Intermittently administered human parathyroid hormone(1-34) treatment increases intracortical bone turnover and porosity without reducing bone strength in the humerus of ovariectomized cynomolgus monkeys. J Bone Miner Res 2001;16(1): 157–165.
9. Parfitt AM. Parathyroid hormone and periosteal bone expansion. J Bone Miner Res 2002;17(10): 1741–1743.
10. Zanchetta JR, Bogado CE, Ferretti JL, Wang O, Wilson MG, Sato M, Gaich GA, Dalsky GP, Myers SL. Effects of teriparatide [recombinant human parathyroid hormone (1-34)] on cortical bone in postmenopausal women with osteoporosis. J Bone Miner Res 2003;18(3):539–543.
11. Uusi-Rasi K, Samanick LM, Zanchetta JR, Bogado CE, Eriksen EF, Sato M, Beck TJ. Effects of teriparatide [rhPTH(1-34)] treatment on structural geometry of the proximal femur in elderly osteoporotic women. Bone 2005;36:948–958.
12. Paschalis EP, Glass EV, Donley DW, Eriksen EF. Bone mineral and collagen quality in iliac crest biopsies of patients given teriparatide: new results from the fracture intervention trial. J Clin Endocrinol Metab 2005;90:4644–4649.

13. Keaveny TM, Donley DW, Hoffman PF, Mitlak BH, Glass EV, San Martin JA. Effects of teriparatide and alendronate on vertebral strength as assessed by finite element modeling of QCT scans in women with osteoporosis. J Bone Miner Res 2007;21:149–157.
14. Hock J. Basic aspects of PTH in skeletal Health; this book;
15. Lindsay R, Silverman SL, Cooper C, Hanley DA, Barton I, Broy SB, Licata A, Benhamou L, Geusens P, Flowers K, Stracke H, Seeman E. Risk of new vertebral fracture in the year following a fracture. JAMA 2001;285(3):320–323.
16. Neer RM, Arnaud CD, Zanchetta JR, Prince R, Gaich GA, Reginster JY, Hodsman AB, Eriksen EF, Ish-Shalom S, Genant HK, Wang L, Mitlak BH. Effect of parathyroid hormone (1-34) on fractures and bone mineral density in postmenopausal women with osteoporosis. N Engl J Med 2001;344(19): 1434–1441.
17. Gallagher JC, Genant HK, Crans CG, Vargas SJ, Krege JH. Teriparatide reduces the fracture risk associated with increasing number and severity of osteoporotic fractures. J Clin Endocrinol Metab 2005;90(3): 1583–1587.
18. Marcus R, Wang O, Satterwhite J, Mitlak B. The skeletal response to teriparatide is largely independent of age, initial bone mineral density, and prevalent vertebral fractures in postmenopausal women with osteoporosis. J Bone Miner Res 2003;18(1):18–23.
19. Miller PD, Shergy WJ, Body JJ, Chen P, Rohe ME, Krege JH. Long-term reduction of back pain risk in women with osteoporosis treated with teriparatide compared with alendronate. J Rheumatol 2005;32:1556–1562.
20. Miller PD, Schwartz EN, Chen P, Misurski DA, Krege JH. Teriparatide iin postmenopausal women with osteoporosis and mild or moderate renal impairment. Osteoporos Int 2007;18:59–68.
21. Prince R, Sipos A, Hossain A, Syversen U, Ish-Shalom S, Marcinowska E, Halse J, Lindsay R, Dalsky GP, Mitlak BJ, Sustained nonvertebral fragility fracture risk reduction after discontinuation of teriparatide treatment. J Bone Miner Res 2005;20(9):1507–1513.
22. Chen P, Miller PD, Delmas PD, Misurski DA, Krege JH. Change in lumbar spine BMD and vertebral fracture risk reduction in teriparatide-treated postmenopausal women with osteoporosis. J Bone Miner Res 2006;21:1785–1790.
23. Sarkar S, Mitlak BH, Wong M, Stock JL Black DM, Harper KD. Relationship between bone mineral density and incident vertebral fracture risk with raloxifene therapy. J Bone Miner Res 2002;17: 1–20.
24. Cummings SR, Karpf DB, Harris F, Genant HK, Ensrud K, LaCroix AX, Black DM. Improvement in spine bone density and reduction in risk of vertebral fractures during treatment with antiresorptive drugs. Am J Med 2002;112:281–289.
25, Watts NB, Geusens P, Barton IP, Felsenberg D. Relationship between changes in BMD and nonvertebral fracture incidence associated with risedronate: reduction in risk of fracture is not related to change in BMD. J Bone Miner Res 2005;20:2097–2104.
26. Hodsman AB, Hanley DA, Ettinger MP, Bolognese MA, Fox J, Metcalfe AJ, Lindsay R. Efficacy and safety of human parathyroid hormone-(1-84) in increasing bone mineral density in postmenopausal osteoporosis. J Clin Endocrinol Metab 2003;88(11):5212–5220.
27. Fox J, Miller MA, Recker RR, Bare SP, Smith SY, Moreau I. Treatment of postmenopausal osteoporotic women with parathyroid hormone 1-84 for 18 months increases cancellous bone formation and improves cancellous architecture: a study of iliac crest biopsies using histomorphometry and micro computed tomography. J Musculoskelet Neuronal Interact 2005;5(4):356–357.
28. Greenspan SL, Bone HG, Ettinger MP, Hanley DA, Lindsay R, Zanchetta JR, Blosch CM, Mathisen AL, Morris SA, Marriott TB. Effect of recombinant human parathyroid hormone (1-84) on vertebral fracture and bone mineral density in postmenopausal women with osteoporosis: a randomized trial. Ann Intern Med 2007;146:326–339.
29. Kurland ES, Cosman F, McMahon DJ, Rosen CJ, Lindsay R, Bilezikian JP. Parathyroid hormone as a therapy for idiopathic osteoporosis in men: effects on bone mineral density and bone markers. J Clin Endocrinol Metab 2000;85(9):3069–3076.
30. Orwoll ES, Scheele WH, Paul S, Adami S, Syversen U, Diez-Perez A, Kaufman JM, Clancy AD, Gaich GA. The effect of teriparatide [human parathyroid hormone (1-34)] therapy on bone density in men with osteoporosis. J Bone Miner Res 2003;18(1):9–17.

31. Kaufman JM, Orwoll E, Goemaere S, San Martin J, Hossain A, Dalsky GP, Lindsay R, Mitlak BH. Teriparatide effects on vertebral fractures and bone mineral density in men with osteoporosis: treatment and discontinuation of therapy. Osteoporos Int 2004;16(5):510–516.
32. Cosman F, Nieves J, Woelfert L, Formica C, Gordon S, Shen V, Lindsay R. Parathyroid hormone added to established hormone therapy: effects on vertebral fracture and maintenance of bone mass after parathyroid hormone withdrawal. J Bone Miner Res 2001;16(5):925–931.
33. Ettinger B, San Martin J, Crans G, Pavo I. Differential effects of teriparatide on BMD after treatment with raloxifene or alendronate. J Bone Miner Res 2004;19(5):745–751.
34. Cosman F, Nieves J, Zion M, Woelfert L, Luckey M, Lindsay R. Daily and cyclic parathyroid hormone in women receiving alendronate. N Eng J Med 2005;353:566–575.
35. Black DM, Greenspan SL, Ensrud KE, Palermo L, McGowan JA, Lang TF, Garnero P, Bouxsein ML, Bilezikian JP, Rosen CJ. The effects of parathyroid hormone and alendronate alone or in combination in postmenopausal osteoporosis. N Engl J Med 2003;349(13):1207–1215.
36. Finkelstein JS, Hayes A, Hunzelman JL, Wyland JJ, Lee H, Neer RM. The effects of parathyroid hormone, alendronate, or both in men with osteoporosis. N Engl J Med 2003;349(13):1216–1226.
37. Deal C, Omizo M, Schwartz EN, Eriksen EF, Cantor P, Wang J, Glass EV, Myers SL, Krege JH. Combination teriparatide and raloxifene therapy for postmenopausal osteoporosis: results from a 6-month double-blind placebo-controlled trial. J Bone Miner Res 2005;20(11):1905–1911.
38. Misof BM, Roschger P, Cosman F, Kurland ES, Tesch W, Messmer P, Dempster DW, Nieves J, Shane E, Fratzl P, Klaushofer K, Bilezikian J, Lindsay R. Effects of intermittent parathyroid hormone administration on bone mineralization density in iliac crest biopsies from patients with osteoporosis: a paired study before and after treatment. J Clin Endocrinol Metab 2003;88(3):1150–1156.
39. Lindsay R, Scheele WH, Neer R, Pohl G, Adami S, Mautalen C, Reginster JY, Stepan JJ, Myers SL, Mitlak BH. Sustained vertebral fracture risk reduction after withdrawal of teriparatide in postmenopausal women with osteoporosis. Arch Intern Med 2004;164(18):2024–2030.
40. Kurland ES, Heller SL, Diamond B, McMahon DJ, Cosman F, Bilezikian JP. The importance of bisphosphonate therapy in maintaining bone mass in men after therapy with teriparatide [human parathyroid hormone(1-34)]. Osteoporos Int 2004;15:992–997.
41. Lindsay R, Nieves J, Formica C, Henneman E, Woelfert L, Shen V, Dempster D, Cosman F. Randomised controlled study of effect of parathyroid hormone on vertebral-bone mass and fracture incidence among postmenopausal women on oestrogen with osteoporosis. Lancet 1997;350(9077):550–555.
42. Lane NE, Sanchez S, Modin GW, Genant HK, Pierini E, Arnaud CD. Bone mass continues to increase at the hip after parathyroid hormone treatment is discontinued in glucocorticoid-induced osteoporosis: results of a randomized controlled clinical trial. J Bone Miner Res 2000;15(5):944–951.
43. Black DM, Bilezikian JP, Ensrud KE, Greenspan SL, Palermo L, Hue T, Lang TF, McGowan JA, Rosen CJ. One year of alendronate after one year of parathyroid hormone (1-84) for osteoporosis. N Engl J Med 2005;353(6):555–565.
44. Harper KD, Krege JH, Marcus R, Mitlak BH. Comments on initial experience with teriparatide in the United States. Curr Med Res Opin 2006;22:1927.
45. Vahle JL, Long GG, Sandusky G, Westmore M, Ma YL, Sato M. Bone neoplasms in F344 rats given teriparatide [rhPTH(1-34)] are dependent on duration of treatment and dose. Toxicol Pathol 2004;32(4):426–438.
46. Jimenez C, Kim W, Al Sagier F, El Naggar A, Sellin R, Berry D, Gagel RF. Primary hyperparathyroidism and osteosarcoma: examination of a large osteosarcoma cohort identifies unique characteristics. J Bone Miner Res 2003;18(Suppl 2):LB6.
47. Tashjian AH Jr, Gagel RF. Teriparatide [human PTH(1-34)]: 2.5 years of experience on the use and safety of the drug for the treatment of osteoporosis. J Bone Min Res 2006;21:354–365.
48. Harper KD, Krege JH, Marcus R, Mitlak BH. Osteosarcoma and teriparatide? J Bone Miner Res 2007;22:334.
49. Horwitz MJ, Tedesco MB, Gundberg C, Garcia-Ocana A, Stewart AF. Short-term, high-dose parathyroid hormone-related protein as a skeletal anabolic agent for the treatment of postmenopausal osteoporosis. J Clin Endocrinol Metab 2003;88(2):569–575.
50. Black DM, Rosen CJ. Parsimony with PTH: is a single weekly injection of PTH superior to a larger cumulative dose given daily? J Bone Miner Res 2002;17(Suppl 1):SA367.

51. Heaney RP, Recker RR. Combination and sequential therapy for osteoporosis. N Engl J Med 2005;353(6):624–625.
52. Cosman F, Nieves JW, Zion M, Barbuto N, Lindsay R. Effects of PTH rechallenge 1 year after the first PTH course in patients on long-term alendronate. J Bone Min Res 2005;20(Suppl I):1079. Nashville, Tenn. Sept. 23–27.
53. Gowen M, Stroup GB, Dodds RA, James IE, Votta BJ, Smith BR, Bhatnagar PK, Lago AM, Callahan JF, DelMar EG, Miller MA, Nemeth EF, Fox J. Antagonizing the parathyroid calcium receptor stimulates parathyroid hormone secretion and bone formation in osteopenic rats. J Clin Invest 2000;105(11): 1595–1604.

23 Screening for Osteoporosis

Margaret L. Gourlay, MD, MPH

CONTENTS

Key Words: Aged, bone density, fracture, mass screening, osteoporosis, postmenopausal/diagnosis, risk factors

INTRODUCTION

The burden of fracture will increase with growth of the elderly population, and by 2020 an estimated half of Americans over 50 years of age may be at risk of fractures from osteoporosis and low bone density *(1)*. Osteoporosis screening has been proposed to identify and treat individuals at high risk of fracture in an effort to reduce fracture-related morbidity and mortality. Mass osteoporosis screening (large-scale screening of whole population groups) is not likely to be cost-effective in any setting *(2)*, so more selective approaches to disease detection have been investigated.

This chapter reviews the elements of a rational screening program, current evidence-based approaches to osteoporosis screening, and future research that would support development of a cost-effective osteoporosis screening protocol. The chapter focuses on women with primary (postmenopausal and age-related) osteoporosis, since the best evidence on screening is available for this group. Patients with secondary osteoporosis and men are discussed separately (see "Screening in Special Populations").

GENERAL PRINCIPLES OF SCREENING

Screening is the early diagnosis of pre-symptomatic disease among well individuals in the general population *(3)*. The decision to screen depends on more than the availability of

From: *Contemporary Endocrinology: Osteoporosis: Pathophysiology and Clinical Management*
Edited by: R. A. Adler, DOI 10.1007/978-1-59745-459-9_23,

a screening test. The natural history and epidemiology of the disease, economic and health policy issues, and benefits versus risks of screening must also be carefully considered. Wilson and Jungner *(4)* proposed the following criteria for a rational screening program (abbreviated below):

1. The condition sought should be an important health problem.
2. There should be an accepted treatment for patients with recognized disease and an agreed upon policy on whom to treat.
3. There should be a recognizable latent or early symptomatic stage, and the natural history of the condition, including development from latent to declared disease, should be adequately understood.
4. There should be a suitable test or examination that is acceptable to the population.
5. The cost of case-finding (including diagnosis and treatment of patients diagnosed) should be economically balanced in relation to possible expenditure on medical care as a whole.

Despite the apparent simplicity of these requirements, screening is widely misunderstood and misused and potential harms of screening are underappreciated *(5)*. Because screening is conducted on apparently healthy, asymptomatic individuals, every adverse outcome of screening is iatrogenic and entirely preventable. Thus, a screening program should only be initiated if the disease meets fundamental screening criteria, and patients and health care providers are ready to accept all arms of the "screening cascade," including adverse outcomes from all types of test results (Fig. 1). Even true-positive tests are only helpful if treatment is more effective at an early stage of disease, rather than later when symptoms first become apparent.

Although osteoporosis meets most of Wilson and Junger's criteria, the best strategy for screening for patients at risk of fracture is still uncertain. This chapter includes a discussion of several strategies in practice or proposed by early 2007.

RESEARCH ON OSTEOPOROSIS SCREENING APPROACHES

A population-based randomized, controlled trial of osteoporosis screening is unlikely to be feasible. However, most screening programs currently implemented for other disorders are not based on evidence from RCTs. Well-done observational studies of screening can help inform a successful screening program if the potential effects of patient self-selection bias (volunteer bias), lead-time bias, and length bias are carefully considered *(6)*. For osteoporosis, the highest level of evidence for screening may come from cohort studies; for example, Kern et al. *(7)* conducted a nonconcurrent cohort study of bone density screening in men and women aged 65 and older participating in a population-based cardiovascular study. Hip bone density screening was associated with 36% fewer incident hip fractures over 6 years compared with usual medical care, but confounding in the study was difficult to characterize. Case–control studies would probably be less helpful due to confounding and bias in selection of cases and controls.

This section describes an analytic framework for osteoporosis screening research and reviews two categories of evidence in the framework: evidence on risk factor assessment and evidence on bone density screening.

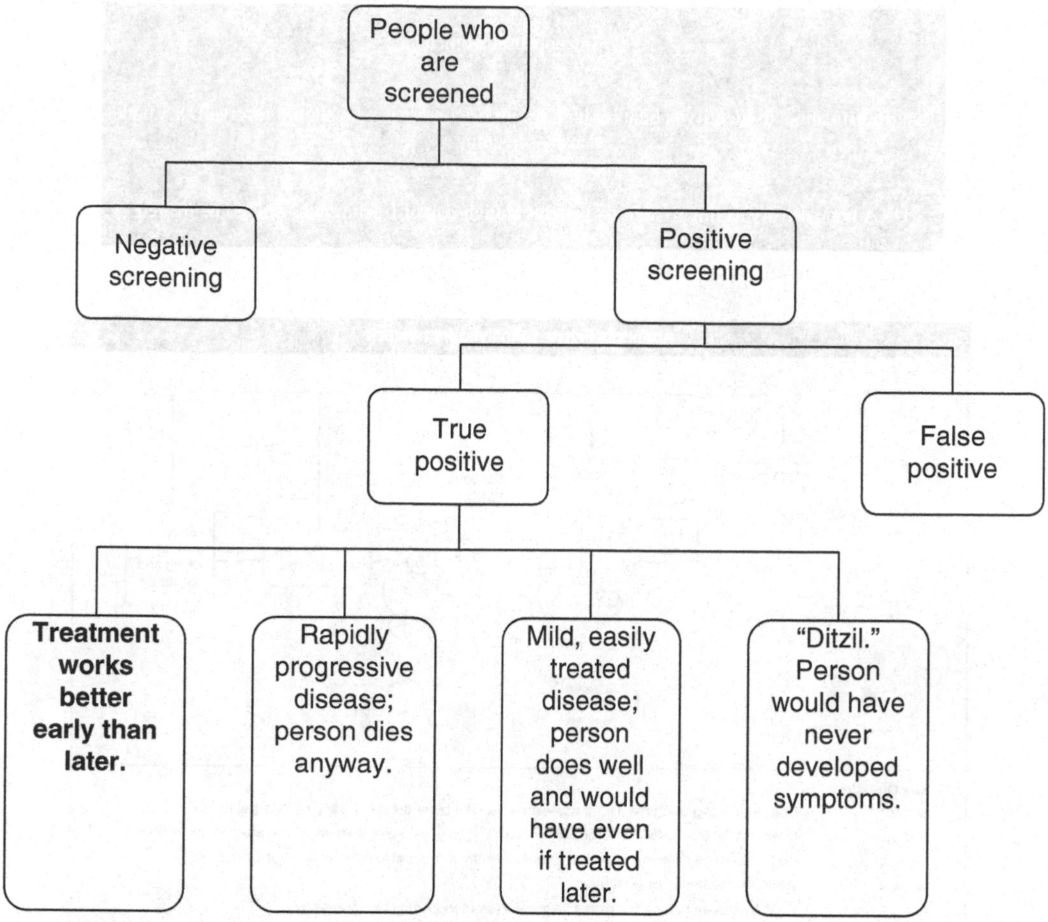

Fig. 1. The screening cascade (slide from Russell Harris, MD, MPH, Third US Preventive Services Task Force).

Analytic Framework for Screening

In 2002, the US Preventive Services Task Force (USPSTF) published an analytic framework for osteoporosis screening as a basis for its age-based screening guidelines for postmenopausal women in the general population *(8)* (Fig. 2). The analytic framework was divided into key questions in a chain of logic that evidence must support to link screening to improved health outcomes. Regarding key question #1, no randomized trial has shown direct evidence that screening reduces fractures, and such a trial is probably not feasible *(9)*. The Task Force proposed two other key questions regarding indirect evidence on risk stratification methods (key question #2) and dual energy X-ray absorptiometry (DXA) bone density testing (key question #3) to support screening for osteoporosis in postmenopausal women. Most screening research to date has focused on a two-step process involving these questions, i.e.:

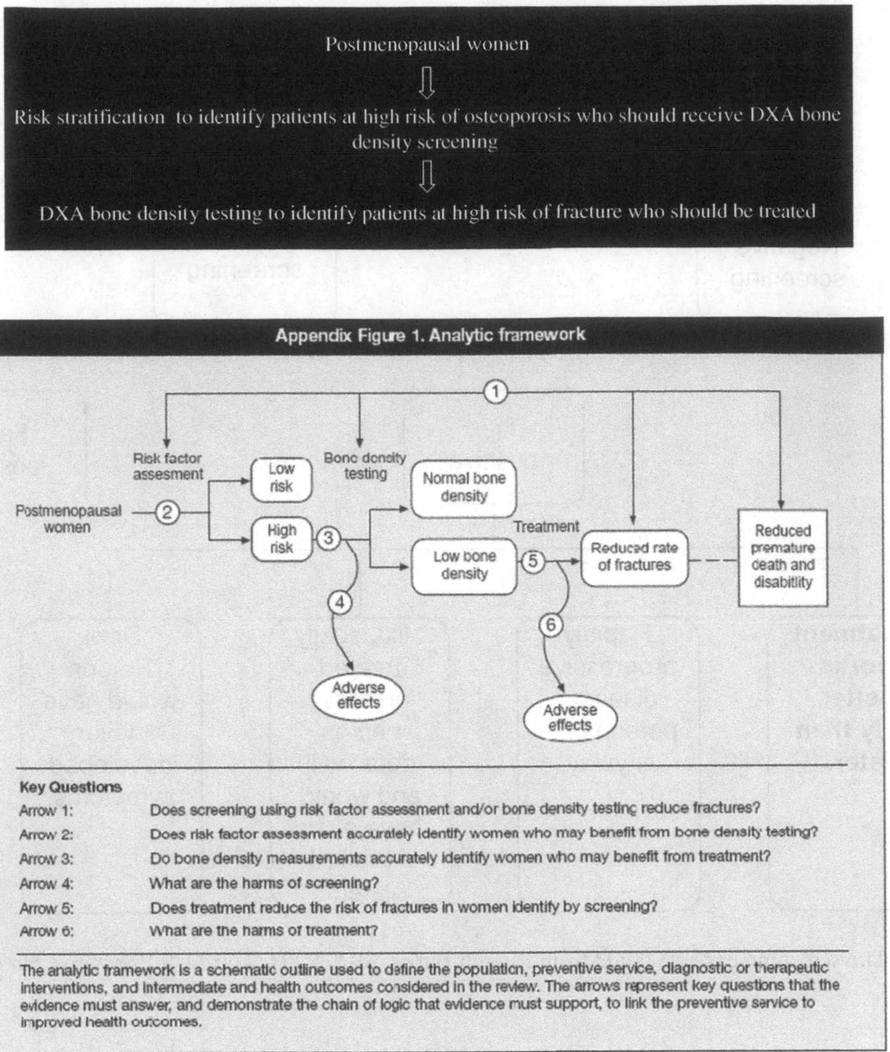

Fig. 2. US Preventive Services Task Force Osteoporosis Screening Analytic Framework *(85)*.

Observational data on risk factor assessment, other risk stratification methods, and bone density testing are described below.

Risk Factor Assessment Before Screening

Although the USPSTF supported the use of risk factor assessment in an osteoporosis screening program, the most useful risk factors and method to apply risk assessment are uncertain. Two types of risk factor assessment have been investigated:

1. Osteoporosis risk assessment to decide which patients should have DXA bone density testing. This has been examined in diagnostic accuracy studies of osteoporosis risk assessment tools.
2. Fracture risk assessment used as an adjunct to bone density testing to decide which patients should be treated. This has been examined in modeling studies with varied approaches and

results, i.e., while several modeling studies have supported use of risk factors to predict fracture *(10–12)*, a 2006 decision analysis indicated that use of risk factors might be less cost-effective than mass bone density screening alone in women aged 70–80 *(13)*. The World Health Organization developed a new "absolute fracture probability algorithm" from a model that incorporates risk factor data from a number of different international data sets. This treatment decision aid was released in 2008.

There is little consensus regarding the best risk factors to use, or whether the same risk factors should be used for each purpose above. The discussion in this section focuses on the first purpose: osteoporosis risk assessment to help guide the decision to screen.

An exhaustive assessment of osteoporosis risk factors is time consuming in a busy primary care practice; therefore, several risk assessment tools have been developed for easy use in clinical settings *(14–18)* (Table 1). These tools were designed to help target bone density testing to women who are most likely to benefit from central (hip and lumbar spine) bone density screening. All of the tools include age and weight, since these variables are the strongest predictors of osteoporosis in postmenopausal women *(19)*.

Osteoporosis Self-Assessment Tool (OST)

The OST was developed from data on 860 community-dwelling postmenopausal women aged 45–88 years (mean age 62.3 years) recruited from 21 clinics in 8 Asian countries *(14)*. This index, based only on age and weight, is the simplest of all osteoporosis risk assessment tools developed to date. A cut point of −1 (≤ -1 is high risk) yielded a sensitivity of 91% and specificity of 45% to detect femoral neck osteoporosis in the development cohort. The OST has been validated in populations of women from Japan (in the original study), the United States *(20)*, Belgium *(21)*, and the Netherlands *(20)* and has shown discriminative ability equivalent to more complex risk tools. Due to its simplicity and good performance, the OST may have the best potential for use in clinical practice *(22,23)*.

Osteoporosis Risk Assessment Instrument (ORAI)

The ORAI development cohort included 926 women aged 45 years and older (mean age 62.8 years) randomly selected using an age and region-stratified sampling frame in the Canadian population *(15)*. The development cohort was predominantly white (94.9%) and postmenopausal (88.3%). The final instrument was based on age, weight, and current estrogen use. Using a score threshold of 9 (≥ 9 is high risk), the tool had a sensitivity of 90.0% and specificity of 45.1% to detect women with low bone density (femoral neck or lumbar spine bone mineral density value of ≥ 2 SDs below the mean for young Canadian women), and a sensitivity of 97.0% and specificity of 41.3% to detect women with osteoporosis in the development cohort. Results were similar in a validation cohort drawn from the same study population ($n = 450$). Cadarette further validated the ORAI in two comparative studies of osteoporosis decision rules in Canadian study populations *(24,25)*.

Simple Calculated Osteoporosis Risk Estimation (SCORE)

The SCORE development cohort included 1279 postmenopausal women aged 45 years and older (mean age 61.5 years) recruited by investigators at 106 US academic and community-based multispecialty centers *(17)*. Participating study sites were 50% family medicine, geriatric or general internal medicine clinics, 20% endocrinology, 20% rheumatology, and 10% gynecology clinics. The development cohort had limited ethnic diversity

Table 1
Published Sensitivity (Sn) and Specificity (Sp) for Osteoporosis Risk Assessment Tools

Tool	*Study*	*Participants*	*Subgroup*	*Outcome*	*"High-risk" score cut point*	*Sn (%)*	*Sp (%)*
OST	Koh et al. *(14)*	Community-dwelling postmenopausal Asian women	Development cohort (*n*=860), validation cohort (*n*=1123)	FN T-score ≤ –2.5, same	≤–1, same	91, 98	45, 29
	Geusens et al. *(20)*	Postmenopausal women from United States (*n*=1102) and the Netherlands	–	FN T-score ≤–2.5	<2	88	52
ORAI	Cadarette et al. *(15)*	Community-dwelling Canadian women, 88% postmenopausal	Development cohort (*n*=926), validation cohort (*n*=450)	FN or LS T-score ≤–2.0, same	≥9, same	90, 93.3	45.1, 46.4
	Cadarette et al. *(24)*	Community-dwelling postmenopausal Canadian women (*n*=2365)	–	FN T-score, <–2.0	≥9	94.2	31.9
	Geusens et al. *(20)*	Postmenopausal women from United States (*n*=1102) and the Netherlands	–	FN T-score, ≤–2.0	>8	82	58

SCORE	Lydick et al. *(17)*	Women recruited from general medicine and subspecialty clinics at a US site, 90% postmenopausal	Development cohort (n=1424), validation cohort (n=259)	FN T score, ≤–2.0, same	≥6, same	89.4, 91	49.7, 40
	Cadarette et al. *(24)*	Community-dwelling postmenopausal Canadian women (n=2365)	–	FN T-score, <–2.0	≥6	97.5	20.8
	Geusens et al. *(20)*	Postmenopausal women from United States (n=1102) and the Netherlands	–	FN T-score, ≤–2.0	>7	80	65
OSIRIS	Ben Sedrine et al. *(16)*	Postmenopausal white-women aged 60–80 (n=1303)	–	FN, total hip or LS T-score <–2.5	≤1	78.5	51.4

FN, femoral neck; LS, lumbar spine.

(89% white, 6% African American, 3% Latino, 3% others or missing). The final scoring system included these factors: age, weight, estrogen use, race, history of rheumatoid arthritis, and history of nontraumatic fractures. Using a threshold score of 6 (≥6 is high risk), the tool had a sensitivity of 90% and specificity of 47% to detect low bone density (femoral neck bone density T-score ≤–2.0) in the development cohort. The SCORE was subsequently tested in data from studies of postmenopausal women in the United States *(20)*, Canada *(24)*, Belgium *(21,26)*, and the Netherlands *(20)*.

Osteoporosis Index of Risk (OSIRIS)

The WHO Collaborating Center for Public Health Aspects of Rheumatic Diseases in Liège, Belgium developed the osteoporosis index of risk (OSIRIS) based on data from 1303 postmenopausal white women aged 60–80 years seen consecutively at an outpatient osteoporosis center between January and December 1999 *(16)*. Women who had taken pharmacological agents for osteoporosis except for hormone therapy, calcium, or vitamin D were excluded. The final index was based on these variables: age, body weight, current hormone therapy use, and history of previous low impact fracture. Using a threshold score of +1 (>+1 is low risk), the sensitivity and specificity of the OSIRIS to detect osteoporosis were 78.5 and 51.4%, respectively. The OSIRIS was subsequently validated in a study of 889 postmenopausal women from France *(27)*.

Other Risk Stratification Methods

Peripheral Bone Density Testing

Peripheral (forearm or heel) bone density is measured by peripheral DXA, which offers the advantages of measurement by a portable densitometer, lower cost, and operation by a less skilled operator than is necessary for central DXA. However, as stated by the International Society for Clinical Densitometry, "there is a lack of consensus on how results from peripheral sites should be interpreted and the capacity of peripheral measurements to identify patients with low central BMD remains debated *(28)*." Because peripheral bone density measures at the heel and forearm may be discordant with central (hip and lumbar spine) measures, and because WHO diagnostic criteria for osteoporosis generally refer to central measures, peripheral measurements alone are insufficient for a comprehensive study of osteoporosis screening. However, peripheral DXA has been studied as a method to help select patients who are likely to benefit from central DXA *(29,30)*.

Bone Quantitative Ultrasound

Although bone quantitative ultrasound has been shown to predict osteoporotic fractures independent of bone mineral density *(31,32)*, its possible role in screening is uncertain. Bone ultrasound has been studied as a method to identify high-risk patients who should have diagnostic central DXA testing. A 2006 meta-analysis of 25 studies examined post-test probabilities of central osteoporosis using calcaneal ultrasound T-score cut points of –0.5, –1.0, and –1.5 in women aged 50 years and older *(33)*. At these cut points, sensitivity and specificity did not definitively rule out or rule in osteoporosis by WHO DXA criteria [e.g., for the quantitative ultrasound index parameter T-score threshold of *–1*, sensitivity was *79%* (95% CI, *69–86%*) and specificity was *58%* (CI, *44–70%*); for T-score threshold of 0, sensitivity was 93% (CI, *87–97%*) but specificity decreased to *24%*

(CI, *10–47%*)]. A 2005 cost-effectiveness analysis of bone quantitative ultrasound in 115 women aged 40–80 referred from general practices in the United Kingdom showed that ultrasound pre-screening would only be cost-effective if performed at a cost substantially less than 16 British pounds (estimated unit cost for 2001–2002) *(34)*.

Barriers to Implementation of Osteoporosis Risk Stratification Methods

Some studies of osteoporosis risk assessment tools have shown favorable results, but insufficient evidence currently exists to support their implementation in primary care settings. The diagnostic accuracy of osteoporosis risk assessment tools in studies of postmenopausal women has been reasonably good (area under the receiver operating characteristic curves ranged from 0.71 to 0.81); however, different studies have used different cut points to achieve optimal sensitivity and specificity *(20,22)*. Such cut point adjustments are not possible in clinical settings where the prevalence of risk factors and osteoporosis in the entire patient population is unknown. Future studies need to test the tools in larger primary care populations to evaluate test performance and determine appropriate score cut points for routine use in postmenopausal women in primary care settings. The OST risk assessment tool (based only on age and weight) should also be further tested in men, since only a few small studies have indicated that the OST may have good diagnostic accuracy in elderly men *(35)*.

Similarly, studies of peripheral DXA and bone ultrasound have used varying "high-risk" T-score cut points in different patient populations. These machines also lack widely accepted reference standards like the NHANES III bone density tables that are available for central DXA measures *(36,37)*. Peripheral bone density screening devices should not be used for risk stratification in clinical settings unless standard cut points and appropriate reference data become available.

Bone Density Screening

Screening strategies are currently based on the operational definition of osteoporosis, which is a central (hip or lumbar spine) bone density T-score ≤ –2.5 (World Health Organization diagnostic criteria) *(38)*. The T-score is a standard deviation score that compares the patient's bone mineral density to the mean value in a reference population of young, healthy adults. This score has been shown to predict fracture in large prospective studies of postmenopausal women *(39,40)*.

Although the WHO diagnostic criteria were designed for postmenopausal women, they were never intended to be a recommendation for screening of all women at or after menopause, and a T-score diagnosis of osteoporosis was not meant to be the sole basis for initiating treatment *(41)*. As mentioned earlier, the WHO absolute fracture probability algorithm and other approaches to fracture risk assessment have incorporated bone density T-scores and risk factors for fracture to help guide treatment decisions.

OSTEOPOROSIS SCREENING GUIDELINES

US Preventive Services Task Force Screening Guidelines

In 2002, the US Preventive Services Task Force published age-based screening guidelines for the general population *(8)* based on a systematic review of key questions in an analytic framework for osteoporosis screening (Fig. 2). For women aged 65 and older, the Task Force recommended routine bone density testing to screen for osteoporosis (grade B recommendation). Medicare covers screening every 2 years for women in this age range, and the National Committee for Quality Assurance has used bone density testing or prescription for a drug to treat or prevent osteoporosis within 6 months after a fracture as a performance measure for health care in women aged 67 years and older *(42)*.

Since osteoporosis is less common in younger age groups, widespread screening would not be cost-effective. For this reason, the Task Force recommended risk assessment to help guide the decision to order a bone density test in women aged 60–64 years. Evidence was inconclusive regarding the benefit of routine osteoporosis screening in postmenopausal women under the age of 60 (grade C recommendation) *(8)*. Similarly, a 2006 analysis by Sanders et al. *(43)* found that fracture prevention was not cost-effective for women aged 50–59. The Task Force also mentioned that insufficient data exist to recommend an optimal screening interval or to develop evidence-based screening guidelines for non-white women.

Publication of the next Task Force report on osteoporosis screening is anticipated in 2010. (personal communication, Russell Harris, MD, MPH, Third US Preventive Services Task Force).

National Osteoporosis Foundation Guidelines

The National Osteoporosis Foundation (NOF) developed the Clinician's Guide to Prevention and Treatment of Osteoporosis, most recently updated in 2008 *(44)* (Table 2). The National Osteoporosis Foundation (NOF) developed the Physician's Guide to Prevention and Treatment of Osteoporosis, most recently updated in 2003 *(44)* (Table 2). The guide was developed by an expert committee in collaboration with a multispecialty

Table 2.
Screening recommendations from the National Osteoporosis Foundation Guidelines for the Prevention and Treatment of Osteoporosis *(44)*

The NOF recommends bone density testing in these categories of patients:
1. In women age 65 and older and men age 70 and older.*
2. In postmenopausal women and men age 50–70, when you have concern based on their risk factor profile.**
3. To those who have suffered a fracture, to determine degree of disease severity.

*Medicare currently covers BMD testing for the following individuals age 65 and older:
Estrogen deficient women at clinical risk for osteoporosis
Individuals with vertebral abnormalities
Individuals receiving, or planning to receive, long-term glucocorticoid (steroid) therapy
Individuals with primary hyperparathyroidism
Individuals being monitored to assess the response or efficacy of an approved osteoporosis drug therapy

Medicare permits individuals to repeat BMD testing every 2 years.

** Risk factors included in the WHO fracture risk assessment model: current age, gender, personal history of a fracture, femoral neck BMD, low body mass index (kg/m^2), use oral glucocorticoid therapy, secondary osteoporosis (e.g., rheumatoid arthritis), parental history of hip fracture, current smoking, alcohol intake 3 or more drinks per day.

council of medical experts in the field of bone health. Recommendations were primarily based on evidence from controlled clinical trials; they were not reported to be based on a systematic review of the literature.

European Case-Finding Approach

Kanis has compared a European case-finding approach to more inclusive US osteoporosis screening recommendations *(45)* (Fig. 3). In a 2005 position paper, he compared a case-finding strategy currently implemented in several European countries *(46)* to a mass bone density screening program for all women aged 65 (supported in some US guidelines) and a screening policy based on a program using "pre-screening" with risk assessment

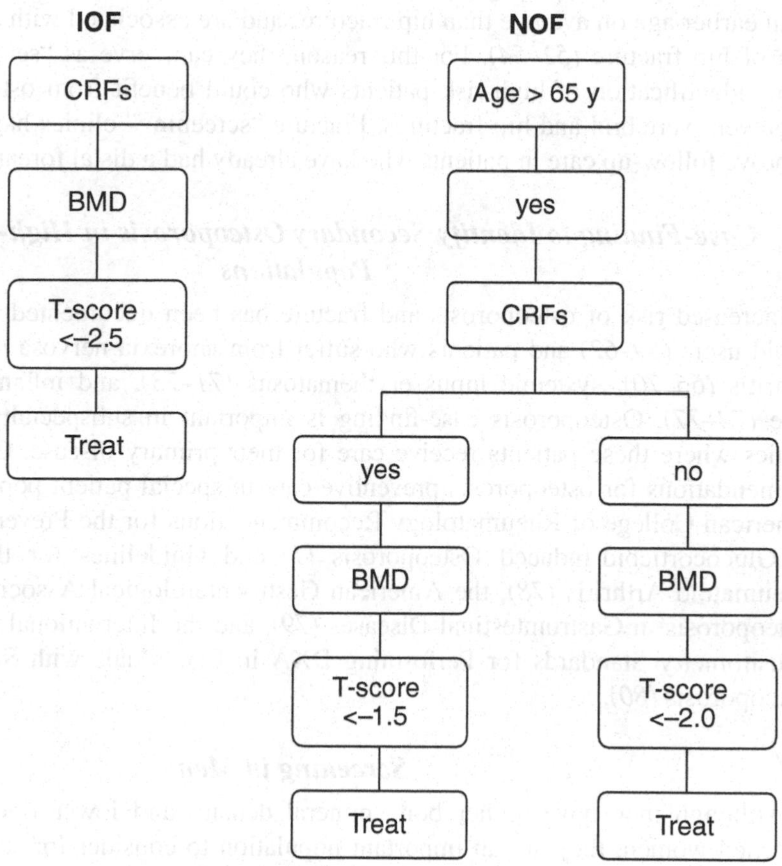

IOF International Osteoporosis Foundation
NOF National Osteoporosis Foundation
CRF clinical risk factor
BMD bone mineral density

Fig. 3. Comparison of case-finding/screening strategies of the International Osteoporosis Foundation and National Osteoporosis Foundation (US). Slide from John Kanis, MD, International Osteoporosis Foundation World Congress on Osteoporosis, Plenary Lecture "WHO Criteria for Indications to Treatment," June 2006 *(87)*.

before bone density testing *(47)*. The risk factors used in the latter strategy were age, BMI, previous fragility fracture, maternal history of any fragility fracture, smoking, long-term use of corticosteroids, and secondary causes of osteoporosis. The risk assessment/pre-screening strategy was more efficient than the other two approaches, since the gradient of fracture risk per standard deviation in risk score was higher than with the use of BMD alone; this improved the sensitivity of screening without sacrificing specificity.

SCREENING IN SPECIAL POPULATIONS

Fracture Clinics

Numerous studies have documented inadequate osteoporosis preventive care for patients even after they sustain a fragility fracture *(48–51)*. Distal forearm (Colle's) fractures occur at an earlier age on average than hip fractures and are associated with a higher subsequent rate of hip fracture *(52–54)*. For this reason, they can serve as "sentinel" fractures that allow identification of high-risk patients who could benefit from osteoporosis treatment to prevent vertebral and hip fractures. Fracture "screening" clinics have been designed to improve follow-up care in patients who have already had a distal forearm fracture *(55–58)*.

Case-Finding to Identify Secondary Osteoporosis in High-Risk Disease Populations

Increased risk of osteoporosis and fracture has been documented in chronic corticosteroid users *(59–62)* and patients who suffer from anorexia nervosa *(63–65)*, rheumatoid arthritis *(66–70)*, systemic lupus erythematosus *(71–73)*, and inflammatory bowel disease *(74–77)*. Osteoporosis case-finding is important in subspecialty and primary care clinics where these patients receive care for their primary disease. Guidelines with recommendations for osteoporosis preventive care in special patient populations include the American College of Rheumatology Recommendations for the Prevention and Treatment of Glucocorticoid-Induced Osteoporosis *(1)* and Guidelines for the Management of Rheumatoid Arthritis *(78)*, the American Gastroenterological Association Guidelines on Osteoporosis in Gastrointestinal Diseases *(79)*, and the International Society for Clinical Densitometry Standards for Performing DXA in Individuals with Secondary Causes of Osteoporosis *(80)*.

Screening in Men

Although men have higher bone mineral density and lower fracture risk than age-matched women, they are an important population to consider for screening due to their higher mortality rate after hip fracture *(81)* and higher likelihood of having potentially modifiable secondary causes of osteoporosis *(82)*. In its 2005 Position Development Conference Report, the International Society for Clinical Densitometry *(83)* recommended bone density testing in men aged 70 and older in the general population. This report was developed based on literature searches of PubMed, EMBASE, and MEDLINE performed by ISCD subcommittee members using a modified method used in Cochrane Reviews and the proposed official positions developed by the subcommittees were reviewed by an expert panel. In a 2002 guideline statement, the ISCD also recommended bone density testing for men with prior fragility fractures or conditions widely recognized to increase risk of bone loss and fracture, e.g., hypogonadism, corticosteroid treatment, hyperparathyroidism, alcohol abuse, anticonvulsant use, prior gastrectomy *(84)*. The 2008 National Osteoporosis Foundation guidelines recommend screening in men. The Canadian Osteoporosis Society has recommended case-finding and bone density testing in men aged 65 and older.

CLINICAL RECOMMENDATIONS

Since safe and effective treatments are available and since bone density testing is safe and has good accuracy and reliability, osteoporosis screening will probably continue to increase despite insufficient evidence to support a specific protocol. The following clinical recommendations for screening are based on the non-systematic evidence review conducted for this chapter in fall 2006:

1. Current evidence-based guidelines support routine central (hip and lumbar spine) bone density screening in women aged 65 and older.
2. Although some observational studies of osteoporosis risk assessment tools have shown favorable results, current evidence is inadequate to support clinical use of these tools for risk stratification before central bone density screening. Clarification of the role of risk assessment would strengthen the evidence base for an osteoporosis screening program.
3. Case-finding for secondary osteoporosis is practiced in high-risk disease subgroups such as chronic glucocorticoid users and patients with rheumatoid arthritis, collagen vascular disease, or inflammatory bowel disease.
4. Although osteoporosis affects fewer men than women, men should be considered for screening because of their high rates of fracture-related morbidity and mortality. The National Osteoporosis Foundation and International Society of Clinical Densitometry recommend bone density screening in men aged 70 and older.

ACKNOWLEDGMENTS

I acknowledge Robert Adler, MD and Russell Harris, MD, MPH for their thoughtful suggestions for this chapter.

REFERENCES

1. US Department of Health and Human Services. Bone health and osteoporosis: a report of the Surgeon General. Rockville, MD: US Department of Health and Human Services, Office of the Surgeon General, 2004.
2. Melton L Johnell O Lau E Mautalen C Seeman E. Osteoporosis and the global competition for health care resources. J Bone Miner Res 2004;19:1055–1058.
3. Sackett D Straus S Richardson W Rosenberg W Haynes R. Diagnosis and screening. In: Evidence-based medicine: how to practice and teach EBM 2nd ed. New York: Harcourt, 2000:261.
4. Wilson JMG Jungner G. Principles and practice of screening for disease. WHO public health paper no. 34. Geneva: World Health Organization, 1968.
5. Grimes D Schulz K. Uses and abuses of screening tests. Lancet 2002;359:881–884.
6. Hennekens C Buring J. Screening. In: Mayrent S ed. Epidemiology in medicine. Philadelphia: Lippincott Williams & Wilkins, 1987:327–347.
7. Kern L Powe N Levine M Fitzpatrick A Harris T Robbins J et al. Association between screening for osteoporosis and the incidence of hip fracture. Ann Intern Med 2005;142:173–181.
8. USPSTF. Screening for osteoporosis in postmenopausal women: recommendations and rationale. Ann Intern Med 2002;137:526–528.

9. Cummings S. Bone density screening: a new level of evidence? Ann Intern Med 2005;142:217–219.
10. Black D Steinbuch M Palermo L Dargent-Molina P Lindsay R Hoseyni M et al. An assessment tool for predicting fracture risk in postmenopausal women. Osteoporos Int 2001;12:519–528.
11. De Laet C Oden A Johansson H Johnell O Jonsson B Kanis J. The impact of use of multiple risk indicators for fracture on case-finding strategies: a mathematical approach. Osteoporos Int 2005;16: 313–318.
12. Melton L Atkinson E Khosla S Oberg A Riggs B. Evaluation of a prediction model for long-term fracture risk. J Bone Miner Res 2005;20:551–556.
13. Schott A, Ganne C, Hans D, Monnier G, Gauchoux R, Krieg M, et al. Which screening strategy using BMD measurements would be most cost effective for hip fracture prevention in elderly women? A decision analysis based on a Markov model. Osteoporos Int 2007;18:143–151.
14. Koh L Ben Sedrine W Torralba T Kung A Fujiwara S Chan S et al. A simple tool to identify Asian women at increased risk of osteoporosis. Osteoporos Int 2001;12:699–705.
15. Cadarette S Jaglal S Kreiger N McIsaac W Darlington G Tu J. Development and validation of the Osteoporosis Risk Assessment Instrument to facilitate selection of women for bone densitometry. CMAJ 2000;162:1289–1294.
16. Ben Sedrine W Chevallier T Zegels B Kvasz A Micheletti M-C, Gelas B et al. Development and assessment of the Osteoporosis Index of Risk (OSIRIS) to facilitate selection of women for bone densitometry. Gynecol Endocrinol 2002;16:245–250.
17. Lydick E Cook K Turpin J Melton M Stine R Byrnes C. Development and validation of a simple questionnaire to facilitate identification of women likely to have low bone density. Am J Man Care 1998;4:37–48.
18. Black DM Palermo L Abbott T Johnell O. SOFSURF: a simple, useful risk factor system can identify the large majority of women with osteoporosis [abstract]. Bone 1998;23(Suppl 4):S605, Abstract SA333.
19. Wildner M Peters A Raghuvanshi V Hohnloser J Siebert U. Superiority of age and weight as variables in predicting osteoporosis in postmenopausal white women. Osteoporos Int 2003;14:950–956.
20. Geusens P Hochberg M van der Voort D Pols H van der Klift M Siris E et al. Performance of risk indices for identifying low bone density in postmenopausal women. Mayo Clin Proc 2002;77:629–637.
21. Richy F Gourlay M Ross P Sen S Radican L De Ceulaer F et al. Validation and comparative evaluation of the osteoporosis self-assessment tool (OST) in a Caucasian population from Belgium. QJM 2004;97: 39–46.
22. Gourlay M Miller W Richy F Garrett J Hanson L Reginster J-Y. Performance of osteoporosis risk assessment tools in postmenopausal women aged 45 to 64 years. Osteoporos Int 2005;16:921–927.
23. Rud B Jensen J Mosekilde L Nielsen S Hilden J Abrahamsen B. Performance of four clinical screening tools to select peri- and early postmenopausal women for dual X-ray absorptiometry. Osteoporos Int 2005;16:764–772.
24. Cadarette S Jaglal S Murray T McIsaac W Joseph L Brown J. Evaluation of decision rules for referring women for bone densitometry by dual-energy x-ray absorptiometry. JAMA 2001;286:57–63.
25. Cadarette S McIsaac W Hawker G Jaakkimainen L Culbert A Zarifa G et al. The validity of decision rules for selecting women with primary osteoporosis for bone mineral density testing. Osteoporos Int 2004;15:361–366.
26. Ben Sedrine W Devogelear JP Kaufman J-M, Goemaere S Depresseux G Zegels B et al. Evaluation of the Simple Calculated Osteoporosis Risk Estimation (SCORE) in a sample of white women from Belgium. Bone 2001;29:374–380.
27. Reginster J Ben Sedrine W Viethel P Micheletti M Chevallier T Audran M. Validation of OSIRIS a prescreening tool for the identification of women with an increased risk of osteoporosis. Gynecol Endocrinol 2004;18:3–8.
28. Picard D Brown J Rosenthall L Couturier M Levesque J Dumont M et al. Ability of peripheral DXA measurement to diagnose osteoporosis as assessed by central DXA measurement. J Clin Densitom 2004;7:111–118.
29. Barr R Adebajo A Fraser W Halsey J Kelsey C Stewart A et al. Can peripheral DXA measurements be used to predict fractures in elderly women living in the community? Osteoporos Int 2005;16:1177–1183.

30. Williams E Daymond T. Evaluation of calcaneus bone densitometry against hip and spine for diagnosis of osteoporosis. Br J Radiol 2003;76:123–128.
31. Stewart A Kumar V Reid D. Long-term fracture prediction by DXA and QUS: a 10-year prospective study. J Bone Miner Res 2006;21:413–418.
32. Huopio J Kroger H Honkanen R Jurvelin J Saarikoski S Alhava E. Calcaneal ultrasound predicts early postmenopausal fractures as well as axial BMD. A prospective study of 422 women. Osteoporos Int 2004;15:190–195.
33. Nayak S Olkin I Liu H Grabe M Gould M Allen E et al. Meta-analysis: accuracy of quantitative ultrasound for identifying patients with osteoporosis. Ann Intern Med 2006;144:831–841.
34. Sim M Stone M Phillips C Cheung W Johansen A Vasishta S et al. Cost effectiveness analysis of using quantitative ultrasound as a selective pre-screen for bone densitometry. Technol Health Care 2005;13: 75–85.
35. Adler R Tran M Petkov V. Performance of the Osteoporosis Self-assessment Screening Tool for osteoporosis in American men. Mayo Clin Proc 2003;78:723–727.
36. Looker A Johnston C Jr, Wahner H Dunn W Calvo M Harris T et al. Prevalence of low femoral bone density in older US women from NHANES III. J Bone Miner Res 1995;10(5):796–802.
37. Looker A Wahner H Dunn W Calvo M Harris T Heyse S et al. Updated data on proximal femur bone mineral levels of US adults. Osteoporos Int 1998;8:468–489.
38. World Health Organization. Assessment of osteoporotic fracture risk and its role in screening for post-menopausal osteoporosis. WHO Technical report series no. 843. Geneva: World Health Organization, 1994.
39. Marshall D Johnell O Wedel H. Meta-analysis of how well measures of bone mineral density predict occurrence of osteoporotic fractures. BMJ 1996;312:1254–1259.
40. Stone K Seeley D Lui L Cauley J Ensrud K Browner W et al. BMD at multiple sites and risk of fracture of multiple types: long-term results from the Study of Osteoporotic Fractures. J Bone Miner Res 2003;18:1947–1954.
41. Leslie W Adler R Fuleihan G Hodsman A Kendler D McClung M et al. Application of the 1994 WHO classification to populations other than postmenopausal Caucasian women: the 2005 ISCD official positions. J Clin Densitom 2006;9:22–30.
42. National Committee for Quality Assurance (NCQA). HEDIS 2006. Health plan employer data & information set. Vol. 2, Technical specifications. Washington (DC): National Committee for Quality Assurance (NCQA); 2005. 350 p. http://www.qualitymeasures.ahrq.gov/summary/summary.aspx?ss=1&doc_id=5759 , accessed November 7, 2006.
43. Sanders K Nicholson G Watts J Pasco J Henry M Kotowicz M et al. Half the burden of fragility fractures in the community occur in women without osteoporosis. When is fracture prevention cost-effective? Bone 2006;38:694–700.
44. National Osteoporosis Foundation. The clinician's guide to prevention and treatment of osteoporosis. 1999, updated 2008. http://www.nof.org/. Accessed August 13, 2009.
45. Kanis J Torgerson D Cooper C. Comparison of the European and USA practice guidelines for osteoporosis. Trends Endocrinol Metab 2000;11:28–32.
46. European Commission. Report on osteoporosis in the European Community – action on prevention. Luxembourg Office for Official Publications of the European Communities, 1998;112 pp.
47. Kanis J Johnell O. Requirements for DXA for the management of osteoporosis in Europe. Osteoporos Int 2005;16:229–238.
48. Kamel H. Secondary prevention of hip fractures among the hospitalized elderly: are we doing enough? J Clin Rheumatol 2005;11:68–71.
49. Feldstein A Nichols G Elmer P Smith D Aickin M Herson M. Older women with fractures: patients falling through the cracks of guideline-recommended osteoporosis screening and treatment. J Bone Joint Surg Am 2003;85-A:2294–2302.
50. Khan S de Geus C Holroyd B Russell A. Osteoporosis follow-up after wrist fractures following minor trauma. Arch Intern Med 2001;161:1309–1312.
51. Freedman K Kaplan F Bilker W Strom B Lowe R. Treatment of osteoporosis: are physicians missing an opportunity? J Bone Joint Surg Am 2000;82-A:1063–1070.

52. Cuddihy M Gabriel S Crowson C Fallon W Melton L III. Forearm fractures as predictors of subsequent osteoporotic fractures. Osteoporos Int 1999 (9): 469–475.
53. Honkanen R Tuppurainen M Kroger H Alhava E Puntila E. Associations of early premenopausal fractures with subsequent fractures vary by sites and mechanisms of fractures. Calcif Tissue Int 1997;60:327–331.
54. Rothberg A Matshidze P. Perimenopausal wrist fracture – an opportunity for prevention and management of osteoporosis. S Afr Med J 2000;90:1121–1124.
55. Majumdar S Rowe B Folk D Johnson J Holroyd B Morrish D et al. A controlled trial to increase detection and treatment of osteoporosis in older patients with a wrist fracture. Ann Intern Med 2004;141: 366–373.
56. Astrand J Thorngren K Tagil M. One fracture is enough! Experience with a prospective and consecutive osteoporosis screening program with 239 fracture patients. Acta Orthop 2006;77:3–8.
57. Brankin E Mitchell C Munro R Service LO. Closing the osteoporosis management gap in primary care: a secondary prevention of fracture programme. Curr Med Res Opin 2005;21:475–482.
58. Ashe M Khan K Guy P Kruse K Hughes K O′ brien P et al. Wristwatch-distal radial fracture as a marker for osteoporosis investigation: a controlled trial of patient education and a physician alerting system. J Hand Ther 2004;17:324–328.
59. van Staa T Leufkens H Cooper C. The epidemiology of corticosteroid-induced osteoporosis: a meta-analysis. Osteoporos Int 2002;13:777–787.
60. van Staa T Leufkens H Abenhaim L Zhang B Cooper C. Oral corticosteroids and fracture risk: relationship to daily and cumulative doses. Rheumatology (Oxford) 2000;39:1383–1389.
61. Kanis J Johansson H Oden A Johnell O De Laet C Melton I et al. A meta-analysis of prior corticosteroid use and fracture risk. J Bone Miner Res 2004;19:893–899.
62. Naganathan V Jones G Nash P Nicholson G Eisman J Sambrook P. Vertebral fracture risk with long-term corticosteroid therapy: prevalence and relation to age, bone density, and corticosteroid use. Arch Intern Med 2000;160:2917–2922.
63. Zipfel S Seibel M Lowe B Beumont P Kasperk C Herzog W. Osteoporosis in eating disorders: a follow-up study of patients with anorexia and bulimia nervosa. J Clin Endocrinol Metab 2001;86: 5227–5233.
64. Grinspoon S Thomas E Pitts S Gross E Mickley D Miller K et al. Prevalence and predictive factors for regional osteopenia in women with anorexia nervosa. Ann Intern Med 2000;133:790–794.
65. Biller B Saxe V Herzog D Rosenthal D Holzman S Klibanski A. Mechanisms of osteoporosis in adult and adolescent women with anorexia nervosa. J Clin Endocrinol Metab 1989;68:548–554.
66. Lane N Pressman A Star V Cummings L Nevitt M Group TSoOFR. Rheumatoid arthritis and bone mineral density in elderly women. J Bone Miner Res 1995;10:257–263.
67. Haugeberg G Uhlig T Falch J Halse J TK K. Bone mineral density and frequency of osteoporosis in female patients with rheumatoid arthritis. Arthritis Rheum 2000;43:522–530.
68. Haugeberg G Uhlig T Falch J Halse J Kvien T. Reduced bone mineral density in male rheumatoid arthritis patients. Arthritis Rheum 2000;43:2776–2784.
69. Laan R Buijs W Verbeek A Draad M Corstens F van de Putte L et al. Bone mineral density in patients with recent onset rheumatoid arthritis: influence of disease activity and functional capacity. Ann Rheum Dis 1993;52:21–26.
70. Gough A Lilley J Eyre S Holder R Emery P. Generalised bone loss in patients with early rheumatoid arthritis. Lancet 1994; 344:23–27.
71. Lee C Almagor O Dunlop D Manzi S Spies S Chadha A et al. Disease damage and low bone mineral density: an analysis of women with systemic lupus erythematosus ever and never receiving corticosteroids. Rheumatology (Oxford) 2006;45:53–60.
72. Bultink I Lems W Kostense P Dijkmans B Voskuyl A. Prevalence of and risk factors for low bone mineral density and vertebral fractures in patients with systemic lupus erythematosus. Arthritis Rheum 2005;52:2044–2050.
73. Yee C Crabtree N Skan J Amft N Bowman S Situnayake D et al. Prevalence and predictors of fragility fractures in systemic lupus erythematosus. Ann Rheum Dis 2005;64:111–113.
74. Kornbluth A Hayes M Feldman S Hunt M Fried-Boxt E Lichtiger S et al. Do guidelines matter? Implementation of the ACG and AGA osteoporosis screening guidelines in inflammatory bowel disease (IBD) patients who meet the guidelines′ criteria. Am J Gastroenterol 2006;101:1546–1550.

75. van Staa T Cooper C Brusse L Leufkens H Javaid M Arden N. Inflammatory bowel disease and the risk of fracture. Gastroenterology 2003;125:1591–1597.
76. Loftus EJ Crowson C Sandborn W Tremaine W O′Fallon W Melton Lr. Long-term fracture risk in patients with Crohn′s disease: a population-based study in Olmsted County, Minnesota. Gastroenterology 2002;123:468–475.
77. Pollak R Karmeli F Eliakim R Ackerman Z Tabb K Rachmilewitz D. Femoral neck osteopenia in patients with inflammatory bowel disease. Am J Gastroenterol 1998;93:1483–1490.
78. American College of Rheumatology Subcommittee on Rheumatoid Arthritis Guidelines. Guidelines for the management of rheumatoid arthritis: 2002 update. Arthritis Rheum 2002; 46: 328–346.
79. American Gastroenterological Association. American Gastroenterological Association medical position statement: guidelines on osteoporosis in gastrointestinal diseases. Gastroenterology 2003;124:791–794.
80. Khan A Hanley D Bilezikian J Binkley N Brown J Hodsman A et al. Standards for performing DXA in individuals with secondary causes of osteoporosis. J Clin Densitom 2006;9:47–57.
81. Center J Nguyen T Schneider D Sambrook P Eisman J. Mortality after all major types of osteoporotic fracture in men and women: an observational study. Lancet 1999;353:878–882.
82. Poor G Atkinson E O′Fallon W Melton Lr. Predictors of hip fractures in elderly men. J Bone Miner Res 1995;10:1900–1907.
83. Binkley N Bilezikian J Kendler D Leib E Lewiecki E Petak S. Official positions of the International Society for Clinical Densitometry and executive summary of the 2005 Position Development Conference. J Clin Densitom 2006;9:4–14.
84. Binkley N Schmeer P Wasnich R Lenchik L. What are the criteria by which a densitometric diagnosis of osteoporosis can be made in males and non-Caucasians (ISCD position statement)? J Clin Densitom 2002;5(Suppl):S19–S27.
85. Nelson H Helfand M Woolf S Allan J. Screening for postmenopausal osteoporosis: a review of the evidence for the US Preventive Services Task Force. Ann Intern Med 2002;137:529–541.
86. NIH consensus development panel on osteoporosis prevention, diagnosis and therapy. Osteoporosis prevention, diagnosis and therapy. JAMA 2001;285:785–795.
87. Kanis J. WHO criteria for indications to treatment. Osteoporos Int 2006;17(Suppl 2):S1.

24 Osteoporosis in Men

Robert A. Adler

Contents

Summary

To many in the general public and in the health-care field as well, osteoporosis is a disorder of older white women. For example, advertising of osteoporosis treatments aimed at consumers always features postmenopausal women. Most studies of osteoporosis in the medical literature have focused on postmenopausal women. Then why devote a chapter to osteoporosis in men? The answer is that while men have fewer fractures than women and the fractures usually occur about 10 years later in life, morbidity and mortality outcomes are worse in men than women. Almost 30% of osteoporotic fractures occur in men *(1)*, resulting in a considerable economic burden. There are gender differences in the causes of osteoporosis, and more studies are now providing insight into osteoporosis in men. Thus, the purpose of this chapter is to review what we know about the epidemiology and pathophysiology of osteoporosis in men and provide, before evidence-based guidelines are established, some framework for evaluation and treatment.

Key Words: Osteoporosis, men, gender differences, fracture risk, bone mineral density

EPIDEMIOLOGY OF OSTEOPOROSIS IN MEN

In most general terms, men fracture about 10 years later in life than women and have about half the fracture risk overall compared to women. The first fact is illustrated by the Rotterdam Study of hip fracture *(2)*, in which the incidence of hip fracture for men aged 80–84 was similar to that of women aged 75–79. Of interest is the fact that life expectancy

From: *Contemporary Endocrinology: Osteoporosis: Pathophysiology and Clinical Management*
Edited by: R. A. Adler, DOI 10.1007/978-1-59745-459-9_24,

for men is increasing faster than that for women; thus there will be more men living long enough to suffer with a hip fracture. As another way to look at the overall epidemiology of osteoporosis in men, studies from Sweden *(3)* have listed the 10-year risk of an "osteoporotic" fracture for men at different ages. An osteoporotic fracture was defined as a low trauma fracture of the spine, the forearm, the proximal humerus, or the hip. At age 50, a man had a 10-year risk of such a fracture of about 3.3% (about 0.8% for hip fracture alone). The risk rose to 4.9% (1.2%) at age 60, 7.6% (3.4%) at age 70, and 13.1% (7.6%) at age 80. For this specific general population, 10-year fracture risk of men was about half of that of women in the same population at any given age. The 10-year risk of fracture has now been formalized in the FRAX™ calculation (see below). In another population *(4)*, that of Dubbo Australia, the lifetime fracture risk for a man at age 60 was about 30%. There may be ethnic differences as well. For example, in the Baltimore Men's Osteoporosis Study *(5)*, prevalence of vertebral fractures on spine radiographs was considerably higher in white men, compared to black men. Finally, the third National Health and Nutrition Examination (NHANES III) survey of bone mineral density of the hip *(6)* defined osteoporosis by dual-energy X-ray absorptiometry (DXA). Using a male normative database, the survey estimated that 1–2 million American men have osteoporosis and 8–13 million have low bone mass. For this study, the authors defined osteoporosis as a hip bone BMD that was at least 2.5 standard deviations below the mean of normal young men. There are controversies about the DXA definition of osteoporosis in men (see below), but regardless of the exact definition, the numbers are impressive. Unlike many other disorders, osteoporosis is asymptomatic until there is a "bone event," a fracture. Thus, for men as for women, osteoporosis is a silent disorder. In addition, because men are thought not to be at risk for osteoporosis *(7)*, there is little screening for osteoporosis and prevention of bone events in men (see below). Finally, there is evidence that men do worse after a fracture: with a higher mortality rate *(8)* and greater need for long-term care facility placement after hip fracture. Thus, this generally neglected area of medicine needs more research as well as dissemination of present and future knowledge of the disorder.

PATHOPHYSIOLOGY OF OSTEOPOROSIS IN MEN

The classification devised years ago by Riggs and Melton *(9)* divides involutional osteoporosis into Type 1, which occurs in women soon after menopause; Type 2, which occurs after age 70; and secondary osteoporosis. A modification of this classification for

Table 1
Classification of Osteoporosis in Men

Type	*Age*	*Usual presentation*	*Associations*
Type 1 primary	Forties to sixties	Vertebral fracture	Increased U_{Ca} Low IGF-I Low bioavail. E_2 Low free vit. D
Type 2 primary	Seventies and older	Hip fracture	Aging Other risk factors?
Secondary	Any	Any OP fracture	See Table 2

men is shown in Table 1. Although men would obviously not fit into the category of postmenopausal osteoporosis, it is clear that men may get osteoporosis during middle age. This is usually manifested by vertebral fractures found in radiographs of a man who complains of back pain. Sometimes the findings are incidental; the fractures may be noted when the patient gets a routine chest X-ray, for example. Type II osteoporosis is found in aging women and men, with the ratio of women to men much lower than in Type I. The final type of osteoporosis is secondary osteoporosis, which is thought to characterize a larger proportion of men with osteoporosis than women with osteoporosis *(10)*.

At least some of the men with Type 1 primary osteoporosis appear to have one of several distinct syndromes. While we still classify these men as having primary osteoporosis, it may eventually be possible to classify these patients as having specific kinds of secondary osteoporosis. For now, the syndrome that has been characterized *(11)* for the longest time is that associated with hypercalciuria. Many of these men will have kidney stones, but all will have excess urinary calcium and therefore negative calcium balance over time. Some of these men will respond to thiazide diuretics. The second type of idiopathic osteoporosis is a very interesting syndrome of low serum IGF-I levels with normal growth hormone secretion *(12)*. The low IGF-I is thought to be due to a variable region of the *IGF-1* gene *(13)*. Another group of men with idiopathic osteoporosis has been found to have low bioavailable estradiol levels *(14)*. Their male offspring appear to be affected as well as are other male members of the family, but the specific genetic abnormality is not known. A new syndrome of low free vitamin D has been tentatively characterized *(15)*. There has been an interesting report *(16)* of increased mast cells found in the marrow of men with osteoporosis, without evidence of systemic mastocytosis. At this point it is not known how common these different syndromes are. Nonetheless, when younger men present with X-ray evidence of a compression fracture or with low bone density, these syndromes should be kept in mind. It has not yet become standard of care to do biochemical tests other than 24-h urine calcium measurement in young men with vertebral fractures. While serum IGF-I is readily available, interpretation must be made with caution. Bioavailable estradiol levels are not easily obtained in clinical practice, although both bioavailable estradiol and bioavailable testosterone can be calculated using the sex steroid level, sex hormone-binding globulin, and serum albumin *(17)*. Finally, performing a standard osteoporosis evaluation (which includes a measure of urinary calcium excretion) should be adequate for choosing therapy for middle-aged men with osteoporosis. If specific treatments for certain varieties of Type 1 osteoporosis become available, then more comprehensive evaluation will be indicated.

Type II osteoporosis is associated with aging. It is not clear whether the risk factors for osteoporosis in men are the same as in women, but there is evidence that low body weight, excess alcohol intake, low vitamin D, and chronic diseases may be risk factors for this kind of osteoporosis. In a recent study *(18)* of men referred to a metabolic bone clinic, most of the men had low levels of 25-hydroxyvitamin D (see also Chapters 12 and 13). Not every population studied will have a high prevalence of 25-hydroxyvitamin D. For example, in the Rancho Bernardo Study *(19)* and a population at 37° South Latitude in Auckland, New Zealand *(18)*, vitamin D insufficiency was not common. On the other hand, in a study from Florida *(20)*, winter 25-hydroxyvitamin D levels were low and were about the same in middle-aged men and women. Finally, in a study from Portland, Oregon *(21)*, many male and female medical residents had low serum 25-hydroxyvitamin D levels. Thus, because the prevalence of vitamin D insufficiency may vary among patient groups, serum 25-hydroxyvitamin D measurements are important in the evaluation of the man with osteoporosis (see below).

Another finding in many men with osteoporosis after age 70 is a low serum testosterone level. Indeed, in men older than 70 years, it is common to find testosterone levels below the normal range of normal young men *(22)*. The question is, is there any connection between the low serum testosterone level and the low bone mineral density noted in these men? Studies from the Mayo Clinic *(23)* have shown that declining serum testosterone levels of aging is not particularly well correlated with bone mineral density in older men. On the other hand, serum bioavailable estradiol is more strongly associated with bone density in older men. Estradiol is formed by aromatization of testosterone. Recently men enrolled in the Osteoporosis Fractures in Men Study (MrOS) have been evaluated carefully *(24)*. In this large group of generally healthy men at least 65 years old, the prevalence of osteoporosis by DXA was twice as great in the men with low testosterone levels compared to those with normal testosterone levels. When the men were divided by BMD measurements, those men with osteoporosis had lower total testosterone and lower total estradiol levels than the men with normal BMD. Thus, there is evidence in men that both testosterone and estradiol have an impact on the prevalence of osteoporosis. Studies of men who lack aromatase enzymes *(25)* provide evidence that estradiol may actually be more important than testosterone in the accretion of peak bone mass in boys and young men. When testosterone therapy is given to a man with hypogonadism, some of the testosterone is converted to estradiol. Thus, when testosterone increases bone density *(26)*, some of the effect may be mediated through conversion to estradiol (see also Chapters 16 and 17).

Table 2
Some Important Causes of Secondary Osteoporosis in Men

Oral glucocorticoid therapy
Androgen withdrawal therapy for prostate cancer
Chronic obstructive pulmonary disease
Primary testicular failure
Secondary hypogonadism
Disorders of mobility such as spinal cord injury, multiple sclerosis, Parkinson's disease, stroke
Alcoholism
Multiple myeloma
Gastrectomy
Surgery for obesity
Organ transplantation
Rheumatoid arthritis
Celiac disease and other causes of malabsorption
Hyperthyroidism
Hyperparathyroidism
Inflammatory bowel disease

Secondary osteoporosis is very important in men *(10)*, and as discussed below, it is important to look for secondary causes when evaluating a man with osteoporosis. The most important secondary cause of osteoporosis in men and women is glucocorticoid-induced osteoporosis (see Chapter 26). Indeed, the patient at lowest risk for primary osteoporosis, the young African-American man, may develop osteoporosis if he is treated with oral glucocorticoid agents for an inflammatory disorder or to prevent organ transplant rejection. Primary or secondary hypogonadism (see Chapter 17) may lead to low bone density, which responds to testosterone replacement *(26)*. Note that this is different from the mild decrease in free testosterone observed in aging men. Some other causes of secondary osteoporosis are listed in Table 2, but there are many potential causes of secondary osteoporosis *(27)*. Most of these apply to both women and men. One increasingly important cause of secondary osteoporosis in men is that associated with androgen deprivation therapy for prostate cancer *(28–30)*. There may be different interpretations of the definitions of primary and secondary osteoporosis. For example, some experts believe that hypercalciuria is a risk factor for osteoporosis rather than a cause of a particular kind of primary osteoporosis. Whatever be the classification, searching for such risk factors or causes is important in men.

EVALUATION OF THE MAN WITH OSTEOPOROSIS OR AT RISK FOR OSTEOPOROSIS

Osteoporosis is a disorder that has no symptoms until there is a "bone event," a fracture. Thus, the man with osteoporosis may present with a fracture, or an asymptomatic compression fracture may be noted incidentally on a lateral chest X-ray obtained for other reasons. The International Society for Clinical Densitometry suggests that men over age 70 should be screened by DXA for osteoporosis *(31)*, but there are no guidelines for this recommendation based on evidence that such screening will lead to fewer fractures (see Chapter 25). Recently, the American College of Physicians published *(32)* guidelines for screening men, based on an evidence synthesis *(33)* prepared for the Department of Veterans Affairs. In addition, the new NOF Guidelines *(34)* include suggestions for screening in men. The FRAX™ calculator *(34)* can be used for men after converting the male database *T* score provided by most DXA machines to a female normative database *T* score. The use of different normative databases is discussed below. The fracture risk calculation can be done on the National Osteoporosis Foundation website *(34)*. When men are identified as having osteoporosis, either by fragility fracture or from a DXA (with or without the FRAX™ calculation), they require evaluation. As outlined in Table 3, much of the evaluation can be accomplished by history and physical examination. Laboratory testing need not be extensive for most men. As stated above, assessing the younger man for the reported syndromes of idiopathic osteoporosis is not usually done, although measurement of urinary calcium is necessary. Importantly, men with low IGF-1 syndrome of Type I osteoporosis respond well to teriparatide therapy (see below). There are no studies comparing bisphosphonate response in men with Type I vs. Type II osteoporosis, but it is reasonable to suspect that all will respond. Many of the causes of secondary osteoporosis will be revealed by careful history and physical examination, but measuring thyroid function tests, serum or urine protein electrophoresis, and gonadal function tests (LH, FSH, testosterone, prolactin) may

Table 3
Evaluation of the Man with Osteoporosis

History
Physical examination, including height, genital exam
Complete blood count (and sometimes serum/urine electrophoresis)
Serum chemistries: calcium, albumin, phosphate, creatinine, alkaline phosphatase
Testosterone, LH, FSH (prolactin)
24-hour urine calcium (or spot urine calcium/creatinine ratio)
25-hydroxyvitamin D
Serum PTH particularly if serum calcium is high or low
TSH and free T4
Consider SHBG for calculation of bioavailable sex steroids
DXA of spine, hip, and forearm
X-ray of thoracic and lumbar spines or vertebral fracture analysis

be helpful in many men. In addition, not only will 24-h urine calcium measurements identify men with hypercalciuria, but hypocalciuria may signify malabsorption and/or vitamin D insufficiency. Measurement of renal function, serum calcium, serum albumin (needed to calculate a corrected serum calcium), and 25-hydroxyvitamin D is also important. Renal osteodystrophy may mimic osteoporosis (or have osteoporosis as a part of it), and some osteoporosis drugs are potentially nephrotoxic. Elevated serum calcium may signify hyperparathyroidism; a low serum calcium may be due to malabsorption. Thus, mostly simple, widely available testing will provide valuable information.

BONE DENSITY MEASUREMENT IN MEN

The reader is directed to Chapters 2–4 on the use of diagnostic tools to diagnose osteoporosis in general. Dual-energy X-ray absorptiometry (DXA) is the most commonly used measurements of bone mass and has been used to define osteoporosis in men. There are a few points that require discussion at this time. The manufacturers of DXA machines supply a normal male database, to which a given man can be compared. Is this the proper way to diagnose osteoporosis in men, or should a female database be used? Some argue *(35)* that the female database should be used because osteoporosis was defined as a bone density 2.5 standard deviations below that of the normal young white female. While there is some evidence that women and men fracture at the same absolute bone mineral density, there is also evidence that men fracture at a higher absolute BMD *(35–37)*. Men generally have larger bones than women. As pointed out by Lang (Chapter 2), bones from women and men with similar volumetric density will have different areal bone density by DXA: the larger male bone will have a higher BMD. Thus, using a female database decreases the number of men who would be diagnosed as having osteoporosis, some of it due to the artifact caused by larger bones. In addition, hip bone density predicts a smaller proportion of the fracture patients in men compared to women *(2)*. Using more stringent criteria for osteoporosis (the female database) would identify even fewer patients. In addition, it is important to note that degenerative spine changes that spuriously raise the spine BMD are more common in older men than in women. For this reason, some experts *(38–40)* have recommended using forearm BMD, done by DXA at the time that spine and hip are measured, for the diagnosis of osteoporosis in men. While the distal one-third radius has been advocated for the diagnosis of osteoporosis in women, it is not clear which site is best for men. It has been known for some time that forearm bone density predicts fracture well in men *(41)*. Men with a distal forearm fracture have lower BMD than do age-matched controls *(42)*; men over age 60 who have previously fractured the wrist have about double the chance of another fracture, compared to those who have not fractured *(43)*. On the other hand, an ankle fracture in this population did not predict future fractures.

The clinical recommendation of this author is to routinely measure spine, hip, and forearm in men, particularly in older men. In some centers, the DXA technician can determine if the spine BMD will be adequate and forearm is not necessary. However, it has been shown that more men will be diagnosed with osteoporosis if forearm is routinely added to spine and hip *(39,40)*. I also believe that the preponderance of evidence favors using the male normative database for men. A very recent study *(44)* from Belgium demonstrates how a national male database can be developed. As will be seen below, all recent studies of osteoporosis treatment have used DXA inclusion criteria based on a male database. However, it must be stated that using forearm BMD to define osteoporosis for treatment has not been used. Nonetheless, forearm BMD predicts fracture as does previous forearm fracture *(41)*.

The American College of Physicians presented the first evidence-based guidelines *(32)* suggesting which men should be screened with BMD. The International Society for Clinical Densitometry recommends that men over age 70 be screened for osteoporosis *(31)*. While this is reasonable, there may be men under 70 years of age who would benefit from having the diagnosis of osteoporosis made early, and it is likely that some men over 70 are not at risk. In postmenopausal women, a performance measure for osteoporosis will be a bone density test by age 65 – and some women will be tested much earlier than 65 based on risk factors. What are risk factors for men that should lead to an earlier DXA measurement? All can agree that oral glucocorticoid therapy or another important cause of secondary osteoporosis would be an indication for earlier DXA. What about other risk factors or screening tests? When we used a heel densitometer and an osteoporosis questionnaire to find men at risk in a pulmonary clinic *(45)*, two conclusions could be made: (1) weight- and age-predicted BMD by DXA better than heel ultrasound with or without the questionnaire; (2) men sick enough to be referred to a pulmonary specialist need a DXA because the prevalence of osteoporosis was high. In response to these findings, we and others *(46–48)* have used the OST screening tool to identify men at risk for osteoporosis. OST, first developed for Asian women *(49)*, is a formula based on weight and age only that predicts DXA. We found that it worked well in a population of mostly white men (with different cutoff values than that for women). Sinnott et al. *(50)* found that the formula also worked well for African-American men, although cutoff values were slightly different. As described in Chapter 23, the place of screening tests for identifying patients at risk for osteoporosis is not completely established. Indeed, data for men are less robust than that for women. Nonetheless, it is impossible to perform DXA tests on all older men. Thus, there must be continued exploration of ways to identify men at risk for fracture. There is at least one study *(51)* demonstrating that screening for osteoporosis leads to fewer fractures. This study must be duplicated in a large population of men.

TREATMENT OF OSTEOPOROSIS IN MEN

For the man with a fragility fracture or for one who has been found to have osteoporosis by DXA test, treatment is indicated. The argument can be made that treatment of osteoporotic men is more important than in women because a man with a hip fracture has a higher likelihood of dying than does a woman *(8)*. Although there are fewer studies of calcium and vitamin D in men, most experts believe that it is important to use calcium and vitamin D supplements as part of the treatment plan. There is nothing known to make calcium and vitamin D less important in men than women, although in one population, men were less likely to be vitamin D deficient than women *(19)*. On the other hand, as noted above, in other male populations *(18,21,52)*, vitamin D insufficiency or deficiency was very common.

Bisphosphonates

Not many years ago, there would have been little to write about treatment of male osteoporosis, but now there is good quality evidence that medications used for osteoporosis in women work well in men also. In postmenopausal women, oral bisphosphonates are the most commonly used therapy for osteoporosis. The same group of agents can also be used for men; both alendronate and risedronate are FDA approved to treat osteoporosis in men. Other bisphosphonates, such as oral etidronate, oral and intravenous ibandronate, intravenous pamidronate, and intravenous zoledronic acid, have been used off-label for male osteoporosis. The first rigorous study of modern bisphosphonate therapy in men was reported by Orwoll et al. *(53)*. In it, men (with osteoporosis defined by DXA using a male normative database or with a prevalent fracture) were randomized to receive daily alendronate or placebo plus calcium and vitamin D for 2 years. The men who received alendronate had greater increases in spine and hip bone density, a smaller decrease in height, and fewer vertebral fractures on X-ray. Of note, about one-third of the men had low serum testosterone levels and appeared to respond to alendronate as well as the men with normal serum testosterone levels. More recently, Ringe et al. *(54)* reported on a 1-year study of risedronate in similar men. Despite the short duration of the study, there was a dramatic decrease in morphometric vertebral fractures (relative decrease of 60%) in the men who received risedronate. One concern about these two reports is that the studies were too small to determine if bisphosphonates decrease clinical fractures. Interestingly, a study in older men who have suffered a stroke helps to decrease this concern. Sato et al. *(55)* randomized 280 Japanese men aged 65 to receive either risedronate or placebo. These post-CVA men were then followed for 18 months. Bone density increased in the risedronate group and decreased in the placebo group. More importantly, there was a statistically significant decrease in the number of hip fractures in the men who had been treated with risedronate. What is remarkable about this study is that the men did not necessarily have osteoporosis at baseline and the dose of risedronate used (2.5 mg daily) is half that of the dose used in the United States. Thus, while bisphosphonates clearly decrease clinical fractures in women, this study from Japan provided evidence that clinical fractures can be prevented in men as well. While multiple randomized controlled trials of anti-osteoporosis agents that show clinical fracture efficacy would be ideal, the cost and the difficulty of such trials prevent an evidence-based answer for this clinical question. The conclusion from what data we have is that bisphosphonates are effective drugs for osteoporosis in men, and the conclusions from studies in women (see Chapter 20) likely apply to men.

While there are no specific data with ibandronate, pamidronate, and zoledronic acid in men with osteoporosis, the studies in women and studies in specific groups [for example, in transplant osteoporosis *(56)* and glucocorticoid-induced osteoporosis *(57)*] suggest that these drugs will work in men with primary osteoporosis. In a study *(58)* of men and women after hip fracture, zoledronic acid decreased the incidence of further fractures. In addition, both zoledronic acid *(59)* and alendronate *(60)* can prevent osteoporosis in men undergoing androgen withdrawal therapy for prostate cancer. Zoledronic acid is now FDA-approved for men.

Parathyroid Hormone Preparations

The only FDA-approved anabolic agent for osteoporosis is teriparatide (see Chapter 22). It is FDA approved for men with osteoporosis, an indication based on studies in men. The earliest study of men by Slovik *(61)* showed that the first 34 amino acid fragments of parathyroid hormone could increase spine bone density. In a larger study of men with idiopathic osteoporosis *(62)*, teriparatide (PTH 1–34) had a dramatic effect on bone mineral density. After 18 months of teriparatide, the spine BMD increased 13.5% in this group of men with a mean age of 50. In a much larger study *(63)*, Orwoll et al. reported on teriparatide use in a group of men with bone density at least 2 standard deviations below the normal young male mean. After treatment for a median of 11 months, those men treated with the FDA-approved dose of 20 μg daily had an increase in spine BMD of 5.9 and 1.5% in the femoral neck. Finkelstein et al. *(64)* reported that alendronate given simultaneously blunted the anabolic effects of teriparatide in men. Much more effective in increasing bone density in men is the sequential use of a bisphosphonate after a course of teriparatide, as reported by Kurland et al. *(65)* and Kaufman et al. *(66)*.

Other Treatments for Osteoporosis

Some of the other treatments for osteoporosis have been studied in women but not extensively or at all in men. Thus, there may be only evidence in women to base treatment on. Not surprisingly, there are several small trials of testosterone effects on BMD in men with specific causes of hypogonadism and in men with the modest decrease in circulating testosterone levels with aging. The former category refers to men with testicular or hypothalamic/pituitary disorders that lead to clearly low levels of testosterone *(67)*. In such men, there are studies to show that testosterone increases bone mineral density *(26,68)*. For men with hypogonadism associated with glucocorticoid therapy, Reid et al. *(69)* showed a 5% increase in spine BMD after testosterone treatment. In the category of men with mildly diminished testosterone levels associated with aging, there is less information. Snyder et al. *(70)* showed that those men with the lowest BMD had the greatest response to testosterone therapy. In a 3-year study, Amory et al. *(71)* demonstrated that testosterone could increase spine bone density by about 10%. It is important to note that there are no testosterone studies large enough to demonstrate any sort of fracture risk reduction. In addition, the long-term prostate and cardiovascular safety of testosterone is unknown. A full review of this subject is beyond the scope of this chapter (see also Chapter 17), but suffice it to say that in the studies of alendronate and risedronate, a significant proportion of the subjects had low testosterone levels. We know from these studies that such men responded well to bisphosphonates and the use of these drugs is associated with lower fracture risk. As reviewed in Chapter 21, long-term use of bisphosphonates appears to be generally safe.

Treatment: Summary and Conclusions

Although there are fewer and smaller studies of osteoporosis treatment in men than in women, several important points can be gleaned. First, all of the major studies chose men at risk using a normal male database for DXA testing. Second, all bisphosphonate studies used calcium and vitamin D in addition to alendronate or risedronate therapy. [The Sato study *(55)* in men with stroke did not.] Third, teriparatide worked as well in men as in women, at least in terms of increasing BMD. Fourth, testosterone increases bone density but its effect on fracture rate and its long-term safety are not established. Thus, for most patients, bisphosphonates are the drugs to use, in conjunction with calcium and vitamin D. For the patient with very low bone density and/or clinical fractures, a case can be made to treat him with teriparatide first for 18–24 months followed by long-term treatment with a bisphosphonate. There are no discontinuation studies in men. Thus, we must extrapolate from studies in women (e.g., *(72)*) that at least 5 years of bisphosphonate therapy is necessary before considering a drug holiday. Finally, it must be restated that men with hip fracture do worse than women: more die of complications and more lose independence. Thus, diagnosis of men with osteoporosis is very important. A study from Sweden *(73)* demonstrated that bisphosphonate therapy was cost-effective in men. It is obvious that more knowledge is necessary to choose those men who will most likely benefit from diagnosis and treatment. It is hoped that longitudinal studies such as MrOS will lead to the insight that is needed to find men at risk and get them to appropriate treatment.

REFERENCES

1. Burge R, Dawson-Hughes B, Solomon DH, Wong JB, King A, Tosteson A. Incidence and economic burden of osteoporosis-related fractures in the United States 2005–2025. J Bone Miner Res 2007;22: 465–475.
2. Schuit SCE, van der Klift M, Weel AEAM, de Laet CEDH, Burger H, Seeman E, Hofman A, Uitterlinden AG, van Leeuwen JPTM, Pols HAP. Fracture incidence and association with bone mineral density in elderly men and women: the Rotterdam Study. Bone 2004;34:195–202.
3. Kanis JA, Johnell O, Oden A, Sernbo I, Redlund-Johnell I, Dawson A, de Laet C, Jonsson B. Long-term risk of osteoporotic fracture in Malmo. Osteoporos Int 2000;11:669–674.
4. Jones G, Nguyen T, Sambrook PN, Kelly PJ, Gilbert C, Eisman JA. Symptomatic fracture incidence in elderly men and women: the Dubbo Osteoporosis Epidemiology Study (DOES). Osteoporos Int 1994;4:277–282.
5. Tracy JK, Meyer WA, Grigoryan M, Fan B, Flores RH, Genant HK, Resnik C, Hochberg MC. Racial differences in the prevalence of vertebral fractures in older men: the Baltimore Men's Osteoporosis Study. Osteoporos Int 2006;17:99–104.
6. Looker AC, Orwoll ES, Johnston CC Jr, Lindsay RL, Wahner HW, Dunn WL, Calvo MS, Harris TB, Heyse SP. Prevalence of low femoral bone density in older U.S. adults from NHANES III. J Bone Miner Res 1997;12:1761–1768.
7. Adler RA. The need for increasing awareness of osteoporosis in men. Clin Cornerstone 2006;8(Suppl 3):S7–S13.
8. Block JE, Stubbs H. Hip fracture-associated mortality reconsidered. Calcif Tissue Int 1997;61:84.
9. Riggs BL, Melton LJ III. Involutional osteoporosis. N Engl J Med 1986;314:1676–1686.
10. Painter SE, Kleerekoper M, Camacho PM. Secondary osteoporosis: a review of the recent evidence. Endocr Pract 2006;12:436–445.

11. Kurland ES, Rosen CJ, Cosman F, McMahon D, Chan F, Shane E, Lindsay R, Dempster D, Bilezikian JP. Insulin-like growth factor-I in men with idiopathic osteoporosis. J Clin Endocrinol Metab 1997;82: 2799–2805.
12. Zerwekh JE, Sakhaee K, Breslau NA, Gottschalk F, Pak CY. Impaired bone formation in male idiopathic osteoporosis: further reduction in the presence of concomitant hypercalciuria. Osteoporos Int 1992;2: 128–134.
13. Rosen CJ, Kurland ES, Vereault D, Adler RA, Rackoff PJ, Craig WY, Witte S, Rogers J, Bilezikian JP. Association between serum insulin growth factor-I (IGF-I) and a simple sequence repeat in IGF-I gene: implications for genetic studies of bone mineral density. J Clin Endocrinol Metab 1998;83:2286–2290.
14. Van Pottelburgh I, Goemaere S, Zmierczak H, Kaufman JM. Perturbed sex steroid status in men with idiopathic osteoporosis and their sons. J Clin Endocrinol Metab 2004;89:4949–4953.
15. Al-oanzi ZH, Tuck SP, Raj N, Harrop JS, Summers GD, Cook DB, Francis RM, Datta HK. Assessment of vitamin D status in male osteoporosis. Clin Chem 2006;52:248–254.
16. Brumsen C, Papapoulos SE, Lentjes EG, Kluin PM, Hamdy NA. A potential role for the mast cell in the pathogenesis of idiopathic osteoporosis. Bone 2002;2002:556–561.
17. http://www.issam.ch/freetesto.htm. Accessed August 14, 2008
18. Ryan C, Petkov VI, Adler RA. Osteoporosis in men: value of laboratory testing. J Bone Miner Res 2005;20(Suppl1):S165, #SA380.
19. Bolland MJ,Grey AB, Ames RW, Mason BH, Horne AM, Gamble GD, Reid IR. Determinants of vitamin D status in older men living in a subtropical climate. Osteoporos Int 2006;17:1742–1748.
20. Saquib N, von Muhlen D, Garland CF, Barrett-Connor E. Serum 25-hydroxyvitamin D, parathyroid hormone, and bone mineral density in men: The Rancho Bernardo study. Osteoporos Int 2006;17:1734–1741.
21. Haney EM, Stadler D, Bilziotes MM. Vitamin D insufficiency in internal medicine residents. Calcif Tissue Int 2005;76:11–16.
22. Mohr BA, Guay AT, O'Donnell AB, McKinlay JB. Normal, bound and nonbound testosterone levels in normally ageing men: results from the Massachusetts Male Aging Study. Clin Endocrinol 2005;62:64–73.
23. Khosla S, Melton LJ III, Atkinson EJ, O'Fallon WM, Klee GG, Riggs BL. Relationship of serum sex steroid levels and bone turnover markers with bone mineral density in men and women: a key role for bioavailable estrogen. J Clin Endocrinol Metab 1998;83:2266–2274.
24. Fink HA, Ewing SK, Ensrud KE, Barrett-Connor E, Taylor BC, Cauley JA, Orwoll ES, Osteoporotic Fractures in Men Study Group. Association of testosterone and estradiol deficiency with osteoporosis and rapid bone loss in older men. J Clin Endocrinol Metab 2006;91:3908–3915.
25. Carani C, Qin K, Simoni M, Faustini-Fustini M, Serpente S, Boyd J, Korach KS, Simpson ER. Effect of testosterone and estradiol in a man with aromatase deficiency. N Engl J Med 1997;337:91–95.
26. Behre HM, Kliesch S, Leifke E, et al. Long-term effect of testosterone therapy on bone mineral density in hypogonadal men. J Clin Endocrinol Metab 1997;82:2386–2390.
27. Fitzpatrick LA. Secondary causes of osteoporosis. Mayo Clin Proc 2002;77:453–468.
28. Mittan D, Lee S, Miller E, Perez RC, Basler J, Bruder JM. Bone loss following hypogonadism in men with prostate cancer treated with GnRH analogs. J Clin Endocrinol Metab 2002;87:3656–3661.
29. Shaninian VB, Kuo Y-F, Freeman JL, Goodwin JS. Risk of fracture after androgen deprivation for prostate cancer. N Engl J Med 2005;352:154–164.
30. Adler RA. Cancer treatment-induced bone loss. Curr Opin Endocrinol Diabetes Obes 2007;14:442–445.
31. International Society for Clinical Densitometry: ISCD Official Positions. Available at http://www.iscd.org/Visitors/positions/OfficialPositionsText.cfm, Accessed March 5, 2007.
32. Qaseem A, Snow V, Shekelle P, Hopkins R, Forbes MA, Owens DK. Screening for osteoporosis in men: a clinical practice guideline from the American College of Physicians. Ann Intern Med 2008;148:680–684.
33. Liu H, Paige NM, Goldzweig CL, Wong E, Zhou A, Suttorp MJ, Munjas B, Orwoll E, Shekelle P. Screening for osteoporosis in men: a systematic review for an American College of Physicians guideline. Ann Intern Med 2008;148:685–701.
34. http://www.nof.org. Accessed August 27, 2008.
35. Seeman E, Bianchi G, Khosla S, Kanis JA, Orwoll E. Bone fragility in men – where are we? Osteoporos Int 2006;17:1577–1583.
36. Selby PL, Davies M, Adams JE. Do men and women fracture bones at similar bone densities? Osteoporos Int 2000;11:153–157.

37. Cauley JA, Fullman RL, Stone KL, Zmuda JM, Bauer DC, Barrett-Connor E, Ensrud K, Lau EMC, Orwoll ES, MrOS Research Group. Factors associated with the lumbar spine and proximal femur bone mineral density in older men. Osteoporos Int 2005;16:1525–1537.
38. Vallarta-Ast N, Krueger D, Binkley N. Densitometric diagnosis of osteoporosis in men. J Clin Densitom 2002;5:383–389.
39. Bruder JM, Ma JZ, Basler JW, Welch MD. Prevalence of osteopenia and osteoporosis by central and peripheral bone mineral density in men with prostate cancer during androgen-deprivation therapy. Urology 2006;67:152–155.
40. Petkov VI, Williams MI, Via PS, Adler RA. Dual energy x-ray absorptiometry (DXA) of forearm in men: radius versus total. J Bone Miner Res 2004;19(Suppl 1):S234, #SU125.
41. Melton LJ III, Atkinson EJ, O'Connor MK, O'Fallon WM, Riggs BL. Bone density and fracture risk in men. J Bone Miner Res 1998;13:1915–1923.
42. Tuck SP, Raj N, Summers GD. Is distal forearm fracture in men due to osteoporosis? Osteoporos Int 2002;13:630–636.
43. Ettinger B, Ray GT, Pressman AR, Gluck O. Limb fractures in elderly men as indicators of subsequent fracture risk. Arch Intern Med 2003;163:2741–2747.
44. Goemaere S, Vanderschueren D, Kaufman J-M, Reginster J-Y, Boutsen Y, Poriau S, Callens J, Raeman F, Depresseux G, Borghs H, Devogelaer J-P, Boonen S, Belgian Bone Club Network on Male Osteoporosis in Europe. Dual energy x-ray absorptiometry-based assessment of male patients using standardized bone density values and a national reference database. J Clin Densitom 2007;10:25–33.
45. Adler RA, Funkhouser HL, Petkov VI, Elmore BL, Via PS, McMurtry CT, Adera T. Osteoporosis in pulmonary clinic patients: does point-of-care screening predict central dual-energy x-ray absorptiometry? Chest 2003;123:2012–2018.
46. Adler RA, Tran MT, Petkov VI. Performance of the osteoporosis self-assessment tool for osteoporosis in American men. Mayo Clin Proc 2003;78:723–727.
47. Hochberg MC, Tracy JK, van der Klift M, Pols H. Validation of a risk index to identify men with an increased likelihood of osteoporosis. J Bone Miner Res 2002;17(Suppl 1):S231, #SA095.
48. Lynn Hs, Woo J, Leung PC, Barrett-Connor EL, Nevitt MC, Cauley JA, Adler RA, Orwoll ES, Osteoporosis in Men (MrOS) Study. An evaluation of osteoporosis screening tools for the osteoporotic fractures in men (MrOS) study. Osteoporos Int 2008;19:1087–1092.
49. Koh LK, Ben Sedrine W, Torralba TP, Kung A, Fujiwara S, Chan SP, Huang QR, Rajatanavin R, Tsai KS, Park HM, Reginster JY, Osteoporosis Self-Assessment Tool for Asians (OSTA) Research Group. A simple tool to indentify Asian women at increased risk of osteoporosis. Osteoporos Int 2001;12:669–705.
50. Sinnott B, Kukreja S, Barengolts E. Utility of screening tools for the prediction of low bone mass in African-American men. Osteoporos Int 2006;17:684–692.
51. Newman ED, Ayoub WT, Starkey RH, Diehl JM, Wood GC. Osteoporosis disease management in a rural health care population: hip fracture reduction and reduced costs in postmenopausal women after 5 years. Osteoporos Int 2003;14:146–151.
52. Levis S, Gomez A, Jimenez C, Veras L, Ma F, Lai S, Hollis B, Roos BA. Vitamin D deficiency and seasonal variation in an adult South Florida population. J Clin Endocrinol Metab 2005;90:1557–1562.
53. Orwoll E, Ettinger M, Weiss S, Miller P, Kendler D, Graham J, Adami S, Weber K, Lorenc R, Pietschmann P, Vandormael K, Lombardi A. Alendronate for the treatment of osteoporosis in men. N Engl J Med 2000;343:604–610.
54. Ringe JD, Faber H, Farahmand P, Dorst A. Efficacy of risedronate in men with primary and secondary osteoporosis: results of a 1-year study. Rheumatol Int 2006;26:427–431.
55. Sato Y, Iwamoto J, Kanoko T, Satoh K. Risedronate sodium therapy for prevention of hip fracture in men 65 years or older after stroke. Arch Intern Med 2005;165:1743–1748.
56. Crawford BAL, Kam C, Pavlovic J, Byth K, Handelsman DJ, Angus PW, McCaughan GW. Zoledronic acid prevents bone loss after liver transplantation. Ann Intern Med 2006;144:239–248.
57. Boutsen Y, Jamart J, Esselinckx W, Devogelaer JP. Primary prevention of glucocorticoid-induced osteoporosis with intravenous pamidronate and calcium: a prospective controlled 1-year study comparing a single infusion, an infusion given once every 3 months, and calcium alone. J Bone Miner Res 2001;16:104–112.
58. Lyles KW, Colon-Emereic CS, Magaziner JS, et al. Zoledronic acid and clinical fractures and mortality after hip fracture. N Engl J Med 2007;357:1799–1809.

59. Smith MR, Eastham J, Gleason DM, Shasha D, Tchekmedyian S, Zinner N. Randomized controlled trial of zoledronic acid to prevent bone loss in men receiving androgen deprivation therapy for nonmetastatic prostate cancer. J Urol 2003;169:2008–2012.
60. Bruder JM, Ma JZ, Basler J, Katselnik D. Effects of alendronate on bone mineral density in men with prostate cancer treated with androgen deprivation therapy. J Clin Densitom 2006;9:431–437.
61. Slovik DM, Neer RM, Potts JT Jr. Short-term effects of synthetic parathyroid hormone – (1–34) administration on bone mineral metabolism in osteoporotic patients. J Clin Invest 1981;68:1261–1271.
62. Kurland ES, Cosman F, McMahon DJ, Rosen CJ, Lindsay R, Bilezikian JP. Parathyroid hormone as a therapy for idiopathic osteoporosis in men: effects on bone mineral density and bone markers. J Clin Endocrinol Metab 2000;85:3069–3076.
63. Orwoll ES, Scheele WH, Paul S, Adami S, Syversen U, Diez-Perez A, Kaufman J-M, Clancy AD, Gaich GA. The effect of teriparatide [Human Parathyroid Hormone (1–34)] therapy on bone density in men with osteoporosis. J Bone Miner Res 2003;18:9–17.
64. Finkelstein JS, Leder BZ, Burnett SA, Wyland JJ, Lee H, de al Paz AV, Gibson K, Neer RN. Effects of teriparatide, alendronate, or both on bone turnover in osteoporotic men. J Clin Endocrinol Metab 2006;91:2882–2887.
65. Kurland ES, Heller SL, Diamond B, McMahon DJ, Cosman F, Bilezikian JP. The importance of bisphosphonate therapy in maintaining bone mass in men after therapy with teriparatide [human parathyroid hormone (1–34)]. Osteoporos Int 2004;15:992–997.
66. Kaufman JM, Orwoll E, Goemaere S, San Martin J, Hossain A, Dalsky GP, Lindsay R, Mitlak BH. Teriparatide effects on vertebral fractures and bone mineral density in men with osteoporosis. Osteoporos Int 2005;16:510–516.
67. Adler RA, Fracture syndromes in men. Adv Osteoporotic Fract Manag 2005;3:112–117.
68. Katznelson L, Finkelstein JS, Schoenfeld DA, Rosenthal DI, Anderson EJ, Klibanski A. Increase in bone density and lean body mass during testosterone administration in men with acquired hypogonadism. J Clin Endocrinol Metab 1996;81:4358–4365.
69. Reid IR, Wattie DJ, Evans MC, Stapleton JP. Testosterone therapy in glucocorticoid-treated men. Arch Intern Med 1996;156:1173–1177.
70. Snyder PJ, Peachey H, Berlin JA, Hannoush P, Haddad G, Dlewati A, Santanna J, Loh L, Lenrow DA, Holmes JH, Kapoor SC, Atkinson LE, Strom BL. Effects of testosterone in hypogonadal men. J Clin Endocrinol Metab 2000;85:2670–2677.
71. Amory JK, Watts NB, Easley KA, Sutton PR, Anawalt BD, Matsumoto AM, Bremner WJ, Tenover JL. Exogenous testosterone or testosterone plus finasteride increases bone mineral density in older men with low serum testosterone. J Clin Endocrinol Metab 2004;89:503–510.
72. Black DM, Schwartz AV, Ensrud KE, Cauley JA, Levis S, Quandt SA, Satterfield S, Wallace RB, Bauer DC, Palermo L, Wehren LE, Lombardi A, Santora AC, Cummings SR, FLEX Research Group. Effects of continuing or stopping alendronate after 5 years of treatment. The Fracture Intervention Trial long-term extension (FLEX): a randomized trial. JAMA 2006;296:2927–2938.
73. Borgstrom F, Johnell O, Jonsson B, Zethraeus N, Sen SS. Cost effectiveness of alendronate for the treatment of male osteoporosis in Sweden. Bone 2004;34:1064–1071.

25 Glucocorticoid-Induced Osteoporosis

Michael Maricic, MD

CONTENTS

Key Words: Glucocorticoid-induced osteoporosis, exogenous glucocorticoids, bone mineral density, glucocorticoid-induced bone loss, parathyroid hormone, bone remodeling, hyperparathyroidism, gonadotopin secretion, hypogonadism

INTRODUCTION

Harvey Cushing first described the association between excess endogenous glucocorticoids and fractures in 1932 *(1)*. By 1954, a few years after the introduction of prednisone to treat rheumatoid arthritis, the deleterious skeletal effects of exogenous glucocorticoids were reported *(2)*. Glucocorticoid-induced bone loss is now the most common form of secondary osteoporosis and fractures are glucocorticoids' most common adverse effect *(3)*. They are among the most common iatrogenic complications of clinical practice as glucocorticoids are used by 0.5–2.5% of adults *(4)*. Concomitant factors including the underlying disease for which patients are treated, age, baseline bone mineral density (BMD), the hormonal status of the patient, and individual differences in sensitivity to glucocorticoid also play a role in whether or not the patient will develop osteoporosis and fractures.

PATHOGENESIS OF GLUCOCORTICOID-INDUCED BONE LOSS

Glucocorticoids have both direct and indirect effects on bone and affect both bone formation and resorption. Among the indirect effects, glucocorticoids cause a decrease

From: *Contemporary Endocrinology: Osteoporosis: Pathophysiology and Clinical Management*
Edited by: R. A. Adler, DOI 10.1007/978-1-59745-459-9_25,

in intestinal calcium absorption and an increase in the urinary excretion of calcium. Although secondary hyperparathyroidism had been thought to play a role in GIOP, elevated parathyroid hormone levels are not consistently found and histomorphometric analysis of bone biopsies from patients with GIOP reveal decreased bone remodeling rather than the increased remodeling seen with secondary hyperparathyroidism *(5)*. Glucocorticoids inhibit gonadotopin secretion leading to hypogonadism. Enhanced bone resorption ensues, at least in part due to enhanced secretion of cytokines such as interleukin-6, tumor necrosis factor alpha, and macrophage-colony stimulating factor (M-CSF) *(6)*.

Bone resorption is coupled with bone formation. A critical system involved in this coupling is the RANK-L (receptor activator of nuclear factor-κB ligand)-RANK-OPG (osteoprotegerin) system. RANK-L is secreted by osteoblasts, then binds to and activates its receptor RANK on the surface of osteoclast precursors and induces osteoclastogenesis *(7)*. OPG is a natural inhibitor of RANK-L, preventing RANK-L from binding to its osteoclast receptor. Glucocorticoids increase the expression of RANK-L and M-CSF *(8)* and decrease OPG expression in osteoblasts and stromal cells. The consequence of these changes is an initial increase in the number of osteoclasts capable of resorbing bone. Eventually, glucocorticoids deplete the population of osteoblasts as described below, which leads to decreased RANK-L and M-CSF expression by osteoblasts with a consequent decrease in osteoblast number *(9)*.

The most significant mechanism of glucocorticoid-induced bone loss is decreased bone formation. Glucocorticoid exposure leads to a decrease in the number of osteoblasts, both by decreasing osteoblast formation and increasing osteoblast apoptosis *(10)*. Pluripotent bone marrow stromal cells have the ability to differentiate into a number of cells of the mesenchymal lineage, including either osteoblasts or adipocytes. Glucocorticoids shift the differentiation of pluripotent stromal cells away from osteoblasts toward the adipocyte lineage through regulation of nuclear factors of the CAAT enhancer-binding protein family and by induction of peroxisome proliferator-activated receptor γ2 *(11)*. Glucocorticoids also suppress canonical Wnt/β-catenin signaling, a key regulator of osteoblastogenesis *(12)*. The bone morphogenetic protein (BMP) pathway involved in stimulating osteoblast differentiation and bone formation is also suppressed by glucocorticoids *(13)*.

In addition to their effects on osteoblastogenesis, glucocorticoids also have effects on bone matrix (inhibition of type I collagen synthesis and increased collagenase production) *(14)* and on skeletal growth factors (they down regulate transcription of the insulin growth factor I (IGF I) gene and its binding proteins *(15)*.

Osteocytes are thought to participate in the detection and healing of bone microdamage. Accelerated apoptosis of osteocytes could lead to bone microdamage and diminished bone quality and strength independent of BMD *(16)*. Increased osteocyte apoptosis has been documented in patients with GIOP *(17)*.

GLUCOCORTICOID EFFECTS ON BONE MINERAL DENSITY

Glucocorticoids affect both trabecular and cortical bone mass, however, bone loss is usually most marked in trabecular bone, due to its high surface area and high metabolic activity. Declines of lumbar spine bone mineral density (BMD) of 8.2% within 20 weeks have been detected by quantitative computed tomography (QCT), a sensitive measure of trabecular bone density *(18)*. After glucocorticoid discontinuation, the trabecular lumbar spine BMD increased by 5.2%. A number of studies have shown that bone loss is similar in men and women (both postmenopausal and premenopausal women). Fractures are more likely to occur in those with the lowest baseline bone mass, thus most studies demonstrate highest fracture rates in postmenopausal women.

GLUCOCORTICOID EFFECTS ON FRACTURE RISK

Glucocorticoid use increases the risk of both vertebral and nonvertebral fractures. In a study using an administrative claims database in the United States, Steinbuch compared fracture risk in glucocorticoid users to age and sex-matched controls *(19)*. The adjusted relative risk (RR) among users of glucocorticoids compared to controls was 2.92 for vertebral, 1.68 for nonvertebral, 1.87 for hip, and 1.75 for any fracture. The combined effect of higher dose, longer duration, and continuous pattern further increased RR estimates to 7-fold for hip and 17-fold for vertebral fractures.

Kanis et al. *(20)* studied the relationship between use of glucocorticoids and fracture risk in a meta-analysis of data from seven cohort studies of 42,000 men and women. Both current and past use of corticosteroids was an important predictor of fracture risk that was independent of prior fracture and BMD. No significant difference in risk was seen between men and women. For osteoporotic fracture, the range of relative risk was 2.63–1.71 and for hip fracture 4.42–2.48.

The largest study examining the relationship between oral glucocorticoid use and fractures was the United Kingdom General Practice Database (GPDP) study reported by van Staa et al. *(21)*. This study compared the relative rates of fracture in 244,235 patients receiving oral glucocorticoids to age and sex-matched controls. An average daily dose of prednisolone of 5 mg/day significantly increased the risk of spine and hip fractures. The most important risk for fracture in GIOP is the daily rather than the cumulative dose of oral glucocorticoids. The risk of nonvertebral fracture increases exponentially for daily doses over 20 mg prednisolone/day *(22)*. Fracture risk rises within 3 months of starting glucocorticoids and falls after discontinuation within 1 year of stopping therapy. However, this increased risk does not fall back to baseline *(21)*, so that even prior users of glucocorticoids have an increased fracture risk irrespective of BMD *(20)*.

Several epidemiological studies have reported increased risk of lower BMD and fracture in patients using inhaled glucocorticoids *(23,24)*. Whether this is due to the glucocorticoids themselves or the underlying disease is controversial. A large cohort study performed by van Staa et al. *(24)* using the GPDB suggests that users of other respiratory medications other than inhaled glucocorticoids also have an increased risk of fracture suggesting that the excess risk appears to be related to the underlying respiratory disease rather than to inhaled glucocorticoid.

Other concomitant factors play a role in bone loss and fractures including the underlying disease state for which glucocorticoids are given, individual differences in sensitivity to glucocorticoids, and the age and hormonal status of the patient. Although men and women are both susceptible to GIOP, the highest fracture rates are seen in postmenopausal women.

BMD Threshold for Fractures in Glucocorticoid-Induced Osteoporosis

The World Health Organization (WHO) criteria for the densitometric diagnosis of osteoporosis (*T*-score < –2.5) were developed based on the relationship of the prevalence of fractures in postmenopausal Caucasian females to the prevalence of *T*-scores below a certain level in the same population *(25)*. The same type of large epidemiological study does not exist for glucocorticoid-treated patients.

To answer the question of whether or not fracture rates occur at a higher bone density or *T*-score in patients on glucocorticoids, van Staa et al. *(26)* analyzed the relationship between BMD and vertebral fracture in postmenopausal women taking glucocorticoids. He compared the incidence of fracture in the placebo groups from the risedronate prevention *(27)* and treatment *(28)* trials to the 1-year fracture risk of postmenopausal women not taking glucocorticoids in three other trials. In the BMD threshold analysis, even though the women taking glucocorticoids were younger (64.7 versus 74.1 years old), had higher mean lumbar *T*-score (–1.8 versus –2.6), femoral neck *T*-score (–1.9 versus –2.6), and less prevalent fractures (42.9 versus 58.3%) than the non-glucocorticoid users, the risk of fracture was higher in the GC users than the non-GC users[adjusted RR 5.7 (CI 2.57–12.54)]. Thus, fracture incidence was markedly higher in the glucocorticoid users at any given level of BMD. This data is one of the reasons for the recommendation of therapeutic intervention in GIOP at *T*-score levels of –1 or lower by the American College of Rheumatology *(29)* and of –1.5 or lower by the United Kingdom societies *(30)*.

Nonpharmacologic Interventions

The use of systemic glucocorticoids should be minimized whenever possible. Nonpharmacologic interventions such as smoking and alcohol cessation and fall risk assessment should be offered to all patients. Exercise to improve lower extremity strength and balance is particularly important in glucocorticoid-treated patients where myopathy and an increased risk of falls are common. Calcium and vitamin D should be considered necessary but not sufficient for patients receiving chronic glucocorticoids, as they do not reduce fracture risk equal to the degree compared with bisphosphonates. Recommended calcium doses are at least 1200–1500 mg/day. Vitamin D should be administered in doses from 400 to 800 IU daily.

A 2-year trial of 65 rheumatoid arthritis patients treated chronically with low-dose prednisone (approximately 5 mg/day) randomized to 1000 mg of calcium carbonate and 500 IU of ergocalciferol versus placebo demonstrated that those given the daily supplements gained 0.7 and 0.9% annually in lumbar spine and greater trochanter bone mineral density (BMD) compared to losses of –2.0 and –0.9% at these sites in the placebo group *(31)*. A meta-analysis on the effectiveness of treatments for GIOP concluded that calcium plus vitamin D was more effective than no treatment or calcium alone at the lumbar spine *(32)*. A recent meta-analysis of active vitamin D_3 analogues in GIOP found that they preserve bone density more effectively than no treatment, plain vitamin D_3, and/or calcium *(33)*. Bisphosphonates, however, were found to be more effective in preserving bone and decreasing the risk of vertebral fractures than active vitamin D_3 analogues.

BISPHOSPHONATES

Bisphosphonates are currently the preferred treatment for GIOP. Most trials have examined their efficacy on BMD as the primary endpoint; however, post hoc analyses consistently support an effect on fracture reduction (mainly in the group at highest risk – postmenopausal women). In the United States, risedronate (5 mg/day) is approved by the Food and Drug Administration (FDA) for the prevention and/or treatment of GIOP and alendronate (5 mg/day for males and premenopausal females and 10 mg/day for postmenopausal females not receiving estrogen therapy) is approved for treatment. Although commonly utilized in clinical practice, neither weekly alendronate nor risedronate have been approved for GIOP. The package labeling for risedronate does state that 35 mg once weekly "may be considered" for prevention of GIOP.

In studies of patients receiving glucocorticoids, daily alendronate, daily risedronate, and cyclic etidronate have demonstrated significant increases in BMD at both the hip and spine, and reductions in vertebral fracture risk (all compared to calcium and vitamin D alone). In the alendronate GIOP trial reported by Saag, there were too few patients with new vertebral fractures after 1 year, so that fracture reduction was not significant *(34)*. After 2 years, a significant reduction of 89% in vertebral fractures was demonstrated *(35)*. A pooling of the risedronate prevention and treatment studies demonstrated a significant 70% reduction in vertebral fractures after 1 year compared to calcium and vitamin D alone *(36)*. Cyclic etidronate was demonstrated to reduce the risk of new vertebral fractures by 85% over 1 year compared to placebo *(37)*.

A meta-regression analysis *(38)* comparing the efficacy of therapies used for the treatment of glucocorticoid-induced osteoporosis determined that bisphosphonates were the most effective class of drugs to preserve vertebral BMD, with an effect size of 1.03 (95% CI, 0.85–1.17) compared to vitamin D (0.46, CI 95%, 0.27–0.62), or calcitonin (0.51, CI 95%, 0.33–0.67) therapy. When combined with vitamin D, the effect size of bisphosphonates further increased to 1.31 (1.07–1.50).

In patients for whom a contraindication to oral bisphosphonates exists, parenteral bisphosphonates including pamidronate and zoledronic acid could be considered (neither is FDA approved for GIOP at this time). In a primary prevention study of 32 patients being started on prednisone ≥10 mg/day, patients were randomized to receive either an intravenous infusions of 90 mg pamidronate at baseline, an infusion of 90 mg at baseline followed by 30 mg pamidronate given every 3 months for 1 year or placebo infusions (all groups received calcium carbonate 800 mg/day). BMD changes at the lumbar spine were +1.7, +2.3, and –4.6% and at the total hip were +1.0, +2.6, and –2.2% for the three respective groups. The differences between the placebo and both pamidronate groups were statistically significant *(39)*.

A single infusion of 4 mg zoledronic acid has been demonstrated in non-glucocorticoid-treated postmenopausal females to increase BMD and reduce markers of bone resorption for up to 12 months *(40)*. Zoledronic acid has not yet been approved for GIOP, however, a trial is currently underway.

Both intravenous and oral formulations of ibandronate have been studied and ibandronate is now approved for daily oral use in the treatment of postmenopausal osteoporosis. A trial of 115 patients receiving long-term glucocorticoids (average daily dose 10 mg prednisone) were randomized to receive either 500 mg of calcium and 1 μg of alfacalcidiol daily or calcium and infusions of 2 mg intravenous ibandronate every 3 months *(41)*. At 3 years, BMD was increased 13.3 % at the lumbar spine and 5.2 % at the femoral neck in the ibandronate group compared to alfacalcidiol group (2.6 and 1.9%, respectively). Although not specifically powered to detect a reduction in fracture risk, the incidence of new vertebral fractures in the alfacalcidiol group (22.8%) was statistically greater than in the ibandronate group (8.6%) a 62% relative risk reduction ($p=0.043$). Intravenous ibandronate is not currently approved nor marketed.

PARATHYROID HORMONE (PTH)

Parathyroid hormone is not approved for the treatment of glucocorticoid-induced osteoporosis, however, its potential for stimulating and/or prolonging the life span of osteoblasts suggests that it may have an important role in GIOP. A study of teriparatide (human recombinant parathyroid hormone 1–34) as monotherapy for GIOP is currently underway.

A 12-month trial of females with low bone mass (T-score ≥ -2.5) who were on long-term estrogen and glucocorticoids (mean 8.5 mg of prednisone daily for an average of 13 years) was performed to compare the additive effects of subcutaneous daily human parathyroid hormone (1–84) with placebo *(42)*. Both groups received 1500 mg calcium and 800 IU vitamin D per day. BMD at the lumbar spine was significantly greater in the combination of PTH and estrogen group (11% increase by dual-energy X-ray absorptiometry and 33% by quantitative CT scanning) compared to the estrogen-alone group at 12 months). Increases in femoral neck BMD were significant in the combination group at 24 months. The effect on BMD was sustained for 1 year following the discontinuation of PTH and the continuation of estrogen *(43)*.

Among other contraindications to teriparatide, it should not be given to children or young adults with open epiphyses.

OTHER THERAPIES

Other pharmacologic options for the prevention of bone loss include nasal spray calcitonin and hormone therapy or selective estrogen receptor modulators in women and testosterone in men. Studies of calcitonin in GIOP are limited with conflicting data on its ability to prevent bone loss *(44)* and no studies demonstrating fracture risk reduction. No studies currently exist examining the role of SERMS in GIOP. A few small studies of hormone therapy in GIOP have been performed. In one trial of postmenopausal women receiving prednisone for rheumatoid arthritis, those randomized to hormone therapy had a significant (3.4%) increase in their lumbar spine BMD compared with controls. There was no significant change in femoral neck BMD in either group *(45)*. Similar small studies of testosterone replacement in GIOP have been performed *(46)*, demonstrating increases in BMD of 5% at 1 year in hypogonadal asthmatic men treated with testosterone compared to controls. Increases in lean body mass (reflecting muscle mass) were also demonstrated in the testosterone treated men.

Due to the increased risks of breast cancer and cardiovascular disease associated with hormone therapy *(47)*, recommendations for its use as a primary treatment for osteoporosis cannot be made. Similar arguments could be made for testosterone replacement where the long-term adverse effects are unknown *(48)*. These therapies are most likely to be appropriate in the patient on glucocorticoids where deficiencies of these hormones lead to vasomotor symptoms, loss of libido, etc., and where specific replacement could enhance the patient's quality of life for reasons other than osteoporosis.

GUIDELINES FOR THE PREVENTION AND TREATMENT OF GIOP

Based in part on the knowledge that the most rapid loss of bone density is observed upon initiating prednisone therapy. The American College of Rheumatology Ad Hoc Guidelines Committee *(29)* recommends prophylactic bisphosphonates for all new glucocorticoid users expected to continue prednisone ≥5 mg/day for more than 3 months. For prevalent glucocorticoid users receiving prednisone doses of ≥5 mg/day who have a *T*-score below –1.0, the ACR also recommends bisphosphonate therapy. Caution is advised in premenopausal women and counseling regarding appropriate contraception is advised. For prevalent glucocorticoid users who have a *T*-score above –1.0, follow-up BMD measurement annually or biannually is recommended. Nonpharmacologic interventions outlined above are also recommended for all patients.

The United Kingdom Royal College of Physicians, National Osteoporosis Society and Bone and Tooth Society recommends pharmacologic intervention at a *T*-score of –1.5 or lower in patients on chronic oral glucocorticoids *(30)*. They recommend taking an aggressive approach in older patients and in those with a history of prior fracture and suggest that treatment to reduce risk of fracture should be initiated at the same time as the glucocorticoid therapy without the need for assessment of bone mineral density.

Likewise, in situations where bone mass measurement is impractical or unavailable, the Department of Veterans Affairs recommends empiric therapy with bisphosphonates when doses of prednisone ≥7.5 mg/day are prescribed for longer than 3 months *(49)*.

None of these guidelines specifically address patients using inhaled glucocorticoids, however, based on the data that patients with chronic lung disease receiving either glucocorticoid or non-glucocorticoid inhalers are at increased risk of fracture *(23,24)*, measurement of BMD in these patients would seem appropriate with treatment determined by their overall risk factor profile.

Although markers of bone formation and resorption predict fracture risk in chronic glucocorticoid users *(50)*, their clinical utility in GIOP remains investigational.

Table 1 provides the author's recommended approach to patients on or beginning glucocorticoid therapy.

CONCLUSIONS

Considerable advances have been made over the past 10 years in the recognition and treatment of GIOP. The possibility of less frequent intravenous bisphosphonates and anabolic agents such as parathyroid hormone raise the potential of more effective therapies in the future. However, despite the knowledge of the fracture risk associated with glucocorticoids, the availability of effective prophylaxis, and treatment and published guidelines, measurement of bone density and institution of medications to prevent bone loss are suboptimal *(51)*, including among specialty physicians *(52)*. Continued education, dissemination of guidelines, and other innovative approaches will be necessary to make a more substantial impact on this disorder.

Table 1
Recommendations for the Prevention and Treatment of GIOP

Minimize dose of systemic glucocorticoids whenever possible
Nonpharmacologic interventions, such as smoking and alcohol cessation, minimization of alcohol intake, fall avoidance strategies, and balance/lower extremity strengthening exercises should be recommended
A daily intake of calcium (1200–1500 mg/day) and serum vitamin D (400–800 IU/day) should be given
Initiate bisphosphonate therapy [risedronate (5 mg/day) or alendronate (5 mg/day in men and premenopausal women or 10 mg/day in postmenopausal women not on estrogen therapy] in patients beginning prednisone ≥5 mg/day for more than 3 months. For prevalent glucocorticoid users receiving prednisone doses of ≥5 mg/day who have a *T*-score below –1.0, initiate bisphosphonate therapy
Consider parathyroid hormone or intravenous bisphosphonates (neither is FDA approved for GIOP) if patients have contraindications to, do not tolerate or fail oral bisphosphonate therapy
Consider estrogen or testosterone replacement where indicated for quality of life issues, but not as primary therapy in lieu of bisphosphonates
Monitor BMD by DXA after 6–12 months, depending on the dose of glucocorticoids and severity of baseline bone loss

REFERENCES

1. Cushing H. The basophil adenomas of the pituitary body and their clinical manifestations (pituitary basophilism). Bull John Hopkins Hosp 1932;50:137–195.
2. Curtis PH, Clark WS, Herndon CH. Vertebral fractures resulting from prolonged cortisone and corticotropin therapy. JAMA 1954;156:467–469.
3. Saag KG, Koehnke R, Caldwell JR, et al. Low dose long-term corticosteroid therapy in rheumatoid arthritis: an analysis of serious adverse events. Am J Med 1994;96(2):115–123.
4. van Staa TP, Cooper C, Abenhaim L, et al. Utilization of oral corticosteroids in the United Kingdom. Q J Med 2000;93:105–111.
5. Carbonare LD, Bertoldo F, Valenti MT, Zenari S, Zanatta M, et al. Histomorphometric analysis of glucocorticoid-induced osteoporosis. Micron 2005;36:645–652.
6. Weitzmann MN, Racifici R. Estrogen deficiency and bone loss: an inflammatory tale. J Clin Invest 2006;116:1186–1194.
7. Hofbauer LC, Gori F, Riggs BL, et al. Stimulation of osteoprotegerin ligand and inhibition of osteoprotegerin production by glucocorticoids in human osteoblastic lineage cells: potential paracrine mechanisms of glucocorticoid-induced osteoporosis. Endocrinology 1999;140:4382–4389.
8. Alesci S, De Martino MU, Illias I. Glucocorticoid-induced osteoporosis: from basic mechanisms to clinical aspects. Neuroimmunomodulation 2005;12:1–19.
9. Canalis E. Glucocorticoid-induced osteoporosis: pathophysiology. In: Maricic M, Gluck O, eds. Bone disease in rheumatology. New York: Lippincott, 2005:105–110.
10. Weinstein RS, Jilka RL, Parfitt AM, et al. Inhibition of osteoblastogenesis and promotion of apoptosis of osteoblasts and osteocytes by glucocorticoids: Potential mechanisms of their deleterious effects on bone. J Clin Invest 1998;102:274–282.
11. Pereira RC, Delany AM, Canalis E. Effects of cortisol and bone morphogenetic protein-2 on stromal cell differentiation: correlation with CCAAT-enhancer binding protein expression. Bone 2002;30:685–691.

12. Ohnaka K, Tanabe M, Kawate H, et al. Glucocorticoid suppresses the canonical Wnt signal in human osteoblast. Biochem Biophys Res Commun 2005;329:177–181.
13. Leclerc N, Lupen CA, Ho VV. Gene expression profiling of glucocorticoid-inhibited osteoblasts. J Mol Endocrinol 2004;33(1):175–193.
14. Delany AM, Jeffrey JJ, Rydziel S, et al. Cortisol increases interstitial collagenase expression in osteoblasts by post-transcriptional mechanisms. J Biol Chem 1995;270:26607–26612.
15. Delany AM, Durant D, Canalis E. Glucocorticoid suppression of IGF I transcription in osteoblasts. Mol Endocrinol 2001;15:1781–1789.
16. Weinstein RS, Powers CC, Parfitt AM, et al. Preservation of osteocyte viability by bisphosphonates contributes to bone strength in glucocorticoid-treated mice independently of BMD: an unappreciated determinant of bone strength. J Bone Miner Res 2002;17(Suppl 1):S156.
17. Weinstein RS, Jilka RL, Parfitt M, et al. Inhibition ofosteoblastogenesis and promotion of apoptosis of osteoblasts and osteocytes by glucocorticoids: potential mechanisms of their deleterious effects on bone. J Clin Invest 1998;102:274–282.
18. Laan RF, van Riel PL, van de Putte LB, et al. Low-dose prednisone induces rapid reversible axial bone loss in patients with rheumatoid arthritis. Ann Intern Med 1993;119(10):963–968.
19. Steinbuch M, Thomas E, Youket E, et al. Oral glucocorticoid use is associated with an increased risk of fracture. Osteoporos Int 2004:15:323–328.
20. Kanis JA, Johannson H, Oden A, et al. A meta-analysis of prior corticosteroid use and fracture risk. J Bone Miner Res 2004;19:893–899.
21. van Staa T, Leufkens H, Abenhaim L, et al. Use of oral corticosteroids and risk of fractures. J Bone Miner Res 2000;15(6):993–1000.
22. van Staa TP, Leufkens HMG, Abenhaim L, Zhang B, et al. Oral corticosteroids and fracture risk: relationship to daily and cumulative doses. Rheumatology 2000;39:1383–1389.
23. Hubbard RB, Smith CJP, Smeeth L, et al. Inhaled corticosteroids and hip fracture: a population-based case-control study. Am J Respir Crit Care Med 2002;166:1563–1566.
24. van Staa TP, Leufkens HGM, Cooper C. Use of inhaled corticosteroids and risk of fractures. J Bone Miner Res 2001;3:581–588.
25. World Health Organization. Asscssment of fracture risk and its application to screening for post-menopausal osteoporosis. Technical report series 843. Geneva:WHO, 1994.
26. Van Staa TP, Laan RF, Barton IP, et al. Bone density threshold and other predictors of vertebral fracture in patients receiving oral glucocorticoid therapy. Arthritis Rheum 2003;48(11):3224–3229.
27. Cohen S, Levy RM, Keller M, et al. Risedronate therapy prevents corticosteroid-induced bone loss: A twelve-month, multicenter, randomized, double-blind, placebo-controlled, parallel-group study. Arthritis Rheum 1999;42(11):2309–2318.
28. Reid DM, Hughes R, Laan RF. Efficacy and safety of daily risedronate in the treatment of corticosteroid-induced osteoporosis in men and women: a randomized trial. J Bone Miner Res 2000;15: 1006–1013.
29. American College of Rheumatology Ad Hoc Committee on Glucocorticoid-Induced Osteoporosis. Recommendation for the prevention and treatment of glucocorticoid-induced osteoporosis. Arthritis Rheum 2001;44:1496–1503
30. Royal College of Physicians, National Osteoporosis Society, Bone and Tooth Society of Great Britain. Glucocorticoid-induced osteoporosis—guidelines for prevention and treatment. London: Royal College of Physicians, 2002
31. Buckley LM, Leib ES, Cartularo KS, Vacek PM, Cooper SM. Calcium and vitamin D3 supplementation prevents bone loss in the spine secondary to low-dose corticosteroids in patients with rheumatoid arthritis. Ann Intern Med. 1996;125:961–968.
32. Amin S, LaValley MP, Simms RW, et al. The role of vitamin D in corticosteroid-induced osteoporosis: a meta-analytic approach. Arthritis Rheum 1999;42:1740–1751.
33. de Nijs RNJ, Jacobs JWG, Algra A., et al. Prevention and treatment of glucocorticoid-induced osteoporosis with active vitamin D3 analogues: a review with meta-analysis of randomized controlled trials including organ transplantation studies. Osteoporos Int 2004;15:589–602
34. Saag KG, Emkey R, Schnitzer T, et al. Alendronate for the treatment and prevention glucocorticoid-induced osteoporosis. N Engl J Med 1998;339:292–299.

35. Adachi JD, Saag K, Emkey R, et al. Effects of alendronate for two years on BMD and fractures in patients receiving glucocorticoids. Arthritis Rheum 2001;44:202–211.
36. Wallach S, Cohen S, Reid DM, et al. Effects of risedronate treatment on bone density an vertebral fracture in patients on corticosteroid therapy. Calcif Tissue Int 2000;67:277–285.
37. Adachi JD, Bensen WG, J. Brown, et al. Intermittent etidronate therapy to prevent corticosteroid induced osteoporosis. N Engl J Med 337;1997:382–387.
38. Amin S, LaValley MP, Simms RW, et al. The comparative efficacy of drug therapies used for the management of corticosteroid-induced osteoporosis: a meta-regression. J Bone Miner Res 2002;17:1512–1526.
39. Boutsen Y, Jamart J, Esselinckx W, et al. Primary prevention of glucocorticoid-induced osteoporosis with intravenous pamidronate and calcium: a prospective controlled 1-year study comparing a single infusion, an infusion given once every 3 months, and calcium alone. J Bone Miner Res 2001;16(1):104–112.
40. Reid IR, Brown JP, Burckhardt P, et al. Intravenous zoledronic acid in postmenopausal women with low bone mineral density. N Engl J Med 2002;346:653–661.
41. Ringe JD, Dorst A, Faber H, Ibach K, et al. Intermittent intravenous ibandronate injections reduce vertebral fracture risk in corticosteroid-induced osteoporosis: results from a long-term comparative study. Osteoporos Int 2003;14(10):801–807.
42. Lane NE, Sanchez S, Modin GW, et al. Parathyroid hormone treatment can reverse corticosteroid-induced osteoporosis. Results of a randomized controlled clinical trial. J Clin Invest 1998;102(8):1627–1633.
43. Lane NE, Sanchez S, Modin GW, et al. Bone mass continues to increase at the hip after parathyroid hormone treatment is discontinued in glucocorticoid induced osteoporosis: results of a randomized controlled clinical trial. J Bone Miner Res 2000;15(5):944–951.
44. Healey JH, Paget SA, Williams-Russo P, et al. A randomized controlled trial of salmon calcitonin to prevent bone loss in corticosteroid-treated temporal arteritis and polymyalgia rheumatica. Calcif Tissue Int 1996;58:73–80.
45. Hall GM, Daniels M, Doyle DV, et al. Effect of hormone replacement therapy on bone mass in rheumatoid arthritis patients treated with and without steroids. Arthritis Rheum 1994;37:1499–1505.
46. Reid IR, Wattie DJ, Evans MC, et al. Testosterone therapy in glucocorticoid-treated men. Arch Intern Med 1996;156:1173–1177.
47. Rossouw JW, Anderson GL, Prentice RL, et al. Risks and benefits of estrogen plus progestin in healthy post-menopausal women: principal results from the women's health initiative randomized controlled trial. JAMA 2002;288:321–333.
48. Rhoden EL, Morgentaler A. Risks of testosterone-replacement therapy and recommendations for monitoring. N Engl J Med 2004;350:482–492.
49. Adler RA, Hochberg MC. Suggested guidelines for evaluation and treatment of glucocorticoid-induced osteoporosis for the 'partment of Veterans Affairs. Arch Intern Med 2003;163(21):2619–2624.
50. van Staa T, Eastell R, Barton IP, et al. The value of bone turnover markers in the prediction of vertebral fracture in patients using oral glucocorticoids. J Bone Min Res 2003;18:(S2):S66.
51. Curtis JR, Westfall AO, Allison JJ, et al. Longitudinal patterns in the prevention of osteoporosis in Glucocorticoid-treated patients. Arthritis Rheum 2005;52:2485–2494.
52. Solomon DH, Katz JN, Jacobs JP, et al. Management of glucocorticoid-induced osteoporosis in patients with rheumatoid arthritis. Arthritis Rheum 2002;46:3136–3142.

26 Transplantation Osteoporosis

Emily Stein, MD and Elizabeth Shane, MD

CONTENTS

Key Words: Transplantation osteoporosis, cyclosporine, transplantation immunology, short-term graft, patient survival, tacrolimus, glucocorticoid-induced osteoporosis, bone loss, fragility fractures, immunosuppressive agents, bone and mineral metabolism, skeletal effects

INTRODUCTION

The introduction of cyclosporine to transplantation immunology in the early 1980s resulted in marked improvement in short-term graft and patient survival and ushered in a new era for patients with end-stage renal, hepatic, cardiac, pulmonary, and hematopoietic disease. The addition of cyclosporine, and later tacrolimus, to post-transplantation immunosuppression regimens permitted the use of lower doses of glucocorticoids (GCs). Therefore, it was initially expected that glucocorticoid-induced osteoporosis would be less of a problem in the cyclosporine era. During the past two decades, however, it has become clear that organ transplant recipients managed with cyclosporine and probably tacrolimus sustain rapid bone loss and fragility fractures *(1–4)*. Moreover, transplantation-related bone loss and fractures may become increasingly prevalent as more patients continue to undergo organ transplantation each year and survival continues to improve *(5)*. This review will summarize our current understanding of the effects of the most commonly prescribed immunosuppressive agents on bone and mineral metabolism. The epidemiology, natural history, and pathogenesis of bone loss and fracture after various types of organ transplantation will be reviewed. Recommendations for prevention of the acute phase of bone loss after

From: *Contemporary Endocrinology: Osteoporosis: Pathophysiology and Clinical Management*
Edited by: R. A. Adler, DOI 10.1007/978-1-59745-459-9_26,

organ transplantation, and treatment of established osteoporosis in organ transplantation candidates and recipients will be summarized.

SKELETAL EFFECTS OF IMMUNOSUPPRESSIVE DRUGS

The Bone-Remodeling System

Transplantation osteoporosis, as with most adult metabolic bone diseases, is the result of alterations in the bone-remodeling system, an orderly progression of events by which bone cells remove old bone tissue and replace it with new. Thus, it is helpful to review the orderly sequence of events that constitutes normal bone remodeling, in order to understand the pathogenesis of transplantation osteoporosis. The two main processes by which remodeling occurs are known as resorption *(6)* and formation *(7)*. Conceptually, these processes are somewhat akin to the repair of cracks and potholes that develop in surfaces of highways. Remodeling occurs on the surfaces of both cancellous and cortical bone. The first step is activation of macrophage precursors to form osteoclasts, giant multinucleated cells that excavate or resorb a cavity on the bone surface. Osteoclasts express receptors for receptor activator of NFκB ligand (RANKL) produced by osteoblasts, calcitonin, prostaglandins, calcium, and vitronectin (integrin $\alpha_1\beta_3$). In general, approximately 0.05 mm^3 of bone tissue is resorbed by each osteoclast, leaving small resorption pits on the bone surface called Howship's lacunae. This process takes approximately 2–3 weeks. After a brief rest period known as the reversal phase, local mesenchymal bone marrow stem cells differentiate into osteoblasts that are attracted to the empty resorption pits. There they accumulate as clusters of plump cuboidal cells along the bone surface. Osteoblasts have two major functions. They produce the proteins, both collagenous and non-collagenous, that constitute the matrix of the newly formed bone. Osteoblasts are also responsible for mineralization of the matrix or osteoid after an approximately 10-day period during which the osteoid has matured. Osteoblasts express receptors for parathyroid hormone, estrogens, vitamin D_3, cell adhesion molecules (integrins), and several cytokines. The complete remodeling cycle at each remodeling site requires approximately 3–6 months. This process serves to replace old, micro-damaged bone with new, mechanically stronger bone. RANKL, RANK, and osteoprotogerin (OPG) are three members of the tumor necrosis factor (TNF) ligand and receptor-signaling family that are final effectors of bone resorption *(8,9)*. RANKL is expressed in osteoblasts and bone marrow stromal cells. When sufficient concentrations of macrophage colony stimulating factor (mCSF) are present, binding of RANKL to RANK, which is expressed on surfaces of osteoclast lineage cells, through cell-to-cell contact, results in rapid differentiation of osteoclast precursors in bone marrow to mature osteoclasts, increased osteoclast activity, and reduced apoptosis of mature osteoclasts. RANKL is neutralized by binding to OPG, another member of the TNF-receptor superfamily secreted by cells of the osteoblast lineage. Competitive binding of RANKL to either RANK or OPG regulates bone remodeling by increasing (RANK) or decreasing (OPG) osteoclastogenesis. Immunosuppressants exert their effects on bone remodeling by interacting with the RANK/RANKL/OPG system *(10)*.

In normal adults, bone remodeling results in no net change in bone mass. Bone loss develops in any situation in which bone remodeling becomes "uncoupled," such that the rate of resorption exceeds the rate of formation. This most often occurs when the rate of resorption is so elevated that it is beyond the capacity of the osteoblasts to restore the original amount of bone volume. However, bone loss may also develop in the setting of depressed bone formation, such that even normal amounts of resorbed bone cannot be replaced. It is very likely that transplantation-related bone loss results from both a primary decrease in the rate of bone formation and a primary increase in the rate of resorption *(1,11)*.

Glucocorticoids

Glucocorticoids (GCs), an integral component of most transplant immunosuppression regimens, are notorious for causing osteoporosis (see Chapter 23). Prednisone or methylprednisolone may be prescribed in high doses (50–100 mg of prednisone or its equivalent daily) immediately after transplantation and during episodes of severe rejection, with gradual reduction over weeks to months. Total exposure varies with the organ transplanted, the number and management of rejection episodes, and the practice of individual transplantation programs.

GCs cause bone loss and fractures by mechanisms summarized in Table 1 and several recent reviews *(12–14)*. The main effect is an immediate and profound inhibition of bone formation by decreasing osteoblast recruitment and differentiation, synthesis of type I collagen, and induction of apoptosis of osteoblasts and osteocytes both in vitro and in vivo *(15)*. These effects are reflected biochemically by low serum levels of osteocalcin, a major non-collagenous bone matrix protein secreted by osteoblasts. Indirect effects include inhibition of growth hormone secretion and decreased production or bioactivity of certain skeletal growth factors (IGF-1, PGE_2, and TGF-β), actions that also reduce bone formation.

GCs also increase bone resorption, through both direct effects on osteoclasts and indirect effects. GCs *directly* increase osteoclast activity by decreasing osteoblast expression of OPG and increasing osteoblast expression of RANKL. In turn, osteoclast maturation is increased and osteoclast apoptosis is decreased. GCs *indirectly* increase resorption by impairing calcium transport across cell membranes, causing reduced intestinal calcium absorption, increased urinary calcium losses, and negative calcium balance. Secondary hyperparathyroidism may result, although it is unlikely that it plays a major role in the pathogenesis of associated bone loss *(16)*. GCs also cause hypogonadotrophic hypogonadism and reduced secretion of adrenal androgens and estrogens, which may also be associated with increases in bone resorption. These contrasting effects of GCs upon bone formation (decreased) and resorption (increased) prevent osteoblasts from replacing the increased amount of bone resorbed at each remodeling site, and rapid bone loss ensues. The magnitude of glucocorticoid stimulatory effects on resorption is less profound than their inhibitory effects on formation; moreover, the effects on resorption are transitory, generally limited to the first 6–12 months. Glucocorticoid-induced myopathy may also contribute to bone loss by altering gravitational forces on the skeleton, reducing weight-bearing activity and mobility, and to fracture rates by increasing the propensity for falls.

Patients taking GCs generally sustain significant bone loss *(13,14)*. Bone loss occurs in all races, at all ages, and in both genders. However, postmenopausal, Caucasian women are at greater risk for fracture than other groups, because glucocorticoid-related bone loss is superimposed upon that already sustained because of aging and estrogen deficiency. In general, bone loss is most rapid during the first 12 months and is directly related to dose and duration of therapy. Areas of the skeleton rich in cancellous bone (ribs, vertebrae, and distal

Table 1
Glucocorticoid Actions that Contribute to Bone Loss

Inhibit bone formation – most important effects that result in a 30% reduction in amount of bone replaced in each remodeling cycle

- Reduce osteoblast numbers
  - Decrease osteoblast replication and differentiation
- Shorten osteoblast life span
  - Increase apoptosis of osteoblasts and osteocytes
- Inhibit osteoblast function
  - Reduce synthesis of type I collagen
  - Decrease synthesis of bone matrix proteins and osteocalcin
- Decrease synthesis of IGF-I and inhibit IGF-II receptor expression in osteoblasts – local anabolic regulators that increase type I collagen synthesis

Stimulate bone resorption – effects on resorption are minor and limited to first 6–12 months

- *Directly* increase osteoclast activity
  - Decrease osteoblast expression of osteoprotegerin (OPG)
  - Increase osteoblast expression of RANKL
  - Increase osteoclast maturation and decrease apoptosis
- *Indirectly* increase resorption
  - Decrease production of gonadal hormones
  - Decrease intestinal calcium absorption
  - Increase urinary calcium excretion
  - Increase secretion of parathyroid hormone

ends of long bones) and the cortical rim of the vertebral body are most severely affected and also fracture most frequently.

In recent years, there has been a trend toward more rapid lowering of glucocorticoid doses after transplantation or rejection episodes and an increase in the use of alternative drugs to treat rejection *(17–20)*. In more recently transplanted patients who have received lower doses of steroids, significant bone loss still occurs although it may be less rapid than previously documented *(21–24)*. Moreover, it should be noted that even rather small doses of GCs are associated with increased fracture risk. A large retrospective general practice database study found that doses of prednisolone as low as 2.5 mg daily were associated with a significant 55% increase in the relative risk of spine fractures; doses between 2.5 and 7.5 mg daily were associated with a 2.6-fold increase in the risk of spine fracture and a 77% increase in the risk of hip fracture *(25)*. Thus, even in those programs that have embraced the use of lower doses of GCs, there is still sufficient exposure in the initial year to cause significant bone loss.

Cyclosporines

Cyclosporine (CsA) is a small fungal cyclic peptide. Its activity depends upon the formation of a heterodimer consisting of cyclosporine and its cycloplasmic receptor, cyclophilin. This cyclosporine–cyclophilin heterodimer then binds to calcineurin *(26)*. CsA, and similarly tacrolimus, inhibits the phosphatase activity of calcineurin through interaction with distinct domains on the calcineurin subunit *(27)*. Calcineurin may regulate both osteoblast *(28)* and osteoclast differentiation *(29)*. Although the gene for calcineurin, which is integral to the immunosuppressive action of CsA, has been identified in osteoclasts and extracted whole rat bone, it does not appear to be altered by CsA administration *(30)*.

Animal studies suggest that CsA has effects on bone and mineral metabolism that may contribute to bone loss after organ transplantation (Table 2) *(11,31)*. When administered to rodents in doses higher than those currently used to prevent allograft rejection, CsA causes rapid and severe cancellous bone loss *(32,33)*, characterized histologically by marked increase in bone resorption. In contrast to the effects of GCs, bone formation is increased in CsA-treated animals, although insufficiently to compensate for the increase in resorption. The stimulatory effects of CsA on osteoclast formation are likely mediated via T lymphocytes *(34–36)*. CsA also increases gene expression of osteocalcin and bone-resorbing cytokines, such as IL-1 and IL-6 *(37)*. Parathyroid hormone (PTH) may facilitate CsA-induced bone loss *(38)*. Drugs that inhibit bone resorption, including estrogen, raloxifene, calcitonin, and alendronate, prevent or attenuate CsA-induced bone loss in the rat *(39–42)*. Similarly, 1,25 dihydroxyvitamin D and prostaglandin E2 also prevent bone loss in CsA-treated rats *(43,44)*. In contrast, testosterone *(29)* does not ameliorate bone loss *(45)*.

Table 2
Skeletal Effects of Cyclosporine (and Tacrolimus)*

Increase expression of bone resorbing cytokines
Increase expression of osteocalcin
Increase bone resorption
Increase bone formation
Cause rapid, severe cancellous bone loss
Effects mediated by T lymphocytes
PTH may have permissive effect
Bone loss prevented by antiresorptive agents, 1,25 dihydroxyvitamin D

*These effects based primarily on animal studies.

Studies examining the effects of CsA on the human skeleton have yielded conflicting results. Several have shown that kidney transplant patients receiving cyclosporine in a steroid-free regimen did not lose bone *(46–48)*. In contrast, a small study of kidney transplant recipients detected no difference in bone loss between those who received CsA monotherapy and those who received azathioprine and prednisolone *(49)* and a recent prospective study found that cumulative CsA dose was associated with bone loss in the 2 years following transplant, independent of the effect of GCs *(50)*.

Tacrolimus (FK506)

FK506 is a macrolide that binds to an immunophilin FK binding protein and blocks T-cell activation in a manner similar to CsA. FK506 has been shown to cause bone loss in the rat model comparable to that observed with CsA *(51)* and accompanied by similar biochemical and histomorphometric alterations (Table 2). In humans, rapid bone loss has been documented after both cardiac *(52)* and liver transplantation *(53)*, when tacrolimus is used for immunosuppression. However, other studies suggest that FK506 may cause less bone loss than CsA in humans *(54,55)*, likely because lower doses of GCs are required for immunosuppression. It remains unclear whether FK506 confers any benefit over cyclosporine with regard to fracture incidence.

Sirolimus (Rapamycin)

Rapamycin is a macrocyclic lactone. Although it is structurally similar to FK506 and binds to the same binding protein, the mechanism by which rapamycin induces immunosuppression is distinct from both FK506 and CsA. When combined with low-dose CsA, rapamycin was bone sparing in rat studies *(56)*. In a recent open label studies, markers of bone turnover (N-telopeptide and osteocalcin) were higher in kidney transplant recipients who received CsA rather than sirolimus: unfortunately BMD was not measured, so it remains unclear whether this translated into lower rates of bone loss *(57)*. However, combining immunosuppressive agents in lower doses may provide hope for achieving adequate immunosuppression while protecting the skeleton.

Azathioprine, Mycophenolate Mofetil, and Other Drugs

Short-term administration of azathioprine is associated with decreases in serum osteocalcin but does not cause bone loss in the rat model *(58)*. No adverse effects of azathioprine administration alone on bone mass have been reported in human subjects. In the past, azathioprine was frequently used in combination with prednisone and CsA or FK506 to prevent organ rejection. However, it has largely been supplanted by mycophenolate mofetil, which does not have deleterious effects on bone in the rat *(59)*. The skeletal effects of other immunosuppressant agents, such as mizoribine, deoxyspergualin, brequinar sodium, leflunomide, and azaspirane, are unclear.

EFFECT OF TRANSPLANTATION ON BONE AND MINERAL METABOLISM

Bone Loss Before Transplantation

In many cases, individuals with chronic diseases severe enough to warrant organ transplantation have already sustained considerable bone loss *(60–62)* (Table 3). The majority of candidates for organ transplantation have one or more accepted risk factors for osteoporosis, including debilitation, loss of mobility and physical inactivity, poor nutrition, and cachexia. They are commonly exposed to drugs known to cause bone loss, such as GCs, heparin, loop diuretics, excessive doses of thyroid hormone, and anticonvulsants. Postmenopausal women are estrogen deficient, as are many chronically ill premenopausal, women. Similarly, men with chronic illness often have hypogonadotrophic hypogonadism. When the disease is present during childhood or adolescence, as is the case with cystic

Table 3
Osteoporosis, Fractures, and Bone Loss in Candidates for Solid Organ Transplantation

Type of transplant	*Prevalence before transplantation*	
	Osteoporosis[a] (%)	*Fractures (%)*
Kidney[b]	8–49	Vertebral: 3–21, Peripheral: 35
Heart	8–10	Vertebral: 18–50
Liver	8–43	Vertebral: 20–25
Lung	30–35	Vertebral: 14–49

Adapted from Cohen and Shane *(1)*.
[a]Accepted definitions included BMD (by dual x-ray absorptiometry) of the spine and/or hip with *Z* score –2 or *T* score≤–2.5.
[b]Definition of osteoporosis also included BMD of predominantly cortical sites such as the femoral shaft or proximal radius that are adversely affected by excessive PTH secretion.

fibrosis or congenital heart disease, peak bone mass, which is attained during adolescence, may be low. Therefore, in caring for organ transplant candidates, it is essential to consider the possibility that bone mass may be reduced before transplantation. Consideration of particular issues related to transplantation of specific organs follows.

Kidney and Kidney–Pancreas Transplantation

Skeletal Status Before Transplantation

In patients with severe chronic kidney disease (CKD) or end-stage renal disease (ESRD), disturbances in calcium and phosphate metabolism, decreased calcitriol synthesis, increased synthesis and secretion of PTH, metabolic acidosis, and defective bone mineralization result in the complex form of bone disease known as renal osteodystrophy *(63)*. Some form of renal osteodystrophy is almost universal in patients who undergo kidney transplantation. A given individual may have high bone turnover, due to hyperparathyroidism with or without osteitis fibrosa, low turnover or adynamic bone disease, osteomalacia, or "mixed" renal osteodystrophy, a combination of one or more of the aforementioned lesions. Type I diabetes, hypogonadism secondary to uremia, and diseases, such as systemic lupus erythematosus, common in patients with CKD and ESRD, also adversely affect the skeleton. Several drugs used routinely in the management of patients with renal disease, such as loop diuretics, calcium-containing phosphate binders, can also affect bone and mineral metabolism. In addition, some kidney transplant candidates may have had previous exposure to GCs or cyclosporine as therapy for immune complex nephritis or other diseases and thus may already have sustained significant bone loss prior to transplantation.

Measurement of BMD by dual energy X-ray absorptiometry (DXA) is of limited utility in patients with ESRD as it does not distinguish among the various types of renal osteodystrophy and more importantly, does not discriminate between patients with and without fractures *(64)*. That being said, several cross-sectional studies have documented that osteoporosis and low bone mass are present in a significant proportion of patients on chronic dialysis (Table 3) *(65–67)*.

Not surprisingly, the risk of fracture in patients with ESRD is greatly elevated. Risk of all fractures has estimated at 4.4–14 times greater than that of the general population *(68,69)*. Vertebral fractures were present in 21% of Japanese hemodialysis patients *(70)*. In one study, 34% of 68 hemodialysis patients had a history of previous fracture *(71)*. In another prospective study, the incidence of fractures was 0.1 fractures per dialysis year in patients with osteitis fibrosa and 0.2 fractures per dialysis year in patients with adynamic bone disease *(72)*. Recently, we have appreciated that hip fractures are also 2-fold more common in patients with moderate-to-severe CKD, who do not yet require dialysis *(73)* than in those with normal kidney function.

Risk factors for low bone mineral density and fractures include female gender, Caucasian race, hyperparathyroidism, adynamic bone disease, secondary amenorrhea, type I diabetes, older age, duration of dialysis, peripheral vascular disease, prior kidney transplant *(74)*, and diabetic nephropathy *(61)*.

Prevalence of Osteoporosis in Kidney Transplant Recipients

Low BMD measurements have been reported in several cross-sectional studies of patients who have undergone kidney transplantation *(2,3,75–77)* (Table 4), although again the prognostic significance of low BMD is unclear in such patients. For example, lumbar spine (LS) BMD was below the "fracture threshold" in 23% of 65 renal transplant recipients studied an average of 4 years after transplantation *(78)*; female gender, postmenopausal status and cumulative prednisone dose were independent predictors of low BMD. Similarly, LS BMD was more than two standard deviations below age- and sex-matched controls (Z score >–2.0) in 41% of patients studied 6–195 months after renal transplantation *(79)* and was directly related to increasing time since transplantation and PTH concentrations. LS and femoral neck (FN) bone density were more than two standard deviations below age- and sex-matched controls in 28.6 and 10.5% of 70 kidney transplant recipients studied an average of 8 years after transplantation *(80)* and was particularly prevalent in women. In a recent study of male renal transplant recipients, only 17% had normal BMD, 30% had osteoporosis at the hip or LS, 41% including the DR; bone resorption markers were elevated in 48% *(81)*. Other studies have shown similar results *(47,82,83)*.

Bone Loss After Kidney Transplantation

Prospective longitudinal studies have documented high rates of bone loss after kidney transplantation (Table 4), particularly during the first 6–18 months after grafting. Julian et al. *(84)* were the first to report that LS BMD decreased by 6.8% at 6 months and by 8.8% at 18 months after transplantation. At 18 months, BMD was below the "fracture threshold" in 10 of 17 patients. Several prospective studies have confirmed this pattern of bone loss *(21,85–91)*, in which the rate of bone loss is greatest during the first 6 months after transplantation and at sites where cancellous bone predominates, such as the LS. The rate of LS bone loss varies between 3 and 10%. There may be a gender difference in the site at which bone is lost *(74,85,87)*; men have been shown to lose more bone at the proximal femur than women in the first few months after transplantation.

The pathogenesis of bone loss after renal transplantation is complex. The majority of studies have found that glucocorticoid dose correlates positively with bone loss. Men and

Table 4
Osteoporosis, Fractures, and Bone Loss After Solid Organ and Bone Marrow Transplantation

Type of transplant	*Prevalence after transplantation*		*Bone loss: first*	*Fracture incidence (%)*
	Osteoporosis[a] (%)	*Fractures (%)*	*post-transplant year (%)*	
Kidney[b]	11–56	Vertebral: 3–29, peripheral: 11–22	Spine: 4–9, hip: 8	Vertebral: 3–10, peripheral: 10–50
Heart	25–50	Vertebral: 22–35	Spine: 2.5–8%, hip: 6–11%	10–36
Liver	30–46	Vertebral: 29–47	Spine: 0–24, hip: 2–4	Vertebral: 24–65
Lung	57–73	42	Spine: 1–5%, hip: 2–5	18–37
Bone marrow	4–15	5	Spine: 2–9, hip: 6–11%	1–16

Adapted from Cohen et al. *(1)*.
[a]Accepted definitions included BMD (by dual x-ray absorptiometry) of the spine and/or hip with *Z* score$\leq$–2 or *T* score$\leq$–2.5.
[b]Definition of osteoporosis also included BMD of predominantly cortical sites such as the femoral shaft or proximal radius that are adversely affected by excessive PTH secretion.

premenopausal women may be at lower risk and postmenopausal women at higher risk. There is also some evidence in the literature to support a role for cyclosporine in the pathogenesis of the high turnover state often apparent in renal transplant recipients by 1 year after renal transplantation.

Bone Histology After Kidney Transplantation

Before transplantation, hyperparathyroidism is the most common lesion on bone biopsy. However, by 6 months after transplantation, glucocorticoid effects predominate, with osteoblast dysfunction and decreased mineral apposition *(84,92)*. In long-term kidney transplant recipients, bone biopsy results are more heterogeneous and include osteoporosis, osteomalacia, and osteitis fibrosa. An increase in osteoblastic activity and mineralization defects were common *(93)*.

Fracture After Kidney Transplantation

Fractures are very common after renal transplantation (Table 5) and affect appendicular sites (feet, ankles, long bones, hips) more commonly than axial sites (spine, ribs) *(81)*. One study determined that non-vertebral fractures are 5-fold more common in males aged 25–64, and 18- and 34-fold more common in females aged 25–44 and 45–64, respectively, who have had a renal transplant than they are in the normal population *(94)*. Prevalent vertebral or appendicular fractures were identified in 24% of long-term kidney transplant subjects *(77)*. Vertebral fractures have been reported in 3–10% of nondiabetic patients after renal transplantation *(47,80)*. A cohort study involving 101,039 subjects found that patients who underwent kidney transplant had a 34% greater risk of hip fracture than those who remained on dialysis *(61)*.

Fractures are particularly common in patients who receive kidney or kidney–pancreas transplants for diabetic nephropathy *(95–98)*. In a retrospective study of 35 kidney–pancreas recipients, approximately half had sustained from one to three symptomatic, nonvertebral fractures by the end of the third post-transplant year *(95)*.

Mineral Metabolism and Bone Turnover After Kidney Transplantation

The changes in biochemical indices of mineral metabolism and bone turnover after renal transplantation are fairly consistent *(84,99)*. PTH levels, usually elevated before transplantation, frequently remain high for some time after transplantation and may never completely normalize *(100)*. Hypercalcemia and hypophosphatemia, related to persistent parathyroid hyperplasia and elevated PTH levels, occur commonly during the first few months. Persistent elevations in fibroblast growth factor-23 (FGF-23) after transplant have recently been hypothesized to be related to post-transplant hypophosphatemia *(101)*. In most patients, these biochemical abnormalities are mild and resolve within the first year. In long-term transplant recipients, persistent elevations in PTH may be associated with reduced hip BMD *(100)*. Calcitriol production by the transplanted kidney may be inadequate to suppress PTH secretion by hyperplastic parathyroid tissue *(102)*, and treatment calcitriol may prevent hyperparathyroidism after renal transplantation *(103)*. Vitamin D deficiency is common and severe in patients after kidney transplantation. In one study *(104)*, the mean serum level of 25-hydroxyvitamin D (25OHD) was 10 ng/ml and one-third of patients had undetectable levels. Transplant recipients had significantly lower levels than age-matched controls *(104)*.

Cardiac Transplantation

SKELETAL STATUS BEFORE TTRANSPLANTATION

Risk factors common in patients with end-stage cardiac failure that may predispose to bone loss before transplantation include exposure to tobacco, alcohol, and loop diuretics; physical inactivity; hypogonadism; and anorexia which may contribute to dietary calcium deficiency. Hepatic congestion and prerenal azotemia may also affect mineral metabolism, causing mild secondary hyperparathyroidism. Although on average bone density of patients awaiting cardiac transplantation may not differ significantly from normal, it has been observed that approximately 8–10% fulfill World Health Organization criteria for osteoporosis (Table 3) *(60,105–107,23)*.

PREVALENCE OF OSTEOPOROSIS IN HEART TRANSPLANT RECIPIENTS

Osteoporosis and fractures constitute a major cause of morbidity after cardiac transplantation. In cross-sectional studies, the prevalence rate of vertebral fractures in cardiac transplant recipients (Table 4) ranges between 18 and 50% and moderate-to-severe bone loss is present in a substantial proportion of subjects at both the LS and the FN *(94,105–118)*. In a cross-sectional study of long-term cardiac transplant recipients, osteopenia or osteoporosis (*T* score less than –1.0) were found in 66% at the FN and 26% at the LS *(119)*. Perhaps related to a failure to achieve peak bone mass, adults who receive cardiac transplants as adolescents have significantly lower BMD at LS, FN, and distal radius than age-matched controls *(120)*.

BONE LOSS AFTER HEART TRANSPLANTATION

The pattern of bone loss after cardiac transplantation is similar to that observed after renal. Prospective longitudinal studies have documented rates of bone loss ranging from 2.5 to 11%, predominantly during the first 3–12 months after transplantation (Table 4) *(52,121–128)*. Although GCs affect the predominantly cancellous bone of the vertebrae to a greater extent than other sites, there is as much or more bone loss at the hip, a site with more cortical bone than the vertebral bodies *(23,125)*. Moreover, while bone loss at the LS slows or stops after the first 6 months, FN bone loss continues during the second half of the first year after transplantation *(23,125)*. There are very few longitudinal data available on the pattern of bone loss after the first year. However, our data suggest that the rate of bone loss slow or stops in the majority of patients, with some recovery at the LS noted during the third year of observation *(23,125)*. Bone loss also slows at the hip after the first year; however, in contrast to the spine, there has been no significant recovery by the fourth post-transplant year. The results of a recent study suggest that there may be less bone loss than suggested in literature from the 1980s and early 1990s *(23)*.

FRACTURE AFTER HEART TRANSPLANTATION

Fragility fractures are most common during the phase of rapid bone loss that characterizes the first post-transplant year (Table 3). In a prospective observational longitudinal study, 36% of patients (54% of the women and 29% of the men) suffered one or more fractures of the vertebrae, ribs, and hip in the first year despite daily supplementation with calcium (1,000 mg) and vitamin D (400 IU) *(129)*. The mean time to first fracture was 4 months, with most patients sustaining their initial fracture during the first 6 months. Lower pretransplant BMD and female gender were associated with a trend toward increased fracture risk. In men, however, it was the rate of bone loss after transplantation rather than the pretransplant bone density that was associated with fracture risk. Many patients fractured who had normal BMD pretransplant and thus it was not possible to predict who would fracture either on the basis of pretransplant BMD or any other demographic or biochemical parameter *(129)*. Two European studies of cardiac transplant recipients reported similar fracture incidence with approximately 30–33% sustaining vertebral fractures during the first 3 years *(130)*. The risk of a vertebral fracture was higher in those patients who had LS *T* scores below –1.0 (hazard ratio 3.1) *(130)*.

In a more recent interventional study, the incidence of vertebral fractures during the first post-transplant year in patients who received only calcium and vitamin D was only 14%, suggesting fracture rates may be lower than in the past *(23)*. However, clinical experience suggests that fractures remain a very common and sometimes devastating complication of heart transplantation. A complete bone evaluation including BMD measurements before or immediately after transplantation, as well as aggressive intervention to prevent bone loss and fractures are needed in all patients regardless of age, sex, or pretransplant bone density.

Mineral Metabolism and Bone Turnover After Heart Transplantation

Biochemical changes after cardiac transplantation include sustained increases in serum creatinine *(125,127,131)* and decreases in 1,25 dihydroxyvitamin D concentrations *(125)*. On an average, serum testosterone concentrations decrease in men with recovery by the sixth post-transplant month *(125,127,131)*. Serum osteocalcin falls precipitously and there is a sharp increase in markers of bone resorption (hydroxyproline and pyridinium crosslink excretion) during the first 3 months with return to baseline levels by the sixth month *(125,127,131)*. This biochemical pattern coincides with the period of most rapid bone loss and highest fracture incidence and suggests that the early post-transplant period is associated with uncoupling of formation from resorption, and restitution of coupling when glucocorticoid doses are lowered. There is also evidence for a high bone turnover state later in the post-transplant course perhaps due to cyclosporine, characterized by elevations in both serum osteocalcin and urinary excretion of resorption markers *(107,109,110,116,117,126,127,131)*. The increased bone turnover may be due in part to secondary hyperparathyroidism related to renal impairment *(110)*. Thus biochemical changes later in the post-transplant course may be mediated, at least in part, by cyclosporine A-induced renal insufficiency, although other etiologies cannot be excluded.

Liver Transplantation

Skeletal Status Before Transplantation

Patients with liver failure have multiple risk factors that may predispose to low bone mineral density before transplantation and fracture after transplantation *(132–134)*. Many patients with end-stage liver disease who are listed for liver transplantation have prevalent osteoporosis (Table 3), as evidenced by low bone mineral density (BMD) and fragility fractures *(135,136)*. Osteoporosis and abnormal mineral metabolism have been described in association with alcoholic liver disease, hemochromatosis, steroid-treated autoimmune chronic active hepatitis, postnecrotic cirrhosis, and particularly in chronic cholestatic liver diseases such as biliary cirrhosis *(137–139)*. A study of 58 patients with cirrhotic end-stage liver disease referred for liver transplantation *(136)* reported that 43% had osteoporosis (defined as *Z* score>2 SD below age-matched controls or presence of vertebral fractures). Serum 25-OHD, 1,25(OH)$_2$D, intact PTH, and osteocalcin (a marker of bone formation) were lower, and urinary hydroxyproline excretion (a marker of bone resorption) was higher in cirrhotic patients than controls. Male patients had lower serum testosterone levels than controls. A study of 56 liver transplant recipients revealed that 23% had osteoporosis that antedated transplantation *(140)*. In a recent study of 360 liver transplant candidates, 38% had osteoporosis and 39% had osteopenia *(141)*.

Histomorphometric studies have found that bone formation is decreased in patients with primary biliary cirrhosis and is reflected by low serum osteocalcin levels *(142–144)*. Another study found biochemical evidence of both decreased bone formation and increased bone resorption in patients with chronic liver disease *(135)*. However, while serum osteocalcin appears to be a valid marker of bone formation in cholestatic liver disease, the utility of collagen-related markers of bone turnover has recently been called into question. In fibrotic liver diseases, the synthesis of type I collagen is markedly increased. Guanabens et al. *(142)* have found that collagen-related bone turnover markers appear influenced by liver, rather than bone, collagen metabolism and do not reflect skeletal turnover in patients with liver disease. Serum osteocalcin and tartrate-resistant acid phosphatase (TRAP) may be more valid markers of bone-remodeling activity in this clinical situation.

Bone Loss and Fracture After Liver Transplantation

Osteoporosis is also common after liver transplantation, as detailed in several recent reviews *(62,145)*. The natural history of bone loss following liver and cardiac transplantation appears similar *(130)*. Rates of bone loss and fracture vary considerably after liver transplantation (Table 3), but were often extremely high, particularly in studies published before 1995 *(130,140,146–153)*, in which LS BMD fell by 2–24%, primarily in the initial few months after liver transplantation. Bone loss appears to stop after 3–6 months with gradual improvement by the second and third post-transplant years. Eastell et al. *(146)* reported that bone mass recovers and bone histology normalizes with increasing survival time after transplantation, and other investigators have shown that there is improvement in BMD in long-term liver transplant recipients *(154)*. This, however, has not been a uniform finding and other studies have found continued losses rather than recovery *(148,155)*.

More recent studies have found smaller amounts of bone loss. Keogh et al. *(156)* reported that femoral neck BMD fell by 8% and LS BMD by 2% after liver transplantation. Ninkovic et al. *(22)* found only a 2.3% loss at the femoral neck, with preservation of LS BMD 1 year after liver transplant. Floreani et al. *(157)* found increases in BMD at 1 year. Smallwood et al. *(158)* reported in a cross-sectional study that lower bone mass following liver transplant was associated with older age, female gender, cholestatic liver disease, and higher prednisone dose. A recent retrospective study found that women receiving cumulative glucocorticoid doses greater than 3,500 mg had lower FN BMD at 1 and 2 years following liver transplant than other patients *(159)*. Guichelaar et al. followed 360 patients after liver transplant. Higher rates of LS bone loss occurred in patients with primary sclerosing cholangitis, current smokers, younger age, higher baseline BMD, shorter duration of liver disease, and ongoing cholestasis *(141)*.

Fracture incidence is also highest in the first year and ranges from 24 to 65%, the latter in a group of women with primary biliary cirrhosis. The vertebrae and ribs are the most common fracture sites. Again, fracture rates appear to be considerably lower in more recent studies *(22)*. Whether type of liver disease at baseline predicts fractures is controversial. Some authors report more bone loss and fractures in patients with primary sclerosing cholangitis *(141)* and alcoholic cirrhosis *(160)*. Glucocorticoid exposure and markers of bone turnover do not reliably predict bone loss or fracture risk. Older age and pre-transplant BMD at the FN and LS were predictive of post-transplant fractures in recent prospective studies *(22,161)*. Vertebral fractures prior to transplant have been shown to predict post-transplant vertebral fractures *(130,162)*. In re-transplanted patients, those with primary biliary cirrhosis and those with previous fragility fractures are at increased risk. These patients may always be at risk for fractures as survival rates and duration increase.

Mineral Metabolism and Bone Turnover After Liver Transplantation

Studies of calciotropic hormone levels and bone turnover markers after liver transplantation are limited. Compston et al. *(163)* reported a significant rise in serum intact PTH during the first 3 months after liver transplantation, although levels did not exceed the upper limit of the normal range. Significant increases in PTH during the first 3–6 months after transplant have been observed by other authors as well *(157,161)*. In contrast, intact PTH levels have been reported to be within the normal range in liver transplant recipients in other studies *(148,151,164)*.

With respect to bone turnover, markers of bone formation (osteocalcin and carboxy-terminal peptide of type I collagen) and resorption are higher in liver transplant recipients than in normal controls in most *(164,151,165,166)*, though not all studies *(167)*. OPG and RANK-L levels are significantly elevated in the first 2 weeks following liver transplant *(168)*. The balance of the data thus suggests that low bone turnover observed in many patients with liver failure converts to a high turnover state that persists indefinitely after liver transplantation.

As is the case with renal and cardiac transplantation, the independent role of GCs and calcineurin inhibitors in the pathogenesis of bone disease in liver transplant patients is difficult to assess since single drug therapy is uncommon. The mechanism of bone loss after liver transplantation has been studied by transiliac crest bone biopsy after tetracycline labeling in 21 patients, evaluated before and 3 months after transplantation. Before transplantation, a low turnover state was observed, with decreased wall width and erosion depth. Postoperative biopsies showed high turnover with increased formation rates and activation frequency, and a trend toward increased indices of resorption *(169)*, which may have been related to the concomitant increase in PTH concentrations *(163)* or alternatively to calcineurin inhibitors.

Lung Transplantation

SKELETAL STATUS BEFORE LUNG TRANSPLANTATION

Hypoxemia, tobacco use, and prior glucocorticoid therapy are frequent attributes of candidates for lung transplantation and may contribute to the pre-transplant bone loss (Table 3), particularly common in these patients *(170,171)*. Cystic fibrosis (CF), a common reason for lung transplantation, is itself associated with osteoporosis and fractures due to pancreatic insufficiency, vitamin D deficiency and calcium malabsorption, and hypogonadism *(172–174)*. A greatly increased rate of all fractures and severe kyphosis has been reported in adults with cystic fibrosis *(172)*. We have observed that vitamin D deficiency is extremely common in CF patients, despite supplementation; bone density was significantly lower in the vitamin D-deficient patients *(173)*. Two cross-sectional studies have found that low bone mass and osteoporosis are present in 45–75% of candidates for lung transplantation *(170,171)*. In both, glucocorticoid exposure was inversely related to BMD. Vertebral fracture prevalence was 29% in patients with emphysema and 25% in patients with CF *(170,171)*. Low bone mass is also common in patients with primary pulmonary hypertension prior to lung transplantation; in a retrospective study, 61% had osteopenia at the FN and 72% at the LS. BMD at the FN correlated with functional measures, walking distance, and pulmonary vascular resistance *(175)*. A recent cross-sectional study of patients with diffuse parenchymal lung disease presenting for lung transplantation found that 13% had osteoporosis and 57% osteopenia. Low BMD was associated with lower body mass index and Hispanic ethnicity *(176)*.

BONE LOSS AND FRACTURE AFTER LUNG TRANSPLANTATION

Few studies have prospectively evaluated patients after lung transplantation (Table 3). A study of 12 patients demonstrated an average 4% decrease in LS BMD during the first 6 months despite calcium and 400 IU of vitamin D *(177)*. Two men sustained multiple vertebral fractures. Another study documented decreases of approximately 5% in both LS and femoral neck BMD during the first 6–12 months after lung transplantation and fractures developed in 18% of 28 patients *(178)*. In a retrospective analysis of 33 lung transplant recipients, who had survived at least 1 year after grafting, BMD was markedly decreased and 42% had vertebral fractures *(179)*. In a 10-year follow-up study of lung transplant recipients, of the 28 (29%) of patients who survived, 11% had prevalent osteoporotic fractures *(180)*. Our experience suggests that as many as 37% of lung transplant recipients suffer fragility fractures and significant bone loss during the first post-transplant year despite antiresorptive therapy *(181)*.

Risk factors for fracture and bone loss include female gender, low pretransplant LS BMD, pretransplant glucocorticoid therapy, and higher bone turnover after transplantation. Some studies have found that bone loss correlates with GC dose *(178)*, but others have not found this relationship *(181)*. Bone turnover markers are elevated following lung transplant. Increased osteoclastic and decreased osteoblastic activity have been observed in post-transplant bone biopsies of CF patients *(182)*.

Bone Marrow Transplantation

BMT is performed with increasing frequency and for expanding indications. In preparation for transplantation, patients receive myeloablative therapy (alkylating agents and/or total body irradiation) and commonly develop profound and frequently permanent hypogonadism, which could certainly cause bone loss. After transplantation, patients may receive GCs, methotrexate, or cyclosporine A, alone or in combination. The pathogenesis of osteoporosis after allogenic BMT is complex, related to many factors including the effects of treatment and effects on the stromal cell compartment of the bone marrow *(76,183,184)*. Low BMD was first reported after BMT by Kelly et al. *(185)*. Since then several cross-sectional studies have confirmed low total body BMD *(186)* or bone mineral content (BMC) *(187)* (by DXA) and LS BMD (by computed tomography) *(188)* in bone marrow transplant recipients (Table 4). However, in one study, only those who were less than 18 years old at the time of transplantation were affected, perhaps because of a failure to achieve optimal bone mass and smaller bone size *(186)*. Two studies have documented that bone mass is low in hypogonadal women after bone marrow transplantation *(189,190)* and that hormone replacement therapy is associated with significant increases in BMD *(189,190)*.

With respect to natural history of bone loss after BMT, a study of nine adults undergoing 6 months of high-dose glucocorticoid and CsA therapy for graft-versus-host disease (GVHD) observed significant LS bone loss *(191)*. Ebeling et al. *(192)* found that low BMD antedates BMT, particularly in subjects with prior glucocorticoid exposure and that post-transplant bone loss is particularly severe in patients who undergo allogeneic BMT, probably because of their increased propensity for GVHD. Valimaki et al. followed a group of patients who had undergone allogeneic BMT for 6 months (n=44) and 12 months (n=36) after grafting. Although some received calcium and vitamin D and some received calcitonin, there was no discernable difference in rates of bone loss; therefore the groups were combined. BMD decreased by approximately 6% at the LS and 7% at the FN *(193)*. Kang et al. *(194)* found that LS BMD decreased by 2.2% and FN BMD by 6.2% during the first year. Similarly, Kashyap et al. *(195)*found that LS BMD decreased by 3.0% and femoral neck BMD by 11.6% during the first 12–14 months. There appears to be little bone loss after the first year *(188)*. The significant bone loss that occurs in the femoral neck does not appear be regained *(196)*.

Bone turnover markers are consistent with the pattern of decreased formation and increased resorption *(193)* observed in other forms of transplantation during the first 3 months, a pattern consistent with uncoupling of formation from resorption. After 3 months, there was recovery of bone formation markers and generally elevated turnover during the latter half of the year *(193)*. Similar elevations of bone turnover markers have also been observed by other investigators after BMT *(188,197,198,184,194)*. Rates of FN bone loss are lower after autologous BMT, about 4%. LS BMD returns to baseline, while FN bone loss persists for 2 years *(199)*.

Cellular or cytokine-mediated abnormalities in bone marrow function after BMT may affect bone turnover and BMD *(200)*. Osteoblastic differentiation is reduced by damage from high-dose chemotherapy, total body irradiation, and treatment with GCs and/or CsA. Colony forming units-fibroblasts (CFU-f) are reduced for up to 12 years following BMT *(183,201)*. Long-term survivors have been shown to have persistent abnormalities in bone turnover and vitamin D *(202)*.

Avascular necrosis (AVN) is common, occurring in 10–20% of allo-BMT survivors, at a median of 12 months following transplant *(192,201)*. The most important risk factor for the development of avascular necrosis is GC treatment of chronic GVHD. AVN may be related to decreased numbers of bone marrow CFU-f in vitro, but does not appear to be related to BMD *(203)*.

Evaluation and Management of Candidates for Transplantation

EVALUATION

There are now abundant data documenting the high prevalence of bone disease in candidates for all types of transplantation. Therefore the possibility of significant bone disease should be addressed before transplantation so that potentially treatable abnormalities of bone and mineral metabolism may be addressed and the skeletal condition of the patient optimized before transplantation (Table 5). Risk factors for osteoporosis should be assessed. These include a family history of osteoporosis, history of adult low-trauma fractures, medical conditions (thyrotoxicosis, renal disease, rheumatological, and intestinal disorders), unhealthy lifestyle choices (physical inactivity, dietary calcium and vitamin D deficiency, excessive caffeine and alcohol intake, tobacco use), and exposure to certain drugs (diphenylhydantoin, lithium, loop diuretics, glucocorticoids, prolonged, and large doses of heparin, thyroid hormone). Additional risk factors important in women include premature menopause, postmenopausal status, anorexia nervosa, or prolonged episodes of amenorrhea. In men, it is important to exclude hypogonadism. A physical examination should focus upon findings that suggest hypogonadism, thyrotoxicosis, and Cushing's syndrome. Risk factors for falling (poor impaired vision, hearing, balance and muscle strength, psychotropic drugs) should also be assessed.

BMD of the spine and hip is the most important test to obtain before transplantation. Radiographs of the thoracic and lumbar spine are also important because the risk of future fracture is greater in patients with prevalent vertebral fractures. A battery of biochemical tests is unnecessary if the BMD is normal and supplementation with calcium and vitamin

Table 5
Skeletal Evaluation of the Candidate for Organ Transplantation

In all candidates:

- Assess risk factors for osteoporosis, including menstrual history, history of low-trauma fractures
- Measure bone densitometry (BMD) of spine and hip by DXA
- Obtain thoracic and lumbar spine radiographs

If BMD testing reveals osteoporosis or if there are prevalent vertebral or non-vertebral fractures:

- Serum electrolytes, BUN creatinine, calcium, parathyroid hormone, 25-hydroxyvitamin D, thyroid function tests (see text)
- In men, serum total and/or testosterone, FSH, and LH
- Urine for calcium and creatinine

D is planned. However, if the pretransplant BMD is low, a thorough biochemical evaluation can alert the physician to the etiology of low bone mass and guide appropriate therapy, targeted to the cause. In such instances, the biochemical evaluation should include a chemistry panel (serum electrolytes, creatinine, calcium, albumin, phosphorus, alkaline phosphatase), thyroid function tests, intact PTH, and serum 25-OHD. In men, total and free testosterone, FSH, and LH concentrations should be obtained. Markers of bone formation (serum osteocalcin and bone-specific alkaline phosphatase) and resorption (urinary deoxypyridinoline, C- or N-telopeptide excretion) can also be measured to assess bone turnover status.

Although pretransplant BMD does not reliably predict fracture in individual patients, low pretransplant BMD probably increases fracture risk, particularly in postmenopausal women. Individuals awaiting transplantation who meet World Health Organization criteria for diagnosis of osteoporosis (*T* score<–2.5), osteopenia or low bone mass (*T* score between –1.0 and –2.5) should be evaluated and treated similarly to others with, or at risk, for osteoporosis (Table 5).

While on the waiting list for transplantation, transplant patients should receive rehabilitation therapy as tolerated to maximize conditioning and physical fitness. All transplant candidates should receive the at least the recommended daily allowance of vitamin D (400–1,000 IU), or as necessary to maintain the serum 25-OHD level above 30 ng/ml (80 nmol/ml) and elemental calcium (1,000–1,500 mg, depending on dietary intake and menopausal status). Calcium citrate is preferred as many of these patients take proton pump inhibitors before or after transplantation, which can reduce intestinal calcium absorption. Hormone replacement therapy should be considered in premenopausal amenorrheic women after BMT, provided there are no contraindications to such therapy. The risks of HRT probably outweigh the benefits as a treatment for bone loss in postmenopausal women after transplantation. Hypogonadal men should also be offered testosterone replacement. Generally accepted guidelines for gonadal hormone replacement should apply to these patients.

Patients who are found to have osteoporosis before transplantation should begin antiresorptive therapy with a bisphosphonate. The pretransplant waiting period is often long enough (1–2 years) for significant improvement in BMD before transplantation. Patients with renal osteodystrophy should be managed in accordance with accepted clinical guidelines *(63)*. A discussion of this topic is beyond the scope of this chapter.

After transplantation, monitoring serum and urine indices of mineral metabolism is less crucial, although it may be useful to detect developing conditions that may contribute to bone loss (vitamin D deficiency or renal insufficiency with secondary hyperparathyroidism. Serum (and urinary) calcium must be monitored frequently if pharmacologic doses of vitamin D or its active 1-hydroxylated metabolites are used, in order to detect hypercalciuria or hypercalcemia. Measurement of BMD should be performed at 6-month intervals for the first 2 years and annually thereafter, particularly if the patient remains on GCs. Bone biopsy may be necessary in the kidney transplant recipient since many experts remain reluctant to use bisphosphonates in patients with adynamic bone disease. Although transiliac crest bone biopsy remains a research tool, more histomorphometric studies would be very helpful in confirming theories of the pathogenesis of transplantation osteoporosis.

Prevention of Transplantation Osteoporosis

The major principles that have been demonstrated consistently after kidney, liver, heart, lung, and bone marrow transplantation and that should guide therapy of transplantation osteoporosis are as follows:

- Rates of bone loss are most rapid immediately after transplantation.
- Fractures also occur very early after transplantation, sometimes within only a few weeks of grafting.
- Fragility fractures develop both in patients with low and those with normal pre-transplant BMD.
- Prevention of the rapid bone loss that during the first few months after transplantation is likely to be considerably more effective in reducing the morbidity from fractures than waiting for fractures to occur before initiating therapy.
- Therefore, preventive strategies should be instituted immediately after transplantation both in patients with normal pretransplant BMD and those with low BMD who have not been treated previously (Table 6).
- The long-term transplant recipient with established osteoporosis and/or fractures should not be neglected (Table 7).

There are several prospective controlled randomized studies for prevention and treatment of transplantation osteoporosis in the literature, although the quality of these studies varies. The recommendations provided herein are also based upon experience with glucocorticoid-induced osteoporosis. Available therapies of transplantation osteoporosis

Table 6
Primary Prevention of Bone Loss in Transplant Recipients

- Measure BMD before or immediately after transplantation and every 6 months for 2 years
- Consider pharmacologic therapy in all patients with low bone mass (*T* score between –1.0 and –2.5) or osteoporosis (*T* score<–2.5)
- Endeavor to use the lowest dose of glucocorticoids possible
    - Consider alternative therapies for rejection
- Calcium intake of 1500 mg/d both before and after transplantation
- Vitamin D intake of 400–1,000 IU, or as needed to maintain serum 25-OHD concentrations above 30 ng/ml (80 nmol/ml)
- Physical rehabilitation program both before and after transplantation
- Replace gonadal steroids in hypogonadal premenopausal women and men
- Begin antiresorptive therapy, preferably a bisphosphonate, before transplantation in patients with antecedent osteoporosis or low bone mass
- Begin antiresorptive therapy, preferably a bisphosphonate, immediately after transplantation in patients with normal or low bone mass and continue for at least the first year

Table 7
Management of the Long-Term Organ Transplant Recipient

In all patients:

- Assess risk factors for osteoporosis
- BMD of spine and hip by DXA
- Thoracic and lumbar spine radiographs
- Calcium intake of 1,500 mg/d both before and after transplantation
- Vitamin D intake of 400–1,000 IU, or as needed to maintain serum 25-OHD concentrations above 30 ng/ml (80 nmol/ml)
- Physical rehabilitation program.

If BMD testing reveals osteoporosis or there are prevalent vertebral fractures:

- Serum electrolytes, BUN creatinine, calcium, parathyroid hormone, 25-hydroxyvitamin D, thyroid function tests
- In men, serum total and/or testosterone, FSH, and LH
- Urine for calcium and creatinine
- Replace gonadal steroids in hypogonadal women and men, if appropriate
- Begin antiresorptive therapy, preferably a bisphosphonate
- These recommendations should not be applied to kidney transplant recipients, in whom the risk of the adynamic bone lesion is high and benefits of bisphosphonates are controversial

include antiresorptive drugs (bisphosphonates, calcitonin, and estrogen), as well as analogues of vitamin D and gonadal hormone replacement (Table 8). Since resorption markers increase after transplantation and correlate directly with rates of bone loss *(99)*, attempts to prevent post-transplantation bone loss, and hopefully fractures, by inhibition of bone resorption are a logical approach.

BISPHOSPHONATES

Bisphosphonates act by inhibiting osteoclastic bone resorption. This class of drugs is most commonly used to treat post-menopausal osteoporosis. However, they have also been used successfully both to prevent and to treat glucocorticoid-induced bone loss and bone loss in transplant recipients. Both alendronate and risedronate have been approved by the FDA for prevention and treatment of GC-induced osteoporosis. Since transplantation osteoporosis can be considered one form of glucocorticoid-induced osteoporosis and since cyclosporine and tacrolimus-induced bone loss are characterized experimentally by increases in both formation and resorption, bisphosphonates offer considerable hope for prevention of transplantation osteoporosis.

Several *(164,204–216)* studies suggest that intravenous bisphosphonates can prevent bone loss and fractures after transplantation. Intravenous pamidronate administered in repeated doses has been shown to prevent bone loss at the LS and FN in kidney *(205,216)*, heart *(209,214)*, liver *(217)*, and lung *(208,213)* transplant recipients. In a small, open but randomized clinical trial, intravenous pamidronate was administered to kidney transplant

Table 8
Specific Therapies for Transplantation Osteoporosis

Bisphosphonates
Etidronate, Pamidronate, Alendronate, Risendronate, Ibandronate, Zoledronic acid
Vitamin D
Parent vitamin D (high dose)
25-OHD (Calcidiol)
1,25(OH)$_2$D (Calcitriol)
1-α-calcidiol
Hormone replacement therapy
Estrogen
Testosterone
Calcitonin

recipients at time of grafting and again 1 month later *(204)*, completely preventing LS and FN bone loss. In contrast, LS BMD fell by 6.4% and FN BMD by 9% in the control subjects. The benefits of this intervention were still apparent 4 years after transplantation, especially at the FN *(205)*. Coco et al. *(216)* compared kidney transplant recipients who received intravenous pamidronate at the time of transplantation and at 1, 2, 3, and 6 months afterward, along with calcium and calcitriol, to those treated with calcium and calcitriol alone. There was no bone loss in the patients who received pamidronate, while the other group sustained losses of 4–6%. Bone biopsies performed 6 months after therapy, however, revealed a high incidence of adynamic bone disease. Aris et al. *(208)*, in a randomized, controlled but nonblinded trial demonstrated that intravenous pamidronate (30 mg every 3 months for 2 years) was associated with 8% increases in spine and hip BMD in patients who underwent lung transplantation for CF. Unfortunately, however, fracture rates were very high and did not differ between the two treatment groups. A retrospective study suggested that treatment with intravenous pamidronate before and every 3 months after liver transplantation prevented symptomatic vertebral fractures in liver transplant recipients who had osteoporosis before transplantation *(218)*. In contrast, a more recent prospective study in liver transplant patients found that bone loss at the FN was not prevented with pamidronate, which was given as a single infusion as long as 3 months before grafting. There was no LS bone loss in either group and fracture rates did not differ *(217)*. In two large prospective studies of patients after allogenic BMT, intravenous pamidronate prevented LS bone loss and reduced proximal femoral bone loss *(219,220)*. Some bone loss at the proximal femur still occurred, however, despite doses up to 90 mg one study *(220)*. The lack of efficacy may be related to a failure of pamidronate to inhibit matrix metalloproteinase (MMP)-mediated bone resorption or to reverse defects in osteoblast function after BMT *(221)*.

Recent randomized trials with the more potent intravenous bisphosphonates, zoledronic acid and ibandronate, have shown significant protective effects on BMD at 6 and 12 months in recipients of liver *(210,222)* and kidney *(211,215)* transplants. Crawford et al. *(222)* administered repeated doses of zoledronic acid before and at 1, 3, and 6 months following liver transplantation. Zoledronic acid prevented bone loss at the LS, FN, and total hip (TH), compared with placebo. One year after transplantation, the effects at the FN and TH persisted, but an increase in LS BMD in the placebo group abolished the significant difference at the spine *(222)*. Intravenous zoledronic acid (4 mg) given 12 months after BMT prevented spinal and femoral bone loss *(223)*. Zoledronic acid has also been shown to increase ex vivo growth of bone marrow CFU-f, perhaps improving osteoblast recovery and increasing osteoblast numbers after BMT.

Clinical trials have also been performed with oral bisphosphonates. In terms of primary prevention of bone loss immediately after transplantation, several studies have compared alendronate with calcitriol. A randomized trial comparing alendronate (10 mg daily) with calcitriol (0.25 μg twice daily) treatment in patients starting immediately after cardiac transplant found that both regimens prevented bone loss at the lumbar spine and hip 1 year after transplant, compared with a reference group receiving only calcium and vitamin D *(23)*. Although alendronate and calcitriol were discontinued during the second year after cardiac transplant, BMD remained stable *(224)*. Kidney transplant patients treated with alendronate (10 mg daily), calcitriol (0.25 μg daily), and calcium carbonate (2 g daily) had marked increases in LS BMD compared to decreases in those who received only calcium and calcitriol *(225)*. Another recent trial found similar improvements in LS BMD in patients treated with alendronate or risedronate following kidney transplant *(226)*.

Long-term cardiac transplant patients treated with clodronate also had improvements in BMD *(227)*. A trial of long-term kidney transplant patients who were started on alendronate, calcitriol, and calcium or only calcitriol and calcium approximately 5 years after transplantation, documented significant improvements in LS and FN BMD in the alendronate group. BMD in the other group was stable *(228)*. Two recent meta-analyses of bisphosphonate trials in kidney transplant recipients found that bisphosphonates effectively prevented bone loss at the LS and FN *(229,230)*. Alendronate has been shown to prevent bone loss *(231)* after liver transplant as well *(160)*. In BMT recipients, risedronate given 12 months after BMT improved BMD at the spine and prevented loss at femoral neck *(232)*.

Once weekly or monthly dosing regimens, now widely used and of equal efficacy to daily regimens in postmenopausal osteoporosis *(233)*, are very useful in transplant patients who have many gastrointestinal symptoms and take large numbers of medications. For such patients, the requirement to take oral bisphosphonates first thing in the morning and wait 30–60 min before eating or taking other medications is particularly inconvenient. In two recent studies, weekly alendronate (70 mg) has improved BMD in liver *(234)* and kidney transplant recipients *(231)*.

At present, bisphosphonates constitute the most promising approach to the prevention of transplantation osteoporosis. As with other forms of therapy, many issues remain to be resolved. These include whether or not they actually prevent fractures, since most studies have been under-powered to address this important issue. Thus, we are still unsure of the optimal drug and route of administration, whether continuous or intermittent (cyclical) therapy should be used, at what level of renal impairment these drugs should be avoided, whether they are safe in renal transplant recipients with adynamic bone disease, and whether they are beneficial in the setting of pediatric transplantation.

VITAMIN D AND ANALOGS

Administration of vitamin D or its analogs is often recommended after transplantation *(235)*. There are several potential mechanisms by which vitamin D and its analogues may influence post-transplantation bone loss. They may overcome GC-induced decreases in intestinal calcium absorption, reduce secondary hyperparathyroidism, promote differentiation of osteoblast precursors into mature cells, or influence the immune system and potentiate the immunosuppressive action of cyclosporine *(236–238)*.

Since most of the observational studies of bone loss after organ transplantation have included at least 400 IU of parent vitamin D in the post-transplant regimen, it is clear that the RDA for vitamin D is not sufficient to prevent transplantation osteoporosis. In two recent studies, parent vitamin D, in doses of 800 IU daily *(239)* or 25,000 IU monthly *(24)* did not prevent bone loss after kidney transplantation.

Active forms of vitamin D may be more effective. Calcidiol (25-OHD) prevents bone loss and increases LS BMD after cardiac transplantation *(240)*. Alfacalcidol (1-α-OHD) prevents or attenuates bone loss at the LS and FN when given immediately after kidney transplantation *(241–243)*. Several investigators have studied the effects of calcitriol in transplant recipients. The results have been contradictory, although some studies have found beneficial effects at doses greater than 0.5 μg per day. Henderson et al. reported that calcitriol (0.5μ g/d) prevented spine and hip bone loss during the first 6 months after heart or lung transplantation and was as effective as cyclic etidronate *(244)*. Calcitriol given during the first year after kidney transplantation was associated with an increase in LS, FN, and forearm BMD *(50)*. In a stratified, placebo controlled randomized study, heart and lung transplant recipients received calcitriol or placebo for 12 or 24 months after transplantation *(245)*. While LS bone loss was equivalent between groups, FN bone loss at 24 months was reduced only in the group that received calcitriol for the entire period. Although these results suggest that the protective effects of calcitriol are not sustained after cessation of treatment, we found no bone loss when we discontinued calcitriol after the first post-transplant year *(224)*. In another study of renal transplant recipients, intermittent calcitriol and calcium prevented TH but not LS bone loss *(246)*. In contrast, studies of long-term kidney *(247)* and heart transplant patients *(248)* have failed to find any benefit of calcitriol. Stempfle et al. *(118)* found that the addition of a small dose to calcitriol (0.25 μg/d) to calcium supplementation and gonadal steroid replacement offered no benefit with regard to bone loss or fracture prevention after cardiac transplantation.

Hypercalcemia and hypercalciuria are the major side effects of therapy of these agents. Either may develop suddenly and at any time during the course of treatment. Thus, frequent urinary and serum monitoring may be required. If hypercalcemia occurs, it must be recognized and reversed promptly because of the adverse effects on renal function and the life-threatening potential of a severely elevated serum calcium concentration. Supplemental calcium and any vitamin D preparations should be discontinued until the calcium normalizes. Although one may be tempted to permanently discontinue pharmacologic doses of vitamin D or its metabolites in view of the necessary serial monitoring and potential dangers, one might also recommence therapy at a lower dose. However, given the requirement for serial monitoring and the narrow therapeutic window with respect to hypercalcemia and hypercalciuria, we regard pharmacologic doses of vitamin D and its analogues as adjunctive rather than primary therapy for the prevention and treatment of transplantation osteoporosis.

Calcitonin

Calcitonin has long been used to treat Paget's disease of bone, a disease characterized by focal areas of high bone turnover. Both injectable and inhaled calcitonins have been used successfully to treat glucocorticoid-induced bone loss in humans *(249)*. However, calcitonin is not consistently useful in preventing bone loss and fractures after transplantation. Most studies show no benefit *(164,206,250)*, although a recent retrospective study found that patients who received intranasal calcitonin after cardiac transplant had less LS bone loss during the first 3 years than those who had not *(251)*. In summary, calcitonin is relatively ineffective in preventing bone loss after transplantation, and we would not recommend its use.

Estrogen

Some studies have found that HRT does protect the skeleton in postmenopausal women after liver *(252)*, lung *(213)*, and bone marrow transplantation *(189)*. In premenopausal women with amenorrhea following BMT, hormone replacement therapy should be administered, provided that there are no contraindications. Continuous rather than cyclical therapy is preferred after transplantation, as estrogen enhances hepatic metabolism of cyclosporine (and presumably FK506) and theoretically may compromise immunosuppression. Whether this occurs in patients is not known. Premenopausal amenorrheic women often begin menstruating after transplantation and estrogen therapy may often be discontinued 3–6 months after surgery. HRT is probably associated with more risk than benefit in postmenopausal women after transplantation and should not be used to treat bone loss in this population.

Testosterone

Hypogonadism is common in men with chronic illness. Moreover, the suppressive effects of cyclosporine A and glucocorticoids on the hypothalamic–pituitary–gonadal axis often lower serum testosterone levels. Although testosterone usually normalizes by 6–12 months after transplantation *(125,131)*, approximately 25% of men evaluated 1–2 years after transplantation will have biochemical evidence of hypogonadism. Hypogonadism is known to cause osteoporosis in men. Moreover, men with low serum testosterone concentrations have been shown to lose bone more rapidly after cardiac transplantation *(125,131)*. Fahrleitner et al. treated hypogonadal male transplant patients with intravenous ibandronate. The patients had improved BMD at 1 year if they were also treated with testosterone compared with those who were not replaced *(253)*.

In general, men who are truly hypogonadal should be treated with testosterone. Potential benefits of testosterone therapy include increased lean body mass and hemoglobin and improved BMD. Potential risks include prostatic hypertrophy, abnormal liver enzymes, and acceleration of hyperlipidemia in patients already prone to atherosclerosis from hypertension, diabetes, glucocorticoid, and CsA therapy. Therefore it is necessary to monitor serum lipids and liver enzymes, and perform regular prostate examinations in men receiving testosterone.

Resistance Exercise

A few small studies have examined the effects of resistance exercise on BMD following heart *(254)* and lung *(255)* transplantation. Resistance exercise led to significant improvements in LS BMD when used alone, and in combination with alendronate. The interpretation of these findings is limited, however, by the extremely small numbers of subjects enrolled and the method used to measure BMD (lateral spine) which is highly variable, leading to a percent change much greater than typically reported.

New Therapeutic Options

Discussion of new advances in immune therapy that will prevent organ rejection but spare bone are beyond the scope of this article. At the present time, using the lowest possible dosages of glucocorticoid and calcineurin phosphatase inhibitors offers the best option. Currently, the most exciting areas of investigation involve anabolic agents that stimulate bone formation, in particular PTH (1–34) or PTH (1–84), as well as RANKL antagonists and cathepsin K inhibitors.

SUMMARY AND CONCLUSIONS

There has been tremendous progress in elucidating the natural history and pathogenesis of transplantation osteoporosis. It is now clear that a substantial proportion of candidates for solid organ and bone marrow transplantation already have osteoporosis. Prospective longitudinal studies have provided definitive evidence of rapid bone loss and a high incidence of fragility fractures, particularly during the first post-transplant year. Vertebral fractures occur both in patients with low and in those with normal pretransplant BMD, so that it is impossible to predict fracture risk in the individual patient. Early post-transplantation bone loss (before 6 months) is associated with biochemical evidence of uncoupled bone turnover, with increases in markers of resorption and decreases in markers of formation. Later in the post-transplantation course (after 6 months), concomitant with tapering of glucocorticoid doses, bone formation recovers, and the biochemical pattern is more typical of a high turnover osteoporosis. More recent studies suggest that rates of bone loss and fracture are lower than they were before 1995. However, the rates of bone loss and fracture following transplantation remain unacceptably high. Bisphosphonates are the most consistently effective agents for the prevention and treatment of bone loss in organ transplant recipients. Patients should be assessed before transplantation and receive treatment for prevalent osteoporosis, if present. Primary prevention therapy should be initiated immediately after transplantation, as the majority of bone loss occurs in the first few months after grafting. Long-term transplant recipients should be monitored and treated for bone disease as well. With proper vigilance, early diagnosis, and treatment, transplant osteoporosis is a preventable disease.

REFERENCES

1. Cohen A, Ebeling P, Sprague S, Shane E. Transplantation osteoporosis. In: Favus M, ed. Primer on the metabolic bone diseases and disorders of bone and mineral metabolism. Washington, DC: American Society for Bone and Mineral Research; 2006:302–309.
2. Cohen A, Shane E. Osteoporosis after solid organ and bone marrow transplantation. Osteoporos Int 2003;14(8):617–630.

3. Epstein S, Shane E. Transplantation osteoporosis. In: Marcus R, Feldman D, Kelsey J, eds. Osteoporosis. San Diego: Academic Press; 2001:327–340.
4. Maalouf NM, Shane E. Osteoporosis after solid organ transplantation. J Clin Endocrinol Metab 2005;90(4):2456–2465.
5. Marks WH, Wagner D, Pearson TC, et al. Organ donation and utilization, 1995–2004: entering the collaborative era. Am J Transplant 2006;6(5 Pt 2):1101–1110.
6. Ross F. Osteoclast biology and bone resorption. In: Favus M, ed. Primer on the metabolic bone diseases and other disorders of bone and mineral metabolism. Washington, DC: American Society for Bone and Mineral Research; 2006:30–35.
7. Aubin J, Lian J, Stein G. Bone formation: maturation and functional activities of osteoblast lineage cells. In: Favus M, ed. Primer on the metabolic bone diseases and other disorders of bone and mineral metabolism. Washington, DC: American Society for Bone and Mineral Research; 2006:20–29.
8. Gori F, Hofbauer LC, Dunstan CR, Spelsberg TC, Khosla S, Riggs BL. The expression of osteoprotegerin and RANK ligand and the support of osteoclast formation by stromal-osteoblast lineage cells is developmentally regulated. Endocrinology 2000;141(12):4768–4776.
9. Hofbauer LC, Khosla S, Dunstan CR, Lacey DL, Boyle WJ, Riggs BL. The roles of osteoprotegerin and osteoprotegerin ligand in the paracrine regulation of bone resorption. J Bone Miner Res 2000;15(1):2–12.
10. Hofbauer LC, Shui C, Riggs BL, et al. Effects of immunosuppressants on receptor activator of NF-kappaB ligand and osteoprotegerin production by human osteoblastic and coronary artery smooth muscle cells. Biochem Biophys Res Commun 2001;280(1):334–339.
11. Epstein S. Post-transplantation bone disease: the role of immunosuppressive agents on the skeleton. J Bone Miner Res 1996;11:1–7.
12. Mazziotti G, Angeli A, Bilezikian JP, Canalis E, Giustina A. Glucocorticoid-induced osteoporosis: an update. Trends Endocrinol Metab 2006;17(4):144–149.
13. Sambrook P. Glucocorticoid-induced osteoporosis. In: Favus M, ed. Primer on the metabolic bone diseases and other disorders of bone and mineral metabolism. Washington, DC: American Society for Bone and Mineral Research; 2006:296–302.
14. van Staa TP. The pathogenesis, epidemiology and management of glucocorticoid-induced osteoporosis. Calcif Tissue Int 2006;79(3):129–137.
15. Weinstein R, Jilka R, Parfitt M, Manolagas S. Inhibition of osteoblastogenesis and promotion of apoptosis of osteoblasts and osteocytes by glucocorticoids: potential mechanisms of their deleterious effects on bone. J Clin Invest 1998;102: 274–282.
16. Rubin MR, Bilezikian JP. Clinical review 151: the role of parathyroid hormone in the pathogenesis of glucocorticoid-induced osteoporosis: a re-examination of the evidence. J Clin Endocrinol Metab 2002;87(9):4033–4041.
17. Gaston RS. Current and evolving immunosuppressive regimens in kidney transplantation. Am J Kidney Dis 2006;47(4 Suppl 2):S3–S21.
18. Paterson AM, Yates SF, Nolan KF, Waldmann H. The new immunosuppression: intervention at the dendritic cell-T-cell interface. Curr Drug Targets Immune Endocr Metabol Disord 2005;5(4):397–411.
19. Pescovitz MD. B cells: a rational target in alloantibody-mediated solid organ transplantation rejection. Clin Transplant 2006;20(1):48–54.
20. Regazzi MB, Alessiani M, Rinaldi M. New strategies in immunosuppression. Transpl Proc 2005;37(6):2675–2678.
21. Mikuls TR, Julian BA, Bartolucci A, Saag KG. Bone mineral density changes within six months of renal transplantation. Transplantation 2003;75(1):49–54.
22. Ninkovic M, Love S, Tom BD, Bearcroft PW, Alexander GJ, Compston JE. Lack of effect of intravenous pamidronate on fracture incidence and bone mineral density after orthotopic liver transplantation. J Hepatol 2002;37(1):93–100.
23. Shane E, Addesso V, Namerow PB, et al. Alendronate versus calcitriol for the prevention of bone loss after cardiac transplantation. N Engl J Med 2004;350(8):767–776.
24. Wissing KM, Broeders N, Moreno-Reyes R, Gervy C, Stallenberg B, Abramowicz D. A controlled study of vitamin D3 to prevent bone loss in renal-transplant patients receiving low doses of steroids. Transplantation 2005;79(1):108–115.
25. Van Staa TP, Leufkens HG, Abenhaim L, Zhang B, Cooper C. Use of oral corticosteroids and risk of fractures. J Bone Miner Res 2000;15(6):993–1000.

26. Kahan BD. Cyclosporine. N Engl J Med 1989;321: 1725–1738.
27. Suthanthiran M, Strom TB. Renal transplantation. N Engl J Med 1994;331:365–376.
28. Sun L, Blair HC, Peng Y, et al. Calcineurin regulates bone formation by the osteoblast. Proc Natl Acad Sci USA 2005;102(47):17130–17135.
29. Sun L, Peng Y, Zaidi N, et al. Evidence that calcineurin is required for the genesis of bone-resorbing osteoclasts. Am J Physiol Renal Physiol 2007;292(1):F285–F291.
30. Awumey E, Moonga B, Sodam B, et al. Molecular and functional evidence for calcineurin alpha and beta isoforms in the osteoclasts. Novel insights into the mode of action of cyclosporine A. Biochem Biophys Res Commun 1999;254:148–252.
31. Tamler R, Epstein S. Nonsteroid immune modulators and bone disease. Ann NY Acad Sci 2006;1068:284–296.
32. Movsowitz C, Epstein S, Fallon M, Ismail F, Thomas S. Cyclosporin A *in vivo* produces severe osteopenia in the rat: effect of dose and duration of administration. Endocrinology 1988;123:2571–2577.
33. Movsowitz C, Epstein S, Ismail F, Fallon M, Thomas S. Cyclosporin A in the oophorectomized rat: unexpected severe bone resorption. J Bone Miner Res 1989;4:393–398.
34. Buchinsky FJ, Ma Y, Mann GN, et al. T lymphocytes play a critical role in the development of cyclosporin A-induced osteopenia. Endocrinology 1996;137(6):2278–2285.
35. Rucinski B, Liu CC, Epstein S. Utilization of cyclosporine H to elucidate the possible mechanisms of cyclosporine A induced osteopenia in the rat. Metabolism 1994;43:1114–1118.
36. Zahner M, Teraz F, Pacifici R. T cells mediate a stimulatory effect of cyclosporine A on human osteoclastogenesis while immature osteoclast precursors are directly regulated by glucocorticoids. J Bone Miner Res 1997;12(Suppl 1):198.
37. Marshall I, Isserow JA, Buchinsky FJ, Paynton BV, Epstein S. Expression of Interleukin 1 and interleukin 6 in bone from normal and cyclosporine treated rats. In: XIIth international conference on calcium regulating hormones, Melbourne, Australia; 1995.
38. Epstein S, Dissanayake A, Goodman GR, et al. Effect of the interaction of parathyroid hormone and cyclosporine A on bone mineral metabolism in the rat. Calcif Tissue Int 2001;68:240–247.
39. Bowman A, Sass D, Marshall I, et al. Raloxifene analog (Ly 117018-HCL) ameliorates cyclosporin A induced osteopenia. J Bone Miner Res 1995;10 (Suppl 1):350.
40. Joffe I, Katz I, Jacobs T, et al. 17 beta estradiol prevents osteopenia in the oophorectomized rat treated with cyclosporin A. Endocrinology 1992;130:1578–1586.
41. Sass DA, Bowman AR, Marshall I, et al. Alendronate prevents cyclosporin-induced osteopenia in the rat. Bone 1997;21:65–70.
42. Stein B, Halloran P, Reinhardt T, et al. Cyclosporin A increases synthesis of 1,25 dihydroxyvitamin D3 in the rat and mouse. Endocrinology 1991;128:1369–1373.
43. Epstein S, Schlosberg M, Fallon M, Thomas S, Movsowitz C, Ismail F. 1,25 dihydroxyvitamin D3 modifies cyclosporine induced bone loss. Calcif Tissue Int 1990;47:152–157.
44. Katz IA, Jee WSS, Joffe I, et al. Prostaglandin E2 alleviates cyclosporin A-induced bone loss in the rat. J Bone Miner Res 1992;4:1191–1200.
45. Bowman AR, Sass DA, Dissanayake IR, et al. The role of testosterone in cyclosporine-induced osteopenia. J Bone Miner Res 1997;12(4):607–615.
46. Ponticelli C, Aroldi A. Osteoporosis after organ transplantation. Lancet 2001;357(9268):1623.
47. Grotz WH, Mundinger A, Gugel B, Exner V, Kirste G, Schollmeyer PJ. Bone fracture and osteodensitometry with dual energy x-ray absorptiometry in kidney transplant recipients. Transplantation 1994;58:912–915.
48. McIntyre HD, Menzies B, Rigby R, Perry-Keene DA, Hawley CM, Hardie IR. Long-term bone loss after renal transplantation: comparison of immunosuppressive regimens. Clin Transplant 1995;9(1):20–24.
49. Cueto-Manzano AM, Konel S, Crowley V, et al. Bone histopathology and densitometry comparison between cyclosporine a monotherapy and prednisolone plus azathioprine dual immunosuppression in renal transplant patients. Transplantation 2003;75(12):2053–2058.
50. Josephson MA, Schumm LP, Chiu MY, Marshall C, Thistlethwaite JR, Sprague SM. Calcium and calcitriol prophylaxis attenuates posttransplant bone loss. Transplantation 2004;78(8):1233–1236.
51. Cvetkovic M, Mann GN, Romero DF, et al. The deleterious effects of long term cyclosporin A, cyclosporin G and FK506 on bone mineral metabolism *in vivo*. Transplantation 1994;57:1231–1237.

52. Stempfle HU, Werner C, Echtler S, et al. Rapid trabecular bone loss after cardiac transplantation using FK506 (tacrolimus)-based immunosuppression. Transpl Proc 1998;30(4):1132–1133.
53. Park KM, Hay JE, Lee SG, et al. Bone loss after orthotopic liver transplantation: FK 506 versus cyclosporine. Transpl Proc 1996;28(3):1738–1740.
54. Goffin E, Devogelaer JP, Lalaoui A, et al. Tacrolimus and low-dose steroid immunosuppression preserves bone mass after renal transplantation. Transpl Int 2002;15(2–3):73–80.
55. Monegal A, Navasa M, Guanabens N, et al. Bone mass and mineral metabolism in liver transplant patients treated with FK506 or cyclosporine A. Calcif Tissue Int 2001;68:83–86.
56. Goodman G, Dissanayake I, Sodam B, et al. Immunosuppressant use without bone loss- Implications for bone loss after transplantation. J Bone Miner Res 2001;16:72–78.
57. Campistol JM, Holt DW, Epstein S, Gioud-Paquet M, Rutault K, Burke JT. Bone metabolism in renal transplant patients treated with cyclosporine or sirolimus. Transpl Int 2005;18(9):1028–1035.
58. Bryer HP, Isserow JA, Armstrong EC, et al. Azathioprine alone is bone sparing and does not alter cyclosporine A induced osteopenia in the rat. J Bone Miner Res 1995;10:132–138.
59. Dissanayake IR, Goodman GR, Bowman AR, et al. Mycophenolate mofetil; a promising new immunosuppressant that does not cause bone loss in the rat. Transplantation 1998;65: 275–278.
60. Shane E, Mancini D, Aaronson K, et al. Bone mass, vitamin D deficiency and hyperparathyroidism in congestive heart failure. Am J Med 1997;103:197–207.
61. Ball AM, Gillen DL, Sherrard D, et al. Risk of hip fracture among dialysis and renal transplant recipients. JAMA 2002;288(23):3014–3018.
62. Hay JE. Osteoporosis in liver diseases and after liver transplantation. J Hepatol 2003;38(6):856–865.
63. Martin K, Al-Aly Z, Gonzalez E. Renal osteodystrophy. In: Favus M, ed. Primer on the metabolic bone diseases and other disorders of bone and mineral metabolism. Washington, DC: American Society for Bone and Mineral Research; 2006:359–366.
64. Jamal SA, Chase C, Goh YI, Richardson R, Hawker GA. Bone density and heel ultrasound testing do not identify patients with dialysis-dependent renal failure who have had fractures. Am J Kidney Dis 2002;39(4):843–849.
65. Lechleitner P, Krimbacher E, Genser N, et al. Bone mineral densitometry in dialyzed patients: quantitative computed tomography versus dual photon absorptiometry. Bone 1994;15(4):387–391.
66. Stein M, Packham D, Ebeling P, Wark J, GJ B. Prevalence and risks factors for osteopoenia in dialysis patients. Am J Kidney Dis 1996;28:515–522.
67. Taal MW, Masud T, Green D, Cassidy MJ. Risk factors for reduced bone density in haemodialysis patients. Nephrol Dial Transplant 1999;14(8):1922–1928.
68. Coco M, Rush H. Increased incidence of hip fractures in dialysis patients with low serum parathyroid hormone. Am J Kidney Dis 2000;36(6):1115–1121.
69. Mittalhenkle A, Gillen DL, Stehman-Breen CO. Increased risk of mortality associated with hip fracture in the dialysis population. Am J Kidney Dis 2004;44(4):672–679.
70. Atsumi K, Kushida K, Yamazaki K, Shimizu S, Ohmura A, Inoue T. Risk factors for vertebral fractures in renal osteodystrophy. Am J Kidney Dis 1999;33(2):287–293.
71. Kohlmeier M, Saupe J, Schaefer K, Asmus G. Bone fracture history and prospective bone fracture risk of hemodialysis patients are related to apolipoprotein E genotype. Calcif Tissue Int 1998;62(3):278–281.
72. Piraino B, Chen T, Cooperstein L, Segre G, Puschett J. Fractures and vertebral bone mineral density in patients with renal osteodystrophy. Clin Nephrol 1988;30(2):57–62.
73. Nickolas TL, McMahon DJ, Shane E. Relationship between moderate to severe kidney disease and hip fracture in the United States. J Am Soc Nephrol 2006;17(11):3223–3232.
74. Ahn HJ, Kim HJ, Kim YS, et al. Risk factors for changes in bone mineral density and the effect of antiosteoporosis management after renal transplantation. Transpl Proc 2006;38(7):2074–2076.
75. Shane E. Transplantation osteoporosis. In: Orwoll E, Bliziotes M, eds. Osteoporosis: pathophysiology and clinical management. Totowa, NJ: Humana Press; 2003:537–567.
76. Shane E, Epstein S. Transplantation Osteoporosis. Transpl Rev 2001;15(1):11–32.
77. Braga Junior JW, Neves RM, Pinheiro MM, et al. Prevalence of low trauma fractures in long-term kidney transplant patients with preserved renal function. Braz J Med Biol Res 2006;39(1):137–147.
78. Wolpaw T, Deal CL, Fleming-Brooks S, Bartucci MR, Schulak JA, Hricik DE. Factors influencing vertebral bone density after renal transplantation. Transplantation 1994;58(11):1186–1189.

79. Bagni B, Gilli P, Cavallini A, et al. Continuing loss of vertebral mineral density in renal transplant recipients. Eur J Nucl Med 1994;21:108–112.
80. Pichette V, Bonnardeaux A, Prudhomme L, Gagne M, Cardinal J, Ouimet D. Long-term bone loss in kidney transplant recipients: a cross-sectional and longitudinal study. Am J Kidney Dis 1996;28:105–114.
81. Roe SD, Porter CJ, Godber IM, Hosking DJ, Cassidy MJ. Reduced bone mineral density in male renal transplant recipients: evidence for persisting hyperparathyroidism. Osteoporos Int 2005;16(2): 142–148.
82. Boot AM, Nauta J, Hokken-Koelega ACS, Pols HAP, Ridder MAJd, Keizer-Schrama SMPF. Renal transplantation and osteoporosis. Arch Dis Child 1995;72:502–506.
83. Cueto-Manzano A, Konel S, Hutchinson AJ, et al. Bone loss in long term renal transplantation. Histopathology and densitometry analysis. Kidney Int 1999;55:2021–2029.
84. Julian BA, Laskow DA, Dubovsky J, Dubovsky EV, Curtis JJ, Quarrles LD. Rapid loss of vertebral bone density after renal transplantation. N Engl J Med 1991;325:544–550.
85. Almond MK, Kwan JTC, Evans K, Cunningham J. Loss of regional bone mineral density in the first 12 months following renal transplantation. Nephron 1994;66:52–57.
86. Gallego R, Oliva E, Vega N, et al. Steroids and bone density in patients with functioning kidney allografts. Transpl Proc 2006;38(8):2434–2437.
87. Horber FF, Casez JP, Steiger U, Czerniack A, Montandon A, Jaeger PH. Changes in bone mass early after kidney transplantation. J Bone Miner Res 1994;9:1–9.
88. Kwan JTC, Almond MK, Evans K, Cunningham J. Changes in total body bone mineral content and regional bone mineral density in renal patients following renal transplantation. Miner Electrolyte Metab 1992;18:166–168.
89. Techawathanawanna N, Avihingsanon Y, Praditpornsilpa K, et al. The prevalence and risk factors of osteoporosis in Thai renal-transplant patients. J Med Assoc Thai 2005;88(Suppl 4):S103–S109.
90. Torregrosa JV, Campistol JM, Montesinos M, et al. Factors involved in the loss of bone mineral density after renal transplantation. Transpl Proc 1995;27(4):2224–2225.
91. Yun YS, Kim BJ, Hong TW, Lee CG, Kim MJ. Changes of bone metabolism indices in patients receiving immunosuppressive therapy including low doses of steroids after transplantation. Transpl Proc 1996;28:1561–1564.
92. Monier-Faugere M, Mawad H, Qi Q, Friedler R, Malluche HH. High prevalence of low bone turnover and occurrence of osteomalacia after kidney transplantation. J Am Soc Nephrol 2000;11:1093–1099.
93. Rolla D, Ballanti P, Marsano L, et al. Bone disease in long-term renal transplant recipients with severe osteopenia: a cross-sectional study. Transplantation 2006;81(6):915–921.
94. Ramsey-Goldman R, Dunn JE, Dunlop DD, et al. Increased risk of fracture in patients receiving solid organ transplants. J Bone Miner Res 1999;14(3):456–463.
95. Chiu MY, Sprague SM, Bruce DS, Woodle ES, Thistlethwaite JR Jr, Josephson MA. Analysis of fracture prevalence in kidney-pancreas allograft recipients. J Am Soc Nephrol 1998;9(4):677–683.
96. Nisbeth U, Lindh E, Ljunghall S, Backman U, Fellstrom B. Fracture frequency after kidney transplantation. Transpl Proc 1994;26:1764.
97. Nisbeth U, Lindh E, Ljunghall S, Backman U, Fellstrom B. Increased fracture rate in diabetes mellitus and females after renal transplantation. Transplantation 1999;67(9):1218–1222.
98. Smets YF, de Fijter JW, Ringers J, Lemkes HH, Hamdy NA. Long-term follow-up study on bone mineral density and fractures after simultaneous pancreas-kidney transplantation. Kidney Int 2004;66(5): 2070–2076.
99. Kulak C, Shane E. Transplantation osteoporosis: biochemical correlates of pathogenesis and treatment. In: Seibel M, Robins S, Bilezikian J, eds. Dynamics of bone and cartilage metabolism: principles and clinical applications, 2nd ed. San Diego: Elsevier; 2006:701–716.
100. Akaberi S, Lindergard B, Simonsen O, Nyberg G. Impact of parathyroid hormone on bone density in long-term renal transplant patients with good graft function. Transplantation 2006;82(6): 749–752.
101. Pande S, Ritter CS, Rothstein M, et al. FGF-23 and sFRP-4 in chronic kidney disease and post-renal transplantation. Nephron Physiol 2006;104(1):p23–p32.
102. Fleseriu M, Licata AA. Failure of successful renal transplant to produce appropriate levels of 1,25-dihydroxyvitamin D. Osteoporos Int 2007;18(3):363–368.

103. Uyar M, Sezer S, Arat Z, Elsurer R, Ozdemir FN, Haberal M. 1,25-dihydroxyvitamin D(3) therapy is protective for renal function and prevents hyperparathyroidism in renal allograft recipients. Transpl Proc 2006;38(7):2069–2073.
104. Querings K, Girndt M, Geisel J, Georg T, Tilgen W, Reichrath J. 25-hydroxyvitamin D deficiency in renal transplant recipients. J Clin Endocrinol Metab 2006;91(2):526–529.
105. Anijar JR, Szejnfeld VL, Almeida DR, Fernandes AR, Ferraz MB. Reduced bone mineral density in men after heart transplantation. Braz J Med Biol Res 1999;32(4):413–420.
106. Cohen A, Shane E. Bone disease in patients before and after cardiac transplantation. In: Compston JE, Shane E, eds. Bone disease of organ transplantation. Burlington, MA: Elsevier Academic Press; 2005:287–301.
107. Lee AH, Mull RL, Keenan GF, et al. Osteoporosis and bone morbidity in cardiac transplant recipients. Am J Med 1994;96:35–41.
108. Garlicki AM, Orchowski F, Myrdko T, et al. Measurement of radial bone mineral density in patients after heart transplantation. Ann Transpl 1996;1(4):32–34.
109. Glendenning P, Kent GN, Adler BD, et al. High prevalence of osteoporosis in cardiac transplant recipients and discordance between biochemical turnover markers and bone histomorphometry. Clin Endocrinol (Oxf) 1999;50(3):347–355.
110. Guo C, Johnson A, Locke T, Eastell R. Mechanism of bone loss after cardiac transplantation. Bone 1998;22:267–271.
111. Hetzer R, Albert W, Hummel M, et al. Status of patients presently living 9 to 13 years after orthotopic heart transplantation. Ann Thorac Surg 1997;64(6):1661–1668.
112. Meys E, Terreaux-Duvert F, Beaume-Six T, Dureau G, Meunier PJ. Bone loss after cardiac transplantation: effects of calcium, calcidiol and monofluorophosphate. Osteoporos Int 1993;3(6):322–329.
113. Muchmore JS, Cooper DKC, Ye Y, Schlegel VJ, Zudhi N. Loss of vertebral bone density in heart transplant patients. Transpl Proc 1991;23:1184–1185.
114. Olivari MT, Antolick A, Kaye MP, Jamieson SW, Ring WS. Heart transplantation in elderly patients. J Heart Transpl 1988;7(4):258–264.
115. Pavie A, Dorent R, Reagan M, et al. La Pitie heart transplantation: 30-year single center clinical experience. Clin Transpl 1998:311–314.
116. Rich GM, Mudge GH, Laffel GL, LeBoff MS. Cyclosporine A and prednisone-associated osteoporosis in heart transplant recipients. J Heart Lung Transpl 1992;11:950–958.
117. Shane E, Rivas MDC, Silverberg SJ, Kim TS, Staron RB, Bilezikian JP. Osteoporosis after cardiac transplantation. Am J Med 1993;94:257–264.
118. Stempfle HU, Werner C, Echtler S, et al. Prevention of osteoporosis after cardiac transplantation: a prospective, longitudinal, randomized, double-blind trial with calcitriol. Transplantation 1999;68(4): 523–530.
119. Chou NK, Su IC, Kuo HL, Chen YH, Yang RS, Wang SS. Bone mineral density in long-term Chinese heart transplant recipients: a cross-sectional study. Transpl Proc 2006;38(7):2141–2144.
120. Cohen A, Addonizio LJ, Lamour JM, et al. Osteoporosis in adult survivors of adolescent cardiac transplantation may be related to hyperparathyroidism, mild renal insufficiency, and increased bone turnover. J Heart Lung Transpl 2005;24(6):696–702.
121. Berguer DG, Krieg MA, Thiebaud D, et al. Osteoporosis in heart transplant recipients: a longitudinal study. Transpl Proc 1994;26(5):2649–2651.
122. Cremer J, Struber M, Wagenbreth I, et al. Progression of steroid-associated osteoporosis after heart transplantation. Ann Thorac Surg 1999;67(1):130–133.
123. Henderson NK, Sambrook PN, Kelly PJ, et al. Bone mineral loss and recovery after cardiac transplantation [letter]. Lancet 1995;346(8979):905.
124. Sambrook PN, Kelly PJ, Keogh A, et al. Bone loss after cardiac transplantation: a prospective study. J Heart Lung Transpl 1994;13:116–121.
125. Shane E, Rivas M, McMahon DJ, et al. Bone loss and turnover after cardiac transplantation. J Clin Endocrinol Metab 1997;82(5):1497–1506.
126. Thiebaud D, Krieg M, Gillard-Berguer D, Jaquet A, Goy J, Burckhardt P. Cyclosporine induces high turnover and may contribute to bone loss after heart transplantation. Eur J Clin Invest 1996;26: 549–555.

127. Valimaki MJ, Kinnunen K, Tahtela R, et al. A prospective study of bone loss and turnover after cardiac transplantation: effect of calcium supplementation with or without calcitonin. Osteoporos Int 1999;10(2):128–136.
128. Van Cleemput J, Daenen W, Nijs J, Geusens P, Dequeker J, Vanhaecke J. Timing and quantification of bone loss in cardiac transplant recipients. Transpl Int 1995;8(3):196–200.
129. Shane E, Rivas M, Staron RB, et al. Fracture after cardiac transplantation: a prospective longitudinal study. J Clin Endocrinol Metab 1996;81:1740–1746.
130. Leidig-Bruckner G, Hosch S, Dodidou P, et al. Frequency and predictors of osteoporotic fractures after cardiac or liver transplantation: a follow-up study. The Lancet 2001;357:342–347.
131. Sambrook PN, Kelly PJ, Fontana D, et al. Mechanisms of rapid bone loss following cardiac transplantation. Osteoporosis Int 1994;4:273–276.
132. Idilman R, de Maria N, Uzunalimoglu O, van Thiel DH. Hepatic osteodystrophy: a review. Hepatogastroenterology 1997;44(14):574–581.
133. Maalouf NM, Sakhaee K. Treatment of osteoporosis in patients with chronic liver disease and in liver transplant recipients. Curr Treat Options Gastroenterol 2006;9(6):456–463.
134. Ninkovic M, Love SA, Tom B, Alexander GJ, Compston JE. High prevalence of osteoporosis in patients with chronic liver disease prior to liver transplantation. Calcif Tissue Int 2001;69(6):321–326.
135. Crosbie OM, Freaney R, McKenna MJ, Hegarty JE. Bone density, vitamin D status, and disordered bone remodeling in end- stage chronic liver disease. Calcif Tissue Int 1999;64(4):295–300.
136. Monegal A, Navasa M, Guanabens N, et al. Osteoporosis and bone mineral metabolism in cirrhotic patients referred for liver transplantation. Calcif Tissue Int 1997;60:148–154.
137. Hay JE, Guichelaar MM. Evaluation and management of osteoporosis in liver disease. Clin Liver Dis 2005;9(4):747–766, viii.
138. Marignani M, Angeletti S, Capurso G, Cassetta S, Delle Fave G. Bad to the bone: the effects of liver diseases on bone. Minerva Med 2004;95(6):489–505.
139. Pares A, Guanabens N. Treatment of bone disorders in liver disease. J Hepatol 2006;45(3):445–453.
140. Hussaini SH, Oldroyd B, Stewart SP, et al. Regional bone mineral density after orthotopic liver transplantation. Eur J Gastroenterol Hepatol 1999;11(2):157–163.
141. Guichelaar MM, Kendall R, Malinchoc M, Hay JE. Bone mineral density before and after OLT: long-term follow-up and predictive factors. Liver Transpl 2006;12(9):1390–1402.
142. Guanabens N, Pares A, Alvarez L, et al. Collagen-related markers of bone turnover reflect the severity of liver fibrosis in patients with primary biliary cirrhosis. J Bone Miner Res 1998;13:731–738.
143. Hodgson SF, Dickson ER, Eastell R, Eriksen EF, Bryant SC, Riggs BL. Rates of cancellous bone remodeling and turnover in osteopenia associated with primary biliary cirrhosis. Bone 1993;14: 819–827.
144. Hodgson SF, Dickson ER, Wahner HW, Johnson KA, Mann KG, Riggs BL. Bone loss and reduced osteoblast function in primary biliary cirrhosis. Ann Intern Med 1985;103(6(Pt 1)):855–860.
145. Compston JE. Osteoporosis after liver transplantation. Liver Transpl 2003;9(4):321–330.
146. Eastell R, Dickson RE, Hodgson SF, et al. Rates of vertebral bone loss before and after liver transplantation in women with primary biliary cirrhosis. Hepatology 1991;14:296–300.
147. Haagsma EB, Thijn CJP, Post JG, Slooff MJH, Gisp CH. Bone disease after liver transplantation. J Hepatol 1988;6:94–100.
148. Hawkins FG, Leon M, Lopez MB, et al. Bone loss and turnover in patients with liver transplantation. Hepato-Gastroenterol 1994;41:158–161.
149. Lopez MB, Pinto IG, Hawkins F, et al. Effect of liver transplantation and immunosuppressive treatment on bone mineral density. Transpl Proc 1992;24:3044–3046.
150. McDonald JA, Dunstan CR, Dilworth P, et al. Bone loss after liver transplantation. Hepatology 1991;14:613–619.
151. Meys E, Fontanges E, Fourcade N, Thomasson A, Pouyet M, Delmas P. Bone loss after orthotopic liver transplantation. Am J Med 1994;97:445–450.
152. Navasa M, Monegal A, Guanabens N, et al. Bone fractures in liver transplant patients. Br J Rheumatol 1994;33:52–55.
153. Porayko MK, Wiesner RH, Hay JE, et al. Bone disease in liver transplant recipients: incidence, timing, and risk factors. Transpl Proc 1991;23(1 Pt 2):1462–1465.

154. Feller RB, McDonald JA, Sherbon KJ, McCaughan GW. Evidence of continuing bone recovery at a mean of 7 years after liver transplantation. Liver Transpl Surg 1999;5(5):407–413.
155. Giannini S, Nobile M, Ciuffreda M, et al. Long-term persistence of low bone density in orthotopic liver transplantation. Osteoporos Int 2000;11(5):417–424.
156. Keogh JB, Tsalamandris C, Sewell RB, et al. Bone loss at the proximal femur and reduced lean mass following liver transplantation: a longitudinal study. Nutrition 1999;15(9):661–664.
157. Floreani A, Mega A, Tizian L, et al. Bone metabolism and gonad function in male patients undergoing liver transplantation: a two-year longitudinal study. Osteoporos Int 2001;12(9):749–754.
158. Smallwood GA, Burns D, Fasola CG, Steiber AC, Heffron TG. Relationship between immunosuppression and osteoporosis in an outpatient liver transplant clinic. Transpl Proc 2005;37(4):1910–1911.
159. Shah SH, Johnston TD, Jeon H, Ranjan D. Effect of chronic glucocorticoid therapy and the gender difference on bone mineral density in liver transplant patients. J Surg Res 2006;135(2): 238–241.
160. Millonig G, Graziadei IW, Eichler D, et al. Alendronate in combination with calcium and vitamin D prevents bone loss after orthotopic liver transplantation: a prospective single-center study. Liver Transpl 2005;11(8):960–966.
161. Monegal A, Navasa M, Guanabens N, et al. Bone disease after liver transplantation: a long-term prospective study of bone mass changes, hormonal status and histomorphometric characteristics. Osteoporos Int 2001;12(6):484–492.
162. Ninkovic M, Skingle SJ, Bearcroft PW, Bishop N, Alexander GJ, Compston JE. Incidence of vertebral fractures in the first three months after orthotopic liver transplantation. Eur J Gastroenterol Hepatol 2000;12(8):931–935.
163. Compston J, Greer S, Skingle S, et al. Early increase in plasma parathyroid hormone level following liver transplantation. J Hepatol 1996;25:715–718.
164. Valero M, Loinaz C, Larrodera L, Leon M, Morena E, Hawkins F. Calcitonin and bisphosphonate treatment in bone loss after liver transplantation. Calcif Tissue Int 1995;57:15–19.
165. Abdelhadi M, Eriksson SA, Ljusk Eriksson S, Ericzon BG, Nordenstrom J. Bone mineral status in end-stage liver disease and the effect of liver transplantation. Scand J Gastroenterol 1995;30(12): 1210–1215.
166. Watson RG, Coulton L, Kanis JA, et al. Circulating osteocalcin in primary biliary cirrhosis following liver transplantation and during treatment with ciclosporin. J Hepatol 1990;11(3):354–358.
167. Rabinowitz M, Shapiro J, Lian J, Bloch GD, Merkel IS, Thiel DHV. Vitamin D and osteocalcin levels in liver transplant recipients. is osteocalcin a reliable marker of bone turnover in such cases? J Hepatol 1992;16:50–55.
168. Fabrega E, Orive A, Garcia-Unzueta M, Amado JA, Casafont F, Pons-Romero F. Osteoprotegerin and receptor activator of nuclear factor-kappaB ligand system in the early post-operative period of liver transplantation. Clin Transpl 2006;20(3):383–388.
169. Vedi J, Greer S, Skingle S, et al. Mechanism of bone loss after liver transplantation: a histomorphometric analysis. J Bone Miner Res 1999;14(2):281–287.
170. Aris R, Neuringer I, Weiner M, Egan T, Ontjes D. Severe osteoporosis before and after lung transplantation. Chest 1996;109:1176–1183.
171. Shane E, Silverberg SJ, Donovan D, et al. Osteoporosis in lung transplantation candidates with end stage pulmonary disease. Am J Med 1996;101:262–269.
172. Aris RM, Renner JB, Winders AD, et al. Increased rate of fractures and severe kyphosis: sequelae of living into adulthood with cystic fibrosis. Ann Intern Med 1998;128:186–193.
173. Donovan DS Jr, Papadopoulos A, Staron RB, et al. Bone mass and vitamin D deficiency in adults with advanced cystic fibrosis lung disease. Am J Respir Crit Care Med 1998;157(6 Pt 1):1892–1899.
174. Ott SM, Aitken ML. Osteoporosis in patients with cystic fibrosis. Clin Chest Med 1998;19(3):555–567.
175. Tschopp O, Schmid C, Speich R, Seifert B, Russi EW, Boehler A. Pretransplantation bone disease in patients with primary pulmonary hypertension. Chest 2006;129(4):1002–1008.
176. Caplan-Shaw CE, Arcasoy SM, Shane E, et al. Osteoporosis in diffuse parenchymal lung disease. Chest 2006;129(1):140–146.
177. Ferrari SL, Nicod LP, Hamacher J, et al. Osteoporosis in patients undergoing lung transplantation. Eur Respir J 1996;9:2378–2382.

178. Spira A, Gutierrez C, Chaparro C, Hutcheon MA, Chan CK. Osteoporosis and lung transplantation: a prospective study. Chest 2000;117(2):476–481.
179. Aringer M, Kiener H, Koeller M, et al. High turnover bone disease following lung transplantation. Bone 1998;23:485–488.
180. Rutherford RM, Fisher AJ, Hilton C, et al. Functional status and quality of life in patients surviving 10 years after lung transplantation. Am J Transpl 2005;5(5):1099–1104.
181. Shane E, Papadopoulos A, Staron RB, et al. Bone loss and fracture after lung transplantation. Transplantation 1999;68:220–227.
182. Haworth CS, Webb AK, Egan JJ, et al. Bone histomorphometry in adult patients with cystic fibrosis. Chest 2000;118(2):434–439.
183. Banfi A, Podesta M, Fazzuoli L, et al. High-dose chemotherapy shows a dose-dependent toxicity to bone marrow osteoprogenitors: a mechanism for post-bone marrow transplantation osteopenia. Cancer 2001;92(9):2419–2428.
184. Lee WY, Cho SW, Oh ES, et al. The effect of bone marrow transplantation on the osteoblastic differentiation of human bone marrow stromal cells. J Clin Endocrinol Metab 2002;87(1):329–335.
185. Kelly PJ, Atkinson K, Ward RL, Sambrook PN, Biggs JC, Eisman JA. Reduced bone mineral density in men and women with allogeneic bone marrow. Transplantation 1990;50:881–883.
186. Bhatia S, Ramsay NK, Weisdorf D, Griffiths H, Robison LL. Bone mineral density in patients undergoing bone marrow transplantation for myeloid malignancies. Bone Marrow Transpl 1998;22(1):87–90.
187. Nysom K, Holm K, Michaelsen KF, et al. Bone mass after allogeneic BMT for childhood leukaemia or lymphoma. Bone Marrow Transpl 2000;25(2):191–196.
188. Kauppila M, Irjala K, Koskinen P, et al. Bone mineral density after allogeneic bone marrow transplantation. Bone Marrow Transpl 1999;24(8):885–889.
189. Branco CC, Rovira M, Pons F, et al. The effect of hormone replacement therapy on bone mass in patients with ovarian failure due to bone marrow transplantation. Maturitas 1996;23:307–312.
190. Castaneda S, Carmona L, Carjaval I, Arranz B, Diaz A, Garcia-Vadillo A. Reduction of bone mass in women after bone marrow transplantation. Calcif Tiss Int 1997;60:343–347.
191. Stern JM, Chestnut CH 3rd, Bruemmer B, et al. Bone density loss during treatment of chronic GVHD. Bone Marrow Transpl 1996;17:395–400.
192. Ebeling P, Thomas D, Erbas B, Hopper L, Szer J, Grigg A. Mechanism of bone loss following allogeneic and autologous hematopoietic stem cell transplantation. J Bone Miner Res 1999;14:342–350.
193. Valimaki M, Kinnunen K, Volin L, et al. A prospective study of bone loss and turnover after allogeneic bone marrow transplantation: effect of calcium supplementation with or without calcitonin. Bone Marrow Transpl 1999;23:355–361.
194. Kang MI, Lee WY, Oh KW, et al. The short-term changes of bone mineral metabolism following bone marrow transplantation. Bone 2000;26(3):275–279.
195. Kashyap A, Kandeel F, Yamauchi D, et al. Effects of allogeneic bone marrow transplantation on recipient bone mineral density: a prospective study. Biol Blood Marrow Transpl 2000;6(3A):344–351.
196. Lee WY, Kang MI, Baek KH, et al. The skeletal site-differential changes in bone mineral density following bone marrow transplantation: 3-year prospective study. J Korean Med Sci 2002;17(6):749–754.
197. Carlson K, Simonsson B, Ljunghall S. Acute effects of high dose chemotherapy followed by bone marrow transplantation on serum markers of bone metabolism. Calcif Tissue Int 1994;55:408–411.
198. Withold W, Wolf H, Kollbach S, Heyll A, Schneider W, Reinauer H. Monitoring of bone metabolism after bone marrow transplantation by measuring two different markers of bone turnover. Eur J Clin Chem Clin Biochem 1996;34:193–279.
199. Gandhi MK, Lekamwasam S, Inman I, et al. Significant and persistent loss of bone mineral density in the femoral neck after haematopoietic stem cell transplantation: long-term follow-up of a prospective study. Br J Haematol 2003;121(3):462–468.
200. Lee WY, Kang MI, Oh ES, et al. The role of cytokines in the changes in bone turnover following bone marrow transplantation. Osteoporos Int 2002;13(1):62–68.
201. Tauchmanova L, Serio B, Del Puente A, et al. Long-lasting bone damage detected by dual-energy x-ray absorptiometry, phalangeal osteosonogrammetry, and *in vitro* growth of marrow stromal cells after allogeneic stem cell transplantation. J Clin Endocrinol Metab 2002;87(11):5058–5065.

202. Kananen K, Volin L, Tahtela R, Laitinen K, Ruutu T, Valimaki MJ. Recovery of bone mass and normalization of bone turnover in long-term survivors of allogeneic bone marrow transplantation. Bone Marrow Transpl 2002;29(1):33–39.
203. Tauchmanova L, De Rosa G, Serio B, et al. Avascular necrosis in long-term survivors after allogeneic or autologous stem cell transplantation: a single center experience and a review. Cancer 2003;97(10): 2453–2461.
204. Fan S, Almond MK, Ball E, Evans K, Cunningham J. Pamidronate therapy as prevention of bone loss following renal transplantation. Kidney Int 2000;57:684–690.
205. Fan SL, Kumar S, Cunningham J. Long-term effects on bone mineral density of pamidronate given at the time of renal transplantation. Kidney Int 2003;63(6):2275–2279.
206. Garcia-Delgado I, Prieto S, Fragnas LG, Robles E, Rufilanchas T, Hawkins F. Calcitonin, editronate and calcidiol treatment in bone loss after cardiac transplantation. Calcif Tissue Int 1997;60:155–159.
207. Shane E, Rodino MA, McMahon DJ, et al. Prevention of bone loss after heart transplantation with antiresorptive therapy: a pilot study. J Heart Lung Transpl 1998;17(11):1089–1096.
208. Aris RM, Lester GE, Renner JB, et al. Efficacy of pamidronate for osteoporosis in patients with cystic fibrosis following lung transplantation. Am J Respir Crit Care Med 2000;162(3 Pt 1):941–946.
209. Bianda T, Linka A, Junga G, et al. Prevention of osteoporosis in heart transplant recipients: a comparison of calcitriol with calcitonin and pamidronate. Calcif Tissue Int 2000;67:116–121.
210. Hommann M, Abendroth K, Lehmann G, et al. Effect of transplantation on bone: osteoporosis after liver and multivisceral transplantation. Transpl Proc 2002;34(6):2296–2298.
211. Grotz W, Nagel C, Poeschel D, et al. Effect of ibandronate on bone loss and renal function after kidney transplantation. J Am Soc Nephrol 2001;12(7):1530–1537.
212. Arlen DJ, Lambert K, Ioannidis G, Adachi JD. Treatment of established bone loss after renal transplantation with etidronate. Transplantation 2001;71(5):669–673.
213. Trombetti A, Gerbase MW, Spiliopoulos A, Slosman DO, Nicod LP, Rizzoli R. Bone mineral density in lung-transplant recipients before and after graft: prevention of lumbar spine post-transplantation-accelerated bone loss by pamidronate. J Heart Lung Transpl 2000;19(8):736–743.
214. Krieg M, Seydoux C, Sandini L, et al. Intravenous pamidronate as a treatment for osteoporosis after heart transplantation: a prospective study. Osteoporosis Int 2001;12:112–116.
215. Haas M, Leko-Mohr Z, Roschger P, et al. Zoledronic acid to prevent bone loss in the first 6 months after renal transplantation. Kidney Int 2003;63(3):1130–1136.
216. Coco M, Glicklich D, Faugere MC, et al. Prevention of bone loss in renal transplant recipients: a prospective, randomized trial of intravenous pamidronate. J Am Soc Nephrol 2003;14(10):2669–2676.
217. Pennisi P, Trombetti A, Giostra E, Mentha G, Rizzoli R, Fiore CE. Pamidronate and osteoporosis prevention in liver transplant recipients. Rheumatol Int 2007;27(3):251–256.
218. Reeves H, Francis R, Manas D, Hudson M, Day C. Intravenous bisphosphonate prevents symptomatic osteoporotic vertebral collapse in patients after liver transplantation. Liver Transpl Surg 1998; 4:404–409.
219. Kananen K, Volin L, Laitinen K, Alfthan H, Ruutu T, Valimaki MJ. Prevention of bone loss after allogeneic stem cell transplantation by calcium, vitamin D, and sex hormone replacement with or without pamidronate. J Clin Endocrinol Metab 2005;90(7):3877–3885.
220. Grigg AC, Shuttleworth P, Reynolds J, et al. Pamidronate therapy for one year after allogeneic bone marrow transplantation (AlloBMT) reduces bone loss from the lumbar spine, femoral neck and total hip. Blood 2004;104:A2253.
221. Ebeling PR. Defective osteoblast function may be responsible for bone loss from the proximal femur despite pamidronate therapy. J Clin Endocrinol Metab 2005;90(7):4414–4416.
222. Crawford BA, Kam C, Pavlovic J, et al. Zoledronic acid prevents bone loss after liver transplantation: a randomized, double-blind, placebo-controlled trial. Ann Intern Med 2006;144(4):239–248.
223. Tauchmanova L, Ricci P, Serio B, et al. Short-term zoledronic acid treatment increases bone mineral density and marrow clonogenic fibroblast progenitors after allogeneic stem cell transplantation. J Clin Endocrinol Metab 2005;90(2):627–634.
224. Cohen A, Addesso V, McMahon DJ, et al. Discontinuing antiresorptive therapy one year after cardiac transplantation: effect on bone density and bone turnover. Transplantation 2006;81(5):686–691.
225. Kovac D, Lindic J, Kandus A, Bren AF. Prevention of bone loss in kidney graft recipients. Transpl Proc 2001;33(1–2):1144–1145.

226. Nowacka-Cieciura E, Cieciura T, Baczkowska T, et al. Bisphosphonates are effective prophylactic of early bone loss after renal transplantation. Transpl Proc 2006;38(1):165–167.
227. Ippoliti G, Pellegrini C, Campana C, et al. Clodronate treatment of established bone loss in cardiac recipients: a randomized study. Transplantation 2003;75(3):330–334.
228. Giannini S, Dangel A, Carraro G, et al. Alendronate prevents further bone loss in renal transplant recipients. J Bone Miner Res 2001;16(11):2111–2117.
229. Mitterbauer C, Schwarz C, Haas M, Oberbauer R. Effects of bisphosphonates on bone loss in the first year after renal transplantation – a meta-analysis of randomized controlled trials. Nephrol Dial Transpl 2006;21(8):2275–2281.
230. Palmer SC, Strippoli GF, McGregor DO. Interventions for preventing bone disease in kidney transplant recipients: a systematic review of randomized controlled trials. Am J Kidney Dis 2005;45(4): 638–649.
231. Toro J, Gentil MA, Garcia R, et al. Alendronate in kidney transplant patients: a single-center experience. Transpl Proc 2005;37(3):1471–1472.
232. Tauchmanova L, Selleri C, Esposito M, et al. Beneficial treatment with risedronate in long-term survivors after allogeneic stem cell transplantation for hematological malignancies. Osteoporos Int 2003;14(12):1013–1019.
233. Schnitzer T, Bone HG, Crepaldi G, et al. Therapeutic equivalence of alendronate 70 mg once-weekly and alendronate 10 mg daily in the treatment of osteoporosis. Alendronate Once-Weekly Study Group. Aging (Milano) 2000;12(1):1–12.
234. Atamaz F, Hepguler S, Karasu Z, Kilic M, Tokat Y. The prevention of bone fractures after liver transplantation: experience with alendronate treatment. Transpl Proc 2006;38(5):1448–1452.
235. Sambrook P. Alfacalcidol and calcitriol in the prevention of bone loss after organ transplantation. Calcif Tissue Int 1999;65(4):341–343.
236. Briffa NK, Keogh AM, Sambrook PN, Eisman JA. Reduction of immunosuppressant therapy requirement in heart transplantation by calcitriol. Transplantation 2003;75(12):2133–2134.
237. Lemire JM. Immunomodulatory role of 1,25 Dihydroxyvitamin D3. J Cell Biochem 1992;49:26–31.
238. Lemire JM, Archer DC, Reddy GS. Dihydroxy-24-oxo-16-ene-vitamin D3, a renal metabolite of the vitamin D analog 1,25-dihydroxy-16ene-vitamin D3, exerts immunosuppressive activity equal to its parent without causing hypercalcemia *in vivo*. Endocrinology 1994;135:2818–2821.
239. Al-Gabri S, Zadrazil J, Krejci K, Horak P, Bachleda P. Changes in bone mineral density and selected metabolic parameters over 24 months following renal transplantation. Transpl Proc 2005;37(2): 1014–1019.
240. Cohen A, Sambrook P, Shane E. Management of bone loss after organ transplantation. J Bone Miner Res 2004;19(12):1919–1932.
241. El-Agroudy AE, El-Husseini AA, El-Sayed M, Ghoneim MA. Preventing bone loss in renal transplant recipients with vitamin D. J Am Soc Nephrol 2003;14(11):2975–2979.
242. De Sevaux RG, Hoitsma AJ, Corstens FH, Wetzels JF. Treatment with vitamin D and calcium reduces bone loss after renal transplantation: a randomized study. J Am Soc Nephrol 2002;13(6): 1608–1614.
243. El-Agroudy AE, El-Husseini AA, El-Sayed M, Mohsen T, Ghoneim MA. A prospective randomized study for prevention of postrenal transplantation bone loss. Kidney Int 2005;67(5):2039–2045.
244. Henderson K, Eisman J, Keogh A, et al. Protective effect of short-tem calcitriol or cyclical etidronate on bone loss after cardiac or lung transplantation. J Bone Miner Res 2001;16(3):565–571.
245. Sambrook P, Henderson NK, Keogh A, et al. Effect of calcitriol on bone loss after cardiac or lung transplantation. J Bone Miner Res 2000;15(9):1818–1824.
246. Torres A, Garcia S, Gomez A, et al. Treatment with intermittent calcitriol and calcium reduces bone loss after renal transplantation. Kidney Int 2004;65(2):705–712.
247. Cueto-Manzano AM, Konel S, Freemont AJ, et al. Effect of 1,25-dihydroxyvitamin D3 and calcium carbonate on bone loss associated with long-term renal transplantation. Am J Kidney Dis 2000;35(2):227–236.
248. Stempfle HU, Werner C, Siebert U, et al. The role of tacrolimus (FK506)-based immunosuppression on bone mineral density and bone turnover after cardiac transplantation: a prospective, longitudinal, randomized, double-blind trial with calcitriol. Transplantation 2002;73(4):547–552.

249. Cranney A, Welch V, Adachi JD, et al. Calcitonin for the treatment and prevention of corticosterid-induced osteoporosis. Cochrane Database Syst Rev 2000;(2):CD001983. Review.
250. Grotz W, Rump AL, Niessen H, et al. Treatment of osteopenia and osteoporosis after kidney transplantation. Transplantation 1998;66:1004–1008.
251. Kapetanakis EI, Antonopoulos AS, Antoniou TA, et al. Effect of long-term calcitonin administration on steroid-induced osteoporosis after cardiac transplantation. J Heart Lung Transpl 2005;24(5): 526–532.
252. Isoniemi H, Appelberg J, Nilsson CG, Makela P, Risteli J, Hockerstedt K. Transdermal oestrogen therapy protects postmenopausal liver transplant women from osteoporosis. A 2-year follow-up study. J Hepatol 2001;34(2):299–305.
253. Fahrleitner A, Prenner G, Tscheliessnigg KH, et al. Testosterone supplementation has additional benefits on bone metabolism in cardiac transplant recipients receiving intravenous bisphosphonate treatment: a prospective study. J Bone Miner Res 2002;17(Suppl. 1):S388.
254. Braith RW, Magyari PM, Fulton MN, et al. Comparison of calcitonin versus calcitonin + resistance exercise as prophylaxis for osteoporosis in heart transplant recipients. Transplantation 2006;81(8):1191–1195.
255. Braith RW, Conner JA, Fulton MN, et al. Comparison of alendronate vs alendronate plus mechanical loading as prophylaxis for osteoporosis in lung transplant recipients: a pilot study. J Heart Lung Transpl 2007;26(2):132–137.

27 Adherence, Compliance, and Persistence with Osteoporosis Therapies

Valentina I. Petkov and Melissa I. Williams

CONTENTS

SUMMARY

Medication adherence is particularly important in osteoporosis. While the terms adherence, compliance, and persistence may be confusing, the fact remains that many patients with osteoporosis do not take therapy as directed or for the prolonged period of time needed to treat this disorder. It is clear from studies of large populations that patients with osteoporosis must take about 75–80% of treatments in order to have fracture risk reduction. Unfortunately most patients have stopped therapy by 1–2 years after the original prescription. Strategies to improve persistence have only been modestly successful. Suggestions for increasing adherence are provided.

Key Words: Adherence, compliance, persistence, osteoporosis, prescriptions, dosing schedules

Medication adherence is a common problem in the treatment of many chronic medical conditions. In fact, it is estimated that approximately 14% of all written prescriptions are not filled, and an additional 13% are filled but not taken *(1)*. A variety of factors including age, ethnicity, comorbidities, and number of medications can affect patient adherence with prescribed regimens *(2)*. Adherence is also affected by dosing schedules and administration requirements. Strategies to improve adherence have been only marginally successful.

From: *Contemporary Endocrinology: Osteoporosis: Pathophysiology and Clinical Management*
Edited by: R. A. Adler, DOI 10.1007/978-1-59745-459-9_27,

In the treatment of chronic asymptomatic conditions such as dyslipidemia and hypertension, fewer than 40% of patients are adherent to their prescribed medications at the end of 1 year *(3,4)*. These conditions are not unlike osteoporosis in that they are often silent in nature, lacking patient-apparent symptoms. Osteoporosis is also characterized by the fact that patients cannot easily observe or feel the benefits of therapy because there are no quick and easily measured outcomes. For these reasons, improving compliance with osteoporosis therapies may be more difficult than achieving blood pressure control or serum lipid lowering. For patients with hypertension or hyperlipidemia, it is relatively easy to demonstrate improved outcomes through lowered blood pressure readings or blood cholesterol levels in response to treatment. In addition, there is no tangible reinforcement factor as is seen in conditions like diabetes or asthma, in which symptoms often remind the patient of the need to take medications *(2)*. Hence, it is not surprising that adherence to osteoporosis therapy is particularly poor. In fact, one study reported that compliance rates at 1 year were below 25% *(5)*. A growing amount of evidence suggests that there are multiple factors associated with adherence and patient's perceptions, which play a role in persistence with osteoporosis therapies. Efforts to evaluate and improve rates of both compliance and persistence are increasing, especially because optimal patient outcomes including fracture reduction have been associated with adherence to osteoporosis therapy.

ADHERENCE, COMPLIANCE, AND PERSISTENCE: DEFINITIONS

The definitions of the terms compliance, adherence, and persistence have changed over time. Compliance and adherence have been frequently used as synonyms, and only recently the term persistence was introduced. All three terms have evolved from an increasing awareness that improved definitions are needed in order to accurately depict this problem within health care. Persistence is easier to define, while some controversy exists in differentiating compliance and adherence. Very simply, persistence is associated with the duration of treatment or the length of time a medication is taken. The term compliance became popular in the 1970s and was defined as "the extent to which a person's behavior in terms of taking medications, following diets, or executing lifestyle changes coincides with medical or health advice" *(6)*. More recently, compliance has come under scrutiny with some arguing that the term is too simplistic in its attempt to identify or describe the complexity of medication misuse. The term adherence evolved out of the concern that compliance did not address some of the social, behavioral, and economic reasons that an individual deviates from medical advice. Lutfey and Wishner *(6)* suggest that using the term "noncompliant" focuses the blame on patient-specific characteristics or behaviors and neglects that which practitioners, the medical system, and the patient–practitioner interaction contribute or fail to contribute. It has been suggested that switching to adherence represents a paradigm shift, focusing on the broader implications of how health care is delivered. Conceptually, adherence differs from compliance in that it incorporates the autonomy of patients. It captures the increasing complexity of medical care by characterizing patients as independent, intelligent people who take an active, voluntary role in defining and pursuing goals for their medical treatment and health care *(6)*. Compliance, a more concrete term, is used frequently in research and is generally defined as the percentage of the prescribed medication taken during the time a patient was persistent. Compliance has also been used to describe the correctness of taking the medication as it has been prescribed. Using the example of oral bisphosphonates like alendronate or risedronate, patients should administer the medication in the morning after an overnight fast, with water only, waiting at least 30 min before lying down, eating, drinking, or taking other medications *(7)*. A patient who does not follow these administration guidelines may be characterized as "noncompliant." Still, while it appears that these terms continue to evolve, most agree that adherence is the broader term and generally comprises the concepts of both compliance and persistence *(8–15)*.

COMPLIANCE AND PERSISTENCE WITH OSTEOPOROSIS THERAPIES

Compliance and persistence with osteoporosis medications have been assessed in numerous studies that utilized administrative databases (e.g., Federal government and managed care organization claims, private health insurance plan claims, pharmacy refill history records). The validity, methodology, advantages, and disadvantages of this type of study are controversial *(16,17)*. Compliance is most frequently expressed as the medication possession ratio (MPR), calculated as the percent of days of available medication while a patient is persistent (e.g., the number of days for which a medication was dispensed in a given fill {numerator} divided by the number of actual days between the two fills {denominator}). The MPR estimates drug availability or that which was prescribed and acquired by the patient. It implies but does not necessarily mean that the drug was taken by the patient or that proper administration occurred. Using the MPR, most studies report the percent of patients with a compliance (MPR) cutoff of 80%. This value is clinically relevant for osteoporosis because patients who meet or exceed that value have been shown to experience fewer fractures. Other studies use an MPR cutoff of 66% or report a mean compliance rate for a predefined time interval, which is usually 1, 2, 3, or 5 years after initiation of treatment.

Most commonly, persistence is reported as the percent of patients who have no gaps in treatment longer than 1, 2, or 3 months in duration. The evaluation of persistence with osteoporosis medications often utilizes database resources, in particular pharmacy refill records. While refill history represents an objective measure of compliance and persistence, some concern exists about whether refill information is an acceptable indicator of patient medication use. In an attempt to determine the agreement and validity of such data, Curtis et al. compared refill histories with self-reported use of osteoporosis medications in 6282 glucocorticoid users. Patients with prescriptions for a bisphosphonate, calcitonin, or raloxifene in a US managed care database were evaluated *(18)*. Agreement between refill history and patient recall ranged from $\kappa = 0.64$ (95% CI 0.53–0.75) (calcitonin) to 0.80 (0.76–0.84) (alendronate). The positive predictive value of a filled prescription in the pharmacy database in the prior 6 months exceeded 90% compared to the reference standard of self-reported current bisphosphonate use. However, the 6-month interval of pharmacy data failed to capture more than 25% of self-reported current bisphosphonate users. The optimal interval of pharmacy data to distinguish between current and past bisphosphonate users was 120–180 days. This study suggested that there is agreement between pharmacy data and self-reported compliance; however, the generalizability of the study results is limited to the survey responders only ($N = 2363$).

Studies of both compliance and persistence with osteoporosis treatments have consistently demonstrated suboptimal to poor adherence in different populations and settings *(5,19–24)*. Table 1 summarizes the results from studies that utilized administrative

Table 1
Summary of Studies that Utilized Administrative Databases to Determine Compliance and Persistence with Osteoporosis (OP) Medications

Author, reference	*Database used*	*Patient characteristics*	*OP meds*	*Mean compliance*	*Percentage of patients with compliance <80%*	*Percentage of patients not persistent*
Lo et al. *(25)*	Kaiser Permanente CA	13,455 women >45 years	Alendronate, QW			49.6% refill gap >60 days at 1 year
Siris et al. *(30)*	Two claims DB from 100 health plans (45 employers)	35,537 women ≥45 years	Alendronate, risedronate		57%	80% refill gap >30 days at 2 years
Weycker et al. *(21)*	49 US health plans	18,822 women ≥45 years	Bisphosphonates, calcitonin, raloxifene, estrogen		47% at 3 months; 70% at 1 year; 84% at 3 years	47% refill gap ≥90 days at 1 year; 77% refill gap ≥90 days at 3 years
Solomon et al. *(23)*	Medicare	40,002 women and men ≥ 65 years	Bisphosphonates, calcitonin, raloxifen, estrogen			45.2% at 1 year; 52.1% at 5 years
Cramer et al. *(31)*	30 health-care plans	2741 women >45 years	Alendronate, risedronate	69.2% QW, 57.6% QD		56% refill gap >30 days QW at 1 year; 68 % refill gap >30 days QD at 1 year

Papaioannou et al. *(32)*	CANDOO DB	1967 women and men; mean age 65 years	Etidronate, alendronate, hormone repl Tx			10% Etdr at 1 year; 22% Aln at 1 year; 20% HRT at 1 year; 56% HRT at 6 years
Caro et al. *(33)*	Saskatchewan health data files	11,249 women; mean age 68 years	Etidronate, estrogen, alendronate	70%	50.6%	40% at 2 years
McCombs et al. *(5)*	Large health insurer in CA	58,109 patients	Single HRT, two HRT, bisphosphonates, raloxifene	73%, 81%, 68%, 61%		77% at 1year; 69% at 1 year; 76% at 1 year; 82% at 1 year
Recker et al. *(34)*	Large US retail pharmacy database (14,000 pharmacies)	211,319 women	Bisphos, QW, Bisphos, QD	65%, 54%	55%, 79%	
Huybrechts et al. *(35)*	US managed care database	38,120 women	Bisphosphonates, HRT	65%	66%	

databases. In these, mean compliance varied between 54 and 81%. The percent of patients with satisfactory compliance (MPR > 80%) ranged between 16 and 53%. First-time prescriptions were not refilled at appropriate intervals or even at all. Lo et al. reported that 29% of women who were prescribed weekly alendronate filled the prescription only once *(25)*.

Persistence failure was also widespread with approximately 50% of the patients discontinuing therapy 1 year after treatment initiation. Many patients had refill gaps that exceeded 60 days usually within the first 12 months of therapy. Other studies report similar data and have characterized the rate of decline. Clearly, it appears that the most rapid increase in discontinuation rates occurs during the first year of osteoporosis treatment with a relative stabilization over time *(21,24)*.

Although the available literature focuses mainly on compliance and persistence in women with postmenopausal osteoporosis, limited research in patients with other types of osteoporosis (i.e., glucocorticoid-induced, male, transplantation osteoporosis) showed suboptimal compliance and persistence with osteoporosis therapies *(26,27)*. In a recent study, Hansen et al. reported that 59% of male veterans were adherent at 1 year and only 54% were adherent at 2 years *(28)*. In our own Veterans Affairs Medical Center, 1- and 2-year adherence is somewhat higher (R.A. Adler, personal communication).

Compliance and Persistence with Different Types of Osteoporosis Medications

One of the major factors attributed to patient adherence with any medication is the type of drug, the ease of administration, and the potential side effects it may cause. Many investigators have evaluated the impact of such factors with various agents used to treat osteoporosis.

Most studies have attempted to use retrospective data to compare rates of compliance and persistence. Solomon et al. *(23)* reported that in a retrospective cohort of >40,000 patients, those starting raloxifene were more compliant than those starting other osteoporosis therapies including bisphosphonates, hormone replacement therapy (HRT), and calcitonin. On the other hand, Segal et al. *(29)* described a >20% discontinuation rate among postmenopausal women taking either daily alendronate or raloxifene during the first 6 months of therapy. In 58% of patients, the reason for discontinuation was due to noncompliance rather than actual side effects. Patient perceptions of therapy were largely the cause for discontinuation. A fear of side effects was the most common reason determined in the raloxifene group (30%), while the inconvenience caused by medication use was most notable in the alendronate group (14.3%). In another study, McCombs et al. *(5)* reviewed the claims data for over 58,000 patients and reported that 1-year compliance rates were below 25% for all osteoporosis therapies, including estrogen, estrogen–progestin, raloxifene, and bisphosphonate medications. The average duration of continuous therapy or MPR was 221 days for raloxifene, 245 for bisphosphonates (including alendronate, etidronate, and risedronate), 262 for estrogen only, and 292 for estrogen–progestin combinations.

Similar results can be found when looking back at studies of hormone replacement therapy (HRT) prior to the results of the Women's Health Initiative. At that time, hormone replacement therapy played a significant role in the prevention of osteoporosis. Like other treatments, however, many studies found that compliance with hormone replacement therapy was suboptimal. In one study, Marwick *(36)* reported that 27% of over 1500 women enrolled in the Harvard Community Health Plan who received a new prescription for HRT terminated treatment in the first 100 days and 40% stopped within 1 year. Another study of over 3800 Medicaid recipients demonstrated that only 17% of postmenopausal women continued therapy during a 35-month observational period *(37)*. Others note that patients either have interrupted therapy or never began therapy due to side effects or concerns associated with pharmacologic actions *(38,39)*. Patients who were considered new users of HRT were noted to discontinue therapy altogether; some as early as 100 days. Overall, 1-year compliance rates were dismal. Faulkner et al. enrolled over 28,000 40–59-year-old women taking either estrogen only or estrogen–progestin combinations *(40)*. The authors found that 54.4% were noncompliant with an MPR of less than 0.75 at 12 months. Noncompliance was more common in younger patients as well as those whose prescriber was not a gynecologist or an obstetrician.

As the only nonantiresorptive agent on the market, teriparatide has demonstrated significant effects on bone mineral density and reductions in fracture risk during clinical trials. Unfortunately, very few studies have chosen to evaluate the adherence of teriparatide as a primary outcome in real-world practice. While little data have been published on compliance, one study did demonstrate a very high persistence rate in a UK population. Arden et al. also reported that of 1104 patients, 87% were continuing treatment with teriparatide at 1 year *(41)*. These data are significant in light of other osteoporosis therapies which are associated with less appealing adherence rates. Yet, we believe that the paucity of studies is far more enlightening than the actual results described. Some investigators have concluded that patients demand far greater benefits than the drug is able to confer, especially in light of the fact that the medication is administered as a daily subcutaneous injection *(42)*.

Equally important in the osteoporosis armamentarium is calcium and vitamin D supplementation. Unfortunately, few studies have examined compliance and persistence with these pharmacologic agents. Physicians and patients with osteoporosis from Austria, the United Kingdom, and Mexico were asked to rate the importance of calcium and vitamin D on a scale of 1–10, with the value 1 meaning not important and 10 meaning extremely important *(43)*. The percentage of physicians from these countries who rated the importance of calcium and vitamin D as 9 or 10 was 86, 28, and 46%, respectively. Overall, 50% of patients reported taking calcium and vitamin D. Of these, 47% reported taking supplements on a "daily" basis and 46% reported taking them on a "regular" basis. As important, providers should discuss the use of these over-the-counter supplements with their patients just as they would discuss prescription medications. Unfortunately, in this same study, 19% of patients reported that they had no discussions with their physicians about calcium, while 39% reported no discussion about vitamin D.

Ultimately, adherence with all osteoporosis therapies is poor. Several recent review articles *(44–47)* also share our view.

DETERMINANTS OF COMPLIANCE AND PERSISTENCE

From a practical standpoint, it is important to be able to recognize factors associated with acceptable and poor adherence and the magnitude of their contribution. Modifiable determinants can be targeted with specially designed programs or through individualized patient care. Almost every study on compliance and persistence with osteoporosis therapies has tried to elucidate these factors. A common problem in all available resources evaluating osteoporosis treatment adherence is the limited number of determinants included in these studies. Much of the research was performed using commercially available pharmacy, institutional or health insurance databases, which rarely contain individual patient characteristics. Patient surveys have the potential to examine a greater number of factors, but the results are limited to only those who respond, which at best is 40–60%. Furthermore, the determinants of osteoporosis treatment compliance and persistence reported in the literature have accounted for a very modest proportion of the variability. This suggests that either compliance is dependent on a much larger number of factors or that the most important factors were excluded from the models.

Solomon et al. *(23)* determined that the following characteristics independently predicted compliance: female sex, younger age, fewer comorbid conditions, using fewer nonosteoporosis medications, bone mineral density testing before and after initiating a medication, a fracture before and after initiating a medication, and nursing home residence during the 12 months before initiating therapy. Still, these factors explained only about 6% of the variance. In another study, predictors of compliance were assessed in patients who discontinued weekly bisphosphonate therapy. Overall, 1-year discontinuation rates were 50% with approximately one-third of women filling only a single prescription for alendronate. According to the authors, those who had prior exposure to high-dose glucocorticoids, those who had gastrointestinal diagnoses or a high number of different classes of prescription medications prescribed to them were more likely to stop treatment. Among those who were more compliant were patients who had a prior BMD test or who had taken hormone replacement therapy in the past *(25)*.

A telephone survey in the United Kingdom of women 50 years and older showed that factors associated with adherence were fracture history, less dissatisfaction with bisphosphonate therapy, and fewer concerns about bisphosphonate medication. Specifically, concerns about treatment included fears of addiction, worries about taking the medication for a long period of time, and the perception that side effects could be worse than the outcome of osteoporosis itself. Interestingly, these were different from factors associated with persistence in which dosage interval (weekly preferred over daily), a shorter duration of disease, and frequent pain were most important *(48)*.

Dosing Regimen and Compliance

The dosing regimen of osteoporosis medications varies from daily intake to yearly administration. Oral bisphosphonates can be given daily, weekly, or monthly. It is expected that a less frequent regimen would be associated with better compliance and persistence. Several studies comparing daily to weekly bisphosphonate use have confirmed improved yet suboptimal adherence with once a week administration *(31,34,49–51)*. Records from a very large cohort of 211,319 women 50 years of age or older were obtained from a retail pharmacy prescription database. The persistence after 1 year of treatment was 56.7% with weekly dosing and 39.0% with daily dosing *(50)*. Panning-van Beest et al. *(52)* found persistence with weekly alendronate to be 51.9% after 1 year of treatment and with daily etidronate and risedronate to be only 30.1–42.2% among 2124 women from the Netherlands. Other studies have demonstrated that weekly dosing is better than monthly regimens. Gold et al. *(53)* reported that adherence with weekly risedronate versus monthly ibandronate measured by MPR was significantly higher (72.7 vs. 52.8%). In addition, persistence with weekly risedronate was significantly longer (144 vs. 100 days). The authors attributed the better rates to patient knowledge of each medication's proven fracture efficacy. Richards et al. reported that 45% of surveyed UK subjects ($N = 2485$, >55 years, 90% female) would prefer daily dosing with minimal administration inconvenience, 20% weekly dosing with moderate administration inconvenience, and 30% a monthly dose *(54)*. When informed about differences in fracture efficacy with weekly and monthly bisphosphonates, a significantly greater proportion (82%) of women preferred a weekly bisphosphonate with proven fracture efficacy at the spine and hip over a monthly bisphosphonate with proven fracture efficacy only at the spine *(55)*. Studies comparing different dosing regimens should be interpreted with caution because the source of study funding may not be unbiased.

Another important aspect of the dosing regimen which is crucial in order to optimize outcomes is proper drug administration. The oral bisphosphonates have limited absorption in the gastrointestinal tract *(56)*. To assure adequate bioavailability, these medications should be taken on an empty stomach, first thing in the morning, with a full glass of tap water, at least 30–60 min before any other medications, food, or beverages are consumed. Bioavailability is significantly reduced by 60% if taken with coffee or orange juice and up to 85% if taken concurrently or within 2 h of a meal. Noncompliance with administration guidelines is common. Mersfelder et al. *(57)* reported in patients prescribed alendronate that the biggest mistake was taking other medications at the same time as the bisphosphonate. In a UK study, 26% of those treated with risedronate did not take the drug properly, most frequently not staying upright, leading to more gastrointestinal adverse events *(58)*.

Compliance and Osteoporosis Clinical Outcomes [Fractures, Bone Mineral Density (BMD), and Bone Turnover Markers (BTM)]

What is the minimum level of compliance that is still associated with benefits of osteoporosis treatment in terms of positive effect on BMD, bone turnover markers, and fracture rates? In controlled trials, compliance and persistence are generally maintained in order to insure that outcomes can be attributed to the medication intervention. Antifracture efficacy in osteoporosis trials has been established through controlled conditions that usually assure high medication compliance. Unfortunately, compliance to this extent is not found in actual practice and therefore decreases the likelihood of fracture reduction in real-world patients. Quite a few studies based on insurance claims and pharmacy databases have demonstrated the impact of compliance on fracture rates *(5,33,35,59)*. In one of the largest observational trials to date, the authors analyzed data on over 35,000 women at least 45 years old with a diagnosis of osteoporosis and prescriptions for alendronate or risedronate. Patients who were refill compliant (MPR > 80%) and persistent (no refill gaps >30 days in 24 months of follow-up) demonstrated reductions of 20–45% in total, vertebral, and hip fractures. The minimal compliance level that was associated with fracture reduction was 50%. There was a steeper decline in fracture risk with compliance exceeding 75%. A strong positive relationship was observed between compliance refill and fracture reduction rates, the benefit of which did not plateau but continued to improve to the maximum level of compliance at 100% *(30)*.

In a similar study, Caro et al. *(33)* demonstrated a 16% greater reduction in fracture rates in compliant patients. This association was maintained even after controlling for other patient characteristics that independently predict future fracture occurrence.

Similarly, Huybrechts et al. *(35)* found a 17% (95% CI 9–25%) increase in fracture rates in osteoporotic women with low medication compliance.

Certainly, there appears to be a relationship between therapeutic drug interventions and fracture protection. Yet it is worthwhile to consider how some patients benefit from fracture reduction in the placebo arm of controlled clinical trials. In some studies, subjects who were compliant with the placebo had better clinical outcomes than noncompliant ones. This observation could be due to a "placebo effect" because patients who believed they would get well indeed got well, or perhaps it may be attributed to improved adherence to medications as part of a healthy lifestyle, particularly calcium and vitamin D *(47,60)*.

Few studies examined the effect of compliance on bone mineral density (BMD) or bone turnover markers (BTM). Tanko et al. tested eight different dosing regimens of daily or weekly ibandronate simulating inadequate dosing with some of the regimens *(61)*. The authors showed that the suppression of BTM is a function of cumulative dose and suggested the use of bone turnover markers to detect suboptimal dosing as a consequence of poor compliance.

Trends in Compliance with Osteoporosis Therapies

Have compliance and persistence with osteoporosis treatments changed over time?

One might expect that compliance would improve with an increase in osteoporosis awareness by providers and patients. If this theory were true, then factors such as an increase in the number of actively publicized medications and direct-to-consumer marketing should have a positive impact. Unfortunately, there has not been an overwhelming positive improvement observed over the past decade. Discontinuation rates and nonadherence were compared in Canadian women 70 years or older who started antiresorptive treatment for osteoporosis between 1998–2001 and 2002–2004. Although the discontinuation rate was significantly lower in the more recent time frame, the magnitude of difference was not impressive. At 6 months, discontinuation occurred in 45.8% of women in the 1998–2001 cohort and 39.4% of women in the 2002–2004 cohort. At 1 year, there was even a smaller degree of difference, 57.5 and 52.2%, respectively *(24)*.

It is well known that there is a cyclical pattern to lifestyle behaviors such as dieting and exercise, use of preventive medications, and treatment of chronic diseases that have few or no symptoms. Patients initiate and discontinue healthy behaviors and medications multiple times *(54,62,63)*. About one-third of women who discontinued weekly alendronate (gap in refill ≥60 days) restarted treatment within 6 months *(24)*. Brookhart et al. *(64)* examined the rate of restarting osteoporosis treatment after prolonged discontinuation. Out of 40,002 Medicare beneficiaries enrolled in Pharmaceutical Assistance Contract for the Elderly (PACE), 67% had lapses in osteoporosis drug use greater than 60 days. In this cohort, 30% restarted treatment within 6 months after discontinuation and 50% within 2 years. It is important to determine which characteristics are associated with re-initiating treatment so that modifiable ones can be targeted in intervention programs. Clinical and laboratory tests measuring the effect of the medication (i.e., cholesterol, bone turnover markers, BMD) are usually associated with better compliance and persistence and result in a higher probability of restarting the medication. In the PACE study, factors associated with restarting osteoporosis treatment were younger age, female sex, history of previous fracture, recent hip fracture, discharge from nursing home, and bone mineral density testing *(64)*.

Economic Implications of Noncompliance and Nonpersistence

The cost-effectiveness of osteoporosis treatment was examined in studies using modeling and simulation techniques applied to the populations of several Western European countries and Canada *(65–69)*. Generally, fracture prevention with bisphosphonates was found to be cost-effective, particularly in older women and in those with previous fractures. McCombs et al. reported several economic implications of noncompliance with osteoporosis treatment (hormone replacement therapy, raloxifene, alendronate, etidronate, and risedronate) in a study of 56,000 women enrolled in a major California health-care plan *(5)*. Compliant patients used fewer physician services, outpatient care services, and inpatient hospital services as compared to noncompliant ones. Another study by Huybrechts et al. found a 37% (95% CI 32–43%) increased risk in all-cause hospitalizations and higher monthly costs for all medical services in noncompliant osteoporosis patients ($600 vs. $340) *(35)*. Quite simply, adherence with osteoporosis medications reduces the financial burden in more ways than just preventing fracture-related health-care visits.

OPPORTUNITIES AND STRATEGIES TO IMPROVE COMPLIANCE

Numerous interventions for enhancing patient adherence to medications for treatment of chronic conditions have been tested in randomized controlled clinical trials (RCT). A review of RCTs by McDonald et al. *(70)* showed that as many as one half of the interventions did not produce any significant change in adherence and only one-third of those that did show improvement had an impact on clinical outcomes. These interventions can be summarized as follows: (1) patient education (oral and written materials, educational programs, and seminars), (2) increased communication and counseling (manual or automated telephone follow-up, computer assisted compliance monitoring, follow-up letters, frequent office visits), (3) more convenient regimens such as simplified dosing, (4) active patient involvement in their care (self-monitoring of blood pressure, glucose, pulmonary function), (5) use of reminders (appointment and refill reminders, reminders to take medications placed at a common area in a patient's home such as refrigerator magnets, dose-dispensing units of medications, pillboxes, and medication charts), and (6) rewards and reinforcement of good compliance. Frequently, these interventions have been used in combination. While complex and labor intensive, these interventions have had a modest effect on patient compliance *(70)*. Although poor compliance and persistence with osteoporosis treatments are widely documented and recognized, research studies examining methods and strategies to improve compliance with osteoporosis therapies are relatively scarce. Clowes et al. showed that monitoring therapy by a nurse with or without assessment of bone resorption markers increased compliance by 57% and average length of treatment (persistence) by 25% compared to no monitoring *(71)*. The intervention included a nurse follow-up office visit at 12, 24, and 36 weeks after initiation of treatment. The nurse used a structured interview containing six open-ended questions related to the patient's well-being, problems with their osteoporosis medication (raloxifene), and adverse events. No direct questions on medication compliance were raised during the follow-up. All patients' questions were answered. In addition to the nurse follow-up, a third group received a urinary NTX with graph interpretation. In this study, adding bone markers did not improve compliance and persistence beyond the nurse follow-up alone; however, the improved compliance and persistence (assessed by an electronic device counting the number of times the medication container was opened) were reflected in a significant increase in BMD at 1 year of treatment compared to the control group.

In other clinical trials, strategies involving education through written materials were attempted. Guilera et al. utilized an educational leaflet with general osteoporosis information which was distributed to a group of patients starting raloxifene. This particular intervention did not improve compliance at 6 or 12 months *(72)*. Others have attempted to provide information on bone mineral density and bone turnover markers to enhance adherence in their patients. Pickney et al. found that regardless of BMD results or age, many patients do not continue the medication initially prescribed *(73)*. Reinforcement of compliance using BTMs has influenced persistence with treatment but only if the response was good (i.e., decrease >30%). BTM follow-up did not have any impact on persistence in patients with stable (±30%) or poor responses (>30% increase) *(74)*. These results strongly suggest that patients need proof and assurance that therapy works in order to persist. Follow-up BMD evaluation and BTM testing may be important tools for keeping patients with low bone density motivated; however, more clinical trials are needed to establish evidence-based recommendations.

Early trials evaluating compliance alluded to patient preference as a factor in maintaining adherence. Richards et al. suggested that various dosing regimens (daily, weekly, monthly) may be associated with improved compliance *(54)*. A recent survey conducted in 3000 women with postmenopausal osteoporosis (1500 of them currently on treatment) from four European countries and Mexico examined patients' preferences regarding osteoporosis medications *(75)*. The most important characteristic was the effectiveness of a medication to reduce fracture risk, followed by side effect profile. Out-of-pocket costs, dosing frequency, formulation, time on the market, and dosing procedure were less important considerations among respondents from most countries.

In the absence of proven strategies to enhance compliance, health-care providers should focus on assessing and addressing compliance on an individual level. In an editorial, Rosenow called for including compliance assessments as "the sixth vital sign" along with the four classical ones and the fifth sign, pain *(76)*. Patient and family education, especially with a new diagnosis, and efficient patient–provider communication that takes into account cultural, ethnic, language, intellectual, and financial circumstances are essential for building understanding, trust, and commitment. Physicians should attempt to stratify the likelihood of a patient being noncompliant and develop a plan for dealing with the issue. This could include more frequent office visits; telephone follow-up, practical advice, and tools (magnets and other reminders, medication charts, pill boxes, proper instructions and labeling of the medication container, involvement of a significant other in patient care, etc.). Unfortunately, the relatively constricted time of clinician–patient interactions makes attaining long-term persistence more challenging. Selecting medications with simplified dosing regimens or provider-controlled administration may be ideal for the noncompliant patient. In that respect, a new bisphosphonate, zoledronic acid, may be a true asset in the battle with osteoporosis medication noncompliance because it is given in a 15-min intravenous infusion once a year *(77)*. Still, this approach requires that the patient seek medical care annually and providers remember to prescribe it. It also does not alleviate the problem that patients must be compliant with calcium and vitamin D therapy.

In conclusion, adherence with osteoporosis medications is poor in the vast majority of patients who would benefit from treatment. Compliance and persistence with medication therapy are critical to achieving optimal outcomes, including fracture risk reduction. Unfortunately, it is not possible to predict which patients will be nonadherent, and strategies have been only moderately successful. As a result, an assessment of both compliance and persistence with osteoporosis medications, dietary supplements, and lifestyle behaviors should be conducted routinely and addressed individually in patients with osteoporosis. Until providers address the issue of adherence in each patient with osteoporosis, we are unlikely to decrease the gap between fracture risk reduction and that which is observed in actual practice.

REFERENCES

1. Berg JS, Dischler J, Wagner DJ, Raia JJ, Palmer-Shevlin N. Medication compliance: a healthcare problem. Ann Pharmacother 1993;27(9 Suppl.):S1–S24.
2. Siegel D, Lopez J, Meier J. Antihypertensive medication adherence in the Department of Veterans Affairs. Am J Med 2007;120(1):26–32.
3. Benner JS, Glynn RJ, Mogun H, Neumann PJ, Weinstein MC, Avorn J. Long-term persistence in use of statin therapy in elderly patients. JAMA 2002;288(4):455–461.
4. Chapman RH, Benner JS, Petrilla AA, Tierce JC, Collins SR, Battleman DS, et al. Predictors of adherence with antihypertensive and lipid-lowering therapy. Arch Intern Med 2005;165(10):1147–1152.
5. McCombs JS, Thiebaud P, McLaughlin-Miley C, Shi J. Compliance with drug therapies for the treatment and prevention of osteoporosis. Maturitas 2004;48(3):271–287.
6. Lutfey KE, Wishner WJ. Beyond "compliance" is "adherence". Improving the prospect of diabetes care. Diabetes Care 1999;22(4):635–639.
7. Reginster JY, Rabenda V, Neuprez A. Adherence, patient preference and dosing frequency: understanding the relationship. Bone 2006;38 (4 Suppl. 1):2–6.
8. Shea SC. Improving medication adherence: how to talk with patients about their medications. Philadelphia, PA: Walther Kluwer Health Inc., 2006.
9. World Health Organization. Adherence to long-term therapies: evidence for action. Geneva, Switzerland: World Health Organization, 2003.
10. Burke LE, Ockene IS. Compliance in healthcare and research. Armonk, NY: Futura Publishing Company Inc., 2001.
11. Sackett DL, Haynes RB. Compliance with therapeutic regimens. Baltimore, MD: The Johns Hopkins University Press, 1976.
12. Desmond J, Copeland LR. Communicating with today's patient: essentials to save time, decrease risk, and increase patient compliance. New York, NY: John Wiley & Sons, 2000.
13. Haynes RB, Taylor DW, Sacket DL. Compliance in health care. Baltimore, MD: The Johns Hopkins University Press, 1979.
14. Barofski I. Medication compliance: a behavioral management approach. Thorofare, NJ: Charles B. Slack Inc., 1977.
15. Weibert Robert T, Dee Donald A. Improving patient medication compliance. Oradel, NJ: Medical Economics Company, 1980.
16. Sikka R, Xia F, Aubert RE. Estimating medication persistency using administrative claims data. Am J Manag Care 2005;11(7):449–457.
17. Dezii CM. Persistence with drug therapy: a practical approach using administrative claims data. Manag Care 2001;10(2):42–45.
18. Curtis JR, Westfall AO, Allison J, Freeman A, Kovac SH, Saag KG. Agreement and validity of pharmacy data versus self-report for use of osteoporosis medications among chronic glucocorticoid users. Pharmacoepidemiol Drug Saf 2006;15(10):710–718.
19. Downey TW, Foltz SH, Boccuzzi SJ, Omar MA, Kahler KH. Adherence and persistence associated with the pharmacologic treatment of osteoporosis in a managed care setting. South Med J 2006;99(6): 570–575.
20. Tosteson AN, Grove MR, Hammond CS, Moncur MM, Ray GT, Hebert GM, et al. Early discontinuation of treatment for osteoporosis. Am J Med 2003;115(3):209–216.

21. Weycker D, Macarios D, Edelsberg J, Oster G. Compliance with drug therapy for postmenopausal osteoporosis. Osteoporos Int 2006;17(11):1645–1652.
22. Zafran N, Liss Z, Peled R, Sherf M, Reuveni H. Incidence and causes for failure of treatment of women with proven osteoporosis. Osteoporos Int 2005;16(11):1375–1383.
23. Solomon DH, Avorn J, Katz JN, Finkelstein JS, Arnold M, Polinski JM, et al. Compliance with osteoporosis medications. Arch Intern Med 2005;165(20):2414–2419.
24. Blouin J, Dragomir A, Ste-Marie LG, Fernandes JC, Perreault S. Discontinuation of antiresorptive therapies: a comparison between 1998–2001 and 2002–2004 among osteoporotic women. J Clin Endocrinol Metab 2007;92(3):887–894.
25. Lo JC, Pressman AR, Omar MA, Ettinger B. Persistence with weekly alendronate therapy among postmenopausal women. Osteoporos Int 2006;17(6):922–928.
26. Yood RA, Harrold LR, Fish L, Cernieux J, Emani S, Conboy E, et al. Prevention of glucocorticoid-induced osteoporosis: experience in a managed care setting. Arch Intern Med 2001;161(10):1322–1327.
27. Curtis JR, Westfall AO, Allison JJ, Freeman A, Saag KG. Channeling and adherence with alendronate and risedronate among chronic glucocorticoid users. Osteoporos Int 2006;17(8):1268–1274.
28. Hansen KE, Swenson ED, Baltz B, Schuna AA, Jones AN, Elliott ME. Adherence to alendronate in male veterans. Osteoporos Int 2008;19:349–356.
29. Segal E, Tamir A, Ish-Shalom S. Compliance of osteoporotic patients with different treatment regimens. IMAJ 2003;5:859–862.
30. Siris ES, Harris ST, Rosen CJ, Barr CE, Arvesen JN, Abbott TA, et al. Adherence to bisphosphonate therapy and fracture rates in osteoporotic women: relationship to vertebral and nonvertebral fractures from 2 US claims databases. Mayo Clin Proc 2006;81(8):1013–1022.
31. Cramer JA, Amonkar MM, Hebborn A, Altman R. Compliance and persistence with bisphosphonate dosing regimens among women with postmenopausal osteoporosis. Curr Med Res Opin 2005;21(9): 1453–1460.
32. Papaioannou A, Ioannidis G, Adachi JD, Sebaldt RJ, Ferko N, Puglia M, et al. Adherence to bisphosphonates and hormone replacement therapy in a tertiary care setting of patients in the CANDOO database. Osteoporos Int 2003;14(10):808–813.
33. Caro JJ, Ishak KJ, Huybrechts KF, Raggio G, Naujoks C. The impact of compliance with osteoporosis therapy on fracture rates in actual practice. Osteoporos Int 2004;15(12):1003–1008.
34. Recker RR, Gallagher R, MacCosbe PE. Effect of dosing frequency on bisphosphonate medication adherence in a large longitudinal cohort of women. Mayo Clin Proc 2005;80(7):856–861.
35. Huybrechts KF, Ishak KJ, Caro JJ. Assessment of compliance with osteoporosis treatment and its consequences in a managed care population. Bone 2006;38(6):922–928.
36. Marwick C. Hormone combination treats women's bone loss. JAMA 1994;272(19):1487.
37. Kotzan JA, Martin BC, Wade WE. Persistence with estrogen therapy in a postmenopausal Medicaid population. Pharmacotherapy 1999;19(3):363–369.
38. Cano A. Compliance to hormone replacement therapy in menopausal women controlled in a third level academic centre. Maturitas 1994;20(2–3):91–99.
39. Bjorn I, Backsrom T. Drug related negative side-effects is a common reason for poor compliance in hormone replacement therapy. Maturitas 1999;32(2):77–86.
40. Faulkner DL, Young C, Hutchins D, McCollam JS. Patient noncompliance with hormone replacement therapy: a nationwide estimate using a large prescription claims database. Menopause 1998;5(4):226–229.
41. Arden NK, Earl S, Fisher DJ, Cooper C, Carruthers S, Goater M. Persistence with teriparatide in patients with osteoporosis: the UK experience. Osteoporos Int 2006;17(11):1626–1629.
42. Fraenkel L, Gulanski B, Wittink D. Patient willingness to take teriparatide. Patient Educ Couns 2007;65(2):237–244
43. Resch H, Walliser J, Phillips S, Wehren LE, Sen SS. Physician and patient perceptions on the use of vitamin D and calcium in osteoporosis treatment: a European and Latin American perspective. Curr Med Res Opin 2007.
44. Cramer JA, Silverman S. Persistence with bisphosphonate treatment for osteoporosis: finding the root of the problem. Am J Med 2006;119(4 Suppl. 1):S12–S17.
45. Cramer JA, Gold DT, Silverman SL, Lewiecki EM. A systematic review of persistence and compliance with bisphosphonates for osteoporosis. Osteoporos Int 2007.

46. Gold DT, Silverman S. Review of adherence to medications for the treatment of osteoporosis. Curr Osteoporos Rep 2006;4(1):21–27.
47. Seeman E, Compston J, Adachi J, Brandi ML, Cooper C, Dawson-Hughes B, et al. Non-compliance: the Achilles' heel of anti-fracture efficacy. Osteoporos Int 2007;18(6):711–719.
48. Carr AJ, Thompson PW, Cooper C. Factors associated with adherence and persistence to bisphosphonate therapy in osteoporosis: a cross-sectional survey. Osteoporos Int 2006;17(11):1638–1644.
49. Cramer JA, Lynch NO, Gaudin AF, Walker M, Cowell W. The effect of dosing frequency on compliance and persistence with bisphosphonate therapy in postmenopausal women: a comparison of studies in the United States, the United Kingdom, and France. Clin Ther 2006;28(10):1686–1694.
50. Ettinger MP, Gallagher R, MacCosbe PE. Medication persistence with weekly versus daily doses of orally administered bisphosphonates. Endocr Pract 2006;12(5):522–528.
51. Kendler D, Kung AW, Fuleihan G, Gonzalez Gonzalez JG, Gaines KA, Verbruggen N, et al. Patients with osteoporosis prefer once weekly to once daily dosing with alendronate. Maturitas 2004;48(3): 243–251.
52. Penning-van Beest FJ, Goettsch WG, Erkens JA, Herings RM. Determinants of persistence with bisphosphonates: a study in women with postmenopausal osteoporosis. Clin Ther 2006;28(2):236–242.
53. Gold DT, Safi W, Trinh H. Patient preference and adherence: comparative US studies between two bisphosphonates, weekly risedronate and monthly ibandronate. Curr Med Res Opin 2006;22(12):2383–2391.
54. Richards JB, Cherkas LF, Spector TD. An analysis of which anti-osteoporosis therapeutic regimen would improve compliance in a population of elderly adults. Curr Med Res Opin 2007;23(2):293–299.
55. Keen R, Jodar E, Iolascon G, Kruse HP, Varbanov A, Mann B, et al. European women's preference for osteoporosis treatment: influence of clinical effectiveness and dosing frequency. Curr Med Res Opin 2006;22(12):2375–2381.
56. Gertz BJ, Holland SD, Kline WF, Matuszewski BK, Freeman A, Quan H, et al. Studies of the oral bioavailability of alendronate. Clin Pharmacol Ther 1995;58(3):288–298.
57. Mersfelder T, Armitstead JA, Ivey MF, Cedars M. A medication use evaluation of alendronate: compliance with administration guidelines. Pharm Pract Manag Q 1999;18(4):50–58.
58. Hamilton B, McCoy K, Taggart H. Tolerability and compliance with risedronate in clinical practice. Osteoporos Int 2003;14(3):259–262.
59. Gold DT, Martin BC, Frytak JR, Amonkar MM, Cosman F. A claims database analysis of persistence with alendronate therapy and fracture risk in post-menopausal women with osteoporosis. Curr Med Res Opin 2007;23(3):585–594.
60. Granger BB, Swedberg K, Ekman I, Granger CB, Olofsson B, McMurray JJ, et al. Adherence to candesartan and placebo and outcomes in chronic heart failure in the CHARM programme: double-blind, randomised, controlled clinical trial. Lancet 2005;366(9502):2005–2011.
61. Tanko LB, Mouritzen U, Lehmann HJ, Warming L, Moelgaard A, Christgau S, et al. Oral ibandronate: changes in markers of bone turnover during adequately dosed continuous and weekly therapy and during different suboptimally dosed treatment regimens. Bone 2003;32(6):687–693.
62. Brookhart MA, Patrick AR, Schneeweiss S, Avorn J, Dormuth C, Shrank W, et al. Physician follow-up and provider continuity are associated with long-term medication adherence: a study of the dynamics of statin use. Arch Intern Med 2007;167(8):847–852.
63. Brownell KD, Rodin J. Medical, metabolic, and psychological effects of weight cycling. Arch Intern Med 1994;154(12):1325–1330.
64. Brookhart MA, Avorn J, Katz JN, Finkelstein JS, Arnold M, Polinski JM, et al. Gaps in treatment among users of osteoporosis medications: the dynamics of noncompliance. Am J Med 2007;120(3):251–256.
65. Stevenson M, Lloyd JM, De Nigris E, Brewer N, Davis S, Oakley J. A systematic review and economic evaluation of alendronate, etidronate, risedronate, raloxifene and teriparatide for the prevention and treatment of postmenopausal osteoporosis. Health Technol Assess 2005;9(22):1–160.
66. Brecht JG, Kruse HP, Mohrke W, Oestreich A, Huppertz E. Health–economic comparison of three recommended drugs for the treatment of osteoporosis. Int J Clin Pharmacol Res 2004;24(1):1–10.
67. Goeree R, Blackhouse G, Adachi J. Cost-effectiveness of alternative treatments for women with osteoporosis in Canada. Curr Med Res Opin 2006;22(7):1425–1436.
68. Johnell O, Jonsson B, Jonsson L, Black D. Cost effectiveness of alendronate (fosamax) for the treatment of osteoporosis and prevention of fractures. Pharmacoeconomics 2003;21(5):305–314.

69. Borgstrom F, Carlsson A, Sintonen H, Boonen S, Haentjens P, Burge R, et al. The cost-effectiveness of risedronate in the treatment of osteoporosis: an international perspective. Osteoporos Int 2006;17(7): 996–1007.
70. McDonald HP, Garg AX, Haynes RB. Interventions to enhance patient adherence to medication prescriptions: scientific review. JAMA 2002;288(22):2868–2879.
71. Clowes JA, Peel NF, Eastell R. The impact of monitoring on adherence and persistence with antiresorptive treatment for postmenopausal osteoporosis: a randomized controlled trial. J Clin Endocrinol Metab 2004;89(3):1117–1123.
72. Guilera M, Fuentes M, Grifols M, Ferrer J, Badia X. Does an educational leaflet improve self-reported adherence to therapy in osteoporosis? The OPTIMA study. Osteoporos Int 2006;17(5):664–671.
73. Pickney CS, Arnason JA. Correlation between patient recall of bone densitometry results and subsequent treatment adherence. Osteoporos Int 2005;16(9):1156–1160.
74. Delmas PD, Vrijens B, Eastell R, Roux C, Pols HA, Ringe JD, et al. Effect of monitoring bone turnover markers on persistence with risedronate treatment of postmenopausal osteoporosis. J Clin Endocrinol Metab 2007;92(4):1296–1304.
75. Duarte JW, Bolge SC, Sen SS. An evaluation of patients′ preferences for osteoporosis medications and their attributes: the PREFER-international study. Clin Ther 2007;29(3):488–503.
76. Rosenow EC, III. Patients′ understanding of and compliance with medications: the sixth vital sign? Mayo Clin Proc 2005;80(8):983–987.
77. Black DM, Delmas PD, Eastell R, Reid IR, Boonen S, Cauley JA, et al. Once-yearly zoledronic acid for treatment of postmenopausal osteoporosis. N Engl J Med 2007;356(18):1809–1822.

Subject Index

From: *Contemporary Endocrinology: Osteoporosis: Pathophysiology and Clinical Management*
Edited by: R. A. Adler, DOI 10.1007/978-1-59745-459-9,